EDITION 5

COMMUNITY/PUBLIC
HEALTH NURSING

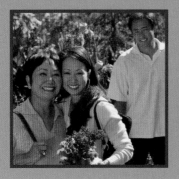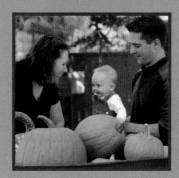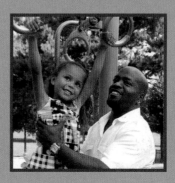

Promoting the Health of Populations

Mary A. Nies, PhD, RN, FAAN, FAAHB
Carol Grotnes Belk Endowed Chair in Nursing and Professor
Adjunct Professor Department of Public Health Sciences
College of Health and Human Services
University of North Carolina at Charlotte
Charlotte, North Carolina

Melanie McEwen, PhD, RN
Associate Professor
University of Texas Health Science Center at Houston
School of Nursing
Houston, Texas

ELSEVIER
SAUNDERS

ELSEVIER
SAUNDERS

3251 Riverport Lane
St. Louis, Missouri 63043

COMMUNITY/PUBLIC HEALTH NURSING:
PROMOTING THE HEALTH OF POPULATIONS

ISBN: 978-1-4377-0860-8

Notices

Knowledge and best practice in this field are constantly changing. As new research and experience broaden our understanding, changes in research methods, professional practices, or medical treatment may become necessary.

Practitioners and researchers must always rely on their own experience and knowledge in evaluating and using any information, methods, compounds, or experiments described herein. In using such information or methods they should be mindful of their own safety and the safety of others, including parties for whom they have a professional responsibility.

With respect to any drug or pharmaceutical products identified, readers are advised to check the most current information provided (i) on procedures featured or (ii) by the manufacturer of each product to be administered, to verify the recommended dose or formula, the method and duration of administration, and contraindications. It is the responsibility of practitioners, relying on their own experience and knowledge of their patients, to make diagnoses, to determine dosages and the best treatment for each individual patient, and to take all appropriate safety precautions.

To the fullest extent of the law, neither the Publisher nor the authors, contributors, or editors, assume any liability for any injury and/or damage to persons or property as a matter of products liability, negligence or otherwise, or from any use or operation of any methods, products, instructions, or ideas contained in the material herein.

Library of Congress Cataloging-in-Publication Data
Community/public health nursing: promoting the health of populations/[edited by] Mary A. Nies, Melanie McEwen. – Ed. 5.
   p.; cm.
   Includes bibliographical references and index.
   ISBN 978-1-4377-0860-8 (hardcover: alk. paper) I. Community health nursing. I. Nies, Mary A. (Mary Albrecht) II. McEwen, Melanie.
   [DNLM: 1. Community Health Nursing. 2. Health Promotion. 3. Public Health Nursing. WY 106]
   RT98.S9 2011
   610.73'43–dc22

                                                            2010028212

Acquisitions Editor: Nancy O'Brien
Developmental Editor: Carlie Irwin
Publishing Services Manager: Anne Altepeter
Project Manager: Cindy Thoms
Senior Book Designer: Kim Denando

Working together to grow
libraries in developing countries

www.elsevier.com | www.bookaid.org | www.sabre.org

ELSEVIER   BOOK AID International   Sabre Foundation

Printed in China

Last digit is the print number: 9 8 7 6 5 4 3 2 1

COMMUNITY/PUBLIC
HEALTH NURSING

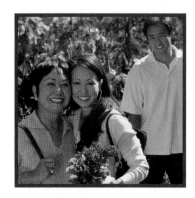
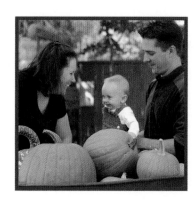
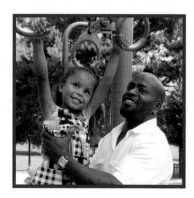

Promoting the Health of Populations

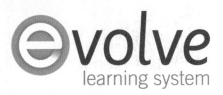

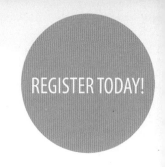

REGISTER TODAY!

To access your Student Resources, visit:

http://evolve.elsevier.com/nies

Evolve Student Resources for Nies & McEwen: *Community/Public Health Nursing,* 5th edition offer the following features:

- **Quiz**

  Multiple-choice review questions with instant scoring and feedback at the click of a button

- **Case Studies**

  Real-life clinical situations to help you develop your assessment and critical thinking skills, with answers provided

- **Glossary**

  Key Terms and their definitions, with search engine. Also available as flashcards

- **WebLinks**

  Link to hundreds of websites carefully chosen to supplement the content of the textbook

- **Resource Tools**

  Materials such as assessment tools and detailed tables that supplement the chapter content

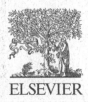

ELSEVIER

To Phil Yankovich, my husband, companion, and best friend, whose love, caring, and true support are always there for me. He provides me with the energy I need to pursue my dreams.

To Kara Nies Yankovich, my daughter, for whom I wish a happy and healthy life. Her energy, joy, and enthusiasm for life give so much to me.

To Earl and Lois Nies, my parents, for their never-ending encouragement and lifelong support. They helped me develop a foundation for creative thinking, new ideas, and spirited debate.

Mary A. Nies

To my husband, Scott McEwen, whose love, support, and encouragement have been my foundation for the past thirty years. I can't wait to see what happens during the next thirty!

Melanie McEwen

AUTHOR BIOGRAPHIES

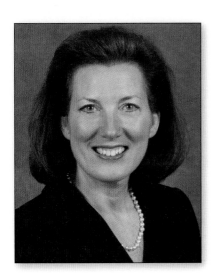

Mary A. Nies

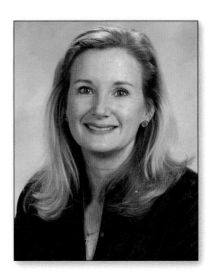

Melanie McEwen

Mary A. Nies, PhD, RN, FAAN, FAAHB, is the Carol Grotnes Belk Endowed Chair in Nursing and Adjunct Professor for the Department of Public Health Sciences in the College of Health and Human Services at the University of North Carolina at Charlotte. Dr. Nies received her diploma from Bellin School of Nursing in Green Bay, Wisconsin; her BSN from University of Wisconsin, Madison; her MSN from Loyola University, Chicago; and her PhD in Public Health Nursing, Health Services, and Health Promotion Research at the University of Illinois, Chicago. She completed a postdoctoral research fellowship in health promotion and community health at the University of Michigan, Ann Arbor. She is a fellow of the American Academy of Nursing and a fellow of the American Academy of Health Behavior. Dr. Nies co-edited *Community Health Nursing: Promoting the Health of Aggregates,* which received the 1993 Book of the Year award from the *American Journal of Nursing.* Her program of research focuses on the outcomes of health promotion interventions for minority and nonminority populations in the community. Her research is involved with physical activity and obesity prevention for populations, especially women. Her work also includes consulting in the areas of public and community health and health promotion education, practice, and research.

Melanie McEwen, PhD, RN, is an Associate Professor at the University of Texas Health Science Center at Houston School of Nursing. Dr. McEwen received her BSN from the University of Texas School of Nursing in Austin; her Master's in Community and Public Health Nursing from Louisiana State University Medical Center in New Orleans; and her PhD in Nursing at Texas Woman's University. Dr. McEwen has been a nursing educator for more than 22 years and is also the co-author of *Community–Based Nursing: An Introduction* (Saunders, 2009) and co-author/editor of *Theoretical Basis for Nursing* (Lippincott, 2011).

CONTRIBUTORS

Carrie L. Abele, PhD, RN
Assistant Professor
School of Nursing
Oakland University
Rochester, Michigan
*Chapter 13 , Cultural Diversity and
    Community Health Nursing*
Chapter 33, Home Health and Hospice

Linda Thompson Adams, DrPH, RN, FAAN
Dean and Professor
School of Nursing
Oakland University
Rochester, Michigan
*Chapter 12, Policy, Politics, Legislation,
    and Community Health Nursing*

Patricia M. Burbank, DNSc, RN
Professor
College of Nursing
The University of Rhode Island
Kingston, Rhode Island
*Chapter 7, Community Health Planning,
    Implementation, and Evaluation*

Mary Brecht Carpenter, RN, BSN, MPH
Adolescent Health Consultant
School Nurse
Loudoun County Public Schools
Ashburn, Virginia
Chapter16, Child and Adolescent Health

Holly B. Cassells, PhD, MPH, RN
Professor
School of Nursing and Health
    Professions
University of the Incarnate Word
San Antonio, Texas
Chapter 5, Epidemiology
Chapter 6, Community Assessment

Tom H. Cook, PhD, RN, FNP
Assistant Professor
School of Nursing
Vanderbilt University
Nashville, Tennessee
*Chapter 2, Historical Factors: Community
    Health Nursing in Context*

Nancy Diacon, DNP, RN, PMHCNS-BC
Manager of Education and Staff
    Development
The Menninger Clinic
Houston, Texas
*Chapter 24, Populations Affected
    by Mental Illness*

Stacy Drake, MSN, MPH, RN, D-ABMDI
Clinical Nursing Instructor
School of Nursing
University of Texas Health Science Center
Houston, Texas
*Chapter 31, Forensic and Correctional
    Nursing*

Nellie S. Droes, RN, BSN, DNSc
Associate Professor
College of Nursing
East Carolina University
Greenville, North Carolina
Chapter 22, Homeless Populations

Anita W. Finkelman, MSN, RN
Nurse Consultant
Chapter 10, The Health Care System

**Susan Rumsey Givens, BSN, RNC,
    MPH, LCCE**
Childbirth Educator
Mount Carmel St. Ann's Hospital
Westerville, Ohio
Chapter 16, Child and Adolescent Health

Lori A. Glenn, RN, MS, CNM
Instructor
McAuley School of Nursing
College of Health Professionals
University of Detroit Mercy
Detroit, Michigan
Chapter 17, Women's Health

Deanna E. Grimes, DrPH, RN, FAAN
Professor
School of Nursing
University of Texas Health Science Center
Houston, Texas
Chapter 25, Communicable Disease

**Karen Leavitt Grow, BSN, RN, CCM,
    CPHM**
Manager, Case Management
Sierra Surgery Hospital
Carson City, Nevada
Chapter 9, Case Management

Diane C. Hatton, RN, CS, DNSc
Professor and Associate Director for
    Research
School of Nursing
San Diego State University
San Diego, California
Chapter 22, Homeless Populations

Jean Cozad Lyon, PhD, APN
Interim CEO
Sierra Surgery Hospital
Carson City, Nevada
Chapter 9, Case Management

**Jane S. Mahoney, PhD, RN,
    PMHCNS-BC**
Director of Nursing Practice
    and Research
The Menninger Clinic
Assistant Professor
College of Medicine
Baylor University
Houston, Texas
*Chapter 24, Populations Affected by Mental
    Illness*

Diane C. Martins, PhD, RN
Assistant Professor
College of Nursing
The University of Rhode Island
Kingston, Rhode Island
*Chapter 3, Thinking Upstream: Nursing
    Theories and Population-Focused Nursing
    Practice*
*Chapter 7, Community Health Planning,
    Implementation, and Evaluation*

Cathy D. Meade, PhD, RN, FAAN
Senior Member
Health Outcomes and Behavior
    Professor
Department of Oncologic Sciences
Moffitt Cancer Center
Tampa, Florida
Chapter 8, Community Health Education

Carrie Morgan, MSN, CFNP
Instructor
Department of Nursing
Western Kentucky University
Bowling Green, Kentucky
Chapter 11, Economics of Health Care
Chapter 18, Men's Health

Marilyn R. Mouradjian, MSN, RN
Visiting Professor
School of Nursing
Oakland University
Rochester, Michigan
Chapter 26, Substance Abuse

Julie Cowan Novak, DNSc, RN, CPNP, FAANP
Associate Dean, Practice and Engagement
Joseph and Thelma Crow Endowed Professor
Director, University of Texas Health Science
    Center San Antonio Student Health Center
    and University of Texas Nursing Clinical
    Enterprise
University of Texas Health Science Center
    San Antonio School of Nursing
San Antonio, Texas
*Chapter 15, Globalization and International
    Health*

Catherine A. Pourciau, RN, MSN, FNP-C
Louisiana State University Health Sciences
    Center
Baton Rouge, Louisiana
Chapter 27, Violence
Chapter 29, School Health

Bridgette Crotwell Pullis, PhD, RN
Assistant Professor of Nursing
The University of Texas Health Science Center
Houston, Texas
*Chapter 4, Health Promotion and Risk
    Reduction*
Chaper 14, Environmental Health

Bonnie Rogers, PhD, COHN-S, FAAN
Director, Occupational Health Program
School of Public Health
University of North Carolina – Chapel Hill
Chapel Hill, North Carolina
Chapter 30, Occupational Health

Mary Ellen Trail Ross, DrPH, RN, CS
Assistant Professor
Department of Nursing Systems
University of Texas Health Science Center
Houston, Texas
Chapter 19, Senior Health

Patti J. Shoe, RN, MSN, FNP-C
Lecturer and Interim NP Coordinator
College of Health and Human Services
University of North Carolina at Charlotte
Charlotte, North Carolina
Chapter 23, Rural and Migrant Health

Beverly Cook Siegrist, EdD, MS, RN, CNE
Professor
School of Nursing
Western Kentucky University
Bowling Green, Kentucky
Chapter 20, Family Health
Chapter 32, Faith Community Nursing

Angela Snow, PhD, RN
Nurse Consultant
*Chapter 31, Forensic and Correctional
    Nursing*

Edith B. Summerlin, PhD, RN
Instructor
School of Nursing
University of Texas Health Science Center
Houston, Texas
Chapter 19, Senior Health
*Chapter 28, Natural and Man-Made
    Disasters*

Patricia L. Thomas, PhD, RN
Assistant Professor and Coordinator
Clinical Nurse Leader Program
McAuley School of Nursing
University of Detroit Mercy
Detroit, Michigan
Chapter 23, Rural and Migrant Health

Deborah M. Tierney, MS, RN, CPNP-PC
Instructor
School of Nursing
Oakland University
Rochester, Michigan
*Chapter 12, Policy, Politics, Legislation,
    and Community Health Nursing*

Linda L. Treloar, PhD, RN, NP-C
Professor of Nursing
Scottsdale Community College
Scottsdale, Arizona
*Chapter 21, Populations Affected
    by Disabilities*

Elaine C. Vallette, DrPH, RN
Dean, Nursing and Allied Health
Baton Rouge Community College
Baton Rouge, Louisiana
Chapter 27, Violence
Chapter 29, School Health

ANCILLARY AUTHORS

Jacqueline L. Burchum, DNSc, APRN, BC
Assistant Professor
College of Nursing
University of Tennessee Health Science
    Center
Memphis, Tennessee
Annotated Learning Objectives
Annotated Lecture Outlines

Penny Leake, PhD, RN
Associate Professor
Department of Nursing
Luther College
Decorah, Iowa
PowerPoint Slides
Teaching Strategies

Melanie McEwen, PhD, RN
Associate Professor
University of Texas Health Science Center
School of Nursing
Houston, Texas
Quiz

Virginia Nehring, PhD, RN
Professor Emeritus
College of Nursing and Health
Wright State University
Dayton, Ohio
Test Bank

REVIEWERS

Alice Susan Bidwell, BSN, MSN, EdD, RN-BC, CS
Professor and Chair, MSN Program
School of Health Professions
Marymount University
Arlington, Virginia

Mary Lashley, PhD, APRN, RN, BC
Professor
College of Health Professions
Towson University
Towson, Maryland

Lynn M. Leon, MSN, RN
Associate Professor
School of Nursing
Malone University
Canton, Ohio

Brenda Talley, PhD, RN, NEA-BC
Associate Professor
School of Nursing
Georgia Southern University
Statesboro, Georgia

Fatma Youssef, RN, MPH, DNSc
Professor
School of Health Professions
Marymount University
Arlington, Virginia

More money is spent per capita for health care in the United States than in any other country ($7400 in 2007). However, many countries have far better indices of health, including traditional indicators such as infant mortality rates and longevity for both men and women than does the United States. The United States is one of the few industrialized countries in the world that lacks a program of national health services or national health insurance. Although the United States spent 16.2% of its gross domestic product on health care expenditures in 2007, a record high of $2.2 trillion, around 16.0% of the population had no health care coverage.

The greater the proportion of money put into health care expenditures in the United States, the less money there is to improve education, jobs, housing, and nutrition. Over the years, the greatest improvements in the health of the population have been achieved through advances in public health using organized community efforts, such as improvements in sanitation, immunizations, and food quality and quantity. The greatest determinants of health are still equated with factors in the community, such as education, employment, housing, and nutrition. Although access to health care services and individual behavioral changes are important, they are only components of the larger determinants of health, such as social and physical environments.

UPSTREAM FOCUS

The traditional focus of many health care professionals, known as a downstream focus, has been to deliver health care services to ill people and to encourage needed behavioral change at the individual level. The focus of community health nursing has traditionally been on health promotion and illness prevention by working with individuals and families within the community. A shift is needed to an upstream focus, which includes working with aggregates and communities in activities such as organizing and setting health policy. This focus will help aggregates and communities work to create options for healthier environments with essential components of health, including adequate education, housing, employment, and nutrition and provide choices that allow people to make behavioral changes, live and work in safe environments, and access equitable and comprehensive health care.

Grounded in the tenets of public health nursing and the practice of public health nurses such as Lillian Wald, this fifth edition of *Community/Public Health Nursing: Promoting the Health of Populations* builds on the earlier works by highlighting an aggregate focus in addition to the traditional areas of family and community health and thus promotes upstream thinking. The primary focus is on the promotion of the health of aggregates. This approach includes the family as a population and addresses the needs of other aggregates or population subgroups. It conceptualizes the individual as a member of the

family and as a member of other aggregates, including organizations and institutions. Furthermore, individuals and families are viewed as a part of a population within an environment (i.e., within a community).

An aggregate is made up of a collective of individuals, be it family or another group that, with others, make up a community. This text emphasizes the aggregate as a unit of focus and how aggregates that make up communities promote their own health. The aggregate is presented within the social context of the community, and students are given the opportunity to define and analyze environmental, economic, political, and legal constraints to the health of these populations.

Community/public health nursing has been determined to be a synthesis of nursing and public health practice with goals to promote and preserve the health of populations. Diagnosis and treatment of human responses to actual or potential health problems is the nursing component. The ability to prevent disease, prolong life, and promote health through organized community effort is from the public health component. Community health nursing practice is responsible to the population as a whole. Nursing efforts to promote health and prevent disease are applied to the public, which includes all units in the community, be they individual or collective (e.g., person, family, other aggregate, community, or population).

PURPOSE OF THE TEXT

In this text, the student is encouraged to become a student of the community, learn from families and other aggregates in the community how they define and promote their own health, and learn how to become an advocate of the community by working with the community to initiate change. The student is exposed to the complexity and rich diversity of the community and is shown evidence of how the community organizes to meet change.

The use of language or terminology by clients and agencies varies in different parts of the United States, and it may vary from that used by government officials. The contributors of this text are a diverse group from various parts of the United States. Their terms vary from chapter to chapter and vary from those in use in local communities. For example, some authors refer to African-Americans, some to blacks, some to European-Americans, and some to whites. The student must be familiar with a range of terms and, most important, know what is used in his or her local community.

Outstanding features of this fifth edition include its provocative nature as it raises consciousness regarding the social inequalities that exist in the United States and how the market-driven health care system contributes to prevention of the realization of health as a right for all. With a focus on social justice, this text emphasizes society's responsibility for the protection of all human life to ensure that all people have their basic needs met, such as adequate health protection and income. Increased attention to the need for reform of the systems of health reimbursement has enhanced the recognition of the need for population-focused care, or care that covers all people residing within geographic boundaries, rather than only those populations enrolled in insurance plans. Working toward providing health promotion and population-focused care to all requires a dramatic shift in thinking from individual-focused care for the practitioners of the future. The future paradigm for health care is demanding that the focus of nursing move toward population-based interventions if we are to forge toward the goals established in *Healthy People 2020*.

This text is designed to **stimulate critical thinking and challenge students to question and debate issues.** Complex problems demand complex answers; therefore the student is expected to *synthesize prior biophysical, psychosocial, cultural, and ethical arenas of knowledge.* However, experiential knowledge is also necessary and the student is challenged to *enter new environments within the community* and gain new sensory, cognitive, and affective experiences. The authors of this text have integrated the concept of **upstream thinking**, introduced in the first edition, throughout this fifth edition as an important conceptual basis for nursing practice of aggregates and the community. The student is introduced to the individual and aggregate roles of community health nurses as they are engaged in a collective and interdisciplinary manner, working **upstream**, to facilitate the community's promotion of its own health. Students using this text will be better prepared to work with aggregates and communities in health promotion and with individuals and families in illness. Students using this text will also be better prepared to see the need to take responsibility for participation in organized community action targeting inequalities in arenas such as education, jobs, and housing and to participate in targeting individual health-behavioral change. These are important shifts in thinking for future practitioners who must be prepared to function in a population-focused health care system.

The text is also designed to increase the **cultural awareness and competency** of future community health nurses as they prepare to address the needs of culturally diverse populations. Students must be prepared to work with these growing populations as participation in the nursing workforce by ethnically and racially diverse people continues to lag. Various models are introduced to help students understand the growing link between social problems and health status, experienced disproportionately by diverse populations in the United States, and understand the methods of assessment and intervention used to meet the special needs of these populations.

The goals of the text are to provide the student with the ability to assess the complex factors in the community that affect individual, family, and other aggregate responses to health states and actual or potential health problems; and to help students use this ability to plan, implement, and evaluate community/public health nursing interventions to increase contributions to the promotion of the health of populations.

MAJOR THEMES RELATED TO PROMOTING THE HEALTH OF POPULATIONS

This text is built on the following major themes:

- A social justice ethic of health care in contrast to a market justice ethic of health care in keeping with the philosophy of public health as "health for all"
- A population-focused model of community/public health nursing as necessary to achieve equity in health for the entire population
- Integration of the concept of *upstream thinking* throughout the text and other appropriate theoretical frameworks related to chapter topics
- The use of population-focused and other community data to develop an assessment, or profile of health, and potential and actual health needs and capabilities of aggregates
- The application of all steps in the nursing process at the individual, family, and aggregate levels
- A focus on identification of needs of the aggregate from common interactions with individuals, families, and communities in traditional environments
- An orientation toward the application of all three levels of prevention at the individual, family, and aggregate levels
- The experience of the underserved aggregate, particularly the economically disenfranchised, including cultural and ethnic groups disproportionately at risk of developing health problems

Themes are developed and related to promoting the health of populations in the following ways:

- The commitment of community/public health nursing is to an equity model; therefore community health nurses work toward the provision of the unmet health needs of populations.
- The development of a population-focused model is necessary to close the gap between unmet health care needs and health resources on a geographic basis to the entire population. The contributions of intervention at the aggregate level work toward the realization of such a model.
- Contemporary theories provide frameworks for holistic community health nursing practice that help the students conceptualize the reciprocal influence of various components within the community on the health of aggregates and the population.
- The ability to gather population-focused and other community data in developing an assessment of health is a crucial initial step that precedes the identification of nursing diagnoses and plans to meet aggregate responses to potential and actual health problems.
- The nursing process includes, in each step, a focus on the aggregate, assessment of the aggregate, nursing diagnosis of the aggregate, planning for the aggregate, and intervention and evaluation at the aggregate level.
- The text discusses development of the ability to gather clues about the needs of aggregates from complex environments, such as during a home visit, with parents in a waiting room of a well-baby clinic, or with elders receiving hypertension screening, and to promote individual,

collective, and political action that addresses the health of aggregates.

- Primary, secondary, and tertiary prevention strategies include a major focus at the population level.
- In addition to offering a chapter on cultural influences in the community, the text includes data on and the experience of underserved aggregates at high risk of developing health problems and who are most often in need of community health nursing services (i.e., low and marginal income, cultural, and ethnic groups) throughout.

ORGANIZATION

The text is divided into eight units. *Unit 1, Introduction to Community Health Nursing*, presents an overview of the concept of health, a perspective of health as evolving and as defined by the community, and the concept of community health nursing as the nursing of aggregates from both historical and contemporary mandates. Health is viewed as an individual and collective right, brought about through individual and collective/political action. The definitions of public health and community health nursing and their foci are presented. Current crises in public health and the health care system and consequences for the health of the public frame implications for community health nursing. The historical evolution of public health, the health care system, and community health nursing is presented. The evolution of humans from wanderers and food gatherers to those who live in larger groups is presented. The text also discusses the influence of the group on health, which contrasts with the evolution of a health care system built around the individual person, increasingly fractured into many parts. Community health nurses bring to their practice awareness of the social context; economic, political, and legal constraints from the larger community; and knowledge of the current health care system and its structural constraints and limitations on the care of populations. The theoretical foundations for the text, with a focus on the concept of upstream thinking, and the rationale for a population approach to community health nursing are presented. Recognizing the importance of health promotion and risk reduction when striving to improve the health of individuals, families, groups, and communities, this unit concludes with a chapter elaborating on those concepts. Strategies for assessment and analysis of risk factors and interventions to improve health are described.

Unit 2, The Art and Science of Community Health Nursing, describes application of the nursing process—assessment, planning, intervention, and evaluation—to aggregates in the community using selected theory bases. The unit addresses the need for a population focus that includes the public health sciences of biostatistics and epidemiology as key in community assessment and the application of the nursing process to aggregates to promote the health of populations. Application of the art and science of community health nursing to meeting the needs of aggregates is evident in chapters that focus on community health planning and evaluation, community health education, and case management.

Unit 3, Factors That Influence the Health of the Community, examines factors and issues that can both positively and negatively affect health. Beginning with an overview of the health care delivery system, this unit examines the importance of economics and health care financing on the health of individuals, families, and populations. Health policy and legislation are also discussed, focusing on how policy is developed and the effect of past and future legislative changes on how health care is delivered in the United States. Cultural diversity and associated issues are described in detail, showing the importance of consideration of culture when developing health interventions in the community. The influence of the environment on the health of populations is considered, and the reader is led to recognize the multitude of external factors that influence health. This unit concludes with an examination of various aspects of global health and describes features of the health care systems and patterns of health and illness in developing and developed countries.

Unit 4, Aggregates in the Community, presents the application of the nursing process to address potential health problems identified in large groups, including children and adolescents, women, men, families, and seniors. The focus is on the major indicators of health (e.g., longevity, mortality, and morbidity), types of common health problems, use of health services, pertinent legislation, health services and resources, selected applications of the community health nursing process to a case study, application of the levels of prevention, selected roles of the community health nurse, and relevant research.

Unit 5, Vulnerable Populations, focuses on those aggregates in the community considered vulnerable: persons with disabilities, the homeless, those living in rural areas including migrant workers, and persons with mental illness. Chapters address the application of the community health nursing process to the special service needs in each of these areas. Basic community health nursing strategies are applied to promoting the health of these vulnerable high-risk aggregates.

Unit 6, Population Health Problems, focuses on health problems that affect large aggregates and their service needs as applied in community health nursing. These problems include communicable disease, violence and associated issues, substance abuse, and a chapter describing nursing care during disasters.

Unit 7, Community Health Settings, focuses on selected sites or specialties for community health: school health, occupational health, faith community health, and home health and hospice. Finally, forensic nursing, one of the more recently added sub-specialty areas of community health nursing, is presented in this unit, combined with correctional nursing content.

SPECIAL FEATURES

The following features are presented to enhance student learning:

- **Learning objectives.** Learning objectives set the framework for the content of each chapter.

- **Key terms.** A list of key terms for each chapter is provided at the beginning of the chapter. The terms are highlighted in blue within the chapter. The definitions of these terms are found in the Glossary located on the book's Evolve website.
- **Chapter outline.** The major headings of each chapter are provided at the beginning of each chapter to help locate important content.
- **Theoretical frameworks.** The use of theoretical frameworks common to nursing and public health will aid the student in application of familiar and new theory bases to problems and challenges in the community.
- *Healthy People 2020.* Goals and objectives of *Healthy People 2020* are presented in a special box throughout the text. (The updated *Heatlhy People 2020* information is new to this edition and based on the proposed objectives.)
- **Upstream thinking.** This theoretical construct is integrated into chapters throughout the text.
- **Case studies and application of the nursing process at individual, family, and aggregate levels.** The use of case studies and **clinical examples** throughout the text is designed to ground the theory, concepts, and application of the nursing process in practical and manageable examples for the student.
- **Research highlights.** The introduction of students to the growing bodies of community health nursing and public health research literature are enhanced by special boxes devoted to specific research studies.
- **Boxed information.** Summaries of content by section, clinical examples, and other pertinent information are presented in colored text to aid the students' learning by focusing on major points, illustrating concepts, and breaking up sections of "heavy" content.
- **Learning activities.** Selected learning activities are listed at the end of each chapter to enable students to enhance learning about the community and cognitive experiences.
- **Photo novellas.** Numerous stories in photograph form depicting public health care in a variety of settings and with different population groups.
- **Ethical insights boxes.** These boxes present situations of ethical dilemmas or considerations pertinent to particular chapters.

NEW CONTENT IN THIS EDITION

- Recognition of the essential aspect of **health promotion and risk reduction** when providing care to individuals, families, and groups in the community, this edition focuses attention on those concepts and presents related strategies and interventions in a new chapter.
- Reflecting the need for enhanced education and information related to spiritiuality, the chapter titled Faith

Community Health stresses various aspects of spiritual care as it describes nursing care provided through parish or congregational practices.
- New and timely information on **emerging infections** (e.g., H1N1, SARS, West Nile virus) and changing recommendations (e.g., pediatric immunization schedule) are given in the Communicable Disease chapter.
- Most chapters contain new or updated **Research Highlights boxes** highlighting timely, relevant examples of the topics from recent nursing literature and **Ethical Insights boxes** that emphasize specific ethical issues.

TEACHING AND LEARNING PACKAGE

Evolve website: The website at **http://evolve.elsevier.com/ nies/** is devoted exclusively to this text. It provides materials for both instructors and students.
- **For Instructors:** Annotated learning objectives, annotated lecture outlines, teaching strategies, PowerPoint lecture slides, image collection, and 750 test bank questions with alternative item questions.
- **For Students:** Quiz with multiple-choice questions with answers and correct answer rationales, Case Studies with questions and answers, Glossary, WebLinks, and Resource Tools (supplemental material).

ACKNOWLEDGMENTS

Community/Public Health Nursing: Promoting the Health of Populations could not have been written without sharing the experiences, thoughtful critique, and support of many people: individuals, families, groups, and communities. We give special thanks to everyone who made significant contributions to this book.

We are indebted to our contributing authors whose inspiration, untiring hours of work, and persistence have continued to build a new era of community health nursing practice with a focus on the population level. We thank the community health nursing faculty and students who welcomed the previous editions of the text and responded to our inquiries with comments and suggestions for the fifth edition. These people have challenged us to stretch, adapt, and continue to learn throughout our years of work. We also thank our colleagues in our respective work settings for their understanding and support during the writing and editing of this edition.

Finally, an enormous "thank you" to Elsevier editors Carlie Irwin, Nancy O'Brien, and Linda Thomas. Their energy, enthusiasm, encouragement, direction, and patience were vital to this project.

Mary A. Nies
Melanie McEwen

CONTENTS

UNIT 4   AGGREGATES IN THE COMMUNITY

UNIT 5   VULNERABLE POPULATIONS

Health: A Community View

Melanie McEwen, Mary A. Nies

Additional Material for Study, Review, and Further Exploration

evolve WEBSITE

http://evolve.elsevier.com/Nies

- Quiz
- Case Studies
- Glossary
- WebLinks

OBJECTIVES

Upon completion of this chapter, the reader will be able to do the following:

1. Compare and contrast the public health nursing definitions of health.
2. Define and discuss the focus of public health.
3. List the three levels of prevention, and give one example of each.
4. Explain the difference between public/community health nursing practice and community-based nursing practice.
5. Describe the purpose of *Healthy People 2020*, and give examples of the focus areas that encompass national health objectives.
6. Discuss the community/public health nursing practice in terms of public health's core functions and essential services.
7. Discuss community/public health nursing interventions as explained by the Intervention Wheel.

KEY TERMS

aggregates
community health
community health nursing
disease prevention
health

health promotion
population
population-focused nursing
primary prevention
public health

public health nursing
secondary prevention
tertiary prevention

OUTLINE

Community/public health nurses are in a position to assist the U.S. health care system in the transition from a disease-oriented system to a health-oriented system. Costs of caring for the sick account for the majority of escalating health care dollars, which increased from 5.7% of the gross domestic product in 1965 to 16% in 2006 (National Center for Health Statistics [NCHS], 2009). National annual health care expenditures reached $2.106 billion in 2006, or an astonishing $7026 per person.

U.S. health expenditures reflect a focus on the care of the sick. In 2006, $0.31 of each health care dollar supported hospital care, $0.21 supported physician services, and $0.10 was spent on prescription drugs (double the percentage since 1980). Although the majority of these funds provided care for the sick, less than $0.03 of every health care dollar backed preventive public health activities (NCHS, 2009). Despite high hospital and physician expenditures, U.S. health indicators rate considerably below the health indicators of many other countries. This reflects the severe disproportion of funding for preventive services and social and economic opportunities. Furthermore, the health status of the population within the United States varies markedly across areas of the country and among groups. For example, the economically disadvantaged and many cultural and ethnic groups have poorer overall health status compared with middle class Caucasians.

Nurses constitute the largest group of health care workers; therefore they are instrumental in creating a health care delivery system that will meet the health-oriented needs of the people. According to a recent survey of registered nurses (RNs) conducted by the Health Resources and Services Administration, about 62% of approximately 2.6 million employed RNs in the United States worked in hospitals during 2008 (down from 66.5% in 1992). This survey also found that about 14.2%, approximately 400,000, of all RNs worked in home, school, or occupational health settings; 10.5% worked in ambulatory care settings; and 5.3% worked in nursing homes or other extended care facilities (U.S. Department of Health and Human Services, Health Resources and Services Administration, Bureau of Health Professions [USDHHS, HRSA, BHP], 2010).

Between 1980 and 2008, the number of nurses employed in community, health, and ambulatory care settings more than doubled (USDHHS, HRSA, BHP, 2010). The decline in the percentage of nurses employed in hospitals and subsequent increase in nurses employed in community settings indicates a shift in focus from illness and institutional-based care to a focus on health promotion and preventive care. This shift will likely continue into the future as alternative delivery systems, such as ambulatory and home care, will employ more nurses (Gaines, Jenkins, and Ashe, 2005; Inglis, 2004; Way and MacNeil, 2007).

Community/public health nursing is the synthesis of nursing practice and public health practice. The major goal of community health nursing is to preserve the health of the community and surrounding populations by focusing on health promotion and health maintenance of individuals, families, and groups within the community. Thus,

community/public health nursing is associated with health and the identification of populations at risk rather than with an episodic response to patient demand.

The mission of public health is social justice, which entitles all people to basic necessities such as adequate income and health protection and accepts collective burdens to make this possible. Public health, with its egalitarian tradition and vision, conflicts with the predominant U.S. model of market justice that only entitles people to what they have gained through individual efforts. Although market justice respects individual rights, collective action and obligations are minimal. An overinvestment in technology and curative medical services within the market justice system has stifled the evolution of a health system designed to protect and preserve the health of the population. There is a need for an ethic of social justice, for it is society's responsibility, rather than the individual's, to meet the basic needs of all people. Thus there is a need for public funding of prevention efforts to enhance the health of our population.

Current U.S. health policy advocates changes in personal behaviors that might predispose individuals to chronic disease or accident. This policy promotes exercise, healthy eating, tobacco cessation, and moderate consumption of alcohol. However, simply encouraging the individual to overcome the effects of unhealthy activities lessens focus on collective behaviors necessary to change the determinants of health stemming from such factors as air and water pollution, workplace hazards, and unequal access to health care. Because living arrangements, work/school environment, and other sociocultural constraints affect health and well-being, public policy must address societal and environmental changes, in addition to lifestyle changes, that will positively influence the health of the entire population.

With ongoing changes in the health care system and increased employment in community settings, there will be greater demands on community health nurses to broaden their public health perspective. The Code of Ethics of the American Nurses Association (ANA) (2001) promotes social reform by focusing on health policy and legislation to positively affect accessibility, quality, and cost of health care. Community and public health nurses, therefore, must align themselves with public health programs that promote and preserve the health of populations by influencing sociocultural issues such as human rights, homelessness, violence, and stigma of illness. This allows nurses to be positioned to promote the health, welfare, and safety of all individuals.

This chapter examines health from a population-focused, community-based perspective. Therefore it requires understanding of how people identify, define, and describe related concepts. The following section explores six major ideas:

1. Definitions of "health" and "community"
2. Determinants of health and disease
3. Indicators of health and disease
4. Definition and focus of public and community health
5. Description of a preventive approach to health
6. Definition and focus of "public health nursing," "community health nursing," and "community-based nursing"

DEFINITIONS OF HEALTH AND COMMUNITY

Health

The definition of health is evolving. The early, classic definition of health by the World Health Organization (WHO) set a trend toward describing health in social terms, rather than in medical terms. Indeed, the WHO (1958, p. 1) defined health as "a state of complete physical, mental, and social well-being and not merely the absence of disease or infirmity."

Social means "of or relating to living together in organized groups or similar close aggregates" (*American Heritage College Dictionary*, 1997, p. 1291) and refers to units of people in communities who interact with each other. "Social health" connotes community vitality and is a result of positive interaction among groups within the community with an emphasis on health promotion and illness prevention. For example, community groups may sponsor food banks in churches and civic organizations to help alleviate problems with hunger and nutrition. Other community groups may form to address problems of violence and lack of opportunity, which can negatively affect social health.

In the mid-1980s, the WHO expanded the definition of health to include the following socialized conceptualization of health:

> The extent to which an individual or group is able, on the one hand, to realize aspirations and satisfy needs; and, on the other hand, to change or cope with the environment. Health is, therefore, seen as a resource for everyday life, not the objective of living; it is a positive concept emphasizing social and personal resources, and physical capacities. (WHO, 1986, p. 73)

Saylor (2004) pointed out that the WHO definition considers several dimensions of health. These include physical (structure/function), social, role, mental (emotional and intellectual), and general perceptions of health status. It also conceptualizes health from a macro perspective, as a resource to be used rather than a goal in and of itself.

The nursing literature contains many varied definitions of health. For example, health has been defined as "a state of well-being in which the person is able to use purposeful, adaptive responses and processes physically, mentally, emotionally, spiritually, and socially" (Murray, Zentner, and Yakimo, 2009, p. 53); "actualization of inherent and acquired human potential through goal-directed behavior, competent self-care, and satisfying relationships with others" (Pender, Murdaugh, and Parsons, 2006, p. 22); and a state of a person that is characterized by soundness or wholeness of developed human structures and of bodily and mental functioning (Orem, 2001).

The variety of characterizations of the word illustrates the difficulty in standardizing the conceptualization of health. Commonalities involve description of "goal-directed" or "purposeful" actions, processes, responses, or behaviors and possessing "soundness," "wholeness," and/or "well-being." Problems can arise when the definition involves a unit of analysis. For example, some authors use the individual or "person" as the unit of analysis and exclude the community.

Others may include additional concepts, such as adaptation and environment, in health definitions and then present the environment as static and requiring human adaptation, rather than as changing and enabling human modification.

For many years, community and public health nurses have favored Dunn's (1961) classic concept of wellness, in which family, community, society, and environment are interrelated and have an impact on health. From his viewpoint, illness, health, and peak wellness are on a continuum; health is fluid and changing. Consequently, within a social environment, the state of health depends on the goals, potentials, and performance of individuals, families, communities, and societies.

Community

The definitions of *community* are also numerous and variable. Baldwin and colleagues (1998) outlined the evolution of the definition of community by examining definitions that appeared in community health nursing texts. They determined that, before 1996, definitions of community focused on geographical boundaries, combined with social attributes of people. Through citing several sources from the later part of the decade, the authors observed that geographical location became a secondary characteristic in the discussion of what defines a community.

In recent nursing literature, community has been defined as "a collection of people who interact with one another and whose common interests or characteristics form the basis for a sense of unity or belonging" (Allender, Rector, and Warner, 2009, p. 6); "a group of people who share something in common and interact with one another, who may exhibit a commitment with one another and may share a geographic boundary" (Lundy and Janes, 2009, p. 16); "a group of people who share common interests, who interact with each other, and who function collectively within a defined social structure to address common concerns" (Clark, 2008, p. 27); and "a locality-based entity, composed of systems of formal organizations reflecting society's institutions, informal groups and aggregates" (Shuster and Goeppinger, 2008, p. 344).

Maurer and Smith (2009) further addressed the concept of community and identified four defining attributes: people, place, interaction, and common characteristics, interests, or goals. Combining ideas and concepts, in this text, community is seen as a group or collection of locality-based individuals, interacting in social units and sharing common interests, characteristics, values, and/or goals.

Maurer and Smith (2009) noted that there are two main types of communities: geopolitical communities and phenomenological communities. Geopolitical communities are those most traditionally recognized or imagined when considering the term *community*. Geopolitical communities are defined or formed by both natural and manmade boundaries and include cities, counties, states, and nations. Other commonly recognized geopolitical communities are school districts, census tracts, zip codes, and neighborhoods. Phenomenological communities, on the other hand, refer to relational, interactive groups. In phenomenological communities, the place or setting is more abstract, and people share a group perspective or identity based on culture, values, history, interests, and goals. Examples of phenomenological communities would be schools, colleges, and universities; churches, synagogues, and mosques; and various groups or organizations.

A community of solution is a type of phenomenological community. A community of solution is a collection of people who form a group specifically to address a common need or concern. The Sierra Club, whose members lobby for the preservation of natural resource lands, and a group of disabled people who challenge the owners of an office building to obtain equal access to public buildings, education, jobs, and transportation are examples. These groups or social units work together to realize a level of potential "health" and to address identified actual and potential health threats and health needs.

Population and *aggregate* are related terms that are often used in public health and community health nursing. Population is typically used to denote a group of people having common personal or environmental characteristics. It can also refer to all of the people in a defined community (Maurer and Smith, 2009). Aggregates are subgroups or subpopulations that have some common characteristics or concerns (Clark, 2008). Depending on the situation, needs, and practice parameters, community health nursing interventions may be directed toward a community (e.g., residents of a small town), a population (e.g., all elders in a rural region), or an aggregate (e.g., pregnant teens within a school district).

DETERMINANTS OF HEALTH AND DISEASE

The health status of a community is associated with a number of factors such as health care access, economic conditions, social and environmental issues, and cultural practices, and it is essential for the community health nurse to understand the determinants of health and recognize the interaction of the factors that lead to disease, death, and disability. It has been estimated that individual behaviors and environmental factors are responsible for about 70% of all premature deaths in the United States (USDHHS, 2000). Indeed, individual biology and behaviors influence health through their interaction with each other and with the individual's social and physical environments. In addition, policies and interventions can improve health by targeting detrimental or harmful factors related to individuals and their environment. Figure 1-1 depicts the interaction of these determinants and shows how health is influenced.

In a seminal work, McGinnis and Foege (1993) described what they termed "actual causes of death" in the United States. Leading the list was smoking, which was implicated in almost 20% of the annual deaths in the United States—approximately 400,000 individuals. Diet and activity patterns were deemed to account for about 14% of deaths (about 300,000 per year), and alcohol was implicated in about 5% of all deaths because of its association with accidents, suicides, homicides, and cirrhosis and chronic liver disease. Although all of these causes of mortality are related to individual lifestyle choices, they can also be strongly influenced by population-focused policy

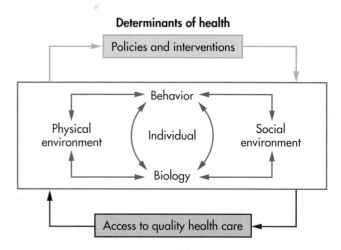

FIGURE 1-1 *Healthy People 2010*—Determinants of health.

efforts and education. For example, the prevalence of adult smoking has fallen dramatically during the past two decades, largely because of legal efforts (e.g., laws prohibiting sale of tobacco to minors and much higher taxes), organizational policy (e.g., smoke-free workplaces), and education. Likewise, recent concerns about the widespread increase in incidence of overweight and obesity have led to population-based measures to address the issue (e.g. removal of soft drink and candy machines from schools, regulations prohibiting certain types of fats from processed foods).

In another important writing, McKeown (2003) observed that health has improved over the past 100 years largely because people become ill less often. He noted that, at the population level, health can be largely attributed to higher standards of living, better nutrition, a healthier environment, and having fewer children. Furthermore, public health efforts, such as immunization, and medical care, including management of acute episodic illnesses (e.g., pneumonia, tuberculosis) and chronic disease (e.g., cancer, heart disease), have also contributed significantly to the increase in life expectancy (Rothstein, 2003).

Community and public health nurses should understand these concepts and appreciate that health and illness are influenced by a web of factors, some that can be changed (e.g., individual behaviors such as tobacco use, diet, activity) and some that cannot (e.g., genetics, age, gender). Other factors (e.g., physical and social environment) will require changes that may need to be accomplished from a policy perspective. Community health nurses must work with policy makers and community leaders to identify patterns of disease and death and to advocate for activities and policies that promote health at the individual, family, and community levels.

INDICATORS OF HEALTH AND ILLNESS

A variety of health indicators are used by health providers, policy makers, and community health nurses to measure the health of the community. Local or state health departments, the Centers for Disease Control and Prevention, and the National Center for Health Statistics provide morbidity, mortality, and other health status–related data. State and local health departments are responsible for collecting morbidity and mortality data and forwarding the information to the appropriate federal-level agency, which is often the Centers for Disease Control and Prevention. Some of the more commonly reported indicators are life expectancy, infant mortality, age-adjusted death rates, and cancer incidence rates.

Indicators of mortality illustrate the health status of a community and/or population because changes in mortality reflect a number of social, economic, health service, and related trends (Torrens, 2008). These data may be useful in analyzing health patterns over time, comparing communities from different geographical regions or comparing different aggregates within a community.

When developing the national health objectives for *Healthy People 2010*, a total of 10 leading health indicators were identified that reflected the major public health concerns in the United States (*Healthy People* box). They include individual behaviors (e.g., physical activity, overweight, and obesity), physical and social environmental factors (e.g., environmental quality, injury, and violence), and health systems issues (e.g., access to health care). Each of these indicators can affect the health of individuals and communities, and they can be correlated with leading causes of morbidity and mortality. For example, tobacco use is linked to heart disease, stroke, and cancer; substance abuse is linked to accidents, injuries, and violence; irresponsible sexual behaviors can lead to unwanted pregnancy, as well as sexually transmitted diseases, including human immunodeficiency virus/acquired immunodeficiency syndrome (HIV/AIDS); and lack of access to health care can contribute to poor pregnancy outcomes, untreated illness, and disability.

 HEALTHY PEOPLE

Leading Health Indicators

- Physical activity
- Overweight and obesity
- Tobacco use
- Substance abuse
- Responsible sexual behavior
- Mental health
- Injury and violence
- Environmental quality
- Immunization
- Access to health care

From US Department of Health and Human Services: *Healthy People 2010 objectives*, Washington, DC, 2000, The Author.

Community health nurses should be aware of health patterns and health indicators within their practice. Nurses should ask many questions, including the following: What are the leading causes of death and disease among various groups served? How do infant mortality rates and teenage pregnancy rates in this community compare with regional, state, and national rates? What are the most serious communicable disease threats? What are the most common environmental risks?

The community health nurse may identify areas for further investigation and intervention through an understanding of health, disease, and mortality patterns. For example, if a school nurse learns that the teenage pregnancy rate

in his or her community is higher than regional and state averages, he or she should address the problem with school officials, parents, and students. Likewise, if an occupational health nurse discovers an apparent high rate of chronic lung disease in an industrial facility, he or she should work with company management, employees, and state and federal officials to identify potential harmful sources. Finally, if a public health nurse works in a state-sponsored AIDS clinic and recognizes an increase in the number of women testing positive for HIV, he or she should report all findings to the designated agencies. The nurse should then participate in investigative efforts to determine what is precipitating the increase and work to remedy the identified threats or risks.

DEFINITION AND FOCUS OF PUBLIC HEALTH AND COMMUNITY HEALTH

C. E. Winslow is known for the following classic definition of public health:

> Public health is the Science and Art of (1) preventing disease, (2) prolonging life, and (3) promoting health and efficiency through organized community effort for:
> (a) sanitation of the environment,
> (b) control of communicable infections,
> (c) education of the individual in personal hygiene,
> (d) organization of medical and nursing services for the early diagnosis and preventive treatment of disease, and
> (e) development of the social machinery to ensure everyone a standard of living adequate for the maintenance of health, so organizing these benefits as to enable every citizen to realize his birthright of health and longevity. (Hanlon, 1960, p. 23)

A key phrase in this definition of public health is "through organized community effort." The term public health connotes organized, legislated, and tax-supported efforts that serve all people through health departments or related governmental agencies.

The public health nursing tradition, begun in the late 1800s by Lillian Wald and her associates, clearly illustrates this phenomenon (Wald, 1971, see Chapter 2). After moving into the immigrant community to provide care for individuals and families, these early public health nurses saw that neither administering bedside clinical nursing nor teaching family members to deliver care in the home adequately addressed the true determinants of health and disease. They resolved that collective political activity should focus on advancing the health of aggregates and improving social and environmental conditions by addressing the social and environmental determinants of health, such as child labor, pollution, and poverty. Wald and her colleagues impacted the health of the community by organizing the community, establishing school nursing, and taking impoverished mothers to testify in Washington, DC (Wald, 1971).

In a key action, the Institute of Medicine (1988) identified the following three primary functions of public health: *assessment, assurance,* and *policy development.* Box 1-1 depicts each of the three primary functions and describes them briefly. All nurses working in community settings should develop knowledge and skills related to each of these primary functions.

The term community health extends the realm of public health to include organized health efforts at the community level through both government *and* private efforts. Participants include privately funded agencies such as the American Heart Association or the American Red Cross. A variety of private and public structures serve community health efforts.

Public health efforts focus on prevention and promotion of population health at the federal, state, and local levels. These efforts at the federal and state levels concentrate on providing support and advisory services to public health structures at the local level. The local level structures provide direct services to communities through two avenues:

- Community health services, which protect the public from hazards such as polluted water and air, tainted food, and unsafe housing
- Personal health care services such as immunization and family planning services, well-infant care, and sexually transmitted disease (STD) treatment

Personal health services may be part of the public health effort and often target the populations most at risk and in need of services. Public health efforts are multidisciplinary because they require people with many different skills. Community health nurses work with a diverse team of public health professionals, including epidemiologists, local health officers, and health educators. Public health science methods that assess biostatistics, epidemiology, and population needs provide a method of measuring characteristics and health indicators and disease patterns within a community. In 1994, the American Public Health Association drafted a list of ten essential public health services, which the U.S. Department of Health and Human Services (USDHHS, 1997) later adopted. This list appears in Box 1-2.

PREVENTIVE APPROACH TO HEALTH

Health Promotion and Levels of Prevention

Contrasting with "medical care," which focuses on disease management and "cure," public health efforts focus on health promotion and disease prevention. Health promotion activities enhance resources directed at improving well-being, whereas disease prevention activities protect people from disease and the effects of disease. Leavell and Clark (1958) identified three levels of prevention commonly described in nursing practice: primary prevention, secondary prevention, and tertiary prevention (Figure 1-2 and Table 1-1).

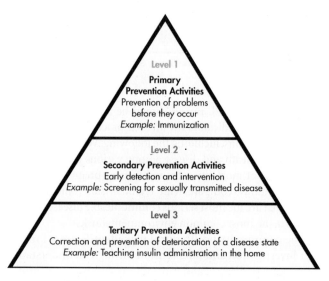

FIGURE 1-2 The three levels of prevention.

TABLE 1-1   EXAMPLES OF LEVELS OF PREVENTION AND CLIENTS SERVED IN THE COMMUNITY

DEFINITION OF CLIENT SERVED*	LEVEL OF PREVENTION		
	PRIMARY (HEALTH PROMOTION AND SPECIFIC PREVENTION)	SECONDARY (EARLY DIAGNOSIS AND TREATMENT)	TERTIARY (LIMITATION OF DISABILITY AND REHABILITATION)
Individual	Dietary teaching during pregnancy Immunizations	HIV testing Screening for cervical cancer	Teaching new clients with diabetes how to administer insulin Exercise therapy after stroke Skin care for incontinent patients
Family (two or more individuals bound by kinship, law, or living arrangement and with common emotional ties and obligations [see Chapter 20])	Education or counseling regarding smoking, dental care, or nutrition Adequate housing	Dental examinations Tuberculin testing for family at risk	Mental health counseling or referral for family in crisis (e.g., grieving or experiencing a divorce) Dietary instructions and monitoring for family with overweight members
Group or aggregate (interacting people with a common purpose or purposes)	Birthing classes for pregnant teenage mothers AIDS and other STD education for high school students	Vision screening of first-grade class Mammography van for screening of women in a low-income neighborhood Hearing tests at a senior center	Group counseling for grade school children with asthma Swim therapy for physically disabled elders at a senior center Alcoholics Anonymous and other self-help groups Mental health services for military veterans
Community and populations (aggregate of people sharing space over time within a social system [see Chapter 6]; population groups or aggregates with power relations and common needs or purposes)	Fluoride water supplementation Environmental sanitation Removal of environmental hazards	Organized screening programs for communities (e.g., health fairs) VDRL screening for marriage license applicants in a city Lead screening for children by school district	Shelter and relocation centers for fire or earthquake victims Emergency medical services Community mental health services for chronically mentally ill Home care services for chronically ill

AIDS, Acquired immunodeficiency syndrome; *HIV,* human immunodeficiency virus; *STD,* sexually transmitted disease; *VDRL,* Venereal Disease Research Laboratory.
*Note that terms are used differently in literature of various disciplines. There are not any clear-cut definitions; for example, families may be referred to as an aggregate, and a population and subpopulations may exist within a community.

Primary prevention relates to activities directed at preventing a problem before it occurs by altering susceptibility or reducing exposure for susceptible individuals. Primary prevention consists of two elements: general health promotion and specific protection. Health promotion efforts enhance resiliency and protective factors and target essentially well populations. Examples include promotion of good nutrition, provision of adequate shelter, and encouraging regular exercise. Specific protection efforts reduce or eliminate risk factors and include such measures as immunization and water purification (Keller et al., 2004a; McEwen and Pullis, 2008).

Secondary prevention refers to early detection and prompt intervention during the period of early disease pathogenesis. Secondary prevention is implemented after a problem has begun but before signs and symptoms appear and targets those populations who have risk factors (Keller et al., 2004a). Mammography, blood pressure screening, scoliosis screening, and Papanicolaou smears are examples of secondary prevention.

Tertiary prevention targets populations that have experienced disease or injury and focuses on limitation of disability and rehabilitation. Aims of tertiary prevention are to keep health problems from getting worse, to reduce the effects of disease

and injury, and to restore individuals to their optimal level of functioning (Keller et al., 2004b; McEwen and Pullis, 2009). Examples include teaching how to perform insulin injections and disease management to a patient with diabetes, referral of a patient with spinal cord injury for occupational and physical therapy, and leading a support group for grieving parents.

Much of community health nursing practice is directed toward preventing the progression of disease at the earliest period or phase feasible using the appropriate level(s) of prevention. For example, when applying "levels of prevention" to a client with HIV/AIDS, a nurse might perform the following interventions:

- Educate students on the practice of sexual abstinence or "safer sex" by using barrier methods (primary prevention)
- Encourage testing and counseling for clients with known exposure or who are in high-risk groups; provide referrals for follow-up for clients who test positive for HIV (secondary prevention)
- Provide education on management of HIV infection, advocacy, case management, and other interventions for those who are HIV positive (tertiary prevention) (McEwen and Pullis, 2008).

The concepts of prevention and population-focused care figure prominently in a conceptual orientation to nursing practice referred to as "thinking upstream." This orientation is derived from an analogy of patients falling into a river upstream and being rescued downstream by health providers overwhelmed with the struggle of responding to disease and illness. The river as an analogy for the natural history of illness was first coined by McKinlay (1979), with a charge to health providers to refocus their efforts toward preventive and "upstream" activities. In a description of the daily challenges of providers to address health from a preventive versus curative focus, McKinlay differentiates the consequences of illness (*downstream* endeavors) from its precursors (*upstream* endeavors). The author then charges health providers to critically examine the relative weight of their activities toward illness response versus the prevention of illness.

A population-based perspective on health and health determinants is critical to understanding and formulating nursing actions to prevent disease. By examining the origins of disease, nurses identify social, political, environmental, and economic factors that often lead to poor health options for both individuals and populations. The call to refocus the efforts of nurses "upstream, where the real problems lie" (McKinlay, 1979) has been welcomed by community health nurses in a variety of practice settings. For these nurses, this theme provides affirmation of their daily efforts to prevent disease in populations at risk in schools, work sites, and clinics throughout their local communities and in the larger world.

⚖ ETHICAL INSIGHTS

Inequities: Distribution of Resources

In the United States, inequities in the distribution of resources pose a threat to the common good and a challenge for community and public health nurses. Factors that contribute to wide variations in health disparities include education, income, and occupation. Lack of health insurance is a key factor in this issue, as about 20% of non-elderly adults and 25% of children in the United States are uninsured. Lack of insurance is damaging to population health, as low-income, uninsured individuals are much less likely than nonpoor insured individuals to receive timely physical examinations and preventive dental care.

Public health nurses are regularly confronted with the consequences of the fragmented health care delivery system. They diligently work to improve the circumstances for populations who have not had adequate access to resources largely because of who they are and where they live.

Ethical questions commonly encountered in community and public health nursing practice include the following: Should resources (e.g., free or low-cost immunizations) be offered to all, even those who have insurance that will pay for the care? Should public health nurses serve anyone who meets financial need guidelines, regardless of medical need? Should the health department provide flu shots to persons of all ages or just those most likely to be severely affected by the disease? Should illegal aliens or persons working on "green cards" receive the same level of health care services that are available to citizens?

Social justice in health care is a goal for all. To this end, community and public health nurses must face the challenges and dilemmas related to these and other questions as they assist individuals, families, and communities deal with the uneven distribution of health resources.

From Ervin NE, Bell SE: Social justice issues related to uneven distribution of resources, *J N Y State Nurses Assoc* 35(1):8-13, 2004.

Prevention Versus Cure

Spending additional dollars for cure in the form of health care services does not improve the health of a population, whereas spending money on prevention does improve health. Feldstein (2007) and others (Sultz and Young, 2006; Torrens, 2008) note that there is an absence of convincing evidence that indicates that the amount of money expended for health care improves the health of a population. The real determinants of health, as mentioned, are prevention efforts that provide education, housing, food, a decent minimal income, and safe social and physical environments. The United States spends nearly one seventh of the nation's wealth on health care or "cure" for individuals; this could possibly divert money away from the needed resources and services that make a greater impact on health (McKeown, 2003; NCHS, 2008).

U.S. policy makers have not committed to achieving these important health outcomes for the poor, vulnerable, and uninsured populations. With a limited health workforce and monetary resources, the United States cannot continue to spend vast amounts on health care services when the investment fails to improve health outcomes. In industrialized countries, life expectancy at birth is not related to the level of health care expenditures; in developing countries, longevity is closely related to the level of economic development and the education of the population (Feldstein, 2007; Sultz and Young, 2006).

A continued overexpansion of the current health care system could actually be detrimental to the health of a population. This may deter a large investment of the country's wealth in education and other developmental efforts that positively impact health. Managed care organizations (MCOs) focus on prevention; therefore they have determined that the rate of health care cost increases have slowed among employees of large firms (Koch, 2008). Prevention programs may help reduce costs for those enrolled in MCOs, but it is unclear who will provide these services for the uninsured, poor, and other vulnerable populations. In addition, who will provide adequate schooling, housing, meals, wages, and a safe environment for the disadvantaged? Reductions in health care spending would decrease the effects of economic disparities by allowing investments in sufficient housing, jobs, nutrition, and safe environments.

Healthy People 2020

In 1979, the U.S. Department of Health and Human Services published a national prevention initiative titled *Healthy People: The Surgeon General's Report on Health Promotion and Disease Prevention*. The 1979 version established goals that would reduce mortality among infants, children, adolescents and young adults, and adults and increase independence among older adults. In 1990, the mortality of infants, children, and adults declined sufficiently to meet the goal. Adolescent mortality did not reach the 1990 target, and data systems were unable to adequately track the target for older adults (USDHHS, 2000).

♥ HEALTHY PEOPLE 2020

Topic Areas

- Access to health services
- Adolescent health
- Arthritis, osteoporosis, and chronic back conditions
- Blood disorders and blood safety
- Cancer
- Chronic kidney disease
- Diabetes
- Disability and secondary conditions
- Early and middle childhood
- Educational and community-based programs
- Environmental health
- Family planning
- Food safety
- Genomics
- Global health
- Health communication and health IT
- Healthcare-associated infections
- Hearing and other sensory or communication disorders
- Heart disease and stroke

- HIV
- Immunization and infectious diseases
- Injury and violence prevention
- Maternal, infant, and child health
- Medical product safety
- Mental health and mental disorders
- Nutrition and weight status
- Occupational safety and health
- Older adults
- Oral health
- Physical activity and fitness
- Public health infrastructure
- Quality of life and well-being
- Respiratory diseases
- Sexually transmitted diseases
- Social determinants of health
- Substance abuse
- Tobacco use
- Vision

From U.S. Department of Health and Human Services: *Healthy People 2020 draft objectives*, Washington, DC, 2009. Accessed April 6, 2010 from www.healthypeople.gov/hp2020/objectives/files/Draft2009objectives.pdf.

Published in 1989, *Healthy People 2000* built on the first Surgeon General's report. *Healthy People 2000* contained the following broad goals (USDHHS, 1989):

1. Increase the span of healthy life for Americans.
2. Reduce health disparities among Americans.
3. Achieve access to preventive services for all Americans.

The purpose of *Healthy People 2000* was to provide direction for individuals wanting to change personal behaviors and to improve health in communities through health promotion policies. The report assimilated the broad approaches of health promotion, health protection, and preventive services and contained more than 300 objectives organized into twenty-two priority areas. Although many of the objectives fell short, the initiative was extremely successful in raising providers' awareness of health behaviors and health promotional activities. States, local health departments, and private sector health workers used the objectives to determine the relative health of their community and set goals for the future.

Healthy People 2010 emerged in January 2000. It expanded on the objectives from *Healthy People 2000* through a broadened prevention science base, an improved surveillance and data system, and a heightened awareness and demand for preventive health services. This reflects changes in demographics, science, technology, and disease. *Healthy People 2010* listed the following broad goals:

Goal 1: Increase quality and years of healthy life.
Goal 2: Eliminate health disparities.

The first goal moved beyond the idea of increasing life expectancy to incorporate the concept of health-related quality of life (HRQOL). This concept of health includes aspects of physical and mental health and their determinants and measures functional status, participation, and well-being. HRQOL expands the definition of health—beyond simply opposing the negative concepts of disease and death—by integrating mental and physical health concepts (USDHHS, 2000).

The third version of the Nation's health objectives, *Healthy People 2020*, was published in 2010. *Healthy People 2020* is divided into 38 "Topic Areas" and contains numerous new objectives and updates for hundreds of objectives from the previous editions. The focus areas are listed in the *Healthy People 2020* box. The objectives can help guide health promotion activities and can be used to aid in community-wide initiatives (USDHHS, 2010). All health care practitioners, particularly those working in the community, should review the *Healthy People 2020* objectives and focus on the relevant areas in their practice. Practitioners should incorporate these objectives into programs, events, and publications whenever possible and should use them as a framework to promote healthy cities and communities. Selected relevant objectives are presented throughout this book to acquaint future community health nurses with the scope of the *Healthy People 2020* initiative and to enhance awareness of current health indicators and national goals (see www.healthypeople.gov for more information).

DEFINITION AND FOCUS OF PUBLIC HEALTH NURSING, COMMUNITY HEALTH NURSING, AND COMMUNITY-BASED NURSING

The terms *community health nursing* and *public health nursing* are often synonymous or interchangeable. Like the practice of community/public health nursing, the terms are evolving. In the past debates and discussions, definitions of "community health nursing" and "public health nursing" indicate similar yet distinctive ideologies, visions, or philosophies of nursing. These concepts and a third related term—*community-based nursing*—are discussed in this section.

Public and Community Health Nursing

Public health nursing has frequently been described as the synthesis of public health and nursing practice. Freeman (1963) provided a classic definition of public health nursing:

Public health nursing may be defined as a field of professional practice in nursing and in public health in which technical nursing, interpersonal, analytical, and organizational skills are applied to problems of health as they affect the community. These skills are applied in concert with those of other persons engaged in health care, through comprehensive nursing care of families and other groups and through measures for evaluation or control of threats to health, for health education of the public, and for mobilization of the public for health action. (p. 34)

Through the 1980s and 1990s, most nurses were taught that there was a distinction between "community health nursing" and "public health nursing." Indeed, "public health nursing" was seen as a subspecialty nursing practice generally delivered within 'official' or governmental agencies. In contrast, "community health nursing" was considered to be a broader and more general specialty area that encompassed many additional subspecialties (e.g., school nursing, occupational health nursing, forensic nursing, home health). In 1980, the American Nurses Association (ANA) defined community health nursing as "the synthesis of nursing practice and public health practice applied to promoting and preserving the health of populations" (p. 2). This viewpoint noted that a community health nurse directs care to individuals, families, or groups; this care, in turn, contributes to the health of the total population.

Most recently, the ANA has revised the standards of practice for this specialty area (ANA, 2007). In the updated standards, the designation was again "public health nursing," and the ANA used the definition presented by the American Public Health Association's Committee on Public Health Nursing (1996). Thus, public health nursing is defined as "the practice of promoting and protecting the health of populations using knowledge from nursing, social, and public health sciences" (ANA/APHA, 1996, p. 5). The ANA (2007) elaborated by explaining that public health nursing practice "is population-focused, with the goals of promoting health and preventing

RESEARCH HIGHLIGHTS

Public Health Nurse Job Satisfaction

A study of 192 public health nurses was conducted to describe the characteristics and relationships of organizational structure and job satisfaction among public health nurses. The researchers found that the nurses in the study reported "moderate" levels of job satisfaction. Factors identified that increased job satisfaction were more years of experience at the health department and improved vertical and horizontal decision-making opportunities. Other factors that nurses indicated would improve their job satisfaction were better pay, more input, and better role clarity. The researchers concluded that job satisfaction improves when supervisors and subordinates consult together concerning job tasks and decisions, and when individuals are involved with peers in decision making.

Campbell SL, Fowles ER, Weber BJ: Organizational structure and job satisfaction in public health nursing, *Public Health Nurs* 21(6):564-571, 2004.

disease and disability for all people through the creation of conditions in which people can be healthy" (p. 5).

Some nursing authors will continue to use *community health nursing* as a global or umbrella term and *public health nursing* as a component or subset. Others, as stated, use the terms interchangeably. This book will use the terms interchangeably.

Community-Based Nursing

The term *community-based nursing* has been identified and defined in recent years to differentiate it from what has traditionally been seen as community and public health nursing practice. Community-based nursing practice refers to "application of the nursing process in caring for individuals, families and groups where they live, work or go to school or as they move through the health care system" (McEwen and Pullis, 2008, p. 6). Community-based nursing is setting-specific, and the emphasis is on acute and chronic care and includes such practice areas as home health nursing and nursing in outpatient or ambulatory settings.

Zotti, Brown, and Stotts (1996) compared community-based nursing and community health nursing and explained that the goals of the two are different. Community health nursing emphasizes preservation and protection of health, and community-based nursing emphasizes managing acute or chronic conditions. In community health nursing, the primary client is the community; in community-based nursing, the primary clients are the individual and the family. Finally, services in community-based nursing are largely direct, and, in community health nursing, services are both direct and indirect.

Community and Public Health Nursing Practice

Community and public health nurses practice disease prevention and health promotion. It is important to note that community health nursing practice is collaborative and is based in research and theory. It applies the nursing process to the care of individuals, families, aggregates, and the community. Table 1-2 presents the Standards for Public Health Nursing (ANA, 2007).

As discussed, the core functions of public health are assessment, policy development, and assurance. In 2003, the Quad Council closely examined the core functions and developed a set of public health nursing competencies; these are summarized in Table 1-3 (Quad Council, 2003). Current and future community health nurses should study these competencies to understand the practice parameters and skills required for public health practice.

POPULATION-FOCUSED PRACTICE AND COMMUNITY/PUBLIC HEALTH NURSING INTERVENTIONS

Community/public health nurses must use a population-focused approach to move beyond providing direct care to individuals and families. Population-focused nursing concentrates on specific groups of people and focuses on health promotion and disease prevention, regardless of geographical location (Baldwin et al., 1998). In short, population-focused practice (Minnesota Department of Health, 2003):

- Focuses on the entire population
- Is based on assessment of the populations' health status

TABLE 1-2 STANDARDS OF PUBLIC HEALTH NURSING PRACTICE

Standards of Care

Standard 1. Assessment	The public health nurse collects comprehensive data pertinent to the health status of populations
Standard 2. Population diagnosis and priorities	The public health nurse analyzes the assessment data to determine the population diagnoses and priorities
Standard 3. Outcomes identification	The public health nurse identifies expected outcomes for a plan that is based on population diagnoses and priorities
Standard 4. Planning	The public health nurse develops a plan that reflects best practices by identifying strategies, action plans, and alternatives to attain expected outcomes
Standard 5. Implementation	The public health nurse implements the identified plan by partnering with others
	5a. Coordination—coordinates programs, services, and other activities to implement the identified plan
	5b. Health education and health promotion—employs multiple strategies to promote health, prevent disease, and ensure a safe environment for populations
	5c. Consultation—provides consultation to various community groups and officials to facilitate the implementation of programs and services
	5d. Regulatory activities—identifies, interprets, and implements public health laws, regulations and policies
Standard 6. Evaluation	The public health nurse evaluates the health status of the population

Standards of Professional Performance

Standard 7. Quality of practice	The public health nurse systematically enhances the equality and effectiveness of nursing practice
Standard 8. Education	The public health nurse attains knowledge and competency that reflects current nursing and public health practice
Standard 9. Professional practice evaluation	The public health nurse evaluates one's own nursing practice in relation to professional practice standards and guidelines, relevant statutes, rules, and regulations
Standard 10. Collegiality and professional relationships	The public health nurse establishes collegial partnerships while interacting with representatives of the population, organizations, and health and human services professionals, and contributes to the professional development of peers, students, colleagues, and others
Standard 11. Collaboration	The public health nurse collaborates with the representatives of the population, organizations, and health and human services professionals in providing for and promoting the health of the population
Standard 12. Ethics	The public health nurse integrates ethical provisions in all areas of practice
Standard 13. Research	The public health nurse integrates research findings in practice
Standard 14. Resource utilization population	The public health nurse considers factors related to safety, effectiveness, cost, and impact on practice and in the planning and delivery of nursing and public health programs, policies, and services
Standard 15. Leadership	The public health nurse provides leadership in nursing and public health

From American Nurses Association: *Public health nursing: scope and standards of practice,* Silver Spring, MD, 2007, American Nurses Publishing. © 2007 by American Nurses Association. Reprinted with permission. All rights reserved.

TABLE 1-3 SUMMARY OF PUBLIC HEALTH NURSING COMPETENCIES

DOMAIN	COMMUNITY AND PUBLIC HEALTH NURSING COMPETENCIES
1. Analytic assessment skills	Defines a problem
	Determines appropriate use and limitation of data
	Selects and defines variables relevant to defined public health problems
	Identifies relevant and appropriate data and information sources
	Evaluates the integrity and comparability of data and identifies gaps in data sources
	Applies ethical principles to the collection, maintenance, use, and dissemination of data and information
	Partners with communities to attach meaning to data
	Obtains and interprets information regarding risks and benefits to the community
	Applies data collection processes, information technology, and computer systems storage/retrieval strategies
	Recognizes how the data illuminate ethical, political, scientific, economic, and overall public health issues
2. Policy development/ program planning skills	Collects, summarizes, and interprets information relevant to an issue
	States policy options and writes clear and concise policy statements
	Identifies, interprets, and implements public health laws, regulations, and policies related to specific programs
	Articulates the health, fiscal, administrative, legal, social, and political implications of policy options
	States the feasibility and expected outcomes of each policy option
	Utilizes current techniques in decision analysis and health planning
	Decides on the appropriate course of action
	Develops a plan to implement policy, including goals, outcome and process objectives, and implementation steps
	Translates policy into organizational plans, structures, and programs
	Prepares and implements emergency response plans
	Develops mechanisms to monitor and evaluate programs for effectiveness and quality

(Continued)

TABLE 1-3   SUMMARY OF PUBLIC HEALTH NURSING COMPETENCIES—Cont'd

DOMAIN	COMMUNITY AND PUBLIC HEALTH NURSING COMPETENCIES
3. Communication skills	Communicates effectively Solicits input from individuals and organizations Advocates for public health programs and resources Leads and participates in groups to address specific issues Uses the media, advanced technologies, and community networks to communicate information Presents accurate demographic, statistical, programmatic, and scientific information for professional and lay audiences Listens to others in an unbiased manner; respects others' points of view; promotes the expression of diverse opinions and perspectives
4. Cultural competency skills	Utilizes appropriate methods for interacting sensitively, effectively, and professionally with persons from diverse cultural, socioeconomic, educational, racial, ethnic, and professional backgrounds and with persons of all ages and lifestyle preferences Identifies the role of cultural, social, and behavioral factors in determining the delivery of public health services Develops and adapts approaches to problems that consider cultural differences Understands the dynamic forces contributing to cultural diversity Understands the importance of a diverse public health workforce
5. Community dimensions of practice skills	Establishes and maintains linkages with key stakeholders Utilizes leadership, team building, negotiation, and conflict resolution skills to build community partnerships Collaborates with community partners to promote the health of the population Identifies how public and private organizations operate within a community Accomplishes effective community engagements Identifies community assets and resources Develops, implements, and evaluates a community public health assessment Describes the role of government in the delivery of community health services
6. Basic public health sciences skills	Identifies the individual's and organizations' responsibilities within the context of the Essential Public Health Services and core functions Defines, assesses, and understands the health status of populations, determinants of health and illness, factors contributing to health promotion and disease prevention, and factors influencing the use of health services Understands the historical development, structure, and interaction of public health and health Identifies and applies basic research methods used in public health Applies the basic public health sciences, including behavioral and social sciences, biostatistics, epidemiology, environmental public health, and prevention of chronic and infectious diseases and injuries Identifies and retrieves current relevant scientific evidence Identifies the limitations of research and the importance of observations and interrelationships Develops a lifelong commitment to rigorous critical thinking
7. Financial planning and management skills	Develops and presents a budget Manages programs within budget constraints Applies budget processes Develops strategies for budget priorities Monitors program performance Prepares proposals for funding from external sources Applies basic human relationship skills to the management of organizations, motivation of personnel, and resolution of conflicts Manages information systems for collection, retrieval, and use of data for decision making Negotiates and develops contracts and other documents for the provision of population-based services Conducts cost-effectiveness, cost-benefit, and cost utility analyses
8. Leadership and systems thinking skills	Creates a culture of ethical standards within organizations and communities Helps create key values and shared vision and uses these principles to guide action Identifies internal and external issues that may impact delivery of essential public health services Facilitates collaboration with internal and external groups to ensure participation of key stakeholders Promotes team and organizational learning Contributes to development, implementation, and monitoring of organizational performance standards Uses the legal and political system to effect change Applies theory of organizational structures to professional practice

From Quad Council of Public Health Nursing Organizations: *Public health nursing competencies,* Washington, DC, 2003, Quad Council.

- Considers the broad determinants of health
- Emphasizes all levels of prevention
- Intervenes with communities, systems, individuals, and families

Whereas community and public health nurses may be responsible for a specific subpopulation in the community (e.g., a school may be responsible for its pregnant teenagers), population-focused practice is concerned with many distinct and overlapping community subpopulations. The goal of population-focused nursing is to promote healthy communities.

Population-focused community health nurses would not have exclusive interest in one or two subpopulations but would focus on the many subpopulations that make up the entire community. A population focus involves concern for those who do, and for those who do not, receive health services. A population focus also involves a scientific approach to community health nursing: an assessment of the community or population is necessary and basic to planning, intervention, and evaluation for the individual, family, aggregate, and population levels.

Community health nursing practice requires the following types of data for scientific approach and population focus: (1) the epidemiology, or body of knowledge, of a particular problem and its solution and (2) information about the community. Each type of knowledge and its source appear in Table 1-4. To determine the overall patterns of health in a population, data collection for assessment and management decisions within a community should be ongoing, not episodical.

Community Health Interventions

Community health nurses focus on the care of individuals, groups, aggregates, and populations in many settings, including homes, clinics, and schools. In addition to interviewing clients and assessing individual and family health, community health nurses must be able to assess an aggregate's health needs and resources and identify its values. Community health nurses must also work with the community to identify and implement programs that meet health needs and evaluate the effectiveness of programs after implementation. For example, school nurses were once only responsible for running first-aid stations. Now they are actively involved in assessing the needs of their population and defining programs to meet those needs through activities such as health screening and group health education and promotion. The activities of school nurses may be as varied as designing health curricula with a school and community advisory group, leading support groups for elementary school children with chronic illness, and monitoring the health status of teenage mothers.

Similarly, occupational health nurses are no longer required to simply maintain an office or dispensary. They are involved in many different types of activities. These activities might include maintaining records of workers exposed to physical or chemical risks, monitoring compliance with Occupational Safety and Health Administration standards, teaching classes on health issues, and leading support group discussions for workers with health-related problems.

Private associations, such as the American Diabetes Association, employ community health nurses for organizational ability and health-related skill. Other community health nurses work with multidisciplinary groups of professionals, serve on boards of voluntary health associations such as the American Heart Association, and are members of health planning agencies and councils.

The Public Health Intervention Wheel

The Public Health Intervention Model was initially proposed in the late 1990s by nurses from the Minnesota Department of Health to describe the breadth and scope of public health nursing practice (Keller et al., 1998). This model was later revised and termed the *Intervention Wheel* (Figure 1-3) (Keller et al., 2004a; Keller et al., 2004b), and it has become increasingly recognized as a framework for community and public health nursing practice.

The Intervention Wheel contains three important elements: (1) it is population-based; (2) it contains three levels of practice (community, systems, and individual/family); and (3) it identifies and defines 17 public health interventions. The levels of practice and interventions are directed at improving population health (Keller et al., 2004a). Within the Intervention Wheel, the 17 health interventions are grouped into five "wedges." These interventions are actions taken on behalf of communities, systems, individuals, and families to improve or protect health status. Table 1-5 provides definitions.

The Intervention Wheel is further dissected into levels of practice in which the interventions may be directed at an entire population within a community, a system that would affect the health of a population, and/or the individuals and families within the population. Thus each intervention can and should be applied at each level. For example, within the intervention "disease investigation," a systems-level intervention might be the community health nurse working with the state health department and federal vaccine program to coordinate a response to cases of measles in a migrant population. A population- or community-level intervention for "screening" would be when public health nurses work with area high schools to give each student a profile of his or her health to promote nutritional and physical activity lifestyle changes to improve the student's health.

TABLE 1-4	INFORMATION USEFUL FOR POPULATION FOCUS	
TYPE OF INFORMATION	**EXAMPLES**	**SOURCES**
Demographic data	Age, gender, race/ethnicity, socioeconomic status, education level	Vital statistic data (national, state, county, local); census
Groups at high risk	Health status and health indicators of various subpopulations in the community (e.g., children, elders, those with disabilities)	Health statistics (morbidity, mortality, natality); disease statistics (incidence and prevalence)
Services/ providers available	Official (public) health departments; health care providers for low-income individuals and families; community service agencies and organizations (e.g., Red Cross, Meals on Wheels)	City directories; phone books; local or regional social workers; low-income providers lists; local community health nurses (e.g., school nurses)

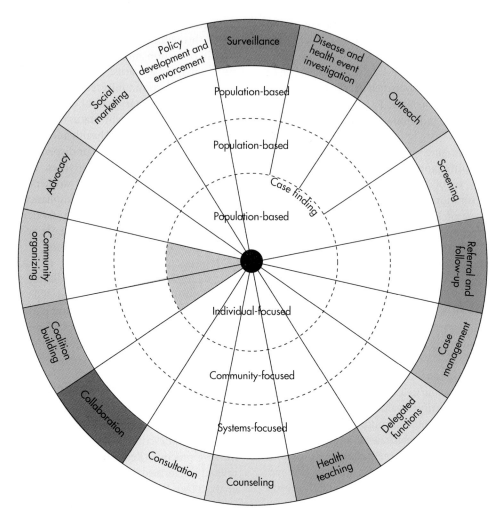

FIGURE 1-3 Public Health Intervention Wheel. (Minnesota Department of Health Center for Public Health Nursing.)

Finally, an individual-level implementation of the intervention "referral and follow-up" would be a nurse who receives a referral to care for an individual with a diagnosed mental illness who would require regular monitoring of his medication compliance to prevent rehospitalization (Keller et al., 2004b).

COMMUNITY HEALTH NURSING, MANAGED CARE, AND HEALTH REFORM

Shifts in reimbursement and the growth of managed care have revitalized the notion of population-based care. MCOs use financial incentives and organizational structures to increase efficiency and decrease health care costs. The foundation for managed care is management of health care for an enrolled group of individuals. This group of enrollees is the population covered by the plan who receive health services from managed care plan providers (Koch, 2008).

An understanding of enrolled populations and health care patterns is essential for managing health care services and resources effectively. Most MCOs have become sophisticated in identifying key subgroups within the population of enrollees

at risk for health problems. Typically, managed care systems target subgroups according to characteristics associated with risk or use of expensive services, such as selected clinical conditions, functional status, and past service use patterns.

In March 2010, President Obama signed the Patient Protection and Affordable Care Act (PL 111-148) into law. Although the law will not be fully implemented for several years and challenges to aspects of it are anticipated, it is intended to expand insurance coverage for most of those currently uninsured in the country and to help control health care costs. Expansion of coverage will be accomplished through requiring individuals to purchase health insurance for themselves and their families, and requiring employers of more than 50 people to offer health insurance to employees. Public programs (i.e., Medicaid and CHIPS) will be expanded to cover health care for those who cannot afford to buy their own insurance. Cost containment will be accomplished through many activities including efforts to control waste, fraud, and abuse and simplification of administration. Finally, the act seeks to improve overall health of the population by encouraging prevention and wellness initiatives (Kaiser Family Foundation, 2010).

TABLE 1-5	PUBLIC HEALTH INTERVENTIONS AND DEFINITIONS
PUBLIC HEALTH INTERVENTION	**DEFINITION**
Surveillance	Describes and monitors health events through ongoing and systematic collection, analysis, and interpretation of health data for the purpose of planning, implementing, and evaluating public health interventions
Disease and other health event investigation	Systematically gathers and analyzes data regarding threats to the health of populations, ascertains the source of the threat, identifies cases and others at risk, and determines control measures
Outreach	Locates populations of interest or populations at risk and provides information about the nature of the concern, what can be done about it, and how services can be obtained
Screening	Identifies individuals with unrecognized health risk factors or asymptomatic disease conditions
Case finding	Locates individuals and families with identified risk factors and connects them with resources
Referral and follow-up	Assists individuals, families, groups, organizations, and/or communities to identify and access necessary resources to prevent or resolve problems or concerns
Case management	Optimizes self-care capabilities of individuals and families and the capacity of systems and communities to coordinate and provide services
Delegated functions	Direct care tasks that a registered professional nurse carries out under the authority of a health care practitioner as allowed by law
Health teaching	Communicates facts, ideas, and skills that change knowledge, attitudes, values, beliefs, behaviors, and practices of individuals, families, systems, and/or communities
Counseling	Establishes an interpersonal relationship with a community, a system, and a family or individual, with the intention of increasing or enhancing their capacity for self-care and coping
Consultation	Seeks information and generates optional solutions to perceived problems or issues through interactive problem solving with a community system and family or individual
Collaboration	Commits two or more persons or an organization to achieve a common goal through enhancing the capacity of one or more of the members to promote and protect health
Coalition building	Promotes and develops alliances among organizations or constituencies for a common purpose
Community organizing	Helps community groups to identify common problems or goals, mobilize resources, and develop and implement strategies for realizing the goals they collectively have set
Advocacy	Pleads someone's cause or acts on someone's behalf, with a focus on developing the community, system, and individual or family's capacity to plead their own cause or act on their own behalf
Social marketing	Utilizes commercial marketing principles and technologies for programs designed to influence the knowledge, attitudes, values, beliefs, behaviors, and practices of the population of interest
Policy development and enforcement	Places health issues on decision makers' agendas, acquires a plan of resolution, and determines needed resources, resulting in laws, rules, regulations, ordinances, and policies. Policy enforcement compels others to comply with laws, rules, regulations, ordinances, and policies

From Keller LO, Strohschein S, Lia-Hoagberg B, Schaffer MA: *Population-based public health interventions: Practice-based and evidence-supported. Part I*, Minnesota Department of Health, Center for Public Health Nursing, 2004a.

The purpose of public health is to improve the health of the public by promoting healthy lifestyles, preventing disease and injury, and protecting the health of communities. In the past, shrinking public health resources have supported personal health services over community health. In public health practice, the community is the population of interest. With the proposed changes to health care financing, the personal health care system will be under increasing pressure to provide the services that health departments previously provided. Traditionally served by public health, the most vulnerable populations will pose tremendous challenges for private health care providers. Public health will be responsible for partnering with private providers to care for these populations.

Providing population-based care requires a dramatic shift in thinking from individual-based care. Some of the practical demands of population-based care are the following:

1. It must be recognized that populations are not homogeneous; therefore it is necessary to address the needs of special subpopulations within populations.
2. High-risk and vulnerable subpopulations must be identified early in the care delivery cycle.
3. Nonusers of services often become high-cost users; therefore, it is essential to develop outreach strategies.

4. Quality and cost of all health care services are linked together across the health care continuum. (Kaiser Family Foundation, 2010.)

Nurses in community and public health have an opportunity to share their expertise regarding population-based approaches to health care for groups of individuals across health care settings. Today, health care practitioners require additional skills in assessment, policy development, and assurance to provide community public health practice and population-based service. Health care professionals should focus attention toward promoting healthy lifestyles, providing preventive and primary care, expanding and ensuring access to cost-effective and technologically appropriate care, participating in coordinated and interdisciplinary care, and involving patients and families in the decision-making process (Pew Health Professions Commission, 1994). Public health nurses must work in partnership with colleagues in managed care settings to improve community health. Partnerships may address information management, cultural values, health care system improvement, and the physical environment roles in health and may require complex negotiations to share data across boundaries. The partners may need to develop new community assessment strategies to augment epidemiological methods that often mask the context or meaning of the human experience of vulnerable populations.

SUMMARY

Knowledge and skills enable community health nurses to work in diverse community settings ranging from the isolated rural area to the crowded urban ghetto. To meet the health needs of the population, the community health nurse must work with many individuals and groups within the community. The community health nurse must develop sensitivity to these groups and respect the community and its established method of problem management. This will enable the nurse to become more proficient in helping the community improve overall health.

LEARNING ACTIVITIES

1. Interview several community health nurses and several clients regarding their definitions of health. Share the results with your classmates. Do you agree with their definitions? Why or why not?
2. Interview several community health nurses regarding their opinions on the focus of community health nursing. Do you agree?
3. Ask several neighbors or consumers of health care about their views of the role of public health and community health nursing. Share your results with your classmates.
4. Become familiar with *Healthy People 2020* (www. Healthypeople.gov). Review objectives from several of the topic areas covered. How does your community compare with groups, aggregates, and populations described? What objectives should be targeted for your community?

REFERENCES

Allender JA, Rector C, Warner K: *Community health nursing: promoting and protecting the public's health*, ed 7, Philadelphia, 2009, Lippincott Williams & Wilkins.

American Heritage College Dictionary, ed 3, New York, 1997, Houghton Mifflin.

American Nurses Association: *A conceptual model of community health nursing*, Pub No CH-10, Kansas City, MO, 1980, The Association.

American Nurses Association: *Code of ethics*, Kansas City, MO, 2001, The Association.

American Nurses Association: *Public health nursing: scope and standards of practice*, Silver Spring, MD, 2007, American Nurses Publishing.

American Public Health Association: *Ad hoc committee on public health nursing: the definition and role of public health nursing practice in the delivery of health care*, Washington, DC, 1996, The Association.

Baldwin JH, et al.: Population-focused and community-based nursing: moving toward clarification of concepts, *Public Health Nurs* 15(1):12–18, 1998.

Clark MJ: *Community health nursing: advocacy for population health*, ed 5, Upper Saddle River, NJ, 2008, Prentice Hall.

Dunn HL: *High level wellness*, Arlington, VA, 1961, RW Beatty.

Feldstein PJ: *Health policy issues: an economic perspective*, ed 4, Chicago, 2007, Health Administration Press.

Freeman RB: *Public health nursing practice*, ed 3, Philadelphia, 1963, Saunders.

Gaines C, Jenkins S, Ashe W: Empowering nursing faculty and students for community service, *J Nurs Educ* 44(11):522–525, 2005.

Hanlon JJ: *Principles of public health administration*, ed 3, St. Louis, 1960, Mosby.

Inglis T: Nursing trends: nurses have more employment options than ever, *AJN Career Guide* 104(1):25–32, 2004.

Institute of Medicine: *The future of public health*, Washington, DC, 1988, National Academy Press.

Kaiser Family Foundation: *Summary of the new health reform law*. Pub # 8061. Menlo Park, CA.

Author. 2010. Accessed April 6, 2010 from www. kff.org/healthreform/8061.cfm.

Keller LO, Strohschein S, Lia-Hoagberg B, et al.: Population-based public health interventions: a model for practice, *Public Health Nurs* 15(3):207–215, 1998.

Keller LO, Strohschein S, Lia-Hoagberg B, Schaffer MA: Population-based public health interventions: practice-based and evidence-supported. Part I, *Public Health Nurs* 21(5):453–468, 2004a.

Keller LO, Strohschein S, Schaffer MA, Lia-Hoagberg B: Population-based public health interventions: innovations in practice, teaching and management. Part II, *Public Health Nurs* 21(5):469–487, 2004b.

Koch A: Private health insurance and managed care. In Williams SJ, Torrens PR, editors: *Introduction to health services*, ed 7, Clifton Park, NY, 2008, Thomson/Delmar.

Leavell HR, Clark EG: *Preventive medicine for the doctor in his community*, New York, 1958, McGraw-Hill.

Lundy KS, Janes S: *Community health nursing: caring for the public's health*, ed 2, New York, 2009, Jones and Bartlett.

Maurer FA, Smith CM: *Community/public health nursing practice: health for families and populations*, ed 4, St. Louis, 2009, Saunders.

McEwen M, Pullis B: *Community-based nursing: an introduction*, ed 3, St. Louis, 2008, Saunders.

McGinnis MJ, Foege W: Actual causes of death in the United States, *JAMA* 270(18):2207–2212, 1993.

McKeown T: Determinants of health. In Lee PR, Estes CL, editors: *The nation's health*, ed 7, Boston, 2003, Jones and Bartlett.

McKinlay JB: A case for refocusing upstream: the political economy of illness. In Jaco EG, editor: *Patients, physicians, and illness*, ed 3, New York, 1979, The Free Press.

Minnesota Department of Health: *Definitions of population based practice*, 2003, The Author: http://www.health.state.mn.us/divs/cfh/ophp/

resources/docs/population-based-practice_ definition.pdf.

Muecke MA: Community health diagnosis in nursing, *Public Health Nurs* 1:23–35, 1984.

Murray RB, Zentner JP, Yakimo R: *Health promotion strategies through the life span*, ed 8, Upper Saddle River, NJ, 2009, Prentice Hall.

National Center for Health Statistics: *Health, United States*, Hyattsville, MD, 2008, The Author, 2009: www.cdc.gov/nchs/data/ hus/hus08.pdf. Accessed May 2, 2009.

Orem DE: *Nursing: concepts of practice*, ed 6, St. Louis, 2001, Mosby.

Pender NJ, Murdaugh CL, Parsons MA: *Health promotion in nursing practice*, ed 5, Upper Saddle River, NJ, 2006, Prentice Hall.

Pew Health Professions Commission: *Current issues in health professions: education and workforce reform*, University of California, San Francisco, 1994, The Author.

Quad Council of Public Health Nursing Organizations: *Public health nursing competencies*, Washington, DC, 2003, Quad Council.

Rothstein WG: Trends in mortality in the twentieth century. In Lee PR, Estes CL, editors: *The nation's health*, ed 7, Sudbury, MA, 2003, Jones and Bartlett.

Saylor C: The circle of health: a health definition model, *J Holist Nurs* 22(2):98–115, 2004.

Shi L, Singh DA: *Delivering health care in America: a systems approach*, ed 4, Boston, 2008, Jones and Bartlett.

Shuster GR, Goeppinger J: Community as client: assessment and analysis. In Stanhope M, Lancaster J, editors: *Public health nursing: population-centered health care in the community*, ed 7, St. Louis, 2008, Mosby.

Sultz HA, Young KM: *Health care USA: Understanding its organization and delivery*, ed 5, Sudbury, MA, 2006, Jones and Bartlett.

Torrens PR: Understanding health systems: the organization of health care in the United States. In Williams SJ, Torrens PR, editors:

Introduction to health services, ed 7, Clifton Park, NY, 2008, Thomson/Delmar.

U.S. Department of Health and Human Services: *Healthy People 2000 objectives*, Washington, DC, 1989, The Author.

U.S. Department of Health and Human Services: *Healthy People 2010 objectives*, Washington, DC, 2000, The Author.

U.S. Department of Health and Human Services, Health Resources and Services Administration, The registered nurse population: Initial findings 2008 national sample survey of registered nurses, The Author, 2010. Accessed April 6, 2010 from http://bhpr.hrsa.gov/healthworkforce/rnsurvey/initialfindings2008.pdf.

U.S. Department of Health and Human Services, Public Health Service: *The public health workforce: an agenda for the 21st century*, Washington, DC, 1997, The Author.

Wald LD: *The house on Henry Street*, New York, 1971, Dover Publications.

Way M, MacNeil M: Baccalaureate entry to practice: a systems review, *J Contin Educ Nurs* 38(4):164–169, 2007.

World Health Organization: The first 10 years of the World Health Organization, *Chron WHO* 1:1–2, 1958.

World Health Organization: A discussion document on the concept and principles of health promotion, *Health Promot* 1:73–78, 1986.

Zotti ME, Brown P, Stotts RC: Community-based nursing versus community health nursing: What does it all mean? *Nurs Outlook* 44(5):211–217, 1996.

Historical Factors: Community Health Nursing in Context

Tom H. Cook

Additional Material for Study, Review, and Further Exploration

evolve WEBSITE

http://evolve.elsevier.com/Nies

- Quiz
- Case Studies
- Glossary
- WebLinks

OBJECTIVES

Upon completion of this chapter, the reader will be able to do the following:

1. Describe the impact of aggregate living on population health.
2. Identify approaches to aggregate health from pre–recorded historic to present times.
3. Understand historical events that have influenced a holistic approach to population health.
4. Compare the application of public health principles to the nation's major health problems at the turn of the twentieth century (i.e., acute disease) with that at the beginning of the twenty-first century (i.e., chronic disease).
5. Describe two leaders in nursing who had a profound impact on addressing aggregate health.
6. Discuss major contemporary issues facing community health nursing, and trace the historical roots to the present.

KEY TERMS

Edwin Chadwick
district nursing
Elizabethan Poor Law
Flexner Report
health visiting
House on Henry Street

Edward Jenner
Robert Koch
Joseph Lister
Florence Nightingale
pandemic
Louis Pasteur

Sanitary Revolution
Lemuel Shattuck
John Snow
stages in disease history
Lillian Wald

OUTLINE

This chapter presents an overview of selected historical factors that have influenced the evolution of community health and explains current health challenges for community health nursing. This text examines the evolving health of Western populations from pre–recorded historic to recent times, the evolution of modern health care and the role of public health nursing, the consequences for the health of aggregates, and the challenges for community health nursing.

EVOLUTION OF HEALTH IN WESTERN POPULATIONS

The study of humankind's evolution has seldom taken into consideration the interrelationship among an individual's health, an individual's environment, and the nature and size of the individual's aggregate. Medical anthropologists use paleontological records and disease descriptions of primitive societies to speculate on the interrelationship of early humans, probable diseases, and environment (Armelagos and Dewey, 1978). Historians have also documented the existence of public health activity (i.e., an organized community effort to prevent disease, prolong life, and promote health) since before recorded historic times. The following section describes how aggregates and early public health efforts impact the health of Western populations.

Aggregate Impact on Health

Polgar (1964) defined the following stages in disease history of humankind: hunting and gathering stage, settled villages stage, preindustrial cities stage, industrial cities stage, and present stage (Figure 2-1). In these stages, increased population, increased population density, and imbalanced human ecology resulted in changes in cultural adaptation. Humans caused this ecological imbalance by altering their environment to accommodate group living. This imbalance had a marked consequence on aggregate health.

Although these stages are associated with the evolution of civilization, it is important to note that the information is limited by cultural bias. For example, the stages depict the evolution of Western civilization from the perspective of the Western world. They consist of overlapping historical time periods, which anthropologists widely debate. However, the stages of human disease do provide a frame of reference to aid in determining the relationship among humans, disease, and environment from pre–recorded historic to present day. The stages chronicle the initiation of each stage in the Western world, but it is important to realize that each stage still exists in civilization today. For example, Australian aborigines continue to hunt and gather food, and settled villages are common in third-world countries.

The community nurse must be aware that populations from each stage represent a great variety of people with distinct cultural traditions and a broad range of health care practices and beliefs. For example, a nurse currently practicing in an American community may have to plan care for immigrants or refugees from a settled village or a preindustrial city. Community nurses must recognize that the environment, the aggregate's health risks, and the host culture's strengths and contributions affect the health status of each particular aggregate. For example, the Hispanic Health and Nutrition Examination Survey (HHANES) collected data between 1982 and 1984 and found that perinatal outcomes among women born in Mexico worsen in correspondence to the length of time they live in the United States (Guendelman et al., 1990). Whereas Mexico's cultural orientation protects mothers from the risk-associated behaviors of drinking and smoking, Mexican descendants born in the United States are more likely to engage in unhealthy behaviors and practices common to other Americans.

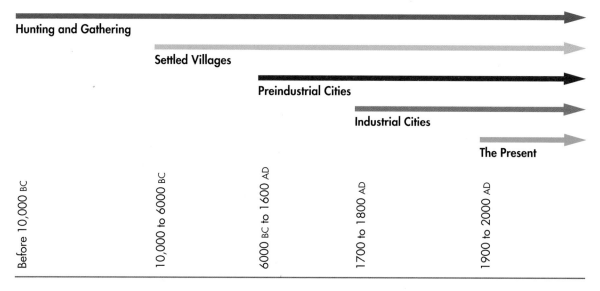

FIGURE 2-1 Stages in the disease history of humankind. Stages overlap and time periods are widely debated in the field of anthropology. Some form of each stage remains evident in the world today.

Hunting and Gathering Stage

During the Paleolithic period, or Old Stone Age, nomadic and seminomadic people engaged in hunting and gathering. Generations of small aggregate groups wandered in search of food for 2 million years. Armelagos and Dewey (1978) reviewed how their size, density, and relationship to the environment probably affected their health. These groups may have avoided many contagious diseases because the scattered aggregates were small, nomadic, and separated from other aggregates. Under these conditions, disease would not spread between the groups. Evidently the disposal of human feces and waste was not a great problem; the nomadic people most likely abandoned the caves they used for shelter once waste accumulated.

Settled Village Stage

Small settlements were characteristic of the Mesolithic period, or Middle Stone Age, and the Neolithic period, or New Stone Age. Wandering people became sedentary and formed small encampments and villages. The concentration of people in these small areas caused new problems. For example, people began to domesticate animals and live close to their herds, which probably transmitted diseases such as salmonella, anthrax, Q fever, and tuberculosis (TB) (Polgar, 1964). These stationary people also domesticated plants, which may have reduced the range of consumable nutrients and may have led to deficiency diseases. They had to secure water and remove wastes, which often resulted in the cross-contamination of the water supply and the spread of waterborne diseases such as dysentery, cholera, typhoid, and hepatitis A.

Preindustrial Cities Stage

In preindustrial times, large urban centers formed to support the expanding population. Populations inhabited smaller areas; therefore preexisting problems expanded. For example, the urban population had to resource increased amounts of food and water and remove increased amounts of waste products. Some cultures developed elaborate water systems. For instance, the Aztec king Ahuitzotl had a stone pipeline built to transport spring water to the inhabitants of Mexico City (Duran, 1964). However, waste removal via the water supply led to diseases such as cholera. With the development of towns, rodent infestation increased and facilitated the spread of plague. People had more frequent close contact with each other; therefore the transmission of diseases spread by direct contact increased, and diseases such as mumps, measles, influenza, and smallpox became endemic (Polgar, 1964). A population must reach a certain size to maintain a disease in endemic proportions (Table 2-1); for example, approximately 1 million people are needed to sustain measles at an endemic level (Cockburn, 1967).

Industrial Cities Stage

Industrialization caused urban areas to become denser and more heavily populated. Increased industrial wastes, air and water pollution, and harsh working conditions took a toll on health. During the eighteenth and nineteenth centuries, there

TABLE 2-1	DISEASE DEFINITIONS
DISEASE	**DEFINITION**
Endemic	Diseases that are always present in a population (e.g., colds and pneumonia)
Epidemic	Diseases that are not always present in a population but flare up on occasion (e.g., diphtheria and measles)
Pandemic	The existence of disease in a large proportion of the population: a global epidemic (e.g., HIV, AIDS, and annual outbreaks of influenza type A)

was an increase in respiratory diseases such as TB, pneumonia, and bronchitis and in epidemics of infectious diseases such as diphtheria, smallpox, typhoid fever, typhus, measles, malaria, and yellow fever (Armelagos and Dewey, 1978). Furthermore, imperialism spread epidemics to susceptible populations throughout the world because settlers, traders, and soldiers moved from one location to another, introducing communicable diseases into native population groups.

Present Stage

Although infectious diseases no longer account for a majority of deaths in the Western world, they continue to cause many deaths in the non-Western world. They also remain prevalent among low-income populations and some racial and ethnic groups in the West. Western diseases such as cancer, venous disorders, heart disease, obesity, and diabetes rarely develop in people from nonindustrial communities. These diseases usually appear when cultures adopt Western customs (Burkitt, 1978). Western diseases also seem to emerge when cultures transition into urban environments. Epidemiological studies suggest that common disease factors are changes in diet (i.e., increases in refined sugar and fats and lack of fiber) and environmental and occupational hazards. An increase in population and population density also increases mental and behavioral disorders (Garn, 1963).

The disease patterns and environmental demands changed when wandering, hunting, and gathering aggregates grew into large populations and became sedentary. Humans had to adapt to an overpopulated, largely urban existence with marked consequences for health; the leading causes of death changed from infectious disease to chronic illnesses.

Evolution of Early Public Health Efforts

Traditionally, historians believed that organized public health efforts were eighteenth- and nineteenth-century activities associated with the Sanitary Revolution. However, modern historians have shown that organized community health efforts to prevent disease, prolong life, and promote health have existed since before recorded historic times.

Public health efforts developed slowly over time. The following sections briefly trace the evolution of organized public health and highlight the periods of pre–recorded historic times (i.e., before 5000 BC), classical times (i.e., 3000 to 200 BC), the Middle Ages (i.e., 500 to 1500 AD), the

Renaissance (i.e., fifteenth, sixteenth, and seventeenth centuries), the eighteenth century, and the nineteenth century. However, it is important to note that, like the disease history of humankind, public health efforts exist in various stages of development throughout the world. The following brief history encapsulates a Western view of organized public health efforts.

Pre–Recorded Historic Times

From the early remains of human habitation, we recognize that early nomadic humans became domesticated and tended to live in increasingly larger groups. Aggregates ranging from family to community inevitably shared episodes of life, health, sickness, and death. Whether based on superstition or sanitation, health practices evolved to ensure the survival of many aggregates. For example, primitive societies used elements of medicine (e.g., voodoo), isolation (e.g., banishment), and fumigation (e.g., smoke) to manage disease and thus protect the community for thousands of years (Hanlon and Pickett, 1990).

Classical Times

In the early years of 3000 to 1400 BC, the Minoans devised ways to flush water and construct drainage systems. Circa 1000 BC, the Egyptians constructed elaborate drainage systems, developed pharmaceutical preparations, and embalmed the dead. Pollution is an ancient problem. Exodus reported that "all the waters that were in the river stank," and in Leviticus the Hebrews formulated the first written hygiene code. This hygiene code protected water and food by creating laws that governed personal and community hygiene such as contagion, disinfection, and sanitation.

Greece. Greek literature contains accounts of communicable diseases such as diphtheria, mumps, and malaria. The Hippocratic book *On Airs, Waters and Places,* a treatise on the balance between humans and their environment, may have been the only volume on this topic until the development of bacteriology in the late nineteenth century (Rosen, 1958). Diseases that were always present in a population, such as colds and pneumonia, were called endemic. Diseases that were occasionally present, such as diphtheria and measles, were called epidemic. The Greeks emphasized the preservation of health, or good living, which the goddess Hygeia represented, and curative medicine, which the goddess Panacea personified. Human life had to be in balance with environmental demands; therefore the Greeks weighed the importance of exercise, rest, and nutrition according to age, sex, constitution, and climate (Rosen, 1958).

Rome. Although the Romans readily adopted Greek culture, they far surpassed Greek engineering by constructing massive aqueducts, bathhouses, and sewer systems. For example, at the height of the Roman empire, Rome provided its 1 million inhabitants with 40 gallons of water per person per day, which is comparable with modern consumption rates (Rosen, 1958). However, inhabitants of the overcrowded Roman slums did not share in public health amenities such as sewer systems and latrines.

> ## BOX 2-1   ROMANS PROVIDED PUBLIC HEALTH SERVICES
>
> The Romans provided public health services that included the following (Rosen, 1958):
> - A water board to maintain the aqueducts
> - A supervisor of the public baths
> - Street cleaners
> - Supervision of the sale of food

The Romans also observed and addressed occupational health threats. In particular, they noted the pallor of the miners, the danger of suffocation, and the smell of caustic fumes (Rosen, 1958) (Box 2-1). For protection, miners devised safeguards by using masks made of bags, sacks, membranes, and bladder skins.

In the early years of the Roman Republic, priests were believed to mediate diseases and often dispensed medicine. Public physicians worked in designated towns and earned money to care for the poor. In addition, they were able to charge wealthier patients a service fee. Much like a modern health maintenance organization (HMO) or group practice, several families paid a set fee for yearly services. Hospitals, surgeries, infirmaries, and nursing homes appeared throughout Rome. In the fourth century, a Christian woman named Fabiola established a hospital for the sick poor. Others repeated this model throughout medieval times.

Middle Ages

The decline of Rome, which occurred circa 500 AD, led to the Middle Ages. Monasteries promoted collective activity to protect public health, and the population adopted protective measures such as building wells and fountains, cleaning streets, and disposing of refuse. The commonly occurring communicable diseases were measles, smallpox, diphtheria, leprosy, and bubonic plague. Physicians had little to offer in the management of diseases such as leprosy. The church took over by enforcing the hygienic codes from Leviticus and establishing isolation and leper houses, or leprosaria (Rosen, 1958).

A pandemic is the existence of disease in a large proportion of the population. One such pandemic, the bubonic plague, ravaged much of the world in the fourteenth century. This plague, or Black Death, claimed close to half the world's population at that time (Hanlon and Pickett, 1990). For centuries, medicine and science did not recognize that fleas, which were attracted to the large number of rodents that inhabited urban areas, were transmitters of plague. Modern public health practices such as isolation, disinfection, and ship quarantines emerged in response to the bubonic plague (Box 2-2).

During the Middle Ages, clergymen acted as physicians and treated kings and noblemen. Monks and nuns provided nursing care in small houses designated as structures similar to today's small hospitals. Medieval writings contained information on hygiene and addressed such topics as housing, diet, personal cleanliness, and sleep (Rosen, 1958).

BOX 2-2 HUMAN PLAGUE CASES DOCUMENTED IN THE UNITED STATES

Plague is an acute, often fatal bacterial infection that is endemic and occasionally epidemic in Africa, Asia, and South America. The bite of infectious fleas spreads plague. Sanitary precautions ensure a low frequency of human plague in the United States. America averages 13 cases of plague each year, and most of these cases occur in New Mexico, California, Texas, and Colorado. In 2006, thirteen cases of human plague were reported and resulted in two fatalities in the United States. This is the largest number of reported cases in the United States since 1994. Control measures include public education and plague surveillance in rodents and rodent predators. When this surveillance detects plague, local health care providers and the public should receive an alert about possible risks.

From Centers for Disease Control and Prevention: Human plague—four states, 2006, *MMWR Morb Mortal Wkly Rep* 55(34):940-943, 2006.

LIFE IN AN ENGLISH HOUSEHOLD IN THE SIXTEENTH CENTURY

In the following account, Erasmus described how life in the sixteenth century must have affected health (Hanlon and Pickett, 1990):

As to floors, they are usually made with clay, covered with rushes that grow in the fens and which are so seldom removed that the lower parts remain sometimes for twenty years and has in it a collection of spittle, vomit, urine of dogs and humans, beer, scraps of fish and other filthiness not to be named. (p. 25)

Such accounts appeared in literature throughout the nineteenth century.

The Renaissance

Although the cause of infectious disease remained undiscovered, two events important to public health occurred during the Renaissance. In 1546, Girolamo Fracastoro presented a theory that infection was a cause and epidemic was a consequence of the "seeds of disease." Also, in 1676, Anton van Leeuwenhoek described microscopic organisms but did not associate them with disease (Rosen, 1958).

The Elizabethan Poor Law, enacted in England in 1601, held the church parishes responsible for providing relief for the poor. This law governed health care for the poor for more than two centuries and became a prototype for later U.S. laws.

Eighteenth Century

Great Britain. The eighteenth century was marked by imperialism and industrialization. Sanitary conditions remained a great problem. During the Industrial Revolution, a gradual change in industrial productivity occurred. The industrial boom sacrificed many lives for profit. In particular, it forced poor children into labor. Under the Elizabethan Poor Law, parishes established workhouses to employ the poor. Orphaned and poor children were wards of the parish;

therefore the parish forced these young children to labor in parish workhouses for long hours (George, 1925). At 12 to 14 years of age, a child became a master's apprentice. Those apprenticed to chimney sweeps reportedly suffered the worst fate because their masters forced them into chimneys at the risk of being burned and suffocated.

Vaccination was a major discovery of the times. In 1796, Edward Jenner observed that people who worked around cattle were less likely to have smallpox. He discovered that immunity to smallpox resulted from an inoculation with the cowpox virus. Jenner's contribution was significant because approximately 95% of the population suffered from smallpox and approximately 10% of the population died of smallpox during the eighteenth century. Frequently, the faces of those who survived the disease were scarred with pockmarks.

Although Europeans such as Hume, Voltaire, and Rousseau and Americans such as Adams, Jefferson, and Franklin were expounding liberal views on human nature, the Sanitary Revolution's public health reforms were beginning to take place throughout Europe and England. In the eighteenth century, scholars used survey methods to study community health problems (Rosen, 1958). The survey mapped "medical topographies," which were geographical factors related to regional health and disease. A health education movement provided books and pamphlets on health to the middle and upper classes, but it neglected "economic factors" and was not concerned with the working classes (Rosen, 1958).

Nineteenth Century

Communicable diseases ravaged the population that lived among unsanitary conditions, and many lives were lost. For example, in the mid-1800s, typhus and typhoid fever claimed two times more lives each year than the Battle of Waterloo (Hanlon and Pickett, 1990).

Edwin Chadwick called attention to the consequences of unsanitary conditions that resulted in health disparities that shortened the life span of the laboring class in particular. Chadwick contended that death rates were high in large industrial cities such as Liverpool, where more than half of all children born of working-class parents died by age 5. Laborers lived an average of 16 years. In contrast, tradesmen lived 22 years, and the upper classes lived 36 years (Richardson, 1887). In 1842, Chadwick published his famous *Report on an Inquiry Into the Sanitary Conditions of the Labouring Population of Great Britain*. The report furthered the establishment of the General Board of Health for England in 1848. Legislation for social reform followed, which concerned child welfare; factory management; education; and care for the elderly, sick, and mentally ill. Clean water, sewers, fireplugs, and sidewalks emerged as a result.

In 1849, a pathologist named Rudolf Virchow argued for social action—bettering the lives of the people through improving economic, social, and environmental conditions—to attack the root social causes of disease. He proposed "a theory of epidemic disease as a manifestation of social and cultural maladjustment" (Rosen, 1958, p. 86). He further argued that the public was responsible for the health of the people; social and economic conditions heavily affected health and disease; efforts to promote health and fight disease must be social, economic, and medical; and the study of social and economic determinants of health and disease would yield knowledge to guide appropriate action.

In 1849, these principles were embodied in a public health law submitted to the Berlin Society of Physicians and Surgeons (Rosen, 1958). According to this document, public health has as its objectives (1) the healthy mental and physical development of the citizen, (2) the prevention of all dangers to health, and (3) the control of disease. Public health cares for society as a whole by considering the general physical and social conditions that may adversely affect health and protects each individual by considering those conditions that prevent the individual from caring for his or her health. These "conditions" may fit into one of the following major categories: conditions that give the individual the right to request assistance from the state (e.g., poverty and infirmity), and conditions that give the state the right and obligation to interfere with the personal liberty of the individual (e.g., transmissible diseases and mental illness).

In 1854, an English physician, anesthetist, and epidemiologist named John Snow demonstrated that cholera was transmissible through contaminated water. In a large population afflicted with cholera, he shut down the community's water resource by removing the pump handle from a well and carefully documented changes as the number of cholera cases fell dramatically (Rosen, 1958).

United States. In the United States during the nineteenth century, waves of epidemics continued to spread. Diseases such as yellow fever, smallpox, cholera, typhoid fever, and typhus particularly impacted the poor. These illnesses spread because cities grew and the poor crowded into inadequate housing with unsanitary conditions.

Lemuel Shattuck, a Boston bookseller and publisher with an interest in public health, organized the American Statistical Society in 1839 and issued a *Census of Boston* in 1845. The census showed high overall mortality and very high infant and maternal mortality rates. Living conditions for the poor were inadequate, and communicable diseases were widely prevalent (Rosen, 1958). Shattuck's 1850 *Report of the Sanitary Commission of Massachusetts* outlined the findings and recommended modern public health reforms that included keeping vital statistics and providing environmental, food, drug, and communicable disease control information. Shattuck called for well-infant, well-child, and school-aged–child health care; mental health care; vaccination; and health education. Unfortunately, the report fell on deaf ears, and little was done to improve population health for many years. For example, a state board of health was not formed until 19 years after the report was issued. Around the same time, the National Institute, a Washington, DC, scientific organization, asked the newly formed American Medical Association (AMA) to establish a committee to uniformly collect vital statistics, which the AMA did, beginning in 1848.

ADVENT OF MODERN HEALTH CARE

Early public health efforts evolved further in the mid-nineteenth century. Administrative efforts, initial legislation, and debate regarding the determinants of health and approaches to health management began to appear on a social, economic, and medical level. The advent of "modern" health care occurred around this time, and nursing made a large contribution to the progress of health care. The following sections discuss the evolution of modern nursing, the evolution of modern medical care and public health practice, the evolution of the community caregiver, and the establishment of public health nursing.

Evolution of Modern Nursing

Florence Nightingale, the woman credited with establishing "modern nursing," began her work during the mid-nineteenth century. Historians remember Florence Nightingale for contributing to the health of British soldiers during the Crimean War and establishing nursing education. However, most historians failed to recognize her remarkable use of public health principles and distinguished scientific contributions to health care reform (Cohen, 1984; Grier and Grier, 1978). The following review of Nightingale's work emphasizes her concern for environmental determinants of health; her focus on the aggregate of British soldiers through emphasis on sanitation, community assessment, and analysis; the development of the use of graphically depicted statistics; and the gathering of comparable census data and political advocacy on behalf of the aggregate.

Nightingale was from a wealthy English family, was well educated, and traveled extensively. Her father tutored her in mathematics and many other subjects. Nightingale later studied with Adolphe Quetelet, a Belgian statistician. Quetelet influenced her profoundly and taught her the discipline of social inquiry (Goodnow, 1933). Nightingale also had a passion for hygiene and health. In 1851, at the age of 31 years, she trained in nursing with Pastor Fliedner at Kaiserswerth Hospital in Germany. She later studied the organization and discipline of the Sisters of Charity in Paris. Nightingale wrote extensively and published her analyses of the many nursing systems she studied in France, Austria, Italy, and Germany (Dock and Stewart, 1925).

In 1854, Nightingale responded to distressing accounts of a lack of care for wounded soldiers during the Crimean War. She and forty other nurses traveled to Scutari, which was part of the Ottoman Empire at the time. Nightingale was accompanied by lay nurses, Roman Catholic sisters, and Anglican sisters. Upon their arrival, they learned that the British army's management method for treating the sick and wounded had created conditions that resulted in extraordinarily high death rates among soldiers. One of Nightingale's greatest achievements was improving the management of ill and wounded soldiers.

Nightingale faced an assignment in The Barrack Hospital, which had been built for 1700 patients. In 4 miles of beds, she found 3000 to 4000 patients separated by only 18 inches of space (Goodnow, 1933).

During the Crimean War, cholera and "contagious fever" were rampant. An equal number of men died of disease and battlefield injury (Cohen, 1984). Nightingale found that allocated supplies were bound in bureaucratic red tape; for example, supplies were "sent to the wrong ports or were buried under munitions and could not be got" (Goodnow, 1933, p. 86).

Nightingale encountered problems reforming the army's methods for care of the sick because she had to work through eight military affairs departments related to her assignment. She sent reports of the appalling conditions of the hospitals to London and in response immediately set up diet kitchens and a laundry and provided food, clothing, dressings, and laboratory equipment with government money and donated funds (Dock and Stewart, 1925).

Major reforms occurred during the first 2 months of her assignment. Aware that an interest in keeping social statistics was emerging, Nightingale realized that her most forceful argument would be statistical in nature. She reorganized the methods of keeping statistics and was the first to use shaded and colored coxcomb graphs of wedges, circles, and squares to illustrate the preventable deaths of soldiers. Nightingale compared the deaths of soldiers in hospitals during the Crimean War with the average annual mortality in Manchester and with the deaths of soldiers in military hospitals in and near London at the time (Figure 2-2). Through her reforms she also showed that, by the end of the war, the death rate among ill soldiers during the Crimean War was no higher than that among well soldiers in Britain (Cohen, 1984). Indeed, Nightingale's careful statistics revealed that the death rate for treated soldiers decreased from 42% to 2%. Furthermore, she established community services and activities to improve the quality of life for recovering soldiers. These included rest and recreation facilities, study opportunities, a savings fund, and

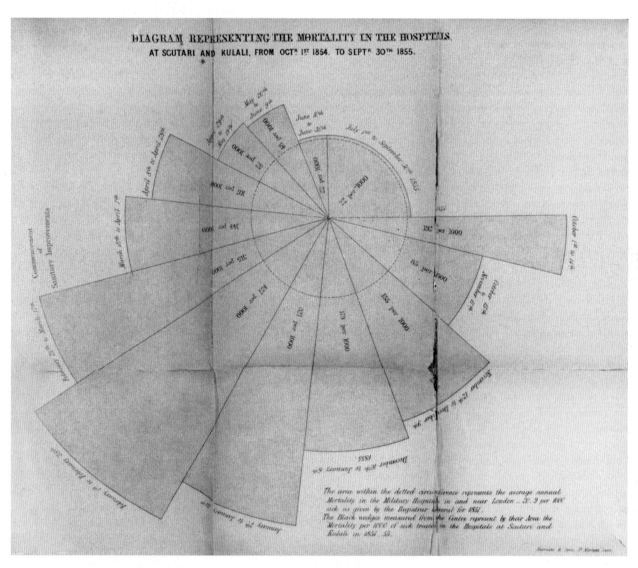

FIGURE 2-2 *A,* Coxcomb charts by Florence Nightingale. (From Nightingale F: *Notes on matters affecting the health, efficiency and hospitalization of the British army,* London, 1858, Harrison and Sons.)

(Continued)

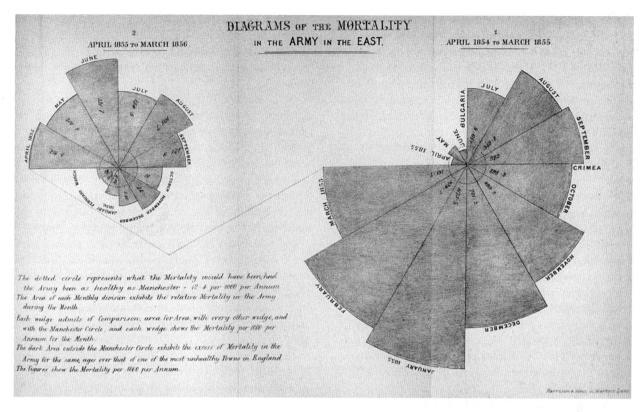

FIGURE 2-2—cont'd *B,* Photographs of large, foldout charts from an original preserved at the University of Chicago Library. (Public domain; courtesy University of Chicago Library.)

a post office. She also organized care for the families of the soldiers (Dock and Stewart, 1925).

After returning to London at the close of the war in 1856, Nightingale devoted her efforts to sanitary reform. At home, she surmised that if the sanitary neglect of the soldiers existed in the battle area, it probably existed at home in London. She prepared statistical tables to support her suspicions (Table 2-2).

In one study comparing the mortality of men aged 25 to 35 years in the army barracks of England with that of men

TABLE 2-2	NIGHTINGALE'S CRIMEAN WAR MORTALITY STATISTICS: NURSING RESEARCH THAT MADE A DIFFERENCE		
YEAR	**DEATHS THAT WOULD HAVE OCCURRED IN HEALTHY DISTRICTS AMONG MALES OF THE SOLDIERS' AGES***	**ACTUAL DEATHS OF NONCOMMISSIONED OFFICERS AND MEN**	**EXCESS OF DEATHS AMONG NONCOMMISSIONED OFFICERS AND MEN**
1839	763	2914	2151
1840	829	3300	2471
1841	857	4167	3310
1842	888	5052	4164
1843	914	5270	4356
1844	920	3867	2947
1845	911	4587	3676
1846	930	5125	4195
1847	981	4232	3251
1848	987	3213	2226
1849	954	4052	3098
1850	919	3119	2200
1851	901	2729	1828
1852	915	3120	2205
1853	920	3392	2472
Total	13,589	58,139	44,550

From Grier B, Grier M: Contributions of the passionate statistician, *Res Nurs Health* 1:103-109, 1978. Copyright ©1978 by John Wiley & Sons, Inc. Reprinted by permission of John Wiley & Sons, Inc.
Number of deaths of noncommissioned officers and men also shows the number of deaths that would have occurred if the mortality were 7.7 per 1000—such as it was among Englishmen of the soldiers' age in healthy districts, in the years 1849 to 1853—which fairly represent the average mortality.
*The exact mortality in the healthy districts is 0.0077122, using the logarithm of 3.8871801.

the same age in civilian life, Nightingale found the mortality of the soldiers was nearly twice that of the civilians. In one of her reports, she stated that "our soldiers enlist to death in the barracks" (Kopf, 1978, p. 95). Further, she believed that allowing a young soldier to die needlessly of unsanitary conditions was equivalent to taking him out, lining him up, and shooting him (Kopf, 1978). She was very political and did not keep her community assessment and analysis to herself. Nightingale distributed her reports to members of Parliament and to the medical and commanding officers of the army (Kopf, 1978). Prominent male leaders of the time challenged her reports. Undaunted, she rewrote them in greater depth and redistributed them.

In her efforts to compare the hospital systems in European countries, Nightingale discovered that each hospital kept incomparable data and that many hospitals used various names and classifications for diseases. She noted that these differences prevented the collection of similar statistics from larger geographical areas. These statistics would create a regional health-illness profile and allow for comparison with other regions. She printed common statistical forms that some hospitals in London adopted on an experimental basis. A study of the tabulated results revealed the promise of this strategy (Kopf, 1978) (Box 2-3).

Nightingale continued the development and application of statistical procedures, and she won recognition for her efforts. The Royal Statistical Society made her a fellow in 1858, and the American Statistical Association made her an honorary member in 1874 (Kopf, 1978).

In 1861, Nightingale lobbied officials to add two areas of data collection to the census. She asked officials to include the number of sick and infirm in the population and data depicting the housing of the population (Kopf, 1978). She stated the following:

The connection between the health and the dwellings of the population is one of the most important that exists. The "diseases" can be approximated also. In all the more important—such as smallpox, fevers, measles, heart disease, etc., all those which affect the national health, there will be very little error. Where there is error, in these things, the error is uniform…and corrects itself. (p. 98)

BOX 2-3 NIGHTINGALE'S USE OF STATISTICAL METHODS IN COMMUNITY ASSESSMENT

London's Southeastern Railway planned to remove St. Thomas' Hospital to increase the railway's right-of-way between London Bridge and Charing Cross. Nightingale applied her statistical method to the health needs of the community by conducting a *community assessment*. She plotted the cases served by the hospital, analyzed the proportion by distance, and calculated the probable impact on the community if the hospital was relocated to the proposed site. In her view, hospitals were a part of the wider community that served the needs of humanity. Kopf (1978) noted that this method of health planning and matching resources to the needs of the population was visionary and was not reapplied until the twentieth century.

Although census officials did not adopt her recommendations linking illness and housing to health, Nightingale's suggestions were visionary. According to Kopf (1978), only a few countries currently gather census data on sickness and housing.

Nightingale also stressed the need to use statistics at the administrative and political levels to direct health policy. Noting the ignorance of politicians and those who set policy regarding the interpretation and use of statistics, she emphasized the need to teach national leaders to use statistical facts.

In addition to her contributions to nursing and her development of nursing education, Nightingale's credits include the application of statistical information toward an understanding of the total environmental situation (Kopf, 1978). Population-based statistics have marked implications for the development of public health and public health nursing. Grier and Grier (1978, p. 103) recognized Nightingale's contributions to statistics and stated that "Her name occurs in the index of many texts on the history of probability and statistics…in the history of quantitative graphics…and in texts on the history of science and mathematics." Specifically, these authors showed that Nightingale's research *preceded* later works, such as the use of correlation in 1880, the *t*-test in 1908, and the subsequent development of the chi-square, contingency table analysis, and analysis of variance. In contrast to Nightingale's research, these newer tests aided in judging the relevance of data when the numbers were few and the effects were small.

It is interesting to note that the paradigm for nursing practice and nursing education that evolved through Nightingale's work did not incorporate her emphasis on statistics and a sound research base. It is also curious why nursing education did not consult her writings and stress the importance of determining health's social and environmental determinants until much later.

Establishment of Modern Medical Care and Public Health Practice

To place Nightingale's work in perspective, it is necessary to consider the development of medical care in light of common education and practice during the late nineteenth and early twentieth centuries. Goodnow (1933) called this time a "dark age." Medical sciences were underdeveloped, and bacteriology was unknown. Few medical schools existed at the time, so apprenticeship was the path to medical education. The majority of physicians believed in the "spontaneous generation" theory of disease causation, which stated that disease organisms grew from nothing (Najman, 1990). Typical medical treatment included bloodletting, starving, using leeches, and prescribing large doses of metals such as mercury and antimony (Goodnow, 1933).

Nightingale's uniform classification of hospital statistics noted the need to tabulate the classification of diseases in hospital patients and the need to note the diseases patients contracted in the hospital. These diseases, such as gangrene and septicemia, were later called *iatrogenic* diseases (Kopf, 1978). Considering the lack of surgical sanitation in hospitals at the time, it is not surprising that iatrogenic infection was rampant. For example, Goodnow (1933) illustrates the following unsanitary operating procedures:

> Before an operation the surgeon turned up the sleeves of his coat to save the coat, and would often not trouble to wash his hands, knowing how soiled they soon would be! The area of the operation would sometimes be washed with soap and water, but not always, for the inevitability of corruption made it seem useless. The silk or thread used for stitches or ligatures was hung over a button of the surgeon's coat, and during the operation a convenient place for the knife to rest was between his lips. Instruments… used for…lancing abscesses were kept in the vest pocket and often only wiped with a piece of rag as the surgeon went from one patient to another. (pp. 471-472)

During the nineteenth century, the following important scientists were born: Louis Pasteur in 1822, Joseph Lister in 1827, and Robert Koch in 1843. Their research also had a profound impact on health care, medicine, and nursing. Pasteur was a chemist, not a physician. While experimenting with wine production in 1854, he proposed the theory of the existence of germs. Although his colleagues ridiculed him at first, Koch applied his theories and developed his methods for handling and studying bacteria. Subsequently, Pasteur's colleagues gave him acknowledgment for his work.

Lister, whose father perfected the microscope, observed the healing processes of fractures. When the bone was broken but the skin was not, he noted that recovery was uneventful. However, when both the bone and the skin were broken, fever, infection, and even death were frequent. He found the proposed answer to his observation through Pasteur's work. Something outside the body entered the wound through the broken skin causing the infection (Goodnow, 1933). Lister's surgical successes eventually improved when he soaked the dressings and instruments in mixtures of carbolic acid (i.e., phenol) and oil.

In 1882, Koch discovered the causative agent for cholera and the tubercle bacillus. Pasteur discovered immunization in 1881 and the rabies vaccine in 1885. These discoveries were significant to the development of public health and medicine. However, physicians accepted these discoveries slowly (Rosen, 1958). For example, TB was a major cause of death in late nineteenth century America and often plagued its victims with chronic illness and disability. It was a highly stigmatized disease, and most physicians thought it was a hereditary, constitutional disease associated with poor environmental conditions. Hospitalization for TB was rare because the stigma caused families to hide their infected relatives. Without treatment, the communicability of the disease increased. Common treatment was a change of climate (Rosen, 1958). Although Koch had announced the discovery of the tubercle bacillus in 1882, it was 10 years before the emergence of the first organized community campaign to stop the spread of the disease.

The case of puerperal (i.e., childbirth) fever illustrates another example of slow innovation stemming from scientific discoveries. Although Pasteur showed that Streptococcus caused puerperal fever, it was years before physicians accepted his discovery. However, medical practice eventually changed, and physicians no longer delivered infants after performing autopsies in puerperal fever cases without washing their hands (Goodnow, 1933).

Debate over the causes of disease occurred throughout the nineteenth century. Scientists discovered organisms during the latter part of the century, which supported the theory that specific contagious entities caused disease. This discovery challenged the earlier, miasmic theory that environment and atmospheric conditions caused disease (Greifinger and Sidel, 1981). The new scientific discoveries had a major impact on the development of public health and medical practice. The emergence of germ theory of disease focused diagnosis and treatment on the individual organism and the individual disease.

State and local governments felt increasingly responsible for controlling the spread of bacteria and other microorganisms. A community outcry for social reform forced state and local governments to take notice of the deplorable living conditions in the cities. In the New York City riots of 1863, the populace expressed their disgust for overcrowding; filthy streets; lack of provisions for the poor; and lack of adequate food, water, and housing for the people. Local boards of health formed and took responsibility for safeguarding food and water stores and managed the sewage and quarantine operation for victims of contagious diseases (Greifinger and Sidel, 1981).

The New York Metropolitan Board of Health formed in 1866, and state health departments formed shortly thereafter. States built large public hospitals that treated TB and mental disease with rest, diet, and quarantine. In 1889, the New York City Health Department recommended the surveillance of TB and TB health education, but physicians did not welcome either recommendation (Rosen, 1958). Despite their objections, the New York City Health Department required institutions to report cases of TB in 1894 and required physicians to do the same in 1897.

In the later part of the nineteenth century, the National Tuberculosis Association attempted to control TB by "enlisting community support and action through a systematic and organized campaign of public health education" (Rosen, 1958, p. 390). Many voluntary health organizations followed with organized efforts to "further community health through education, demonstrating ways of improving health services, advancing related research or legislation, and guarding and representing the public interest in this field" (Rosen, 1958, p. 384).

In 1883, The Johns Hopkins University Medical School in Baltimore, Maryland, formed under the German model that promoted medical education on the principles of scientific discovery. In the United States, the Carnegie Commission appointed Abraham Flexner to evaluate medical schools throughout the country based on the German model. In 1910, the Flexner Report outlined the shortcomings of U.S. medical schools that did not use this model. Within a few years, the report caused philanthropic organizations such as the

BOX 2-4   SCIENTIFIC THEORY/SINGLE
AGENT THEORY

The emphasis on the use of scientific theory, or single agent theory, in medical care developed into a focus on disease and symptoms rather than a focus on the prevention of disability and care for the "whole person." The old-fashioned family doctor viewed patients in relation to their families and communities and apparently helped people cope with problems in personal life, family, and society. American medicine adopted science with such vigor that these qualities faded away. Science allowed the physician to deal with tissues and organs, which were much easier to comprehend than the dynamics of human relationships or the complexities of disease prevention. Many physicians made efforts to integrate the various roles, but society was pushing toward academic science.

Rockefeller and Carnegie Foundations to withdraw funding of these schools, which ensured the closure of scientifically "inadequate" medical schools (Greifinger and Sidel, 1981). A "new breed" of physicians emerged who had been taught that germ theory was the "single agent theory" of disease causation (Greifinger and Sidel, 1981, p. 132) (Box 2-4).

Philanthropic foundations continued to influence health care efforts. For example, the Rockefeller Sanitary Commission for the Eradication of Hookworm formed in 1909. Hookworm was an occupational hazard among Southern workers. The discovery of preventive efforts to eradicate hookworm kept the workers healthy and thus proved to be a great industrial benefit. The model was so successful that the Rockefeller Foundation established the first school of public health, The Johns Hopkins School of Hygiene and Public Health, in 1916. The focus of this institution was the preservation and improvement of individual and community health and the prevention of disease through multidisciplinary efforts. The faculty came from a broad range of sciences including biological, physical, social, and behavioral. Foundations made additional efforts, which led to the formation of the International Health Commission, schools of tropical medicine, and medical research institutes in foreign ports.

Community Caregiver

The traditional role of the community caregiver or the traditional healer has nearly vanished. However, medical and nurse anthropologists who have studied primitive and Western cultures are familiar with the community healer and caregiver role (Leininger, 1976; Logan and Hunt, 1978). The traditional healer is common in non-Western, ancient, and primitive societies (Hughes, 1978). The healer may have taken various forms (e.g., shaman, midwife, herbalist, or priest). Although traditional healers have always existed, professionals and many people throughout industrialized societies may overlook or minimize their role. The role of the healer is often integrated with other institutions of society including religion, medicine, and morality. The notion that one person acts alone in healing may be foreign to many societies; healers can be individuals, kin, or entire societies (Hughes, 1978).

Societies retain folk practices because they offer repeated success. Most cultures have a pharmacopoeia and maintain therapeutic and preventive practices. One fourth to one half of folk medicines are empirically effective, and many modern drugs are based on the medicines of primitive cultures (e.g., eucalyptus, coca, and opium) (Hughes, 1978).

Folk healing practices may be beneficial to the "patient" and may be socially cohesive; healing rituals and sessions frequently involve the patient and the patient's family and neighbors. When the healer allows the patient to participate in his or her own treatment and to involve his or her family and neighbors, the healer may apply the "treatment" to a whole group, or aggregate (Hughes, 1978).

Since ancient times, cultural practices have affected health. The late nineteenth and early twentieth century practice of midwifery illustrates modern medicine's encroachment over traditional healing in many Western cultures (Ehrenreich and English, 1973; Smith, 1979). For example, traditional midwifery practices made women rise out of bed within 24 hours of delivery to help "clear" the lochia; throughout the mid-1900s, modern medicine recommended keeping women in bed (Smith, 1979).

HISTORICAL METHODOLOGY FOR NURSING RESEARCH

Historiography is the methodology of historical research. It involves specialized techniques, principles, and theories that pertain to historical matters. Historical research involves interpreting history and contributing to understanding through data synthesis. It relies on existing sources or data and requires the researcher to gain access to sources such as libraries, librarians, and databases.

Historical research should be descriptive. It should answer the questions of who, what, when, where, how, and the interpretive why. Historians reconstruct an era using primary sources and interpret the story from that perspective. Historical research in nursing will enhance the understanding of current nursing practice and will help prepare for the future.

From Lusk B: Historical methodology for nursing research, *Image J Nurs Sch* 29:3555-3560, 1997.

Establishment of Public Health Nursing

Public health nursing as a holistic approach developed in the late nineteenth and early twentieth centuries. Public health nursing and community health nursing evolved from home nursing practice, community organizations, and political interventions on behalf of aggregates.

England

Public health nursing developed from providing nursing care to the sick poor and providing information and channels of community organization that enable the poor to improve their own health status.

District Nursing. District nursing, which stemmed from public health nursing, developed in England. Between 1854 and 1856, the Epidemiological Society of London developed a plan that trained selected poor women to provide nursing care to the community's sick poor. The society theorized that nurses belonging to their patient's social class would be more effective caregivers and that more nurses would be available in the community (Rosen, 1958).

A similar plan implemented in Liverpool in 1859 was more successful. After experiencing the excellent care a nurse gave his sick wife in his home, William Rathbone strongly believed that nurses could offer the same care throughout the community. He developed a plan that divided the community into 18 districts and assigned a nurse and a social worker to each district. This team met the needs of their communities in nursing, social work, and health education. The community widely accepted the plan. To further strengthen it, Rathbone consulted Nightingale about educating the district nurses. She assisted him by providing training for the district nurses, referring to them as "health nurses." The model was successful, and eventually voluntary agencies on the national level adopted the plan (Rosen, 1958).

Health Visiting. Health visiting to provide information for improved health is a parallel service based on the district nursing tradition. The Ladies Section of the Manchester and Salford Sanitary Association originated health visiting in Manchester in 1862. Health pamphlets alone had little effect; therefore this service enlisted home visitors to distribute health information to the poor.

In 1893, Nightingale pointed out that the district nurse should be a health teacher and a nurse for the sick in the home. She believed that teachers should educate "health missioners" for this purpose. However, the model charged the district nurse with providing care for the sick in the home and the health visitor with providing health information in the home. Eventually, government agencies sponsored health visitors, medical health officers supervised them, and the municipality paid them. Thus a collaborative model developed between government and voluntary agencies and exists in the United States today.

United States

In the United States, public health nursing also developed from the British traditions of district nursing and home nursing. In 1877, the Women's Board of the New York City Mission sent a graduate nurse named Frances Root into homes to provide care for the sick. The innovation spread, and nursing associations, later called visiting nurse associations, were implemented in Buffalo in 1885 and in Boston and Philadelphia in 1886.

In 1893, nurses Lillian Wald and Mary Brewster established a district nursing service on the Lower East Side of New York City called the House on Henry Street. This was a crowded area teeming with unemployed and homeless immigrants who needed health care. This organization, later called the Visiting Nurse Association of New York City, played an important role in establishing public health nursing in the United States. Box 2-5 contains Wald's compelling account of her early exposure to the community where she identified public health nursing needs.

Wald described a range of services that evolved from the House on Henry Street. Nurses provided home visits, and patients paid carfare or a cursory fee. Physicians were consultants to Henry Street, and families could arrange a visit by calling the nurse directly or a physician could call the nurse on the family's behalf. The nursing service adopted the philosophy of meeting the health needs of aggregates, which included the many evident social, economic, and environmental determinants of health. By necessity, this involved an aggregate approach that empowered people of the community.

Helen Hall, who later directed the House on Henry Street, wrote that the settlement's role was "one of helping people to help themselves" (Wald, 1971) through the development of centers of social action aimed at meeting the needs of the community and the individual. Community organization led to the formation of a great variety of programs including youth clubs, a juvenile program, sex education for local schoolteachers, and support programs for immigrants. A community studies department carried out systematic community assessments "so that we could tell our neighbors' story where it would do the most good" (Wald, 1971, p. vi). Mothers from the settlement went to Washington, DC, and testified about raising children in "decaying tenements." Neighbors of the settlement entered a democratic process that took them from the steps of city hall to the nation's capital to speak out on behalf of the needs of the aggregate. They spoke out for necessities such as traffic lights, schools, garbage collection services, unemployment insurance, and health care. The Children's Bureau and the Social Security Act Legislation formed as a result of these efforts. The testimony had an impact on the formation of Medicare in 1963.

Aggregate programs such as school nursing were based on individual observations and interventions. Wald reported the following incident that preceded her successful trial of school nursing (1971):

I had been downtown only a short time when I met Louis. An open door in a rear tenement revealed a woman standing over a washtub, a fretting baby on her left arm, while with her right she rubbed at the butcher's aprons which she washed for a living.

"Louis," she explained, "was bad." He did not "cure his head of lice and what would become of him, for they would not take him into the school because of it." Louis said he had been to the dispensary many times. He knew it was awful for a twelve-year-old boy not to know how to read the names of the streets on the lamp-posts, but "every time I go to school Teacher tells me to go home."

It needed only intelligent application of the dispensary ointments to cure the affected area, and in September, I had the joy of securing the boy's admittance to school for the first time in his life. The next day, at the noon recess, he fairly rushed up our five flights of stairs in the Jefferson Street tenement to spell the elementary words he had acquired that morning. (pp. 46-47)

BOX 2-5   LILLIAN WALD: *THE HOUSE ON HENRY STREET*

The following highlights from *The House on Henry Street*, published in 1915, bring Lillian Wald's experience to life:

A sick woman in a squalid rear tenement, so wretched and so pitiful that, in all the years since, I have not seen anything more appalling, determined me, within half an hour, to live on the East Side.

I had spent two years in a New York training-school for nurses.... After graduation, I supplemented the theoretical instruction, which was casual and inconsequential in the hospital classes twenty-five years ago, by a period of study at a medical college. It was while at the college that a great opportunity came to me.

While there, the long hours "on duty" and the exhausting demands of the ward work scarcely admitted freedom for keeping informed as to what was happening in the world outside. The nurses had no time for general reading; visits to and from friends were brief; we were out of the current and saw little of life saved as it flowed into the hospital wards. It is not strange, therefore that I should have been ignorant of the various movements which reflected the awakening of the social conscience at the time.

Remembering the families who came to visit patients in the wards, I outlined a course of instruction in home nursing adapted to their needs, and gave it in an old building in Henry Street, then used as a technical school and now part of the settlement. Henry Street then as now was the center of a dense industrial population.

From the schoolroom where I had been giving a lesson in bedmaking, a little girl led me one drizzling March morning. She had told me of her sick mother, and gathering from her incoherent account that a child had been born, I caught up the paraphernalia of the bedmaking lesson and carried it with me.

The child led me over broken roadways—there was no asphalt, although its use was well established in other parts of the city—over dirty mattresses and heaps of refuse—it was before Colonel Waring had shown the possibility of clean streets even in that quarter—between tall, reeking houses whose laden fire-escapes, useless for their appointed purpose, bulged with household goods of every description. The rain added to the dismal appearance of the streets and to the discomfort of the crowds which thronged them, intensifying the odors which assailed me from every side. Through Hester and Division Street we went to the end of Ludlow; past odorous fishstands, for the streets were a market-place, unregulated, unsupervised, unclean; past evil-smelling, uncovered garbage-cans; and—perhaps worst of all, where so many little children played—past the trucks brought down from more fastidious quarters and stalled on these already overcrowded streets, lending themselves inevitably to many forms of indecency.

The child led me on through a tenement hallway, across a court where open and unscreened closets were promiscuously used by men and women, up into a rear tenement, by slimy steps whose accumulated dirt was augmented that day by the mud of the streets, and finally into the sickroom.

All the maladjustments of our social and economic relations seemed epitomized in this brief journey and what was found at the end of it. The family to which the child led me was neither criminal nor vicious. Although the husband was a cripple, one of those who stand on street corners exhibiting deformities to enlist compassion, and masking the begging of alms by a pretense at selling; although the family of seven shared their two rooms with boarders—who were literally boarders, since a piece of timber was placed over the floor for them to sleep on—and although the sick woman lay on a wretched, unclean bed, soiled with a hemorrhage two days old, they were not degraded human beings, judged by any measure of moral values.

In fact, it was very plain that they were sensitive to their condition, and when, at the end of my ministrations, they kissed my hands (those who have undergone similar experiences will, I am sure, understand), it would have been some solace if by any conviction of the moral unworthiness of the family I could have defended myself as a part of a society which permitted such conditions to exist. Indeed, my subsequent acquaintance with them revealed the fact that, miserable as their state was, they were not without ideals for the family life, and for society, of which they were so unloved and unlovely a part.

That morning's experience was a baptism of fire. Deserted were the laboratory and the academic work of the college. I never returned to them. On my way from the sickroom to my comfortable student quarters my mind was intent on my own responsibility. To my inexperience it seemed certain that conditions such as these were allowed because people did not know, and for me there was a challenge to know and to tell. When early morning found me still awake, my naive conviction remained that, if people knew things—and "things" meant everything implied in the condition of this family—such horrors would cease to exist, and I rejoiced that I had had a training in the care of the sick that in itself would give me an organic relationship to the neighborhood in which this awakening had come.

To the first sympathetic friend to whom I poured forth my story, I found myself presenting a plan which had been developing almost without conscious mental direction on my part.

Within a day or two a comrade from the training-school, Mary Brewster, agreed to share in the venture. We were to live in the neighborhood as nurses, identify ourselves with it socially, and, in brief, contribute to it our citizenship.

I should like to make it clear that from the beginning we were most profoundly moved by the wretched industrial conditions which were constantly forced upon us....I hope to tell of the constructive programmes that the people themselves have evolved out of their own hard lives, of the ameliorative measures, ripened out of sympathetic comprehension, and finally, of the social legislation that expresses the new compunction of the community. (pp. 1-9)

From Wald L: *The house on Henry Street,* New York, 1971, Dover Publications (original work published 1915, Henry Holt).

Overcrowded schools, an uninformed and uninterested public, and an unaware department of health all contributed to this social health neglect. Wald and the nursing staff at the settlement kept anecdotal notes on the sick children teachers excluded from school. One nurse found a boy in school whose skin was desquamating from scarlet fever and took him to the president of the Department of Health in an attempt to place physicians in schools. A later program had physicians screen children in school for 1 hour each day.

Twentieth Century. In 1902, Wald convinced Dr. Lederle, Commissioner of Health in New York City, to try a school nursing experiment. Henry Street loaned a public health nurse named Linda Rogers to the New York City Health Department to work in a school (Dock and Stewart, 1925). The experiment was successful, and schools adopted nursing on a widespread basis. School nurses performed physical assessments, treated minor infections, and taught health to pupils and parents.

In 1909, Wald mentioned the efficacy of home nursing to one of the officials of the Metropolitan Life Insurance Company. The company decided to provide home nursing to its industrial policyholders, and soon the United States and Canada used the program successfully (Wald, 1971).

The increasing demand for public health nursing was hard to satisfy. In 1910, the Department of Nursing and Health formed at the Teachers College of Columbia University in New York City. A course in visiting nursing placed nurses at the Henry Street settlement for fieldwork. In 1912, the newly formed National Organization for Public Health Nursing elected Lillian Wald its first president. This organization was open to public health nurses and to those interested in public health nursing. In 1913, the Los Angeles Department of Health formed the first Bureau of Public Health Nursing (Rosen, 1958). That same year, the Public Health Service appointed its first public health nurse.

At first, many public health nursing programs used nurses in specialized areas such as school nursing, TB nursing, maternal-child health nursing, and communicable disease nursing. In recent years, more generalized programs have become acceptable. Efforts to contain health care costs include reducing the number of hospital days. With the advent of shortened hospital stays, private home health agencies provide home-based illness care across the United States.

With a current focus on cost containment and the provision of health care services under managed care, change is taking place in the traditional models of public health nursing and visiting nursing in voluntary home health agencies. The focus of care is increasing within the community; therefore new models that use nursing in the community to contain costs are appearing with variation among states and areas within a state. For example, some models may focus on providing care to populations that subscribe to HMOs (Graff et al., 1995; Shamansky, 1995), whereas others focus on specialized areas such as communicable diseases.

CONSEQUENCES FOR THE HEALTH OF AGGREGATES

An understanding of the consequences of the health care delivery system's impact on aggregate health is necessary to form conclusions about community health nursing from a historical perspective. Implications for the health of aggregates relate to new causes of mortality (i.e., *Hygeia*, or good living, vs. *Panacea*, or curative medicine) and additional theories of disease causation.

Twenty-First Century
New Causes of Mortality
Since the end of the twentieth century, the focus of disease in Western societies has changed from mostly infectious diseases to chronic diseases. Increased food production and better nutrition during the nineteenth and early twentieth centuries contributed to the decline in infectious disease–related deaths. Other factors include better sanitation through water purification, sewage disposal, improved food handling, and milk pasteurization. According to McKeown (1981) and Evans, Barer, and Marmor (1994), "modern" medicine such as antibiotics and immunization had little effect on health until well into the twentieth century. Indeed, improved vaccination programs began in the 1920s, and powerful antibiotics came into use after 1935.

The advent of chronic disease in Western populations puts selected aggregates at risk, and those aggregates need health education, screening, and programs to ensure occupational and environmental safety. Too often modern medicine focuses on the single cause of disease (i.e., germ theory) and treating the acutely ill. Therefore health providers have treated the chronically ill with an acute care approach although preventive care, health promotion, and restorative care are necessary to combat escalating rates of chronic disease. This expanded approach may develop under new systems of cost containment.

Hygeia versus Panacea
The Grecian Hygeia (i.e., healthful living) versus Panacea (i.e., cure) dichotomy still exists today. Although the change in the nature of health "problems" is certain, the roles of individual and collective activities in the prevention of illness and premature death are slow to evolve. Consequently, "complex life-threatening disorders are better understood; on the other hand, inadequate numbers of professionals have been trained to specialize in the treatment of the common, uncomplicated health problems that account for 90 percent of visits to doctors" (Lee, Brown, and Red, 1981, p. 197).

In 1997, about two thirds of the active physicians in the United States were specialists (U.S. Department of Health and Human Services, Health Resources and Services Administration, Bureau of Health Professions [USDHHS/HRSA/BHP], 1999). Medical education is increasingly responsible for training primary care physicians (e.g., internal medicine, obstetrics-gynecology, family medicine, and pediatrics) to meet the growing need for primary care. This need for primary care providers and the phenomenal growth of managed care calls for more advanced practice nurses in primary care positions. In addition to primary care, Hygeia requires a coordinated system that addresses health problems holistically using multiple approaches and planning outcomes for aggregates and populations. A redistribution of interest and

BOX 2-6   A MODEL OF DISTRICT NURSING

In rural New England, an ethnohistorical study of public health nursing's development unexpectedly found a model of population-based nursing that may meet the nation's current and future health concerns (Dreher, 1984). The study collected data from public records; the census; direct observations; and interviews with town residents, public officials, medical care providers, and active and retired public health nurses. The health model of the 1920s used a district nurse, or "town hall" nurse, which exists today. The findings showed that the district nurse provided health education and services to people in four neighboring towns. The district nurse's activities were under local administration, and property tax revenues paid for the services; patients and third-party reimbursement did not contribute funds. The district nurse provided a full range of community nursing services to people in need, whether or not the patients were able to pay or were covered by insurance. The nurse performed school nursing, health promotion and prevention, and home health care. The district nurse held weekly office hours in the town halls of the four communities, performed blood pressure screening, and gave routine parenteral medications and health counseling. Mobility was not an issue because the district nurse performed home visits for patients confined to their homes. The district nurse conducted routine screening in schools and planned and carried out programs that addressed identified needs. The annual cost per visit from the district nurse was far less than the nurse services from a nearby home health agency. This model exemplifies a way of addressing the nation's health problems through prevention, promotion, and maintenance care.

resources to address the major determinants of health, such as food, housing, education, and a healthy social and physical environment, is necessary (Evans, Barer, and Marmor, 1994; Lamarche, 1995) (Box 2-6).

Additional Theories of Disease Causation

The germ theory of disease causation is a unicausal model that evolved in the late nineteenth century. Najman (1990) reviewed the following theories of disease causation: the multicausal view, which considers the environment multidimensional, and the general susceptibility view, which considers stress and lifestyle factors. Najman contended that each theory accounts for some disease under some conditions, but no single theory accounts for all disease. Other factors such as literacy and nutrition may reduce infectious disease morbidity and mortality to a greater extent than medical interventions alone (Najman, 1990).

SOCIAL CHANGES AND COMMUNITY HEALTH NURSING

Several social and political changes have occurred in the United States that have affected the development of community health nursing practice. During the twentieth century, the health of the aggregate client, nursing, health, and environment have been influenced by the development of health insurance, the rise of discrimination and racism, the development of feminism, population-based training, and in the twenty-first

century effects of terrorism in America. The following material reviews each of these developments and highlights their importance to community health nursing practice.

Changes in health insurance changed the landscape of health care delivery. The greatest health concerns at the beginning of the twentieth century were lost wages associated with sickness. The cost of health care was so low there was little understanding of the need for health insurance. Between 1900 and 1920 there was little technology. Treatments available at the time, including surgery, were often performed in private homes. Industrialization and organized labor worked on providing health insurance to its workers.

During the 1920s and 1930s, the costs of health care increased. As the population moved from rural to urban living, the number of large private homes, the delivery point for health care, decreased. Increased technology and the acceptance of medicine as a science and the closure of several medical schools during the 1920s increased the demand and therefore raised the cost of health care (Faulkner, 1960; Rosenberg, 1987).

As hospitals began to organize, they formed the American Hospital Association, whose leaders encouraged the development of health insurance plans. During the 1930s, health insurance plans that were unique to individual hospitals merged under the name of Blue Cross (Eilers, 1963; Anderson, 1944; Thomasson, 2002). Increases in medical technology and the fact that employers began to offer health insurance in place of employee compensation during and after World War II further supported the growth of private health insurance (Health Insurance Institute, 1966). Federal and state movements during the 1960s supported the development of federal and state health insurance for the poor and the elderly populations (Oliver, Lee, and Lipton, 2004). Most of health care is paid for using either public or private insurance plans. Services covered by many insurance plans often do not include community-based health care.

Discrimination and racism have affected the development of community health in America (Gamble, 1997; Pernick, 1997). The American Nurses Association Position Statement on Discrimination and Racism in Health Care (1998) states that "differential access to resources limits basic and preventive health care to members of some groups. An equal distribution of health care resources results in morbidity and mortality rates that vary substantially among racial and ethnic categories and economic classes." Current community health initiatives need to be developed to address historical traditions and practices to ensure the absence of both discrimination and racism in current health care practice.

The historical concept of feminism can be traced to the eighteenth century. Although feminism means many things to different people, the philosophy of feminism embraces gender issues, economics, politics, and the humanities. Its basic premise is that people are inherently equal and deserve equal opportunities. In health care, feminism focuses on reproductive freedom for women. Feminists, regardless of focus, support the equality of all and are united against innate stereotypes.

Feminism has affected community health care delivery in two important ways. The feminist perspective has encouraged the involvement of people, especially women, in all dimensions of economic life. Employment and career opportunities based on talent, not gender, provide women with multiple career opportunities. Nursing as a career is but one health career opportunity for women, as well as men. And second, the feminist perspective of equality is in direct opposition to discrimination in health care delivery.

Today's nurse also plays a significant role in providing care to populations traumatized by natural disasters, genocide, and the care of new refugees. A major nursing role as client advocate is needed to optimize care when working with those suffering trauma. Nurses often join with multiple care providers who literally change the world for traumatized populations.

The current effect of terrorism against the United States is a recent historical event that will affect public health nursing practice well into the twenty-first century. In response to terrorism against the United States on September 11, 2001, the community health system is considered a resource in this country's arsenal against terrorist activities that can positively affect the nation's health. *Bioterrorism preparedness* are new buzzwords in health care. It is the responsibility of community health leaders to successfully enable the nation's health system to respond to any future bioterrorist attack. There are vulnerable areas of defense that remain within the U.S. public health response efforts, which need continual attention (The Century Foundation, 2005). In the event of future terrorism against the United States, increased numbers of community health practitioners would be needed to distribute vaccines and antibodies in an emergency. Additionally, public health laboratories would require additional capabilities to respond to a chemical terrorism threat, increased electronic tracking of disease outbreak information, and adequate crisis response plans by state. Currently, community health priorities are being met with limited and often inadequate resources (Trust for America's Health, 2009).

VIEWING IMMIGRANTS AS ASSETS: A GLIMPSE INTO AUSTRALIA'S PUBLIC HEALTH HISTORY

Like the United States and Canada, Australia is a land of immigration with its own unique public health history. In 1788—18 years after Captain Cook claimed the continent for Britain— the British began using Australia as a settlement for England's convicts and continued doing so until 1825. From 1826 to 1850, Australia held England's excess population. After 1850, the living conditions in England improved significantly and caused the level of British immigration to drop dramatically. Populating the Australian colony turned into a public health disaster for England because the journey was a difficult 6 to 8 months at sea.

The first few convict fleets barely survived the journey. By the time the immigrants arrived in Australia, they were plagued with disease and unable to build a settlement. British historical records show that the second English fleet contained 1260 convicts. By the time the fleet reached Australia, 267 convicts perished. Shortly after arriving, 124 of the survivors died in the Sydney hospital. For

the next 25 years, the surviving convicts were limited in their ability to help England build a settlement because they were starved and diseased. Overcrowding and reduced food and water rations made the journey difficult to survive. These poor travel conditions were related to the overall negligence and corruption of the private contractors who put priority on valuable cargo.

The British authorities realized that they needed to ensure the convicts' safe arrival. William Redfern, the assistant surgeon and former convict of New South Wales, advised Governor Macquarie to regulate the shipping contractors and supervise the convicts' health. Redfern recommended placing a convict surgeon aboard each ship to improve traveling conditions. Specifically, he recommended that the surgeons air out passenger cabins and bedding daily, make more drinking water available, provide full rations and articles of comfort, install bathing and cleaning facilities, and regularly fumigate the ship with nitric or muriatic acid. After Macquarie installed these regulations, the death rate among convicts on ships to Australia plummeted between 1788 and 1868; it was much lower in comparison with the passenger deaths on similar private fleets making the shorter trip from Europe to North America.

The Australian government believed that it was even more important that settlers, rather than convicts, arrive healthy and ready to work; therefore these public health standards were extended to ships that carried assisted immigrants. The Australian government prepaid the fares for assisted immigrants. Regulations from London mandated that surgeons and matrons be responsible for the hygiene, medical care, welfare, and discipline of the passengers. This measure, called the Passenger Act, created a marked improvement in the health of young children and all immigrants by placing a doctor and nurse aboard each ship. The British Board of Trade controlled the health conditions on all passenger ships and made the passage to Australia seem safe, more like returning from a vacation, where immigrants felt better than when they left their home port (Jupp, 1990).

This glimpse into Australia's immigration policy exemplifies one development in the history of public health. Whether it coerced the convicts or assisted passage for settlers, the Australian government populated its country through the belief that immigrants are assets and proved that the health of immigrants is a public responsibility.

Data from Jupp J: Two hundred years of immigration. In Reid J, Trompf R, editors: *The health of immigrant Australia*, Orlando, Fla, 1990, Harcourt Brace.

CHALLENGES FOR COMMUNITY AND PUBLIC HEALTH NURSING

Community health nurses face the challenge of promoting the health of populations. They must accomplish this with an "inclusive" understanding of the multiple causes of morbidity and mortality. The specialization of medicine and nursing has affected the delivery of nursing and medical care. Well-prepared nurses must be aware of the increased technological advances specialization has instigated. These advances resulted in an increase in the number and percentage of advanced practice nurses in the past two decades. In 1996, 6.3% of RNs in the United States were master's prepared (USDHHS, 1999), and most of these advanced practice nurses were specialists. However, the past decade has also seen an increase in the number and percentage of nurses working in community settings. In 1996, approximately 40% of all nurses worked in community settings such as occupational health, public health departments, physicians' offices, and schools (USDHHS, 1999).

The community need for a bimodal focus on prevention, health promotion, and home care may become more widespread with the changing patterns of reimbursement. Holistic care requires multiple dimensions and must have more attention in the future. During the turn of the century, an ethnohistorical study of public health nursing in rural New England examined the cost-benefit ratios of the population-based district nurse (Dreher, 1984). The district nurse provided preventive, curative, and health-maintenance services. Dreher proposed that such a model might better address the nation's health problems.

The need for education in community health nursing calls for a primary care curriculum that prepares students to meet the needs of aggregates through community strategies that include an understanding of statistical data and epidemiology. Such a curriculum would move the focus from the individual to a broader population approach. Strategies would promote literacy, nutrition programs, prevention of overweight in school-aged children, decent housing and income, education, and safe social and physical environments.

Health care services to individuals alone cannot solve today's health problems. All health care workers must learn to work with and on behalf of aggregates and help them build a constituency for the consumer issues they face.

A *population focus* for nursing addresses the health of all in the population through the careful gathering of information and statistics. A population focus will better enable community health nurses to contribute to the ethic of social justice by emphasizing society's responsibility for health (Beauchamp, 1986). Helping aggregates to help themselves will empower people and create avenues for addressing their concerns.

The history of community health nursing provides insight into the dilemmas faced in contemporary times. Duffus (1938) stated the following about Wald's work:

> The "case" element in these early reports of Wald got less and less emphasis; she instinctively went behind the symptoms to appraise the whole individual, saw that one could not understand the individual without understanding the family, saw that the family was in the grip of larger social and economic forces which it could not control. (p. 51)

Health care historians have reconstructed the history of health in Western populations by carefully sifting, weighing, and determining the importance of written fragments of "the facts." The historian's values and theories influence the writing of our past.

Traditionally, historians believed nonphysician healers were inauthentic "amateurs" who were marginal to "the maintenance of the physical health and well-being of society" (Versluysen, 1980, p. 176). This characterization was especially apparent for women healers. However, healers typically practiced in the home until the late nineteenth century. They were often invisible, yet represented an extensive system of care delivery. Contemporary historians who are often

feminists are now researching the healers' accounts of home care that earlier historians have overlooked, such as diaries, health manuals, and letters (Newbern, 1994).

According to Versluysen (1980), historians also tended to mention a few heroines within typical feminine stereotypes. For example, Nightingale's lifelong intellectual endeavors and marked achievements considerably expanded the profile of this remarkable woman beyond the typical focus on her 2 years in Crimea and her role in founding modern nursing education. She was a health statistician, a prolific writer and scientist, a radical environmental sanitarian, and a reformer of both the British Army medical care system and the sanitary policy in India.

In addition, historians have also neglected the social and environmental contexts of health and medical care. These dimensions are necessary to place health care in a broader context. Historians need this broad context to grasp the state of public health and public health efforts during specific periods.

EXAMPLE OF HISTORICAL NURSING RESEARCH

In response to public health problems, public health and community health nursing evolved in Louisiana between 1835 and 1927. Yellow fever epidemics in the early 1800s provided the early impetus for nursing growth. A nursing service called the Howard Association began in 1833 and provided food, medicine, and nursing care for yellow fever victims. Natural disasters, such as the Mississippi River flood in 1927, also caused the enhancement of accessible public health efforts.

Maternal and child care was another important area for early community and public health nursing efforts. In 1916, the state board of health employed the first public health nurse to reduce infant and maternal mortality, improve the health of preschool and school-aged children, and decrease the mortality and morbidity of communicable diseases.

From Hanggi-Myers LJ: *The origins and history of the first public health/community health nurses in Louisiana: 1835-1927,* Dissertation Abstracts, New Orleans, 1996, Louisiana State University Medical Center.

SUMMARY

Western civilization evolved from the Paleolithic period to the present, and people began to live in increasingly closer proximity to each other; therefore, they experienced a change in the nature of their health problems.

In the mid-nineteenth and early twentieth centuries, public health efforts and the precursors of modern and public health nursing began to improve societal health. Nursing pioneers such as Nightingale in England and Wald in the United States focused on the collection and analysis of statistical data, health care reforms, home nursing, community empowerment, and nursing education. They established the groundwork for today's community health nursing.

Modern community health nurses must grapple with an array of philosophical controversies that affect their practice. These controversies include different opinions about what "intervention" means, a focus on both the individual and the aggregate, discrimination, feminism, the potential for additional terrorism in America, and the best way to solve the critical problem of runaway health care costs.

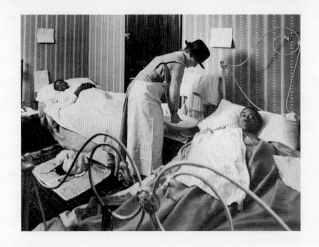

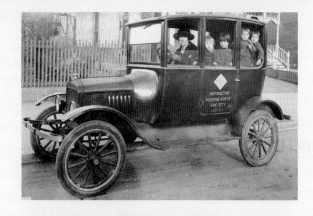

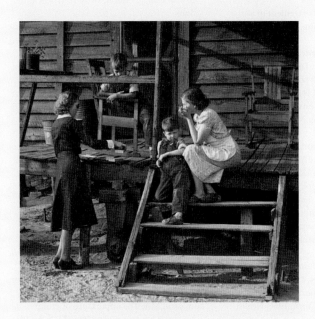

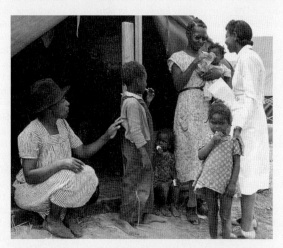

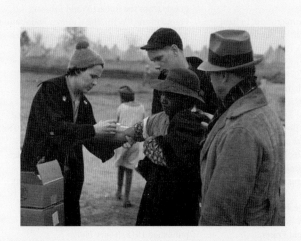

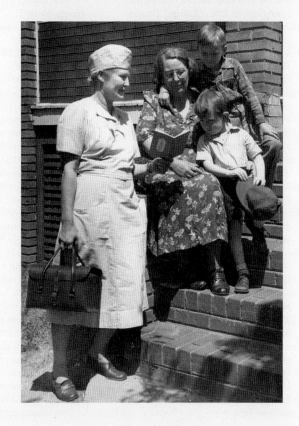

LEARNING ACTIVITIES

1. Research the history of the health department or Visiting Nurse Association in a particular city or county.
2. Find two recent articles about Florence Nightingale. After reading the articles, list Nightingale's contributions to public health, public health nursing, and community health nursing.
3. Discuss with peers how Lillian Wald's approach to individual and community health care provides an understanding

of how to facilitate the empowerment of aggregates in the community.
4. Obtain copies of early articles from nursing journals (e.g., *American Journal of Nursing* dates from 1900). Discuss the health problems, medical care, and nursing practice these articles illustrated.
5. Collect copies of early nursing textbooks. Discuss the evolution of thoughts on pathology, illness management, and health promotion.

REFERENCES

American Nurses Association: *Position Statement on Discrimination and Racism in Health Care*, 1998. Retrieved January 26, 2010, www.nursingworld.org/position/ethics/race.aspx.

Anderson OW: *State enabling legislation for non-profit hospital and medical plans*, Ann Arbor, MI, 1944, University of Michigan Press.

Armelagos GK, Dewey JR: Evolutionary response to human infectious diseases. In Logan MH, Hunt EE, editors: *Health and the human condition*, North Scituate, MA, 1978, Duxbury Press.

Beauchamp DE: Public health as social justice. In Mappes T, Zembaty J, editors: *Biomedical ethics*, ed 2, New York, 1986, McGraw-Hill.

Burkitt DP: Some diseases characteristic of modern western civilization. In Logan MH, Hunt EE, editors: *Health and the human condition*, North Scituate, MA, 1978, Duxbury Press.

The Century Foundation, New York: 2005, (January 13, 2005).

Cockburn TA: The evolution of human infectious diseases. In Cockburn T, editor: *Infectious diseases: their evolution and eradication*, Springfield, IL, 1967, Charles C Thomas.

Cohen IB: Florence Nightingale, *Sci Am* 250:128–137, 1984.

Dock LL, Stewart IM: *A short history of nursing: From the earliest times to the present day*, New York, 1925, Putnam.

Dreher M: District nursing: the cost benefits of a population-based practice, *Am J Public Health* 74:1107–1111, 1984.

Duffus RL: *Lillian Wald: neighbor and crusader*, New York, 1938, Macmillan.

Duran FD: *The Aztecs: the history of the Indies of New Spain*, New York, 1964, Orion Press (Translated, with notes, by D Heyden and F Horcasitas).

Ehrenreich B, English D: *Witches, midwives, and nurses: a history of women healers*, Old Westbury, NY, 1973, The Feminist Press.

Eilers RD: *Regulation of Blue Cross and Blue Shield plans*, Homewood, IL, 1963, Richard D. Irwin.

Evans RG, Barer ML, Marmor TR: *Why are some people healthy and others not? The determinants of health of populations*, Hawthorne, NY, 1994, Aldine de Gruyter.

Fairman PL: *Analysis of the image of nursing and nurses as portrayed in fictional literature from 1850 to 1995*, Dissertation Abstracts, 1996 University of San Francisco.

Faulkner EJ: *Health insurance*, New York, 1960, McGraw-Hill.

Gamble VN: Under the shadow of Tuskegee: African Americans and health care, *Am J Public Health* 87(11):1773–1778, 1997.

Garn SM: Culture and the direction of human evolution, *Hum Biol* 35:221–236, 1963.

George MD: *London life in the XVIIIth century*, New York, 1925, Knopf.

Goodnow M: *Outlines of nursing history*, Philadelphia, 1933, Saunders.

Graff WL, et al: Population management in an HMO: new roles for nursing, *Public Health Nurs* 12:213–221, 1995.

Greifinger RB, Sidel VW: American medicine: charity begins at home. In Lee P, Brown N, Red I, editors: *The nation's health*, San Francisco, 1981, Boyd and Fraser.

Grier B, Grier M: Contributions of the passionate statistician, *Res Nurs Health* 1:103–109, 1978.

Guendelman S, et al: Generational differences in perinatal health among the Mexican American population: findings from HHANES 1982–84, *Am J Public Health* 80(Suppl.):61–65, 1990.

Hanggi-Myers LJ: *The origins and history of the first public health/community health nurses in Louisiana: 1835–1927*, Dissertation Abstracts, New Orleans, 1996, Louisiana State University Medical Center.

Hanlon JJ, Pickett GE: *Public health administration and practice*, ed 9, St. Louis, 1990, Mosby.

Health Insurance Institute: *Source book of health insurance data, 1960*, New York, 1966, Health Insurance Institute.

Hughes CC: Medical care: ethnomedicine. In Logan MH, Hunt EE, editors: *Health and the human condition*, North Scituate, MA, 1978, Duxbury Press.

Jupp J: Two hundred years of immigration. In Reid J, Trompf R, editors: *The health of immigrant Australia*, Orlando, FL, 1990, Harcourt Brace.

Kopf EW: Florence Nightingale as statistician, *Res Nurs Health* 1:93–102, 1978.

Lamarche PA: Our health paradigm in peril, *Public Health Rep* 110:556–560, 1995.

Lee PR, Brown N, Red I, editors: *The nation's health*, San Francisco, 1981, Boyd and Fraser.

Leininger M: *Transcultural health care issues and conditions*, Philadelphia, 1976, FA Davis.

Logan MH, Hunt EE, editors: *Health and the human condition*, North Scituate, MA, 1978, Duxbury Press.

McKeown T: Determinants of health. In Lee P, Brown N, Red I, editors: *The nation's health*, San Francisco, 1981, Boyd and Fraser.

Najman JM: Theories of disease causation and the concept of a general susceptibility: a review, *Soc Sci Med* 14A:231–237, 1990.

Newbern VB: Women as caregivers in the South: 1900–1945, *Public Health Nurs* 11:247–254, 1994.

Nightingale F: *Notes on matters affecting the health, efficiency and hospitalization of the British army*, London, 1858, Harrison and Sons.

Oliver TR, Lee PR, Lipton HL: A political history of Medicare and prescription drug coverage, *Milbank Q* 82(2):283–354, 2004.

Pernick MS: Eugenics and public health in American history, *Am J Public Health* 87(11):1767–1772, 1997.

Polgar S: Evolution and the ills of mankind. In Tax S, editor: *Horizons of anthropology*, Chicago, 1964, Aldine.

Richardson BW: *The health of nations: a review of the works of Edwin Chadwick*, vol 2, London, 1887, Longmans, Green.

Rosen G: *A history of public health*, New York, 1958, MD Publications.

Rosenberg CE: *The care of strangers*, New York, 1987, Basic Books.

Shamansky SL: A longer-than-usual editorial about population-based managed care, *Public Health Nurs* 12:211–212, 1995.

Smith FB: *The people's health 1830–1910*, London, 1979, Croom Helm.

Thomasson MA: The importance of group coverage: how tax policy shaped U.S. health insurance, *Explorations in Economic History* 39:233–253, 2002.

Trust for America's Health; report funded by grants from the Robert Wood Johnson Foundation (RWJF), the Bauman Foundation, and the New York Community Trust: 2009. Retrieved March 24, 2010 from www.healthyamericans.org.

U.S. Department of Health and Human Services, Health Resources and Services Administration, Bureau of Health Professions: *United States health workforce personnel factbook*, Rockville, MD, 1999, The Author.

Versluysen MC: Old wives' tales? Women healers in English history. In Davies C, editor: *Rewriting nursing history*, Totowa, NJ, 1980, Barnes & Noble.

Wald L: *The house on Henry Street*, New York, 1971, Dover Publications (original work published 1915, Henry Holt).

Thinking Upstream: Nursing Theories and Population-Focused Nursing Practice

*Diane C. Martins**

Additional Material for Study, Review, and Further Exploration

evolve WEBSITE

http://evolve.elsevier.com/Nies

- Quiz
- Case Studies
- Glossary
- WebLinks

OBJECTIVES

Upon completion of this chapter, the reader will be able to do the following:

1. Describe different theories and their application to community/public health nursing.
2. Differentiate between upstream interventions, which are designed to alter the precursors of poor health, and downstream interventions, which are

characterized by efforts to modify individuals' perceptions of health.

3. Critique a theory in regard to its relevance to population health issues.
4. Explain how theory-based practice achieves the goals of community/public health nursing by protecting and promoting the public's health.

KEY TERMS

conservative scope of practice
critical theoretical perspective
health belief model (HBM)

macroscopic
microscopic
Milio's framework for prevention

self-care deficit theory
theory
upstream thinking

OUTLINE

It seems as though many community health problems are so complex, so multifaceted, and so deep that it is impossible for a nurse to make substantial improvements in health. Although we see persons in whom cancer, cardiovascular disease, or pulmonary disease has just been diagnosed, we know that their diseases began years or even decades ago. In many cases, genetic risks for diseases are interwoven with social, economic, and environmental risks in ways that are difficult to understand and more difficult to change. In the face of all these challenges, how can we as nurses hope to affect the health of the public in a significant way? How can the actions we take today reduce the current burden of illness and prevent illness in the next generation of citizens?

When nurses work on a complex community health problem, they need to think strategically. They need to know where to focus their time, energy, and programmatic resources. Most likely they will be up against health problems that have

*The author would like to acknowledge the contribution of Patricia G. Butterfield, who wrote this chapter for the previous edition.

existed for years, with other layers of foundational problems that may have existed for generations. If nurses use organizational resources in an unfocused manner, they will not solve the problem at hand and may create new problems along the way. If they do not build strong relationships with community partners (e.g., parent groups, ministers, local activists), they will fail. If nurses are unable to advocate for their constituencies in a scientifically responsible, logical, and persuasive manner, they will fail. In the face of these challenges and many more, how can nurses succeed in their goal to improve public health?

Fortunately, there are road maps for success. Some of those road maps can be found by reading a nursing history book or an archival work that tells the story of a nurse who succeeded in improving health by leveraging diplomacy skills or neighborhood power; Lillian Wald is one example of such a nurse. Other road maps may be found in "success stories" that provide an overview of how a nurse approached a problem, mobilized resources, and moved strategically to promote change. This chapter addresses another road map for success: the ability to think conceptually, almost like a chess player, to formulate a plan to solve complex problems. Thinking conceptually is a subtle skill that requires you to understand the world at an abstract level, seeing the manifestations of power, oppression, justice, and access as they exist within our communities. Most of all, thinking conceptually means that you develop a "critical eye" for the community and understand how change happens at micro and macro levels.

This chapter begins with a brief overview of nursing theory followed by a discussion of the scope of community health nursing in addressing population health concerns. Several theoretical approaches are compared to demonstrate how different conceptualizations can lead to different conclusions about the range of interventions available to the nurse.

THINKING UPSTREAM: EXAMINING THE ROOT CAUSES OF POOR HEALTH

I am standing by the shore of a swiftly flowing river and hear the cry of a drowning man. I jump into the cold waters. I fight against the strong current and force my way to the struggling man. I hold on hard and gradually pull him to shore. I lay him out on the bank and revive him with artificial respiration. Just when he begins to breathe, I hear another cry for help. I jump into the cold waters. I fight against the strong current, and swim forcefully to the struggling woman. I grab hold and gradually pull her to shore. I lift her out onto the bank beside the man and work to revive her with artificial respiration. Just when she begins to breathe, I hear another cry for help. I jump into the cold waters. Fighting again against the strong current, I force my way to the struggling man. I am getting tired, so with great effort I eventually pull him to shore. I lay him out on the bank and try to revive him with artificial respiration. Just when he begins to breathe, I hear another cry for help. Near exhaustion, it occurs to

me that I'm so busy jumping in, pulling them to shore, applying artificial respiration that I have no time to see who is upstream pushing them all in....(Adapted from a story told by Irving Zola as cited in McKinlay JB: A case for refocusing upstream: the political economy of illness. In Conrad P, The sociology of health and illness: critical perspectives, New York, 2008, Macmillan, pp. 578-591.)

In his description of the frustrations in medical practice, McKinlay (1979) used the image of a swiftly flowing river to represent illness. In this analogy, doctors are so busy rescuing victims from the river that they fail to look upstream to see who is pushing patients into the perilous waters. There are many things that could cause a patient to fall (get pushed) into the waters of illness, such as tobacco company products, companies that profit from selling products high in saturated fats, the alcoholic beverage industry, the beauty industry, exposure to environmental toxins, or occupationally induced illnesses. Manufacturers of illness are what push clients into the river. Cigarette companies are a good example of a manufacturer of illness—their product causes a change for the worse in the health status of their consumers, and they take little to no responsibility for it. McKinlay used this analogy to illustrate the ultimate futility of "downstream endeavors," which are characterized by short-term, individual-based interventions, and challenged health care providers to focus more of their energies "upstream, where the real problems lie" (McKinlay, 1979, p. 9). Downstream health care takes place in our emergency departments, critical care units, and many other health care settings focused on illness care. Upstream thinking actions focus on modifying economic, political, and environmental factors that are the precursors of poor health throughout the world. Although the story cites medical practice, it is equally fitting to the dilemmas of nursing practice. Although nursing has a rich history of providing preventive and population-based care, the current health system emphasizes episodic and individual-based care. This system has done little to stem the tide of chronic illnesses to which 70% of American deaths can be attributed (Centers for Disease Control and Prevention, 2004).

HISTORICAL PERSPECTIVES ON NURSING THEORY

Many scholars agree that Florence Nightingale was the first nurse to formulate a conceptual foundation for nursing practice. Nightingale believed that clean water, clean linens, access to adequate sanitation, and quiet would improve health outcomes, and she put these beliefs into practice during the Crimean War (Bostidge, 2008). However, in the years after her leadership, nursing practice became largely atheoretical and was based primarily on reacting to the immediacy of patient situations and the demands of medical staff. Thus, hospital and medical personnel defined the boundaries of nursing practice. Once nursing leaders saw that others were defining their profession, they became proactive in advancing the theoretical and scientific foundation of nursing practice.

Some of the early nursing theories were extremely narrow and depicted health care situations that involved only one nurse and one patient. Family members and other health professionals were noticeably absent from the context of care. Historically, this characterization may have been an appropriate response to the constraints of nursing practice and the need to emphasize the medically dependent activities of the nursing profession.

Although somewhat valuable, theories that address health from a microscopic, or individual, rather than a macroscopic, or global/social, perspective have limited applicability to community/public health nursing. Such perspectives are inadequate because they do not address social, political, and environmental factors that are central to an understanding of communities. More recent advances in nursing theory development address the dynamic nature of health-sustaining and/or health-damaging environments and address the nature of a collective (e.g., school, worksite) versus an individual client.

HOW THEORY PROVIDES DIRECTION TO NURSING

The goal of theory is to improve nursing practice. Chinn and Kramer (2008) stated that using theories or parts of theoretical frameworks to guide practice best achieves this goal. Students often find theory intellectually burdensome and cannot see the benefits to their practice of something so seemingly obscure. Theory-based practice guides data collection and interpretation in a clear and organized manner; therefore it is easier for the nurse to diagnose and address health problems. Through the process of integrating theory and practice, the student can focus on factors that are critical to understanding the situation. The student also has an opportunity to analyze the realities of nursing practice in relation to a specific theoretical perspective, in a process of ruling in and ruling out the fit of particular concepts (Schwartz-Barcott et al., 2002). Barnum (1998) stated, "A theory is like a map of a territory as opposed to an aerial photograph. The map does not give the full terrain (i.e., the full picture); instead it picks out those parts that are important for its given purpose" (p. 1). Using a theoretical perspective to plan nursing care guides the student in assessing a nursing situation and allows the student "to plan and not get lost in the details or sidetracked in the alleys" (J. M. Swanson, personal communication to P. Butterfield, May 1992).

As with other abstract concepts, different nursing authors have defined and interpreted theory in different ways. Several authors' definitions of theory are listed in Box 3-1. The lack of uniformity among these definitions reflects the evolution of thought and the individual differences in the understanding of relationships among theory, practice, and research. The definitions also reflect the difficult job of describing complex and diverse theories within the constraints of a single definition. Reading several definitions can foster an appreciation for the richness of theory and help the reader identify one or two particularly meaningful definitions. Within the profession,

BOX 3-1 DEFINITIONS OF THEORY PROPOSED BY NURSING THEORISTS

- "A systematic vision of reality; a set of interrelated concepts that is useful for prediction and control" (Woods and Catanzaro, 1988, p. 568).
- "A conceptual system or framework invented for some purpose; and as the purpose varies so too must the structure and complexity of the system" (Dickoff and James, 1968, p. 19).
- "A creative and rigorous structuring of ideas that projects a tentative, purposeful, and systematic view of phenomena" (Chinn and Kramer, 1999, p. 51).
- "A set of ideas, hunches, or hypotheses that provides some degree of prediction and/or explanation of the world" (Pryjmachuk, 1996, p. 679).
- "Theory organizes the relationships between the complex events that occur in a nursing situation so that we can assist human beings. Simply stated, theory provides a way of thinking about and looking at the world around us" (Torres, 1986, p. 19).

definitions of theory typically refer to a set of concepts and relational statements and the purpose of the theory. This chapter presents theoretical perspectives that are congruent with a broad interpretation of theory and correspond with the definitions proposed by Dickoff and James (1968), Torres (1986), and Chinn and Kramer (2008).

MICROSCOPIC VERSUS MACROSCOPIC APPROACHES TO THE CONCEPTUALIZATION OF COMMUNITY HEALTH PROBLEMS

Each nurse must find her or his own way of interpreting the complex forces that shape societies to understand population health. The nurse can best achieve this transformation by integrating population-based practice and theoretical perspectives to conceptualize health from a macroscopic versus microscopic perspective. Table 3-1 differentiates between these two approaches to conceptualizing health problems.

It is helpful to use the example of a target to understand the concept of microscopic versus macroscopic. The individual is the bull's-eye; this center contains the health problem of interest (e.g., pediatric exposure to lead compounds). In this context, a microscopic approach to assessment would focus exclusively on individual children with lead poisoning. Nursing interventions would focus on the identification and removal of lead sources in the home. However, the nurse can broaden his or her view of this problem by addressing individual health threats and by examining interpersonal and intercommunity factors that perpetuate lead poisoning on a national scale. This approach would include the bull's-eye and the concentric circles that extend from the center of the target. A macroscopic approach to lead exposure may incorporate the following activities: examining trends in the prevalence of lead poisoning over time, estimating the percentage of older homes in a neighborhood that may contain lead pipes or lead-based paint surfaces, and locating industrial sources of lead emissions. These efforts usually involve the

TABLE 3-1	MICROSCOPIC VERSUS MACROSCOPIC APPROACHES TO THE DELINEATION OF COMMUNITY HEALTH NURSING PROBLEMS	
MICROSCOPIC APPROACH	**MACROSCOPIC APPROACH**	
Examines individual, and sometimes family, responses to health and illness	Examines interfamily and intercommunity themes in health and illness	
	Delineates factors in the population that perpetuate the development of illness or foster the development of health	
Often emphasizes behavioral responses to individual's illness or lifestyle patterns	Emphasizes social, economic, and environmental precursors of illness	
Nursing interventions are often aimed at modifying individual's behavior through changing his or her perceptions or belief system	Nursing interventions may include modifying social or environmental variables (i.e., working to remove care barriers and improving sanitation or living conditions)	
	May involve social or political action	

collaborative efforts of nurses from school, occupational, and other community settings. Doty (1996) noted that macro-level perspectives provide nurses with the conceptual tools that empower clients to make health decisions based on their own interests and the interests of the community at large.

One common dilemma in community health practice is the tension between working on behalf of individuals and working on behalf of a population. For many nurses, this tension is exemplified by the need to reconcile and prioritize multiple daily tasks. Population-directed actions are often more global than the immediate demands of ill people; therefore they may sink to the bottom of the priority list. A community health nurse or nursing administrator may plan to spend the day on a community project directed at preventive efforts, such as screening programs, updating the surveillance program, or meeting with key community members about a specific preventive program. However, the nurse may actually end up spending the time responding to the emergency of the day. This type of reactive rather than proactive nursing practice prevents progress toward "big picture" initiatives and population-based programs. When faced with multiple demands, nurses must be vigilant in devoting a sustained effort toward population-focused projects. Daily pressures can easily distract the nurse from population-based nursing practice. Several nursing organizations focus on this population while one organization, the Quad Council of Public Health Nursing, coordinates the four public health/community health nursing organizations. The four organizations include:

- Public Health Nursing Section of the American Public Health Association (APHA)
- Association of Community Health Nurse Educators (ACHNE)
- Association of State and Territorial Directors of Nursing (ASTDN)
- American Nurses Association (ANA)

The organizations emphasize "systems thinking" in daily practice and the importance of improving health through the design and implementation of population-based interventions (APHA, 2009).

A theoretical focus on the individual can preclude understanding of a larger perspective. Dreher (1982) used the term conservative scope of practice in describing frameworks that focus energy exclusively on intrapatient and nurse-patient factors. She stated that such frameworks often adopt

psychological explanations of patient behavior. This mode of thinking attributes low compliance, missed appointments, and reluctant participation to problems in patient motivation or attitude. Nurses are responsible for altering patient attitudes toward health rather than altering the system itself, "even though such negative attitudes may well be a realistic appraisal of health care" (Dreher, 1982, p. 505). This perspective does not entertain the possibility of altering the system or empowering patients to make changes.

ASSESSING A THEORY'S SCOPE IN RELATION TO COMMUNITY HEALTH NURSING

Theoretical scope is especially important to community health nursing because there are many levels of practice within this specialty area. For example, a home health nurse who is caring for ill people after hospitalization has a very different scope of practice than a nurse epidemiologist or health planner. Unless a given theory is broad enough in scope to address health and the determinants of health from a population perspective, the theory will not be very useful to community health nurses. Although the past 25 years yielded much advancement in the development of nursing theory, there continues to be a lack of clarity about community health nursing's theoretical foundation (Batra, 1991). Applying the terms *microscopic* and *macroscopic* to health situations may help nurses fill this void and stimulate theory development in community health nursing.

Although the concept of macroscopic is similar to the upstream analogy, the term *macroscopic* refers to a broad scope that incorporates many variables to aid in understanding a health problem. Upstream thinking would fall within this domain. Viewing a problem from this perspective emphasizes the variables that precede or play a role in the development of health problems. Macroscopic is the broad concept, and upstream is a more specific concept. These related concepts and their meanings can help nurses develop a critical eye in evaluating a theory's relevance to population health.

REVIEW OF THEORETICAL APPROACHES

The differences among theoretical approaches demonstrate how a nurse may draw very diverse conclusions about the reasons for client behavior and the range of available interventions. The following section uses two theories to exemplify individual microscopic approaches to community health nursing problems; one originates within nursing and one is based in social psychology. Two other theories demonstrate the examination of nursing problems from a macroscopic perspective; one originates from nursing and another has roots in phenomenology. The format for this review is as follows:

1. The individual is the focus of change (i.e., microscopic).
   a. Orem's self-care deficit theory of nursing
   b. The health belief model (HBM)
2. Thinking upstream: Society is the focus of change (i.e., macroscopic).
   a. Milio's framework for prevention
   b. Critical theoretical perspective

The Individual Is the Focus of Change
Orem's Self-Care Deficit Theory of Nursing

In 1958, Dorothea Orem, a staff and private duty nurse who later was a faculty member at Catholic University of America, began to formalize her insights about the purpose of nursing activities and why individuals required nursing care (Eben et al., 1986; Fawcett, 2001). Her theory is based on the assumption that self-care needs and activities are the primary focus of nursing practice. Orem outlined her self-care deficit theory of nursing and stated that this general theory is actually a composite of the following related constructs: the theory of self-care deficits, which provides criteria for identifying those who need nursing; the theory of self-care, which explains self-care and why it is necessary; and the theory of nursing systems, which specifies nursing's role in the delivery of care and how nursing helps people. Major concepts from Orem's self-care deficit theory are listed in Box 3-2.

BOX 3-2   CONCEPTS FROM OREM'S SELF-CARE DEFICIT THEORY

- *Self-care:* "The production of actions directed to self or to the environment in order to regulate one's functioning in the interest of one's life, integrated functioning, and well-being."
- *Therapeutic self-care demand:* "The measures of care required at moments in time in order to meet existent requisites for regulatory action to maintain life and to maintain or promote health, development, and general well-being."
- *Self-care agency:* "The complex capability for action that is activated in the performance of the actions or operations of self-care."
- *Self-care deficit:* "A relationship between self-care agency and therapeutic self-care demand in which self-care agency is not adequate to meet the known therapeutic self-care demand."
- *Nursing agency:* "The complex capability for action that is activated by nurses in their determination of needs for, design of, and production of nursing for people with a range of types of self-care deficits."
- *Nursing system:* "A continuing series of actions produced when nurses link one way or a number of ways of helping to meet their own actions or the actions of people under care that are directed to meet these persons' therapeutic self-care demands or to regulate their self-care agency."

From Orem DE: *Nursing: concepts of practice*, ed 6, New York, 2001, Mosby, p 31.

The basic concepts of this theory evolved from observing the chronology of illness in hospitalized patients. The self-care deficit theory is based on the premise that nursing is a response to a sick person's inability to administer self-care. Nursing assumes the role of providing some or all self-care activities on the patient's behalf (Orem, 2001). This focus makes the content and scope of the theory most useful to nurses practicing within an institutional setting. Orem briefly specified the role of population-based nursing in the sixth edition of her book, *Nursing: Concepts of Practice* (2001). However, some of her concepts are so specific to an individual orientation to disease that applying them to a population can be awkward at best. Individual patient deficits (and nurses' efforts to address them) are central to this theory; thus, its ability to inform community-level problems and health promotion strategies is limited.

Application of self-care deficit theory. During a discussion about theory-based initiatives, a British occupational health nurse lamented over her nursing supervisor's intention to adopt Orem's self-care deficit theory. She was frustrated and argued that much of the model's assumptions seemed incongruous with the realities of her daily practice. Kennedy (1989) maintained that the self-care deficit theory assumes that people are able to exert purposeful control over their environments in the pursuit of health; however, people may have little control over the physical or social aspects of their work environment. On the basis of this thesis, she concluded that the self-care model is incompatible with the practice domain of occupational health nursing.

Kennedy exemplified the dissonance that nurses feel when a particular theory is inappropriately imposed in a work setting. Although it is easy to recognize the importance of Orem's concepts to many arenas of nursing practice, it is also apparent that her perspective would not lend itself well to understanding the diverse health needs of people in a worksite. Kennedy (1989) clearly articulated this position when she stated that "the many facets of the occupational health nurse's role may 'fit in comfortably with Orem's self-care model.' But will Orem's model fit into the many facets of the occupational health nurse's role? That is the key question we should be asking" (p. 354).

The Health Belief Model

The second theory that focuses on the individual as the locus of change is the health belief model (HBM). The model evolved from the premise that the world of the perceiver determines action. The model had its inception during the late 1950s when America was breathing a collective sigh of relief after the development of the polio vaccine. When some people chose not to bring themselves or their children into clinics for immunization, social psychologists and other public health workers recognized the need to develop a more complete understanding of factors that influence preventive health behaviors. Their efforts resulted in the HBM.

Kurt Lewin's work lent itself to the model's core dimensions. He proposed that behavior is based on current dynamics confronting an individual rather than prior experiences (Maiman and Becker, 1974). Figure 3-1 outlines the variables and

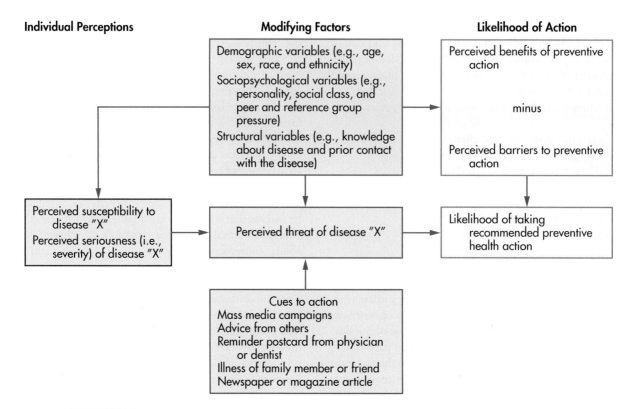

FIGURE 3-1 Variables and relationships in the HBM. (Redrawn from Rosenstock IM: Historical origins of the health belief model. In Becker MH, editor: *The health belief model and personal health behavior,* Thorofare, NJ, 1974, Charles B Slack).

relationships in the HBM. The health belief model is based on the assumption that the major determinant of preventive health behavior is disease avoidance. The concept of disease avoidance includes perceived susceptibility to disease "X," perceived seriousness of disease "X," modifying factors, cues to action, perceived benefits minus perceived barriers to preventive health action, perceived threat of disease "X," and the likelihood of taking a recommended health action. Disease "X" represents a particular disorder that a health action may prevent. It is important to note that actions that relate to breast cancer will be different from those relating to measles. For example, in breast cancer, a cue to action may involve a public service advertisement encouraging women to make an appointment for a mammogram. However, for measles, a cue to action may be news of a measles outbreak in a neighboring town.

Application of the HBM. Over the years, a number of authors have proposed broadening the scope of the HBM to address health promotion and illness behaviors (Kirscht, 1974; Pender, 1987) and to merge its concepts with other theories that describe health behavior (Cummings, Becker, and Malie, 1980). The following section contains a brief personal account of the author's perceptions addressing the strengths and limitations of the model.

During my nursing education classes at the undergraduate level, I was exposed to a large number of nursing theories. The HBM was probably my least favorite. Most of the content was interesting, but I found it difficult applying the concepts to patients in the community and home setting. The model's focus on compliance was something that nurses with a critical theoretical perspective would have difficulty applying in their own clinical practice. My perception of the model changed a few years ago when my younger brother had pancreatic cancer diagnosed. This experience allowed me to see how the HBM could offer some insight into an individual's health behaviors. It helped me organize ideas about why people choose to accept or reject the instructions of well-intended nurses and doctors. Concepts such as perceived seriousness, perceived susceptibility, and cue to action afforded new insights into the dynamics of health decision making. I began to apply the model's concepts to guide my work with my family. My brother who became ill had smoked much of his life. Another brother also smoked. My family members believed that you are destined to follow a path of life and death, but this experience clearly modified their health beliefs. Until this point, my family members did not quit smoking because they did not perceive the susceptibility and seriousness of smoking; they belonged to a reference group that disdained most traditional medical practices and favored inaction over action. During the next several weeks, my siblings requested information on strategies that would help them quit smoking and hopefully decrease their chances for the development of cancer.

Over the years, I have become more skilled in assessing and identifying patient needs and issues and have gained a better appreciation for the strengths and limitations that any theoretical framework imposes on a situation.

Limitations of the HBM. The HBM places the burden of action exclusively on the client. It assumes that only those clients who have distorted or negative perceptions of the specified disease or recommended health action will fail to act. In practice, this model focuses the nurse's energies on interventions designed to modify the client's distorted perceptions.

The HBM offers an explanation of health behaviors that is similar to a mechanical system. Consulting the HBM, a nurse may induce compliance by using model variables as catalysts to stimulate action. For example, an intervention study based on HBM precepts sought to increase follow-up in clients with hypertension by increasing their perceived susceptibility and seriousness of the dangers of hypertension (Jones, Jones, and Katz, 1987). The study provided patients with education over the telephone or in the emergency department and resulted in a dramatic increase in compliance. However, they noted that several patient groups, in particular, a group of patients without child care, failed to respond to the intervention. Studies such as these, which have been conducted by behavioral researchers for more than 25 years, demonstrate the predictive abilities and the limitations of HBM concepts (Lajunen and Rasanen, 2004; Mirotznik et al., 1998).

The HBM may effectively promote behavioral change by altering patients' perspectives, but it does not acknowledge the health professional's responsibility to reduce or ameliorate health care barriers. The model reflects the type of theoretical perspective that dominated nursing education and behavioral health for many years. The narrow scope of the model is its strength and its limitation: the nurse is not challenged to examine the root causes of health opportunities and behaviors in the communities we serve.

The Upstream View: Society Is the Focus of Change
Milio's Framework for Prevention

Milio's framework for prevention (1976) provides a thought-provoking complement to the HBM and provides a mechanism for directing attention upstream and examining opportunities for nursing intervention at the population level. Nancy Milio outlined six propositions that relate an individual's ability to improve healthful behavior to a society's ability to provide accessible and socially affirming options for healthy choices. Milio used these propositions to move the focus of attention upstream in an attempt to create a framework for initiating upstream policies. She noted that the range of available health choices is critical in shaping a society's overall health status. In addition, she stated that policy decisions in governmental and private organizations shape the range of choices available to individuals. She believed that national-level policy making was the best way to favorably impact the health of most Americans rather than concentrating efforts on imparting information in an effort to change individual patterns of behavior.

Milio (1976) proposed that health deficits often result from an imbalance between a population's health needs and its health-sustaining resources. She stated that the diseases associated with excess (e.g., obesity and alcoholism) afflict affluent societies and the diseases that result from inadequate or unsafe food, shelter, and water afflict the poor. Within this context, the poor in affluent societies may experience the least desirable combination of factors. Milio (1976) cited the socioeconomic realities that deprive many Americans of a health-sustaining environment despite the fact that "cigarettes, sucrose, pollutants, and tensions are readily available to the poor" (p. 436). Propositions proposed by Milio are listed in Table 3-2.

TABLE 3-2 APPLICATION OF MILIO'S FRAMEWORK IN PUBLIC HEALTH NURSING

MILIO'S PROPOSITION SUMMARY	POPULATION HEALTH EXAMPLES
Population health results from deprivation and/or excess of critical health resources.	Individuals and families living in poverty have poorer health status compared with middle and upper class individuals and families.
Behaviors of populations result from selection from limited choices; these arise from actual and perceived options available as well as beliefs and expectations resulting from socialization, education and experience.	Positive and negative lifestyle choices (e.g., smoking, alcohol use, safe sex practices, regular exercise, diet/nutrition; seatbelt use) are strongly dependent on culture, socioeconomic status, and educational level.
Organizational decisions and policies (both governmental and non-governmental) dictate many of the options available to individuals and populations and influence choices.	Health insurance coverage and availability is largely determined and financed by the federal and state governments (e.g., Medicare and Medicaid) and employers (e.g., private insurance); the source and funding of insurance very strongly influences health provider choices and services.
Individual choices related to health promotion or health damaging behaviors is influenced by efforts to maximize valued resources.	Choices and behaviors of individuals are strongly influenced by desires, values and beliefs. For example, the use of barrier protection during sex by adolescents is often dependent on peer pressure and the need for acceptance, love, and belonging.
Alteration in patterns of behavior resulting from decision making of a significant number of people in a population can result in social change.	Some behaviors, such as tobacco use have become difficult to maintain in many settings or situations in response to organizational and public policy mandates. As a result, tobacco use in the United States has dropped dramatically.
Without concurrent availability of alternative health-promoting options for investment of personal resources, health education will be largely ineffective in changing behavior patterns.	Addressing persistent health problems (e.g., overweight/obesity) is hindered because most people are very aware of what causes the problem, but are reluctant to make lifestyle changes to prevent or reverse the condition. Often, 'new' information (e.g., a new diet) or resources (e.g., a new medication) can assist in attracting attention and directing positive behavior changes.

Adapted from Milio, N: A framework for prevention: Changing health-damaging to health-generating life patterns. *American Journal of Public Health,* 66:435-439, 1976.

Personal and societal resources affect the range of health-promoting or health-damaging choices available to individuals. Personal resources include the individual's awareness, knowledge, and beliefs and the beliefs of the individual's family and friends. Money, time, and the urgency of other priorities are also personal resources. Community and national locale strongly influence societal resources. These resources include the availability and cost of health services, environmental protection, safe shelter, and the penalties or rewards for failure to select the given options.

Milio (1976) challenged health education's assumption that knowledge of health-generating behaviors implies an act in accordance with that knowledge. She proposed that "most human beings, professional or nonprofessional, provider or consumer, make the easiest choices available to them most of the time" (p. 435). Health-promoting choices must be more readily available and less costly than health-damaging options for individuals to gain health and for society to improve health status. Milio's framework can enable a nurse to reframe this view by understanding the historic play of social forces that have limited the choices available to the parties involved.

Comparison of the HBM and Milio's conceptualizations of health. Milio's health resources bear some resemblance to the concepts in the HBM. The purpose of the HBM is to provide the nurse with an understanding of the dynamics of personal health behaviors. The HBM specifies broader contextual variables, such as the constraints of the health care system, and their influence on the individual's decision-making processes. The HBM also assumes that each person has unlimited access to health resources and free will. In contrast, Milio based her framework on an assessment of community resources and their availability to individuals. By assessing such factors up front, the nurse is able to gain a more thorough understanding of the resources people actually have. Milio offered a different set of insights into the health behavior arena by proposing that many low-income individuals are acting within the constraints of their limited resources. Furthermore, she investigated beyond downstream focus and population health by examining the choices of significant numbers of people within a population.

Compared with the HBM, Milio's framework provides for the inclusion of economic, political, and environmental health determinants; therefore, the nurse is given broader range in the diagnosis and interpretation of health problems. Whereas the HBM allows only two possible outcomes (i.e., "acts" or "fails to act" according to the recommended health action), Milio's framework encourages the nurse to understand health behaviors in the context of their societal milieu.

Implications of Milio's framework for current health delivery systems. Through its broader scope, Milio's model provides direction for nursing interventions at many levels. Nurses may use this model to assess the personal and societal resources of individual patients and analyze social and economic factors that may inhibit healthy choices in populations. Population-based interventions may include such diverse activities as working to improve the nutritional content of school lunches and encouraging political activity on behalf of health care reform (Hobbs et al., 2004; Milio, 1981).

Overall, current health care delivery systems perform best when responding to people with diagnostic-intensive and acute illnesses. Those people who experience chronic debilitation or have less intriguing diagnoses generally fare worse in the health care system despite efforts by community- and home-based care to "fill the gaps." Nurses in both hospital and community-based systems often feel constrained by profound financial and service restrictions imposed by third-party payers. These third parties often terminate nursing care after the resolution of the latest immediate health crisis and fail to cover care aimed toward long-term health improvements. Many health systems use nursing standards and reimbursement mechanisms that originate from a narrow, compartmentalized view of health.

Personal behavior patterns are not simply "free" choices about "lifestyle" that are isolated from their personal and economic context. Lifestyles are patterns of choices made from available alternatives according to people's socioeconomic circumstances and how easily they are able to choose some over others (Milio, 1981). It is therefore imperative to practice nursing from a broader understanding of health, illness, and suffering.

Critical Theoretical Perspective

Similar to Milio's framework for prevention, critical theoretical perspective uses societal awareness to expose social inequalities that keep people from reaching their full potential. This theoretical perspective is devised from the belief that social meanings structure life through social domination. "A critical perspective can be used to understand the linkages between the health care system and the broader political, economic, and social systems of society" (Waitzkin, 1983, p. 5). According to Navarro (1976), in *Medicine Under Capitalism,* the health care system mirrors the class structure of the broader society. According to Conrad (2008), a critical theoretical perspective is one that does not consider the present structure of health care as sacred. A critical theoretical perspective accepts no truth or fact merely because it has been accepted as such in the past. The social aspects of health and illness are too complex to use only one perspective. This critical theoretical perspective assumes that health and illness entail societal and personal values and that these values have to be made explicit if illness and health care problems are to be satisfactorily dealt with. This perspective is informed by the following values and assumptions:

1. The problems and inequalities of health and health care are connected to the particular historically located social arrangements and the cultural values of society.
2. Health care should be oriented toward the prevention of disease and illness.
3. The priorities of any health care system should be based on the needs of the clients/population and not the health care providers.
4. Ultimately, society itself must be changed for health and medical care to improve (Conrad, 2008).

Proponents of this theoretical approach maintain that social exchanges that are not distorted from power imbalances will stimulate the evolution of a more just society (Allen, Diekelmann, and Benner, 1986). Critical theory assumes that truth standards are socially determined and that no form of scientific inquiry is value free. Allen and colleagues (1986) stated, "One cannot separate theory and value, as the empiricist claims. Every theory is penetrated by value interests" (p. 34).

Application of critical theoretical perspective. Application of a critical theoretical perspective can be seen when health care is used as a form of social control. The social control function in health care is used to get patients to adhere to norms of appropriate behavior. This is done through the medicalization of a wide range of psychological and socioeconomic issues. *Medicalization* is to identify or categorize (a condition or behavior) as being a disorder requiring medical treatment or intervention. Examples include medicalization related to sexuality, family life, aging, learning disabilities, and dying (Conrad, 1975, 1992; Zola, 1972). Medicalization can incorporate many facets of health and illness care from childbirth and allergies to hyperactivity and hospitals that have become dominated by the medical profession and its explanation of health and illness. When social problems are medicalized there is often profit to be made. This can be seen when a patient readily receives a prescription for a medication before the root social cause of the illness is addressed by the health care provider. Using medical treatments for "undesirable behavior" has been implemented throughout history including lobectomies for mental illness and synthetic stimulants for classroom behavior problems.

In this context, the nurse may examine how the concepts of power and empowerment influence access to quality child care (Kuokkanen and Leino-Kilpi, 2000). The nurse may contrast an organization's policies with interviews from workers who believe the organization is an impediment to achieving quality child care. Data analysis may also include an examination of the interests of workers and administration in promoting social change versus maintaining the status quo.

Wild (1993) used critical social theory to analyze the social, political, and economic conditions associated with the cost of prescription analgesics and the corresponding financial burden of clients who require these medications. Wild compared the trends in pharmaceutical pricing with the inflation rates of other commodities. The study stated that pharmaceutical sales techniques, which market directly to physicians, distance the needs of ill clients from the pharmaceutical industry. Wild's analysis specified nursing actions that a downstream analysis would not consider, such as challenging pricing policies on behalf of client groups.

Challenging assumptions about preventive health through critical social theory. The HBM and Milio's prevention model focus on personal health behaviors from a disease avoidance or preventive health perspective; nurses may also analyze this phenomenon using critical social theory. Again, McKinlay's upstream analogy refers to health workers who were so busy fishing sick people out of the river that they did not look upstream to see how they were ending up in the water. Later in the same article, McKinlay (1979) used his upstream analogy to ask the rhetorical question, "How preventive is prevention?" (p. 22). He used this tactic to critically examine different intervention strategies aimed at enhancing preventive behavior. Figure 3-2 illustrates McKinlay's model, which contrasts the different modes of prevention. He linked health professionals' curative and lifestyle modification interventions to a downstream conceptualization of health; the majority of alleged preventive actions fail to alter the process of illness at its origin. Political-economic interventions remain the most effective way to address population determinants of health and ameliorate illness at its source.

McKinlay (1979) further delineated the activities of the "manufacturers of illness—those individuals, interest groups, and organizations which, in addition to producing material goods and services, also produce, as an inevitable byproduct, widespread morbidity and mortality" (pp. 9, 10). The manufacturers of illness embed desired behaviors in the dominant cultural norm and thus foster the habituation of high-risk behavior in the population. Unhealthy consumption patterns are integrated into everyday lives; for example, the American holiday dinner table offers concrete examples of "the binding of at-riskness to culture" (p. 12). The existing health care system, in a misguided attempt to help, devotes its efforts to changing the products of the illness manufacturers

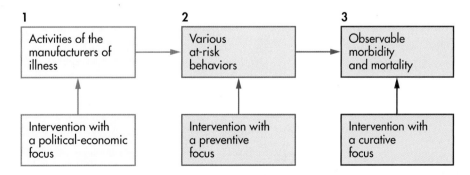

FIGURE 3-2 Continuum of health behaviors and corresponding intervention foci. (From McKinlay JB: A case for refocusing upstream: the political economy of illness. In Proceedings of an American Heart Association Conference: Applying Behavioral Science to Cardiovascular Risk, Seattle, June 17-19, 1979. Reproduced with permission. Copyright © American Heart Association).

and neglects the processes that create the products. The manufacturers of illness include everyday examples such as the tobacco industry, the alcohol industry, and multiple corporations that produce environmental carcinogens.

Waitzkin (1983) continued this theme by asserting that the health care system's emphasis on lifestyle diverts attention from important sources of illness in the capitalist industrial environment and "it also puts the burden of health squarely on the individual rather than seeking collective solutions to health problems" (p. 664). Salmon (1987) supported this position by noting that the basic tenets of Western medicine promote an understanding of individual health and illness factors and obscure the exploration of their social and economic roots. He stated that critical social theory "can aid in uncovering larger dimensions impacting health that are usually unseen or misrepresented by ideological biases. Thus the social reality of health conditions can be both understood and changed" (p. 75).

⚖ ETHICAL INSIGHTS

Social Injustice in Community-Based Practice

Chafey (1996) refers to "putting justice to work in community-based practice" and notes that nursing has a rich historic legacy in social justice activities. Although social justice activities are alive and well in nursing practice, many leaders think that the continuing struggle for resources is taking its toll on the scope of social action within community health systems. In addition, the policies of the current federal administration often emphasize market justice values over social justice values. Market justice refers to the principle that people are entitled to valued ends (e.g., status, income) when they acquire them through fair rules of entitlement. In contrast, social justice refers to the principle that all citizens bear equitably in the benefits and burdens of society (Drevdahl et al., 2001). These are complex concepts and cannot be easily distilled into a clear set of rules or nursing policies. However, in the context of community health nursing, health (and consequently health care) is considered a right rather than a privilege. To the extent that certain citizens, by virtue of their income, race, health needs, or any other attribute, are unable to access health care, our society as a whole suffers. Nurses are well positioned to "stand on the shoulders" of yesterday's nursing leaders and act on behalf of justice in health care access for all citizens.

Nurses in all practice settings face the challenge of understanding and responding to collective health within the context of a health system that allocates resources at the individual level. The Tavistock Group (1999) released a set of ethical principles that summarizes this juxtaposition by noting that "the care of individuals is at the center of health care delivery, but must be viewed and practiced within the overall context of continuing work to generate the greatest possible health gains for groups and populations" (pp. 2, 3). This perspective is an accurate reflection of Western-oriented thought, which generally gives individual health precedence over collective health. Although nurses can appreciate the concept of individual care at the center of health delivery, they should also consider transposing this principle. This allows the nurse to consider a health care system that places the community in the center of health care and holds the goal of generating health gains for individuals. Fortunately, these worldviews of health delivery systems are not mutually exclusive, and nurses can understand the duality of health care needs in individuals and populations.

HEALTHY PEOPLE 2020

The *Healthy People 2020* documents provide health professionals with a broad mandate to save lives by thinking and acting strategically. The *Healthy People 2020* documents are classified into 38 "topic areas" that address specific diseases (e.g., diabetes, cancer, chronic kidney disease), care systems (e.g., health care access), and cross-cutting issues in public health (e.g., persons with disabilities, family planning). Each of the focal areas specified by the Centers for Disease Control and Prevention and in the *Healthy People 2020* documents encompasses a complex and multifaceted problem, one that can be addressed only by "looking upstream." By thinking about the root causes of health problems, we begin to understand the importance of directing nursing efforts toward the antecedents of poor health and lost opportunities. There is simply no other way to bring positive changes to the more than 290 million U.S. and 6 billion global citizens that inhabit our planet.

The following photos present environmental health issues and efforts being taken by nurses to address them.

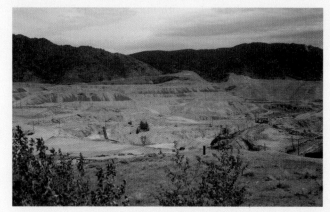

Open mine waste in the rural West can pose a continuing threat to local citizens. Nurses have been involved in advocacy efforts to ensure that citizens receive periodic screening for exposure to lead. Nurses can be active in policy efforts to prevent environmental disasters in the future.

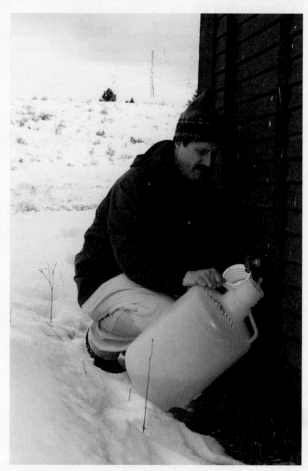

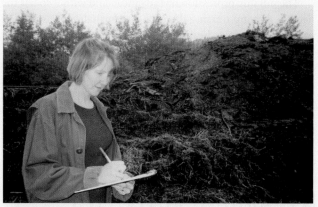

A public health nurse inspects the site of an asphalt spill off of a rural railway car. Hazardous materials spills often occur in remote areas away from health care services. Broad conceptual frameworks allow nurses to think upstream and incorporate environmental risks into the consideration of community health issues.

Citizens can be unaware of biologic and chemical contaminants in their drinking water. Nurses are playing more active roles in water testing and in communicating the results of such tests to community members. When health is conceptualized broadly, nurses understand and view risk in new ways.

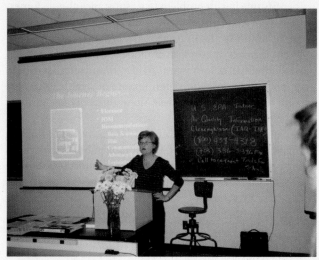

A public health nurse teaches a class on environmental health for local nurses. Environmental health is an important part of community health nursing's expanding practice.

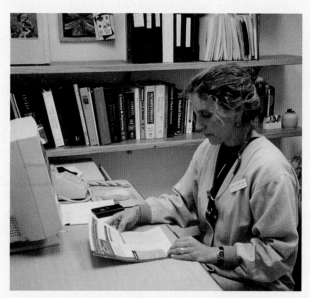

A nurse practitioner reviews educational materials addressing occupational and environmental health risks. By providing guidance for her clients, she is working to reduce risks and empowering her clients to act to reduce their personal and community-based risks.

RESEARCH HIGHLIGHTS

Understanding the Health Experiences of Homeless Populations

How do we understand the health experiences of oppressed populations in the community such as the homeless? Using the lens of the homeless person, a descriptive phenomenological study was conducted. The research question was "What are your experiences with the health care system as a homeless person?" The purposive sample consisted of 15 homeless adults. Four major themes emerged:

1. Living without essential resources compromises health
2. Putting off health care until a crisis arises
3. Encountering barriers to receiving health care to include (a) social triage, (b) feeling labeled and stigmatized, (c) a non-system for health care for the homeless, (d) being treated with disrespect, and (e) feeling invisible to health care providers and
4. Developing underground resourcefulness

Although homeless persons articulated many problems in their health care system encounters, they also described their own resourcefulness and the strategies they employ to manage being marginalized by society and the health care system. Using the critical theoretical perspective, our increased understanding of health care experiences from the homeless persons' view/lens can guide community health nursing emancipatory actions.

From Martins DC: Experiences of homeless people in the health care delivery system: a descriptive phenomenological study, *Public Health Nurs* 25(5):420-430, 2008.

SUMMARY

Nursing and health service literature often focus on health care access issues. This topic is interesting because tremendous disparities for access exist between insured and uninsured people in the United States. Access to care is associated with economic, social, and political factors, and, depending on individual and population needs, it can be a primary determinant of health status and survival. Structural variables, such as race-ethnicity, educational status, gender, and income, may be highly predictive of health status. These types of factors, which are also strongly grounded in the sociopolitical and economic milieu, identify risk factors for poor health and opportunities for community-based interventions.

Community health nurses have been instrumental in making many of the lifesaving advances in sanitation, communicable diseases, and environmental conditions that today's society takes for granted. Community health practice helps develop a broad context of nursing practice because community environments are inherently less restrictive than hospital settings. Clarke and Cody (1994) compared the environmental characteristics in community-based settings with those in hospital-based settings. They proposed that the dynamic nature of community settings lends itself best to the education of professional nurses (Clarke and Cody, 1994).

In a discussion addressing the future of community health nursing, Bellack (1998) differentiates between "nursing in the community" and "nursing with the community." This subtle reframing of the nursing role reinforces the notion that the health agenda originates from natural leaders, church members, local officials, parents, children, teens, and other community members. Forming and advancing a shared vision of health can be a formidable challenge for the nurse; as with any other complex issue, multiple viewpoints are the norm. Even "naming" health problems can be difficult, because different constituents are likely to see issues differently and pursue different lines of reasoning. However, allowing the genesis of change to occur from within the community is the essential challenge of nursing "with" the community. "Nursing with the community" efforts allow the nurse to create agendas that arise from community members rather than those imposed upon community members. Listening, being patient, providing accurate and scientifically sound information, and respecting the experiences of community members are essential to the success of these efforts.

The nursing profession has advanced and with it so has the need to develop nursing theories that formalize the scientific base of community health nursing. The richness of community health nursing comes from the challenge of conceptualizing and implementing strategies that will enhance the health of many people. Likewise, nurses in this practice area must have access to theoretical perspectives that address the social, political, and environmental determinants of population health. The integration of population-based theory with practice gives nurses the means to favorably impact the health of the global community.

LEARNING ACTIVITIES

1. Select a theory or conceptual model. Evaluate its potential for understanding health in individuals, families, a population of 400 children in an elementary school, a community of 50,000 residents, and 2000 workers within a corporate setting.
2. Identify one health problem (e.g., substance abuse, domestic violence, or cardiovascular disease) that is prevalent in the community or city. Analyze the problem using two different theories or conceptual models. One should emphasize individual determinants of health, and another should emphasize population determinants of health. What are some differences in the way these different perspectives inform nursing practice?
3. Review the ANA's definition of community health nursing practice and the APHA's definition of public health nursing practice. What do these definitions indicate about the theoretical basis of community health nursing? How does the theoretical basis of community health nursing practice differ from that of other nursing specialty areas?

REFERENCES

Allen DG, Diekelmann N, Benner P: Three paradigms for nursing research: methodologic implications. In Chinn P, editor: *Nursing research methodology: issues and implementation*, Rockville, MD, 1986, Aspen Publishers.

American Public Health Association (2009) Public Health Nursing Section, *Quad council PHN competencies*, The Author: www.apha.org/membergroups/sections/aphasections/phn/. Accessed May 28, 2009.

Barnum BS: *Nursing theory: analysis, application, evaluation*, ed 5. Philadelphia, PA, 1998, Lippincott.

Batra C: Professional issues: the future of community health nursing. In Cookfair JM, editor: *Nursing process and practice in the community*, St. Louis, 1991, Mosby.

Bellack JP: Community-based nursing practice: necessary but not sufficient, *J Nurs Educ* 37(3):99–100, 1998.

Bostidge M: *Florence Nightingale: the making of an icon*, New York, 2008, Farrar, Straus and Giroux.

Centers for Disease Control and Prevention, (2004) National Center for Chronic Disease Prevention and Health Promotion: Chronic disease prevention, The Author: www.cdc.gov/nccdphp/. Accessed May 28, 2009.

Chafey K: Caring is not enough: ethical paradigms for community-based care, *N HC Perspect Community* 17(1):10–15, 1996.

Chinn PL, Kramer MK: *Theory and nursing: integrated knowledge development*, ed 7, St. Louis, 2008, Mosby.

Clarke PN, Cody WK: Nursing theory-based practice in the home and community: the crux of professional nursing education, *Adv Nurs Sci* 17(2):41–53, 1994.

Conrad P: The discovery of hyperkinesis: notes on the medicalization of deviant behavior, *Soc Probl* 23:12–21, 1975.

Conrad P: Medicalization and social control, *Annual Review of Sociology* 18:209–232, 1992.

Conrad P: *The sociology of heath and illness: critical perspectives*, New York, 2008, Macmillan.

Cummings KM, Becker MH, Malie MC: Bringing the models together: an empirical approach to combining variables to explain health actions, *J Behav Med* 3:123–145, 1980.

Dickoff J, James P: A theory of theories: a position paper, *Nurs Res* 17:197–203, 1968.

Doty R: Alternative theoretical perspectives: essential knowledge for the advanced practice nurse in the promotion of rural family health, *Clin Nurs Specialist* 10(5):217–219, 1996.

Dreher M: The conflict of conservatism in public health nursing education, *Nurs Outlook* 30(9):504–509, 1982.

Drevdahl D, Kneipp S, Canales M, et al: Reinvesting in social justice: a capital idea for public health nursing? *ANS Adv Nurs Sci* 24(2):19–31, 2001.

Eben J, et al: Self-care deficit theory of nursing. In Marriner A, editor: *Nursing theorists and their work*, St. Louis, 1986, Mosby.

Fawcett J: The nurse theorists: 21st-century updates—Dorothea E, Orem, *Nurs Sci Q* 14(1):34–38, 2001.

Hobbs S, Ricketts T, Dodds J, Milio N: Analysis of interest group influence on federal school meals regulations 1992 to 1996, *J Nutr Educ Behav* 36(2):90–98, 2004.

Jones PK, Jones SL, Katz J: Improving follow-up among hypertensive patients using a health belief model intervention, *Arch Intern Med* 147:1557–1560, 1987.

Kennedy A: How relevant are nursing models? *Occup Health* 41(12):352–354, 1989.

Kirscht JP: The health belief model and illness behavior. In Becker MH, editor: *The health belief model and personal health behavior*, Thorofare, NJ, 1974, Charles B. Slack.

Kuokkanen L, Leino-Kilpi H: Power and empowerment in nursing: three theoretical approaches, *J Adv Nurs* 31(1):235–241, 2000.

Lajunen T, Rasanen M: Can social psychological models be used to promote bicycle helmet use among teenagers? A comparison of the health belief model, theory of planned behavior and the locus of control, *J Safety Res* 35(1):115–123, 2004.

Maiman LA, Becker MH: The health belief model: origins and correlates in psychological theory. In Becker MH, editor: *The health belief model and personal health behavior*, Thorofare, NJ, 1974, Charles B. Slack.

McKinlay JB: In Conrad P, editor: *The sociology of health and illness: critical perspectives*, New York, 2008, Macmillan, pp 578–591.

Milio N: A framework for prevention: changing health-damaging to health-generating life patterns, *Am J Public Health* 66:435–439, 1976.

Milio N: *Promoting health through public policy*, Philadelphia, 1981, FA Davis.

Mirotznik J, Ginzler E, Zagon G, et al: Using the health belief model to explain clinic appointment-keeping for the management of a chronic disease condition, *J Community Health* 23(3):195–210, 1998.

Navarro V: *Medicine under capitalism*, New York, 1976, Prodist.

Orem DE: *Nursing: concepts of practice*, ed 6, New York, 2001, Mosby.

Pender NJ: *Health promotion in nursing practice*, ed 2, Norwalk, Conn, 1987, Appleton-Century-Crofts.

Pryjmachuk S: A nursing perspective on the interrelationship between theory, research, and practice, *J Adv Nurs* 23:679–684, 1996.

Salmon JW: Dilemmas in studying social change versus individual change: considerations from political economy. In Duffy M, Pender NJ, editors: *Conceptual issues in health promotion: a report of proceedings of a Wingspread Conference*, Indianapolis, IN, 1987, Sigma Theta Tau.

Schwartz-Barcott D, Patterson BJ, Lusardi P, et al: From practice to theory: tightening the link via three fieldwork strategies, *J Adv Nurs* 39(3):281–289, 2002.

Tavistock Group: A shared statement of ethical principles for those who shape and give health care: a working draft from the Tavistock Group, *Image J Nurs Sch* 31:2–3, 1999.

Torres G: *Theoretical foundations of nursing*, Norwalk, CT, 1986, Appleton-Century-Crofts.

Waitzkin H: A Marxist view of health and health care. In Mechanic D, editor: *Handbook of health, health care, and the health professions*, New York, 1983, Free Press.

Wild LR: Caveat emptor: a critical analysis of the costs of drugs used for pain management, *Adv Nurs Sci* 16:52–61, 1993.

Zola I: Medicine as an institution of social control, *Sociol Rev* 20(4):487–504, 1972.

4

Health Promotion and Risk Reduction

Bridgette Crotwell Pullis, Mary A. Nies

Additional Material for Study, Review, and Further Exploration

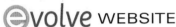 WEBSITE

http://evolve.elsevier.com/Nies
- Quiz
- Case Studies
- Glossary
- WebLinks

OBJECTIVES

Upon completion of this chapter, the reader will be able to do the following:
1. Discuss various theories of health promotion, including Pender's Health Promotion Model, the Health Belief Model, the Transtheoretical Theory, and the Theory of Reasoned Action.
2. Discuss definitions of health.
3. Demonstrate an understanding of the difference between health promotion and health protection.
4. Define risk.
5. Discuss the relationship of risk to health and health promotion activities.
6. Demonstrate an understanding of stratification of risk factors by age, race, and gender.
7. Discuss the influence of various factors on health.
8. List health behaviors for health promotion and disease prevention.
9. Relate the clinical implications of health promotion activities.

KEY TERMS

determinants of health
health
health promotion

health protection
portion distortion
risk

risk communication
risk reduction

OUTLINE

HEALTH PROMOTION AND COMMUNITY HEALTH NURSING

Since its inception, nursing has focused on helping individuals, groups, and communities maintain and protect their health. Florence Nightingale and other nursing pioneers recognized the importance of nutrition, rest, and hygiene in maximizing and protecting one's state of health. Though people are responsible for their health and medical care, they often seek advice from nurses in the community regarding health promotion and to help them make sense of the many, and often competing, recommendations that appear daily on TV, online, in newspapers, and in magazines.

Read the following Clinical Example about Jamie R.:

Clinical Example

Jamie R. is a lifelong athlete. Married with three grown children, she rises at 4:20 each morning to go to the gym to swim for an hour before going to her job as an executive with a large company. A nonsmoker, Jamie rarely drinks alcohol and eats a diet consisting mostly of vegetables, grains, and fruit. Jamie's body mass index is in the normal range, and, though her cholesterol and triglyceride levels are elevated, she does not require medication for this issue. After work, Jamie and her husband relax by walking their two dogs and reading. An early riser, Jamie is in bed by 9:30 almost every night. At 50 years of age, Jamie is youthful and energetic.

We all have friends like Jamie; people who seem to have an endless amount of energy and self-discipline. The rest of us, however, are typically less successful in achieving our health promotion goals.

Green and Kreuter (1991) define **health promotion** as "any combination of health education and related organizational, economic, and environmental supports for behavior of individuals, groups, or communities conducive to health" (p. 2). Parse (1990) states that health promotion is that which is motivated by the desire to increase well-being and to reach the best possible health potential. Jamie exemplifies this motivation to stay in her best health, at least at first glance. Let's look further into Jamie's health history.

When it comes to health practices, Jamie is a study in contradictions. Jamie's father had a myocardial infarction (MI) at the age of 48 years and died of an MI at the age of 50 years. Many of Jamie's paternal relatives have died of heart disease. Jamie's mother and one maternal aunt each had breast cancer diagnosed in their early 50s. Though she has an annual physical by her family doctor and monitors her blood cholesterol and triglycerides, Jamie has never been screened for cardiac disease. Jamie takes the flu vaccine every year but has not had a tetanus-diphtheria vaccine booster in 14 years; though she sees her gynecologist yearly, she has had only one mammogram, 3 years ago.

In skipping annual mammograms and in not pursuing cardiac screening despite her high risk, Jamie is neglecting an important step in maintaining her health—health protection. **Health protection** is those behaviors in which one engages with the specific intent to prevent disease, to detect disease in the early stages, or to maximize health within the constraints of disease (Parse, 1990). Immunizations and cervical cancer screening are examples of health protection activities.

In discussing health promotion, it is helpful to define what is meant by **health**. An early definition defines health as "being sound in body, mind, and spirit: freedom from physical disease or pain" (Merriam-Webster, 2009). As health promotion has become an important strategy to improve health, the way health is defined has shifted from a focus on the curative model to a focus on multidimensional aspects such as the social, cultural, and environmental facets of life and health (Benson, 1996). The well-known definition by the World Health Organization (WHO) states that health is "a state of complete physical, mental and social well-being, and not merely the absence of disease" (WHO, 2009). WHO also states that health is the extent to which an individual or group is able to realize aspirations, to satisfy needs, and to change or to cope with the environment. In this aspect, health is viewed not only as an important goal but as a resource for living (WHO, 1986).

HEALTHY PEOPLE 2020

Healthy People 2020 is the health promotion initiative for the nation. Developed through a consortium and managed by the U.S. Department of Health and Human Services (USDHHS), *Healthy People 2020* "challenges individuals, communities, and professionals, indeed all of us to take specific steps to ensure that good health, as well as long life, are enjoyed by all" (USDHHS, 2009).

The broad goals of *Healthy People 2020* are to attain high quality, longer lives free of preventable disease, disability, injury, and premature death; achieve high equity, eliminate disparities and improve the health of all groups; create social and physical environments that promote good health for all; and promote quality of life, healthy development, and healthy behaviors across all life stages. Objectives toward achieving these goals are organized into 38 topic areas with corresponding priorities for action for each objective. Leading health indicators, or **determinants of health**, in each topic area help track progress toward meeting the goals of *Healthy People 2020*. A list of leading health indicators common across most of the topic areas is found in Table 4-1. Figure 4-1 illustrates the relationships among the determinants of health. The home page for *Healthy People 2020* can be accessed at www.healthypeople.gov/Default.htm.

DETERMINANTS OF HEALTH

Biology is an individual's genetic makeup, family history, and any physical and mental health problems developed in the course of life. Aging, diet, physical activity, smoking, stress, alcohol or drug abuse, injury, violence, or a toxic or infectious agent may produce illness or disability that changes an individual's biology.

Behaviors are the individual's responses to internal stimuli and external conditions. Behaviors interact with biology in a common relationship as one may influence the other. If a person chooses behaviors such as alcohol abuse or smoking, his or her biology may be changed as a result (e.g., liver cirrhosis, chronic obstructive pulmonary disease [COPD]). On the other hand, if an individual has a history of colon cancer in his or her family, the individual may choose to have regular screenings, thereby preventing advanced cancer and possibly death, and changing his or her biology for the better. One's biology may impact behavior; if a person has hypertension or diabetes, he or she may choose to begin an exercise regimen and to eat more healthfully.

Social environment includes interactions and relationships with family, friends, co-workers, and others in the community. Social institutions, such as law enforcement, faith communities, schools, and government agencies, are also part

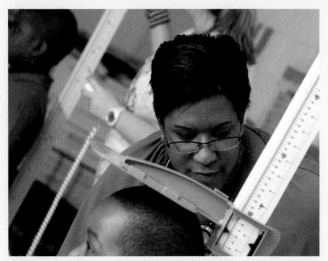

Elementary school screening: A nursing student takes height and weight measurements, which serve as a baseline to measure the growth rate of students.

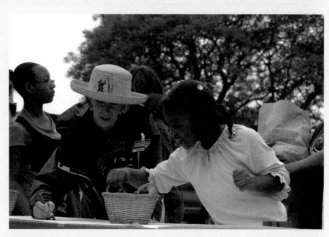

A Veggie Fair in the community teaches children and their parents about the benefits of eating vegetables.

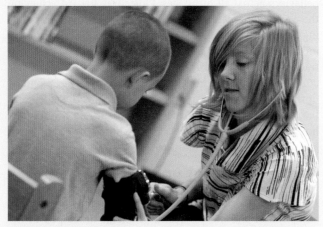

Elementary school screening: A nursing student securely holds the cuff as she takes this little boy's blood pressure.

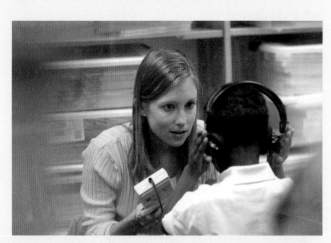

Elementary school screening: A nursing student watches and listens as she gives a hearing test.

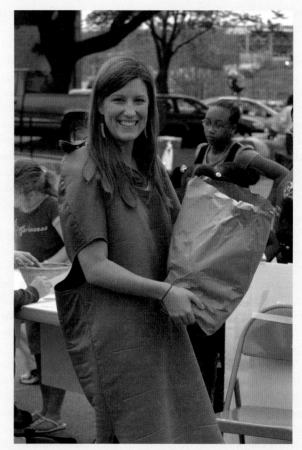

Participants have fun educating children at the Veggie Fair, which will hopefully result in children and their parents enjoying vegetables as a nutritious part of their daily diet.

TABLE 4-1   LEADING HEALTH INDICATORS

FOCUS AREA	PHYSICAL ACTIVITY	OVERWEIGHT AND OBESITY	TOBACCO USE	SUBSTANCE ABUSE	RESPONSIBLE SEXUAL BEHAVIOR	MENTAL HEALTH	INJURY AND VIOLENCE	ENVIRONMENTAL QUALITY	IMMUNIZATION	ACCESS TO HEALTH CARE
Access to quality health services	X	X	X	X	X	X	X		X	X
Arthritis, osteoporosis, and chronic back conditions	X	X					X			
Cancer	X	X	X	X	X			X	X	X
Chronic kidney disease	X	X	X							
Diabetes	X	X	X	X		X			X	X
Disability and secondary conditions	X	X	X	X					X	X
Educational and community-based programs	X	X	X	X	X	X	X	X	X	X
Environmental health				X				X		X
Family planning				X				X		X
Food safety				X				X		X
Health communication	X	X	X	X	X	X	X	X	X	X
Heart disease and stroke	X	X	X	X		X	X	X	X	X
HIV				X	X	X		X	X	X
Immunization and infectious diseases				X		X	X			X
Injury and violence prevention			X	X		X	X			X
Maternal, infant, and child health	X	X	X	X	X	X	X		X	X
Medical product safety					X					
Mental health and mental disorders			X	X	X	X	X	X		
Nutrition and overweight	X	X	X	X		X				
Occupational safety and health				X		X	X	X		
Oral health	X	X	X	X	X	X		X		X
Physical activity and fitness	X	X	X	X	X	X		X		X
Public health infrastructure	X	X	X	X	X	X	X	X		X
Respiratory diseases	X	X	X	X	X	X	X	X	X	X
Sexually transmitted diseases					X					
Substance abuse			X	X	X	X	X			X
Tobacco use			X					X		X
Vision and hearing								X		X

From Office of Disease Prevention and Health Promotion, US Department of Health and Human Services: *Leading health indicators touch everyone, Healthy People 2010,* 2009 (website): www.healthypeople. gov/LHI/Touch_fact.htm. Accessed March 18, 2009.
HIV, Human immunodeficiency virus.

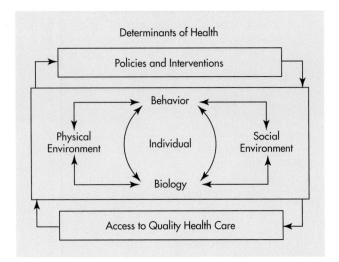

FIGURE 4-1 The relationship among the determinants of health. (From US Department of Health and Human Services: *Healthy people 2010: understanding and improving health,* January 30, 2001 (website): www.healthypeople.gov/Document/tableofcontents.htm#under. Accessed April 22, 2009.)

of the social environment, as well as housing, safety, public transportation, and availability of resources. The social environment has a great impact on the health of individuals, groups, and communities, yet it is complex in nature because of differing cultures and practices.

Physical environment is that which is experienced with the senses; that is smelled, seen, touched, heard, and tasted. The physical environment can impact health negatively or positively. If there are toxic or infectious substances in the environment, this is certainly a negative influence on health. If the environment is clean with areas to recreate and play, this is a good influence on health.

Policies and interventions can have a profound effect on the health of individuals, groups, and communities. Positive effects such as policies against smoking in public places, seatbelt and child restraint laws, litter ordinances, and enhanced health care promote health. Policies are implemented at local, state, and national levels by many agencies such as transportation, health and human services, veterans' affairs, housing, and justice departments.

Access to quality health care: expansion of health care access is essential to decrease health disparities and to increase the quality of life and the quantity of years of healthy life (USDHHS, 2001).

THEORIES IN HEALTH PROMOTION

Health promotion activities are broad in scope and in setting. Community health nurses and their clients engage in health promotion activities in workplace settings, schools, clinics, and communities. The theories that are used most in health promotion are very diverse to accommodate the variety of settings, clients, and activities in community health. A working knowledge of theory is important in understanding why people act as they do and why they may or may not follow

advice given to them by medical professionals, and in helping clients progress from knowledge to behavior change. Some of the most frequently used health promotion theories and models are discussed below.

Pender's Health Promotion Model

Developed in the 1980s and revised in 1996, Pender's Health Promotion Model (HPM) explores the myriad biopsychosocial factors that influence individuals to pursue health promotion activities. The constructs or variables of the HPM are listed and described in Table 4-2. The HPM depicts the complex multidimensional factors with which people interact as they work to achieve optimum health. This model contains seven variables related to health behaviors, as well as individual characteristics that may influence a behavioral outcome.

Pender's model does not include threat as a motivator, as threat may not be a motivating factor for clients in all age groups (Pender et al., 2006). The Health Promotion Model is depicted in Figure 4-2.

Relating the Health Promotion Model for Jamie R. in the Clinical Example on page 51, the experience of having relatives who died of heart disease and cancer has probably increased her desire to engage in healthful behavior. Similarly, her busy schedule and lack of communication with her doctor may be reflected in her lack of desire to have screening or immunizations. Jamie has a habit of engaging in exercise and a high self-efficacy related to her success with exercise in the past. Jamie feels better after exercise, and she receives positive comments from significant others regarding her appearance, also increasing her motivation to exercise. Jamie works out in a lovely gym and is very committed to her workout routine. Jamie has found that by working out first thing in the morning, the competing demands that may keep her from exercising are minimized.

The Health Belief Model

Initially proposed in 1958, the Health Belief Model (HBM) provides the basis for much of the practice of health education and health promotion today. The Health Belief Model was developed by a group of social psychologists to explain why the public failed to participate in screening for tuberculosis (Hochbaum, 1958). Hochbaum and his associates had the same questions that perplex many health professionals today: Why do people who may have a disease reject health screening? Why do individuals participate in screening if it may lead to the diagnosis of disease? Through their work, this group found that information alone is rarely enough to motivate one to act. Individuals must know what to do and how to do it before they can take action. Also, the information must be related in some way to the individual's needs. One of the most widely used conceptual frameworks in health behavior, the Health Belief Model has been used to explain behavior change and maintenance of behavior change and to guide health promotion interventions (Janz, Champion, and Stretcher, 2002).

The Health Belief Model has several constructs: perceived seriousness, perceived susceptibility, perceived benefits of treatment, perceived barriers to treatment, cues to action, and

TABLE 4-2 PENDER'S HEALTH PROMOTION MODEL

INDIVIDUAL CHARACTERISTICS AND EXPERIENCES	EACH PERSON'S UNIQUE CHARACTERISTICS AND EXPERIENCES AFFECT THEIR ACTIONS. THEIR EFFECT DEPENDS ON THE BEHAVIOR IN QUESTION.
Prior related behavior	Prior behaviors influence subsequent behavior through perceived self-efficacy, benefits, barriers, and affects related to that activity. Habit is also a strong indicator of future behavior.
Personal factors	Personal factors that may influence behavior are biologic factors such as age, BMI, strength, and agility; psychological factors include self-esteem, self-motivation, and perceived health status; sociocultural factors include race, ethnicity, acculturation, education, and socioeconomic status.
Behavior specific cognitions and affect	In the HPM, these variables are considered to be very significant in behavior motivation. They are a "core" for intervention because they may be modified through nursing actions. Assessment of the effectiveness of interventions is accomplished by measuring the change in these variables.
Perceived benefits of action	The perceived benefits of a behavior are strong motivators of that behavior. These motivate behavior through intrinsic and extrinsic benefits. Intrinsic benefits include increased energy or decreased appetite. Extrinsic benefits include social rewards such as compliments, or monetary rewards.
Perceived barriers to action	Barriers are perceived unavailability, inconvenience, expense, difficulty or time regarding health behaviors.
Perceived self-efficacy	Self-efficacy is one's belief that he is capable of carrying out a health behavior. If one has high self-efficacy regarding a behavior, one is more likely to engage in that behavior than if one has low self-efficacy.
Activity-related affect	The feelings associated with a behavior will likely affect whether an individual will repeat or maintain the behavior.
Interpersonal influences	In the HPM, these are feelings, thoughts, regarding the beliefs or attitudes of others. Primary influences are family, peers, and health care providers.
Situational influences	These are perceived options available, demand characteristics, and the aesthetic features of the environment where the behavior will take place. For example, a lovely day will increase the probability of one taking a walk; the fire code will prevent one from smoking indoors.
Commitment to a plan of action	Pender states that "commitment to a plan of action initiates a behavioral event" (Pender et al., 2006, p. 56). This commitment will compel one into the behavior until completed unless a competing demand or preference intervenes.
Immediate competing demands and preferences	These are alternative behaviors that one considers as possible optional behaviors immediately prior to engaging in the intended, planned behavior. One has little control over competing demands, but one has great control over competing preferences.
Health-promoting behavior	This is the goal or outcome of the HPM. The aim of health-promoting behavior is the attainment of positive health outcomes.

From Pender N, Murdaugh CL, Parsons MA: *Health promotion in nursing practice*, 5th ed, Upper Saddle River, NJ, 2006, Pearson.
BMI, Body mass index.

self-efficacy. These components are found in Table 4-3. All of these constructs relate to the client's perception. How does the client perceive the seriousness of the condition? His susceptibility to the condition? The benefits of prevention or treatment? The barriers to prevention or treatment? The HBM is depicted in Figure 4-3 (McEwen and Pullis, 2009).

Applying the HBM to Jamie, she may not perceive that she is susceptible to heart disease or breast cancer, or she may not perceive that there is a benefit of screening, or treatment for heart disease or cancer, thus her failure to take up screening for these diseases.

The Transtheoretical Model

The Transtheoretical Model (TTM) combines several theories of intervention, thus the name *transtheoretical*. Table 4-4 lists the core constructs of the model, which also include the constructs of self-efficacy and the processes of change. The Transtheoretical Model is depicted in Figure 4-4.

The Transtheoretical Model is based on the assumption that behavior change takes place over time, progressing through a sequence of stages. It also assumes that each of the stages is both stable and open to change. In other words, one

TABLE 4-3 KEY CONCEPTS AND DEFINITIONS OF THE HEALTH BELIEF MODEL

CONCEPT	DEFINITION
Perceived susceptibility	One's belief regarding the chance of getting a given condition
Perceived severity	One's belief regarding the seriousness of a given condition
Perceived benefits	One's belief in the ability of an advised action to reduce the health risk or seriousness of a given condition
Perceived barriers	One's belief regarding the tangible and psychological costs of an advised action
Cues to action	Strategies or conditions in one's environment that activate readiness to take action
Self-efficacy	One's confidence in one's ability to take action to reduce health risks

From Janz, JK, Champion, VL, & Stretcher, VJ: The health belief model. In Glanz K, Rimer, BK, Lewis, FM editors: *Health behavior and health education: theory, research, and practice*, San Francisco, 2002, Jossey-Bass.

Individual Characteristics
and Experiences

Behavior-specific
Cognitions and Affect

Behavioral
Outcome

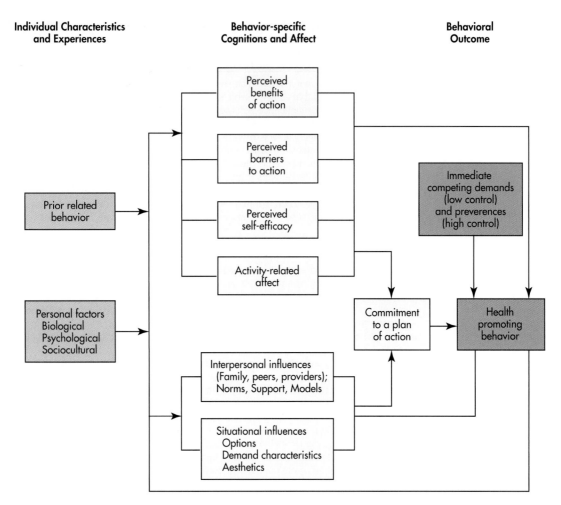

FIGURE 4-2 The Health Promotion Model. (From Pender N: *The University of Michigan School of Nursing, the Health Promotion Model,* 2009 (website): www.nursing.umich.edu/faculty/pender/chart.gif. Accessed March 26, 2009.)

may stop in one stage, progress to the next stage, or return to the previous stage.

The TTM and Change

Change is difficult, even for the most motivated of individuals. People resist change for many reasons. Change may

- Be unpleasant (exercising)
- Require giving up pleasure (eating desserts or watching TV)
- Be painful (insulin injections)
- Be stressful (eating new foods)
- Jeopardize social relationships (gatherings with friends and family involve food)
- Not seem important any more (older individuals or those with the ill effects of lifestyle choices such as diabetes and hypertension)
- Require change in self-image (from couch potato to athlete) (Westberg and Jason, 1996).

Theory of Reasoned Action

Developed by Fishbein and Ajzen, the Theory of Reasoned Action (TRA) attempts to predict a person's intention to perform or not to perform a certain behavior (Montano and Kasprzyk, 2008). The Theory of Reasoned Action is based on the assumption that all behavior is determined by one's behavioral intentions. These intentions are determined by one's attitude regarding a behavior and the subjective norms associated with the behavior (Montano and Kasprzyk, 2008). One's attitude is determined by one's beliefs about the outcomes of performing the behavior, weighted by one's assessment of the outcomes. Consider Jamie R. from the Clinical Example on page 51 for a moment. Jamie must believe strongly that exercise will have positive results, as she rises early and takes time from her busy schedule to work out daily. Conversely, Jamie may believe strongly that routine immunizations or health screenings will have negative results.

One's subjective norm is determined by one's *normative beliefs,* or whether or not important persons in one's life approve or disapprove of the behavior under consideration, weighted by one's motivation to comply with those important persons (Montano and Kasprzyk, 2008). If Jamie believes that her husband or children think that she should get a mammogram, and if she is motivated to comply with their wishes, Jamie will have a positive subject norm regarding getting a mammogram.

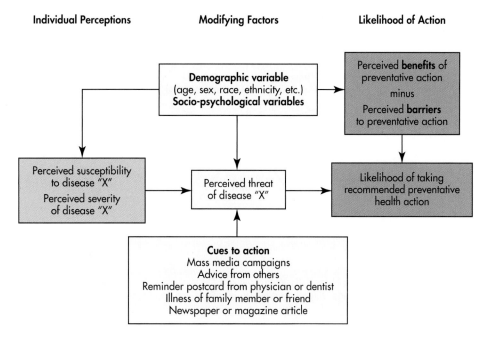

Individual Perceptions   Modifying Factors   Likelihood of Action

FIGURE 4-3 The Health Belief Model. (From Janz, N and Becker, M. "The Health Belief Model: A Decade Later." *Health Education Quarterly.* (1984) 11 (1):1-47.)

TABLE 4-4	THE TRANSTHEORETICAL MODEL
CONSTRUCTS	**DESCRIPTION**
Stages of Change	
Precontemplation	The individual has no intention to take action toward behavior change in the next six months. May be in this phase due to a lack of information about the consequences of the behavior, or due to failure on previous attempts at change.
Contemplation	The individual has some intention to take action toward behavior change in the next six months. Weighing pros and cons to change.
Preparation	The individual intends to take action within the next month, and has taken steps toward behavior change. Has a plan of action.
Action	The individual has changed overt behavior for less than six months. Has changed behavior sufficiently to reduce risk of disease.
Maintenance	The individual has changed overt behavior for more than six months. Strives to prevent relapse. This phase may last months to years.
Decisional Balance	
Pros	The benefits of behavior change
Cons	The costs of behavior change

From Prochaska, J.O., Redding C.A., Evers, K.E. 2008. The Transtheoretical Model and Stages of Change. In Glanz, K., Rimer, B., Viswanath, K. (Eds). *Health behavior and health education: Theory, research, and practice (pp. 97-121).* San Francisco: Josey-Bass.

Recently, the variable of perceived control has been added to the TRA to account for the amount of control an individual may have over whether or not he or she performs the behavior. With the addition of perceived control, the Theory of Planned Behavior was developed (Montano and Kasprzyk, 2008). Figure 4-5 illustrates the TRA and the Theory of Planned Behavior.

RISK AND HEALTH

Oleckno defines risk as "the probability that a specific event will occur in a given time frame" (2002, p. 352). A risk factor is an exposure that is associated with a disease (Friis and Sellers, 2004). Jamie R. from the Clinical Example on page 51 has an increased *risk* of heart disease and cancer. Jamie's *risk factors* include a family history of both of these diseases, work stress, her age, environmental exposures, and gender. There are known risk factors for some diseases, such as smoking and its association with lung cancer, and high blood pressure and heart disease. Some risk factors are assumed, such as cell phones and brain tumors. There are three criteria for establishing a risk factor:

1. The frequency of the disease varies by category, or amount of the factor. Cigarette smokers are more likely to develop lung cancer than nonsmokers and those who smoke heavily are more likely to develop lung cancer than those who smoke little.

2. The risk factor must precede the onset of the disease. Cigarette smokers have lung cancer after they have been smoking for awhile. If smokers had lung cancer before starting to smoke, this would cast doubt on smoking as a risk factor for lung cancer.

3. The association of concern must not be due to any source of error. In any research study, (especially one involving

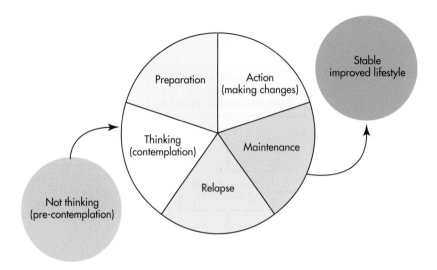

FIGURE 4-4 The Transtheoretical Model. (From Prochaska J, DiClemente C: Transtheoretical therapy: towards a more integrative model of change, *Psychotherapy: Theory, Research and Practice* 19:276-88, 1982.)

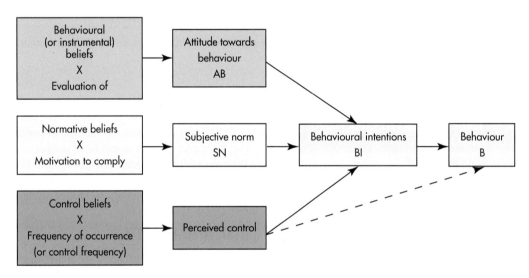

FIGURE 4-5 From Montano, Daniel E. and Kaspryzk, Danuta: Theory of Reasoned Action, Theory of Planned Behavior, and the Integrated Behavioral Model in *Health Behavior and Health Education* by Glanz, K., Rimer, B.K., and Viswanath, K., pp 67-96. 2008, Jossey-Bass: San Francisco.

human behavior) there are many sources of error such as study design, data collection methods, and data analysis.

Other criteria that have been noted in literature include strength of the association, consistency with repetition, specificity, and plausibility (Friis and Sellers, 2004).

In order to determine the health risks to individuals, groups, and populations, a risk assessment may be conducted. A risk assessment is a systematic way of distinguishing the risks posed by potentially harmful exposures. The four main steps of a risk assessment are hazard identification, risk description, exposure assessment, and risk estimation (Savitz, 1998).

THE RELATIONSHIP OF RISK TO HEALTH AND HEALTH PROMOTION ACTIVITIES

Health is directly related to the activities in which we participate, the food we eat, and substances to which we are exposed daily. Where we live and work, our gender, age, and genetic

makeup also impact health. In the assessment of risk regarding health and health promotion activities, there are two types of risks: modifiable risks and nonmodifiable risks. *Modifiable risk factors* are those aspects of a person's health risk over which he or she has control. Examples include smoking, leading a sedentary or active lifestyle, type and amount of food eaten, and the type of activities in which he or she engages (skydiving is riskier than bowling). *Nonmodifiable risk factors* are those aspects of one's health risk over which one has no or little control. Examples include genetic makeup, gender, age, and environmental exposures. A useful tool to help clients assess their family history for possible health risks is available at the U.S. Surgeon General's website at https://family-history.hhs.gov/fhh-web/home.action. This assessment is easy to use and can create a dialogue between family members to discuss family health history. As the nurse assesses the various aspects of a client's health, it is important to evaluate behaviors that have a positive effect on the client's health, not

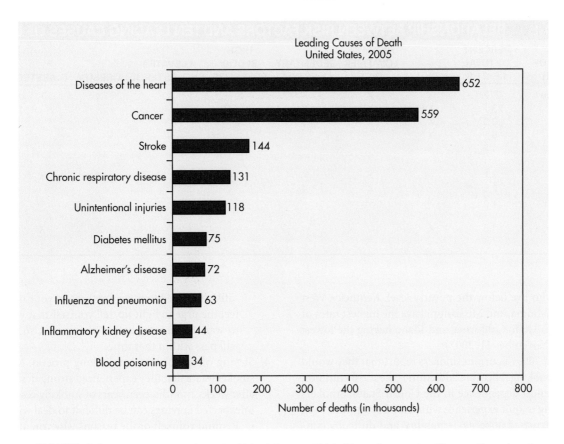

Leading Causes of Death
United States, 2005

FIGURE 4-6 Leading causes of death, United States, 2005. (From Centers for Disease Control and Prevention, National Center for Chronic Disease Prevention, 2008: www.cdc.gov/nccdphp/overview.htm.)

only those behaviors that are detrimental to health. Healthful behaviors such as maintaining an exercise regimen, or following an eating plan, build self-efficacy and self-esteem. Positive health behaviors also provide a foundation on which a nurse can build to address unhealthful behaviors. If a client has been successful at smoking cessation, the confidence and self-efficacy learned from this change can be drawn upon to help him stick to a low-sodium, low-fat diet to address his hypertension.

Risk reduction is a proactive process in which individuals participate in behaviors that enable them to react to actual or potential threats to their health (Pender, 1996). Risk communication is the process through which the public receives information regarding possible or actual threats to health. Risk communication is affected by the way individuals and communities perceive, process, and act on their understanding of risk (Finnigan and Vinswanath, 2008). Individuals, groups, and communities receive information on health risks from many sources besides health care professionals today. The Internet is a newer source of risk communication for many community members. Newspapers, periodicals, radio, TV, and billboards are long-standing sources of health information in public health. Though there are many sources of information on health risks available to the public, quality varies widely in the accuracy of the information presented (Moynihan, et al., 2000; Sopczyk, 2008; Kunst et al., 2002).

Approximately 50% of annual U.S. deaths occur as a result of modifiable or lifestyle factors (McGinnis and Foege, 1993; Mokdab et al., 2004). Figure 4-6 depicts the leading causes of death and the numbers of deaths related to each. Those causes of death with the highest mortality (heart disease, cancer, stroke, and chronic respiratory disease) are all related to lifestyle factors (McGinnis and Foege, 2004). Table 4-5 details the relationship of the leading causes of death and common risk factors.

Tobacco and Health Risk

Smoking cessation is an important step in achieving optimum health. In the United States, smoking is the leading cause of preventable death, accounting for approximately one out of every five deaths or 438,000 people per year. Smoking is a causal factor in cancers of the esophagus, bladder, stomach, oral cavity, pharynx, larynx, cervix, and lung with more than 90% of lung cancers in men and 80% of lung cancers among women attributable to smoking (Centers for Disease Control and Prevention [CDC], November 11, 2007). Smoking also has an economic impact, costing $97.2 billion annually in health care and lost productivity (American Lung Association, nd).

Most smokers are between the ages of 18 and 44 years, and more men smoke than do women. The prevalence of smoking is highest among American Indians and African Americans. Smoking is most common among adults who are less educated

TABLE 4-5 — RELATIONSHIP BETWEEN RISK FACTORS AND TEN LEADING CAUSES OF DEATH

CAUSE OF DEATH	PERCENT OF TOTAL DEATHS	SMOKING	HIGH-FAT, LOW-FIBER DIET	SEDENTARY LIFESTYLE	HIGH BLOOD PRESSURE	ELEVATED CHOLESTEROL	OBESITY	DIABETES	ALCOHOL ABUSE
Heart disease	27.2	X	X	X	X	X	X	X	X
Cancer	23.1	X	X	X			X		X
Stroke	6.3	X	X		X	X	X		
COPD	5.1	X							
Unintentional injury	4.7	X							X
Diabetes	3.1		X	X			X	X	
Alzheimer's	2.8		X	X					
Pneumonia and influenza	2.5	X							
Kidney disease	1.8	X			X	X	X	X	X
Septicemia	1.4						X	X	

and adults who live below the poverty level. Kentucky, West Virginia, Oklahoma, and Mississippi have the highest rates of smokers, with Utah, California, and Idaho having the lowest rates (CDC, November 11, 2007).

More than 70% of current smokers report that they would like to quit smoking. Nicotine addiction is the most common form of chemical dependence in the United States. Smokers who are trying to quit experience withdrawal symptoms such as anxiety, increased appetite, irritability, and difficulty concentrating. These symptoms make quitting difficult, and most people will relapse several times before being able to quit successfully. Nicotine replacement, pharmaceutical alternatives, hypnosis, and acupuncture may be helpful in the attempt to quit smoking. The American Cancer Society recommends these steps to quit smoking:

1. Make the decision to quit. Any change is scary, and smoking cessation is a big change, requiring a long-term commitment.
2. Set a date to quit and choose a plan.
   - Mark the date on your calendar.
   - Tell your family and friends about the date, and ask for their support.
   - Get rid of all tobacco products, ashtrays, and lighters in your environment.
   - Stock up on oral substitutes such as sugarless gum, hard candy, fruit, and carrot sticks.
   - Decide on a plan, and prepare to implement it; register for the stop-smoking class, or see your doctor about nicotine replacement therapy or pharmaceutical alternatives.
   - Practice saying "No thank you, I don't smoke."
   - Think back to your previous attempts to quit, and see what worked and what did not work.
   - If you are taking bupropion or varenicline, take your medication each day of the week leading up to your quit day.
3. Deal with withdrawal through
   - Avoiding temptation
   - Changing your habits. Walk when you are stressed or during breaks. Use hard candy, carrot sticks, or gum to satisfy the need to put something in your mouth. If you feel the urge to light up, tell yourself that you are going to wait 10 minutes before giving in. Usually, the urge will pass within that time.
4. Staying off of tobacco is a lifelong process. Many former smokers state that they experienced strong desires to smoke after weeks, months, even years of smoking cessation. These unexpected cravings can be difficult to deal with.
   - Remind yourself of the reasons why you quit.
   - Wait out the craving. There is no such thing as just one cigarette or just one puff.
   - Avoid alcohol.
   - Begin an exercise program and work on eating a healthy diet to avoid gaining weight (American Cancer Society, 2009).

Information on quitting can be accessed at the CDC website at www.cdc.gov/tobacco/data_statistics/fact_sheets/cessation/cessation2.htm (CDC, April 2008). The American Lung Association also has information on smoking cessation at www.lungusa.org/site/c.dvLUK9O0E/b.33484/k.438A/Quit_Smoking.htm, and the American Cancer Society has a quit-smoking guide at www.cancer.org/docroot/PED/content/PED_10_13X_Guide_for_Quitting_Smoking.asp?from=fast. A resource for teens who are trying to quit smoking is available at www.lungusa.org/site/c.dvLUK9O0E/b.39865/k.1F9F/Teen_Smoking_Reduced_Due_To_Not_On_Tobacco_NOT.htm.

Only 4% to 7% of smokers are able to quit smoking on any attempt without pharmaceutical or other interventions to help them, so nurses must provide information and referrals to help clients access resources to help them to get off and to stay off of tobacco.

Smokeless tobacco also poses a health threat. Commonly called *spit tobacco*, smokeless tobacco is a significant health threat and is not a safe substitute for smoking tobacco. Smokeless tobacco is known to be a cause of cancer and oral health problems and increases the risk of cancer of the oral cavity. Smokeless tobacco causes nicotine addiction and dependence, and adolescents who use smokeless tobacco are more likely to take up smoking (CDC, April 27, 2007).

In the United States, 3% of adults use smokeless tobacco, with far more men (6%) than women (0.4%) being users of smokeless tobacco. It is estimated that 8% of high school students and 3% of middle school students use smokeless tobacco. Smokeless tobacco use is more common among young white males with its heaviest use among those living in the southern or north central states and among blue collar workers, service workers, or laborers, and among the unemployed. American Indian/Alaska Natives are the heaviest users of smokeless tobacco, followed by whites. School nurses are in an important position to intervene early in the use of smokeless tobacco. Most smokeless tobacco use begins in middle school, and interventions to prevent or stop this habit are essential in the school setting (CDC, April 27, 2007).

The clinical implications regarding tobacco use are clear. First, community health nurses must ask about tobacco use at every clinic visit or home visit and look for teachable moments when the client may be interested in discussing his or her tobacco habit (a respiratory illness or a scare with an oral lesion may prompt the client to reconsider the habit). Assess the client's tobacco use: "Do you use tobacco?", "What kind of tobacco (cigarettes, cigars, chewing tobacco, pipe) do you use?", "How much do you smoke (dip, chew)?", "Have you thought about quitting?" Explore with the client why he or she may or may not have considered giving up the tobacco habit, and what options are available to help should he or she desire to quit. Refer the client to smoking cessation websites or other health care professionals for assistance in quitting. Chances are great that the client is very well acquainted with the health risks posed by tobacco, but not the options for helping him or her to quit. Encourage the client to attempt to give up tobacco, and encourage him or her in any attempts to decrease or stop using tobacco.

Alcohol Consumption and Health

Alcohol use is very common in our society. In 2006, 61% of Americans reported being current drinkers, 15% were former drinkers, 24% were lifetime abstainers, and about 5% were heavy drinkers. One in five adults reported drinking five or more drinks per day. Men are more likely (68%) than women (55%) to be current drinkers and to binge drink. Men are also more than twice as likely to suffer death or injury related to drinking. Nationally, women are nearly twice as likely as men to be lifetime abstainers, yet six of every ten women of childbearing age drink alcohol, and a third of these women binge drink. In 2002, one of every ten women reported drinking while pregnant. For both men and women, those aged 25 to 44 years had the highest prevalence of drinking. The drinking prevalence declines at age 44 years and declines steadily with age thereafter. Non-Hispanic white people have the highest drinking prevalence, with non-Hispanic white men being the heaviest drinkers (CDC, September 2006).

Alcohol use, particularly heavy alcohol use, is responsible for many health problems such as liver disease or unintentional injuries. *Excessive alcohol use* is drinking more than two drinks per day on average for men or more than one drink per day for women or *binge drinking,* which is drinking five

or more drinks on a single occasion for men or four or more drinks in a single occasion for women. A drink is any drink containing 0.6 ounces or 1.2 tablespoons of pure alcohol. A drink is

- 12 ounces of beer or wine cooler
- 8 ounces of malt liquor
- 5 ounces of wine
- 1.5 ounces of 80-proof distilled spirits or liquor (gin, rum, vodka, whiskey) (CDC, August 6, 2008)

The *Dietary Guidelines for Americans* (USDHHS, 2005) state that alcohol should be consumed in moderation, no more than one drink per day for women and no more than two drinks per day for men. Persons who should not drink are those who

- Are under 21 years of age
- Are taking medications that can cause harmful reactions when mixed with alcohol
- Are pregnant or trying to become pregnant
- Are recovering from alcoholism or are unable to control the amount that they drink
- Have a medical condition that may be worsened by alcohol
- Are driving or planning to drive or to perform activities requiring coordination and concentration (CDC, August 6, 2008)

Responsible for 79,000 deaths annually, alcohol use is the third leading lifestyle-related cause of death for the nation. In 2005 alone there were more than 1.6 million hospitalizations and more than 4 million emergency department visits for alcohol-related conditions. The short-term risks of alcohol consumption are usually due to binge drinking or excess drinking and include risky sexual behavior, violence, unintentional injuries from motor vehicle accidents, falls, firearms, and drowning. Miscarriage or stillbirth and alcohol poisoning are also possible immediate effects of excessive alcohol use. The long-term risks of alcohol use are neurologic conditions such as dementia and stroke; cardiovascular problems such as MI, hypertension, and cardiomyopathy; psychiatric problems such as depression and anxiety; social problems such as unemployment and family dysfunction; cancer of the mouth, throat, liver, and breast; and liver disease including cirrhosis and hepatitis. Pancreatitis and gastritis are other gastrointestinal consequences of long-term alcohol consumption (CDC, August 6, 2008).

The prevalence of underage drinking declined significantly when states enacted the age 21 minimum legal drinking age, and those states with more stringent drinking laws have a lower prevalence of adult and underage binge drinking. Despite age limits for legal consumption of alcohol, alcohol consumption contributes to more than 46,000 deaths among underage youth annually, with the prevalence of underage drinking being a striking 60%. The prevalence of adult binge drinking behavior is strongly predictive of binge drinking behavior by college students living in the same state (CDC, September 3, 2008a).

Clinical implications for health promotion related to alcohol consumption emphasize prevention of underage drinking and identifying and assisting groups and individuals at risk for alcohol abuse and dependence. A helpful resource for locating and contacting local agencies for alcohol treatment is the National Drug and Alcohol Treatment Referral Routing Service available at 1-800-662-HELP.

Preventing underage drinking is a public health priority. Enforcement of the legal drinking age, as well as enforcement of bans on sales of alcohol to minors, is an important aspect of prevention. Increased excise tax on alcoholic beverages has also been found to decrease underage drinking. Education of both adults and youth regarding alcohol and the myriad of risks posed by underage alcohol consumption must accompany enforcement efforts. The "Too Smart to Start" program targets parents and caregivers of 9- to 13-year-olds. The goal of the program is to increase the percentage of youth and their caregivers who view underage drinking unfavorably (CDC, 2008a).

Diet and Health

Diet is one of the most modifiable of risk factors. A healthy diet contributes to the prevention of such chronic diseases as type 2 diabetes, hypertension, heart disease, and some cancers. Because 17% of U.S. children 2 to 19 years of age are overweight, 66% of U.S. adults are overweight, and 32% are obese (Flegal et al., 2002; Ogden et al., 2006; CDC, April 2, 2009), diet is an important topic in health promotion. Americans are bombarded with nutrition information, resulting in many being confused and having no idea how to apply the information that they have received. As portion sizes get larger, Americans of all ages are spending more time engaged in inactive pursuits such as watching TV or using a computer. Commonly, the terms "portion" and "serving" are misused. A *portion* is the "amount of a single food item served in a single eating occasion." A meal or a snack is a single eating occasion with the amount of green beans or roast beef on your plate being the portion. A *serving* is a "standardized unit of measuring foods" used in dietary guidelines. A cup or an ounce is an example of a serving size (CDC, May 2006).

Though there are many contributing factors to overweight and obesity, controlling one's weight is a matter of balancing caloric intake with physical activity. Too many calories in and too few calories out will eventually result in overweight. Figure 4-7 illustrates this energy balance. One's body weight is determined by a complex interplay among metabolism, genetics, behavior, environment, culture, and socioeconomic status, making the problem of overweight a difficult one to study and to impact (CDC, January 28, 2009).

Mississippi, Alabama, and Tennessee have the highest prevalence of overweight and obese residents in the nation. Mississippi's prevalence of overweight and obesity is 32%, with Alabama and Tennessee each having a prevalence rate of 30%. Only Colorado has a prevalence of overweight and obesity below 20% (CDC, July 24, 2008). Persons aged 45 to 64 years are most likely to be overweight in the United States, with 73% of men and 63% of women being overweight. Obesity rates vary between races and ethnicities. Between 2003 and 2006, 53% of non-Hispanic black women were overweight or obese compared with 32% of non-Hispanic

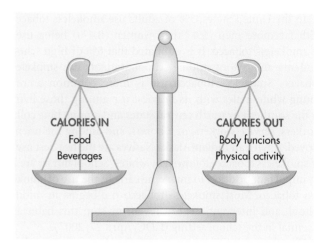

FIGURE 4-7 Caloric balance equation. (From Centers for Disease Control and Prevention: *Overweight and obesity: an overview. Overweight and obesity,* January 28, 2009 [website]: www.cdc.gov/nccdphp/dnpa/obesity/contributing_factors.htm. Accessed April 20, 2009).

white women and 52% of women of Mexican origin. More Hispanic males were overweight than white or non-Hispanic black men (USDHHS, 2009).

Fats are an essential nutrient for energy and serve many purposes in the body, but too much fat in the diet, especially trans fats, saturated fats, and cholesterol, may increase the risk of heart disease (USDHHS, 2005a). In 2007, only a quarter of persons in the United States reported eating the recommended five or more servings of fruits and vegetables per day. Though the benefits of eating a diet rich in fruits and vegetables is well known, this trend is unchanged since 1996 (CDC, November 6, 2008). The CDC has information on incorporating fruits and vegetables into a daily diet at www.fruitsandveggiesmatter.gov/.

Although the same eating plan is not appropriate for everyone, the U.S. Department of Agriculture (USDA) does make some key recommendations regarding a healthy diet based on a 2000 calorie per day intake:

- Select 2 cups of fruit and 2½ cups of vegetables per day. Select a variety of colors and types.
- Consume three or more 1-ounce equivalent servings per day of whole-grain products.
- Consume 3 cups per day of fat-free or low-fat milk or milk products.
- Keep total fat intake to 20% to 35% of caloric intake.
- When choosing fats, emphasize lean meats, beans, poultry, and fat-free or low-fat milk products.
- Limit intake of trans fatty acids or saturated fats.
- Choose fiber-rich fruits and vegetables often.
- Prepare beverages and foods with little added sugar.
- Consume less than 1 teaspoon of salt per day.
- Consume alcoholic beverages moderately—up to one drink per day for women and two drinks per day for men.

Special populations such as pregnant or lactating women, infants, children, older adults, athletic or very active adults, and adolescents have differing nutritional needs. Specific recommendations for these individuals can be accessed at the

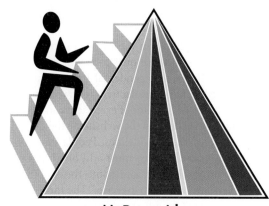

MyPyramid.gov
STEPS TO A HEALTHIER YOU

FIGURE 4-8 MyPyramid logo. (From US Department of Agriculture: *MyPyramid.gov,* April 7, 2009 (website): www.mypyramid.gov/index. html. Accessed April 20, 2009.)

website for the *Dietary Guidelines for Americans:* www.cnpp. usda.gov/Publications/DietaryGuidelines/2005/2005DGPolicy-Document.pdf (USDHHS, 2005b).

The USDA recommends that all Americans go to www. mypyramid.gov/index.html to develop a personalized eating plan based on individual needs and preferences. *MyPyramid* (Figure 4-8) was released in 2005, replacing the Food Guide Pyramid from 1992. This tool helps users easily translate the USDA guidelines into the kinds and amounts of food to eat each day. The pyramid is applicable for children, as well as adults, and is simple (and fun) enough that children can use it themselves (USDA, April 7, 2009).

Studies confirm that eating away from home is associated with an increased likelihood of overweight (McCrory et al., 1999; Schroder, Fito, and Cavas, 2007). Busy families have more opportunities to eat away from home as the number of eateries has increased in recent years. From 1999 to 2004, American families spent 45% of their food budget on foods eaten away from home (The Keystone Center, 2006). Bowman and Vineyard (2004) found that, on a typical day, 30% of 4- to 19-year-olds consumed fast food. The highest consumption of fast food was associated with non-Hispanic black individuals, males, higher household income, older children, and living in the South.

Portions served in restaurants are larger than portions served at home. Convenience foods and prepackaged foods contain larger portion sizes than in the 1970s (CDC, 2008). When presented with a large portion size, individuals often unknowingly eat larger amounts than they would usually eat or than they intend to eat. This phenomenon is called portion distortion and occurs frequently when dining out (Burger, Kern, and Coleman, 2007; Schwartz and Byrd-Bredbenner, 2006). Portion control is an important aspect of weight management, and distortion of portion sizes makes this difficult task harder. There are several reasons why we tend to overeat when we eat away from home: foods presented in restaurants are high energy density (high number of calories for a particular weight of food); restaurant foods are also very palatable,

and there is a wide variety of this great-tasting food to choose from; we want to get more food for our money, so we order the larger entrées (The Keystone Center, 2006).

What about eating away from home? For many people, eating at home all of the time is impossible or impractical, and food is central to many social interactions. In order to consume fewer calories when eating out, one may

- Patronize establishments that offer a variety of food choices and are willing to make substitutions or changes
- Order lower-fat steamed, broiled, baked, roasted, or poached items, or ask that an item be prepared in a lower-calorie way, such as grilled rather than fried
- Choose lower-calorie sauces or condiments, or do without them altogether
- Substitute colorful vegetables for other side dishes (such as French fries)
- Ask for half of the meal to be boxed to take home before the meal is brought to the table
- Share an entrée with someone
- Order a vegetarian meal
- Select a fruit for dessert

To decrease reliance on away-from-home foods, plan ahead and

- Pack healthy snacks to avoid the use of vending machines
- Cook a healthful dinner at home, and make extra to pack for lunch the next day
- Purchase healthful foods when grocery shopping to pack for lunch, such as prepackaged salads, fresh fruits, vegetables, and low-calorie soups
- Bring along nutritious foods for travel or longer excursions that will not spoil, such as fresh fruits and vegetables, or pack a cooler with healthy foods

There are various online communities and other support groups available to help individuals manage their weight. Group support is helpful for some, whereas others prefer to have programs that they can implement on their own. The cost to join a weight-management community ranges from free to moderate in price.

Physical Activity and Health

There are many reasons why people engage in physical activity and exercise: for weight management, increased energy, better appearance; to fit into those favorite jeans; to prevent development or worsening of a chronic health condition; to manage stress; to improve mood and self-esteem; or any combination of these reasons. About 62% of U.S. adults engage in regular leisure-time physical activity with the remaining 38% being physically inactive. About one in eight adults gets some form of vigorous physical activity at least five times per week, with about one fourth of adults participating in some kind of strength-building activity.

Several factors acting individually and in concert can affect the likelihood that one is physically active. Men are a little more likely to engage in leisure physical activity and are more likely to engage in strength training than women. The percentage of adults who engage in leisure-time physical activity decreases with age, from its highest among adults aged 18 to 24 years. White adults and Asian adults are more likely to engage in leisure-time physical activity than are black and Hispanic adults. The percentage of adults participating in leisure-time physical activity increases with level of education, with adults having an advanced degree being twice as likely to engage in some physical activity as high school graduates. The percentage of adults who engage in regular leisure-time physical activity also increases with income level. Adults whose income is four times the federal poverty level are nearly twice as likely to engage in some form of regular leisure-time physical activity as are adults whose income is below the poverty level. Adults living in the southern region of the United States get the least amount of leisure-time physical activity (CDC, September 2006).

As has been previously mentioned, one's surroundings also impact whether one will choose to exercise. The Sightline Institute has ranked cities across the United States for suitability for walking. So, what makes a city walkable?

- A center: a shopping center, park, or main street
- Mixed use, mixed income: businesses are located next to homes at all price points
- Pedestrian-centric design: businesses are close to the street to encourage foot traffic with parking in back
- Density: the city is compact enough to allow businesses to flourish and for public transportation to run frequently
- Parks and public space: there are plenty of public areas in which to gather
- Nearby schools and workplaces: schools and workplaces are close enough that most people can walk from home (The Sightline Institute, 2008)

Research has found that one's environment is a significant factor in health promotion. Adults and adolescents living in neighborhoods with high walkability engage in significantly more walking and cycling than those living in neighborhoods with low walkability (Frank, 2005; Saelens et al., 2003).

How much exercise do I need? What counts as exercise? Nurses in the community hear these questions commonly as they educate the public on the need to increase physical activity. The answers to these questions will depend on the age, physical condition, and gender of the client. The CDC website at www.cdc.gov/physicalactivity/everyone/guidelines/index.html presents the amount of exercise recommended for adults and children. Videos on the website further explain and illustrate the use of these guidelines. People may feel overwhelmed by the idea that they must add one more demand to an already busy schedule, and some think "I'm in such bad shape, I'll never be able to exercise." The most important idea is that one must take a first step to try exercise. Walking, biking, taking the stairs, swimming—there is something for everyone, and *any* exercise is better than none. Exercise may also be broken up into smaller blocks of time during the day if it is not possible or convenient to do it all at once. Physical activity can also be a family affair, with the entire family using the time to reconnect and have fun together.

Sleep

Sleep is an essential component of chronic disease prevention and health promotion, yet 74% of adults report having a sleeping problem one or more nights per week. One quarter of the U.S. population reports that they occasionally do not get enough sleep, 39% report getting less than 7 hours of sleep per night, and 37% report being so sleepy during the day that it interferes with daily activities. Insufficient sleep is associated with diabetes, heart disease, obesity, and depression. Insufficient sleep contributes to 100,000 motor vehicle crashes each year and 15,000 deaths. Sleep requirements change as people age (Figure 4-9), and, depending on life circumstances, one may require more than the minimum hours listed. If a person is so tired or sleepy that it interferes with his or her daily activities, that person probably needs more sleep (National Sleep Foundation, nd).

How Much Sleep Do You Really Need?	
Age	Sleep needs
Newborns (1-2 months)	10.5-18 hours
Infants (3-11 months)	9-12 hours during night and 30-minute to two-hour naps, one to four times a day
Toddlers (1-3 years)	12-14 hours
Preschoolers (3-5 years)	11-13 hours
School-aged children (5-12 years)	10-11 hours
Teens (11-17)	8.5-9.25 hours
Adults	7-9 hours
Older adults	7-9 hours

FIGURE 4-9 How much sleep do we really need? (Used with permission of the National Sleep Foundation: For further information, please visit www.sleepfoundation.org/how-much-sleep-do-we-really-need.)

As we age, sleep is often interrupted by pain, trips to the bathroom, medications, medical conditions, and sleep disorders. In order to get enough sleep, we must plan to set aside enough time for sleep. Preferably, this means that we can awaken naturally, without an alarm clock, ensuring adequate rest. The need for sleep is regulated by two processes. One is the number of hours we are awake. The longer we are awake, the stronger the desire is to sleep. The other process is the circadian biological clock in the brain, the suprachiasmatic nucleus (SCN), that responds to light. This makes us tend to be sleepy at night when it is dark and active during the day when it is light. The circadian rhythm is why we are sleepiest between 2:00 and 4:00 AM and 1:00 and 3:00 PM. The circadian rhythm also regulates the 24-hour cycle of the body. While we sleep, important hormones are released, memory is consolidated, blood pressure is decreased, and kidney function changes (National Sleep Foundation, nd).

Practicing sleep hygiene will help achieve optimum sleep:
1. Avoid caffeine and nicotine close to bedtime.
2. Avoid alcohol as it can cause sleep disruptions.
3. Retire and get up at the same time everyday.
4. Exercise regularly, but finish all exercise and vigorous activity at least 3 hours before bedtime.
5. Establish a regular, relaxing bedtime routine (a warm bath, reading a book).
6. Create a dark, quiet, cool sleep environment.
7. Have a comfortable mattress and bedding.
8. Use the bed for sleep only; do not read, listen to music, or watch TV in bed.
9. Avoid large meals before bedtime. (National Sleep Foundation, nd)

Sleep assessment is an important nursing function. If a client reports snoring, apnea, restlessness, or insomnia, he or she may have a sleep disorder. Recommend keeping a sleep log detailing how many hours are spent in sleep each night and any problems with sleep. If insufficient sleep is causing trouble concentrating or completing daily activities, recommend consulting a doctor, as a sleep disorder may be to blame. A sleep assessment tool and a list of sleep disorders and descriptions of each may be found at the National Sleep Foundation's website at http://www.sleepfoundation.org/article/how-sleep-works/let-sleep-work-you.

SUMMARY

Health promotion is an essential component to ongoing good health and well-being, yet many Americans have difficulty with one or more of the components of health promotion.

Exercise, diet, sleep, and tobacco and alcohol use all affect our health. Nurses, particularly community health nurses, are in a position to assess and counsel clients on their health habits. Community health nurses also possess the unique combination of community familiarity and knowledge and training to impact health at the policy level. As the environment is made safer and more walkable, or with a lower density of available alcohol or fast food, the community as a whole will benefit.

LEARNING ACTIVITIES

1. How has *Healthy People* changed? Get to know the *Healthy People 2020* proposed objectives at www.healthypeople.gov/hp2020/objectives/TopicAreas.aspx. Read over the new objectives and compare them with the *Healthy People 2010* objectives at www.healthypeople.gov/About/.
2. How did Americans do in meeting *Healthy People 2010* objectives? Choose a focus area from *Healthy People 2010*, and access the periodic reviews for *Healthy People 2010* at www.healthypeople.gov/data/PROGRVW/. Was progress made toward achieving the objectives for this focus area? What are the challenges to meeting the objectives? What are the strategies for meeting the objectives? Did the objective change for *Healthy People 2020*?
3. How is your community doing compared with other communities? Prevalence and incidence rates for diseases or health conditions allow us to make comparisons between communities. Rates of activities such as smoking and physical activity allow us to make comparisons between communities regarding other areas of health promotion. Consider a community of which you are a member (e.g., your state, your county, your age group, or your school). Choose a health promotion topic that is of particular importance to your community of interest such as sexual health, obesity, communicable disease, or physical activity. How does your community compare with a similar community in a different area of the state or the country? How does your community compare with a similar community in another part of the world?
4. How do people, groups, and populations meet health goals? Interview someone who is successful at meeting his or her health promotion goals. For example: How did the person manage to keep his or her weight at a healthy level? How did the person stop smoking? How does he or she make time to exercise daily? Does the individual have a philosophy of health that helps him or her stay on track with health promotion goals? How does the individual incorporate health promotion into daily life? What advice does he or she have for others striving to achieve better health?

REFERENCES

American Cancer Society: *Guide to quitting smoking. Prevention and early intervention*, January 12, 2009 (website): www.cancer.org/docroot/PED/content/PED_10_13X_Guide_for_Quitting_Smoking.asp?from=fast. Accessed April 2, 2009.

American Lung Association: *Quit smoking*, nd (website): www.lungusa.org/site/c.

dvLUK9O0E/b.33484/k.438A/Quit_Smoking.htm. Accessed April 2, 2009.

Benson H: *Timeless healing: The power and biology of belief*, New York, 1996, Scribner.

Bowman S, Vineyard B: Fast-food consumers vs non-fast-food consumers: a comparison of their energy intakes, diet quality, and overall weight status, *J Am Coll Nutr* 23:163–168, 2004.

Burger KS, Kern M, Coleman KJ: Characteristics of self-selected portion sizes in young adults [electronic version], *J Am Diet Assoc* 107:611–608, 2007.

Centers for Disease Control and Prevention: *Do increased portion sizes affect how much we eat? Nutrition resources for health professionals*, May 2006 (website): www.cdc.gov/nccdphp/

dnpa/nutrition/pdf/portion_size_research.pdf. Accessed April 20, 2009.

Centers for Disease Control and Prevention: *Health behaviors of adults: United States, 2002–2004*, September 2006 (website): www.cdc.gov/nchs/data/series/sr_10/sr10_230.pdf. Accessed May 5, 2009.

Centers for Disease Control and Prevention: *Smokeless tobacco. Smoking and tobacco use*, April 27, 2007 (website): www.cdc.gov/tobacco/data_statistics/fact_sheets/smokeless/smokeless_tobacco.htm. Accessed April 27, 2009.

Centers for Disease Control and Prevention: *Adult cigarette smoking in the United States: current estimates (updated 2007). Smoking and tobacco use*, November 11, 2007 (website): www.cdc.gov/mmwr/preview/mmwrhtml/mm5644a2.htm. Accessed April 1, 2009.

Centers for Disease Control and Prevention: *Cessation fact sheet. Smoking and tobacco use*, April 2008 (website): www.cdc.gov/tobacco/data_statistics/fact_sheets/cessation/cessation2.htm. Accessed April 2, 2009.

Centers for Disease Control and Prevention: *US obesity trends 1985–2007. Overweight and obesity*, July 24, 2008 (website): www.cdc.gov/nccdphp/dnpa/obesity/trend/maps/index.htm. Accessed April 19, 2009.

Centers for Disease Control and Prevention: *General information on alcohol and health*, August 6, 2008 (website): www.cdc.gov/alcohol/quickstats/general_info.htm. Accessed May 4, 2009.

Centers for Disease Control and Prevention: *Alcohol and public health*, September 3, 2008a (website): www.cdc.gov/alcohol/index.htm. Accessed May 1, 2009.

Centers for Disease Control and Prevention: *Quick stats: age 21 legal minimun drinking age. Alcohol and public health*, September 3, 2008b (website): www.cdc.gov/alcohol/quickstats/mlda.htm. Accessed May 4, 2009.

Centers for Disease Control and Prevention: *Incorporating eaten-away-from-home food into a healthy eating plan. Nutrition resources for health professionals*, December 22, 2008 (website): www.cdc.gov/nccdphp/dnpa/nutrition/pdf/r2p_away_from_home_food.pdf. Accessed April 13, 2009.

Centers for Disease Control and Prevention: *Overweight and obesity: an overview. Overweight and obesity*, January 28, 2009 (website): www.cdc.gov/nccdphp/dnpa/obesity/contributing_factors.htm. Accessed April 20, 2009.

Centers for Disease Control and Prevention: *Overweight prevalence*, April 2, 2009 (website): www.cdc.gov/nchs/fastats/overwt.htm. Accessed April 20, 2009.

Centers for Disease Conrol and Prevention, National Center for Chronic Disease Prevention and Health Promotion: *Fruit and vegetable consumption per day, nationwide—2007. Nutrition information for health professionals*, November 6, 2008 (website): apps.nccd.cdc.gov/5ADaySurveillance/displayV.asp. Accessed April 13, 2009.

Finnigan JR, Vinswanath K: Communication theory and health behavior change. In Glanz KR, Rimer BK, Vinswanath K, editors: *Health behavior and health education*, 4th ed, San Francisco, 2008, Jossey-Bass, pp 363–384.

Flegal K, Carroll O, Johnson: Prevalence and trends among US adults, 1999–2000, *JAMA* 288:1723–1727, 2002.

Frank LS: Linking objectively measured physical activity with objectively measured urban form: findings from SMARTRAQ, *Am J Prev Med* (28):117–125, 2005.

Friis R: *Sellers: Epidemiology for public health practice*, London, 2004, Jones and Bartlett.

Green L, Kreuter M: *Health promotion and planning: an educational and environmental approach*, Mountain View, CA, 1991, Mayfield.

Hochbaum G: *Public participation in medical screening programs: a socio-psychological study*, Washington, DC, 1958, U.S. Public Health Service.

Janz NK, Champion VL, Stretcher VJ: The Health Belief Model. In Glanz K, Rimer BK, Lewis FM, editors: *Health behavior and health education: theory, research, and practice*, San Francisco, 2002, Josey-Bass.

The Keystone Center: *The Keystone forum on away-from-home foods: opportunities for preventing weight gain and obesity*, Washington, DC, 2006, The Keystone Center.

Kunst H, Groot L, Latthe K: Accuracy of information on apparently credible websites: survey of five common health topics, *BMJ* (9):581–582, 2002.

McCrory MA, Fuss PJ, Hays NP, et al: Overeating in America: association between restaurant food consumption and body fatness in healthy adult men and women, *Obes Res* 92:564–571, 1999.

McEwen M, Pullis B: *Community-based nursing: an introduction*, St. Louis, 2009.

McGinnis JM, Foege WH: Actual causes of death in the United States, *JAMA* (270):2207–2212, 1993.

McGinnis JM, Foege WH: The immediate and the important, *JAMA* (291):1263–1264, 2004.

Merriam-Webster Online Dictionary: *Health*, March 2009 (website): www.merriam-webster.com/dictionary/health. Accessed March 23, 2009.

Mokdab AH, Marks JS, Stroup DF, et al: Actual causes of death in the United States 2000, *JAMA* (291).1238–1245, 2004.

Montano D, Kasprzyk D: Theory of reasoned action, theory of planned behavior, and the integrated behavioral model. In Glanz KR, editor: *Health behavior and health education: theory, research, and practice*, 4th ed, San Francisco, 2008, Jossey-Bass, pp 67–96.

Moynihan R, Bero L, Ross-Degnan D, Henry D, et al: Coverage by the news media of the benefits and risks of medications [electronic version], *N Engl J Med* (342):1645–1649, 2000.

National Sleep Foundation: *How much sleep do we really need?*, nd http://www.sleepfoundation.org/article/how-sleep-works/how-much-sleep-do-we-really-need. Accessed January 28, 2010.

Ogden C, Carroll C, Curtin LR, et al: Prevalence of overweight and obesity in the United States, 1999–2004, *JAMA* 295:1545–1599, 2006.

Oleckno W: *Essential epidemiology*, Prospect Heights, Ill, 2002, Waveland Press.

Parse R: Health promotion and prevention: two distinct cosmologies, *Nurs Sci Q* (3):101, 1990.

Pender N: *Health promotion and disease prevention*, 3rd ed, Stamford, CT, 1996, Appleton & Lange.

Pender N, Murdaugh CL, Parsons MA: *Health promotion in nursing practice*, 5th ed, Upper Saddle River, NJ, 2006, Pearson.

Saelens B, Salis JF, Black JB, Chen D, et al: Neighborhood-based differences in physical activity: an environment scale evaluation, *Research and Practice* (93):43–54, 2003.

Savitz DR: Methods in chronic epidemiology. In Brownson R.C., Remington P.L., Davis J.R., editor: *Chronic disease epidemiology and control*, Washington, DC, 1998, American Public Health Association, pp 27–54.

Schroder H, Fito M, Cavas M: Association of fast food consumption with energy intake, diet quality, body mass index, and the risk of obesity in a representative Mediterranean population, *Br J Nutr* 98:1274–1280, 2007.

Schwartz J, Byrd-Bredbrenner C: Portion distortion: typical portion sizes selected by young adults, *J Am Diet Assoc* 106:1412–1418, 2006.

The Sightline Institute: *What makes a city walkable? Walkscore: find a walkable place to live*, 2008 (website): www.walkscore.com/rankings/what-makes-a-city-walkable.shtml Accessed May 10, 2009.

Sopczyk D: Technology in education. In Bastable S, editor: *Nurse as educator*, Sudbury, MA, 2008, Jones and Bartlett, pp 515–555.

U.S. Department of Agriculture: *MyPyramid.gov*, April 7, 2009 (website): www.mypyramid.gov/index.html. Accessed April 20, 2009.

U.S. Department of Health and Human Services: *Healthy people 2010: understanding and improving health*, January 30, 2001 (website): www.healthypeople.gov/Document/tableofcontents.htm#under. Accessed April 22, 2009.

U.S. Department of Health and Human Services: *A healthier you*, 2005a (website): www.health.gov/dietaryguidelines/dga2005/healthieryou/contents.htm. Accessed April 14, 2009.

U.S. Department of Health and Human Services: *Dietary guidelines for Americans 2005*, 2005b (website): www.cnpp.usda.gov/Publications/DietaryGuidelines/2005/2005DGPolicy-Document.pdf. Accessed April 20, 2009.

U.S. Department of Health and Human Services: *Health: United States 2008*, Washington, DC, 2009, US Department of Health and Human Services.

Westberg J, Jason H: Fostering healthy behavior: the process. In Woolf SH, Jonas S, Lawrence RS, editors: *Health promotion and disease prevention in clinical practice*, Baltimore, 1996, Williams and Wilkins.

World Health Organization: Health promotion: a discussion document on the concept and principles, *Public Health Rev* 14:245–254, 1986.

World Health Organization: *Mental health*, 2009 (website): www.who.int/topics/mental_health/en/. Accessed March 23, 2009.

Epidemiology

Holly B. Cassells

OBJECTIVES

Upon completion of this chapter, the reader will be able to do the following:

1. Identify epidemiological models used to explain disease and health patterns in populations.
2. Use epidemiological methods to describe the state of health in a community or aggregate.
3. Calculate epidemiological rates in order to characterize population health.
4. Understand the use of epidemiological methods in primary, secondary, and tertiary prevention.
5. Evaluate epidemiological study designs for researching health problems.

KEY TERMS

age-adjustment of rates	epidemiological triangle	proportionate mortality ratio
age-specific rates	epidemiology	rates
analytic epidemiology	incidence rates	risk
attack rates	morbidity rates	risk factor
cause-and-effect relationship	mortality rates	screening programs
crude rates	natural history of disease	standardization of rates
descriptive epidemiology	person-place-time model	surveillance
ecosocial epidemiology	prevalence rate	web of causation

OUTLINE

Use of Epidemiology in Disease Control and Prevention
Calculation of Rates
    Morbidity: Incidence and Prevalence Rates
    Other Rates
Concept of Risk
Use of Epidemiology in Disease Prevention
    Primary Prevention
    Secondary and Tertiary Prevention

    Establishing Causality
    Screening
    Surveillance
Use of Epidemiology in Health Services
Epidemiological Methods
    Descriptive Epidemiology
    Analytic Epidemiology

Epidemiology is the study of the distribution and determinants of health and disease in human populations (Harkness, 1995) and is the principal science of community health practice. It entails a body of knowledge derived from epidemiological research and specialized epidemiological methods and approaches to scientific research. Community health nurses use epidemiological concepts to improve the health of population groups by identifying risk factors and optimal approaches that reduce disease risk. Epidemiological methods are important for accurate community assessment and diagnosis and in planning and evaluating effective community interventions. This chapter discusses the uses of epidemiology and its specialized methodologies.

USE OF EPIDEMIOLOGY IN DISEASE CONTROL AND PREVENTION

Although epidemiology originated in ancient times, formal epidemiological techniques developed in the nineteenth century. Early applications focused on identifying factors associated with infectious diseases and the epidemic spread of disease in the community. Public health practitioners hoped to improve preventive strategies by identifying critical factors in disease development.

Specifically, investigators attempted to identify characteristics of people who had a disease such as cholera or plague and compared them with characteristics of those who remained healthy. These differences might include a broad range of personal factors such as age, gender, socioeconomic status, and health status. Investigators also questioned whether there were differences in the location or living environment of ill people, compared with healthy individuals, and whether these factors influenced disease development. Finally, researchers examined whether common time factors existed (i.e., when people acquired disease). Use of this person-place-time model organized epidemiologists' investigations of the disease pattern in the community (Box 5-1). This study of the amount and distribution of disease constitutes descriptive epidemiology. Identified patterns frequently indicate possible causes of disease that epidemiologists can examine with more advanced epidemiological methods.

In addition to investigating the person, place, and time factors related to disease, epidemiologists examine complex relationships among the many determinants of disease. This investigation of the causes of disease, or etiology, is called analytic epidemiology.

Even before the identification of bacterial agents, public health practitioners recognized that single factors were insufficient to cause disease. For example, while exploring the cholera epidemics in London in 1855, Dr. John Snow collected data about social and physical environmental conditions that might favor disease development. He specifically examined the contamination of local water systems. Snow also gathered information about people who became ill; this included their living patterns, their water sources, their socioeconomic characteristics, and their health status. A comprehensive database helped him develop a theory about the possible cause of the epidemic. Snow suspected that a single biological agent was responsible for the cholera infection, although the organism, *Vibrio cholerae*, was undiscovered. He compared the death rates among individuals using one source of water with those among people using a different water source. This suggested an association between cholera and water quality.

The epidemiologist examines the interrelationships between host and environmental characteristics and uses an organized method of inquiry to derive an explanation of disease. This model of investigation is called the epidemiological triangle because the epidemiologist must analyze the following three elements: agent, host, and environment (Figure 5-1). The development of disease is dependent on the extent of the host's exposure to an agent, the strength or virulence of the agent, and the host's genetic or immunological susceptibility. Disease is also dependent on the environmental conditions existing at the time of exposure, which include the biological, social, political, and physical environment (Table 5-1). The model implies that the rate of disease will change when the balance among these three factors is altered. By examining each of the three elements, a community health nurse can methodically assess a health problem, determine protective factors, and evaluate the factors that make the host vulnerable to disease.

Conditions linked to clearly identifiable agents such as bacteria, chemicals, toxins, and other exposure factors are readily explained by the epidemiological triangle. However, other models that stress the multiplicity of host and environmental interactions have developed, and understanding of disease has progressed. The "wheel model" is an example of such a model (Figure 5-2). The wheel consists of a hub that represents the host and its human characteristics such as genetic makeup, personality, and immunity. The surrounding wheel represents the environment and comprises biological, social, and physical dimensions. The relative size of each component in the wheel depends on the health problem. A relatively large genetic core represents health conditions associated with heredity. Origins of other health conditions may be more dependent on environmental factors (Mausner and Kramer, 1985). This model subscribes to multiple-causation rather than single-causation disease theory; therefore it is more useful for analyzing complex chronic conditions and identifying factors that are amenable to intervention.

BOX 5-1   PERSON-PLACE-TIME MODEL

Person: "Who" factors, such as demographic characteristics, health, and disease status

Place: "Where" factors, such as geographical location, climate and environmental conditions, and political and social environment

Time: "When" factors, such as time of day, week, or month and secular trends over months and years

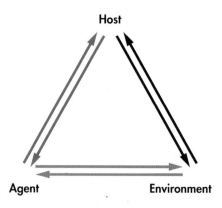

FIGURE 5-1 Epidemiological triangle.

EXAMPLE OF THE EPIDEMIOLOGICAL APPROACH
An early example of the epidemiological approach is John Snow's investigation of a cholera epidemic in the 1850s. He analyzed the distribution of person, place, and time factors by comparing the death rates among people living in different geographical sectors of London.

Snow noted that people using a particular water pump had significantly higher mortality rates resulting from cholera than people using other water sources in the city. Although the cholera organism was yet unidentified, the clustering of disease cases around one neighborhood pump suggested new prevention strategies to public health officials (i.e., that cholera might be reduced in a community by controlling contaminated drinking water sources) (Snow, 1936).

Following the discovery of the causative agents of many infectious diseases, public health interventions eventually resulted in a decline in widespread epidemic mortality, particularly in developed countries. This caused the focus of public health to shift to chronic diseases such as cancer, coronary heart disease, and diabetes during the past few decades. These chronic diseases tend to have multiple interrelated factors associated with their development rather than a single causative agent.

In studying chronic diseases, epidemiologists use methods that are similar to those used in infectious disease investigation, thereby developing theories about chronic disease control. Risk factor identification is of particular importance to chronic disease reduction. Risk factors are variables that

TABLE 5-1   A CLASSIFICATION OF AGENT, HOST, AND ENVIRONMENTAL FACTORS THAT DETERMINE THE OCCURRENCE OF DISEASES IN HUMAN POPULATIONS

AGENTS OF DISEASE—ETIOLOGICAL FACTORS	EXAMPLES
A. Nutritive elements	
Excesses	Cholesterol
Deficiencies	Vitamins, proteins
B. Chemical agents	
Poisons	Carbon monoxide, carbon tetrachloride, drugs
Allergens	Ragweed, poison ivy, medications
C. Physical agents	Ionizing radiation, mechanical
D. Infectious agents	
Metazoa	Hookworm, schistosomiasis, onchocerciasis
Protozoa	Amoebae, malaria
Bacteria	Rheumatic fever, lobar pneumonia, typhoid, TB, syphilis
Fungi	Histoplasmosis, athlete's foot
Rickettsia	Rocky Mountain spotted fever, typhus, Lyme disease
Viruses	Measles, mumps, chicken pox, smallpox, poliomyelitis, rabies, yellow fever, human immunodeficiency virus

HOST FACTORS (i.e., INTRINSIC FACTORS)— SUSCEPTIBILITY OR RESPONSE INFLUENCE EXPOSURE TO AGENT	EXAMPLES
A. Genetic	Cystic fibrosis, Huntington's disease
B. Age	Alzheimer's disease
C. Sex	Rheumatoid arthritis
D. Ethnic group	Tay-Sachs disease, sickle cell disease
E. Physiological state	Fatigue, pregnancy, puberty, stress, nutritional state
F. Prior immunological experience	Hypersensitivity, protection
Active	Prior infection, immunization
Passive	Maternal antibodies, gamma globulin prophylaxis
G. Intercurrent or preexisting disease	Diabetes, liver dysfunction, hypertension
H. Human behavior	Personal hygiene, food handling, diet, interpersonal contact, occupation, recreation, use of health resources, tobacco use

ENVIRONMENTAL FACTORS (i.e., EXTRINSIC FACTORS)—INFLUENCE EXISTENCE OF THE AGENT, EXPOSURE, OR SUSCEPTIBILITY TO AGENT	EXAMPLES
A. Physical environment	Geology, climate
B. Biological environment	
Human populations	Density
Flora	Sources of food, influence on vertebrates and arthropods, as a source of agents
Fauna	Food sources, vertebrate hosts, arthropod vectors
C. Socioeconomic environment	
Occupation	Exposure to chemical agents
Urbanization and economic development	Urban crowding, tension and pressures, cooperative efforts in health and education
Disruption	Wars, floods

Modified from Lilienfeld DE, Stoley PD: *Foundations of epidemiology,* New York, 1994, Oxford University Press.

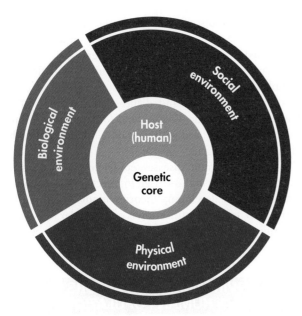

FIGURE 5-2 Wheel model of human-environment interaction. (Redrawn from Mausner JS, Kramer S: *Mausner and Bahn epidemiology: an introductory text,* ed 2, Philadelphia, 1985, Saunders.)

BOX 5-2   CORONARY HEART DISEASE RISK FACTORS SUPPORTED BY EPIDEMIOLOGICAL DATA FROM THE FRAMINGHAM STUDY

- Age
- Gender (male)
- Current cigarette smoking
- Hypertension
- High LDL cholesterol
- Low HDL cholesterol
- (Diabetes)*
- Family history of premature coronary heart disease[†]

From Executive summary of the third report of the National Cholesterol Education Program (NCEP) expert panel on detection, evaluation, and treatment of high blood cholesterol in adults (adult treatment panel III), *JAMA* 285:2486-2497, 2001. *HDL,* High-density lipoprotein; *LDL,* low-density lipoprotein.
*Diabetes is not included in the Framingham Global Risk Score but is now considered to be a coronary heart disease risk equivalent, meaning that persons with diabetes will be treated as intensively as those with coronary heart disease.
[†]Included in NCEP list of major risk factors but not Framingham Global Risk Score.

increase the rate of disease in people who have them (e.g., a genetic predisposition) or in people exposed to them (e.g., an infectious agent or a diet high in saturated fat). Therefore their identification is critical to identifying specific prevention and intervention approaches that effectively and efficiently reduce chronic disease morbidity and mortality. For example, the identification of cardiovascular disease risk factors has suggested a number of lifestyle modifications that could reduce the morbidity risk before disease onset. Primary prevention strategies, such as dietary saturated fat reduction, smoking cessation, and hypertension control, were developed in response to previous epidemiological studies that identified these risk factors (Box 5-2). The web of causation model illustrates the complexity of relationships among causal variables for heart disease (Figure 5-3).

A newer paradigm, ecosocial epidemiology, challenges both the more individually focused risk factor approach to understanding disease origins and the growing interest in molecular epidemiology, exemplified by the sequencing of genes to determine individual susceptibility to various diseases (MacDonald, 2004). This ecological approach emphasizes the role of evolving macro-level socioenvironmental factors, including complex political and economic forces along with microbiological processes, in understanding health and illness. Investigating the context of health will necessitate alternative research approaches, such as qualitative and ecological studies and studies of social institutions and processes. In turn, the examination of social and contextual origins will enlighten the interventions of public health practitioners.

For example, Buffardi and colleagues (2008) analyzed the ecosocial and psychosocial correlates of diagnosis of sexually transmitted infections (STIs) among young adults. Specifically, they examined STI diagnosis within "contextual conditions" including low income, "housing insecurity," childhood physical

or sexual abuse, intimate partner abuse, gang participation, personal history of having been arrested, and drug/alcohol use. It was determined that STIs were statistically associated with housing insecurity, exposure to crime, and having been arrested. Additionally, nearly all of the contextual conditions predicted more lifetime sexual partners and earlier initiation into sexual behavior. The researchers concluded that ecosocial or contextual conditions strongly enhance STI risk by increasing sexual risk behaviors and likelihood of exposure to infection.

In another study, Campbell and others (2009) developed a "comprehensive model" for late-stage diagnosis of breast cancer using data from the national cancer registry. The researchers considered variables of socioeconomic status and poverty indicators, race/ethnicity, and geographical residence (address). They determined that minority and poor women experience more frequent advanced breast cancer at diagnosis. Indeed, both black and Hispanic women are at greater risk for regional and distant-stage diagnosis of breast cancer than white women, and poverty, regardless of race/ethnicity, was strongly associated with the probability of the diagnosis being made at later stages. A final note from the study was that it was important for all researchers to examine health disparities within a "well-defined medical care catchment area."

CALCULATION OF RATES

The community health nurse must analyze data about the health of the community to determine the pattern of disease in a community. The nurse may collect data by conducting surveys or compiling data from existing records (e.g., data from clinic facilities or vital statistics records). Assessment data often are in the form of counts or simple frequencies of events (e.g., the number of people with a specific health condition). Community health practitioners interpret these raw counts by transforming them into rates.

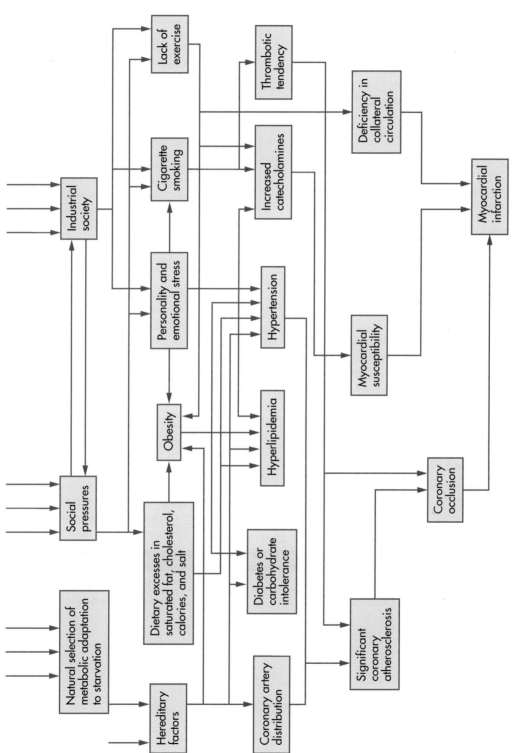

FIGURE 5-3 The web of causation for myocardial infarction: a current view. (From Friedman GD: *Primer of epidemiology*, ed 4, New York, 1994, McGraw-Hill.)

Rates are arithmetic expressions that help practitioners consider a count of an event relative to the size of the population from which it is extracted (e.g., the population at risk). Rates are population proportions or fractions in which the numerator is the number of events occurring in a specified period of time. The denominator consists of those in the population at the specified time period (e.g., per day, per week, or per year). This proportion is multiplied by a constant (k) that is a multiple of 10, such as 1000, 10,000, or 100,000. The constant usually converts the resultant number to a whole number, which is larger and easier to interpret. Thus, a rate can be the number of cases of a disease occurring for every 1000, 10,000, or 100,000 people in the population.

$$\text{Rate} = \frac{\text{Numerator}}{\text{Denominator}} = \frac{\text{Number of health events in a specified period}}{\text{Population in same area in same specified period}} \times k$$

When raw counts are converted to rates, the community health nurse can make meaningful comparisons with rates from other cities, counties, districts, or states; from the nation; and from previous time periods. These analyses assist the nurse in determining the magnitude of a public health problem in a given area and allow more reliable tracking of trends in the community over time (Box 5-3).

Sometimes a ratio is used to express a relationship between two variables. A ratio is obtained by dividing one quantity by another, and the numerator is not necessarily part of the denominator. For example, a ratio could contrast the number of male births to that of female births. Proportions can describe characteristics of a population. A proportion is often a percentage, and it represents the numerator as part of the denominator.

Morbidity: Incidence and Prevalence Rates

The two principal types of morbidity rates, or rates of illness, in public health are incidence rates and prevalence rates. Incidence rates describe the occurrence of new cases of a

TB, Tuberculosis.

disease (e.g., tuberculosis, influenza) or condition (e.g., teen pregnancy) in a community over a period of time relative to the size of the population at risk for that disease or condition during that same time period. The denominator consists of only those at risk for the disease or condition; therefore, known cases or those not susceptible (e.g., those immunized against a disease) are subtracted from the total population (Table 5-2).

$$\text{Incidence rate} = \frac{\text{Number of new cases or events occurring in the population in a specified period}}{\text{Population at risk during same specified period}} \times k$$

The incidence rate may be the most sensitive indicator of the changing health of a community because it captures the fluctuations of disease in a population. Although incidence

TABLE 5-2 EXAMPLES OF RATE CALCULATIONS

MORBIDITY RATES	CRUDE DEATH RATE	SPECIFIC RATES
Incidence Rate $\frac{\text{Number of new cases in given time period}}{\text{Population at risk in same time period}} \times 10{,}000 =$ $\frac{75}{(4000 - 250 \text{ old cases})} = .02$ .02 × 1000 = 20 per 1000 per time period	**Crude Rates** $\frac{\text{Number of deaths in year}}{\text{Total population size}} \times 100{,}000$ $\frac{1720}{200{,}000} = .0086$ .0086 × 100,000 = 860 per 100,000 per year	**Infant Mortality Rate** $\frac{\text{Number of infant deaths} <1 \text{ year of age}}{\text{Number of births in same year}} \times 1000$ $\frac{300}{45{,}000} = .00666$ .00666 × 1000 = 6.66 per 1000 live births
Prevalence Rate $\frac{\text{Number of existing cases}}{\text{Total population}} \times 1000 =$ $\frac{250}{4000} = .0625$ .0625 × 1000 = 62.5 per 1000	**Crude Birth Rate** $\frac{\text{Number of births in year}}{\text{Total population size}} \times 100{,}000$ $\frac{2900}{200{,}000} = .0450$ .0145 × 100,000 = 1450 per 100,000 per year	**Fertility Rate** $\frac{\text{Number of live births}}{\text{Number of women aged 15-44 years}} \times 1000$ $\frac{35{,}000}{500{,}000} = .07$ per women aged 15-44 years .07 × 1000 = 70 per 1000 women aged 15-44 years

rates are valuable for monitoring trends in chronic disease, they are particularly useful for detecting short-term acute disease changes—such as those that occur with infectious hepatitis or measles—when the duration of the disease is typically short.

If a population is exposed to an infectious disease at a given time and place, the nurse may calculate the attack rate, a specialized form of the incidence rate. Attack rates document the number of new cases of a disease in those exposed to the disease. A common example of the application of the attack rate is food poisoning; the denominator is the number of people exposed to a suspect food, and the numerator is the number of people who were exposed and became ill. The nurse can calculate and compare the attack rates of illness among those exposed to specific foods to identify the critical food sources or exposure variables.

A prevalence rate is the number of all cases of a specific disease or condition (e.g., deafness) in a population at a given point in time relative to the population at the same point in time.

$$\text{Prevalence rate} = \frac{\begin{array}{c}\text{Number of existing cases in}\\\text{population at a specified point in time}\end{array}}{\begin{array}{c}\text{Population at same specified point}\\\text{in time}\end{array}} \times k$$

When prevalence rates describe the number of people with the disease at a specific point in time, they are sometimes called point prevalences. For this reason, cross-sectional studies frequently use them. Period prevalences represent the number of existing cases during a specified period or interval of time and include old cases and new cases that develop within the same period of time.

The following factors influence prevalence rates: the number of people who experience a particular condition (i.e., incidence) and the duration of the condition. A nurse can derive the prevalence rate by multiplying incidence by duration ($P = I \times D$). An increase in the incidence rate or the duration of a disease increases the prevalence rate of a disease. With the advent of life-prolonging therapies (e.g., insulin for treatment of type 1 diabetes mellitus), the prevalence of a disease may increase without a change in the incidence rate. Those who survive a chronic disease without cure remain in the "prevalence pot" (Figure 5-4). For conditions such as cataracts, surgical removal permits many people to recover and thereby move out of the prevalence pot. Although the incidence has not necessarily changed, the reduced duration of the disease lowers the prevalence rate of cataracts in the population.

Morbidity rates are not available for many conditions because surveillance of many chronic diseases is not widely conducted. Furthermore, morbidity rates may be subject to underreporting when they are available. Routinely collected birth and death rates, or mortality rates, are more widely available. Table 5-2 provides examples of calculating selected rates.

Other Rates

Numerous other rates are useful in characterizing the health of a population. For example, crude rates summarize the occurrence of births (i.e., crude birth rate), mortality (i.e., crude death rates), or diseases (i.e., crude disease rates) in the general

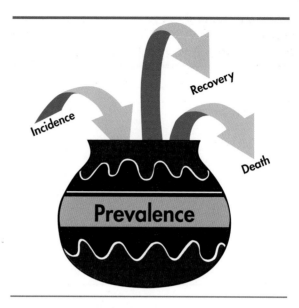

FIGURE 5-4 Prevalence pot: the relationship between incidence and prevalence. (Redrawn from Morton RF, Hebel JR, McCarter RJ: *A study guide to epidemiology and biostatistics,* ed 3, Gaithersburg, MD, 1990, Aspen Publishers.)

population. The numerator is the number of events, and the denominator is the average population size or the population size at midyear (i.e., usually July 1) multiplied by a constant.

The denominators of crude rates represent the total population and not the population at risk for a given event; therefore, these rates are subject to certain biases in interpretation. Crude death rates are sensitive to the number of people at the highest risk for dying. A relatively older population will probably produce a higher crude death rate than a population with a more evenly distributed age range. Conversely, a young population will have a somewhat lower crude death rate. Similar biases can occur for crude birth rates (e.g., higher birth rates in young populations). This distortion occurs because the denominator reflects the entire population and not exclusively the population at risk for giving birth. Age is one of the most common confounding factors that can mask the true distribution of variables. However, many variables, such as race and socioeconomic status, can also bias the interpretation of biostatistical data. Therefore, the nurse may use several approaches for removing the confounding effect of these variables on rates.

Age-specific rates characterize a particular age-group in the population and usually consider deaths and births. Determining the rate for specific subgroups of a population and using a denominator that reflects only that subgroup remove age bias.

$$\text{Age-specific rate} = \frac{\begin{array}{c}\text{Number of cases in a specific age}\\\text{category in population at a}\\\text{specified time}\end{array}}{\begin{array}{c}\text{Population in the same age category at}\\\text{the same specified time}\end{array}} \times k$$

To characterize a total population using age-specific rates, rates for each category must be computed separately. This is because a single summary rate, such as a mean, cannot

TABLE 5-3   COMPARISON OF U.S. MORTALITY RATES—2006 (PRELIMINARY)

DEATH RATE	RATE PER 100,000
Crude death rate	810.3
Age-adjusted death rate	776.4
Age-specific death rates	
Under 1 year (infant)	692.7
1 to 4	28.4
5-14	15.3
15-24	82.0
25-34	106.0
35-44	190.0
45-54	427.1
55-64	890.0
65-74	2062.2
75-84	5117.1
85 and over	13,251.8

From Centers for Disease Control and Prevention, National Center for Health Statistics: Deaths: preliminary data for 2006, *Natl Vital Stat Rep* 56(16):2008: www.cdc.gov/nchs/data/nvsr/nvsr56/nvsr56_16.pdf.

adequately characterize a total population. Specific rates for other variables can be determined in a similar fashion (e.g., race-specific or gender-specific rates) (Table 5-3).

Age-adjustment or standardization of rates is another method of reducing bias when there is a difference between the age distributions of two populations. The nurse uses either the direct method or the indirect standardization method. The direct method selects a standard population, which is often the population distribution of the United States. This method essentially converts age-specific rates for age categories of the two populations to those of the standard population, and it calculates a summary age-adjusted rate for each of the two populations of interest. This enables the nurse to compare the two rates as if both had the standard population's age

structure (i.e., without the prior problem of age distortion). Tables 5-4, 5-5, and 5-6 give examples of the computations.

The second method, indirect standardization, allows the nurse to compare two populations as though they possessed similar age distributions (i.e., it removes the effect of age). This is helpful especially when age-specific rates are unknown or, in direct adjustment, when the nurse must compare many strata. Indirect adjustment involves the calculation of a standardized mortality ratio (SMR), which is a single age-adjusted death ratio that compares the observed deaths with those that would be expected if the population of interest had the mortality experience of the standard population.

$$SMR = \frac{Total\ observed\ deaths}{Total\ expected\ deaths}$$

A ratio of 1 indicates that observed deaths and expected deaths were equal. A ratio greater than 1 indicates that more deaths occurred in the population of interest than expected, based on the standard population's rates. A ratio of less than 1 indicates that fewer deaths occurred in the population of interest than expected based on the standard population's rates. Standardized ratios and rates adjusted using the direct method can be produced for other rates (e.g., birth or morbidity rates) and for other variables (e.g., income or birth weight).

The procedure for calculating a SMR is essentially the reverse of direct standardization (Tables 5-7 and 5-8). First, the nurse applies age-specific rates from a standard population to each age category of the two populations of interest to produce expected deaths for each stratum. The standard population may be the U.S. population, like direct adjustment, or it may be the larger or more stable of the two populations. Second, the nurse divides the actual number of observed deaths by the sum of expected deaths for each population to produce a SMR for each population. Note that age-adjusted rates are actually not "real" death rates; rather, they

TABLE 5-4   DIRECT STANDARDIZATIONS OF MORTALITY RATES BY AGE FOR "SOUTH COMMUNITY" AND "NORTH COMMUNITY"

AGE (YR)	SIZE OF POPULATION (A)	PERCENTAGE OF POPULATION	NUMBER OF DEATHS (B)	AGE-SPECIFIC DEATH RATE PER 1000 (B/A)
South Community*				
<15	5400	30.4	10	1.85/1000
15 to 44	7300	41.1	16	2.19/1000
45 to 64	3400	19.2	38	11.18/1000
>65	1650	9.3	84	50.91/1000
Total	17,750	100	148	
North Community†				
<15	1030	34.2	2	1.94/1000
15 to 44	1500	49.8	4	2.67/1000
45 to 64	407	13.5	4	9.83/1000
>65	75	2.5	4	53.33/1000
Total	3012	100	14	

Step 1: Determine age-specific death rates. Divide the number of deaths by the population size for each age category.

*Crude death rate $= \frac{148}{17,750} = \frac{8.34}{1000}$.

†Crude death rate $= \frac{14}{3012} = \frac{4.64}{1000}$.

TABLE 5-5 DIRECT STANDARDIZATIONS OF MORTALITY RATES

| AGE (YR) | UNITED STATES 1990 | | | SOUTH COMMUNITY* | | NORTH COMMUNITY† | |
	SIZE OF POPULATION	PERCENT OF POPULATION (A)‡	AGE-SPECIFIC DEATH RATE PER 1000 (B₁)	EXPECTED NUMBER OF DEATHS PER 1000 (A × B₁)	AGE-SPECIFIC DEATH RATE PER 1000 (B₂)	EXPECTED NUMBER OF DEATHS PER 1000 (A × B₂)
<15	55,961,000	21.9	1.85	0.405	1.94	0.425
15 to 44	118,490,000	46.5	2.19	1.018	2.67	1.242
45 to 64	48,345,000	19.0	11.18	2.124	9.83	1.868
>65	32,283,000	12.7	50.91	6.466	53.33	6.773
Totals	255,079,000	100		10.013		10.308

Step 2: Compute expected number of deaths by multiplying proportion of United States population by age-specific death rates. Sum expected deaths to produce age-adjusted death rate.

*Age-adjusted mortality rate = $\frac{10,013}{1000}$ (sum of A = B₁)

†Age-adjusted mortality rate = $\frac{10,308}{1000}$ (sum of A = B₂).

‡Convert to decimal before computing product **A × B**.

TABLE 5-6 SUMMARY OF TABLES 5-4 AND 5-5

AREA	CRUDE MORTALITY RATE	AGE-ADJUSTED MORTALITY RATE
South Community	8.34 per 1000	10.013 per 1000
North Community	4.64 per 1000	10.308 per 1000

* When the confounding effect of different age distributions is removed through age adjustment, mortality rates for the two communities are similar.

TABLE 5-8 SMR BASED ON DATA FROM TABLES 5-4 AND 5-7

VARIABLE	SOUTH COMMUNITY	NORTH COMMUNITY
Total observed deaths (from Table 5-4)	148	14
Total expected deaths (totaled from Table 5-7)	124.52	10.21
SMR of death (observed to expected)	1.19	1.37

SMRs of greater than 1 indicate that more deaths were observed in both communities than would be expected on the basis of the mortality experience of the overall U.S. population. When mortality data for the two communities are standardized to a third or standard population, the SMRs indicate a similar mortality experience.

are representations of the experience of populations if their age distributions were similar to the standard population.

The proportionate mortality ratio (PMR) method also describes mortality. It represents the percentage of deaths resulting from a specific cause relative to deaths from all causes. It is often helpful in identifying areas in which public health programs might make significant contributions in reducing deaths. In some situations, a high PMR may reflect a low overall mortality or reduced number of deaths resulting from other causes. Therefore the PMR requires consideration in the context of the mortality experience of the population.

$$PMR = \frac{\text{Number of deaths resulting from a specific cause in a specific time period}}{\text{Total number of deaths in time period}}$$

Table 5-9 summarizes the advantages and disadvantages of crude, specific, and adjusted rates. Numerous other rates assess particular segments of the population. Table 5-10 provides a summary of the major public health rates. A standard epidemiology textbook contains more information.

CONCEPT OF RISK

The concepts of risk and risk factor are familiar to community health nurses whose practices focus on disease prevention. Risk refers to the probability of an adverse

TABLE 5-7 INDIRECT STANDARDIZATION OF MORTALITY RATES

| AGE (YR) | AGE-SPECIFIC U.S. DEATH RATES (A) | POPULATION SIZE (B) | | EXPECTED DEATHS (A × B)/100,000 | |
		SOUTH COMMUNITY	NORTH COMMUNITY	SOUTH COMMUNITY	NORTH COMMUNITY
<15	95.18	5400	1030	5.14	0.98
15 to 44	155.40	7300	1500	11.34	2.33
45 to 64	788.76	3400	407	26.82	3.21
>65	4922.32	1650	75	81.22	3.69

US age-specific mortality rates are multiplied by population of each community to produce expected deaths. These are then summed, and standard mortality ratios are calculated as shown in Table 5-8. Death rates are per 100,000 population.

TABLE 5-9   ADVANTAGES AND DISADVANTAGES OF CRUDE, SPECIFIC, AND ADJUSTED RATES

RATE	ADVANTAGES	DISADVANTAGES
Crude	Actual summary rates Readily calculable for international comparisons (widely used despite limitations)	Populations vary in composition (e.g., age): therefore differences in crude rates are difficult to interpret
Specific	Homogeneous subgroup Detailed rates useful for epidemiological and public health purposes	Cumbersome to compare many subgroups of two or more populations
Adjusted	Summary statements Differences in composition of group "removed," permitting unbiased comparison	Fictional rates Absolute magnitude dependent on chosen standard population Opposing trends in subgroups masked

Modified from Mausner JS, Kramer S: *Mausner and Bahn epidemiology: an introductory text*, ed 2, Philadelphia, 1985, Saunders.

TABLE 5-10   MAJOR PUBLIC HEALTH RATES

RATE DENOMINATOR	RATES	USUAL	FACTOR RATE FOR UNITED STATES, 2005
Total population	Crude birth rate = Number of live births during the year/Average (midyear) population	Per 1000 population	14.0
	Crude death rate = Number of deaths during the year/Average (midyear) population	Per 100,000 population	825.9
	Age-specific death rate = Number of deaths among people of a given age group in 1 yr/Average (midyear) population in specified age group	Per 100,000 population	16.3 (5 to 14 yr) 432 (45 to 54 yr) 2137.1 (65 to 74 yr)
	Cause-specific death rate = Number of deaths from a stated cause in 1 yr/Average (midyear) population	Per 100,000 population	220 (Heart diseases) 188.7 (Malignant neoplasms)
Women aged 15 to 44 yr	Fertility rate = Number of live births during 1 year/Number of women aged 15 to 44 yr in same year	Per 1000 women aged 15 to 44 yr	66.7
Live births	Infant mortality rate = Number of deaths in 1 yr of children younger than 1 yr/Number of live births in same year	Per 1000 live births	6.9
	Neonatal mortality rate = Number of deaths in 1 yr of children younger than 28 days/Number of live births in same year	Per 1000 live births	4.5
	Maternal mortality rate (puerperal) = Number of deaths from puerperal causes in 1 yr/Number of live births in same year	Per 100,000 live births	15.1
Live births and fetal deaths	Fetal death rate = Number of fetal deaths in 1 yr/Number of live births in same year	Per 1000 live births and fetal deaths	6.2*
	Perinatal mortality rate = Number of fetal deaths (>28 wk plus infant deaths <7 days)/Number of live births and fetal deaths (>28 wk during the same year)	Per 1000 live births and fetal deaths	6.7*

Modified from Mausner JS, Kramer S: *Mausner and Bahn epidemiology: an introductory text*, ed 2, Philadelphia, 1985, Saunders. Rates from Centers for Disease Control and Prevention, National Center for Health Statistics: *Health, United States, 2008*: www.cdc.gov/nchs/data/hus/hus08.pdf.
*Rates are for 2003.

event (i.e., the likelihood that healthy people exposed to a specific factor will acquire a specific disease). Risk factor refers to the specific exposure factor, such as cigarette smoke, excessive stress, high noise levels, or environmental chemicals. Frequently, the exposure factor is external to the individual. Risk factors may include fixed characteristics of people, such as age, sex, or genetic makeup. Although these intrinsic factors are not alterable, certain lifestyle changes may reduce the effect of these risk factors. For example, positive dietary practices and exercise regimens may modify the effects of the risk factor of aging for certain health conditions. Specifically, calcium and hormonal supplements may reduce the risk of osteoporosis for susceptible women.

Epidemiologists describe disease patterns in aggregates and quantify the effects of exposure to particular factors on the disease rates. To identify specific risk factors, epidemiologists compare rates of disease for those exposed with those not exposed. One method for comparing two rates is subtracting the rate of nonexposed individuals from the exposed. This measure of risk is called the *attributable risk*; it is the estimate of the disease burden in a population. For example, if the rate of non–insulin-dependent diabetes were 5000 per 100,000 people in the obese population (i.e., those weighing more than 120% of ideal body weight) and 1000 per 100,000 people in the nonobese population, the attributable risk of non–insulin-dependent diabetes resulting from obesity would be

$$4000 \text{ per } 100,000 \text{ people (i.e., } \frac{5000}{100,000} - \frac{1000}{100,000}).$$

This means that 4000 cases per 100,000 people may be attributed to obesity. Thus a prevention program designed to reduce obesity could theoretically eliminate 4000 cases per 100,000 people in the population. Attributable risks are particularly important in describing the potential impact of a public health intervention in a community.

A second measure of the excess risk caused by a factor is the *relative risk ratio*. The relative risk is calculated by dividing the incidence rate of disease in the exposed population by the incidence rate of disease in the nonexposed population. In the previous example, a relative risk of 5 was obtained by dividing 5000/100,000 by 1000/100,000. This risk ratio suggests that an obese individual has a fivefold greater risk of diabetes than a nonobese individual. In general, a relative risk of 1 indicates no excessive risk from exposure to a factor; a relative risk of 1.5 indicates a 50% increase in risk; a relative risk of 2 indicates twice the risk; and a relative risk of less than 1 suggests a factor may have a protective effect associated with a reduced disease rate.

The relative risk ratio forms the statistical basis for the risk factor concept. Relative risks are valuable indicators of the excess risk incurred by exposure to certain factors. They have been used extensively in identifying the major causal factors of many common diseases and direct public health practitioners' efforts to reduce health risks.

Community health nurses may apply the concept of relative risk to suspected exposure variables to isolate risk factors associated with community health problems. For example, a community health nurse might investigate an outbreak of probable food-borne illness. The nurse may compare the incidence rate among those exposed to potato salad in a school cafeteria with the incidence rate among those unexposed. The relative risk calculated from the ratio of these two incidence rates indicates the amount of excess risk for disease incurred by eating the potato salad. A community health nurse might also determine the relative risks for other suspected foods and compare them with the relative risk for potato salad. Attack rates are the calculated incidence rates for foods involved in food-borne illnesses. A food with a markedly higher relative risk than other foods might be the causal agent in a food-borne epidemic. The identification of the causal agent, or specific food, is critical to the implementation of an effective prevention program such as teaching proper food-handling techniques.

USE OF EPIDEMIOLOGY IN DISEASE PREVENTION
Primary Prevention
The central goals of epidemiology are describing the disease patterns, identifying the etiological factors in disease development, and taking the most effective preventive measures. These preventive measures are specific to the stage of disease progression or the natural history of disease, from prepathogenesis through resolution of the disease process. When interventions occur before disease development, they are called *primary prevention*. Primary prevention relies on epidemiological information to indicate those behaviors that are protective, or those that will not contribute to an increase in disease, and those that are associated with increased risk.

Two types of activities constitute primary prevention. Those actions that are general in nature and designed to foster healthful lifestyles and a safe environment are called *health promotion*. Actions aimed at reducing the risk of specific diseases are called *specific protection*. Public health practitioners use epidemiological research to understand practices that are likely to reduce or increase disease rates. For example, numerous research studies have confirmed that regular exercise is an important health promotion activity that has positive effects on general, physical, and mental health. Immunizations exemplify specific protection measures that reduce the incidence of particular diseases.

Secondary and Tertiary Prevention
Secondary prevention occurs after pathogenesis. Those measures designed to detect disease at its earliest stage, namely screening and physical examinations that are aimed at early diagnosis, are *secondary prevention*. Interventions that provide for early treatment and cure of disease are also in this category. Again, epidemiological data and clinical trials determining effective treatments are crucial in disease identification. Mammography, guaiac testing of feces, and the treatment of infections and dental caries are all examples of secondary prevention.

Tertiary prevention includes the limitation of disability and the rehabilitation of those with irreversible disease such as diabetes and spinal cord injury. Epidemiological studies examine risk factors affecting function and suggest optimal strategies in the care of patients with chronic advanced disease.

Establishing Causality
As discussed earlier, a principal goal of classic epidemiology is to identify etiological factors of diseases to encourage the most effective primary prevention activities and develop

treatment modalities. During the last few decades, researchers recognized that many diseases have not one but multiple causes. Epidemiologists who examine disease rates and conduct population-focused research often find multiple factors associated with health problems. For example, cardiovascular disease rates may vary by location, ethnicity, and smoking status. Even infectious diseases often require not only an organism but also certain behaviors or conditions to cause exposure. Determining the extent that these correlates represent associative or causal relationships is important for public health practitioners who seek to prevent, diagnose, and treat disease.

The following six criteria establish the existence of a cause-and-effect relationship:

1. *Strength of association:* Rates of morbidity or mortality must be higher in the exposed group than in the non-exposed group. Relative risk ratios, or odds ratios, and correlation coefficients indicate whether the relationship between the exposure variable and the outcome is causal. For example, epidemiological studies demonstrated an elevated relative risk for heart disease among smokers compared with nonsmokers (Doll and Hill, 1956).

2. *Dose-response relationship:* An increased exposure to the risk factor causes a concomitant increase in disease rate. The risk of heart disease mortality is higher for heavy smokers compared with light smokers (Mattson, Pollack, and Cullen, 1987).

3. *Temporally correct relationship:* Exposure to the causal factor must occur before the effect, or disease. For heart disease, smoking history must precede disease development.

4. *Biological plausibility:* The data must make biological sense and represent a coherent explanation for the relationship. Nicotine and other tobacco-derived chemicals are toxic to the vascular endothelium. In addition to raising low-density lipoprotein (LDL) and decreasing high-density lipoprotein (HDL) cholesterol levels, cigarette smoking causes arterial vasoconstriction and platelet reactivity, which contributes to platelet thrombus formation.

5. *Consistency with other studies:* Varying types of studies in other populations must observe similar associations. Numerous studies of different designs have repeatedly supported the relationship between smoking and heart disease.

6. *Specificity:* The exposure variable must be necessary and sufficient to cause disease; there is only one causal factor. Although specificity may be strong causal evidence, this criterion is less important today. Diseases do not have single causes; they have multifactorial origins.

The exposure variable of smoking is one of several risk factors for heart disease. Few factors are linked to a single condition. Smoking is not specific to heart disease alone. It is a causal factor for other diseases such as lung and oral cancers. Further, smoking is not "necessary and sufficient" to the development of heart disease because there are nonsmokers who also have coronary heart disease. Therefore the causal criterion of specificity more frequently pertains to infectious diseases.

Although these criteria are useful in evaluating epidemiological evidence, it is important to note that causality can never be proved and is always a matter of judgment. In reality, absolute causality is only rarely established. Rather, epidemiologists more commonly refer to suggested causal and associated factors. The effect of confounding variables makes it difficult to ascertain true relationships between the exposure and outcome variables. Confounding variables are independently related to both the dependent variable and the independent variable. Therefore, confounding variables may mask the true relationship between the dependent and independent variables. For example, Brunner and others (2008) explained the need to control physical activity when examining the relationship between dietary patterns and coronary heart disease. This is necessary because studies have shown that physical exercise is independently related to both diet (Sanchez et al., 2007; Williams et al., 2005) and heart disease (Blair and Morris, 2009; Pritchard et al., 2002) in some populations. The apparent association between fat intake and heart disease may be attributable to the difference in physical activity between those with and without heart disease. Those with heart disease may tend to have a higher fat intake and a decreased activity level compared with those without heart disease. The outcome is not solely attributable to dietary fat. On the other hand, Buring and Lee (1995) provided an example in which dietary fat is not a confounding variable despite its relation to physical activity. Dietary fat is not a confounder of the relationship of physical exercise and osteoporosis because dietary fat is not a risk factor for the dependent variable of osteoporosis.

By measuring the confounding variable, the researcher can statistically account for its effect in the analysis (e.g., by using multiple logistical regression analysis or stratification). A biostatistics text contains a discussion of these methods. Alternatively, matching subjects in treatment and control groups with respect to the confounding variable minimizes the effects of the confounder. Again, standardization for variables such as age is another method for managing spurious associations, which makes true relationships more apparent. An understanding of such relationships facilitates the practitioners' interpretation and application of findings.

Screening

Again, a central aim of epidemiology is to describe the course of disease according to person, place, and time. Observations of the disease process may suggest factors that aggravate or ameliorate its progress. This information also assists in determining effective treatment and rehabilitation options (i.e., secondary or tertiary prevention approaches).

The purpose of screening programs is to identify risk factors and diseases in their earliest stages. Screening is usually a secondary prevention activity because indications of disease appear *after* a pathological change has occurred. In all forms of secondary and tertiary prevention, the identification of illness prompts the nurse to consider which forms of upstream prevention could have affected disease development.

Community health nurses commonly conduct screening programs. A community health nurse may devote a large portion of his or her work activities to performing physical examinations, promoting client self-examination, or conducting screening programs in schools, clinics, or community settings. Although these secondary prevention activities are important services that provide vital information on community health status, they focus on detecting existing disease. Nurses should contrast secondary prevention activities with primary prevention and anticipatory guidance, which are hallmarks of community health nursing practice, and which attempt to prevent the development of disease.

There are several guidelines community health nurses should consider for screening programs. First, nurses must plan and execute adequate and appropriate follow-up treatment for patients with disease. Health fairs have been criticized for the lack of consistent follow-up of screening activities. Second, in the planning phase, the nurse should determine whether early disease diagnosis constitutes a real benefit to clients in terms of increased life expectancy or quality of life. Third, a critical prerequisite to screening is the existence of acceptable and medically sound treatment and follow-up. In the past, public health providers have debated the ethical and practical arguments for implementing widespread human immunodeficiency virus (HIV) screening. Concern exists regarding the potential for stigma and discrimination against those who screen positively for a test; therefore, those implementing screening programs should establish procedures for ensuring confidentiality. These procedures, in conjunction with the development of effective antiviral treatments, have encouraged earlier identification of HIV-positive individuals.

A screening program's procedures must also be cost-effective and acceptable to clients. Although colonoscopy is a common and effective screening procedure for colon cancer, it is neither simple nor inexpensive. Although it is recommended periodically for all Americans with no known risk factors beginning at age 50, only about 43% of that group have undergone the procedure (Centers for Disease Control and Prevention [CDC], 2008). Finally, a nurse should consider whether or not to screen a population on the basis of the significant costs for screening programs and procedures, follow-up for clients who test positive, and subsequent medical care (Box 5-4).

When developing a screening program, the community health nurse also must evaluate issues specific to the validity of the screening test. Detecting clients with disease is the purpose of screening, and *sensitivity* is the test's ability to do this correctly. Conversely, *specificity* is the extent to which a test can correctly identify those who do not have disease. To obtain estimates of these two dimensions, the nurse must compare screening results with those of some definitive diagnostic procedure (Mausner and Kramer, 1985). For a given test, the sensitivity and specificity tend to be inversely related to each other. When a test is highly sensitive, individuals without disease may be labeled positive. These false-positive tests may cause stress and worry for clients and require further diagnostic testing to confirm a diagnosis. With a highly sensitive test, specificity may be lower and the test may not detect disease in some clients. These false-negative test results mean that some individuals may receive false reassurance and will not receive follow-up care.

BOX 5-4   GUIDELINES FOR SCREENING PROGRAMS

- Screen for conditions in which early detection and treatment can improve disease outcome and quality of life.
- Screen populations that have risk factors or are more susceptible to the disease.
- Select a screening method that is simple, safe, inexpensive to administer, acceptable to clients, and has acceptable sensitivity and specificity.
- Plan for the timely referral and follow-up of positive cases.
- Identify referral sources that are appropriate, cost-effective, and convenient for clients.

Optimally, a screening test should be maximally sensitive and specific. To a large extent, this depends on the stringency of the cutoff point established for determining a positive disease case. For example, with an established high blood pressure criterion of 140/90 mm Hg, more people will have high blood pressure than with a cutoff of 150/90 mm Hg. The lower cutoff is more sensitive and will lead to more false positives. The higher criterion may be more specific, and, although fewer people will be hypertensive, there will be fewer false-positive cases than with the lower cutoff level. Table 5-11 includes the formula for calculating sensitivity and specificity.

Sensitivity and specificity reflect the *yield* of a screening test, which is the amount of detected disease. One measure of yield is the *positive predictive value* of a test, which is the proportion of true positive results relative to all positive test results. On the basis of Table 5-11, the formula is $\frac{a}{a+b}$. The positive predictive value is dependent on the prevalence of undetected disease in a population. Screening for a rare disease such as phenylketonuria will yield a lower predictive value and more false-positive results. In phenylketonuria, a low predictive value is acceptable because the false-negative result has very serious consequences. The predictive value is also affected by the nature of the screened population. Screening only the individuals at high risk for a disease will produce a higher predictive value and can be a more efficient way to identify those with health problems. For example, diabetes screening in an American Indian, Mexican-American, or African-American adult population should produce a higher predictive value than screening the general adult population.

TABLE 5-11   SENSITIVITY AND SPECIFICITY OF A SCREENING TEST

SCREENING TEST	THOSE WITH DISEASE	THOSE WITHOUT DISEASE
Positive	True positives (a)	False positives (b)
Negative	False negatives (c)	True negatives (d)

$$\text{Sensitivity (in percent)} = \frac{\text{True positives}}{\text{All with disease}} = \frac{(a)}{(a+c)} \times 100.$$

$$\text{Specificity (in percent)} = \frac{\text{True negatives}}{\text{All without disease}} = \frac{(d)}{(b+d)} \times 100.$$

Surveillance

In addition to screening, surveillance is a mechanism for the ongoing collection of community health information. Monitoring for changes in disease frequency is essential to effective and responsive public health programs. Identifying trends in disease incidence or identifying risk factor status by location and population subgroup over time allows the community health nurse to evaluate the effectiveness of existing programs and implement interventions targeted to high-risk groups. Again, identifying new cases for calculating incidence rates is particularly useful in evaluating morbidity trends. However, this form of surveillance data is more difficult to collect, and public health practitioners can access the data only for selected diseases. Prevalence rates, mortality data, risk factor data, and hospital and health service data can help indicate a program's successes or deficiencies.

The CDC coordinates a system of data collection among federal, state, and local agencies. These groups compile numerous sets of data and base some of these data sets on the entire population (e.g., vital statistics data) and other collections on subsamples of the population (e.g., the National Health Interview Survey). The completeness of data reporting is variable because not all diseases are reportable. For example, practitioners are required to report only four sexually transmitted diseases (i.e., acquired immunodeficiency syndrome [AIDS], syphilis, gonorrhea, and chlamydia) to local and state health departments. Furthermore, not all practitioners report cases on a regular basis and not all people with sexually transmitted diseases actually seek care. Studies have indicated that practitioners also underreport childhood communicable diseases, such as chickenpox and mumps. The CDC conducts studies that estimate the magnitude of this underreporting problem.

Practitioners have a continuing need for comprehensive and systematically collected surveillance data that describe the health status of national and local subgroups. They use this information to evaluate the impact of programs on specific groups in a community.

For example, the effectiveness of *Healthy People 2010* and *Healthy People 2020* depends on the availability of reliable baseline and continuing data to characterize health problems and evaluate goal achievement as listed in the *Healthy People 2020* table. *Healthy People 2020* (U.S. Department of Health and Human Services, 2009) recognizes the ongoing need to extend the inclusiveness of such data collection systems. For example, simply documenting children's mortality rates resulting from injury is insufficient for the development of specific methods of injury prevention. Data on the number of injured children and the nature of injury (e.g., motor vehicle accidents, drowning, abuse) across the nation would increase the usefulness of surveillance information.

Nurses need to describe trends in health and illness by a community's locale, demographics, and risk factor status to intervene effectively on behalf of communities. They must compare the data for their locale with those of a relevant neighboring area (e.g., a census tract, city, county, state, or nation) to gain perspective on the magnitude of a local problem. Ideally, the nurse should have access to surveillance data at several different levels over a period of time. In some instances, community health nurses find it necessary to construct their own surveillance systems that are tailored to specific health conditions or programs in a community. These smaller data collection systems help nurses evaluate programs when the data are readily accessible and compatible with data from large city or statewide surveillance systems.

HEALTHY PEOPLE 2020

Objectives for Data Collection and Reporting

PHI HP2020–3: Increase the proportion of population-based *Healthy People 2020* objectives for which national data are available for all major population groups.
PHI HP2020–4: Increase the proportion of *Healthy People 2020* objectives that are tracked regularly at the national level.
PHI HP2020–5: Increase the proportion of *Healthy People 2020* objectives for which national data are released within one year of the end of data collection.
PHI HP2020–13: Increase the percentage of vital events (births, deaths, fetal deaths) reported using the latest U.S. standard certificates of birth and death and the report of fetal death.

From U.S. Department of Health and Human Services: *Healthy People 2020*: 2009 draft objectives. Accessed April 6, 2010 from: www.healthypeople.gov/HP2020/Objectives/TopicAreas.aspx

Clinical Example

In April 1991, a cluster of six neural tube defects (NTDs) occurred in babies born in Brownsville, Texas, within a span of 6 weeks. Further investigation in Cameron County indicated a rate of 27.1 cases per 10,000 live births compared with 14.7 for babies conceived from 1986 to 1989 and compared with the U.S. rate of approximately 8 per 10,000. This rate was more than three times the national rate and represented an increased risk in Hispanic women. This increased risk was partially attributable to cultural and environmental factors, including lower socioeconomic status and migrant farm work. The investigators implemented a surveillance program that included fetuses of less than 20 weeks' gestation, which obtained more accurate population-based data. Additionally, the program implemented folic acid supplementation in Texas counties along the Mexican border. From 1993 to 1996, NTD rates dropped to 13 per 10,000 following supplementation.

Research suggests that 50% to 70% of NTDs may be preventable with folic acid supplementation. This finding supports the fortification of bread and cereal products; in January 1998, the Food and Drug Administration mandated the addition of 140 mcg of vitamin B per 100 g of most grain products. It is estimated that there has been a 24% reduction in the number of NTDs since grain fortification with folic acid began.

Reducing Infant Mortality Rates Using the Perinatal Periods of Risk Model

Infant mortality rates are an accepted indicator for measuring a nation's health. The rate is representative of the health status and social well-being of any nation. Despite decreases in the past 50 years, infant mortality rates in the United States remain higher than in other industrialized countries. Using overall infant mortality rates to determine the effectiveness of interventions does not help communities focus on particular underlying factors contributing to the rates. Targeting interventions to the factors most responsible for the infant mortality rate should help reduce the rate more rapidly and effectively. This study was designed to determine and rank contributing factors to fetal-infant mortality in a specific community using the perinatal periods of risk (PPOR) model.

The PPOR model provides direction, focus, and suggestions for effective interventions. The model helps users identify and rank four factors as they contribute to the overall infant mortality rate: (a) mother's health before and between pregnancies, (b) maternal health care systems, (c) neonatal health care systems, and (d) infant health during the first year of life. The PPOR model is based on two major theoretical constructs: age of fetus-infant at death and birth weight. The PPOR model maps each death in a geographic region based on birth weight and age at death, including fetal, neonatal, and postneonatal periods. The lowest birth weight infant deaths are combined into one cell named the maternal health cell. The three remaining groups are put into cells suggesting the primary preventive focus for that group: maternal health, newborn health, and infant health. Multiple interventions are important in reducing infant mortality, and the PPOR model guides prioritizing interventions based on the cell contributing the most to infant mortality rates.

The PPOR model was used to map fetal-infant mortality for 1995 to 1998 in Tulsa County, Oklahoma, as compared with traditional calculation methods. The overall fetal-infant mortality rate using the PPOR model was 12.7 compared with 7.11 calculated using the traditional method. The PPOR calculation helped clearly distinguish which factor was contributing the most to the overall fetal-infant mortality rate. The maternal health cell was contributing 42% to the overall rate in Tulsa County. Because the highest infant mortality was in the maternal health cell, intervention strategies were designed to promote the health of women prior to and between pregnancies. The PPOR model is a useful tool for community partnerships to use in targeting actions for the population groups contributing most to infant mortality rates.

From Burns PG: Reducing infant mortality rates using the perinatal periods of risk model, *Public Health Nurs* 22(1):2-7, 2005.

Dietary intake alone may be insufficient; therefore, the Centers for Disease Control and Prevention recommend that all women of reproductive age consume 400 mcg (0.4 mg) to 800 mcg (0.8 mg) of folic acid daily from a combination of dietary sources such as cereal or grain products, leafy green vegetables, and vitamin supplements.

Data from Centers for Disease Control and Prevention: *Spina bifida,* 2005: www.cdc.gov/ncbddd/birthdefects/SpinaBifida.htm and Centers for Disease Control and Prevention: Neural tube defects in Texas, *Dis Prev News* 58(2):5-6, 1998; Centers for Disease Control and Prevention: Neural tube defect surveillance and folic acid intervention—Texas-Mexico border, 1993-1998, *MMWR Morb Mortal Wkly Rep* 49(1):1-4, 2000: www.cdc.gov/mmwr/preview/mmwrhtml/mm4901a1.htm.

Again, epidemiologists describe the course of disease over time. These secular trends are changes that occur over years or decades, such as the decline in uterine cancer and the increase in breast cancer. Frequently, epidemiologists document the associated patterns of treatment and intervention. In many instances, studies conducted by clinical epidemiologists provide this information. Cancer registries are a form of surveillance that document the prevalence and incidence of cancer in a community and document its course, treatment, and associated survival rates. The Surveillance, Epidemiology and End Results (SEER) program of the National Cancer Institute compiles national cancer data from existing cancer registries covering approximately 26% of the U.S. population (National Cancer Institute, 2006).

Public health practitioners need to conduct community surveys of population segments to plan for the sector's health. For example, a survey of the disabled population that assesses prevalence may also evaluate the adequacy of present services and project future needs.

USE OF EPIDEMIOLOGY IN HEALTH SERVICES

Presented epidemiological approaches can be used to describe the distribution of disease and its determinants in populations. However, epidemiological principles are also useful in studying population health care delivery and in describing and evaluating the use of community health services. For example, determining the ratio of health care providers to population size helps assess the system's ability to provide care. The clients' reasons for seeking care, the clients' payment methods, and the clients' satisfaction are also informative. Regardless of whether community health nurses or health services researchers collected these data, the information is essential for those who strive to improve clients' access to quality health care.

HEALTH SERVICES EPIDEMIOLOGY

Health services epidemiology focuses on the population's health care patterns. In particular, public health practitioners are concerned with the accessibility and affordability of services and the barriers that may contribute to excess morbidity in at-risk groups. Traditionally, children are a vulnerable group, and they are a particular focus of health services research. Studies examining poverty rates and care access have underscored the need to expand insurance coverage to those who do not have private medical insurance and do not qualify for Medicaid programs or the State Children's Health Insurance Program (SCHIP).

Ultimately, nurses must apply epidemiological findings in the practice arena. It is essential that they incorporate study results into prevention programs for communities and at-risk populations. Further, the philosophy of public health and epidemiology dictates that nurses extend its application into major health policy decisions, because the aim of health policy planning is to achieve positive health goals and outcomes for improved societal health.

A goal of policy development is to bring about desirable social changes. Epidemiological factors, history, politics, economics, culture, and technology influence policy development. The complex interaction of these factors may explain the slow application of epidemiological knowledge. Lung disease in the United States exemplifies the incomplete progress in implementing effective health policy. In the early 1950s, studies identified and conclusively linked cigarette smoking to lung cancer and heart disease (Doll and Hill, 1952). Since the 1950s, protective public policies have included cigarette taxes, cigarette warning labels, smoking restrictions in public areas, smoke-free workplaces, and restrictions on selling tobacco to minors.

In summary, there remain many public policies that public health practitioners and epidemiologists have yet to modify in the interest of improved health. Community health nurses should exercise "societal responsibility" in applying epidemiological findings, but this will require the active involvement of the citizen consumer. Community health nurses collaborating with community members can combine epidemiological knowledge and aggregate-level strategies to affect change on the broadest scale.

EPIDEMIOLOGICAL METHODS

Descriptive Epidemiology

Descriptive epidemiology focuses on the amount and distribution of health and health problems within a population. Its purpose is to describe the characteristics of both people who are protected from disease and those who have a disease. Factors of particular interest include age, sex, ethnicity or race, socioeconomic status, occupation, and family status. Epidemiologists use morbidity and mortality rates to describe the extent of disease and to determine the risk factors that make certain groups prone to acquiring disease.

In addition to "person" characteristics, the place of occurrence describes disease frequency. For example, certain parasitic diseases, such as malaria and schistosomiasis, occur in tropical areas. Other diseases may occur in certain geopolitical entities. For example, gastroenteritis outbreaks often occur in communities with lax water quality standards. Time is the third parameter that helps define disease patterns. Epidemiologists may track incidence rates over a period of days or weeks (e.g., epidemics of infectious disease) or over an extended period of years (e.g., secular trends in the cancer death rate).

These person, place, and time factors can form a framework for disease analysis and may suggest variables associated with high versus low disease rates. Descriptive epidemiology can then generate hypotheses about the cause of disease, and analytic epidemiology approaches can test these hypotheses (Box 5-5).

BOX 5-5   AN EXAMPLE OF DESCRIPTIVE EPIDEMIOLOGY

- The **P**erson-**P**lace-**T**ime **M**odel is illustrated by an outbreak of hepatitis C at an outpatient hemodialysis unit in New York.
  - *Person:* Initially, three patients undergoing hemodialysis were reported to have seroconverted from anti–hepatitis C virus (HCV) negative to anti-HCV positive during a 3-month period. Six additional patients at the facility, of 162 patients, were subsequently determined to have been infected.
  - *Place:* A large, for-profit, outpatient hemodialysis unit that treats 70 to 100 patients per day.
  - *Time:* The cases were diagnosed during the first half of 2008; subsequent epidemiological investigation reviewed data from 2001, notifying previous patients of their need to be tested.

From Centers for Disease Control and Prevention: Hepatitis C virus transmission at an outpatient hemodialysis unit—New York, 2001-2008, *MMWR Morb Mortal Wkly Rep* 58(8):189-194, 2009: www.cdc.gov/mmwr/preview/mmwrhtml/mm5808a2.htm.

Analytic Epidemiology

Analytic epidemiology investigates the causes of disease by determining why a disease rate is lower in one population group than in another. This method tests hypotheses generated from descriptive data and either accepts or rejects them on the basis of analytic research. The epidemiologist seeks to establish a cause-and-effect relationship between a preexisting condition or event and the disease (see previous section on causality). To determine this relationship, the epidemiologist may undertake two major types of research studies, *observational* and *experimental*.

Observational Studies

Epidemiologists frequently use *observational studies* for descriptive purposes, but they also use them to discover the etiology of disease. The investigator can begin to understand the factors that contribute to disease by observing disease rates in groups of people differentiated by experience or exposure. For example, differences in disease rates may occur in the obese compared with the nonobese, in smokers compared with nonsmokers, and in those with high stress levels compared with those with low stress levels. These characteristics (i.e., obesity, smoking, and stress) are called *exposure variables*.

Unlike experimental studies, observational studies do not allow the investigator to manipulate the specific exposure or experience or to control or limit the effects of other extraneous factors that may influence disease development. For example, life stress is related to depression. People with low socioeconomic status also have high depression rates. People with low socioeconomic status frequently experience greater life stresses; therefore, the confounding factor of socioeconomic status makes it more difficult to demonstrate the effect of stress on depression. The three major study designs used in observational research are cross-sectional, retrospective, and prospective studies.

Time Dimension

Present

Sample: Subjects sampled
from population-at-large at
one point in time

Advantages	Disadvantages
Quick to plan and conduct	Cannot calculate relative risk with prevalence data
Relatively inexpensive	Temporal sequence of factor and outcome unknown
May provide preliminary indication of whether an association between a risk factor and disease exists	
Provides prevalence data needed for planning health services	
Hypothesis generating	

FIGURE 5-5 Cross-sectional, or prevalence, study.

Cross-sectional studies. Cross-sectional studies, some-times called *prevalence* or *correlational* studies, examine relationships between potential causal factors and disease at a specific time (Figure 5-5). Surveys that simultaneously collect information about risk factors and disease exemplify this design. For example, the National Health and Nutrition Examination Survey (NHANES) has collected cross-sectional data regarding current dietary practices, physical status, and health in people ranging from 1 to 72 years of age since the early 1970s (CDC, 2009). Data from the NHANES surveys have been analyzed and compared over the years by a number of researchers and provided important health information.

For example, reports using NHANES data showed that nearly 30% of the U.S. adult population had hypertension (CDC, 2007) and that about 12% of residents of New York City had diabetes (Thorpe et al., 2009). NHANES data also showed that the prevalence of metabolic syndrome among American women was almost 23% and increased markedly with age (Cohen et al., 2006). In another work, Arrieta and Russell (2008) examined data from the initial NHANES survey (1971-1975) and follow-up data in that same cohort and were able to conclude that individuals who reported moderate activity levels had significantly reduced mortality over the next 20 years compared with those with low levels of activity.

Although a cross-sectional study can identify associations among disease and specific factors, it is impossible to make causal inferences because the study cannot establish the temporal sequence of events (i.e., the cause preceded the effect). For example, the NHANES was unable to determine whether high salt intake precedes hypertension—thus making it a causal factor—or whether they are unrelated.

Therefore cross-sectional studies have limitations in discovering etiological factors of disease. These studies can help identify preliminary relationships that other analytic designs may explore further; therefore, they are hypothesis-generating studies.

Retrospective studies. Retrospective studies compare individuals with a particular condition or disease with those who do not have the disease. These studies determine whether cases, or a diseased group, differ in their exposure to a specific factor or characteristic relative to controls, or a nondiseased group. To make unambiguous comparisons, investigators select the cases according to explicitly defined criteria regarding the type of case and the stage of disease. Investigators also select a control group from the general population, which is characteristically similar to the cases (Figure 5-6).

Frequently, people hospitalized for diseases that are not under study become controls if they do not share the exposure or risk factor under study. For example, a researcher may select patients with heart disease to be controls in a study of patients with lung cancer. However, this may introduce serious bias because these patients often share the risk factor of smoking. The methods of data collection must be the same for both groups to prevent further introduction of bias into the study. Therefore it is desirable for interviewers to remain unaware of which subjects are cases and which are controls.

In retrospective studies, data collection extends back in time to determine previous exposure or risk factors. Investigators analyze study data by comparing the proportion of subjects with disease, or cases, who possess the exposure or risk factors with the corresponding proportion in the control group. A greater proportion of exposed cases than controls suggests a relationship between the disease and the risk factor.

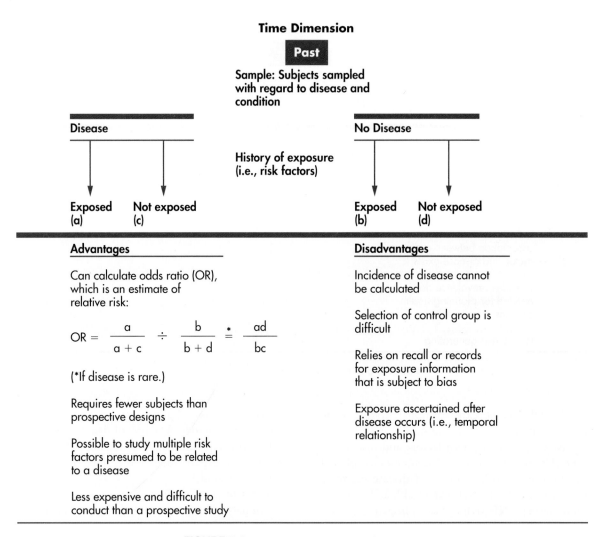

FIGURE 5-6 Retrospective, or case-control, study.

Investigators often use retrospective study designs because these designs address the question of causality better than cross-sectional studies. Retrospective studies also require fewer resources and less data collection time than prospective studies. Many examples of *retrospective,* or *case-control,* studies exist in the literature. One classic example is Doll and Hill's (1952) investigation of risk factors for lung cancer. They compared exposure rates for cases in which lung cancer was diagnosed with those in the control group in whom cancer was diagnosed outside the chest and oral cavity. Doll and Hill recorded detailed smoking histories in all subjects. Compared with the controls, a significantly higher proportion of patients with lung cancer smoked. This study yielded the hypothesis that smoking may be etiologically related to lung cancer.

Prospective studies. Prospective studies monitor a group of disease-free individuals to determine if and when disease occurs (Figure 5-7). These individuals, or the cohort, share a common experience within a defined time period. For example, a birth cohort consists of all people born within a given time period. The study assesses the cohort with respect to an exposure factor associated with the disease and thus classifies it at the beginning of the study. The study then monitors the cohort for disease development. The investigator compares the disease rates for those with a known exposure with rates for those who remain unexposed. The study observes subjects prospectively; therefore it summarizes data collected over time by the incidence rates of new cases (Box 5-6). Again, comparing two incidence rates produces a measure of relative risk.

$$\text{Relative risk} = \frac{\text{Incidence rate among exposed}}{\text{Incidence rate among unexposed}}$$

The relative risk indicates the extent of excess risk incurred by exposure relative to nonexposure. A relative risk of 1 suggests no excess risk resulting from exposure, whereas a relative risk of 2 suggests twice the risk of having disease from exposure.

Prospective studies, or *longitudinal, cohort,* or *incidence* studies, are advantageous because they obtain more reliable information about the cause of disease than do other study methodologies. These studies establish a stronger temporal relationship between the presumed causal factors and the effect than do retrospective and cross-sectional

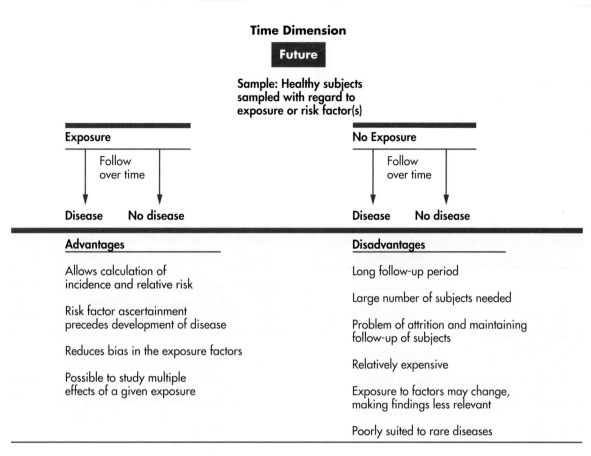

Time Dimension

Future

Sample: Healthy subjects
sampled with regard to
exposure or risk factor(s)

Exposure

Follow
over time

Disease   No disease

No Exposure

Follow
over time

Disease   No disease

Advantages	Disadvantages
Allows calculation of incidence and relative risk	Long follow-up period
Risk factor ascertainment precedes development of disease	Large number of subjects needed
Reduces bias in the exposure factors	Problem of attrition and maintaining follow-up of subjects
Possible to study multiple effects of a given exposure	Relatively expensive
	Exposure to factors may change, making findings less relevant
	Poorly suited to rare diseases

FIGURE 5-7 Prospective, or cohort, study.

studies. Calculations of incidence rates and relative risks provide a valuable indicator of the level of risk that exposure creates.

However, certain disadvantages are inherent in the prospective design. It is costly in terms of resources and staff to monitor a cohort over time, and lengthy studies result in subject attrition. Problems arising from the nature of chronic diseases may compound these logistical dilemmas. Frequently, chronic diseases have long latency periods between exposure and symptom manifestation. Furthermore, the onset of chronic conditions may be sufficiently insidious, which makes it extremely difficult to document the incidence of disease. In

---

⚖ ETHICAL INSIGHTS

The Tuskegee Syphilis Study

In 1932 the U.S. Public Health Service (PHS) began a longitudinal-experimental study of 600 African-American sharecroppers, 399 of whom had syphilis and 201 without the disease. It was conducted in one of the poorest counties of Alabama, and the subjects were unaware that they had syphilis but were told they were being treated for "bad blood." Enticed by the promise of free medical care and meals, the subjects joined the study without knowledge of their disease, its treatment, or the study procedures. The experimental group was initially treated with ineffective doses of the treatments of the time, bismuth or mercury, and later with aspirin. Even when penicillin became available in the late 1940s, they were actively denied treatment. For 40 years, these men were followed by PHS investigators affiliated with the Tuskegee Institute and hospital who claimed to observe the differences in the progression of the disease in blacks, compared with the control group. During the course of the study, many died of syphilis or other causes, numerous wives became infected, and children were born with congenital syphilis. In 1972, a former venereal disease interviewer, Peter Buxtun, blew the whistle on the study, and reports were published in newspapers. Only after the public became outraged about the unethical nature of the study did the Centers for Disease Control and Prevention and the PHS move to end the study. In 1973, the National Association for the Advancement of Colored People (NAACP) won a $10 million class action suit on behalf of the subjects. In 1997, President Bill Clinton formally apologized to the few survivors and their families for the harm inflicted on these men and their families in the name of public health research. The Tuskegee Study raises questions about how a study could proceed without informing and seeking consent of participants, how available treatment could be withheld, and how government researchers could pursue an unethical research plan without periodic review and questioning. Furthermore, the racial and discriminatory issues suggest disturbing questions for researchers and practicing nurses to contemplate, one being that Tuskegee contributes to a legacy of distrust that minorities may harbor toward both the health care delivery system and research programs.

From Centers for Disease Control and Prevention, National Center for HIV/AIDS, Viral Hepatitis, STD, and TB Prevention: *The Tuskegee timeline,* 2005: www.cdc.gov/nchstp/od/tuskegee/time.htm; Infoplease: *The Tuskegee syphilis experiment,* 2005, Pearson Education: www.infoplease.com/ipa/A0762136.html.

addition, many diseases do not have a unifactorial cause (i.e., single variable) because many interacting factors influence disease. These problems do not negate the benefits of prospectively designed epidemiological studies; rather, they suggest a need to carefully plan and tailor the study specifically to the disease and the study's purpose.

The literature contains numerous prospective studies. In many cases, these studies have been instrumental in substantiating causal links between specific risk factors and disease. A classic example is an early Doll and Hill cohort study of lung cancer deaths (1956). Doll and Hill originally completed questionnaires on a cohort of physicians in Great Britain. Next, they classified the subjects according to several variables, emphasizing the number of cigarettes smoked. In 4½ years, they accessed death certificate data. These data revealed a higher mortality rate resulting from lung cancer and coronary thrombosis among smoking physicians compared with nonsmokers. The death rate for heavy smokers was 166 per 100,000 versus 7 per 100,000 for nonsmokers. Combining these two incidence rates in a measure of excess risk indicated that heavy smokers were 23.7 times more likely to develop lung cancer than nonsmokers (Relative risk = $\frac{166}{100,000} \div \frac{7}{100,000}$, or 23.7). These findings in a prospective study provided strong epidemiological support for smoking as a risk factor for lung cancer.

Another well-known prospective study is the Framingham Heart Study, which has followed an essentially healthy cohort of Framingham, Massachusetts, residents for more than 50 years. Findings from the study suggested that serum cholesterol level and other risk factors are associated with the future development of cardiovascular disease (Pencina et al., 2009; Kulminski et al., 2008). The Framingham Study and subsequent "Offspring Studies" helped form the basis for later experimental studies aimed at reducing serum cholesterol through diet modification or drug therapy to ultimately lower the incidence rate of coronary heart disease.

The Nurses' Health Study was initiated in 1976 with 122,000 registered nurses with the intent of examining the long-term consequences of oral contraceptives. The initial cohort still returns questionnaires every 2 years, and data have been collected on diet and nutrition, smoking, hormone use, and menopause, as well as various chronic illnesses. In 1989 the Nurses' Health Study II was initiated to study lifestyle issues, contraception, and illness patterns in younger women, and in 2008 a third study was begun looking at similar issues in another cohort.

These studies continue to monitor nurses' changing health status and risk factors and examine factors associated with the development of numerous health conditions such as breast cancer and heart disease (Nurses' Health Study, 2009). For example, research using Nurses' Health Study data has determined that regular use of nonsteroidal anti-inflammatory drugs (i.e., aspirin) does not reduce the incidence of ovarian cancer (Pinheiro et al., 2009) or breast cancer (Eliassen et al., 2009). Similarly, the nurses' health studies indicated there is no evidence that long-term coffee consumption increases the risk of stroke (Lopez-Garcia et al., 2009), but regular consumption of sugar-sweetened beverages does increase the risk of coronary heart disease (Fung et al., 2009). Last, Whang and others (2009) learned that clinical depression in women was associated with development of coronary heart disease and sudden cardiac death.

Experimental Studies

Another type of analytic study is the experimental design (Figure 5-8). Epidemiological investigations apply experimental methods to test treatment and prevention strategies. The investigator randomly assigns subjects at risk for a particular disease to an experimental or a control group. The investigator observes both groups for the occurrence of disease over time, but only the experimental group receives intervention.

Theoretically, it is possible to introduce an exposure or risk factor as the experimental factor; however, ethical considerations usually prohibit the use of human subjects for these purposes. For example, it is unacceptable to require an experimental group to smoke cigarettes in an experiment; therefore the investigator uses case-control or cohort epidemiological designs. This limitation usually restricts experimental epidemiological studies to prophylactic and therapeutic clinical trials. For example, experimental studies commonly test vaccines and medications for safety and efficacy.

The experimental design is also useful for investigating chronic disease prevention. The Diabetes Prevention Program (DPP) study tested the effect of an intensive behavioral intervention, including both caloric restriction and an increase in physical activity. An average of a 5% weight loss was associated with a 58% reduction in the incidence of type 2 diabetes (DPP Research Group, 2002). The DPP was a primary prevention study, in contrast to the Heart Protection Study, which examined an intervention

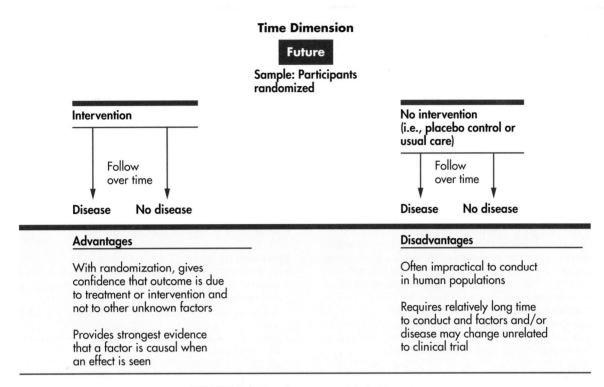

FIGURE 5-8 Experimental, or clinical trial, study.

in subjects with preexisting vascular disease or diabetes. This secondary prevention trial showed that a cholesterol-lowering drug (simvastatin 40 mg), compared with a placebo, reduced the risk of vascular disease (Heart Protection Study Collaborative Group, 2002). Thus experimental studies help determine which of many preventive programs to implement. Although these studies are medical, experimental designs may help evaluate community health nursing interventions. For example, they may help determine the effectiveness of a sex education program in preventing high rates of teenage pregnancy or the feasibility of an AIDS prevention program among intravenous drug users. For 5 years, nurses participated in a randomized trial of telephone interventions directed toward high-risk prenatal clients. The trial's findings were the impetus for several community-based programs to reduce the incidence of preterm and low-birth-weight babies (Moore, 1999).

SUMMARY

Epidemiology offers the community health nurse methods to quantify the extent of health problems in the community and provides a body of knowledge about risk factors and their association with disease. At each step of the nursing process, epidemiological applications support the practice of the community health nurse. Compiling descriptive data from surveys or studies contributes to understanding the community's health level. In assessing community problems, epidemiological rates describe the magnitude of disease and provide support for community diagnoses. Epidemiological studies suggest interventions and their potential efficacy, information that is useful in planning prevention and intervention approaches. Evaluation studies using epidemiological methods, either reported in literature or conducted by community health nurses, are essential for providing optimal research-based care.

CASE STUDY **USING AN EPIDEMIOLOGICAL AND PUBLIC HEALTH APPROACH TO MANAGING A FOOD-BORNE OUTBREAK**

Nurses working in schools, day care centers, camps, and other facilities where food is served must be cognizant of safe food-handling principles. Further, they must be aware of the potential for transmitting disease if proper procedures are not followed. Outbreaks of food-borne illness must be assessed and managed, and often it is the community health nurse who initiates and participates in this process. The following is a scenario in which the nurse utilized the nursing process to analyze and intervene in such an epidemic.

Assessment

On Wednesday, October 4, the school nurse at Greenly Elementary School saw 8 students who complained of abdominal cramping, diarrhea, and fever. Parents of the sick students were called, and the students were sent home. On Thursday, the nurse was alerted to a large number of absent students. Specifically, 62 students and 10 teachers were absent. Most reported diarrhea symptoms. Because the absentee rate of 10% exceeded the average daily

(Continued)

rate of 4% for the 620-student school and because the nurse determined that the large number of diarrhea cases suggested an epidemic, the local public health department was notified. Public health officials arrived at the school and began to assess students still at school and those who were recovering at home. Stool cultures were collected and sent to the state laboratory. Results indicated that the organism causing illness was in most cases *Shigella sonnei,* the most commonly found form of the bacteria. Persons with severe symptoms were referred to their physicians for possible antibiotic therapy. Food histories of meals eaten both at school and outside of school were taken.

Friday saw a continuing increase in absenteeism of students and staff reporting gastrointestinal illness. Public health specialists defined the criteria for identifying cases on the basis primarily of positive laboratory results, symptoms of diarrhea or vomiting, fever with nausea or abdominal pain, or all of these. Cafeteria staff were interviewed, and it was determined that one staff member had had diarrhea over the previous weekend but had returned to work on Monday. Public health staff continued to take dietary histories of affected and unaffected persons and constructed rates of illness for all foods served in the cafeteria beginning on Friday of the previous week. These data are displayed in the following table.

how it should be prevented in the everyday lives of students. Needs of special ages and developmental levels of children were also important. A formal plan of what needed to be done, by whom, and when was drawn up. Research into the nature and prevention of *Shigella* was gathered from the Centers for Disease Control and Prevention and the local health department, among other sources. Health department staff developed a plan to release information to the public about the prevention of gastrointestinal illnesses, as many of these diseases are easily spread and so many students were already ill.

Long-Term Goal
- An absence of cases of infectious diarrhea

Short-Term Goals
- Treatment and recovery of all identified cases of diarrhea
- Implementation of an effective program of hygienic practices among students and staff
- Implementation of a food-handler program for all cafeteria workers
- Adequately inform larger community in order to prevent spread of the epidemic

NUMBER OF EXPOSED BY MEAL AND FOOD ITEM (N = 143)

EXPOSURE VARIABLE (FOOD EATEN)	NUMBER WHO ATE		NUMBER WHO DID NOT EAT		
	ILL (A)	NOT ILL (B)	ILL (C)	NOT ILL (D)	ODDS RATIO*
Ate on Monday	47	60	18	18	0.78
Ate on Tuesday	63	57	3	20	**7.37**
Fajitas	57	52	8	26	**4.56**
Salad	44	21	24	54	**4.7**
Salsa	26	29	40	48	1.07
Tortillas	48	53	16	26	1.47
Beans	29	32	34	48	1.28
Milk	53	56	11	23	1.98
Ate on Wednesday	21	64	43	15	0.11

Modified from Texas Department of Health, *Shigella* outbreak in an elementary school, *Dis Prev News* 55(6):1-3, 1995.
*Odds ratios were calculated with the formula: ad/bd.

From the data, it can be seen that students who ate lunch at school on Tuesday and ate fajitas and salad had higher rates of illness than those who did not. Therefore it was concluded that the outbreak of *Shigella* could be attributed to a food source.

Diagnosis
Determining the likely cause of the outbreak was important in specifying a diagnosis and directing the planning of an intervention. The following diagnosis was formulated:

Increased risk for infectious diarrhea among elementary school children related to inadequate hygiene and food handling practices as evidenced by a 19% increase in reported cases within a 4-day period.

Planning
The school nurse, in conjunction with public health specialists, determined that several groups should be targeted in order to eliminate the further spread of disease. They identified a need to assist families in understanding the nature of the disease, how to care for their children who were ill, and how to prevent the spread at home. Within the school, there was a need to review food-handling practices and the training that cafeteria workers received. Staff, including teachers, also required information about *Shigella* and

Intervention
The school nurse took a central leadership role directing action within the school aimed at staff, students, and student families. Teaching of appropriate hand washing was stressed. Hand-washing supplies and facilities were inspected for soap and running water. Food preparation guidelines were reviewed with staff, and policies regarding remaining at home when ill were reiterated. The health department staff provided technical assistance and made recommendations. They informed community physicians about surveillance and reporting requirements and provided information regarding identifying cases and treatment regimens. Day care centers and preschools were advised to watch for diarrhea outbreaks and to adhere to strict hand-washing and diaper-handling practices, as these facilities tend to be high-risk areas for the transmission of organisms such as *Shigella.* The media were contacted to elicit their help in disseminating correct and useful information to the community.

Evaluation
Immediate evaluation involved monitoring the decline in *Shigella* cases both within the school and in the larger community. The school nurse noted that rates of absenteeism returned to normal on the following Monday. She determined that all classes had

CASE STUDY USING AN EPIDEMIOLOGICAL AND PUBLIC HEALTH APPROACH TO MANAGING A FOOD-BORNE OUTBREAK—cont'd

hygiene instruction within the following 2 weeks and that all teachers had received a flyer with specific information about *Shigella*, its care, and prevention. She observed that bathrooms had filled soap dispensers, that a friendly sign reminding students to wash hands was posted near sinks, and that students were given the opportunity to wash hands before lunch and snacks. The public health department, likewise, continued surveillance activities after encouraging physicians to collect and submit stool cultures for suspected cases and to report cases to the health department. Rates of diarrhea declined rapidly in the week after the school outbreak. The infection did not spread to other schools or community groups. This outcome can be attributed to successful epidemic management, yet surveillance remains critical if the public's health is to be protected.

Levels of prevention

Primary
- Teach students and staff about hand washing and hygienic practices.
- Maintain a system that promotes safe food-handling practices.
- Exclude those with symptoms from school or food handling.

Secondary
- Culture all symptomatic individuals.
- Treat those with advanced diarrhea symptoms with antibiotics.
- Exclude those with positive cultures from food handling, and those with symptoms from school.
- Advise families and individuals in the care of those with diarrhea.

Tertiary
- Treat and counsel those determined to be carriers of *Shigella*.

Information on *Shigella* infections available at www.cdc.gov/nczved/dfbmd/disease_listing/shigellosis_gi.html.

LEARNING ACTIVITIES

1. Compile a database of relevant demographic and epidemiological data for your community by examining census reports, vital statistics reports, city records, and other sources in libraries and agencies.
2. Using numerators from vital statistics and denominators from census data, compute crude death and birth rates for your community.
3. Compare morbidity and mortality rates for your community with those of the state and the nation. Determine whether your community rates are higher or lower, and hypothesize about reasons for any disparities.
4. Consult *Healthy People 2020* to find the national goals for selected causes of morbidity and mortality. Identify groups at an increased risk for these selected diseases. What are the approaches suggested by these documents for reducing the rates of disease? How can this information be useful in planning for your community?

REFERENCES

Arrieta A, Russell LB: Effects of leisure and non-leisure physical activity on mortality in U.S. adults over two decades, *Ann Epidemiol* 18:889–895, 2008.

Blair SN, Morris JN: Healthy hearts—and the universal benefits of being physically active: physical activity and health, *Ann Epidemiol* 19:253–256, 2009.

Brunner EJ, Mosdol A, Witte DR, et al: Dietary patterns and 15-y risks of major coronary events, diabetes, and mortality, *Am J Clin Nutr* 87(5):1414–1421, 2008.

Buffardi AL, Thomas KK, Holmes KK, et al: Moving upstream: ecosocial and psychosocial correlates of sexually transmitted infections among young adults in the United States, *Am J Public Health* 98(5):1128–1136, 2008.

Buring JE, Lee I-M: Annotation: confounding in epidemiologic research, *Am J Public Health* 85:164–165, 1995.

Campbell RT, Li X, Doleck TA, et al: Economic, racial and ethnic disparities in breast cancer in the US: towards a more comprehensive model, *Health & Place* 15:870–879, 2009.

Centers for Disease Control and Prevention: Prevalence of actions to control high blood pressure—20 states, 2005, *MMWR Morb Mortal Wkly Rep* 56:420–423, 2007.

Centers for Disease Control and Prevention: *Colorectal (colon) screening rates*, 2008. www.cdc.gov/cancer/colorectal/statistics/screening_rates.htm.

Centers for Disease Control and Prevention: *About the National Health and Nutrition Examination Survey*, 2009. www.cdc.gov/nchs/nhanes/about_nhanes.htm.

Centers for Disease Control and Prevention, National Center for HIV/AIDS, Viral Hepatitis, STD, and TB Prevention: *The Tuskegee timeline*, 2005: www.cdc.gov/nchstp/od/tuskegee/time.htm.

Cohen A, Pieper CF, Brown AJ, et al: Number of children and risk of metabolic syndrome in women, *J Women's Health* 15:763–772, 2006.

Diabetes Prevention Program Research Group: Reduction in the incidence of type 2 diabetes with lifestyle intervention or metformin, *N Engl J Med* 346:393–403, 2002.

Doll R, Hill AB: Study of the aetiology of carcinoma of the lung, *BMJ* 2:1271–1285, 1952.

Doll R, Hill AB: Lung cancer and other causes of death in relation to smoking, *BMJ* 2:1071–1081, 1956.

Eliassen AH, Chen WY, Spiegelman D, et al: Use of aspirin, other nonsteroidal anti-inflammatory drugs and acetaminophen and risk of breast cancer among premenopausal women in the Nurses' Health Study II, *Arch Intern Med* 169:115–121, 2009.

Friedman GD: *Primer of epidemiology*, ed 4, New York, 1994, McGraw-Hill.

Fung TT, Malik V, Rexrode KM, et al: Sweetened beverage consumption and risk of coronary heart disease in women, *Am J Clin Nutr* 89:1037–1042, 2009.

Harkness G: *Epidemiology in nursing practice*, St. Louis, 1995, Mosby.

Heart Protection Study Collaborative Group: MRC/BHF Heart Protection Study of cholesterol lowering with simvastatin in 20,536 high-risk individuals: a randomized placebo-controlled trial, *Lancet* 360:7–22, 2002.

Kulminski AM, Arbeev KG, Ukraintseva SV, et al: Changes in health status among participants of the Framingham Heart Study from the 1960s to the 1990s, *Ann Epidemiol* 18:696–701, 2008.

Lopez-Garcia E, Rodriguez-Artalejo F, Rexrode KM, et al: Coffee consumption and risk of stroke in women, *Circulation* 119:1116–1123, 2009.

MacDonald MA: From miasma to fractals: the epidemiology revolution and public health nursing, *Public Health Nurs* 21:380–391, 2004.

Mattson ME, Pollack ES, Cullen JW: What are the odds that smoking will kill you? *Am J Public Health* 77:425–431, 1987.

Mausner JS, Kramer S: *Mausner and Bahn epidemiology: an introductory text*, ed 2, Philadelphia, 1985, Saunders.

Moore ML: From randomized trial to community-focused practice, *Image J Nurs Sch* 31:349–354, 1999.

Morton RF, Hebel JR, McCarter RJ: *A study guide to epidemiology and biostatistics*, ed 3, Gaithersburg, MD, 1990, Aspen Publishers.

National Cancer Institute: *Surveillance, epidemiology and end results*, 2006: seer.cancer.gov/csr/1975_2006/about.html.

Nurses' Health Study: *History of the Nurses' Health Study*, 2009. http://www.channing.harvard.edu/nhs/.

Pencina MJ, D'Agostino RB, Larson MG, et al: Predicting the 30-year risk of cardiovascular disease: the Framingham Heart Study, *Circulation* 119:3078–3084, 2009.

Pinheiro SP, Tworoger SS, Cramer DW, et al: Use of nonsteroidal anti-inflammatory agents and incidence of ovarian cancer in 2 large prospective cohorts, *Am J Epidemiol* 169:1378–1387, 2009.

Pritchard JE, Nowson CA, Billington T, et al: Benefits of a year-long workplace weight loss program on cardiovascular risk factors, *Nutrition & Dietetics* 59:87–93, 2002.

Sanchez A, Norman GJ, Sallis JF, et al: Patterns and correlates of multiple risk behaviors in overweight women, *Prev Med* 46:196–202, 2007.

Snow J: *On the mode of communication of cholera*, ed 2, London, 1855, Churchill. (Reproduced in *Snow on cholera*, New York, 1936, Commonwealth Fund).

Thorpe LE, Upadhyay UD, Chamany S, et al: Prevalence and control of diabetes and impaired fasting glucose in New York City, *Diabetes Care* 32(1):57–62, 2009.

U.S. Department of Health and Human Services: *Healthy people 2010*, conference ed, Washington DC, 2000, US Government Printing Office.

Whang W, Kubzansky LD, Kawachi I, et al: Depression and risk of sudden cardiac death and coronary heart disease in women: results from the Nurses' Health Study, *J Am Coll Cardiol* 53:950–958, 2009.

Williams PT, Blanche PJ, Rawlings R, et al: Concordant lipoprotein and weight responses to dietary fat change in identical twins with divergent exercise levels, *Am J Clin Nutr* 82:181–187, 2005.

Community Assessment

Holly B. Cassells

OBJECTIVES

Upon completion of this chapter, the reader will be able to do the following:
1. Discuss the major dimensions of a community.
2. Identify sources of information about a community's health.
3. Describe the process of conducting a community assessment.
4. Formulate community and aggregate diagnoses.
5. Identify uses for epidemiological data at each step of the nursing process.

KEY TERMS

aggregate
census tracts
community diagnosis
community of solution

Healthy Communities
metropolitan statistical areas
needs assessment
social system

vital statistics
windshield survey

OUTLINE

The Nature of Community
    Aggregate of People
    Location in Space and Time
    Social System
Healthy Communities

Assessing The Community: Sources of Data
    Census Data
    Vital Statistics
    Other Sources of Health Data
Needs Assessment
Diagnosing Health Problems

The primary concern of community health nurses is to improve the health of the community. To address this concern, community health nurses use all the principles and skills of nursing and public health practice. This involves using demographic and epidemiological methods to assess the community's health and diagnose its health needs.

Before beginning this process, the community health nurse must define the community. The nurse may wonder how he or she can provide services to such a large and nontraditional "client," but there are smaller and more circumscribed entities that comprise a community than towns and cities. A major aspect of public health practice is the application of approaches and solutions to health problems that ensure the majority of people receive the maximum benefit. To this end, the nurse works to use time and resources efficiently.

Despite the desire to provide services to each individual in a community, the community health nurse recognizes the impracticality of this task. An alternative approach considers the community itself to be the unit of service and works collaboratively with the community using the steps of the nursing process. Therefore, the community is not only the context or place where community health nursing occurs; it is the focus of community health nursing care. The nurse partners with community members to identify community problems and develop solutions to ultimately improve the community's health.

Another central goal of public health practitioners is primary prevention, which protects the public's health and prevents disease development. Chapter 3 discussed how these "upstream efforts" are intended to reduce the pain, suffering, and huge expenditures that occur when significant segments of the population essentially "fall into the river" and require downstream resources to resolve their health problems. In a society greatly concerned about increasingly high health care costs, the need to prevent health problems becomes dire. In addition to reducing the occurrence of disease in individuals, community health nurses must examine the larger aggregate—its structures, environments, and shared health risks—to develop improved upstream prevention programs.

This chapter addresses the first steps in adopting a community- or population-oriented practice. A community health nurse must define a community and describe its characteristics before applying the nursing process. Then, the nurse can launch the assessment and diagnosis phase of the nursing process at the aggregate level and incorporate epidemiological approaches. Comprehensive assessment data are essential to directing effective primary prevention interventions within a community.

Gathering these data is one of the core public health functions identified in the Institute of Medicine's (1988) original report on the future of public health. The community health nurse participates in assessing the community's health and its ability to deal with health needs. With sound data, the nurse makes a valuable contribution to health policy development (Wold et al., 2008).

THE NATURE OF COMMUNITY

Many dimensions describe the nature of community. These include an aggregate of people, a location in space and time, and a social system (Box 6-1).

Aggregate of People

An aggregate is a community composed of people who share common characteristics. For example, members of a community may share residence in the same city, member-

---

BOX 6-1	MAJOR FEATURES OF A COMMUNITY

- Aggregate of people
  The "who": personal characteristics and risks
- Location in space and time
  The "where" and "when": physical location frequently delineated by boundaries and influenced by the passage of time
- Social system
  The "why" and "how": interrelationships of aggregates fulfilling community functions

---

ship in the same religious organization, or similar demographic characteristics such as age or ethnic background. The aggregate of senior citizens, for example, comprises primarily retirees who frequently share common ages, economic pressures, life experiences, interests, and concerns. This group lived through the many societal changes of the past 50 years; therefore, they may possess similar perspectives on current issues and trends. Many elderly people share concern for the maintenance of good health, the pursuit of an active lifestyle, and the security of needed services to support a quality life. These shared interests translate into common goals and activities, which also are defining attributes of a common interest community. Communities also may consist of overlapping aggregates, in which case some community members belong to multiple aggregates.

Many human factors help delineate a community. Health-related traits, or *risk factors,* are one aspect of "people factors" to be considered. People who have impaired health or a shared predisposition to disease may join together in a group, or community, to learn from and support each other. Parents of disabled infants, people with acquired immunodeficiency syndrome (AIDS), or those at risk for a second myocardial infarction may consider themselves a community. Even when these individuals are not organized, the nurse may recognize that their unique needs constitute a form of community, or aggregate.

A community of solution may form when a common problem unites individuals. Although people may have little else in common with each other, their desire to redress problems brings them together. Such problems may include a shared hazard from environmental contamination, a shared health problem arising from a soaring rate of teenage suicide, or a shared political concern about an upcoming city council election. The community of solution often disbands after problem resolution, but it may subsequently identify other common issues.

Each of these shared features may exist among people who are geographically dispersed or in close proximity to each other. However, in many situations, proximity facilitates the recognition of commonality and the development of cohesion among members. This active sharing of features fosters a sense of community among individuals.

Location in Space and Time

Regardless of shared features, geographic or physical location may define communities of people. Traditionally, community is an entity delineated by geopolitical boundaries; this view best exemplifies the dimension of location. These boundaries demarcate the periphery of cities, counties, states, and nations. Voting precincts, school districts, water districts, and fire and police protection precincts set less visible boundary lines.

Census tracts subdivide larger communities. The U.S. Census Bureau uses them for data collection and population assessment. Census tracts facilitate the organization of resident information in specific community geographic locales. In densely populated urban areas, the size of tracts tends to be small; therefore, data for one or more census tracts frequently describe neighborhood residents. Although residents may not be aware of their census tract's boundaries, census tract data help define and describe neighborhood communities.

RESEARCH HIGHLIGHTS

Development of a Dynamic Model to Guide Health Disparities Research

Rew et al. (2009) reported on a 6-year project in which public health nurses were involved with 19 studies to analyze health disparities among low-income, rural, Mexican-American, and American Indian populations. Through a series of projects, the team identified a number of predisposing risk factors and barriers to access and utilization of services that contribute to disparities in health outcomes in the targeted populations. The risk factors they observed included gender, race/ethnicity, low income level, and geographic location. Identified barriers included language, transportation problems, lack of awareness of health problems, a distrust of the health system, cultural beliefs, lack of insurance, and lack of culturally sensitive providers.

The researchers noted several areas or needs for health promotion for the targeted populations. These were related to diabetes, mental health problems, and "life-span issues" (e.g., high rates of adolescent pregnancies, poor diet/nutrition, choice of occupation, end-of-life care). As a result, the researchers suggested a set of health promotion interventions including working to enhance interest in engaging in regular exercise, health promotion during pregnancy, and life-span efforts to prevent injury, focusing on prevention of accidents among infants/small children, elders, and those with occupational risks.

From Rew L, Hoke MM, Horner SD, et al: Development of a dynamic model to guide health disparities research, *Nurs Outlook* 57(3):132-142, 2009.

A *geographic community* can encompass less formalized areas that lack official geopolitical boundaries. A geographic landmark may define neighborhoods (e.g., the East Lake section of town or the North Shore area). A particular building style or a common development era also may identify community neighborhoods. Similarly, a dormitory, a communal home, or a summer camp may be a community because each facility shares a close geographic proximity. Geographic location, including the urban or rural nature of a community, strongly influences the nature of the health problems a community health nurse might find there. Public health is increasingly recognizing that the interaction of humans with the natural environment and with constructed environments, consisting of buildings and spaces for example, is critical to healthy behavior and quality of life. The spatial location of health problems in a geographic area can be mapped with the use of Geographic Information System software, assisting the nurse to identify vulnerable populations and for public health departments to develop programs specific to geographic communities.

Location and the dimension of time define communities. The community's character and health problems evolve over time. Although some communities are very stable, most tend to change with the members' health status and demographics and the larger community's development or

decline. For example, the presence of an emerging young workforce may attract new industry, which can alter a neighborhood's health and environment. A community's history illustrates its ability to change and how well it addresses health problems over time.

Social System

The third major feature of a community is the relationships that community members form with each other. Community members fulfill the essential functions of community by interacting in groups. These functions provide socialization, role fulfillment, goal achievement, and member support. Therefore, a community is a complex social system, and its interacting members comprise various subsystems within the community. These subsystems are interrelated and interdependent (i.e., the subsystems affect each other and affect various internal and external stimuli). These stimuli consist of a broad range of events, values, conditions, and needs.

A health care system is an example of a complex system that consists of smaller, interrelated subsystems. A health care system can also be a subsystem because it interacts with and depends on larger systems such as the city government. Changes in the larger system can cause repercussions in many subsystems. For example, when local economic pressures cause a health department to scale back its operations, this affects many subsystems. The health department may eliminate or reduce programs, limit service to other health care providers, reduce access to groups that normally use the system, and deny needed care to families who constitute subsystems in society. Almost every subsystem in the community must react and readjust to such a financial constraint.

EXAMPLE OF SYSTEMS INTERRELATIONSHIPS

Health problems can have a severe impact on multiple systems. For example, the AIDS epidemic required significant funds for AIDS clients and public AIDS education and prevention. It made unrelenting demands on many communities that were already strapped for funds to meet their citizens' basic health needs. In San Francisco, the allocation of funds for AIDS programs initially reduced funding for other programs, such as immunizations, family planning, and well-child care.

HEALTHY COMMUNITIES

Complex community systems receive many varied stimuli. The community's ability to respond effectively to changing dynamics and meet the needs of its members indicates productive functioning. Examining the community's functions and subsystems provides clues to existing and potential health problems. Examples of a community's functions include the provision of accessible and acceptable health services, educational opportunities, and safe, crime-free environments.

The model in Figure 6-1 suggests assessment dimensions that can help a nurse develop a more complete list of critical community functions. The community health nurse can then prioritize these functions from a particular community's perspective. For example, a study of Americans' views on

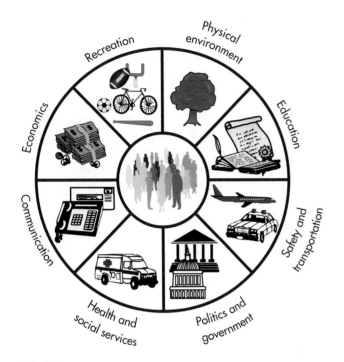

FIGURE 6-1 Diagram of assessment parameters. (From Anderson ET, McFarlane JM: *Community as partner: theory and practice in nursing,* ed 5, Philadelphia, 2008, Lippincott Williams & Wilkins.)

health and healthy communities suggested that the public is more concerned with quality-of-life issues than the absence of disease. Figure 6-2 indicates that the most important determinants of a healthy community are low crime rates and a child-friendly neighborhood environment (Healthcare Forum, 1994).

The movement called Healthy Communities helps community members bring about positive health changes. Involving more than 1400 cities worldwide, the model stresses that interconnectedness among people and among public and private sectors is essential for local communities to address the causes of poor health (Healthy Communties Institute, 2009). Urban communities are encouraged to consider the health consequences of new policies and programs they introduce by conducting Health Impact Assessments (Robert Wood Johnson Foundation, 2010). These assessments of projects such as the potential impact of transit systems and sick leave policies, serve an important function of bringing a public health perspective to urban and civic initiatives. Each community and aggregate presumably will have a unique perspective on critical health qualities. Indeed, a community or aggregate may have divergent definitions of health, differing even from that of the community health nurse (Aronson, Norton, and Kegler, 2007). Nevertheless, nurses and health professionals work with communities in developing effective solutions that are acceptable to residents. Building a community's capacity to address future problems is often referred to as developing *community competence.* The nurse assesses the community's commitment to a healthy future, the ability to foster open communication and to elicit broad participation in problem identification and resolution, the

active involvement of structures such as a health department that can assist a community with health issues, and the extent to which members have successfully worked together on past problems. This information provides the nurse with an indication of the community's strengths and potential for developing long-term solutions to identified problems.

ASSESSING THE COMMUNITY: SOURCES OF DATA

The community health nurse becomes familiar with the community and begins to understand its nature by traveling through the area. The nurse begins to establish certain hunches or hypotheses about the community's health, strengths, and potential health problems through this down-to-earth approach, called "shoe leather epidemiology." The community health nurse must substantiate these initial assessments and impressions with more concrete or defined data before he or she can formulate a community diagnosis and plan.

Community health nurses often perform a community windshield survey by driving or walking through an area and making organized observations. The nurse can gain an understanding of the environmental layout, including geographic features and the location of agencies, services, businesses, and industries, and can locate possible areas of environmental concern through "sight, sense, and sound." The windshield survey offers the nurse an opportunity to observe people and their role in the community. Box 6-2 provides examples of questions to guide a windshield survey assessment. See illustrations depicting an actual "windshield survey" on p. 95.

In addition to direct observational methods, certain public health tools become essential to an aggregate-focused nursing practice. The analysis of demographic information and statistical data provides descriptive information about the population. Epidemiology involves the analysis of these data to discover the patterns of health and illness distribution in a population. Epidemiology also involves conducting research to explain the nature of health problems and identify the aggregates at increased risk. The rest of this section provides data sources and describes how the community health nurse can use demographic and epidemiological data to assess the aggregate.

Census Data

Every 10 years, the U.S. Census Bureau undertakes a massive survey of all American families. In addition to this decennial census, intermediate surveys collect specific types of information. These collections of statistical data describe the population characteristics of the nation within progressively smaller geopolitical entities (e.g., states, counties, and census tracts). The census also describes large metropolitan areas that extend beyond formal city boundaries, called metropolitan statistical areas. These areas consist of a central city with more than 50,000 people and include the associated suburban or adjacent counties, which yields a total metropolitan area with more than 100,000 people. Cities and their

WINDSHIELD SURVEY

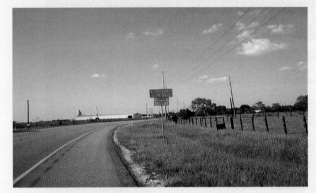

Brookshire is a town of about 3500 in Southeast Texas.

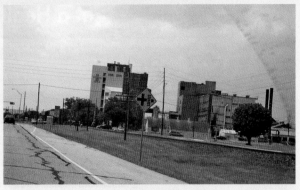

The economy of the town is predominately agriculture and processing.

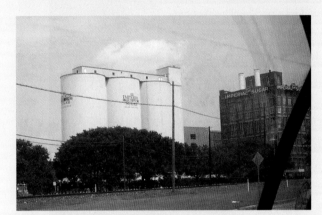

Sugar mills and farms are the source of most jobs.

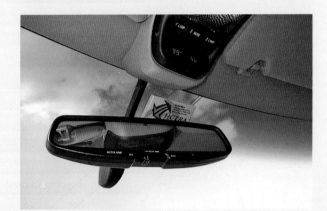

The car's thermometer shows 99 degrees, evidence of a pervasive health threat in the summertime.

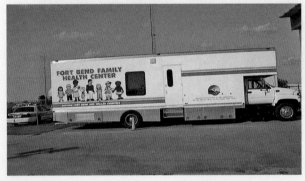

Accessible and affordable health care is a challenge. This van provides services to unskilled workers and area elders.

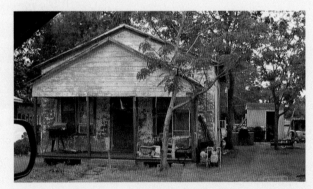

Much of the housing is substandard and suggests low-income families.

Photos courtesy University of Texas Health Science Center at Houston, School of Nursing, Community Health Division.

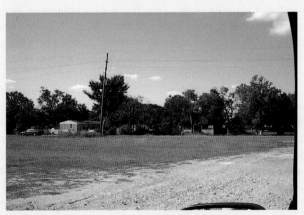

Many people live in small homes on multiple-acre lots.

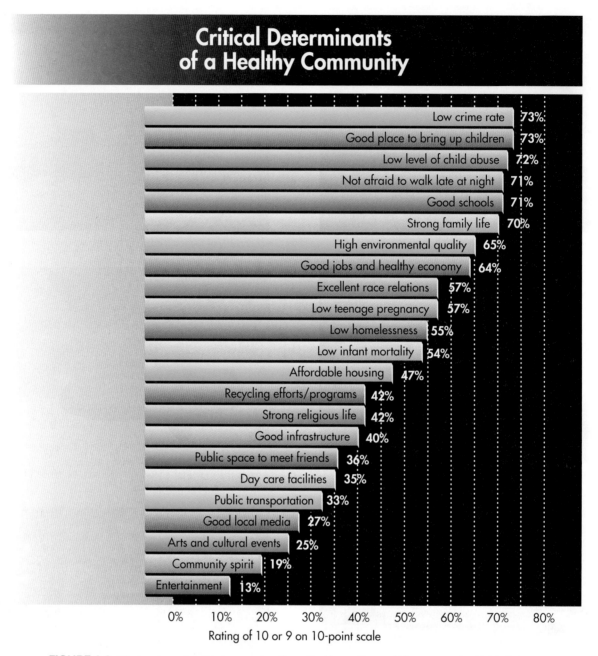

FIGURE 6-2 What makes a healthy community. (From Healthcare Forum: *What creates health? Individuals and communities respond, a national study conducted by DYG, Inc., for the Healthcare Forum*, San Francisco, 1994, The Author.)

associated counties with a population of 1 million or more constitute consolidated statistical areas. A census tract is one of the smallest reporting units. It usually consists of 3000 to 6000 people who share similar characteristics such as ethnicity, socioeconomic status, or housing class.

The census is extremely helpful to community health nurses familiarizing themselves with a new community. The census tabulates many demographic variables including population size, socioeconomic status, housing characteristics, and the distribution of age, sex, race, and ethnicity. Variables that describe the community's health are not part of census data. However, census numbers can be denominators for morbidity and mortality rates (see the Calculation of Rates section

in Chapter 5). Public and university libraries generally maintain archived census data, and all data since the 1990 census, including the most current findings, are available on the Internet at www.census.gov. Computerization of the data allows the nurse to view several variables in combination (e.g., age and ethnicity) and easily construct a community profile.

The nurse analyzes and interprets data by comparing current and local census data with previous data and information from various locations. The nurse can identify the attributes that make each community unique by comparing data for one census unit, such as a census tract or a city, with those of another community or the entire nation. These attributes provide clues to the community's potential vulnerabilities

BOX 6-2   QUESTIONS TO GUIDE COMMUNITY OBSERVATIONS DURING A WINDSHIELD SURVEY

1. Community vitality
- Are people visible in the community? What are they doing?
- Who are the people living in the neighborhood? What is their age range? What is the predominant age (e.g., elderly, preschoolers, young mothers, or school-aged children)?
- What ethnicity or race is most common?
- What is the general appearance of those you observed? Do they appear healthy? Do you notice any obvious disabilities, such as those with walkers or wheelchairs, or those with mental or emotional disabilities? Where do they live?
- Do you notice residents who are well nourished or malnourished, thin or obese, vigorous or frail, unkempt or scantily dressed, or well dressed and clean?
- Do you notice tourists or visitors to the community?
- Do you observe any people who appear to be under the influence of drugs or alcohol?
- Do you see any pregnant women? Do you see women with strollers and young children?

2. Indicators of social and economic conditions
- What is the general condition of the homes you observe? Are these single-family homes or multifamily structures? Is there any evidence of dilapidated housing or of areas undergoing urban renewal? What forms of transportation do people seem to be using? Is there public transit? Are there adequate bus stops with benches and shade? Is transportation to health care resources available?
- Is there public housing? What is its condition?
- Are there any indicators of the kinds of work available to residents? Are there job opportunities nearby, such as factories, small businesses, or military installations? Are there unemployed people visible, such as homeless people?
- Do you see men congregating in groups on the street? What do they look like, and what are they doing?
- Is this a rural area? Are there farms or agricultural businesses?
- Do you note any seasonal workers, such as migrant or day laborers?
- Do you see any women hanging out along the streets? What are they doing?
- Do you observe any children or adolescents out of school during the daytime?
- Do you observe any interest in political campaigns or issues, such as campaign signs?
- Do you see any evidence of health education on billboards, advertisements, signs, radio stations, or television stations? Do these methods seem appropriate for the people you observed?
- What kinds of schools and day care centers are available?

3. Health resources
- Do you notice any hospitals? What kind are they? Where are they located?
- Are there any clinics? Whom do they serve? Are there any family planning services?
- Are there doctors' and dentists' offices? Are they specialists or generalists?
- Do you notice any nursing homes, rehabilitation centers, mental health clinics, alcohol or drug treatment centers, homeless or abused shelters, wellness clinics, health department facilities, family planning services, or pharmacies?
- Are these resources appropriate and sufficient to address the kinds of problems that exist in this community?

4. Environmental conditions related to health
- Do you see evidence of anything that might make you suspicious of ground, water, or air pollutants?
- What is the sanitary condition of the housing? Is housing overcrowded, dirty, or in need of repair? Are windows screened?
- What is the condition of the roads? Are potholes present? Are drainage systems in place? Are there low water crossings, and do they have warning signals? Are there adequate traffic lights, signs, sidewalks, and curbs? Are railroad crossings fitted with warnings and barriers? Are streets and parking lots well lit? Is this a heavily trafficked area, or are roads rural? Are there curves or features that make the roads hazardous?
- Is there handicapped access to buildings, sidewalks, and streets?
- Do you observe recreational facilities and playgrounds? Are they being used? Is there a YMCA or community center? Are there any day care facilities or preschools?
- Are children playing in the streets, alleys, yards, or parks?
- Do you see any restaurants?
- Is food sold on the streets? Are people eating in public areas? Are there trash receptacles and places for people to sit? Are public restrooms available?
- What evidence of any nuisances such as ants, flies, mosquitoes, or rodents do you observe?

5. Social functioning
- Do you observe any families in the neighborhoods? Can you observe their structure or functioning? Who is caring for the children? What kind of supervision do they have? Is more than one generation present?
- Are there any identifiable subgroups related to each other either socially or geographically?
- What evidence of a sense of neighborliness can you observe?
- What evidence of community cohesiveness can you observe? Are there any group efforts in the neighborhood to improve the living conditions or the neighborhood? Is there a neighborhood watch? Do community groups post signs for neighborhood meetings?
- How many and what type of churches, synagogues, or places of worship are there?
- Can you observe anything that would make you suspicious of social problems such as gang activity, juvenile delinquency, drug or alcohol abuse, or adolescent pregnancy?

6. Attitude toward health and health care
- Do you observe any evidence of folk medicine practice, such as a botanical or herbal medicine shop? Are there any alternative medicine practitioners?
- Do you observe that health resources are well utilized or underutilized?
- Is there evidence of preventive or wellness care?
- Do you observe any efforts to improve the neighborhood's health? Do you notice any health fairs? Do you see advertisements for health-related events, clinics, or lectures?

or health risks. For example, a community health nurse may review census reports and discover that a district has many elderly people. This directs the nurse toward further assessment of the social resources (i.e., housing, transportation, and community centers), health resources (i.e., hospitals, nursing homes, and geriatric clinics), and health problems common to aging people. By identifying the trends in the population over time, the community health nurse can modify public health programs to meet the changing needs of the community.

Vital Statistics

The official registration records of births, deaths, marriages, divorces, and adoptions form the basis of data in vital statistics. Every year, city, county, and state health departments aggregate and report these events for the preceding year. When compared with previous years, vital statistics provide indicators of population growth or reduction. In addition to supplying information about the number of births and deaths, registration certificates record the cause of death, which is useful in determining morbidity and mortality trends. Similarly, birth certificates document birth information (e.g., cesarean delivery and teen mothers) and the occurrence of any congenital malformations. This information also is important in assessing the community health status.

⚖️ **ETHICAL INSIGHTS**

Attending to Nondominant Trends: "Hidden Pockets" of Need

Whereas most public health practitioners are attuned to the leading indicators or dominant trends in data, vital statistics or census data can suggest the existence of small "hidden pockets" of people with special needs. One nurse initially assessed her community as in an upper-middle-class bracket. She was surprised to find 20 families living below the poverty level and 3 families living without running water. Although these 20 families made up far less than 1% of the community population, they nevertheless necessitated the attention of the community health nurse. Some may view a focus on such a minority segment as insignificant and in conflict with the "Rule of Utility," which posits "the greatest good for the greatest number." However, community health nursing practice combines principles of beneficence and social justice with utilitarianism, and thus small vulnerable segments of the community are considered legitimate clients of community health nursing. Indeed, social justice not only "gives moral privilege to the needs of the most vulnerable" but also suggests the amelioration of conditions that create social and economic disparities (Boutain, 2005). Furthermore, nurses recognize that this "hidden pocket" is a small piece of the total community and, as such, contributes to its overall health. By attending to these families' health needs, the health of the whole is positively affected.

Other Sources of Health Data

The U.S. Census Bureau conducts numerous surveys on subjects of government interest such as crime, housing, and labor. Results of these surveys, the census reports, and vital statistics reports are usually available through public libraries and on the Internet. The National Center for Health Statistics (NCHS) compiles annual National Health Survey data, which describe health trends in a national sample. The NCHS publishes reports on the prevalence of disability, illness, and other health-related variables. Specifically, the Behavioral Risk Factor Surveillance System is the world's largest telephone survey of U.S. citizens' health behaviors and risk factors. It tracks trends by nation, state, and year, with the goal of identifying emerging health problems. Data also are used to evaluate achievement of health objectives and develop prevention strategies. A user-friendly website allows one to

compile graphs and maps to describe specific risk behaviors by state. See the book's Evolve website at http://evolve.elsevier.com/Nies.

In addition to accessing these important sources of information, community health nurses also can access a broad range of local, regional, and state government reports that contribute to the comprehensive assessment of a population. Local agencies, chambers of commerce, and health and hospital districts collect invaluable information on their community's health. Local health planning agencies also compile and analyze statistical data during the planning process. The community health nurse can use all of these formal and informal resources in learning about a community or aggregate (Table 6-1). Box 6-3 lists additional information about sources of population health data.

Formal data collection does not exist for all community aspects; therefore many community health nurses must perform additional data collection, compilation, and analysis. For example, school nurses regularly use aggregate data from student records to learn about the demographic composition of their population. They conduct ongoing surveys of classroom attendance and causes of illness, which are essential to an effective school health program. Sometimes the nurse must screen the entire school population to discover the extent of a disease. Thus the school nurse is both a consumer of existent data and a researcher who collects new data for the assessment of the school community.

NEEDS ASSESSMENT

The nurse must understand the community's perspective on health status, the services used or required, and concerns. Most official data do not capture this type of information. Data collected directly from an aggregate may be more insightful and accurate; therefore community health nurses sometimes conduct community needs assessments. There are several approaches to gathering subjective data; however, a nurse's careful planning of the process will contribute to its reliability and utility regardless of the method. Box 6-4 presents the required steps in conducting a needs assessment.

Selecting a strategy for collecting needs assessment data is dependent on the size and nature of the aggregate, the purpose for collecting information, and the resources available to the nurse. In some cases, the nurse may survey a small sample of clients to measure their satisfaction with a program. In other situations, a large-scale community needs assessment may help the nurse determine gaps in service. Although the process of needs assessment can indicate a program's strengths and weaknesses, it can also raise expectations for new services on the part of community members (Timmreck, 2003).

A first approach to gathering data is to interview key *community informants*. These may be knowledgeable residents, elected officials, or health care providers. It is essential that the community health nurse recognize that the views of these people may not reflect the views of all residents. A second approach is to hold a *community forum* to discuss selected questions. It is important for the nurse to carefully plan the

TABLE 6-1   COMMUNITY ASSESSMENT PARAMETERS

PARAMETERS	IMPORTANCE TO CHN	SOURCE OF INFORMATION
Geography Topography Climate (e.g., extreme heat or cold)	Influences nature of health problems and access to health care	Almanac Chamber of Commerce
Population Size Demographic character (e.g., aged or young) Trends Migration Density	Describes population served; suggests their health risks and needs Suggests growth or decline Increases stress; may increase exposure to communicable disease	Census documents Chamber of Commerce Local documents
Environment Water (e.g., source; fluoridated) Sewage and waste disposal Air quality (e.g., ozone; pollutants) Food quality and access Housing (e.g., single-family or multifamily dwellings) Animal control (e.g., exposure to rabies and other zoonotic diseases)	Affects quality of life and nature of environmental health problems Reflects community resources Suggests socioeconomic issues	Local and state health departments Newspapers Local environmental action group Census documents
Industry Employment levels Manufacturing White vs. blue collar Income levels	Affects social class, access to health care, and resources Influences nature of health problems	Chamber of Commerce Almanac Employment commission Census documents
Education Schools (e.g., physical plant; playground safety) Types of education Literacy rates Special education Health services Sex education School lunch programs (e.g., nutritious diets) After-school programs Day care Access to higher education	Influences socioeconomic status, access to health care, and ability to read and understand health information	Census documents School districts and nurse
Recreation Parks and playgrounds Libraries Public and private recreation Special facilities	Reflects quality of life, resources available to community, and concern for the young and disadvantaged	Parks and recreation departments Newspapers
Religion Churches and synagogues Denominations Community programs Health-related programs and parish health programs Community organizations	Influences values in community by organizing common interests and concerns Reflects involvement of members, community skills, and resources for community needs	Chamber of Commerce Newspapers Community center newsletters
Communication Newspapers Neighborhood news Radio and television Telephone Internet Hotlines Medical media Public service announcements	Reflects concerns and needs of the community Networks and resources available for health-related use	Local libraries Newspapers Local health department Medical and nursing society
Transportation Intercity and intracity Handicapped Emergency transport	Affects access to services, food, and other resources Reflects resources available to community	Local bus and train service Local hospital emergency service

(Continued)

TABLE 6-1   COMMUNITY ASSESSMENT PARAMETERS—cont'd

PARAMETERS	IMPORTANCE TO CHN	SOURCE OF INFORMATION
Public Services Fire protection Police protection Emergency medical services Rape treatment centers Utilities	Affects community security Reflects available resources	Local police department
Political Organization Structure Method for filing positions Responsibilities of positions Sources of revenue Voter registration	Reflects level of citizen activism, involvement, values, and concerns Mechanism for nurse activism and lobbying	Newspapers Local political party organization Local board of elections Local representatives
Community Development or Planning Activities Major issues	Reflects community needs and concerns Affects level of professionals' involvement in issues	Newspapers Local and state planning board Local community organizations
Disaster Programs American Red Cross Disaster plans Potential sources of disaster	Offers a level of preparedness, coordination, and available resources Influences resources and plans	Local American Red Cross office Local emergency coordinating council Local fire department
Health Statistics Mortality Morbidity Leading causes of death Births	Reflects health problems, trends, and state of community health Affects resources needed and CHN services provided	Local and state health department Health facilities and programs National vital statistics reports NCHS reports *MMWR*
Social Problems Mental health Alcoholism and drug abuse Suicide Crime School dropout Unemployment Gangs	Affects health problems and amounts of required services Influences CHN program priorities	Local and state department of social services Local mental health centers Local hotlines Libraries
Health Manpower Number of physicians, dentists, and nurses per population	Influences available health resources and nature of CHN practice	Local and state health planning agency Health professional organizations Telephone directory Community service director
Health Professional Organizations	Provides support for CHN practice	
Community Services (e.g., cost and eligibility, accessibility, and acceptability) Institutional care (e.g., hospitals and nursing homes) Mental health care Ambulatory care Preventive health services Nursing services Welfare services	Reflect available resources	Local United Way organization Local voluntary service directory County hospital Local health department Telephone directory

CHN, Community health nursing.

meeting in advance to gain the most useful information. The community health nurse can also mail surveys to community members to elicit information from a more diverse group of people who may be unwilling or unable to attend a community forum. *Focus groups* are a third approach; these can be very effective in gathering community views, particularly for remote and vulnerable segments of a community and for those with underdeveloped opinions (Hildebrandt, 1999). Nurses who conduct focus groups must carefully select participants, formulate questions, and analyze recorded sessions. These sessions can produce greater interaction and expression of ideas than surveys and may provide more insight into an aggregate's opinions. In addition to encouraging community participation in the identification of assets and needs, focus groups may lay the groundwork for community involvement in planning the solutions to identified problems (Clark et al., 2003).

BOX 6-3   RETRIEVAL OF DATA

Current data on U.S. population health are stored in many places. Finding the latest statistics at the local, state, or national level can be a challenging experience for a student, community health nurse, graduate student, or nurse researcher. However, statistics provide a necessary comparison in identifying the health status of an aggregate or population in a community. The following guidelines suggest places to begin a search.

Visit the book's Evolve website at http://evolve.elsevier.com/Nies to obtain contact information for the specific agencies listed below.

- *Reference librarian:* The best place to start is in a school or community library or in a large university's health sciences library. Cultivate a relationship with the reference librarian and learn how to access the literature of interest (e.g., government documents) or how to perform computer-guided literature searches.
- *Government documents:* Local libraries have a listing of government depository libraries, which house government documents for the public. If the government document is not available at a local library, ask the reference librarian to contact a regional or state library for an interlibrary loan. The Library of Congress in Washington, DC, has a *Directory of U.S. Government Depository Libraries*.
- *Health: United States, 2008:* This is an annual publication of the NCHS (2008), which reports the latest health statistics for the United States. It presents statistics in areas such as maternal-child health indicators (e.g., prenatal care, low birth weight, and infant mortality), life expectancy, mortality, morbidity (e.g., cancer incidence and survival, AIDS, and

diabetes), environmental health indicators (e.g., air pollution and noise exposure), and health system use (e.g., national health expenditures, health insurance coverage, physician contacts, and diagnostic and surgical procedures). Graphs and tables are easy to read and interpret with accompanying texts. Many statistics include a selected number of years to illustrate trends. Some statistics compare themselves with other countries and U.S. minority populations.

- *Morbidity and Mortality Weekly Report (MMWR):* The Centers for Disease Control and Prevention (CDC) in Atlanta, Georgia, prepares this publication. State health departments compile weekly reports for the publication, which outline the numbers of cases of notifiable diseases such as AIDS, gonorrhea, hepatitis, measles (rubeola), pertussis, rubella, syphilis, tuberculosis, and rabies and reports the deaths in 122 U.S. cities by age. It also reports accounts of interesting cases, environmental hazards, disease outbreaks, or other public health problems. Local and state health departments and many local and health sciences libraries house this weekly publication. A subscription is available at the CDC website, www.cdc.gov/mmwr.
- *CDC:* The CDC compiles information on a range of topics including health behavior, educational and community-based programs, unintentional injuries, occupational safety and health, environmental health, oral health, diabetes and chronic disabling conditions, communicable disease, immunizations, clinical preventive services, and surveillance and data systems. Data are reported in several publications and on the website, www.cdc.gov.

BOX 6-4   STEPS IN THE NEEDS ASSESSMENT PROCESS

1. Identify aggregate for assessment.
2. Identify required information.
3. Select method of data gathering.
4. Develop questionnaire or interview questions.
5. Develop procedures for data collection.
6. Train data collectors.
7. Arrange for a sample representative of the aggregate.
8. Conduct needs assessment.
9. Tabulate and analyze data.
10. Identify needs suggested by data.
11. Develop an action plan.

DIAGNOSING HEALTH PROBLEMS

The next step of the nursing process is synthesizing assessment data into diagnostic statements about the community's health. These statements specify the nature and cause of the actual or potential community health problem and direct the community health nurses' plans to resolve the problem. Muecke (1984) developed a format that assists in writing a community diagnosis. The diagnosis consists of four components: the identification of the health problem or risk, the affected aggregate or community, the etiological or causal statement, and the evidence or support for the diagnosis (Figure 6-3). Each of these components has an important role to play in the nursing process. The problem represents a synthesis of all assessment data. The "among" phrase specifies the aggregate that will be the beneficiary of the nurse's action plan, and whose health is at risk. The "related to" phrase describes the cause of the health

Increased risk of _____
(disability, disease, etc.)

among _____ related to
(community or population)

_____ as demonstrated
(etiological statement)

in _____ .
(health indicators)

FIGURE 6-3 Format for community health diagnosis. (Redrawn from Muecke MA: Community health diagnosis in nursing, *Public Health Nurs* 1:23-35, 1984. Used with permission of Blackwell Scientific Publications.)

problem and directs the focus of the intervention. All plans and interventions will be aimed at addressing this underlying cause. Last, the health indicators are the supporting data or evidence, drawn from the completed assessment. These data can suggest the magnitude of the problem and have a bearing on prioritizing diagnoses. Other factors that assist the nurse in ranking the importance of diagnoses include the emergent nature of the diagnosis, its potential impact on a broad range of community residents, and the community's perceptions of the health issue.

With a clear statement of the problem in the form of a diagnosis, the community health nurse is ready to begin the planning phase of the nursing process. Inherent in this phase is a plan for the intervention and its evaluation. Once again, epidemiological data can be useful as a basis for determining success. By comparing baseline data, national and local data, and other relevant indicators, the nurse can construct benchmarks to gauge achievement of program objectives. This may entail the calculation of incidence rates, if the goal is to reduce the development of disease, or primary prevention. Comparing data with national rates or with prevalence rates found in a local community may be other indicators of success. Reducing the presence of risk factors and documenting patterns of healthy behavior are other objective indices of successful programs.

It is evident that epidemiological data and methods are essential to each phase of the nursing process. The community health nurse compiles a range of assessment data that support the nursing diagnosis. Epidemiological studies support program planning by establishing the effectiveness of certain interventions and their specificity for different aggregates. Finally, epidemiological data are important for the community health nurse's documentation of a program's long-term effectiveness. Box 6-5 provides an evaluation example.

BOX 6-5   EXAMPLE OF OUTCOMES EVALUATION

Fritz et al. (2008) reported on a school-based intervention directed at reducing cigarette smoking among high school–aged adolescents. In this intervention, a team of nurses developed a Computerized Adolescent Smoking Cessation Program (CASCP) consisting of four 30-minute computerized sessions designed to support the student's desire to quit smoking and to decrease the factors that promote continuation of smoking.

In the study, a group of 121 students who were current, self-reported smokers were divided into "experimental" and "control" groups, and the experimental group completed the CASCP program. Outcome evaluation of the data showed that the program was quite effective as 23% of the experimental group quit smoking; this was compared with 5% of the control group. Further, of those who did not quit, nicotine dependence and the number of cigarettes smoked daily decreased in the experimental group. The researchers concluded that the use of a program such as the CASCP can be an effective and inexpensive intervention to help adolescent smokers reduce nicotine dependence and stop smoking.

From Fritz DJ, Gore PA, Hardin SB et al: A computerized smoking cessation intervention for high school smokers, *Pediatr Nurs* 34(1):13-17, 2008.

CASE STUDY

Application of the Nursing Process Assessment and Diagnosis

The following example demonstrates the process of collecting and analyzing data and deriving community diagnoses. It also exemplifies the multiple care levels within which community health nurses function: the individual client, the family, and the aggregate or community levels. In this scenario, the nurse identified an individual client health problem during a home visit, which provided the initial impetus for an aggregate health education program. Data collection expanded from the assessment of the individual to a broad range of literature and data about the nature of the problem in populations. The nurse then formulated a community-level diagnosis to direct the ensuing plan. This was subsequently implemented at the aggregate level and then evaluated.

School nurses frequently address a broad range of student health problems. In the West San Antonio School District, school nurses generally reserve several hours a week for home visits. In a recent case, a teacher expressed concern for a high school junior named "John," whose brother was dying of cancer. In a health class, John shared his personal fears about cancer, which caused his classmates to question their own cancer risks and how they might reduce their risks.

Assessment

The school nurse visited John's family and learned that their 25-year-old son had testicular cancer. Since his diagnosis 1 year earlier, he had undergone a range of therapies that were palliative but not curative; the cancer was advanced at the time of diagnosis. The nurse spent time with the family discussing care, answering questions, and exploring available support for the entire family.

At a school nurse staff meeting, the nurse inquired about her colleagues' experiences with other young clients with this type of cancer. Only one nurse remembered a young man with testicular cancer. The nurses were not familiar with its prevalence, incidence, risk factors, prevention strategies, or early detection approaches. The nurse recognized the high probability that high school students would have similar questions and could benefit from reliable information.

The school nurse embarked on a community assessment to answer these questions. The nurse first collected information about testicular cancer. Second, the nurse reviewed the nursing and medical literature for key articles discussing client care, diagnosis, and treatment. Epidemiological studies provided additional data regarding testicular cancer's distribution pattern in the population and associated risk factors.

The nurse learned that young men aged 20 to 35 years were at the greatest risk. Other major risk factors were not identified. It was learned that healthy young men do not seek testicular cancer screening and regular health care; they may be apprehensive about conditions affecting sexual function. These factors contribute to delayed detection and treatment. Although only an estimated 8400 new cases of testicular cancer were diagnosed in the United States in 2009, it was one of the most common tumors in young men. Furthermore, this cancer is amenable to treatment with early diagnosis (American Cancer Society, 2009).

On the basis of these facts, the nurse reasoned that a prevention program would benefit high school students. However, to perform a comprehensive assessment, it was important that the nurse clarified what students did know, how comfortable they were discussing sexual health, and how much the subject interested them. Therefore the nurse approached the junior and senior high school students and administered a questionnaire to elicit this information. The nurse also queried the health teacher about the amount of pertinent cancer and sexual development information the students received in the classroom. The nurse considered the latter an important prerequisite to dealing with the sensitive subject of sexual health. According to the health teacher, the students did receive instruction about physical development and psychosexual issues. Students expressed a strong desire for more classroom instruction on these subjects and more information on cancer prevention. However, they did not have sufficient knowledge of the beneficial health practices related to cancer prevention and early detection.

CASE STUDY—cont'd

Key Assessment Data
- Health status of John's brother
- Knowledge, coping, and support resources of family
- Testicular cancer, its natural history, treatment and prevention, incidence, prevalence, mortality, and risk factors
- High school students' knowledge about cancer and its prevention
- Students' comfort level discussing sexual health issues

Community

There is an increased risk of undetected testicular cancer among young men related to insufficient knowledge about the disease and the methods for preventing and detecting it at an early stage as demonstrated by high rates of late initiation of treatment.

Planning

Clarifying the problem and its cause helped the nurse direct the planning phase of the nursing process and determine both long-term and short-term goals.

Long-Term Goal
- Students will identify testicular lesions at an early stage and seek care promptly.

Short-Term Goals
- Students will understand testicular cancer and self-detection techniques.
- Students will exhibit comfort with sexual health issues by asking questions.
- Male students will report regular testicular self-examination.

Planning encompassed several activities, including the discovery of recommended health care practices regarding testicular cancer. The nurse also sought to determine the most effective and appropriate educational approaches for male and female high school students. Identifying helpful community agencies was also an essential part of the process. The local chapter of the American Cancer Society provided valuable information, materials, and consultative services. A nearby nursing school's media center and faculty were also very supportive of the program.

After formalizing her objectives and plan, the nurse presented the project to the high school's teaching coordinator and principal. Their approval was necessary before the nurse could implement the project. After eliciting their enthusiastic support, the nurse proceeded with more detailed plans. She selected and developed classroom instruction methods and activities that would maximize high school students' involvement. The nurse also ordered a film and physical models for demonstrating and practicing testicular self-examination. She prepared group exercises designed to relax and assist students in being comfortable with the sensitive subject matter. The nurse scheduled two 40-minute sessions dealing with testicular cancer for the junior-level health class. In a final step of the planning phase, she designed evaluation tools that assessed knowledge levels after each class session and measured the extent to which students integrated these health practices into their lifestyles at the end of their junior and senior years.

The nurse was now ready to proceed with the implementation of a testicular cancer prevention and screening program. She initiated the assessment phase by identifying an individual client and family with a health need, and she extended the assessment to the high school aggregate. Her data collection at the aggregate level, for both the general and local high school populations, assisted in her community diagnosis. The diagnosis directed the development of a community-specific health intervention program and its subsequent implementation and evaluation.

Intervention

The nurse conducted the two sessions in a health education class. At the beginning of the class period, students participated in a group exercise, and the nurse asked them about their knowledge of testicular cancer. The nurse showed a film and led a discussion about cancer screening. In the second session, she demonstrated the self-examination procedure using testicular models and supervised the students while they practiced the procedure on the models. The nurse advised the male students about the frequency of self-examination. With the females, she discussed the need for young men to be aware of their increased risk, drawing a parallel to breast self-examination.

Evaluation

After completing the class sessions, the nurse administered the questionnaires she developed for evaluation purposes. Analysis of the questionnaires indicated that knowledge levels were very high immediately after the classes. Students were pleased with the frank discussion, the opportunity to ask questions, and the clear responses to a sensitive subject. Teachers also offered positive feedback. Consequently, the nurse became a knowledgeable health resource in the high school.

Intermediate-term evaluation occurred at the end of the students' junior and senior years. The nurse arranged a 15-minute evaluation during other classes, which assessed the integration of positive health practices and testicular self-examinations into the students' lifestyles. At the end of the school year, the prevalence of regular self-assessment was significantly lower than knowledge levels. However, 30% of male students reported regularly practicing self-examinations at the end of 1 year, and 70% reported they had performed a self-examination at least once during the past year.

The compilation of incidence data is ideal for long-term evaluation, and it documents the reduction of a community health problem. Testicular cancer is very rare; therefore, incidence data are not reliable and may not be feasible to collect. However, for more prevalent conditions, objective statistics help reveal increases and decreases in disease rates, and these may be related to the strengths and deficiencies of health programs.

Levels of Prevention

The following are examples of the three levels of prevention as applied to this case study.

Primary
- Promotion of healthy lifestyles and attitudes toward sexuality
- Education about sexual health and the care of one's body

Secondary
- Self-examination to detect testicular cancer in its earliest stage
- Referral for medical care as soon as a lump or symptom is discovered
- Medical and surgical care to treat and cure testicular cancer

Tertiary
- Advanced care, including hospice services for those with incurable disease
- Support services and grief counseling to help families cope with loss of a loved one

SUMMARY

Communities form for a variety of reasons and can be homogeneous or heterogeneous in their composition. To help assess the nature of a given community, community health nurses study and interpret data from sources such as local government agencies, census reports, morbidity and mortality reports, and vital statistics. Nurses can gather valuable information about the causes and prevalence of health and disease in a community through epidemiological studies. On the basis of this information, the community health nurse can apply the nursing process, expanding assessment, diagnosis, planning, intervention, and evaluation from the individual client level to a targeted aggregate in the community.

LEARNING ACTIVITIES

1. Walk through a neighborhood, and compile a list of variables that are important to describe with demographic and epidemiological data. Write down hunches or preconceived notions about the nature of the community's population. Compare ideas with the collected statistical data.
2. Walk through a neighborhood, and describe the sensory information (i.e., smells, sounds, and sights). How does each relate to the community's health?
3. Compile a range of relevant demographic and epidemiological data for the community by examining census reports, vital statistics reports, city records, and other library and agency sources.
4. Using the collected data, identify three community health problems, and formulate three community health diagnoses.

REFERENCES

American Cancer Society: *Cancer reference information. Overview: testicular cancer*, 2009, The Author: www.cancer.org/docroot/CRI/CRI_2_1x.asp?rnav=criov&dt=41.

Aronson RE, Norton BL, Kegler MC: "Broad view of health": findings from the California Healthy Cities and Communities Evaluation, *Health Educ Behav* 34(3):441–452, 2007.

Boutain D: Social justice in nursing: a review of the literature. In de Chesnay M, editor: *Caring for the vulnerable*, Boston, 2005, Jones and Bartlett.

Clark MJ, et al: Involving communities in community assessment, *Public Health Nurs* 20:456–463, 2003.

Healthcare Forum: *What creates health? Individuals and communities respond, a national study conducted by DYG, Inc., for the Healthcare Forum*, San Francisco, 1994, The Author.

Healthy Communities Institute. What is the Healthy Cities Movement: 2009: www.healthycommunitiesinstitute.com/ihcf.html.

Hildebrandt E: Focus groups and vulnerable populations: insight into client strengths and needs in complex community health care environments, *Nurs Health Care Perspect* 20(5):256–259, 1999.

Institute of Medicine: *The future of public health*, Washington, DC, 1988, National Academy Press.

Johnson RW: *Foundation: Health Impact Project: About Health Impact Assessment*, 2010. www.healthimpactproject.org/hia.

Muecke MA: Community health diagnosis in nursing, *Public Health Nurs* 1:23–35, 1984.

National Center for Health Statistics: Health: United States, 2008, The Author: www.cdc.gov/nchs/hus.htm.

Timmreck TC: *Planning, program development, and evaluation: a handbook for health promotion, aging, and health services*, ed 2, Boston, 2003, Jones and Bartlett.

Wold SJ, Brown CM, Chastain CD, et al: Going the extra mile: beyond health teaching to political involvement, *Nurs Forum* 43(4):171–176, 2008.

Community Health Planning, Implementation, and Evaluation

*Diane C. Martins, Patricia M. Burbank**

Additional Material for Study, Review, and Further Exploration

evolve WEBSITE

http://evolve.elsevier.com/Nies
- Quiz
- Case Studies
- Glossary
- WebLinks

OBJECTIVES

Upon completion of this chapter, the reader will be able to do the following:

1. Describe the concept "community as client."
2. Apply the nursing process to the larger aggregate within a system's framework.
3. Describe the steps in the health planning model.
4. Identify the appropriate prevention level and system level for nursing interventions in families, groups, aggregates, and communities.
5. Recognize major health planning legislation.
6. Analyze factors that have contributed to the failure of health planning legislation to control health care costs.
7. Describe the community health nurse's role in health planning, implementation, and evaluation.

KEY TERMS

certificate of need (CON)
community as client
health planning
Health Planning Model

Hill-Burton Act
key informant
National Health Planning and
    Resources Development Act

Partnership for Health Program
    (PHP)
Regional Medical Programs
    (RMPs)

OUTLINE

Overview of Health Planning
Health Planning Model
  Assessment
  Planning
  Intervention
  Evaluation
Health Planning Projects
  Successful Projects
  Unsuccessful Projects
  Discussion

Health Planning Federal Legislation
  Hill-Burton Act
  Regional Medical Programs
  Comprehensive Health Planning
  Certificate of Need
  National Health Planning and Resources
    Development Act
  Changing Focus of Health Planning
Nursing Implications

*The authors would like to acknowledge the contribution of Deborah Godfrey Brown, who cowrote this chapter for the previous edition.

Health planning for and with the community is an essential component of community health nursing practice. The term *health planning* seems simple, but the underlying concept is quite complex. Like many of the other components of community health nursing, health planning tends to vary at the different aggregate levels. Health planning with an individual or a family may focus on direct care needs or self-care responsibilities. At the group level, the primary goal may be health education, and, at the community level, health planning may involve population disease prevention or environmental hazard control. The following example illustrates the interaction of community health nursing roles with health planning at a variety of aggregate levels.

Clinical Example

Bianca Tesch is an RN in a suburban high school. During the course of the school year, she noted an increasing incidence of pregnancy-related dropouts. A nurse at the junior high school confirmed a corresponding increase in withdrawal among younger pregnant teenagers. After reviewing information in nursing journals, other professional journals, and the general media, Bianca discovered a national epidemic of unwed pregnant teenagers.

Bianca questioned the reason for the increased pregnancies. Her assessment of the problem included several findings. Sexually active teenagers do not use contraception regularly because they want their actions to seem "spontaneous" and not "planned." Also, a variety of sexual misconceptions led teens to believe they were invulnerable to pregnancy. For example, a typical misconception among female students was "I will not become pregnant if I do not have regular periods or if my boyfriend does not ejaculate inside me." Teenagers also find it difficult or embarrassing to obtain certain contraceptives. The suburb does not have a local family planning clinic, and area physicians are reluctant to counsel teenagers or prescribe contraceptives without parental permission. The nurse also discovered that, several years earlier, a group of parents stopped an attempt by the local school board to establish sex education in the school system. The parents believed this responsibility belonged in the home.

Bianca considered all of these factors in developing her plan of action. She met with teachers, officials, and parents. Teachers and school officials were willing to deal with this sensitive issue if parents could recognize its validity. In meetings, many parents revealed they were uncomfortable discussing sexuality with their teenaged children and welcomed assistance. However, they were concerned that teachers might introduce the mechanics of reproduction without giving proper attention to the moral decisions and obligations involved in relationships. The parents expressed their desire to participate in curriculum planning and to meet with the teachers instead of following a previous plan that required parents to sign a consent form for each teenager. In support of the parents, Bianca asked a nearby metropolitan family planning agency to consider opening a part-time clinic in the suburb. The local school board proposed instituting a home-tutoring program for pregnant teenagers, which would encourage their return to school.

Implementing such a comprehensive plan is time consuming and requires community involvement and resources. The nurse enlisted the aid of school officials and other community professionals. Time will reveal the plan's long-term effectiveness in reducing teen pregnancy.

This example shows how nurses can and should become involved in health planning. Teen pregnancy is a significant health problem and often results in lower education and lower socioeconomic status, which can lead to further health problems. The nurse's assessment and planned interventions involved individual teenagers, parents and families, the school system, and community resources.

This chapter provides an overview of health planning and evaluation from a nursing perspective. It also describes a model for student involvement in health planning projects and a review of significant health planning legislation.

OVERVIEW OF HEALTH PLANNING

One of the major criticisms of community health nursing practice involves the shift in focus from the community and larger aggregate to family caseload management or agency responsibilities. When focusing on the individual or family, nurses must remember that these clients are members of a larger population group or community, and environmental factors influence them. Nurses can identify these factors and plan health interventions by implementing an assessment of the entire aggregate or community. Figure 7-1 illustrates this process.

The concept of "community as client" is not new. Lillian Wald's work at New York City's Henry Street settlement in the late 1800s exemplifies this concept. At the Henry Street settlement, Miss Wald, Mary Brewster, and other public health nurses worked with extremely poor immigrants.

> *The "case" element in Wald's early reports received less and less emphasis; she instinctively went beyond the symptoms to appraise the whole individual. She observed that one could not understand the individual without understanding the family and saw that the family was in the grip of larger social and economic forces, which it could not control (Duffus, 1938).*

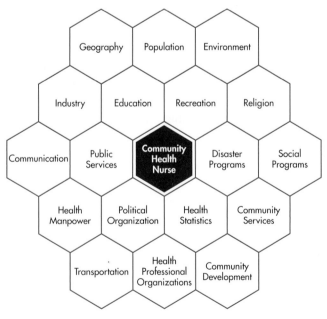

FIGURE 7-1   The community as client. Chapter 6, Table 6-1 (pp. 99-100), provides assessment parameters that help identify the client's assets and needs.

The early beginnings of public health nursing incorporated visits to the homebound ill and applied the nursing process to larger aggregates and communities to improve health for the greatest number of people. Wald's goals, and those of other public health nurses, were health promotion and disease prevention for the entire community (Silverstein, 1985). Health planning at the aggregate or community level is necessary to accomplish these goals.

Through the 1950s, public health nursing adopted Wald's nursing concepts, which focused on mobilizing communities to solve local problems, treat the poor, and improve the environmental conditions that fostered disease. During the 1950s, social changes such as suburbanization, increased family mobility, and enhanced government health expenditures updated nursing roles. Since the mid-1960s, there has been a shift from public health nursing, which emphasizes community care, to community health nursing, which includes all nonhospital nursing activities. New trends constantly emerge through health care reform debates. It has become more important to use nurses as primary care providers in the health care system. A continued shift into the community requires that community health nurses become increasingly visible and vocal leaders of health care reform.

The increased focus on community-based nursing practice yields a greater emphasis on the aggregate becoming the client or care unit. However, the community health nurse should not neglect nursing care at the individual and family levels by focusing on health care only at the aggregate level. Rather, the nurse can use this community information to help understand individual and family health problems and improve their health status. Table 7-1 illustrates the differences in community health nursing practice at the individual, family, and community levels.

However, before nurses can participate in health care planning, they must be knowledgeable about the process and comfortable with the concept of community as client or care focus. It is essential that undergraduate and graduate nursing programs integrate these concepts into the curricula. If basic and advanced nursing education includes health planning, the student becomes aware of the process and the professional involvement opportunities.

Early efforts to provide students with learning experiences in community health investigation included Hegge's (1973) use of learning packets for independent study and Ruybal's opportunities for students to apply epidemiological concepts in community program planning and evaluation (Ruybal, Bauwens, and Fasla, 1975). However, neither of these approaches presented a complete model that incorporated the nursing process into a health planning framework. Several other authors, including Budgen and Cameron (2003) and Shuster and Goeppinger (2008), described the community health planning process. However, none of these models uses practical examples for actual student implementation throughout the entire process.

HEALTH PLANNING MODEL

A model based on Hogue's (1985) group intervention model was developed in response to this need for population focus. The Health Planning Model aims to improve aggregate health and applies the nursing process to the larger aggregate within a systems framework. Figure 7-2 depicts this model. Incorporated into a health planning project, the model can help students view larger client aggregates and gain knowledge and experience in the health planning process. Nurses must carefully consider each step in the process, using this model. Box 7-1 outlines these steps. In addition, Box 7-2 provides the systems framework premises that nurses should incorporate.

Several considerations affect how nurses choose a specific aggregate for study. The community may have extensive or limited opportunities appropriate for nursing involvement.

TABLE 7-1   LEVELS OF COMMUNITY HEALTH NURSING PRACTICE

CLIENT	EXAMPLE	CHARACTERISTICS	HEALTH ASSESSMENT	NURSING INVOLVEMENT
Individual	Lisa McDonald	An individual with various needs	Individual strengths, problems, and needs	Client-nurse interaction
Family	Moniz family	A family system with individual and group needs	Individual and family strengths, problems, and needs	Interactions with individuals and the family group
Group	Boy Scout troop Alzheimer's support group	Common interests, problems, and needs Interdependency	Group dynamics Fulfillment of goals	Group member and leader
Population group	Patients with AIDS in a given state Pregnant adolescents in a school district	Large, unorganized group with common interests, problems, and needs	Assessment of common problems, needs, and vital statistics	Application of nursing process to identified needs
Organization	A work place A school	Organized group in a common location with shared governance and goals	Relationship of goals, structure, communication, patterns of organization to its strengths, problems, and needs	Consultant and/or employee application of nursing process to identified needs
Community	Immigrant neighborhood Anytown, USA	An aggregate of people in a common location with organized social systems	Analysis of systems, strengths, characteristics, problems, and needs	Community leader, participant, and health care provider

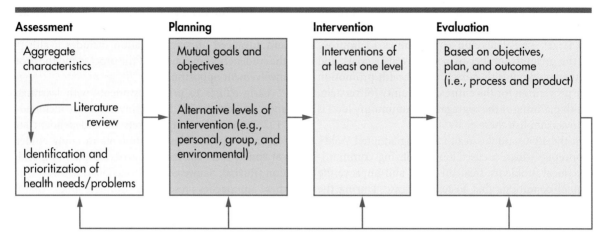

FIGURE 7-2 Health Planning Model.

BOX 7-1   HEALTH PLANNING PROJECT OBJECTIVES

I. Assessment
  A. Specify the aggregate level for study (e.g., group, population group, or organization). Identify and provide a general orientation to the aggregate (e.g., characteristics of the aggregate system, suprasystem, and subsystems). Include the reasons for selecting this aggregate and the method for gaining entry.
  B. Describe specific characteristics of the aggregate.
    1. *Sociodemographic characteristics:* Including age, sex, race or ethnic group, religion, educational background and level, occupation, income, and marital status.
    2. *Health status:* Work or school attendance, disease categories, mortality, health care use, and population growth and population pressure measurements (e.g., rates of birth and death, divorce, unemployment, and drug and alcohol abuse). Select indicators appropriate for the chosen aggregate.
    3. *Suprasystem influences:* Existing health services to improve aggregate health and the existing or potential positive and negative impact of other community-level social system variables on the aggregate. Identify the data collection methods.
  C. Provide relevant information from the literature review, especially in terms of the characteristics, problems, or needs within this type of aggregate. Compare the health status of the aggregate with similar aggregates, the community, the state, and the nation.
  D. Identify the specific aggregate's health problems and needs based on comparative data collection analysis and interpretation

and literature review. Include input from clients regarding their need perceptions. Give priorities to health problems and needs, and indicate how to determine these priorities.

II. Planning
  A. Select one health problem or need, and identify the ultimate goal of intervention. Identify specific, measurable objectives as mutually agreed upon by the student and aggregate.
  B. Describe the alternative interventions that are necessary to accomplish the objectives. Consider interventions at each system level where appropriate (e.g., aggregate system, suprasystem, and subsystems). Select and validate the intervention(s) with the highest probability of success. Interventions may use existing resources, or they may require the development of new resources.

III. Intervention
  A. Implement at least one level of planned intervention when possible.
  B. If intervention was not implemented, provide reasons.

IV. Evaluation
  A. Evaluate the plan, objectives, and outcomes of the intervention(s). Include the aggregate's evaluation of the project. Evaluation should consider the process, product, appropriateness, and effectiveness.
  B. Make recommendations for further action based on the evaluation, and communicate these to the appropriate individuals or system levels. Discuss implications for community health nursing.

BOX 7-2   SYSTEMS FRAMEWORK PREMISES

I. Each system is a goal-directed collection of interacting or interdependent parts, or subsystems.
II. The whole system is continually interacting with and adapting to the environment, or suprasystem.
III. There is a hierarchical structure (suprasystem → system → subsystems).
IV. Each system is characterized by the following:
  A. *Structure:* Arrangement and organization of parts, or subsystems
    1. Organization and configuration (e.g., traditional vs. nontraditional; greater variability [no right or wrong and no proper vs. improper form])
    2. Boundaries (open vs. closed; regulate input and output)
    3. Territory (spatial and behavioral)
    4. Role allocation
  B. *Functions:* Goals and purpose of system and activities necessary to ensure survival, continuity, and growth of system
    1. General

  a. *Physical:* Food, clothing, shelter, protection from danger, and provision for health and illness care
  b. *Affectional:* Meeting the emotional needs of affection and security
  c. *Social:* Identity, affiliation, socialization, and controls
    2. Specific: Each family, group, or aggregate has its own individual agenda regarding values, aspirations, and cultural obligations
  C. *Process and dynamics*
    1. Adaptation: Attempt to establish and maintain equilibrium; balance between stability, differentiation, and growth; self-regulation and adaptation (equilibrium and homeostasis)
      a. *Internal:* Families, groups, or aggregates
      b. *External:* Interaction with suprasystem
    2. Integration: Unity and ability to communicate
    3. Decision making: Power distribution, consensus, accommodation, and authority

Additionally, each community offers different possibilities for health intervention. For example, an urban area might have a variety of industrial and business settings that need assistance, whereas a suburban community may offer a choice of family-oriented organizations such as boys and girls clubs and parent-teacher associations that would benefit from intervention.

A nurse should also consider personal interests and strengths in selecting an aggregate for intervention. For example, the nurse should consider whether he or she has an interest in teaching health promotion and preventive health or in planning for organizational change, whether his or her communication skills are better suited to large or small groups, and whether he or she has a preference for working with the elderly or with children. Thoughtful consideration of these and other variables will facilitate assessment and planning.

Assessment

To establish a professional relationship with the chosen aggregate, a community health nurse must first gain entry into the group. Good communication skills are essential to make a positive first impression. The nurse should make an appointment with the group leaders to set up the first meeting.

The nurse must initially clarify his or her position, organizational affiliation, knowledge, and skills. The nurse should also clarify mutual expectations and available times. Once entry is established, the nurse continues negotiation to maintain a mutually beneficial relationship.

Meeting with the aggregate on a regular basis will allow the nurse to make an in-depth assessment. Determining sociodemographic characteristics (e.g., distribution of age, sex, and race) may help the nurse ascertain health needs and develop appropriate intervention methods. For example, adolescents need information regarding nutrition, abuse of drugs and alcohol, and relationships with the opposite sex. They usually do not enjoy lectures in a classroom environment, but the nurse must possess skills to initiate small-group involvement and participation. An adult group's average educational level will affect the group's knowledge base and its comfort with formal versus informal learning settings. The nurse may find it more difficult to coordinate time and energy commitments if an organization is the focus group, because the aggregate members may be more diverse.

The nurse may gather information about sociodemographic characteristics from a variety of sources. These sources include observing the aggregate, consulting with other aggregate workers (e.g., the factory or school nurse, a Head Start teacher, or the resident manager of a high-rise senior-citizen apartment building), reviewing available records or charts, interviewing members of the aggregate (i.e., verbally or via a short questionnaire), and interviewing a key informant. A key informant is a formal or informal leader in the community who provides data that is informed by his or her personal knowledge and experience with the community.

In assessing the aggregate's health status, the nurse must consider both the positive and negative factors. Unemployment or the presence of disease may suggest specific health problems, but low rates of absenteeism at work or school may suggest a need to focus more on preventive interventions. The specific aggregate determines the appropriate health status measures. Immunization levels are an important index for children, but nurses rarely collect this information for adults. However, the nurse should consider the need for influenza and/or pneumonia vaccines with the elderly. Similarly, the nurse would expect a lower incidence of chronic disease among children, whereas the elderly have higher rates of long-term morbidity and mortality.

The aggregate's suprasystem may facilitate or impede health status. Different organizations and communities provide various resources and services to their members. Some are obviously health related, such as the presence or absence of hospitals, clinics, private practitioners, emergency facilities, health centers, home health agencies, and health departments. Support services and facilities such as group meal sites or Meals on Wheels (MOW) for the elderly and recreational facilities and programs for children, adolescents, and adults are also important. Transportation availability, reimbursement mechanisms or sliding-scale fees, and community-based volunteer groups may determine the use of services. An assessment of these factors requires researching public records (e.g., town halls, telephone directories, and community services directories) and interviewing health professionals, volunteers, and key informants (i.e., someone who is familiar with the community) in the community. The nurse should augment existing resources or create a new service rather than duplicating what is already available to the aggregate.

A literature review is an important means of comparing the aggregate with the norm. For example, children in a Head Start setting, day care center, or elementary school may exhibit a high rate of upper respiratory tract infections during the winter. The nurse should review the pediatric literature and determine the normal incidence for this age range in group environments. Further, the nurse should research potential problems in an especially healthy aggregate (e.g., developmental stresses for adolescents or work or family stresses for adults) or determine whether a factory's experience with work-related injury is within an average range. Comparing the foregoing assessment with research reports, statistics, and health information will help determine and prioritize the aggregate's health problems and needs.

The last phase of the initial assessment is identifying and prioritizing the specific aggregate's health problems and needs. This phase should relate directly to the assessment and the literature review and should include a comparative analysis of the two. Most important, this step should reflect the aggregate's perceptions of need. Depending on the aggregate, the nurse may consult the aggregate members directly or interview others who work with the aggregate (e.g., a Head Start teacher). Interventions are seldom successful if the nurse omits or ignores the clients' input.

During the needs assessment, four types of needs should be assessed. The first is the expressed need or the need expressed by the behavior. This is seen as the demand for services and the market behavior of the targeted population. The second need is normative, which is the lack, deficit, or inadequacy as determined by expert health professionals.

The third type of need is the perceived need expressed by the audience. Perceived needs include the population's wants and preferences. The final need is the relative need, which is the gap showing health disparities between the advantaged and disadvantaged populations (Issel, 2009).

Finally, the nurse must prioritize the identified problems and needs to create an effective plan. The nurse should consider the following factors when determining priorities:

- Aggregate's preferences
- Number of individuals in the aggregate affected by the health problem
- Severity of the health need or problem
- Availability of potential solutions to the problem
- Practical considerations such as individual skills, time limitations, and available resources

In addition, the nurse may further refine the priorities by applying a framework such as Maslow's (1968) hierarchy of needs (i.e., lower-level needs have priority over higher-level needs) or Leavell and Clark's (1965) levels of prevention (i.e., primary prevention may take priority for children, whereas tertiary prevention may take higher priority for the elderly).

Assessment and data collection are ongoing throughout the nurse's relationship with the aggregate. However, the nurse should proceed to the planning stage once the initial assessment is complete. It is particularly important to link the assessment stage with other stages at this step in the process. Planning should stem directly and logically from the assessment, and implementation should be realistic.

An essential component of health planning is to have a strong level of community involvement. The nurse is responsible for advocating for client empowerment throughout the assessment, planning, implementation, and evaluation phase of this process. Community organization reinforces one of the field's underlying premises as outlined by Nyswander (1956): "Start where the people are." Moreover, Labonte (1994) stated that the community is the engine of health promotion and a vehicle of empowerment. He describes five spheres of an empowerment model, that focus on the following levels of social organization: interpersonal (personal empowerment), intragroup (small-group development), intergroup (community collaboration), interorganizational (coalition building), and political action. Attention to collective efforts and support of community involvement and empowerment, rather than focusing on individual efforts, will help ensure that the outcomes reflect the needs of the community and truly make a difference in people's lives.

Labonte's (1994) multilevel empowerment model allows us to consider both macro-level and micro-level forces that combine to create both health and disease. Therefore, it seems that both micro and macro viewpoints on health education provide nurses with multiple opportunities for intervention across a broad continuum. In summary, health education activities that have an "upstream" focus examine the underlying causes of health inequalities through multilevel education and research. This allows nurses to be informed by critical perspectives from education, anthropology, and public health (Israel et al., 2005).

Successful health programs rely on empowering citizens to make decisions about individual and community health. Empowering citizens causes power to shift from health providers to community members in addressing health priorities. Collaboration and cooperation among community members, academicians, clinicians, health agencies, and businesses help ensure that scientific advances, community needs, sociopolitical needs, and environmental needs converge in a humanistic manner.

Planning

Again, the nurse should determine which problems or needs require intervention in conjunction with the aggregate's perception of its health problems and needs, and based on the outcomes of prioritization. Then the nurse must identify the desired outcome or ultimate goal of the intervention. For example, the nurse should determine whether to increase the aggregate's knowledge level and whether an intervention will cause a change in health behavior. It is important to have specific and measurable goals and desired outcomes. This will facilitate planning the nursing interventions and determining the evaluation process.

Planning interventions is a multistep process. First, the nurse must determine the intervention levels (e.g., subsystem, aggregate system, and/or suprasystem). A system is a set of interacting and interdependent parts (subsystems), organized as a whole with a specific purpose. Just as the human body can be viewed as a set of interacting subsystems (e.g., circulatory, neurological, integumentary), a family, a worksite, or a senior high-rise can also be viewed as a system. Each system then interacts with, and is further influenced by, its physical and social environment, or suprasystem (for example, the larger community).

Second, the nurse should plan interventions for each system level, which may center on the primary, secondary, or tertiary levels of prevention. These levels apply to aggregates, communities, and individuals. Primary prevention consists of health promotion and activities that protect the client from illness or dysfunction. Secondary prevention includes early diagnosis and treatment to reduce the duration and severity of disease or dysfunction. Tertiary prevention applies to irreversible disability or damage and aims to rehabilitate and restore an optimal level of functioning. Plans should include goals and activities that reflect the identified problem's prevention level.

Third, the nurse should validate the practicality of the planned interventions according to available personal as well as aggregate and suprasystem resources. Although teaching is often a major component of community health nursing, the nurse should consider other potential forms of intervention (e.g., personal counseling, policy change, or community service development). Input from other disciplines or community agencies may also be helpful. Finally, the nurse should coordinate the planned interventions with the aggregate's input to maximize participation.

Goals and Objectives

Development of goals and objectives is essential. The goal is generally where the nurse wants to be, and the objectives are the steps needed to get there. Measurable objectives are the specific measures used to determine whether or not the nurse is successful in achieving the goal. The objectives are instructions about what the nurse wants the population to be able to do. In writing the objectives, the nurse should use verbs and include specific conditions (how well or how many) that describe to what degree the population will be able to demonstrate mastery of the task.

The objectives may be used to later measure learning outcomes, but the objectives need to be measurable. Objectives may also be referred to as behavioral objectives or outcomes because they describe observable behavior rather than knowledge. An example of the goals and measurable objectives for a city with a high rate of childhood obesity is shown in Box 7-3.

Intervention

The intervention stage may be the most enjoyable stage for the nurse and the clients. The nurse's careful preliminary assessment and planning should help ensure the aggregate's positive response to the intervention. Although implementation should follow the initial plan, the nurse should prepare for unexpected problems (e.g., bad weather, transportation problems, poor attendance, or competing events). If the nurse is unable to complete the intervention, the reasons for its failure should be analyzed. Interventions should be included from a range of strategies including mass media (public service announcements, radio, television, billboards), general information dissemination (e.g., pamphlets, DVDs, CDs, posters), electronic information dissemination (e.g., websites, blogs, tweets, video stream), and public forums (e.g., town meetings, focus groups, discussion groups).

Evaluation

Evaluation is an important component for determining the success or failure of a project and understanding the factors that contributed to its success or failure. The evaluation should include the participant's verbal or written feedback and the nurse's detailed analysis. Evaluation includes reflecting on each previous stage to determine the plan's strengths and weaknesses (*process evaluation*). Process evaluation is also referred to as *formative evaluation*. It allows one to evaluate both positive and negative aspects of each experience honestly and comprehensively and whether the desired outcomes were achieved (*product evaluation*). Product evaluation is summative and can consist of end-of-intervention surveys and other tools that measure whether objectives have been met. *Summative evaluation* is another term for product evaluation and looks at outcomes. Evaluation should include adequacy, efficiency, appropriateness, and cost benefit. During both process and product evaluation, the nurse may ask the following questions:

- Was the assessment adequate?
- Were plans based on an incomplete assessment?
- Did the plan allow adequate client involvement?
- Were the interventions realistic or unrealistic in terms of available resources?
- Did the plan consider all levels of prevention?
- Were the stated goals and objectives accomplished?
- Were the participants satisfied with the interventions?
- Did the plan advance the knowledge level of the aggregate and the nurse?

The intervention may have limited impact if the nurse fails to communicate follow-up recommendations to the aggregate upon completion of the project. Although follow-up activity is not necessary for every plan, most require additional interventions within the aggregate using community agencies and resources. A comprehensive health planning project involves a close working relationship with the aggregate and careful consideration of each step. Long-term evaluation may need to be done by those professionals working continuously with the aggregate, to determine behavior changes and/or changes in health status.

BOX 7-3 **PROGRAM GOALS AND OBJECTIVES FOR REDUCTION OF CHILDHOOD OBESITY**

GOAL: Reduce the rate of childhood obesity in the city of New Bedford.

OBJECTIVES:

1. The percentage of children over the 98th percentile for weight will be reduced to 5%.
2. All the children will be invited to join a 5, 2, 1 program:
   - Five fruits and vegetables per day
   - Two-hour limit on TV, video games, and computer per day
   - One hour of physical activity per day
3. New food pyramid will be taught to all school nurses and health educators by the end of the school year.
4. New food pyramid will be presented and distributed to parents at all the summer health fairs.

RESEARCH HIGHLIGHTS

Cardiorespiratory Health Effects Associated With Volcanic Air Pollution

Recognizing that millions of people live near active volcanoes, Longo (2009) conducted an epidemiological study to provide estimates and qualitative descriptions of cardiorespiratory health effects associated with volcanic air pollution from Kilauea.

Kilauea Volcano is the largest point source for sulfur dioxide in the United States and has released air pollution on nearby communities since 1983. Exposure levels of Kilauea's air pollutants were determined by environmental sampling. Prevalence estimates of cardiorespiratory health effects in adults were measured and compared between an exposed and a nonexposed reference community.

Findings showed that ambient and indoor concentrations of volcanic pollutants were above recommended exposure levels. This significantly increased the incidence of a number of health problems including cough, phlegm, rhinorrhea, sore and dry throat, sinus congestion, wheezing, eye irritation, and diagnosed bronchitis. In addition, 35% of those exposed, mainly current and former smokers and those with chronic respiratory disease, believed that their health was adversely affected by volcanic gases.

From Longo BM: The Kilauea Volcano adult health study, *Nurs Res* 58(1): 23-31, 2009.

HEALTH PLANNING PROJECTS

Successful Projects

Student projects have used this health planning model with group, organization, population group, and community aggregates. Table 7-2 describes interventions with these aggregates at the subsystem, aggregate system, and suprasystem levels.

Textile Industry

Clinical Example

A nursing student studied a textile plant that had approximately 470 employees but did not have an occupational health nurse. The student nurse collected data and identified three major problems or needs by collaborating with management and union representatives. First, the student nurse observed that the most common, costly, and chronic work-related injury in plant workers was lower back injury. Second, some employees had concerns about possible undetected hypertension. Third, the first-aid facilities were disorganized and without an accurate inventory system. The student nurse planned and implemented interventions for all three areas.

On the suprasystem level, the student nurse formulated plans with the company's physicians and lobbied management to enact an employee training program on proper lifting techniques. The student nurse proposed creating specific and concise job descriptions and requirements to facilitate potential employees' medical assessment. In addition, the student nurse organized and clearly labeled the first-aid supplies and developed an inventory system. On the aggregate system level, the student nurse planned and conducted a hypertension screening program. Approximately 85% of the employees underwent screening, and 10 people had elevated blood pressure readings. These 10 people were referred for follow-up care, and hypertension was subsequently diagnosed in several of them.

In evaluating the project, management representatives recognized that a variety of nursing interventions could improve or maintain workers' health. Consequently, management hired the student nurse upon graduation to be the occupational health nurse.

Crime Watch

Clinical Example

Another nursing student was concerned with the rising incidence of crime in a community and organized a crime watch program. The student nurse met periodically with the police and local residents, or aggregate system. Interventions included posting crime watch signs in the neighborhood and establishing more frequent police patrols at the suprasystem level. Evaluation of the program revealed that the residents had increased awareness and concern for neighborhood safety.

Rehabilitation Group

Clinical Example

After working at a senior citizens center for a few weeks, a student nurse began a careful assessment of the center's clients. The student nurse interviewed the center's clients and visited its homebound clients served by social workers and the MOW program. Several of the homebound clients identified a need for socialization and rehabilitation. The center had recently purchased a van equipped to transport handicapped people in wheelchairs, which was a necessary factor in fulfilling this need.

After the student nurse assessed the clients' health and functional status and determined mutual goals, four of these homebound clients expressed a desire to attend a rehabilitation program at the center. The student nurse and the center's management initiated a weekly program based on the clients' needs, which included van transportation, a coffee hour, a noontime meal, an exercise class, and a craft class. Although some members were initially reluctant to participate and one man withdrew from the group, the group ultimately functioned very well. In evaluating this new program, it was clear that the student nurse made progress in meeting the goals of increased socialization and rehabilitation among elders at the center.

Unsuccessful Projects

Project failure is usually caused by problems with one or more steps of the nursing process. Usually the student does not discover problems until the evaluation phase. The following unsuccessful projects illustrate failures at different steps in the nursing process. Table 7-3 summarizes the identified problem areas for these examples.

TABLE 7-2	INTERVENTIONS BY TYPE OF AGGREGATE AND SYSTEM LEVEL	
PROJECT	TYPE OF AGGREGATE	SYSTEM LEVEL FOR INTERVENTION
Rehabilitation group	Group, organization	Subsystem and aggregate system
Textile industry	Population group	Aggregate system and suprasystem
Crime watch	Group, organization, and population group	Aggregate system and suprasystem
Bilingual students (case study)	Community	Aggregate system and suprasystem

TABLE 7-3	UNSUCCESSFUL PROJECTS
PROJECT	PROBLEMATIC STEP OF NURSING PROCESS
Group home for developmentally delayed	Assessment (i.e., mutual identification of health problems and needs)
Safe Rides program	Planning (i.e., mutual identification of goals and objectives)
Manufacturing plant	Evaluation (i.e., recommendations for follow-up) Implementation

Group Home for Developmentally Delayed Adults

Clinical Example

A nursing student worked with an aggregate of six women living in a group home for developmentally delayed citizens. The nursing student observed that the clients were all overweight, and she decided to establish a weight reduction program. She proceeded to meet with the women, chart their weight, and discuss their food choices on a weekly basis. After 8 weeks, her evaluation revealed that none of the women had lost weight and a few had actually gained weight. During the assessment phase the student failed to consider the women's perceptions of need. The women did not consider their weight a priority health problem, and their boyfriends provided positive reinforcement regarding their appearance.

Safe Rides Program

Clinical Example

One student nurse assessed a university student community through a questionnaire and identified a drinking and driving problem. Of those she surveyed, 77% admitted to driving under the influence of alcohol, and 16.5% stated they had been involved in an alcohol-related car accident. After identifying the problem and determining student interest, the student nurse worked with the campus alcohol and drug resource center to plan and implement a program called Safe Rides. In this program, student volunteers would work a hotline and dispatch "on-call" drivers to pick up students who are unsafe to drive.

The student nurse resolved many potential complications before implementation (e.g., liability coverage for all participating individuals and expense funds for gasoline). The student nurse formulated a 12-hour training program that lasted 3 weeks to prepare student volunteers for the Safe Rides program. By the end of the semester, Safe Rides was ready to begin. However, the student nurse graduated at the semester's end, and her commitment was the program's prime motivating force. Although others were committed and involved, the student nurse did not arrange for a replacement to coordinate and continue the program upon her departure. The Safe Rides program required ongoing coordination efforts, and no one fully implemented the program in the student's absence.

Manufacturing Plant

Clinical Example

Even careful planning cannot always eliminate potential obstacles. For example, one student nurse chose to work in an occupational setting involving heavy industry. The occupational health nurse and the nurse's personnel supervisor both approved the student nurse's entry into the organization. After reviewing the literature, working with the nurse for several weeks, and assessing the organization and its employees, the student nurse concluded that back injury risk was a primary problem. She planned to decrease the risk factors involved in back injuries by distributing information about proper body mechanics in a teaching session.

The personnel manager resisted this plan. Although he recognized the need for education, he was initially unwilling to allow employees to attend the session on company time. The student and manager reached a compromise by allowing attendance during extended coffee breaks. The personnel manager, however,

canceled the program before the student nurse could implement the class; negotiations for a new union contract were forming, and there was high probability of a strike. This caused management to deny any changes in the usual routine.

The student nurse proceeded appropriately and received clearance from the proper officials, but she could not anticipate or circumvent union problems. The student nurse could only share her information and concern with the nurse and the personnel manager and encourage them to implement her plan when contract negotiations were complete.

Discussion

Each of these projects attempted to address a particular level of prevention. Most of these examples focused on primary prevention and health promotion because they were student conducted and time limited. Table 7-4 lists these projects and their prevention levels. However, the full-time community health nurse working with an aggregate (e.g., in the occupational health setting) would target interventions for all three levels of prevention at a variety of system levels. It is useful to view nursing interventions with aggregates within a matrix structure to address all intervention opportunities. The matrix in Table 7-5 gives examples of how the occupational health nurse may intervene at all system levels and all prevention levels.

In practice, most interventions occur at the individual level and include all prevention levels. Interventions at the aggregate level are usually less frequent. For many occupational health nurses, time does not allow intervention at the suprasystem level. However, industries are integral parts of the community system. Factors that affect community health also affect employee health and vice versa. Some industries take their reciprocal relationship with the surrounding community quite seriously. For nurses in these industries, interventions at the suprasystem level may become a reality and improve the health of the community and the workers. This is a good example of refocusing upstream by addressing the real source of problems. Although the chosen example is occupational health nursing, any nurse working with aggregate systems can construct a similar matrix for interventions.

These projects illustrate the variety of available opportunities for aggregate health planning. In addition, they exemplify the application of the nursing process within various aggregate

TABLE 7-4	LEVEL OF PREVENTION FOR EACH PROJECT		
PRIMARY PREVENTION	**SECONDARY PREVENTION**	**TERTIARY PREVENTION**
Textile industry	Textile industry	Rehabilitation group
Crime watch	Group home for developmentally delayed	
Manufacturing plant		
Safe Rides program		

TABLE 7-5	OCCUPATIONAL HEALTH: LEVELS OF PREVENTION FOR SYSTEM LEVELS		
SYSTEM LEVEL	**PRIMARY PREVENTION**	**SECONDARY PREVENTION**	**TERTIARY PREVENTION**
Subsystem	Yearly physical examination for each employee	Regular blood pressure monitoring and diet counseling for each employee with elevated blood pressure	Referral for job retraining for employee with a back injury
Aggregate and group system	Incentive program to encourage departments to use safety devices	Weight reduction group for overweight employees	Support group for employees who are recovering from problems with alcohol or drug use
Suprasystem	Health fair open to the community and employees	Counseling and referral of community members with elevated blood pressure or cholesterol on the basis of health fair findings	Media advertising to encourage people with substance abuse problems to seek help and use community resources that provide assistance

types, at different systems levels, and at each prevention level. These examples demonstrate the vital importance of each step of the nursing process.

1. Aggregate assessments must be thorough. The textile industry project exemplifies this point. Assessments should elicit answers to key questions about the aggregate's health and demographic profile and should compare this information with similar aggregates presented in the literature.
2. The nurse must complete careful planning and set goals that the nurse and the aggregate accept. The rehabilitation group project illustrates the importance of mutual planning.
3. Interventions must include aggregate participation and must meet the mutual goals. The Crime Watch project exemplifies this point.
4. Evaluation must include process and product evaluation and aggregate input.

HEALTH PLANNING FEDERAL LEGISLATION

Health planning at the national, state, and local levels is another example of aggregate planning. Planning at any of these levels can be a broader extension of the suprasystem level and affects the individual, family, group, population, and organization levels. Again, upstream change can occur on these levels; for example, individual consumers and consumer groups have protested some managed-care practices at the suprasystem level, because health policy can directly affect patient care.

Historically, nurses have influenced health planning only minimally at the community level, but health planning has a tremendous effect on nurses and nursing practice. It is necessary to understand planning on a suprasystem level; therefore the following section contains a review of past health planning efforts with projections for the future.

Hill-Burton Act

In 1946, Congress passed the Hospital Survey and Construction Act (Hill-Burton Act, PL 79-725) to address the need for better hospital access. This act provided federal aid to states for hospital facilities. A state had to submit a plan documenting available resources and need estimates to qualify for hospital construction and modernization funds under the Hill-Burton Act (Sultz and Young, 2006). In addition, each state had to designate a single agency for the development and implementation of the hospital construction plan. The Hill-Burton Act caused the expenditure of vast sums of money and resulted in an increase in the number of beds, especially in general hospitals. Although the act and its amendments focused only on construction, it improved the quality of care in rural areas and introduced systematic statewide planning (Gourevitch, Caronna, and Kalkut, 2005).

Regional Medical Programs

The Hill-Burton Act provided construction-related planning, but it did not address coordination and care delivery directly. In response to recommendations from Dr. Michael DeBakey's national commission, Heart Disease, Cancer, and Stroke Amendments of 1965 (PL 89-239) were enacted. This legislation was more comprehensive and established regional medical programs.

The Regional Medical Programs (RMPs) intended to make the latest technology for the diagnosis and treatment of heart disease, cancer, stroke, and related diseases available to community health care providers through the establishment of regional cooperative arrangements among medical schools, research institutions, and hospitals. The goals of these cooperative arrangements were to improve the health manpower and facilities available to the communities. The intent was to avoid interfering with methods of financing, hospital administration, patient care, or professional practice.

Although RMPs have been credited with the regionalization of certain services and the introduction of innovative approaches to organization and care delivery, some observers believed the reforms were not comprehensive enough. The RMPs did not partner with the existing federal and state programs; therefore, there were gaps and duplication in service delivery, personnel training, and research (Kovner, 2002).

Comprehensive Health Planning

Congress signed the Comprehensive Health Planning and Public Health Services Amendments of 1966 (PL 89-749) into law to broaden the previous legislation's categorical approach to health planning. Combined with the Partnership for Health Amendments of 1967 (PL 90-174), these amendments created the Partnership for Health Program (PHP). The PHP provided federal grants to states to establish and administer a local agency program to enact local comprehensive health care planning. The PHP's objectives were promoting and ensuring the highest level of health for every person and not interfering with the existing private practice patterns (Shonick, 1995).

To meet these objectives, the PHP formulated a two-level planning system. Under this system, each state had to designate a single health planning agency, or "A" agency. To play a statewide coordinating role, the "A" agency had to partner with an advisory council, which consisted largely of health care consumers. Meanwhile, the local "B" agencies formulated plans to meet designated local community needs, which could be any public or nonprofit private agency or organization. "A" agencies were to encourage the formation of local, comprehensive, health planning "B" agencies, and federal grants were made available for that purpose (Shonick, 1995).

Although the comprehensive health plans were the first of these programs to mandate consumer involvement, they may have failed in their basic intent. The possible failure may have resulted from funding shortage, conflict avoidance in policy formulation and goal establishment, political absence, and provider opposition (e.g., American Medical Association, American Hospital Association, and major medical centers) (Shonick, 1995).

Certificate of Need

In response to increased capital investments and budgetary pressures, state governments developed the idea of obtaining prior governmental approval for certain projects through the use of a certificate of need (CON). New York State passed the first CON law in 1964, which required government approval of hospitals' and nursing homes' major capital investments. Eventually all states supported this CON requirement, and it ultimately became a component of health legislation (PL 93-641). In practice, state CON programs differ in structure and goals. These differences include program focus, decision-making levels, review standard scope, and appeals process exemption (Sultz and Young, 2006).

National Health Planning and Resources Development Act

Given the perceived failure of the comprehensive health planning programs, the federal government focused on a new approach to health planning. The federal government was greatly concerned with the cost of health care, which escalated dramatically following the end of World War II; the uneven distribution of services; the general lack of knowledge of personal health practices; and the emphasis on more costly modalities of care. The National Health Planning and Resources Development Act of 1974 (PL 93-641) combined the strengths of the Hill-Burton Act, RMPs, and the comprehensive health planning program to forge a new system of single-state and area-wide health planning agencies (Harlow, 2006).

The goals and purposes of the new law were an increase in accessibility, acceptability, continuity, and quality of health services; control over the rising costs of health care services; and prevention of unnecessary duplication of health resources. The new law addressed the needs of the underserved and provided quality health care. The provider and consumer were to be involved in planning and improving health services, and it placed the system of private practice under scrutiny.

At the center of the program was a network of local health planning agencies, which developed a health systems plan for their geographic service area. The local agencies then submitted these plans to a state health planning and development agency, which integrated the plans into a preliminary state plan. The state agency presented this preliminary plan to a statewide health coordinating council for approval. The law required that the council consist of at least 16 governor-appointed members and that 50% of these members represent health system agencies and 50% represent consumers. One major function of this council was to prepare a state health plan that reflected the goals and purposes of the act. Once the council formulated a tentative plan, they presented it at public hearings throughout the state for discussion and possible revisions (Thorpe, 2002).

Despite careful deliberations by health planners with input from consumers, not all states accepted the health system plan at the grassroots level. A number of problems were encountered, and, in time, the legislation failed to effect major change in the health care system. A significant problem was that legislation grandfathered the entire health care system (i.e., health care delivery methods did not change). Although legislation mandated consumer involvement in the health system agency, it was often difficult to implement this aspect. Additionally, despite the mandated efforts by CON and required reviews, costs continued to rise, and the health care system remained essentially unchanged (Thorpe, 2002).

Comprehensive Health Reform

The Patient Protection and Affordable Care Act of 2010 includes several elements that involve health planning (Kaiser Family Foundation, 2010). Provisions from that act include:

- Creation of task forces on preventive services and community preventive services to develop, update, and disseminate evidence-based recommendations on health care delivery
- Establishment of the National Prevention, Health Promotion, and Public Health Council, an agency that will be charged with development of a national strategy to improve the nation's health
- Creation of an innovation center within the Centers for Medicare and Medicaid Services
- Development of a national quality improvement strategy that will seek to improve delivery of health care services and population health
- Provision of billions of dollars for funding community health centers, school based clinics and the National Health Service Corps to improve access to care
- Establishment of an Independent Payment Advisory Board to make proposals to reduce the growth in Medicare spending
- Establishment of a workforce advisory committee to develop a national workforce strategy and to suggest ways to enhance the workforce supply by supporting education of health professionals through scholarships and loans

Many of these provisions will not be implemented for several years. Thus, the impact of these changes will not be realized for some time

Health Planning in Public Health

According to Issel (2009), many planning programs to address public health problems began as environmental planning of water and sewer systems. Additional population-based planning became necessary with the advent of immunizations. Blum (1974) was the first to suggest how public health planning should be done. Perspectives on health planning range from systematic problem solving and an epidemiological approach to a social awareness approach.

Beginning in the mid-1980s the Centers for Disease Control and Prevention (CDC) began to develop and promote systematic methods for health planning in public health. These models were important for a structured approach to public health planning.

PATCH. The Planning Approach to Community Health (PATCH) model was based on Green's PRECEDE (Predisposing, Reinforcing, and Enabling factors in Community Education Development and Evaluation) (Green et al., 1980; Green and Kreuter, 2005). This model encouraged the idea that health promotion is a process that enables the population to have more control of its own health. An essential element of the PATCH model is community participation. Another element is the use of data to develop comprehensive health strategies. The PATCH model achieved this through mobilizing the community, collecting health data, selecting health priorities, developing a comprehensive intervention plan, and evaluating the process (Issel, 2009).

APEX-PH Program. The Assessment Protocol for Excellence in Public Health (APEX-PH) began in 1987 as a cooperative project of the American Public Health Association (APHA), the Association of Schools of Public Health (ASPH), the Association of State and Territorial Health Officials (ASTHO), the CDC, the National Association of County and City Health Officials (NACCHO), and the United States Conference of Local Health Officers (USCLHO). The APEX-PH is a voluntary process for organizational and community self-assessment, planned improvements, and continuing evaluation and reassessment. It is a true self-assessment and is intended to be more of a public endeavor involving the community, as well as the public organizations (CDC, 2009).

MAPP. More recently, the CDC and NACCHO have released the MAPP (Mobilizing for Action Through Planning and Partnerships) model. MAPP is a health planning model that helps public health leaders to facilitate community priorities about health issues and identify sources to address them. The first phase of MAPP is to mobilize the community, the second is to guide the community toward a shared vision for long-range planning, and the third is to conduct four assessments. The assessments are identifying community strengths, local health system, health status, and forces of change within the population (NACCHO, 2009).

Changing Focus of Health Planning

Health planning legislation is heavily influenced by the politics of the administration in power at any given time. The Reagan administration encouraged competition within the health care system. During the 1980s, the administration emphasized cost shifting and cost reduction with greater state power, less centralization of functions, and less national control. This approach represented the government's philosophical shift and combined it with a funding cutback from the Omnibus Budget Reconciliation Act in 1981. This resulted in a curtailment on federal

health planning efforts at that time (Mueller, 1993). The cutbacks caused health system agencies to redefine their role, and the federal government recommended eliminating these agencies.

A reduction in federal funding and the influence of medical lobbies caused the closure of some health system agencies. Those that remained open experienced a decrease in staff, a resulting decrease in overall board functioning, and a reordering of priorities. In an effort to compensate for the decrease in federal funding, some health system agencies sought nonfederal funding or built coalitions to provide the necessary power base for change. Although the administration did not renew federal health planning legislation in the 1980s, it used other regulatory approaches to control costs. These included basing payments to Medicare on diagnosis-related groups and, in the 1990s, many individual states requiring their Medicaid recipients to enroll in health maintenance organizations (HMOs).

The Clinton administration's plan for health care reform included mechanisms to revitalize planning at the national level. The failure of Congress to pass the plan in 1994 gave planning efforts back to state and local agencies. As a result, most states have become very involved in various aspects of health planning. Indeed, there is considerable variation as many have statewide health plans, local health plans, and some other type of local health planning (American Health Planning Association [AHPA], 2009).

At the beginning of the twenty-first century, 36 states and the District of Columbia still required CON reviews for selected expenditures that include nursing homes, psychiatric facilities, and expensive equipment (AHPA, 2009). However, within these programs, requirements for approval are more liberal, expedited reviews are conducted, and certain projects are exempted from review, which weakens the CON cost-containment mandate. Newer high-technology services (i.e., lithotripsy, gamma knives, and positron emission tomography) still need CON review in most states. Furthermore, it is anticipated that state CON programs will continue to assume a stronger role because states must increasingly monitor and report the quality, cost, and access to health care that managed care promised.

Health care system and health insurance reform were central issues in the 2008 presidential election. President Obama's election, along with a Democratically controlled Congress, provided the opportunity to make dramatic changes in how health care is managed in the United States. Throughout most of 2009 and into 2010, Congress debated a number of different options, and the Patient Protection and Affordable Care Act became law in March 2010.

With full implementation of the Health Care Act, there should be enhanced emphasis on health promotion/health care and local, community-based approaches to health issues as opposed to emphasis on illness-oriented medical care to help defray costs and improve the overall health of the population. The *Healthy People 2020* objectives support this notion. To help achieve improved health status for all, health planning needs a coordinated approach that combines public and private cooperation with an emphasis on supplies and services. Advances in planning models and the sophistication level of planners will impact future health planning efforts.

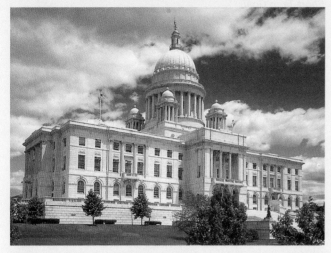

Student nurses can support the health planning process to improve aggregate health care with awareness of, and involvement in, the political process. This can involve following health care legislation at the state and national levels, being an informed voter, contacting legislators on issues of concern, and participating in special events.

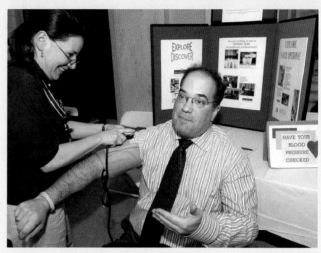

Student nurses attend "Higher Ed Day" at the statehouse to highlight their accomplishments and their participation in the improvement of the health of the state's residents. This student nurse is taking an individual's blood pressure while providing educational information about hypertension identification, referral, and treatment. (Courtesy Michael Salerno.)

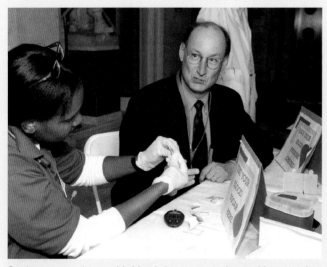

Student nurses also provide blood glucose screenings, with appropriate educational information regarding normal ranges, diet-controlled diabetes, and appropriate referral and treatment when necessary. (Courtesy Michael Salerno.)

Rhode Island Board of Governors
for Higher Education
301 Promenade Street
Providence, Rhode Island 02908–5748

Telephone 401 222-6560
Facsimile 401 222-6111
TDD 401 222-1350

R I B G H E

April 14, 2005

Professor Debby Godfrey Brown
Nursing
University of Rhode Island
White Hall, Room 233
Kingston, RI 02881

Dear Professor Brown:

During the 2004 session of the General Assembly, legislative leaders appropriated $800,000 to increase enrollment in our three nursing programs. This decision proved to be a prudent investment. Your participation in Higher Education Day at the State House received rave reviews. The blood pressure and glucose screenings were services that virtually every legislator and policymaker could identify with. Thank you for your participation and please extend my thanks to the future nurses as well.

Sincerely,

Jack R. Warner

They knew we were here! Positive feedback helps the student nurses to recognize the importance of their participation and nursing actions. In addition, their role modeling can have an influence on other legislation such as funding for their nursing program.

CASE STUDY   APPLICATION OF THE NURSING PROCESS

José Mendez, a bilingual community health nursing student, worked with the school system in a community that had a large Portuguese subsystem. His primary responsibility was for students enrolled in the town's bilingual program. His contacts included the school nurse and the program teachers.

Assessment

José included the specific group of students, the members of the school system's organizational level, and the population group of the town's Portuguese-speaking residents in his assessment of the aggregate's health needs. José identified the subsystem's lack of primary disease prevention, specifically related to hygiene, dental care, nutrition, and lifestyle choices, by observing the children, interviewing teachers and community residents, and reviewing the literature. José's continued assessment and prioritization revealed that the problem was related to a lack of knowledge and not a lack of concern.

Diagnosis
Individual
- Inadequate preparation at home regarding basic hygiene, dental care, nutrition, and healthy lifestyles

Family
- Deficient knowledge regarding basic hygiene, dental care, nutrition, and healthy lifestyles

Community
- Inadequate resources for communicating basics of hygiene, dental care, nutrition, and healthy lifestyles to the Portuguese community

Planning

The teachers and staff of the bilingual program helped contract and set goals, which reinforced the need for mutuality at this step in the process. A variety of alternative interventions were necessary to accomplish the following goals:

Individual
Long-Term Goal
- Students will regularly practice good hygiene, preventive dental care, good nutrition, exercise, and adequate sleep habits.

Short-Term Goal
- Students will learn the basics of good hygiene, preventive dental care, good nutrition, exercise, and adequate sleep habits.

Family
Long-Term Goal
- Families will regularly practice and teach their children good hygiene, preventive dental care, good nutrition, exercise, and adequate sleep habits.

Short-Term Goal
- Families will learn the basics of good hygiene, preventive dental care, good nutrition, exercise, and adequate sleep habits.

Community
Long-Term Goal
- Systematic programs will provide families and their children with education and information regarding the basics of good hygiene, preventive dental care, good nutrition, exercise, and adequate sleep habits.

Short-Term Goal
- Bilingual personnel will translate information into Portuguese, and program teachers will distribute it to families. This information will cover the basics of good hygiene, preventive dental care, good nutrition, exercise, and adequate sleep habits.

Intervention
Sometimes nursing students' projects are more limited than the planning stage's ideal; in this case, interventions assessed only one grade level.

Individual
- The student nurse taught children many healthy lifestyle basics, including nutrition, hygiene, and dental care. Classes presented information in Portuguese and English.

Family
- All parents received a summary of the class content in both languages and in pictures.

Community
- The local teachers communicated the student nurse's activities to their state-level coordinators, and the coordinators incorporated the student nurse's materials into the bilingual program throughout the state.

Evaluation
Individual, Family, Community
This community health planning project had an impact on the individuals in the specific aggregate and had broader implications for the family systems and the community suprasystem. The outcomes, or product, were hugely successful. Mutually identified goals and objectives influenced the development of the process and incorporated input from a variety of sources. The student nurse believed the resources and support for the bilingual program were adequate. Although the student nurse only addressed primary prevention, the continuing nature of the project will allow the teachers, the school nurse, and the families to assess problems related to the program's content. Future implementation may address secondary and tertiary prevention.

Questions:
How would you evaluate this project? How would you determine process and product evaluation? What would you do differently?

NURSING IMPLICATIONS

Nurses must work collaboratively with health planners to improve aggregate health. Nurses can influence health planning at the local and state, or community level by fusing current technology with their knowledge of health care needs and skills gained through working with individuals, families, groups, and population groups. This is an example of "upstream interventions." Indeed, the nurse may become directly involved in the planning process by participating in CON reviews or gaining membership on health planning councils. Even as students, nurses can begin to participate by engaging in aggregate-level projects, such as those outlined in this chapter, and by tracking health care legislation and contacting their legislators about important issues.

Increased nursing involvement is one method of strengthening local and national health planning. Nurses can use the Health Planning Model presented in this chapter to facilitate a systematic approach to improve aggregate health care. Nurses can assess aggregates from small groups through population groups; identify the group's health needs; and perform planning, intervention, and evaluations by applying this model. The health of individuals, families, and groups would improve if nurses reemphasized the larger aggregate.

SUMMARY

Community health nurses are responsible for incorporating health planning into their practice. Nurses' unique talents and skills, augmented by the comprehensive application of the nursing process, can facilitate population health improvement at various aggregate levels. Health planning policy and process constitute part of the knowledge base of the baccalaureate-prepared nurse. Systems theory provides one framework for nursing process application in the community. Interventions are possible at subsystem, system, and suprasystem levels using all three levels of prevention.

LEARNING ACTIVITIES

1. Assess a neighborhood or local community using the following exploratory techniques: Perform a windshield survey by driving through the area and identifying types of houses, schools, churches, health-related agencies, and businesses, and looking for potential environmental and safety hazards. Interview a town hall clerk, a senior citizen at a meal site or day care center, a newspaper reporter, a visiting nurse, a police officer, a social worker, or a school nurse regarding health issues in the community. Call the local, county, or state health department for morbidity and mortality statistics. Try to attend a town council or school committee meeting. Compare and contrast these findings with classmates' findings.

2. Construct a matrix similar to Table 7-5 using interventions from a school setting.

3. In class, identify 10 to 15 questions that will elicit important health information from young adults. Each student must write answers to these questions. Tally the student responses, and draw conclusions from this assessment. Identify problems or potential problem areas, and construct a plan to solve or prevent these problems.

4. Attend a state or local health planning meeting. Observe the number of health care providers and consumers in attendance. Compare the meeting's issues with the goals of improving care quality and reducing health care costs.

REFERENCES

American Health Planning Association: National directory of health planning, policy, and regulatory agencies, ed 20, Falls Church, VA, 2009, AHPA.

Blum HL: *Planning for health*, New York, 1974, Human Sciences Press.

Budgen C, Cameron G: Program planning implementation and evaluation, 2003. In Centers for Disease Control and Prevention, APEXPH, 2009: wonder.cdc.gov/wonder/prevguid/p0000089/p0000089.asp. Accessed May 31, 2009.

Comprehensive Health Planning and Public Health Services Amendments of 1966: PL 89–749, 1966.

Duffus RL: *Lillian Wald: neighbor and crusader*, New York, 1938, Macmillan.

Gourevitch MN, Caronna CA, Kalkut G: Acute care. In Kovner AR, Knickman JR, editors: *Jonas and Kovner's health care delivery system in the United States*, ed 8, New York, 2005, Springer.

Green LW, Kreuter MW: *Health promotion planning: an educational and ecological approach*, ed 4, New York, 2005, McGraw-Hill.

Green LW, Kreuter MW, Deeds SG, et al: *Health education planning: a diagnostic approach*, Palo Alto, CA, 1980, Mayfield Publishing.

Harlow JM: Government and other types of oversight. In Garber KM, editor: *The U.S. health care delivery system: fundamental facts, definitions, and statistics*, Chicago, Ill, 2006, American Hospital Association.

Heart Disease, Cancer, and Stroke Amendments of 1965: PL 89–239, 1965.

Hegge ML: Independent study in community health nursing, *Nurs Outlook* 21:652–654, 1973.

Hogue C: An epidemiologic approach to distributive nursing practice. In Hall JE, Weaver BR, editors: *Distributive nursing practice: a systems approach to community health*, ed 2, Philadelphia, 1985, Lippincott Williams & Wilkins.

Hospital Survey and Construction Act of 1946 (Hill-Burton Act): PL 79–725.

Israel BA, Eng E, Schulz AJ, et al, editors: *Methods in community-based participatory research for health*, San Francisco, 2005, Jossey-Bass.

Issel LM: *Health program planning and evaluation*, ed 2, Sudbury, MA, 2009, Jones and Bartlett.

Kaiser Family Foundation: Focus on Health Reform 2010 - http://www.kff.org/healthreform/upload/8061.pdf2010b

Kovner AR: Hospitals. In Kovner A, Jonas S, editors: *Health care delivery in the United States*, ed 7, New York, 2002, Springer.

Labonte R: Health promotion and empowerment: reflections on professional practice, *Health Educ Q* 21:253–268, 1994.

Leavell HR, Clark EG: *Preventive medicine for the doctor in his community*, New York, 1965, McGraw-Hill.

Maslow AH: *Toward a psychology of being*, New York, 1968, Van Nostrand Reinhold.

Mueller K: *Health care policy in the United States*, Lincoln, NE, 1993, University of Nebraska Press.

National Association of County and City Health Officials (NACCHO): MAPP, 2009: www.naccho.org/topics/infrastructure/MAPP/index.cfm. Accessed May 31, 2009.

National Health Planning and Resources Development Act of 1974: PL 93–641, 1974.

Nyswander DB: Education for health: some principles and their application, *Health Educ Mono* 14:65–70, 1956.

Partnership for Health Amendments of 1967: PL 90–174, 1967.

Ruybal SE, Bauwens E, Fasla MJ: Community assessment: an epidemiological approach, *Nurs Outlook* 23:365–368, 1975.

Shonick W: *Government and health services*, New York, 1995, Oxford University Press.

Shuster GF, Goeppinger J: Community as client: assessment and analysis. In Stanhope M, Lancaster J, editors: *Public health nursing: population-centered health care in the community*, ed 7, St Louis, 2008, Mosby.

Silverstein NG: Lillian Wald at Henry Street: 1893–1895, *ANS Adv Nurs Sci* 7:1–12, 1985.

Sultz HA, Young KM: *Health care USA: understanding its organization and delivery*, ed 5, Boston, 2006, Jones and Bartlett.

Thorpe K: Cost containment. In Kovner A, Jonas S, editors: *Health care delivery in the United States*, ed 7, New York, 2002, Springer.

Community Health Education

Cathy D. Meade

Additional Material for Study, Review, and Further Exploration

evolve WEBSITE

http://evolve.elsevier.com/Nies

- Quiz
- Case Studies
- Glossary
- WebLinks
- Resource Tools
  - 8A: Learning Theories and Their Relationship to Health Education

- 8B: Framework for Developing Health Communications
- 8C: Patient Communication: Testicular Self-Examination (TSE)
- 8D: SMOG Formula for Estimating Readability Grade Level of Printed Text

OBJECTIVES

Upon completion of this chapter, the reader will be able to do the following:

1. Describe the goals of health education within the community setting.
2. Examine the nurse's role in community education within a sociopolitical and cultural context.
3. Select a learning theory, and describe its application to the individual, family, or aggregate.
4. Examine innovative and effective teaching and learning strategies that exemplify community-centered health education for the individual, family, or aggregate.

5. Compare and contrast Freire's approach to health education with an individualistic health education model.
6. Examine the importance of community engagement for having an impact on health disparities.
7. Outline a systematic process for developing culturally and literacy relevant health education materials, messages, media, and programs.
8. Relate and apply factors that enhance the suitability of health education materials, messages, media, and programs for an intended audience.
9. Prepare an appropriate and meaningful teaching plan and evaluation criteria for the individual, family, and group.

KEY TERMS

cognitive theory
community empowerment
community-based participatory methods
culturally effective care

health disparities
health education
health literacy
humanistic theories
learner verification

learning
materials and media
participatory action research (PAR)
problem-solving education
social learning theory

OUTLINE

Connecting with Everyday Realities
Health Education in the Community
Learning Theories, Principles, and Health Education Models
  Learning Theories
  Knowles' Assumptions About Adult Learners
  Health Education Models

Models of Individual Behavior
Model of Health Education Empowerment
Community Empowerment
The Nurse's Role in Health Education
Enhancing Communication
Framework for Developing Health Communications

CONNECTING WITH EVERYDAY REALITIES

The nurse may be tempted to often ask the following questions:

- Why does she keep smoking when she is pregnant?
- Why does the senior not get a follow-up for his fecal occult blood test (FOBT) abnormality?
- Why does this young man not take his diabetic medications (insulin) each day?
- Why are the parents late in immunizing their kids?
- Why won't more women attend the clinic's breast cancer screenings—they're free!
- Why does the community have such an alarming rate of obesity?

Although these questions represent the nurse's intense desire to understand the link between health behavior and health education, they do not yield answers or empower individuals or families. In fact, such questions do not address the root health issues and create a "blaming the victim" approach (Israel et al., 1994). The nurse might reframe the previous questions to better get at the root reasons and, in turn, empower individuals, families, and groups. Instead, ask the following questions:

- What life stressors are getting in the way of the expectant mom from quitting smoking for good? What stage of quitting might she be in? What factors might motivate her to stop?
- What factors might be preventing the senior man from getting a follow-up test (colonoscopy)? Might the colonoscopy procedure be scary? What beliefs might the man have about such tests? Might the instructions be difficult to understand? Does he have money for the prep? What can I do to verify understanding of the situation and better connect with his beliefs, motivations, and current knowledge?
- How does the young man with diabetes prefer to learn? What makes it difficult for him to know when to take his meds? What can I do to better connect the lifesaving instructions about insulin to his everyday activities? Could finances be an issue?
- What types of barriers might prevent the family from getting their kids immunized on time? Do they understand the schedule? Could I do a better job of explaining the importance of childhood immunizations? Might the family be confused about the different types of immunizations, especially in light of media attention about H1N1 (swine flu)? Could a personalized chart record help?
- What kinds of outreach methods might better attract community members to the free cancer screening? In what way could sustained relationships with community stakeholders and community members make a difference? How might I further engage community members in planning health events and screenings?
- What role might I play in developing links with schools, grocery stores, churches, and community centers to reach families with nutrition messages that are easy to understand and that fit their cultural background? What social, physical, cultural, linguistic, or structural factors should be considered when developing health messages?

HEALTH EDUCATION IN THE COMMUNITY

Historically, teaching has been a significant nursing responsibility since Florence Nightingale's (1859) early work. Gardner (1936) emphasized that health teaching is one of the most fundamental nursing principles and that "a nurse, in even the most obscure position must be a teacher of no mean order." There is much support for the nurse's involvement in health education, including the nurse practice acts, professional statements of the American Nurses Association (ANA) (1975), the patient's bill of rights of the American Hospital Association (AHA) (1975), the Joint Commission on Accreditation of Healthcare Organizations (now the Joint Commission, 1995), national standards on culturally and linguistically appropriate services of the Office of Minority Health (OMH) (1999), and the *Healthy People 2020* objectives of the U.S. Department of Health and Human Services (USDHHS) (2000) (see proposed communication objectives at www.healthypeople.gov/hp2020/Objectives/TopicArea.aspx?id=25&TopicArea=Health+Communication+and+Health+IT). Health education is an integral part of the nurse's role in the community for promoting health, preventing disease, and maintaining optimal wellness (Box 8-1). Moreover, the community is a vital link for the delivery of effective and equitable health care and offers the nurse multiple opportunities for providing appropriate health education within the context of a setting that is familiar to community members (Meade et al., 2002a).

The role of the nurse as health educator is especially important in light of the increasing diversity and demographically changing population in the United States, the increasingly technological advancements in health care, and the need to reduce the disconnect between scientific discovery and the delivery of interventions in the community (Freeman, 2004; Chu et al., 2008). More than ever before, health education activities and services are taking place outside the walls of hospitals in such settings as missions, YMCAs, beauty and barber shops, grocery stores, homeless

BOX 8-1   HEALTH EDUCATION ROLES AND ACTIVITIES OF THE NURSE IN THE COMMUNITY

- Advocate
- Caregiver
- Case manager
- Collaborator
- Community care agent
- Consultant
- Counselor
- Culture broker
- Educator
- Facilitator of health-promoting behaviors
- Information agent and broker
- Innovator

- Liaison
- Mediator
- Navigator
- Negotiator
- Policy analyst, policy maker, or change agent
- Promoter of collaborative partnerships
- Promoter of self-care and self-efficacy
- Recognizes dimensions of health choices
- Referral resource
- Researcher
- Sensitizer
- Social activist

Based on data from Clark (2007); Rankin and Stallings (2000); Redman (2006).

shelters, community-based clinics, health maintenance organizations, schools, work sites, senior centers, mobile health units, homes, and Women, Infants, and Children (WIC) sites. At the core of health education is the development of trusting relationships based on nurturing interactions, the use of community-based participatory methods that highlight community strengths, and the creation of sustainable collaborations and partnerships (Gwede et al., 2009; Leung, Yen, and Minkler, 2004; Luque et al., 2010; Martinez et al., 2008; Meade et al., 2009; Minkler, 2005; Olshansky et al., 2005; Smedley et al., 2003).

Health education's goal is to understand health behavior and to translate knowledge into relevant interventions and strategies for health enhancement, disease prevention, and chronic illness management. Health education aims to enhance wellness and decrease disability; attempts to actualize the health potential of individuals, families, communities, and society; and includes a broad and varied set of strategies aimed at influencing individuals within their social environment for improved health and well-being (Green and Kreuter, 2004). The nurse is ideally situated to bring together the necessary skills, knowledge, and community resources to impact the health of the community.

Health education is any combination of learning experiences designed to predispose, enable, and reinforce voluntary behavior conducive to health in individuals, groups, or communities (Green and Kreuter, 2004). Steuart and Kark (1962) state that "health education must achieve its ends through means that leave inviolate the rights of self-determination of the individuals and their community." A major challenge for community health nurse educators is to address the complex and intersecting sociopolitical conditions that affect community health by placing value on the contributions of community members and building on their strengths. The lasting effect of cognitive and behavioral changes relies heavily on learner participation to influence change in health behaviors and practices (Green and Kreuter, 2004; Leung et al., 2004; MacLeod and Zimmer, 2005; Cashman et al., 2008; Wallerstein and Duran, 2006; Kannan et al., 2008). In this manner, nurses alone cannot set individual, family, or community priorities. Rather, learners (community members) must be involved in determining their health education needs and priorities.

Community health education is based on practical, relevant, and scientifically sound methods and widely accessible technology. In the late 1970s, Kleinman (1978) described a social and cultural community health care system that related external factors (e.g., economical, political, and epidemiological) to internal factors (e.g., behavioral and communicative). This view of a sociocultural health care system grounds health education activities within sociopolitical structures, especially within local environmental settings, and views the community as client (Coleman et al., 2009; Giachello et al., 2003; Horowitz et al., 2004; Kobetz et al., 2009; Martyn et al., 2009; Meade et al., 2007; Petersen et al., 2004; Villarruel et al., 2007). As such, because the community level is often the location of health prevention and health intervention programs, it is significant for obtaining positive health outcomes. Moreover, the creation and delivery of relevant health education interventions and communications within the community setting is a national imperative as outlined by *Healthy People 2020*, OMH's Standards for the Provision of Culturally Competent Health Care (1999), and several Institute of Medicine reports (e.g., Nielsen-Bohlman et al., 2004; Smedley et al., 2003). Nurses are uniquely qualified to influence the health and well-being of community members' health behaviors through original and inventive activities that incorporate culturally, linguistically, and educationally relevant health education and outreach communications (Meade et al., 2007; Watters, 2003).

LEARNING THEORIES, PRINCIPLES, AND HEALTH EDUCATION MODELS

Learning Theories

Learning theories are helpful in understanding how individuals, families, and groups learn. The field of psychology provides the basis for these theories and illustrates how environmental stimuli elicit specific responses. Such theories can aid nurses to recognize the mechanisms that potentially modify knowledge, attitude, and behavior. Bigge and Shermis (2004) assert that learning is an enduring change that involves the modification of insights, behaviors, perceptions, or motivations. Although psychology textbooks describe learning theories in great detail, the following broad categories relate to the nursing application in a community setting:

RESEARCH HIGHLIGHTS

Linking Theory to Practice: An Example of a Sexually Transmitted Infection/Human Immunodeficiency Virus Risk Reduction Intervention in a Primary Care Setting

Reducing sexually transmitted infections (STIs)/human immuno-deficiency virus (HIV) is a national imperative. Responding to this priority, the "Sister to Sister: Respect Yourself! Protect Yourself! Because You Are Worth It!" program was created. This counseling theory–based intervention consists of a single 20-minute one-on-one nurse-led intervention and addresses three key themes: family/community, caring, and self-worth. The intervention includes counseling strategies, videos, condom demonstration, and client role-plays to support behavioral change through practice (Jemmott et al., 2008). As background, this educational, skill-based HIV risk-reduction intervention was previously designed and evaluated using a randomized controlled trial among African-American women (Jemmott, Jemmott, and O'Leary, 2007). Based on the Social Cognitive Theory and Theory of Planned Behavior, the curriculum targets risky sexual behaviors and women's control beliefs about factors that would facilitate and/or hinder their abilities to perform them. The nurses evaluated the effectiveness of four theory-based interventions: skill-building vs. information only, and two methods of intervention delivery (one-on-one vs. group) against a control group among a sample of 564 Black women (mean age 27.2 years) seeking outpatient care in a primary care clinic. Primary outcomes were self-reported sexual behaviors, and the secondary outcome was sexually transmitted disease (STD) incidence. Results indicated that the "Sister to Sister" one-on-one brief skill-building and group skill-building interventions were both effective at reducing sexual risk behaviors and STI occurrence, and that these effects lasted at the 12-month follow-up point. Findings showed that the skill-building group intervention did not produce superior outcomes to the one-on-one intervention. Even though the group intervention was lengthier and one might posit that greater benefit would be gained from interactions with other group members, the personalized nature of the one-on-one intervention may have been more customized to meet the specific risks of the women. Thus, the authors concluded that the brief nurse-led one-on-one and group skill-building interventions were effective in reducing STI/HIV sexual risk behaviors and STI incidence. One limitation of the study is that the primary measure was assessed by self-report. Overall, the findings are similar to those of other studies that support the use of cognitive behavioral skill-building interventions for reducing sexual risk behavior among women. Although continued research is necessary to replicate the study with other populations of women in other settings, there is high potential for application for brief nurse-led theory-based interventions for reducing the spread of sexually transmitted HIV infection.

From Jemmott JB et al: Sexually transmitted infection/HIV risk reduction interventions in clinical practice settings, *J Obstet Gynecol Neonatal Nurs* 37:137-145, 2008; and Jemmott LS, Jemmott JB, O'Leary A: A randomized controlled trial of brief HIV/STD prevention interventions for African American women in primary care settings: effects on sexual risk behavior and STD rate, *Am J Public Health* 97:1034-1040, 2007.

stimulus-response (S-R) conditioning (i.e., behavioristic), cognitive, humanistic, and social learning. **Resource Tool 8A** Learning Theories and Their Relationship to Health Education on the book's Evolve website at http://evolve.elsevier.com/Nies outlines these learning theories.

The nurse should remember that theories are not completely right or wrong. Different theories work well in different situations. Knowles (1989) relates that behaviorists program individuals through S-R mechanisms to behave in a certain fashion. Humanistic theories help individuals develop their potential in self-directing and holistic manners. Cognitive theorists recognize the brain's ability to think, feel, learn, and solve problems and train the brain to maximize these functions. Although social learning theory is largely a cognitive theory, it also includes elements of behaviorism (Bandura, 1977b). Social learning theory's premise is based on behavior explaining and enhancing learning through the concepts of efficacy, outcome expectation, and incentives.

Clinical Example
Application of Characteristics of Adult Learners to the Development of a Community Support Group

The following example illustrates the long-standing value of incorporating theoretical underpinnings in the development of community activities designed to meet specific learning needs. It provides a description of how nurses can play an active role in bolstering the community capacity and health of their community. Although this example dates back to the 1980s, it serves as an important reminder of the value of applying learning theories to one's work. As viewed later in this chapter, LUNA (Latinas Unidas por un Nuevo Amanecer, Inc., a nonprofit organization), whose mission is to provide support and offer culturally and linguistically relevant education to Hispanic breast cancer survivors and their families, was created based on similar tenets.

As background, the author and a colleague began a community support group for individuals with amyotrophic lateral sclerosis (ALS), more commonly known as Lou Gehrig's disease based on an identified community need. The support group was open to family members and friends. ALS is an incurable degenerative neuromuscular disease that affects nerve and muscle function and the brain's ability to control muscle movement. Community members provided feedback and identified the need for specific education topics and support for ALS. At that time, southeast Wisconsin did not have a support group. This initial dialogue provided the organizing framework for the inception of the first support group and, based on observations and interactions at the monthly meetings, an illustration of Knowles' assumptions follows:

Need to know: At the first support groups, the facilitator nurses introduce topics by describing the reason for the discussion and rationale for the selected subject (e.g., common concerns of patients and family members and informal assessments based on conversations). To prepare for discussion, group members introduce themselves, and the nurse asks what they hope to learn from the presentation. In some cases, members are unsure why they desire more information on a given topic but indicate that they want to listen. Progression of the disease is variable; therefore the need to know is often facilitated by the nurses and other patients who have already noted the importance of specific learning tasks (e.g., need for assistive walking device, need for financial planning, or need for information on assistive breathing devices).

Self-concept: A comfortable, informal environment allows patients to express feelings, emotions, and frustrations about this disease. Participants are encouraged to express themselves. Participants cultivate mutual respect and trust, and hugs are common as members begin to understand that others share similar situations and concerns. Group members have an opportunity to speak out about ways to manage and cope with their disease (e.g., decisions about life support and feeding tubes). Even if their choices are not the same as others', participants recognize and acknowledge these decisions without imposing their own value judgments. Facilitators and group members become equal partners in the learning process. At the core of the meetings was the formation of therapeutic healing relationships.

Experiences: Some patients and family members have gone through other difficult life experiences and stressors (e.g., other illnesses or deaths in the family) and can help others cope with the management of ALS. Patients share the strengths gained from such experiences with other support group members. Additionally, individuals and family members who are going through varying stages of the disease process can share their experiences (e.g., obtaining home care, selecting a computer, and managing breathing difficulties). They share tips and timesaving strategies with each other and newly diagnosed families and can learn from those experiences.

Readiness to learn: Family members often assume many roles when someone is ill, especially with a chronic illness such as ALS. The redefinition of roles creates new learning opportunities; however, this may hinder learning if it is too overwhelming. For example, the well spouse may assume the roles of caregiver, parent, and financial supporter. It is helpful to identify resources to help the family cope with new roles (e.g., respite care).

Orientation to learning: Learning a variety of psychomotor skills is necessary to care for the patient with ALS (e.g., suctioning, positioning, using a feeding tube, and toileting). The timeframe for learning such skills varies depending on the course of illness. Presenting information about such skills too early in the course of the disease may cause fear and anxiety. Families are often resistant to learning such tasks until the need is apparent. In some cases, this may be evident at a crisis point (e.g., a fall, a choking incident, or severe respiratory distress). However, nurse facilitators introduce these topics slowly by providing information via the support group, newsletter, e-mails, printed brochures, and personal one-on-one discussions.

Motivation: Individuals and families experience a shift in life goals when facing ALS. Such shifts may create learning opportunities aimed at enhancing quality of life, survivorship, and maintaining self-esteem. For example, a college professor with ALS kept his link to the university. He was highly motivated to continue his research work and supervise his graduate students. To continue his academic work, he learned to manage his breathing by using a ventilator, arranging transportation to the university, obtaining nursing care, and creating communication methods by using a computer.

Today, there are more than eight ALS support/caregiver groups in Wisconsin that grew from just a few who recognized an unmet need in the community. The ALS Association (ALSA) Wisconsin Chapter evolved from a local support group and became an official ALSA chapter in 1987. The chapter has four primary goals: (1) provide education, guidance, services, and support to patients with ALS, their families, and their caregivers; (2) promote public awareness of ALS; (3) raise funds for ALS research; and (4) establish an ALS-certified, multidisciplinary clinic to provide the highest level of care to the patients served by the chapter. For more information on services, go to alsawi.org/hopeline.php.

Knowles' Assumptions About Adult Learners

Knowles (1988, 1989) outlined several assumptions about adult learners. He contends that adults, like children, learn better in a facilitative, nonrestrictive, and nonstructured environment. Nurses who are familiar with these assumptions can develop teaching strategies that motivate and interest individuals, families, and groups and encourage active and full participation in the learning process. Nurses can help to create a self-directing, self-empowering learning environment. The following characteristics impact learning: the client's need to know, concept of self, readiness to learn, orientation to learning, experience, and motivation. Table 8-1 expands on these characteristics.

Health Education Models

In addition to learning theories, applying education theories and principles to situations involving individuals, families, and groups illustrates how ideas fit together, offers explanations for health behaviors or actions, and helps direct community nursing interventions. Such theoretical elements form the basis of understanding health behavior. Glanz and colleagues (2008) state that theories give educators the power to assess an intervention's strength and impact, and they serve to enrich, inform, and complement practice. Theoretical frameworks offer nurses an intervention blueprint that promotes learning and provides them with an organized approach to explaining concept relationships (Padilla and Bulcavage, 1991).

> *What the nurse needs is often not a single theory that would explain all that he or she hears, but rather a framework with meaningful hooks and rubrics on which to hang the new variables and insights offered by different theories. With this customized metatheory or framework, the nurse can triage new ideas into categories that have personal utility in his or her practice and everyday realities. (Green, 1998, p. 2)*

Models of Individual Behavior

Two models that explain preventive behavior determinants are the Health Belief Model (HBM), which is presented in Table 8-2 (Becker et al., 1977; Hochbaum, 1958; Kegeles et al., 1965; Rosenstock, 1966), and the Health Promotion Model (HPM) (Pender, Murdaugh, and Parsons, 2005). Both models are multifactorial, are based on value expectancy, and address individual perceptions, modifying factors, and likelihood of action. The HBM is based on social psychology and has undergone much empirical testing to predict compliance on singular preventive measures. The initial purpose of the HBM was to explain why people did not participate in health education programs to prevent or detect disease, in particular, tuberculosis (TB) screening programs (Hochbaum, 1958). Subsequent studies addressed other preventive actions and factors related to adherence to medical regimens (Becker, 1974). Primarily, the HBM is a value expectancy theory that addresses factors that promote health-enhancing behavior. It is disease specific and focuses on avoidance orientation.

TABLE 8-1	CHARACTERISTICS OF ADULT LEARNERS
CHARACTERISTICS	**APPLICATION TO HEALTH EDUCATION**
Need to Know Adults must know why they need to learn.	The nurse explores why individuals, families, and groups want to learn. The nurse helps individuals recognize their need to learn.
Concept of Self Adults have a self-concept that developed from dependence to independence. It moves from other's direction to self-direction. Adults want to be capable of self-direction.	The nurse acknowledges that individuals, families, and groups are able to make choices and decisions. The nurse creates an environment in which patients can express themselves. The nurse recognizes that individuals, families, and groups can learn from their selected actions and can take self-direction and responsibility for such behaviors.
Experience Adults may draw upon many life experiences. Such experiences are enriching and are powerful learning resources.	The nurse assesses individuals, families, and groups for life experiences related to health issues. The nurse helps facilitate connections between previous and present experiences. The nurse allows individuals, families, and groups to share experiences with others in a supportive manner. Experiential methods, problem solving, case methods, and discussion can help uncover the learner's experiences. The nurse clarifies previous and present experiences; this is especially helpful with negative or biased experiences.
Readiness to Learn Developmental tasks and social roles affect readiness to learn. The timing of learning experiences with developmental tasks is important.	The nurse assesses and identifies individual, family, and group roles (e.g., caregivers or single parents) and key developmental tasks. The nurse seeks to understand the impact of roles and tasks on learning. The nurse creates role-modeling experiences.
Orientation to Learning Learning is present oriented and "now" based. Learning is directed to the immediate need and is problem centered.	The nurse assesses the learning needs of individuals, families, and groups on the basis of their priority. The nurse recognizes everyday stresses and hassles and addresses them within their learning context. The nurse provides health information, gives responses to their immediate needs, offers/provides health information, and offers problem-solving skills.
Motivation Internal drivers and factors are powerful motivators (e.g., self-esteem, life goals, quality of life, and responsibility).	The nurse determines individual, family, and group motivators. The nurse assesses for barriers that block motivation (e.g., poor self-esteem or lack of resources) and provides appropriate education, counseling, and referrals.

Modified from Knowles MS: *The making of an adult educator: an autobiographical journey,* San Francisco, 1989, Jossey-Bass; and Knowles MS: *The modern practice of adult education: from pedagogy to andragogy,* Chicago, 1988, Cambridge Press.

TABLE 8-2	HEALTH BELIEF MODEL
COMPONENTS	**EXAMPLE AND EXPLANATION**
Perceived susceptibility	Belief that disease state is present or likely to occur
Perceived severity	Perception that disease state or condition is harmful and has serious consequences
Perceived benefits	Belief that health action is of value and has efficacy
Perceived barriers	Belief that health action would be associated with hindrances (e.g., cost)
Self-efficacy	Belief that actions can be performed to achieve the desired outcome (one's confidence)
Demographics	Age, sex, and ethnicity
Cues to action	Influencing factors to get ready for action (e.g., billboards, reminder cues, newspapers)

For a more detailed description of the HBM, see Becker (1974).

The HBM considers perceived susceptibility, perceived severity, perceived benefits, perceived barriers, and other socio-psychological and structural variables. In an early review of 46 studies using the HBM, perceived benefits were found to be the most powerful predictive element within the model, whereas perceived severity had the lowest associative value (Janz and Becker, 1984). Self-efficacy, or the notion that an individual can act successfully on a given behavior to produce the desired outcome (Bandura, 1977a, 1977b), was later added to the HBM (Rosenstock, Strecher, and Becker, 1988; Strecher et al., 1986).

Champion and Skinner (2008) point out that one of the limitations of the HBM is the variability in measurement of the central HBM constructs, which include the inconsistent measurement of HBM concepts and the lack of establishing validity and reliability of the measures prior to testing. For example, applying similar construct measures across different behaviors, such as barriers for mammography and colonoscopy, may be quite different. Although the past decade has produced some good examples of HBM scale development (Champion, 1999; Champion et al., 2008; Joseph et al., 2007; Rawl et al., 2000), caution should be taken when applying the HBM in multicultural settings. It would be important to determine whether the overall assumptions of the HBM—assumptions related to the value of health and illness—are similar to those of the particular racial/ethnic group under study. Further, checking wording for cultural distinctions is critical to the model's usefulness (Janz, Champion, and Strecher, 2002). Although the HBM identifies an array of variables important in explaining individual health, nurses should view these variables within a larger societal perspective.

Pender's Health Promotion Model (HPM) is a competence or approach-oriented model and, unlike the HBM, does not rely on personal threat as a motivating factor. The HPM brings together a number of constructs from expectancy-value theory and social cognitive theory within a holistic nursing framework (Pender et al., 2005). Gillis (1993) reviewed 23 studies conducted between 1983 and 1992 and reported that Pender's HPM was the most common theoretical framework in health promotion studies. Gillis identified that self-efficacy was the strongest determinant of participation in a health-promoting lifestyle, followed by social support, perceived benefits, perceived barriers, and an individual's definition of health education. Locus of control was the least important determinant, although it is the most studied.

The HPM is meant to provide an organizing framework to explain why individuals engage in health actions. It is applicable across the lifespan and has been used to examine the multidimensional nature of persons interacting with their physical and interpersonal environments, such as bicycle helmet use (Lohse, 2003) or health-promoting behaviors among Hispanics (Hulme et al., 2003), as a causal model of commitment to a plan for exercise in a sample of 400 Korean adults (Shin et al., 2005), and use of hearing protection devices by 703 construction workers (Ronis, Hong, and Lusk, 2006). Table 8-3 lists the main HPM components with behavioral action as the desired output.

The HBM and HPM can assist community health nurses in examining an individual's health choices and decisions for influencing health-related behaviors. The models offer nurses a cluster of variables that provide interesting insights into explaining health behavior. These variables are helpful cues; the nurse should consider them in planning and interacting with health education interventions but not try to fit an individual into all the categories. Simply put, models are aids that guide nurses in assessing patients and in developing, selecting, and implementing relevant educational interventions. In applying the models, a nurse might consider the following questions in relation to his or her own health behavior:

- Do you strive for improved health?
- Are you or your family susceptible to heart disease or obesity?

TABLE 8-3 HEALTH PROMOTION MODEL COMPONENTS AND OUTPUTS

COGNITIVE-PERCEPTUAL FACTORS	EXAMPLE AND EXPLANATION
Importance of health	Perceived value of health to functioning and life
Perceived control of health	Perceived ability to control health (external, internal, or chance)
Perceived self-efficacy	Perceived ability to perform the necessary behaviors to achieve an outcome
Definition of health	Views of what health means for the individual
	May vary from absence of illness to self-actualization
Perceived health status	Perception of how the individual views health
	May range from wellness to illness
Perceived benefits of health-promoting behaviors	Perception of positive outcomes that can occur from health-promoting behavior (e.g., feel fit and toned)
Perceived barriers to health-promoting behaviors	Perception of things that obstruct health-promoting behaviors (e.g., money and transportation)

MODIFYING FACTORS	EXAMPLE AND EXPLANATION
Demographics	Age, sex, and race
Biologic	Weight and body fat
Interpersonal influences	Interactions with family and nurses
Situational factors	Environmental determinants that make health-promoting options available
Behavioral	Previous knowledge or skills
Cues to action	Influencing factors such as internal cues (e.g., good self-image) and external cues (e.g., mass media)

For a more comprehensive description and explanation of the HPM, see Pender et al. (2005).

- Does a family history of cardiovascular disease motivate you or your family to exercise?
- Does looking fit and toned and having energy motivate you to exercise?
- Do work, school, or family responsibilities get in the way of your exercise plans?
- Has a family member, friend, or health professional recently reminded you of the benefits of exercise and encouraged you to start exercising?
- Do you believe you can initiate and incorporate an exercise program into your lifestyle, or do you need external reinforcement and cues?
- Do money, safety, and time pose barriers to planning an exercise program?
- Do you see any benefits to exercise, for example, looking and feeling better and more energized?
- In modifying your health behaviors, how important is exercise compared with other behaviors (e.g., getting relief from work and school stresses, cutting down on snacks, spending quality time with your family)?

Think about these questions and consider your answers. Talk about these issues with a colleague and try to develop an action plan tailored to your own priorities, needs, and capabilities.

Model of Health Education Empowerment

The HBM and HPM focus on individual strategies for achieving optimal health and well-being. The models are similar in that they are multifactorial, are based on the idea of value expectancy, and address individual perceptions, modifying factors, and likelihood of action. Although such approaches may be appropriate in changing individual behaviors, they do not address the complex relationships among social, structural, and physical factors in the environment, such as racism, lack of social support systems, and inaccessible health services (Israel et al., 1998; Smedley et al., 2003). Van Wyk (1999) suggests that nurses cannot assign power and control to the individual within the community but rather that the "power" must be taken on by the individual with the nurse *guiding* the dynamic process. This process includes examining such factors as education, health literacy, gender, and class and recognizing the structural and foundational changes that are needed to elicit change for socially and politically disenfranchised groups. Thus, knowledge is produced in a social context, and it is inextricably bound to relations of power.

An appropriate health education model is one that embraces a broader definition of health and addresses social, political, and economic aspects of health. This view of the health care system as a sociocultural system better grounds health education interventions within the sociopolitical structure, especially within local environmental settings (Goodman et al., 1998; Labonte, 1994). Such a theoretical perspective is congruent with community health education because it supports learner participation and involvement and emphasizes empowerment.

Empowerment and literacy are two concepts that share a common history: The concept of empowerment can be traced back to Paulo Freire, a Brazilian educator in the 1950s who sought to promote literacy among the poorest of the poor, most oppressed members of the population. He based his work on a problem-solving approach to education, which contrasts with the banking education approach that places the learner in a passive role. Problem-solving education allows active participation and ongoing dialogue and encourages learners to be critical and reflective about health issues. Freire suggested that when individuals assume the role of *objects*, they become powerless and allow the environment to control them. However, when individuals become *subjects*, they influence environmental factors that affect their lives and community. Thus community members, or subjects, are the best resources to elicit change (Freire, 2000, 2005).

Freire's methodology, often referred to as critical consciousness, involves not only education but also activism on the part of the educator. The basic tenet of Freire's work centers on empowerment, the contextualization of peoples' daily experiences, and collaborative, collegial dialogue in adult education. Freire's work speaks to a variety of action research applications, including those that relate to improving community health of marginalized populations. Freire's approach to health education increases health knowledge through a participatory group process and emphasizes establishing sustainable lateral relationships. This process explores the problem's nature and addresses the problem's deeper issues. The nurse, or facilitator-educator, is a resource person and is an equal partner with the other group members. Listening is the first phase and is essential to understanding the issues. The exchange of ideas and concerns creates a problem-posing dialogue and identifies root problems or generative themes. The group discusses and explores the problem's root causes. Finally, group members create relevant action plans that are congruent with their own reality (Freire, 2000).

The goal of participatory action research (PAR) is social change. It is consistent with the role and responsibilities of the community nurse (Olshansky et al., 2005) and embraces the use of community-based participatory methods. What this means is that participation and action from stakeholders and important knowledge about conditions and issues gained facilitates strategies reached collectively (e.g., access to care, access to information). In this manner, the value of communities' experiential knowledge is affirmed (Leung et al., 2004). Examples of the use of PAR include Horowitz et al. (2004), who describe the use of combining local and academic expertise to study health disparities and create peer-led classes to improve chronic disease management in East and Central Harlem; Edgren and colleagues (2005), who offered suggestions for involving the community in fighting against asthma; English and colleagues (2004), who developed the REACH 2010 program to build a public health community capacity program with a tribal community in the Southwest; and Giachello et al., (2003), who addressed the disproportionately high rate of diabetes in southeast Chicago through community-led activities.

At the core of empowerment are *information, communication,* and *health education* (World Health Organization [WHO], 1994). When nurses involve individuals, families, and groups in their learning, it validates their role and helps ensure the intervention's relevance (Leung et al., 2004; Meade et al., 2003; Minkler, Wallerstein, and Wilson, 2008; Olshansky et al., 2005). Nurses can use empowerment strategies to help people develop skills in problem solving, critical thinking, networking, negotiating, lobbying, and information seeking to enhance health. Freire's approach may seem similar to health education's emphasis on helping people take responsibility for their health by providing them with information, skills, reinforcement, and support. However, Freire purports that knowledge imparted by the collective group is significantly more powerful than information provided by health educators. Freire's approach attempts to uncover the social and political aspects of problems and encourages group members to define and develop action strategies. Hence, health changes are complex and usually do not have immediate solutions; therefore the term problem *posing*, rather than problem *solving*, may better describe this empowerment process (Minkler, Wallerstein, and Wilson, 2008).

Examples of Empowerment Education and Participatory Methods

1. **López and colleagues (2005)** relate how photovoice was used as a participatory action research method with African-American breast cancer survivors in rural east North Carolina, referred to as the "inspirational images project." The aim of the study was to use this research method to allow women to convey the social and cultural meaning of silence about breast cancer and to voice their survivorship concerns so that relevant interventions could be developed to meet their needs. The task of the women was to take at least six pictures of people, places, or things that they enjoyed in life; significant things they encountered as a survivor; and what was used to cope. Discussion of photographs (e.g., picture of church) led to discussions including a six-step inductive questioning technique suggested by Wallerstein and Bernstein (1988), which helps participants in framing educational strategies:

   - What do you *SEE* in this photograph?
   - What is *HAPPENING* in the photograph?
   - How does this relate to *OUR* lives?
   - *WHY* do these issues exist?
   - How can we become *EMPOWERED* by our new social understanding?
   - What can we *DO* to address these issues?

   The use of photovoice offers an important and creative way to facilitate shared knowledge to achieve social change.

2. **N. Wilson and colleagues (2008)** describe YES! (Youth Empowerment Strategies), an after-school program for underserved elementary and middle school youth. Designed to reduce risky behaviors including drug, alcohol, and tobacco use, YES! combines multiple youth empowerment strategies to bolster youth's capacities and strengths to build problem-solving skills. A number of empowerment education projects including photovoice and social action projects (e.g., awareness campaigns, projects to improve school spirit) were developed that involved members of the intended audience in the planning and implementation.

3. **Luque et al. (2010)** report the use of empowering processes based on Freire's Popular Education principles (Freire, 2000) and Social Cognitive Theory, which focused on the constructs of environment, behavioral capability, observational learning, and self-efficacy (Bandura, 1977a, 1977b) for creating a barbershop training program about prostate cancer. By employing techniques borrowed from empowerment education (Wallerstein and Bernstein, 1988), barbers were engaged in group learning activities and problem-posing exercises around preferences and values related to prostate cancer health. Once the training and curriculum was completed among eight barbers, the team worked closely with the barbers to modify and create a supportive workplace environment for new health education tools (easy-to-read posters, brochures, DVD player, prostate cancer display model) to fuel discussions about prostate cancer health and decision making. Once the barbers were trained, structured surveys with barbershop clients (N = 40) were conducted. Results showed a significant increase in participants' self-reported knowledge of prostate cancer and an increased likelihood of discussing prostate cancer with a health care provider ($P <.001$). In conclusion, the barber-administered pilot intervention appears to be an appropriate and viable communication strategy for promoting prostate knowledge to a priority population in a convenient and familiar setting.

Community Empowerment

Community empowerment is a central tenet of community organization, whereby community members take on greater power to create change. It is based on community cultural strengths and assets. An empowerment continuum acknowledges the value and interdependence of individual and political action strategies aimed at the collective while maintaining the community organization as central (Minkler, Wallerstein, and Wilson, 2008). As such, community organization reinforces one of the field's underlying premises as outlined by Nyswander (1956): "Start where the people are." Meade and Calvo (2001) point out that attention must be given to collective rather than individual efforts to ensure that the outcomes reflect the voices of the community and truly make a difference in people's lives. Further, Labonte (1994) states that the community is the engine of health promotion and a vehicle of empowerment. He describes five spheres of an empowerment model, which focus on the following levels of social organization: interpersonal (personal empowerment), intragroup (small-group development), intergroup (community), interorganizational (coalition building), and political action. A multilevel empowerment model allows us to consider both macro-level and micro-level forces that combine to create both health and disease. Therefore, it seems that both micro and macro viewpoints on health education provide nurses with multiple opportunities for intervention across a broad continuum.

In summary, health education activities that respond to McKinlay's (1979) call to study "upstream," that is, to examine the underlying causes of health inequalities, through multilevel education and research allow nurses to be informed by critical perspectives from education, anthropology, and public health. For more extensive readings on this topic, see *Methods in Community-based Participatory Research for Health* (Israel et al., 2005) and *Community-Based Participatory Research for Health: From Process to Outcomes* (Minkler and Wallerstein, 2008).

To effect change at the community level, nurses must be knowledgeable about key concepts central to community organization (Table 8-4). This approach is an effective methodological tool that enables nurses to partner with the community, identify common goals, develop strategies, and mobilize resources to increase community empowerment, capacity, and community competence. Key concepts inherent in community health education programming are empowerment, principle of participation, issue selection, principle of relevance, social capital, and creation of critical consciousness (Minkler, Wallerstein, and Wilson, 2008).

TABLE 8-4   COMMUNITY ORGANIZATION PRACTICE

KEY CONCEPTS	APPLICATION TO HEALTH EDUCATION (NURSING ACTIONS)
Empowerment Help individuals, families, and groups gain insight and mastery over life situations through problem solving and dialogue	The nurse works with community members in identifying and defining issues and creates mechanisms for discussion and problem solving and identification of other factors that have an impact on everyday lives.
Principle of Relevancy Know what issues are important to community members (these may differ from the issues important to nurses)	The nurse holds town hall meetings and group discussions to allow members to share concerns and important issues. The nurse encourages the community to define issues. The nurse facilitates community members to make decisions about health programs and messages.
Principle of Participation Learn by doing	The nurse encourages group support. The nurse recognizes that active vs. passive participation results in greater likelihood of attitude and behavior changes.
Issue Selection Identify community problems that the community believes are specific, meaningful, and attainable	The nurse uses problem-solving techniques to help group members identify relevant issues vs. troubling problems (e.g., door-to-door surveys and group process activities).
Creation of Critical Consciousness Encourage relationships of equality and mutual respect among group members and educators to identify root problems and generate appropriate action plans	The nurse uses problem-posing dialogue (Freire, 2005) to understand root issues and devises creative and innovative methods to transform situations.
Social Capital Relationships (networks) between community members (i.e., trust, engagement)	The nurse encourages community members to work together to improve social networks: they work together on a particular health gap in their community through partnership activities.

Modified from Minkler M, Wallerstein N, Wilson N: Improving health through community organization and community building. In Glanz K et al., editors: *Health behavior and health education: theory, research and practice,* ed 4, San Francisco, 2008, Jossey-Bass, pp. 288-312.

Keck (1994) indicated that successful community health relies on empowering citizens to make decisions about individual and community health. Empowering citizens causes power to shift from health providers to community members in addressing health priorities. Collaboration and cooperation among community members, academicians, clinicians, health agencies, and businesses help ensure that scientific advances, community needs, sociopolitical needs, and environmental needs converge in a humanistic manner. The development of LUNA (Latinas Unidas por un Nuevo Amanecer, Inc.) in Tampa, Florida, illustrates how the basic tenets of community need and organization fuel the development of a locally initiated group. LUNA represents a grassroots initiative to meet the needs of Hispanic breast cancer survivors and serves as a model for nurses, researchers, and community advocates working with underserved groups of cancer survivors.

Clinical Example

Example of Community Empowerment-Collaboration-Participation: LUNA

In 2002, a Latina nurse (Melba Martinez, RN, BSN), who had had breast cancer diagnosed in 1995, started the first grassroots support group for Latinas with breast cancer in West Central Florida. The group began with five members and within the first year had 38 active members who attended monthly meetings.

The group was initiated in response to an unmet need in the Tampa Bay area, that is, lack of education services for Latinas with breast cancer diagnosed and who primarily spoke Spanish. Over the years, LUNA has created a network of more than 200 Latina survivors and has grown and become *Latinas Unidas por un Nuevo Amanecer,* Inc., a nonprofit organization whose mission is to provide support and offer culturally and linguistically relevant education to Hispanic breast cancer survivors and their families, friends, and caregivers. The organization primarily serves underserved, immigrant, low-income Latinas with limited English proficiency, assists with navigating the health care system, and serves as a community resource. LUNA draws on the tenets of community organization and empowerment fueled by problem-posing education. The three components of the LUNA model are (1) education (e.g., classes and presentations, Spanish cancer information, health care navigation, community outreach), (2) support (e.g., peer to peer, home, hospital and phone visits, communications), and (3) social reintegration (e.g., celebration of life events such as birthdays, cancer camps, walks, and other social events), very similar to the start-up of the ALS Support group previously described.

Outcomes From LUNA

1. Campamento Alegria: The first-ever Spanish-language oncology camp for Latina cancer survivors. A biennial program designed to provide Latinas in whom cancer has been diagnosed a positive and unforgettable experience through a variety of activities that help sustain them through their cancer

journey (Martinez et al., 2008). Campamento Alegria aims to serve 100 women, who would otherwise not have this opportunity to participate in such activities. There are no fees for the patients/survivors for a 3-day/2-night stay at the retreat facility, meals and related activities, orientation, and reunion meeting.

2. Community education and outreach: Attendance at various community events and health fairs to increase breast cancer screening awareness and provide cancer information and resources in Spanish.

3. Ongoing monthly educational support group meetings: Presentations and classes provided by Spanish-speaking health professionals on various survivorship issues and cancer-related topics.

4. Plans to develop a patient navigator program for Latina patients with newly diagnosed cancer.

The process for creating LUNA began with one nurse who, through dedication and dialogue with others in the same situation, began taking charge of the situation based on input from other community members. From both her nursing and personal experiences she knew how hard it was for Hispanic women in whom cancer has been diagnosed to navigate the health care system, how difficult it was to take time for self-care, and how challenging it was for Hispanic women to talk about their fears. She recognized that Latinas with breast cancer should reach out to each other with understanding and compassion in their own language to move toward self-education and self-actualization. Since its inception, LUNA has partnered with various community-based organizations, hospitals, academic centers, churches, and other social support services to create a strong web of support. For example, LUNA has a strong partnership with the Tampa Bay Community Cancer Network (TBCCN), a community network program, funded by the National Cancer Institute's Center to Reduce Cancer Health Disparities, and local hospitals. Together they have worked with researchers to adapt a stress management program for Latinas undergoing chemotherapy. LUNA represents a ground-up effort, which got its start by addressing an unmet need of Hispanic breast cancer survivors. It serves as an excellent model and reminder for nurses, researchers, and community advocates that the best ideas come from the soul. For more information: hispanicbreastcancer.org/ (in Spanish).

"Never doubt that a small group of thoughtful, committed citizens can change the world. Indeed, it is the only thing that ever has."

Margaret Mead

Acknowledgments: Melba Martinez, RN, BSN, and Dinorah (Dina) Martinez, MA, MPH.

THE NURSE'S ROLE IN HEALTH EDUCATION

Although learning theories and health education models provide a useful framework for planning health interventions, the nurse's ability to facilitate the education process and become a partner with individuals and communities is key to the method's application. At the core of health education is the therapeutic and healing relationship between the nurse and individuals, families, and the community. Simply put, nurses hold the process together and are catalysts for change in delivering humanistic care. Nurses activate ideas, offer appropriate interventions, identify resources, and facilitate

group empowerment. Rankin and Stallings (2000) describe the following key characteristics of nurses in facilitating the teacher-learner process: confidence, competence, caring, and communication. It is beyond the scope of this chapter to describe multiple communication techniques in detail, but the reader is reminded about the value of establishing inclusion and trust before delivering the health education content.

Clinical Example

Mr. Chen often visits the neighborhood senior center weekly to play cards and have lunch with several of his longtime friends. Once a month he takes part in the blood pressure clinic offered by the health department. The health department's outreach services offers clinics in community-based centers, and an increased number of community members use this free service on an ongoing basis. Mr. Chen has limited resources, so the clinic provides him with valuable access to health information. On his first visit to the clinic, his blood pressure is 178/88 mm Hg. On his second visit, his reading is 188/94. He states that the city hospital has treated him for high blood pressure for more than 5 years, that doctors prescribed several medications 6 months earlier, and that he received some written materials to read (they were all in English). Although he reads somewhat in English, he tells the nurse that it would have been nice to see materials in his familiar language.

The nurse's assessment reveals that Mr. Chen takes his medication only when he does not "feel so good." He said his doctor advises him to take his medicines regularly, and he states that he takes them faithfully when he does not feel well. He tells the nurse that he remembers getting some booklets about his medications and "blood," but he found them too long and tiring to read. The nurse's educational assessment reveals that Mr. Chen has completed 8 years of schooling, does not read much, enjoys television over print, and prefers to learn from pictures or from other people in groups. He states that he likes to get his health information in English but would prefer to get some materials in Chinese. His low reading skills impact his ability to get health instructions in a meaningful way. He has taken the health instruction literally (e.g., he interprets "take regularly" to mean take consistently when "I don't feel right" vs. take the pills on a regular schedule).

To facilitate learning, the nurse establishes a teaching plan with Mr. Chen's input. This plan involves communicating health instructions in more relevant ways (e.g., using pictures, drawings, mnemonics, videotapes), providing some word cards for him in Chinese, and putting him in touch with county financial resources to assist in buying his medicines. The nurse also establishes a follow-up plan with a bilingual nurse to verify Mr. Chen's understanding of how to take his meds by asking him to repeat back in his own words when/how he takes his meds (teach-back methods). She also plans to develop a series of health education group classes for the seniors about health and wellness, with high blood pressure being one of the topics of discussion.

ENHANCING COMMUNICATION

The critical step of inclusion establishes the base for possible health action; it sets the relationship. The nurse enhances inclusion by greeting individuals, families, and groups in a warm fashion, offering comfort, and attending to immediate concerns or stresses. Education does not begin with the first instructional word. Rather, education begins with establishing an atmosphere conducive to learning, whereby a therapeutic trusting relationship forms the foundation for building a healing relationship. If the nurse attends to inclusion first, individuals, families, and groups begin to trust the nurse and thereby trust the health education message. This trust is evident through active participation and commitment in the education process.

Although Chapter 13 contains a detailed perspective on cultural diversity and community health nursing, it is important to note that the ongoing enhancement and refinement of nursing knowledge and skills for providing culturally effective care is critical to community health education. Nurses are key in responding to diverse community members' everyday health realities with meaningful and understandable information that "fits those realities." This entails taking time to get to know individuals, their families, and their experiences.

Meleis (1999) cogently describes culturally competent care as care that exhibits sensitivity to the differences in individuals based on their vast experiences and responses due to their backgrounds, sexual orientation, socioeconomic status, ethnicity, literacy, and cultural background. She depicts several properties that make up the "essence of health nurses" who deliver culturally competent care. First, they possess an explanatory system that values diversity. This is a system that is not drained by the constant attempt to interpret symbols but rather is energized by the variations. Second, they show expert assessment skills to discern different and similar patterns of responses that help to plan appropriate educational interventions. Third, culturally competent nurses are aware of the diversity of communication patterns and how language and communication influence "trust within the relationship." Culturally effective professionals also recognize how marginalization may increase health risks for individuals and that using the expertise of insiders in the culture is a highly valued skill. Last, nurses who deliver culturally effective care readily acknowledge differences and do not tolerate inequities.

For detailed information on the provision of culturally appropriate health care, consult the OMH's national standards for culturally and linguistically appropriate services (CLAS) (OMH, 1999). The standards reinforce the ability of health care providers and organizations to understand and respond effectively to the cultural and linguistic needs brought by patients and community members to the health care setting. Several standards have particular relevance to community nursing. Standard 1 relates that consumers should receive, from all staff members, effective, understandable, and respectful care that is provided in a manner compatible with their cultural health beliefs and practices and preferred language. Standard 12 states that health care organizations should develop participatory, collaborative partnerships with communities and utilize a variety of formal and informal mechanisms to facilitate community and patient/

ETHICAL INSIGHTS
Ethical Issues Related to Health Education and Health Literacy

- **Health literacy:** Do community members understand the plethora of printed and electronic health messages communicated to them in terms of language, ease of reading, and linguistics? Nurses should assess their roles as educators, information brokers, advocates, facilitators, collaborative problem solvers, and navigators. Nurses should consider the demands of the health care system on client autonomy.
- **Individual vs. collective/societal rights and responsibility for health:** What communication factors should the nurse consider when balancing the health education needs of the individual vs. collective (e.g., family and community)? What communication gaps can be bridged by the development and implementation of culturally, linguistically, and literacy relevant health information?
- **Social justice and equity:** Do all community members enjoy equity in their access to health education and information? Does health information take into account the diversity of a demographically changing country? What type of materials are available for non-English–speaking clients? What strategies, programs, and interventions can be implemented to reduce the discovery to delivery disconnect?
- **Allocation of resources:** In what way do policies promote and/or hinder promotion of health literacy? Do national/local government and corporate/institutional policies impact the availability, accessibility, and equitable distribution of information resources? In what way do current policies reward and support patient education? How can the nurse get involved in shaping and redirecting health policy and moving policy into practice? This includes policies at the institutional, community, local, and national level.
- **Cultural effectiveness:** What skills, knowledge, and experiences are necessary when planning health education within the context of people's history and everyday realities? The nurse should assess his or her abilities to approach health education tasks with confidence, compassion, competence, and cultural humility (Marks, 2009; OMH, 1999).

consumer involvement in designing and implementing CLAS-related activities. For more information, see the OMH website at minorityhealth.hhs.gov.

As each nurse addresses diversity and strives for culturally effective care, it is key that issues are identified and alternatives explored that are empowering and affirming to all involved. This requires self-awareness and recognizing that diversity development, attention to the culturally and linguistically appropriate care, and cultural effectiveness are a process, not a program. In short, cultural competency is an ongoing journey that requires an openness to acknowledge what one does not know and the willingness to seek better ways to get the job done.

Consider also some of the ethical issues that you might confront in the community. As an example, consider the following nursing research study by Strickland and colleagues (1999), who addressed religion in the design and delivery of a culturally and linguistically appropriate cervical health promotion program for eastern Washington's Yakama Indian women. The investigators conducted personal interviews with spiritual leaders and male and female members of the

Wa'Shat Longhouse religion and obtained religious influences by asking questions about life views, communication channels, and leadership. Results showed that program goals must be holistic, teaching methods must include circular symbols, and intentions must be linked with natural communication patterns and must involve elders. Results revealed that storytelling, talking circles, role models, and multiple sensory modalities were important teaching approaches. For example, the circle symbol of unity connected the people and the earth. The group facilitator needs to be an equal learner who respects the wisdom, experiences, and contributions of each member. Also, time is loosely structured among the Yakama; therefore, an educational session may require an entire morning. The investigators also found that, unlike other cultures, the Yakama culture values information directly from the elders over the dissemination of prevention information.

FRAMEWORK FOR DEVELOPING HEALTH COMMUNICATIONS

Within the community, the nurse's intended audience may be an individual, family, group, or many segments of the community. Using a systematic approach to the development, design, and delivery of health education programs, messages and media provide the nurse with an organized, user-friendly approach to health message delivery. Although nurses may use a variety of educational models, theoretical frameworks, and teaching and learning principles, the National Cancer Institute suggests the "Framework for Developing Health Communications" to create a variety of health education messages and programs (USDHHS, 2005).

 See **Resource Tool 8B**, Framework for Developing Health Communications, on the book's Evolve website at http://evolve.elsevier.com/Nies.

This organizing framework has four stages (simplified from six) and is depicted by a circular loop that offers the opportunity for continuous assessment, feedback, and improvement. The framework has been used widely by the author when developing cancer education materials and media on such topics as smoking, prostate cancer, breast and cervical cancer, and stress management (Brandon et al., 2004; Jacobsen et al., 2002; Meade, McKinney, and Barnas, 1994; Meade et al., 2003; Meade et al., 2002a; Quinn et al., 2006; Schapira, Meade, and Nattinger, 1997). This framework can be easily adapted to the design and development of all types of health education topics such as diabetes, hypertension, nutrition, and so forth.

This framework is based on the principles of social marketing, health education, and mass communication theories and relies on intended audience assessment to guide the process. It is highly congruent with Freire's model of empowerment education, which encourages ongoing dialogue with potential consumers and users of health education services. Although this model focuses on communication strategies aimed at the programmatic level, the basic elements are applicable to individual, family, and group systems. The nurse should not expect to apply the model in a linear manner but rather to move back and forth between the stages. These stages mirror the nursing process (assessment, planning, implementation, and evaluation) and provide a sequential path for continuous assessment, feedback, and improvement for achieving a successful communication program.

The ideas contained in this "Framework for Developing Health Communications" model are a practical schema for planning and implementing health education communications programs. Nurses should use the model as a guide to planning health education messages and programs. It is also suggested that the nurse use an organized and systematic approach rather than attempt to fit his or her health education plan into every step (see "Launching a Breast Education and Outreach Screening Program").

Stage I: Planning and Strategy Development

The planning stage provides the foundation for the communication program's planning process and is crucial in setting the stage for communications. Understanding the intended audience's learning needs and targeting the program or message to the audience is key to activating effective health education. This step reinforces Freire's philosophical tenets of ascertaining the intended audience's needs and creating an open dialogue. This stage also reduces expensive alterations once the program is under way.

Questions to Ask

- Who is the intended audience?
- What is known about the audience and from what sources?
- What are the communication and education objectives and goals?
- What evaluation strategies will the nurse use?
- What is the health issue of interest?

Collaborative Actions to Take

- Review available data from health statistics, census data, local sources, libraries, newspapers, and local or community stakeholders.
- Think about and get community partners involved.
- Obtain new data (i.e., interviews and focus groups using problem-posing dialogue format).
- Determine the intended group's needs and perceptions of health problems (i.e., identify audiences). Determine the community's assets and strengths.
  - Physical (e.g., gender, age, health history)
  - Behavioral (e.g., lifestyle characteristics and health-related activities)
  - Demographic (e.g., income, years of schooling, language, and cultural characteristics)
  - Psychographics (e.g., beliefs, values, and attitudes)
- Identify issues behind the issues and identify health knowledge gaps.
- Establish goals and objectives that are specific, attainable, prioritized, and time specific.
- Assess resources (e.g., money, staff, and materials).

LAUNCHING A BREAST EDUCATION AND OUTREACH SCREENING PROGRAM

The H. Lee Moffitt Cancer Center and Research Institute, or Moffitt, formed a partnership with Suncoast Community Health Centers, Inc., or Suncoast, in rural Hillsborough County, Florida. The partnership brought breast cancer education and screening services to Hispanic migrant and seasonal farmworkers and low-income rural women via Moffitt's Lifetime Cancer Screening Mobile Unit. In 1993, a cancer center physician visited Suncoast, which is a federally funded, community-based center located about 30 miles south of Tampa. He was struck by the center's services and impressed with the clinic's dedication to reaching medically underserved populations. Suncoast consists of three comprehensive health care clinics in Plant City, Ruskin, and Dover, Florida, and offers services to Hillsborough County's low-income rural populations, which includes farmworkers. Suncoast provides a range of medical services, but it did not have mammography facilities. Moffitt was expanding its community outreach initiatives through mobile outreach services. Moffitt is a freestanding, private, nonprofit institution located at the University of South Florida campus in Tampa. Moffitt is a National Cancer Institute–designated comprehensive cancer center in Florida and is widely known for state-of-the-art treatment, outpatient and ambulatory services, and advanced screening modalities. After a series of meetings between Suncoast and Moffitt's Lifetime Cancer Screening Center, the groups formed a partnership based on a shared goal, that is, improving the breast health of high-risk and medically underserved women. Both parties determined that the goal was to develop and offer the community culturally appropriate education, accessible mammography service, and follow-up care. This program continues to be a sustainable initiative through the community education and outreach program and has expanded its outreach to other areas within the surrounding catchment area.

Stage II: Developing and Pretesting Concepts, Messages, and Materials

The nurse's decisions in stage I can help guide him or her in selecting appropriate communication channels and producing effective and relevant materials. The nurse must consider how to reach the intended audience and use supporting materials and media. "Channel" refers to how the nurse will reach communication sites (i.e., churches, clinics, missions, nurses, or community-based organizations). "Format" refers to how the nurse will communicate the health message (e.g., through individual or group discussion) (Table 8-5). Materials and media are the program's tools, not the program itself (Table 8-6). Education is a human activity and should not focus on audiovisuals exclusively. To ensure that the messages are relevant and meaningful, the nurse can employ qualitative research methods (pretesting) to obtain feedback about the understandability and acceptability of the materials. Learning now what works and does not work saves time later.

Questions to Ask
- What channels are best?
- What formats should be used?
- Are there existing resources?
- How can the nurse present the message?

DESCRIPTION OF HEALTH ISSUE AND INTENDED AUDIENCE

Despite progress in the fight against cancer, many communities continue to bear a disproportionate share of the cancer burden. Cancer disparities very likely arise from the complex interplay of factors, that is, low socioeconomic status, education level achieved, literacy, social injustice, and poverty, that impede awareness about screening and follow-up care. Together, these factors affect access to care and cancer survival and yield an uneven distribution of cancer morbidity and mortality, which substantially impacts marginalized populations (Albano et al., 2007; Chu et al., 2007; Brookfield et al., 2009; American Cancer Society, 2009). As such, Meade et al. (2009) suggest that, when developing cancer outreach and screening programs, it is absolutely critical to layer on additional levels of understanding of and sensitivity to the social, cultural, and political conditions of home countries, language and literacy needs, basic health care access obstacles, cultural significance of gender and age roles, culturally mediated etiologic perceptions of disease, illness experiences, religiosity, and the sociopolitical nature of immigration situations. Such factors impact health communication and health education.

The lack of mammography screening and education for rural Hillsborough County's medically underserved women represented a health service gap (Meade et al., 2002a). In particular, individuals residing in rural areas, such as Hispanic farmworkers, and in urban areas, such as Haitian women, represent particular subgroups of women who face a number of potential barriers to acceptable mammography services. These barriers may reflect lack of insurance, limited access to health care, lower levels of education and literacy, cultural and linguistic differences, and immigrant status. Educational and communication interventions and tools that address (1) unique value systems, (2) cultural and linguistic factors, and (3) access issues, as well as capitalize on the strengths of the women, are needed (Meade and Calvo, 2001; Meade et al., 2009). Our experiences remind us that women want and need health information about breast health, but they also experience everyday survival issues and struggles. What was required in Hillsborough County was the delivery of a culturally relevant health service in a geographically convenient area. Women aged 40 years and older were eligible for this service. The intended audience was primarily Hispanic migrant and seasonal farmworkers but also included women from diverse ethnic backgrounds who were medically underserved (i.e., Haitian, rural white).

Goal: To prevent premature death and disability from breast cancer through early detection, screening, and culturally and linguistically relevant education.

Objectives: To increase education, mammograms, clinical breast examinations, and follow-up programs among medically underserved women in rural Hillsborough County.

- How will the intended audience react to the message?
- Will the audience understand, accept, and use the message?
- What changes may improve the message?

Collaborative Actions to Take
- Identify messages and materials.
- Decide whether to use existing materials or produce new ones.

TABLE 8-5   TEACHING-LEARNING FORMATS

TEACHING FORMAT	APPLICATION TO HEALTH EDUCATION
Brainstorming session	Allows participants the freedom to generate ideas and discuss them in a group setting. Cultivates creativity. Fosters empowerment to allow members to identify the issue and find solutions.
Community-wide programs	Can reach large numbers of community members through a systematic plan. May include individual or group approaches with a defined intended audience.
Demonstration	Effective in learning perceptual motor skills. Aids in visual identification.
Group discussion	Members can learn from each other and receive support. Nurses can tailor teaching content to group needs. Ideal for groups combining patients and families. Nurses, health professionals, or lay members can lead the groups. Facilitator must be comfortable with group method and familiar with group characteristics.
Lecture	Varying group sizes can use formal oral presentations. Group members share expertise and experiences. Presenter must be comfortable and possess speaking ability. Requires organizational skills and ability to highlight key points in interesting and creative ways. A combination of lecture media may enhance learning. Audience participation is linked to the presenter's speaking style and ability. Audience feedback is limited.
Personal discussion (i.e., individual and one-on-one)	Allows individual assessment and identification of cultural barriers, physical impairments, learning needs, literacy, and anxiety. Promotes the tailoring of health education plans. Ideal to capture "teachable moments." Does not allow sharing and support from others. High cost of staff time.
Role playing	Effective in influencing attitudes and opinions. Encourages problem-solving and critical thinking skills. Enhances learner participation. Some members may be hesitant to become involved.
Task force committee	Joins individuals with diverse backgrounds and expertise to achieve a goal. May represent many interests and perspectives.
Town hall meetings	Can offer shared experience in a familiar setting.

Data from Rankin and Stallings (2000); Redman (2006); USDHHS (2005).

TABLE 8-6   MATERIALS AND MEDIA

MEDIA	CONSIDERATIONS IN HEALTH EDUCATION SETTINGS
Audiotapes	Do not require reading. Portable and small. Individuals can use them at home in a comfortable setting and can replay and use them at their own pace. Economical. Helpful for individuals with visual difficulties or low literacy skills.
Bulletin boards	Inexpensive and easy to develop. Direct attention to a specific message; use few words.
Exhibits and displays	Graphics offer appeal. Placement in high-traffic areas (e.g., waiting rooms and examination rooms reach wide audiences).
Flip charts and chalkboards	Excellent format to enlarge teaching concepts or cue reader to salient points; may add graphics and diagrams. Chalkboards are reusable; flip charts have replacement pads. Inexpensive.
Games and simulations	Involve patients in a fun manner; involve the entire family. Highly effective with children.
Graphics	Can convey important points in salient and visual fashion.
Drawings and visuals	Can aid understanding for low-literacy audiences. Visual messages should be pretested to ensure acceptability and understanding.
Interactive videotapes (i.e., multimedia)	A variety of computer programs, talking touch screens, interactive videodisks, and computer-assisted instructions are available and are undergoing testing. Algorithms and branching decisions aid patients in decision making, problem solving, and fact acquisition (Yost et al., 2009; Woolfe et al., 2005). Interactive patient education is becoming more common via kiosks in waiting rooms. Nurses should assess computer comfort level. Software development may be time intensive and costly.
Models and real objects	Bring the teaching concept to the patient in a familiar way.

TABLE 8-6	MATERIALS AND MEDIA—cont'd
MEDIA	**CONSIDERATIONS IN HEALTH EDUCATION SETTINGS**
Demonstrations	Helpful when conveying psychomotor skills; encourage patient involvement and tactile learning (e.g., penis model for condom placement or breast model to show breast self-examination).
	No reading needed.
Storytelling	Reading is minimal.
	Encourages questions and elicits insights (Werle, 2004).
	Helpful in individual and group instruction.
	Nurses can incorporate models and real objects into displays or fairs.
Overheads	Useful in small- and large-group settings.
	Highlight key points and help patient focus ideas.
	Use of color and advance organizers, large type, and key points is recommended; avoid busy and cluttered overheads.
	Can be prepared in advance.
	Inexpensive.
Photographs, picture books, and slide series (i.e., PowerPoint slides); photo-essay and photovoice	Help promote understanding by showing realistic images and real situations.
	Help patients make connections to their life.
	Photographs may appear alone or in combination with other photographs or slides or placed in an album (Houts et al., 2006; Machtinger et al., 2007; Quinn et al., 2008; Roberts et al., 2009).
	PowerPoint slides are easily updated.
	Helpful for patients with limited literacy skills; offer visual presentation of concepts.
	Effective with an individual and with small groups (i.e., self-study or reflection).
	Easily updated.
Printed materials (brochures, leaflets, or booklets)	Portable, widely available, and economical.
	Useful in reinforcing health concepts and interactions.
	Patients can set and adjust the pace and refer back to information later.
	Can be effective with individuals, families, groups, or community-wide dissemination.
	Materials written at simple levels can be effective and acceptable for both low-level and high-level readers (Doak et al., 1998; Meade and Byrd, 1989).
	Tailored materials are highly effective and are a promising strategy for health education (Hawkins et al., 2008).
	Nurses should assess issues of readability, design, layout, cultural relevance, and appropriateness of content.
Programmed materials, self-help guides, slides, and tape programs	May involve printed materials combined with visuals to allow self-pacing.
	Helpful to learn facts.
	Nurse should assess individual or group to determine whether independent learning style is preferred.
	Storytelling (Larkey et al., 2009).
Teaching cards	Portable, use few words, and offer visual interpretations.
Flashcards	The nurse can create them economically and update them easily.
	Effective with individual, small-group, or family instruction.
Radio and newspapers	Reach large audiences within the community.
	Effective in conveying general health information in a user-friendly manner.
	Nurses can play an active role in disseminating health information.
Television and cable television	Reach large audiences within the community.
	Can help enhance community members' general health and well-being.
	Effective in influencing attitudes and behaviors.
	Offer a familiar medium for viewer to learn about health topics.
	Nurses can play key roles in reaching the community.
Telephones/videophones	Automated phone systems: reminder phone calls (Rubin et al., 2006).
	Telephone coaching (Sepulveda et al., 2008); telenursing (Jönsson and Willman, 2008); smoking cessation (Paul et al., 2004).
Videotapes, DVDs	Combine audio and visual medium to convey realistic images (Meade, 1996).
	Videotapes/DVDs should incorporate a role modeling concept.
	Used in stress management materials (Jacobsen et al., 2002); prostate cancer (Sheehan, 2009); and deaf audiences (Pollard et al., 2009).
	Expensive to produce and update; require access to audiovisual equipment and viewing sites.
	Videotapes/DVDs may be costly to produce and purchase but with computerized digital editing are easily updated.
Online resources (i.e., Internet, simple dial-up services, information, databases, bulletin board chat services, and World Wide Web)	Electronic information sources can link individuals, families, and groups to health.
	Common Internet providers are America Online and EarthLink.
	Can reach large audiences rapidly.
	Must access World Wide Web sites for accuracy, credibility, and relevancy.
	New technologies can help consumers find health information, advice, and support.
Podcasts	Portable video technology that uses media broadcasts and can be accessed via the Internet and viewed on a personal computer or on a handheld device, such as an iPod or an MP3 player (Abreu et al., 2008).

Data from USDHHS (2005).

- Select channels and formats.
- Develop relevant materials with the target audience.
- Pretest the message and materials and obtain audience feedback (e.g., through interviews, questionnaires, focus groups, and readability testing). Pretesting helps ensure comprehension, acceptability, and personal relevance.

SELECTING CHANNELS AND METHODS

Nurses selected a combination of channels to communicate health information about breast cancer, screenings, and early detection methods (e.g., community-based clinics, missions, social service agencies, health events, and fairs). Nurses conducted individual interactions at the mobile site.

Nurses collected a variety of health materials and media about breast cancer from national, state, and local sources and determined that many of the printed materials were not culturally or educationally suited for the individuals the nurses were serving; for example, the materials were geared toward high reading levels, and few Spanish-language or Haitian Creole materials were available.

DEVELOPING MATERIALS

Grants from Avon, National Alliance of Breast Cancer Organizations (NABCO), Susan G. Komen for the Cure Florida Suncoast Affiliate, and National Cancer Institute supported the development of English, Spanish, and Creole materials to educate women about breast health. Additionally, although translators were sporadically present in the mobile unit, it became apparent that bilingual staff was necessary. Ongoing dialogue with community members and clinics helped refine the screening process, the education component, and follow-up services to ensure effectiveness, efficiency, appropriateness, and timely follow-up. All mobile runs and health events now include bilingual and bicultural staff.

Stage III: Implementing the Program

At this stage, the nurse introduces the health education message and program to the intended audience and reviews and revises necessary components. The nurse also analyzes the program and health message for effectiveness and tracks the mechanisms using process evaluation. This type of managing the implementation process examines the procedures and tasks involved in the program or message, such as monitoring media, identifying the intended audience's interim reactions, and addressing internal functioning (e.g., work schedules and expenditures).

Questions to Ask

- How should the health education program/message get launched?
- How do we maintain interest and sustainability?
- How can we use process evaluation?
- What are the strengths of the health program?
- How can we be sure that we keep on track within the timeline and budget?
- How can we find out if we have reached the intended audience?
- How well did each step work (i.e., process evaluation)?
- Are we maintaining good relationships with our partners?

Collaborative Actions to Take

- Work with community organizations, businesses, media, and other health agencies to enhance effectiveness.
- Monitor and track progress.
- Establish process evaluation measures (e.g., follow-up with users of the service, number of community members who used the service, and expenditures).

IMPLEMENTATION

The mass media publicizes the services and disseminates human-interest stories, especially during October—Breast Cancer Awareness Month. The outreach worker posts flyers at a variety of sites (e.g., beauty shops, laundromats, missions, churches, grocery stores, churches, unemployment offices, and community centers). Twice per month, the mobile unit travels to rural areas. There, the staff greet women and answer questions about the mammography procedure and follow-up. Staff consists of the outreach worker, nurse practitioner, and mammography technician.

Stage IV: Assessing Effectiveness and Making Refinements

Outcome evaluation examines whether changes in knowledge, attitudes, and behavior did or did not occur as a result of the program. Together with the process evaluation, the data informs how well the program is functioning and directs modifications. The nurse prepares for a new development cycle using information gained from audience feedback, communication channels, and the program's intended effect. This phase helps to continually refine the health message and respond to the intended audience's needs. New information helps to validate the program's strengths and allows for necessary modifications. Feedback is necessary to continually refine the message and direct new messages, such as those related to human papillomavirus (HPV).

Questions to Ask

- What was learned?
- How can outcome evaluation be used to assess effectiveness?
- What worked well, and what did not work well?
- Has anything changed within the intended audience?
- How might we refine the methods, channels, or formats?
- Overall, what lessons were learned, and what modifications could strengthen the health education activity?

Collaborative Actions to Take

- Conduct outcome evaluations (e.g., randomized experiment, evaluation studies, define data needed for data collection).
- Reassess and revise goals and objectives.
- Modify unsuccessful strategies or activities.
- Generate continual support from businesses, health care agencies, and other community groups for ongoing collaboration and partnerships.
- Provide justification for continuing or ending the program.

Instructions: Think about a target group that you are currently working with and
planning to deliver/create a health education program or message.
Complete the exercise by asking yourself the following questions:

Questions to Ask	Action Plan
• What is the overall intended message/goal? What are my reasons for planning this message? How do I know that it is needed or wanted by the audience?	
• Who is the intended audience? (Write a brief statement describing the characteristics of the group.)	
• What are the benefits of this message to the group?	
• What channels will I use to deliver the message? Provide a rationale.	
• Will I need to create materials? Are there available materials that are appropriate for the group?	
• How will I know if my message gets across to the audience? Did the audience respond? How many people were reached? Who responded?	
• Was there change? What are the reasons the message was or was not effective? What can be modified to strengthen the message?	

FIGURE 8-1 Planning your health education message.

- Summarize the health education program or message in an evaluation report.
- The reader should consider how to plan health education messages or programs using this model. The exercise in Figure 8-1 will help the reader organize ideas systematically.

ASSESSING EFFICIENCY

Process Evaluation: A number of newspaper, television, and radio advertisements publicized the free or low-cost mammography service and highlighted the importance of breast health. Also, several human-interest stories emerged, which communicated the screening services to a wider audience. The on-site service logistics have made continual improvements, most notably in adding a dedicated outreach worker to the program. Since the onset of the program, an increase in the number of staff involved in the program, volunteers, and the number of funded projects that support the program enhanced the breadth and depth of the services. Most notably, the Tampa Bay Community Cancer Network (TBCCN) has increased the number of committed key stakeholders who have identified additional areas of need and outreach (Gwede et al., 2009). As a result of a partner needs assessment, additional cancer education workshops, health events, and festivals have broadened the mammography outreach services.

Additional funding for a Patient Research Navigation Program, a randomized clinical trial, has further augmented outreach efforts. Designed to eliminate barriers to cancer diagnosis and treatment, this project, one of nine in the country (Freund et al., 2008; Wells et al., 2008), is generating new knowledge for the advancement of an evidence-based culturally and literacy appropriate lay navigation program for those who have a breast abnormality by evaluating timeliness to resolution of abnormality and enhancing timeliness to diagnosis and delivery of cancer care. The expectation is that this program will eventually lead to lower cancer mortality among underserved populations in underserved areas in the country, including the Tampa Bay region of Florida. The role of nurses as navigators in the community is a fertile area of research.

In the first few years of operation, a total of 200 women underwent screening, which is a modest number. Assessment revealed that many women failed to appear for breast screenings because they had a "fear of cancer" and were uncertain how to navigate the health care system. Typically, many women from the community did not seek preventive health care; they sought care only for acute illness. Assessment showed that peer outreach was necessary to ensure participation. In 2008 (the last full year of data), more than 1000 women were outreached. Women expressed gratitude for the sensitivity and personal attention given by the peer outreach worker and mobile unit staff. Formal and informal feedback reveals that women respond well to the services and are especially satisfied with the Spanish-language and Haitian Creole educational materials.

Outcome Evaluation: During the program's initial years, fewer than 200 women received screening per year. The number of women screened now approaches more than 1000 per year. The number of community partners has increased considerably, a reflection of enhanced community capacity and awareness. Regular health fairs and health events are scheduled, and continual refinement of services and follow-up are ongoing.

HEALTH EDUCATION RESOURCES

A variety of health education materials and resources are available from local, state, and national organizations and agencies. Such associations provide helpful information about services, educational materials, and links to support groups or self-help groups. Often, printed and electronic materials are available for free or for a nominal cost. Nurses can help individuals, families, and groups access materials, services, or equipment loan programs and become knowledgeable about available community resources. Additionally, identifying gaps in services or resources may help nurses create the necessary services or materials. Some examples of resources follow:

- Local and regional hospitals, clinics, libraries, adult education centers, health education centers, and businesses
- Local and state governmental sources (e.g., health departments and social service agencies); check the Yellow Pages or Internet for listings
- Community-based organizations (i.e., advertised, nonadvertised, and those recommended by community leaders and stakeholders, National Association of Community Health Centers)
- Universities and colleges, community colleges, and academic nursing centers
- Professional organizations (e.g., American Public Health Association, National Association of Hispanic Nurses, National Black Nurses Association, National Student Nurses Association)
- Commercial organizations (e.g., pharmaceutical companies, medical supply companies, and patient and health education companies); printed and electronic sources are often available
- Federal government sources (e.g., National Institutes of Health [NIH]; National Cancer Institute; National Heart, Lung, and Blood Institute; OMH; Centers for Disease Control and Prevention [CDC]; National AIDS Clearinghouse; and Office on Smoking and Health)
- Voluntary agencies and their local affiliates (e.g., American Heart Association, Amyotrophic Lateral Sclerosis Association, Susan G. Komen for the Cure, Lance Armstrong Foundation, American Diabetes Association, American Council for Drug Disorders, American Dairy Council, Alzheimer's Association, and American Lung Association)
- Internet searches
- Medline Plus Health Information (i.e., a service of the National Library of Medicine for patient and consumer information), medlineplus.gov

Can you think of another organization that you or your family recently obtained information from relating to a health need? The book's Evolve website (http://evolve.elsevier.com/Nies/) contains a summary of major organizations and resources. Also, university or college libraries often provide information on beginning and advanced search strategies and are one of the most credible and accessible forms of information. The National Library of Medicine, at www.nlm.nih.gov/hinfo.html, maintains extensive health-related bibliographies and offers links to databases such as Medline Plus Health Information, Household Products Database, Office of the Surgeon General, NIH Senior Health, and more.

The nurse can locate many health resources through a variety of search engines on the Internet. As the Web continues to evolve as a major source of information exchange, an assessment of the quantity, quality, and broad nature of information must be undertaken as well. Key to the plethora of resources is gauging the appropriateness of the materials and media in consideration of literacy (see next section).

Literacy and Health

In her 1944 text, *The Public Health Nurse in the Community*, Rue stated that the community's illiteracy level is an important factor in health program planning. This factor remains a significant issue in planning health education programs and materials. Low literacy is a problem of great magnitude in the United States and has serious implications across the continuum of health care. Consider the following clinical example.

Clinical Example

A 2-year-old has an inner ear infection diagnosed and is prescribed an antibiotic. Her mother understands that her daughter should take the prescribed medication twice a day. After carefully studying the label on the bottle and deciding that it does not tell how to take the medicine, she fills the teaspoon and pours the antibiotic into her daughter's ear (Parker et al., 2003).

Thus, the nurse in a community setting who sees a sick child at the pediatric clinic might ask the following questions:

- Do the parents have an understanding of the names of the medicines for their baby, how they work, and how and when to give them?

- In what manner might teach-back methods (described later in this chapter) help the parents have a good understanding on how to administer the antibiotic?
- Will the parents know what to do if their infant gets a fever?
- Do the parents know how to read a thermometer? Did I show them? Were they able to "show me back"?
- Does the family know who to call and under what conditions, should their baby's condition worsen? Does the family have an understanding of what constitutes *worsen?* Will the parents know what action to take in case of a very high fever at 1:00 AM? Will they have critical literacy skills to manage similar situations?

As background, the conceptual definitions of health literacy have evolved over time. In 1991, "literacy" was operationally defined as the ability to read and write at the fifth-grade reading level in any language and measured according to a continuum (National Literacy Act, 1991). "Health literacy," on the other hand, is about empowerment, that is, having access to information, knowledge, and innovations. It is viewed as increasingly important for social, economic, and health development and is a key public health issue in the delivery of effective safe health care (Eichler, Wieser, and Brugger, 2009; Kickbush, 2001; Mancuso, 2009; Murphy-Knoll, 2007; National Adult Literacy Survey, 2003; Nielsen-Bohlman et al., 2004; Nutbeam, 2008; Peerson and Saunders, 2009). For example, health literacy skills entail knowing when and where to go for health screenings, reading labels on prescription bottles, understanding public health messages about text messaging while driving, completing health insurance forms, recognizing how to read food labels, or being aware of the expectations of clinical trials. The World Health Organization's (1998) definition of health literacy reflects a health promotion orientation and aligns health literacy with skills that enable people to take part more fully in everyday activities "…cognitive and social skills which determine the motivation and ability of individuals to gain access to, understand and use information in ways which promote and maintain health" (www.who.int/hpr/NPH/docs/hp_glossary_en.pdf, p. 10).

The American Medical Association's Report of the Council on Scientific Affairs (1999) defines health literacy as a constellation of skills for performing basic reading tasks required to function in the health care environment for accessing, understanding, and using information to make health decisions and further identified that patients with the most health care needs were often the least able to read and understand information to function successfully in the health care system. The recognition of this topic as a serious health issue subsequently resulted in the naming of a specific objective in the *Healthy People 2010* document (*Healthy People 2020* is currently underway), stating that a public health goal "is to improve the health literacy of persons with inadequate or marginal literacy skills" (Objective 11.2) (USDHHS, 2000). The document goes on to state that low health literacy prevents many individuals from gaining the full benefits of health care and suggests that health literacy is linked to health promotion and preventive behaviors.

Nutbeam (2000) proposes three levels for intervention that have individual and population benefits: (1) functional/basic literacy (focus is on increasing basic reading/writing skills), (2) communicative/interactive literacy (focus is on enhancing abilities to extract information and apply in new settings and with providers), and (3) critical literacy (focus is on advancing skills to analyze information critically and use the information to control and manage life situations). Too often, he asserts, the provider's focus is on basic literacy, rather than on critical literacy. The latter, he asserts, increases community members' empowerment abilities to successfully manage their everyday situations.

In 2004, the Institute of Medicine (IOM) published a landmark report titled *Health Literacy: A Prescription to End Confusion* that relates that millions of U.S. adults are unable to read and act on the plethora of health instructions and messages (Nielsen-Bohlman et al., 2004). The definition of health literacy adopted by the IOM report is consistent with the *Healthy People 2020* document and is as follows: "the capacity to obtain, interpret and understand basic health information and services and the competence to use such information and services to enhance health." The IOM report lists a series of recommendations that offer the nurse a blueprint of action. Several recommendations emphasize the need for clear communication, stress the importance of involving consumers in the development of the health communications process, and relate the need to create culturally and linguistically appropriate health information. For more details on the report and other health literacy–related resources, go to the IOM's website, www.iom.edu/, and search for the term *health literacy.* Pause for a moment now, and consider the skills needed to read the words on this page, the skills needed to assimilate the information, and the skills needed to ultimately apply the information to your interactions with community members.

Paasche-Orlow and Wolf (2007) propose a logic conceptual model that links health literacy to health outcomes by viewing health literacy as a "risk factor to be managed in clinical care." Nutbeam (2008), on the other hand, suggests that health literacy from public health and health promotion perspectives should be conceptualized as an "asset." In this manner, strategies to promote literacy move beyond mere transmission of content to the promotion of skills that develop confidence in how to act on the information. This viewpoint regards health literacy as a critical component of empowerment by improving people's access to health information and their capacity to use it. Moreover, Peerson and Saunders (2009) further recount that implicit in understanding the broad concepts of health literacy is that motivation and behavioral activation must be considered as separate entities. Simply put, having knowledge does not necessarily equate to action. Therefore, the quality of provider interactions and an increased awareness and sensitivity to the possible impact of low literacy on individuals and communities is paramount (Nutbeam, 2008). As such, nurses play pivotal roles in their community outreach and engagement activities for conveying knowledge, deciphering motivations, adapting health education messages, making information accessible, promoting health decisions, and facilitating empowering processes to increase the useful uptake of information.

Early research shows serious disparities between the reading levels of materials and patients' reading skills (Meade, 1999; Meade and Byrd, 1989; Meade, McKinney, and Barnas, 1994; Mohrmann et al., 2000). Additionally, materials often fail to incorporate the intended audience's cultural beliefs, values, languages, and attitudes (Doak et al., 1998; Makosky et al., 2009; Meade et al., 2003; Meade et al., 2009; Nielson-Bohlman et al., 2004; Powe et al., 2007). Studies show that low literacy increases the use of health care services and costs (Eichler, Wieser, and Brugger, 2009; Guerra, Krumholz, and Shea, 2005; Howard, Gazmararian, and Parker, 2005; Nielson-Bohlman et al., 2004); decreases self-esteem and increases shame and stigma (Waite et al., 2008; Wolf et al., 2007); and adversely affects diabetes, medication, and blood pressure control (Davis et al., 2006a; Jahan, 2008; Pandit et al., 2009; Schillinger et al., 2009); and that women who had abnormal Pap smears and who were perceived by their physician to have low literacy were significantly less likely to present for follow-up (Lindau, Basu, and Leitsch, 2006).

Additional studies reveal that health literacy may impact participation in research and pose barriers to obtaining informed consent (Kilbridge et al., 2009; Simon et al., 2009), lead to health care and linguistic isolation that places individuals at risk for the development of health complications (Donelle, Arocha, and Hoffman-Goetz, 2008), and impede patient-provider communication (Sudore et al., 2009).

The past decade has seen unprecedented advances in translating research findings into public health practices to reduce health risks, yet such successes have not been realized by all members of society representing various age, race and ethnic, and socioeconomic groups. It continues to be seen that community members who are unable to read well enough to cope with the persistent reading demands of an increasingly complicated health care system often fall behind more literate groups in adopting and using health education and promotion procedures and interventions (Nutbeam, 2008; Meade et al., 2007; Murphy-Knoll, 2007). Simply put, health instructions not read and interventions poorly understood influence self-care abilities and health and wellness. Although the exact relational mechanisms between literacy and health are unclear, it is known that individuals with very low literacy skills are at an increased risk for poor health, which contributes to health disparities. Paasche-Orlow and Wolf (2007) identify three possible causal points along the health care continuum: access and utilization, patient-provider interactions, and self-care. They point out that the relationship of literacy to health outcomes is not necessarily linear—as people exist within a sociocultural network. A number of systematic reviews of health literacy studies (Dewalt et al., 2004; Eichler, Wieser, and Brugger, 2009; Mancuso, 2009; Nielsen-Bohlman et al., 2004; Paasche-Orlow et al., 2005) show evidence of the high prevalence of limited health literacy, increasingly complex medical systems, and need for high-level navigation skills for self-management of acute and chronic disease and promotion of health. Further, the WHO Commission on Social Determinants (2007) identifies literacy as a key determinant in health inequities. With this said, the nurse is ideally

qualified and skilled to promote health in the community and address health literacy through the implementation of multiple techniques, as explained in the upcoming sections.

The Doaks (Leonard and Cecilia), who brought the literacy issue to the forefront in public health, describe the health community as a written culture. Unfortunately, many written instructions are over the head of patients. There is a serious mismatch between the readability levels of health instructions and the reading skills of patients, but nurses can adapt the literacy levels of their instructions and reduce this mismatch. Techniques to reduce this mismatch are cogently outlined in the book *Teaching Patients With Low Literacy Skills* (Doak, Doak, and Root, 1996), which offers practical suggestions for preparing and evaluating materials. This book is not currently in print, but all chapters can be accessed through the Harvard health literacy website at www.hsph.harvard.edu/healthliteracy/overview.html. The chapter author has used the information contained in this book in the development of educational materials, community-based programs, and research interventions.

What steps can nurses employ to address health literacy in the community setting? Within stage I of the "Framework for Developing Health Communications" model, the nurse can use assessment skills to determine the reading level of the intended audience. For example, the nurse could employ a number of informal and formal assessment measures to assess an individual's literacy skills. Informal measures include asking a series of simple questions to provide a better indication of his or her reading skills. For example: *Do you enjoy reading? What do you read? How often do you read? Where do you get your health information?* Although years of schooling completed can serve as a gauge of literacy, previous studies suggest that a three- to four-grade–level difference often exists between an individual's literacy level and years of education completed. The nurse could ask patients to read a paragraph from a health material aloud. Skilled readers enjoy reading, are fluent readers, understand content, interpret the meaning of words, and look up unfamiliar words. Limited readers read slowly, miss the intended meaning, take words literally, tire quickly from reading, and skip over uncommon words. Also, the nurse should ask the patients a few questions about the information they read. Readers should be able to answer questions about the material's content. Although these strategies are especially helpful with individuals with low literacy, people at all literacy levels prefer and better understand simply written, concise materials and are more motivated by materials that are relevant to their learning needs (Doak et al., 1998; Doak LG et al., 1996).

There has also been ongoing attention to the development of literacy screening questions, but further validation studies are needed before they are implemented in clinical care settings (Mancuso, 2009). Formal instruments that have been used in health care settings to estimate academic skills include the Wide Range Achievement Test, Level IV (Wilkinson & Robertson, 2006) and the Rapid Estimate of Adult Literacy in Medicine (REALM—assesses ability to read common terms in English and is used as a brief literacy-screening tool—Figure 8-2) (Davis et al., 1993;

Rapid Estimate of Adult Literacy in Medicine (REALM)©

Terry Davis, PhD • Michael Crouch, MD • Sandy Long, PhD

Patient's name/
Subject #_____
Date_____ Clinic_____

Reading Level _____   Grade Completed _____
Date of Birth_____
Examiner_____

List 1	List 2	List 3
fat	fatigue	allergic
flu	pelvic	menstrual
pill	jaundice	testicle
dose	infection	colitis
eye	exercise	emergency
stress	behavior	medication
smear	prescription	occupation
nerves	notify	sexually
germs	gallbladder	alcoholism
meals	calories	irritation
disease	depression	constipation
cancer	miscarriage	gonorrhea
caffeine	pregnancy	inflammatory
attack	arthritis	diabetes
kidney	nutrition	hepatitis
hormones	menopause	antibiotics
herpes	appendix	diagnosis
seizure	abnormal	potassium
bowel	syphilis	anemia
asthma	hemorrhoids	obesity
rectal	nausea	osteoporosis
incest	directed	impetigo

Score
List 1 _____
List 2 _____
List 3 _____
Raw Score _____

Directions:
1. Give the patient a laminated copy of the Realm and score answers on an unlaminated copy that is attached to a clipboard. Hold the clipboard at an angle so that the patient is not distracted by your scoring procedure. Say:
"I want to hear you read as many words as you can from this list. Begin with the first word on List 1 and read aloud. When you come to a word you cannot read, do the best you can or say 'blank' and go on to the next word."
2. If the patient takes more than five seconds on a word, say "blank" and point to the next word, if necessary, to move the patient along. If the patient begins to miss every word, have him/her pronounce only known words.
3. Count as an error any word not attempted or mispronounced. Score by marking a plus (+) after each correct word, a check (✓) after each mispronounced word, and a minus (−) after words not attempted. Count as correct any self-corrected words.
4. Count the number of correct words for each list and record the numbers in the "Score" box. Total the numbers and match the total score with its grade equivalent in the table below.

Grade Equivalent

Raw Score	Grade Range
0 to 18	**3rd Grade and Below** Will not be able to read most low literacy materials; will need repeated oral instructions, materials composed primarily of illustrations, or audiotapes or videotapes.
19 to 44	**4th to 6th Grade** Will need low literacy materials; may not be able to read prescription labels.
45 to 60	**7th to 8th Grade** Will struggle with most patient education materials; will not be offended by low literacy materials.
61 to 66	**High School** Will be able to read most patient education materials.

FIGURE 8-2 The Rapid Estimate of Adult Literacy in Medicine (REALM) is a screening instrument to assess an adult patient's ability to read common medical words and lay terms for body parts and illnesses. It is designed to assist medical professionals in estimating a patient's literacy level to use the appropriate level of patient education materials or oral instructions. The test takes 2 to 3 minutes to administer and score. (Reprinted with permission of Dr. Terry Davis, Louisiana State University. From Davis TC et al: Rapid estimate of adult literacy in medicine: a shortened screening instrument, *Fam Med* 25:56-57, 1993.)

Davis et al., 2006b). Although these instruments take only minutes to administer, they are unavailable in Spanish. The Test of Functional Health Literacy in Adults, long and short forms (TOFHLA and S-TOFHLA) (Parker et al., 1995) have been used in a variety of health settings with English-speaking/reading subjects (Cordasco et al., 2009; Schillinger et al., 2006; Ginde et al., 2008; Jackson and Eckert, 2008) and to some degree with Spanish-speaking subjects (Brice et al., 2008). Building on prior work (Chew et al., 2004; Wallace, 2006), Morris and colleagues (2006) developed the Single Item Literacy Screener (SILS): "How often do you need to have someone help when you read instructions, pamphlets, or other written material from your doctor or pharmacy (1 = never; 2 = rarely; 3 = sometimes; 4 = often; 5 = always)?" This particular item was found to be reasonably successful in detecting health literacy (compared with the TOFHLA, but only moderately sensitive). It focuses on only one aspect of health literacy, that is, reading materials. In 2006, Lee and colleagues reported on the Short Assessment of Health Literacy for Spanish-speaking Adults (SAHLSA), which is a word recognition tool that requires the subject to read out loud from a list of 50 medical terms and associate each term to another word of similar meaning. Another short assessment tool was created by Weiss and colleagues (2005) called the Newest Vital Sign (NVS). This tool, available in English and Spanish as a six-question assessment tool based on an ice cream nutrition label, is a quick 3- to 5-minute assessment. Osborn and colleagues (2007) used the NVS and found that it was able to identify patients with limited literacy skills but may misclassify those with adequate literacy according to the REALM and S-TOFHLA.

As one can see, there are many formal tools to measure reading level or word recognition, which in turn may be helpful to gauge an individual's health literacy. Yet, the time to administer them in community-based settings greatly limits their use. Moreover, such formal assessments should be secondary to the nurse's informal and ongoing assessments that allow for verification of understanding about specific health content within a specific context. Thus, Meade and Calvo (2001) suggest asking people a series of simple questions as mentioned previously, including years of schooling, to obtain an overall indication or gauge of health literacy, and employing ongoing learner verification and teach-back methods.

Clearly, ongoing research is needed to develop a relevant health literacy index (Kickbush, 2001; Mancuso, 2009; Nielsen-Bohlman et al., 2004). The promising news here is that health literacy can be realized through health education (Nutbeam, 2009). Key to implementing effective health education strategies is understanding that literacy has distinctive content and context.

Helpful Tips for Effective Teaching

- Assess reading skills using informal and formal methods.
- Determine what your patient wants to know.
- Identify motivating factors for learning new information.

- Stick with the essentials. Limit the number of concepts or key points. Focus on key critical and survival skills.
- Set realistic goals and objectives. Take cues from your patients about what they want to learn and how to help them learn.
- Use clear and concise language. Avoid technical terms if possible. For example, substitute the word *problem* for *complication.* Use the term *high blood pressure* instead of the word *hypertension,* or use the word *chance* instead of *possibility.* Do not needlessly simplify if the intended meaning is lost. Although the words *insulin* and *infection* are polysyllabic words, people with diabetes are often quite familiar with them (Box 8-2).
- Consider developing a glossary or vocabulary list for common words on the health topic. For example, in teaching a family about dental health, create a list of common words about the topic and words that might substitute well (e.g., flossing, toothbrush, cavity, decay, check-ups, x-rays).
- Space your teaching out over time if possible. Incorporate health education activities into other activities. For example, ask women about their smoking habits at each prenatal visit. Relate teaching to their everyday concerns. Introduce HPV education into women's and men's health visits.
- Personalize health messages. Use the active voice. For example, instead of saying, "It is important that patients read labels if they want to cut down on fat and sodium intake," say "Read the labels on foods to know what is in them. This helps to cut down on your fat and salt intake." See **Resource Tool 8C**, Patient Communication: Testicular Self-Examination (TSE), on the book's Evolve website at http://evolve.elsevier.com/Nies.

BOX 8-2   PATIENT COMMUNICATION: PROSTATE CANCER AND TREATMENT OPTIONS

Version A (harder to grasp)
The doctor has recently communicated to the patient that he has localized prostate cancer, commonly labeled stage II. In addition to managing the anxieties associated with a life-threatening illness, patients with this disease must carefully consider the available treatment modalities and account for the potential effect each one may have on quality of life. Patients must seriously evaluate the benefits and adverse side effects of each treatment modality and determine the most efficacious intervention for their lifestyle.

Version B (easier to grasp)
You have just been told that you have early stage prostate cancer. Choosing a treatment is hard, but it is important. Besides dealing with fears that go along with having cancer, you need to know about your treatment options.
- Get to know the benefits and side effects of each treatment.
- Think about how each treatment may affect your life.
- Ask questions. Write them down. Talk with your family.
- Choose the best treatment for you.

- Incorporate methods of illustration, demonstration, and real-life examples. Connect the health message to everyday events and real-life situations.
- Give and get. Review information often. Ask the patient questions before, during, and after teaching.
- Summarize often. Provide the patient with feedback. Obtain feedback from the patient.
- Be creative. Use your imagination to convey difficult concepts (e.g., use picture cards, drawings, objects, DVDs, podcasts, flipcharts, multimedia decision aids, photographs, storytelling).
- Use appropriate resources and materials to enhance teaching and convey ideas (e.g., videotapes, computer-based interactive programs, iPods, and bulletin boards).
- Put patients at ease. Focus on inclusion and trust before delivering content.
- Praise patients, but do not patronize them. Let them know what they are doing right. Focus on their strengths and assets and what they bring to the teaching encounter.
- Be encouraging throughout the educational steps. We all like to be told what we are doing right.
- Allow time for patients and family members to think and ask questions.
- Remember that comprehension and understanding require time and practice. Ongoing feedback helps refocus the teaching encounter and can keep you on track.
- Employ "teach-back" methods. This means asking patients to state in their own words (i.e., teach back) key concepts, decisions, or instructions just discussed (Wilson FL et al., 2008).
- Conduct learner verification (i.e., process that checks suitability of information) to ensure understanding (Table 8-7).
- Evaluate the teaching plan, and keep adding new information to the interaction.

Assess Materials: Become a Wise Consumer and User

Materials are collected, stored, and disseminated within community sites. In many instances, nurses distribute pamphlets, but patients either do not read them or review them only superficially.

> *People of this country have had so much pamphlet materials passed out to them free that some have lost respect for free literature. Health educators may have contributed to this delinquency by passing out health literature carelessly and indiscriminately. The nurse who expects the pamphlet to take the place of the health teacher is employing weak measures in the health education program. (Rue, 1944, p. 215)*

This statement continues to be true today. Moreover, many of today's pamphlets are even more complex and lengthier because of technological advances and health care innovations. Thus, it is important that nurses evaluate health materials, including websites, before they disseminate them to individuals, families, or the general public. Health materials should strengthen previous teaching and be used as an adjunct to health instruction.

Assessing the Relevancy of Health Materials

It is critical that nurses find and use materials, documents, and media that are appropriate for the intended target audience in community health education initiatives. Some questions that the nurse should ask include the following:

- Do the materials match the intended audience?
- Are the materials appealing and culturally and linguistically relevant?
- Do they convey accurate and up-to-date information?
- Are the messages clear and understandable?
- Do the messages promote self-efficacy and motivation?

Figure 8-3 provides an assessment guide for reviewing health materials that this author has used for gauging

TABLE 8-7	COMPONENTS OF LEARNER VERIFICATION (CHECKS THE SUITABILITY OF THE MESSAGE WITH COMMUNITY MEMBERS)	
COMPONENTS	**DESCRIPTION**
Attraction	Readers should be attracted to the message. For example, the cover should stimulate interest, and, when possible, pictures should foster an identification that "tells me that this is important for my situation." *Example: Is this material attractive/pleasing to you?* *Overall, would you be likely to pick up and read this brochure?*
Comprehension	Readers should be able to summarize the main points in their own words, not the vocabulary of the instruction. *Example: What do you feel is the main point?* *Are there any words that you might not understand?*
Acceptance	Readers need to perceive that the information is culturally acceptable for their lifestyle, situation, and background. *Example: Is there anything that bothers you about this booklet?* *In your opinion, who is this booklet for?*
Persuasion	Readers need to feel that the instruction is significant for them. *Example: Do you think that the message in this booklet is important for you?*
Self-efficacy	Is the message doable, and does the reader feel confident in carrying it out? *Example: Do you think you could do what is suggested in this booklet?*

Modified from Doak CC et al. (1996). (Chapter on learner verification can now be accessed at the Harvard health literacy website: www.hsph.harvard.edu/healthliteracy/).

Assessment of Health Education Materials

Name of material/media _____

Author _____

Intended target audience _____

Cost/availability/producer _____

Directions: Assess your printed material using the following tool. Use the rating scale of 1-4 for each item in a major category.   *1 = poor   2 = fair   3 = good   4 = very good   N/A = not applicable.*

For each category, give it an overall category rating of: *(+) effective* or *(−) not effective, (X) unsure*

Category/criteria Comments	Rating 1 = Poor; 2 = Fair; 3 = Good; 4 = Very Good
Format/Layout	
Organizational style	_____
White/black space	_____
Margins	_____
Grouping of elements	_____
Use of headers/advance organizers	_____
Overall category rating of:	
(+) effective _____ (−) not effective _____ (X) unsure _____	
Type	
Size	_____
Style	_____
Spacing	_____
Overall category rating of:	
(+) effective _____ (−) not effective _____ (X) unsure _____	
Verbal Content	
Clarity	_____
Quantity	_____
Relevancy to intended group (e.g., age, gender, race/ethnicity)	_____
Use of active voice	_____
Difficulty/readability level	_____
Grade level	_____
Accuracy	_____
Currency	_____
Overall category rating of:	
(+) effective _____ (−) not effective _____ (X) unsure _____	

Category/criteria	Rating Comments 1 = Poor; 2 = Fair; 3 = Good; 4 = Very Good
Visual Content	
Tone/mood	_____
Clarity	_____
Cueing	_____
Relevancy to intended group (e.g., age, gender, race/ethnicity)	_____
Currency	_____
Accuracy	_____
Detail	_____
Overall category rating of:	
(+) effective _____ (−) not effective _____ (X) unsure _____	
Aesthetic Quality/Appeal	
Attractiveness	_____
Color	_____
Quality of production	_____
Personalized instructions	_____
Overall category rating of:	
(+) effective _____ (−) not effective _____ (X) unsure _____	
Comments:	

Overall, based on your scoring of 1 to 4 and an evaluation of its effectiveness with the intended target audience, how suitable would you rate this educational tool? Circle one.

1 = poor: probably won't work with my intended audience. I would probably not ever use it.

2 = fair: has a low likelihood of success with my intended audience. I would use it rarely and only in combination with other sources.

3 = good: has a good likelihood of being suitable and relevant for about half of my intended audience. I would use it sometimes.

4 = very good: has a high likelihood of being suitable and relevant for most of my intended audience. I would most definitely use it!

FIGURE 8-3 Form for assessing health education materials. (Modified from EPET, 1981; Meade and Calvo, 2001.) Assessment guide to review health materials. (Modified from University of Kentucky: Assessment guide to review health materials, Patient Education Materials Workshop, 1980.)

the appropriateness of materials. The nurse can use this guide in critiquing printed materials. Similarly, the nurse can make slight modifications in assessing other types of health resources (e.g., videotapes/DVDs, websites, and multimedia interactive modules). The tool allows the nurse to review health materials systematically for appropriateness within the intended target audience. The material assessment should focus on the following criteria: format-layout, type, verbal content, visual content, and aesthetic quality.

CASE STUDY APPLICATION OF THE NURSING PROCESS

The following case study and teaching plan provide an example of selected teaching approaches and learning needs for the individual, family, and community.

Emma Jackson, aged 29 years, receives ongoing health care at her neighborhood's community-based clinic, a federally funded community clinic. She visits the nurse practitioner, and the nurse confirms that Mrs. Jackson is 2 months pregnant. She is married and has a 6-year-old son. Emma tells the nurse she smokes and wants to quit, but she has been unable to quit since her last pregnancy. She tells the nurse, "I smoke when I get stressed. I have so many things on my mind." Her husband is also a smoker and has tried to quit at times as well. The nurse refers Mrs. Jackson to a community nursing student named Irene Green for counseling, education, and follow-up.

Assessment

Irene recognizes that smoking during pregnancy is detrimental for the unborn infant, unhealthy for Mrs. Jackson, and harmful for the 6-year-old child who breathes the secondhand smoke (USDHHS, 2004). Irene also knows that smokers often experience stages of readiness in their attempts to quit, and relapse is often part of the process (Prochaska and DiClemente, 1983). She notes that family and community support systems are important.

Irene assesses Mrs. Jackson on an individual level, which follows:
- Smoking history, smoking patterns, and previous attempts to quit
- Support systems (e.g., family, friends, and peers)
- Perceived barriers to quitting
- Perceived benefits to quitting
- Perceived priority in addressing this health issue vs. other everyday stresses
- Perceived effect of smoking behavior on family communication patterns
- Confidence and perceived efficacy in ability to quit

Assessment of other groups includes families, neighborhoods, churches, community organizations, and environmental messages that promote smoking cessation.

Diagnosis
Individual
- Ineffective health maintenance (tobacco use) in response to personal stressors, unawareness of available resources, and insufficient support systems
- Ineffective coping related to inadequate resources and support networks, evidenced by unsuccessful management of stressors
- Decisional conflict related to previous unsuccessful attempts (lack of confidence in ability to quit smoking and stay quit)
- Health-seeking behaviors (desire to quit smoking) for individual and family

Family
- Potential for interrupted family processes related to lack of agreement about household smoking patterns

Community
- Inadequate organized smoking cessation programs and initiatives for populations at risk related to lack of economic resources and community-building coalitions

Planning
Individual
Long-Term Goal
- Mrs. Jackson will quit smoking.

Short-Term Goals
- Mrs. Jackson will recognize that continued smoking is unhealthy for herself, her unborn infant, her young child, and her family.
- Mrs. Jackson will become aware of ways to enhance her confidence during smoking cessation.
- Mrs. Jackson will identify situations and stressors that influence her smoking patterns.
- Mrs. Jackson will learn two strategies to cope with stressful situations and apply those strategies.

Family
Long-Term Goal
- Mr. and Mrs. Jackson will quit smoking and become a smoke-free family.

Short-Term Goals
- Mr. and Mrs. Jackson will acknowledge the benefits of a smoke-free environment.
- Mr. Jackson will recognize the need to quit smoking.
- The couple will recognize the need to support each other in smoking cessation.
- Mr. and Mrs. Jackson will identify and discuss specific supportive actions during the smoking cessation phases. The couple will enlist the support of another person or network.

Community
Long-Term Goals
- The community will support and endorse a smoke-free environment and publicize these efforts through billboards and other media.
- Community agencies and organizations will integrate smoking cessation and relapse programs and messages into their existing health-related activities.
- Cigarette advertising will cease.

Short-Term Goals
- A coalition of community members will develop and implement policies to support smoking cessation and relapse strategies.
- A consortium of health care agencies and community-based organizations will recognize the need to develop partnerships in creating smoking cessation strategies for the community and for high-risk groups.

Intervention
Individual
Planning and interventions encourage expression, promote the use of adaptive coping mechanisms, offer positive reinforcement, disseminate appropriate smoking cessation strategies, and provide culturally and educationally relevant materials and media. The nurse applies the five A's approach to smoking cessation counseling (Ask, Advise, Assess, Assist, and Arrange). Irene offers empowerment strategies to help Mrs. Jackson cope with her smoking cessation attempts and identifies daily hassles and stressors. Irene gives

CASE STUDY   APPLICATION OF THE NURSING PROCESS—cont'd

tailored smoking cessation messages and culturally and educationally appropriate materials and initiates a follow-up plan that is acceptable and doable based on ongoing assessment and feedback (Melvin et al., 2000; Hudmon et al., 2003; USDHHS, 2004; Quinn et al., 2006).

Family

Planning and interventions recognize the need for strong support systems within families. Irene provided education and counseling to promote family self-care and recognized that she must address and incorporate Mr. Jackson's support, or lack thereof, into the care plan. Irene makes links to community resources (e.g., health classes, support groups, and networking with other expectant moms who quit or are attempting to quit) to build Mrs. Jackson's support system.

Community

Planning and interventions implemented on an aggregate level identify key community leaders, agencies, legislators, and lay members who are committed to supporting smoking cessation/relapse initiatives at a sociopolitical level (e.g., creating smoking cessation/relapse initiatives at various community channels). Program initiatives assist community members in defining issues and solutions to the effects of smoking on individuals, families, and community groups. Developing coalitions and partnerships among community-based organizations, health care groups, governmental agencies, and intended audience members through dialogue and increased awareness is essential.

Evaluation

Evaluation is systematic and continuous and focuses on the individual, family, and community.

Individual

An evaluation of Mrs. Jackson's smoking habits occurs within the health system and the community (clinics and WIC). These groups address both process (decrease in number of cigarettes smoked) and outcome (quit or not quit) endpoints. Mrs. Jackson experiences an increase in her coping skills and support system, which is evident in her personalized care plan.
- Irene tailors smoking cessation messages to Mrs. Jackson to fit her everyday life.
- Irene provides Mrs. Jackson with follow-up (e.g., telephone, letter, and follow-up visits).

Family

Care plans include supporting pattern development with family or significant other in smoking cessation initiatives.
- Irene assesses family health patterns and screens for other at-risk behaviors.
- Irene identifies and addresses family support and communication patterns in the care plan.

Community

Irene introduces smoking cessation and relapse programs and smoking prevention initiatives to at least two channels of dissemination (e.g., churches, schools, work sites, and community-based clinics).
- Smoking cessation/relapse messages are infused throughout the community through radio, television, and billboards.
- Community task forces and coalitions demonstrate a collaborative partnership among lay members, community leaders, organizers, and legislators to address smoking-related health issues.

Format/Layout

- Is the information organized clearly? Does it make sense?
- Do headers or advance organizers cue the reader? Headers help the reader visualize what is next.
- Is there a 50% to 50% allocation of white and black space? This gives the reader breathing space.
- Is the information easy to read and uncluttered?

Type

- Is the type or font a readable size? Consider the age of your intended group and whether visual difficulties are likely.

Verbal Content

- Is the information current, accurate, and relevant to the intended group?
- Is the information culturally acceptable?
- Are difficult terms defined?
- Does the text reflect the racial and ethnic diversity of the intended audience?
- What is the reading level?

Visual Content

- Are the graphics accurate, current, and relevant to the intended group?
- Does cueing help the reader connect the printed words and pictures?
- Will the reader understand the intended meanings of the pictures?
- Is the information culturally acceptable?
- Are the pictures on the cover reflective of the material inside?
- Do the pictures reflect the target audience's racial and ethnic diversity?

Aesthetic Quality and Appeal

- Is the material appealing?
- Are there helpful special features (e.g., glossary, space for notes, and useful telephone numbers)?

Assessment of Reading Level

Part of the written material's assessment is reading level. Many formulas are available to estimate the printed text's readability and grade level, including the SMOG readability formula. See **Resource Tool 8D**, SMOG Formula for Estimating Readability Grade Level of Printed Text, on the book's Evolve website at http://evolve.elsevier.com/Nies.

Readability formulas are objective, quantitative tools that measure sentence and word variables. However, they do not consider factors such as motivation, experience, or need for information (Meade and Smith, 1991). They do not determine the effects of visuals or design factors that could influence readability and comprehension of cancer education information (Friedman and Hoffman-Goetz, 2006). These formulas do estimate reading ease and provide guidelines for assessing and rewriting health information. The Flesch-Kincaid Formula (Flesch, 1948) is another broad estimate of reading and is programmed into most computer software programs' grammar editing tools.

Learner Verification

The best way to identify material suitability is to deliver the materials to the intended audience and obtain feedback about acceptability, understanding, and usefulness. Learner verification engages intended members in dialogue and helps uncover unsuitable aspects of the material (i.e., content, visuals, or format) (Doak LG et al., 1996). If the nurse discovers a need for new educational materials or media, he or she may incorporate Freirean principles to produce empowering products. The Freire approach supports learner participation in the development process, ensures that the learner is the active subject of the educational experience, and allows learners to define content and outcomes. Freire's approach focuses on people's experiences and ideas and creates themes to address them.

The process of learner verification helps to identify the likelihood that the message is well suited to the audience. It involves verifying or checking whether certain elements work well together to result in a good match of information for the learner. See Table 8-7 for a description of the specific elements and sample questions associated with each one. For example, the chapter author used a learner verification processes to develop education toolboxes on breast and cervical cancer and prostate cancer for Hispanic migrant and seasonal farmworker and African-American women and men, respectively. Following the conduct of a series of focus groups with members of the intended audience to elicit themes about health, illness, cancer, and prevention, we then conducted a series of learner verification measures. Through a series of systematic questions and interviewing processes, we were able to collect information in the intended audience's own words to help shape and refocus the cancer issues (breast, cervical, and prostate) from their own perspective (African-American men and women and Hispanic men and women farmworkers). Such verifying checks help to assess the understanding of words and pictures; the acceptability of music, narrator, and pictures; the efficacy and persuasion of the message; and overall attractiveness of the tools (e.g., videotape, DVD, flipchart, and booklet). Similarly, this approach was used to adapt smoking-relapse prevention materials for pregnant and postpartum women (Quinn et al., 2006) and recently used to develop educational tools (booklet, DVD, audiotape) as part of a stress management toolkit for Latina women undergoing chemotherapy (Meade, 2009). The use of learner verification fits well within the framework of community-based participatory research methods as outlined earlier in this chapter.

SUMMARY

Teaching is a significant component of community health nursing, and it impacts virtually every nursing activity. The goal of health education is to facilitate a process that allows individuals, families, and groups to make well-informed decisions about health practices. An understanding of learning and the theoretical frameworks that explain behaviors and health actions is inherent in community health education. No single theory explains human behavior; the nurse must apply multiple theories and approaches.

Nurses must be knowledgeable about sociopolitical, cultural, environmental, and ecological forces affecting community health to ensure the success of health education strategies. Health education, which is relevant for an intended group, is based on individual variables and social, structural, political, cultural, and economic factors within the larger community context. Nurses develop relevant teaching interventions by assessing their audience and their characteristics thoroughly and by using an organized and systematic approach to delivering health messages and programs. Implementing social action strategies such as advocating health-promoting lifestyles, creating an environment for problem-posing dialogue, and providing links to appropriate health resources support the philosophy of critical consciousness. Nurses can facilitate the principle of social justice by mastering health information delivery and committing themselves to creating empowerment strategies that equip individuals, families, and communities with knowledge and navigation skills for healthy lifestyles and environments.

Nurses can use a variety of methods, materials, and media to support health education activities, including electronic and web-based information. The nurse should review and evaluate these resources for their cultural, linguistic, and literacy suitability for the intended group. Embracing the notion that health education is an ongoing interactive process influenced by many internal and external factors is key to meeting the needs of individuals, families, and communities. Nurses can make important contributions to the prevention of disease and the promotion of personal and community health with knowledge, spirit, and an ongoing mindset and commitment to empowerment strategies.

LEARNING ACTIVITIES

1. In groups of three to four students, describe how theoretical frameworks help explain health behavior. Identify the strengths and limitations of models that focus on individual health determinants versus models that encompass sociopolitical factors.
2. Discuss the role of the nurse in health education. Outline specific activities and roles that the community nurse can perform with regard to health education issues. Share with each other a particular experience relating to cultural effectiveness that would enhance/impede this role.
3. Identify a specific intended group in the community (e.g., medically underserved, homeless, seniors, pregnant women, new immigrants, deaf children, teens).
   a. Describe the group's characteristics, learning needs, and strengths.
   b. Identify the methods for obtaining this information.
   c. Next, describe the application of Freire's empowerment education model to address health issues.

4. Identify an issue of concern among community members (e.g., obesity, access to care). Discuss sociopolitical issues that impact this health issue. Outline specific community-based participatory activities and roles that the community nurse can perform that might help address this health issue. Identify at least two ways to promote community engagement on this topic.

5. Select a health education brochure or health website. Apply the assessment criteria presented to assess its appropriateness for the intended audience. Evaluate the relative strengths of the printed material or website and potential areas for improvement using learner verification questions.

REFERENCES

Abreu DV, et al: Podcasting: contemporary patient education, *Ear Nose Throat J* 87(208):210–211, 2008.

Albano JD, et al: Cancer mortality in the United States by education level and race, *J Natl Cancer Inst* 99:1384–1394, 2007.

American Cancer Society: *Cancer facts and figures 2009*, Atlanta, 2009, The Author.

Association AM: Ad Hoc Committee on Health Literacy for the Council on Scientific Affairs: Health literacy: report of the council on scientific affairs, *JAMA* 281:552–557, 1999.

Bandura A: Self-efficacy: toward a unifying theory of behavioral change, *Psychol Rev* 84:191–215, 1977a.

Bandura A: *Social learning theory*, Englewood Cliffs, NJ, 1977b, Prentice Hall.

Becker MH, editor: *The health belief model and personal health behavior*, Thorofare, NJ, 1974, Charles B. Slack.

Becker MH, et al: The health belief model and prediction of dietary compliance: a field experiment, *J Health Soc Behav* 18:348–366, 1977.

Bigge ML, Shermis SS: *Learning theories for teachers*, ed 6, Boston, 2004, An Allyn & Bacon Classics Edition.

Brandon TM, et al: Efficacy and cost-effectiveness of minimal intervention to prevent smoking relapse: dismantling the effects of content versus contact, *J Consult Clin Psych* 20:797–808, 2004.

Brice JH, et al: Health literacy among Spanish-speaking patients in the emergency department, *J Natl Med Assoc* 100:1326–1332, 2008.

Brookfield KF, et al: Disparities in survival among women with invasive cervical cancer: a problem of access to care, *Cancer* 115:166–178, 2009.

Cashman SB, et al: The power and the promise: working with communities to analyze data, interpret findings, and get to outcomes, *Am J Public Health* 98:1407–1417, 2008.

Champion VL: Revised susceptibility, benefits, and barriers scale for mammography screening, *Res Nurs Health* 22:341–348, 1999.

Champion VL, et al: Measuring mammography and breast cancer beliefs in African American women, *J Health Psychol* 138:27–37, 2008.

Champion VL, Skinner CS: The health belief model. In Glanz K, Rimer BK, Visnawath K, editors: *Health behavior and education: theory, research, and practice*, ed 4, San Francisco, 2008, Jossey-Bass, pp 45–65.

Chew LD, et al: Brief questions to identify patients with inadequate literacy, *Fam Med* 36:588–594, 2004.

Chu KC, et al: Measures of racial/ethnic health disparities in cancer mortality rates and the influence of socioeconomic status, *J Natl Med Assoc* 99(1092–1100):1102–1104, 2007.

Chu KC, et al: Parallels between the development of therapeutic drugs and cancer health disparity programs: implications for disparities reduction, *Cancer* 113:2790–2796, 2008.

Clark MJD: *Community health nursing: caring for populations*, ed 5, Englewood Cliffs, NJ, 2007, Prentice Hall.

Coleman CL, et al: Development of an HIV risk reduction intervention for older seropositive African American men, *AIDS Patient Care STDS* 8:647–655, 2009.

Cordasco KM, et al: Health literacy and English language comprehension among elderly inpatients at an urban safety-net hospital, *J Health Hum Serv Adm* 32:30–50, 2009.

Davis TC, et al: Rapid estimate of adult literacy in medicine: a shortened screening instrument, *Fam Med* 25:56–57, 1993.

Davis TC, et al: Low literacy impairs comprehension of prescription drug warning labels, *J Gen Intern Med* 21:847–851, 2006a.

Davis TC, et al: Development and validation of the Rapid Estimate of Adolescent Literacy in Medicine (REALM-Teen): a tool to screen adolescents for below-grade reading in health care settings, *Pediatrics* 118:1707–1714, 2006b.

Dewalt DA, et al: Literacy and health outcomes: a systematic review of the literature, *J Gen Intern Med* 19:1228–1239, 2004.

Doak CC, Doak LG, Root JH: *Teaching patients with low literacy skills*, ed 2, Philadelphia, 1996, Lippincott Williams & Wilkins. See Harvard health literacy website: www.hsph.harvard.edu/healthliteracy/overview.html.

Doak CC, et al: Improving comprehension for cancer patients with low literacy skills: strategies for clinicians, *CA Cancer J Clin* 48:151–162, 1998.

Doak LG, et al: Strategies to develop effective cancer education materials, *Oncol Nurs Forum* 23:1305–1312, 1996.

Donelle L, Arocha JF, Hoffman-Goetz L: Health literacy and numeracy: key factors in cancer risk comprehension, *Chronic Dis Can* 29:1–8, 2008.

Edgren KK, et al: Community involvement in the conduct of a health education and research project: community against asthma, *Health Prom Pract* 6:263–269, 2005.

Eichler K, Wieser S, Brugger U: The costs of limited health literacy: a systematic review, *Int J Public Health* 2009 Published online 31 July.

English KC, et al: Intermediate outcomes of a tribal community public health infrastructure assessment, *Ethn Dis* 14:S1-61–S1-69, 2004.

Flesch RR: A new readability yardstick, *J Appl Psychol* 32:221–223, 1948.

Freeman HP: Poverty, culture, and social injustice: determinants of cancer disparities, *CA Cancer J Clin* 54:72–77, 2004.

Freire P: *Pedagogy of the oppressed*, New York, 1970, Herder and Herder (Translated from original manuscript, 1968), New York, 2000, Continuum is the 30th anniversary edition.

Freire P: *Education for critical consciousness*, New York, 1973, Continuum 2005, reprint.

Freund K, et al: National Cancer Institute Patient Navigation Research Program: methods, protocol, and measures, *Cancer* 113:3391–3399, 2008.

Friedman DB, Hoffman-Goetz L: A systematic review of readability and comprehension instruments used for print and web-based cancer information, *Health Educ Behav* 33:352–373, 2006.

Gardner MS: *Public health nursing*, ed 3, New York, 1936, Macmillan (University of Michigan reprint, 2009.)

Giachello AL, et al: Reducing diabetes health disparities through community-based participatory action research: the Chicago southeast diabetes community action coalition, *Pub Health Rep* 118:309–323, 2003.

Gillis AJ: Determinants of a health-promoting lifestyle: an integrative review, *J Adv Nurs* 18:345–353, 1993.

Ginde AA, et al: Multicenter study of limited health literacy in emergency department patients, *Acad Emerg Med* 15:577–580, 2008.

Glanz K, Rimer BK, Viswanath K, editors: *Health behavior and health education: theory, research and practice*, ed 4 San Francisco, 2008, Jossey Bass.

Goodman RM, et al: Identifying and defining the dimensions of community capacity to provide a basis for measurement, *Health Educ Behav* 25:358–378, 1998.

Green L: Introduction to behavior change and maintenance: theory and measurement. In Schumaker S, Schron EB, Ockene JK, editors: *The handbook of health behavior change*, New York, 1998, Springer.

Green LW, Kreuter MW: *Health program planning: an educational and ecological approach*, ed 4, New York, 2004, McGraw-Hill.

Guerra CE, Krumholz M, Shea JA: Literacy and knowledge, attitudes and behavior about mammography in Latinas, *J Health Care Poor Underserved* 16:152–166, 2005.

Gwede C, et al: Exploring disparities and variability in perceptions and self-reported colorectal cancer screening among three ethnic subgroups of US Blacks (in press). No update yet for publication date – it will be published in Oncology Nursing Forum.

Hochbaum GM: *Public participation in medical screening programs: a sociopsychological study, US Public Health Service Pub No 572,* Washington, DC, 1958, US Government Printing Office.

Horowitz CR, et al: Using community-based participatory research to reduce health disparities in East and Central Harlem, *Mt Sinai J Med* 71:368–374, 2004.

Houts PS, et al: The role of pictures in improving health communication: a review of research on attention, comprehension, recall, and adherence, *Patient Educ Couns* 61:173–190, 2006.

Howard DH, Gazmararian J, Parker RM: The impact of low health literacy on the medical costs of Medicare managed care enrollees, *Am J Med* 118:371–377, 2005.

Hudmon KS, et al: Development and implementation of a tobacco cessation training program for students in the health professions, *J Cancer Educ* 18:142–149, 2003.

Hulme PA, et al: Health-promoting lifestyle behaviors of Spanish-speaking Hispanic adults, *J Transcult Nurs* 14:244–254, 2003.

Israel BA, et al: Health education and community empowerment: conceptualizing and measuring perceptions of individual, organization, and community control, *Health Educ Q* 32:149–170, 1994.

Israel BA, et al: Review of community-based research: assessing partnership approaches to improve public health, *Annu Rev Public Health* 19:173–202, 1998.

Israel BA, et al: *Methods in community-based participatory research for health,* San Francisco, 2005, Jossey-Bass.

Jackson RD, Eckert GJ: Health literacy in an adult dental research population: a pilot study, *J Public Health Dent* 68:196–200, 2008.

Jacobsen PB, et al: Efficacy and costs of two forms of stress management training for cancer patients undergoing chemotherapy, *J Clin Oncol* 20:2851–2862, 2002.

Jahan S: Poverty and infant mortality in the Eastern Mediterranean region: a meta-analysis, *J Epidemiol Community Health* 62:745–751, 2008.

Janz NK, Becker MH: The health belief model: a decade later, *Health Educ Q* 11:1–47, 1984.

Janz NK, Champion VL, Strecher VJ: The health belief model. In Glanz K, Rimer BK, Lewis FM, editors: *Health behavior and education: theory, research and practice,* ed 2, San Francisco, 2002, Jossey-Bass, pp 45–66.

Jemmott JB, et al: Sexually transmitted infection/HIV risk reduction interventions in clinical practice settings, *J Obstet Gynecol Neonatal Nurs* 37:137–145, 2008.

Jemmott LS, Jemmott JB, O'Leary A: A randomized controlled trial of brief HIV/STD prevention interventions for African American women in primary care settings: effects on sexual risk behavior and STD rate, *Am J Public Health* 97:1034–1040, 2007.

Joint Commission: *Comprehensive accreditation manual for hospital (CAMH): the official handbook.*

Joint Commission on Accreditation of Healthcare Organizations: *1996 accreditation manual for hospitals,* vol 1, Oak Brook, Ill, 1995, The Author.

Jönsson AM, Willman A: Implementation of telenursing within home healthcare, *Telemed J E Health* 14:57–62, 2008.

Joseph CL, et al: Asthma in Adolescents Research Team, a web-based, tailored asthma management program for urban African-American high school students, *Am J Respir Crit Care Med* 175:888–895, 2007.

Kannan S, et al: A community-based participatory approach to personalized, computer-generated nutrition feedback reports: the Healthy Environments Partnership, *Prog Community Health Partnersh* 2:41–53, 2008.

Keck CW: Community health: our common challenge, *Fam Community Health* 172:1–9, 1994.

Kegeles SS, et al: Survey of beliefs about cancer detection and Papanicolaou tests, *Public Health Rep* 80:815–823, 1965.

Kickbush IS: Health literacy: addressing the health and education divide, *Health Prom Intern* 16:289–297, 2001.

Kilbridge KL, et al: Lack of comprehension of common prostate cancer terms in an underserved population, *J Clin Oncol* 27:2015–2021, 2009.

Kleinman A: Concepts and a model for the comparison of medical systems as cultural systems, *Soc Sci Med* 12:85–93, 1978.

Knowles MS: *The modern practice of adult education: from pedagogy to andragogy,* rev ed, Chicago, 1988, Cambridge Press.

Knowles MS: *The making of an adult educator: an autobiographical journey,* San Francisco, 1989, Jossey-Bass.

Kobetz E, et al: Patnè en Aksyon: addressing cancer disparities in Little Haiti through research and social action, *Am J Public Health* 99:1163–1165, 2009.

Labonte R: Health promotion and empowerment: reflections on professional practice, *Health Educ Q* 21:253–268, 1994.

Larkey LK, et al: Storytelling for promoting colorectal cancer screening among underserved Latina women: a randomized pilot study, *Cancer Control* 16(1):79–87, 2009.

Lee SY, et al: Development of an easy-to-use Spanish health literacy test, *Health Serv Res* 41:1392–1412, 2006.

Leung MW, Yen IH, Minkler M: Community-based participatory research: a promising approach for increasing epidemiology's relevance in the 21st century, *Intern J Epidemiol* 33:499–506, 2004.

Lindau ST, Basu A, Leitsch SA: Health literacy as a predictor of follow-up after an abnormal Pap smear: a prospective study, *J Gen Intern Med* 21:829–834, 2006.

Lohse JL: A bicycle safety education program for parents of young children, *J Sch Nurs* 19:100–110, 2003.

Lopéz EDS, et al: Photovoice as a community-based participatory action method. In Israel BA, Eng E, Schulz AJ, Parker EA, editors: *Methods in community-based participatory research for health,* San Francisco CA, 2005, Jossey-Bass, pp 326–358.

Luque JS, Rivers B, Kambon M, Brookins R, Green BL, Meade CD: Barbers against prostate cancer: A feasibility study for training barbers to deliver prostate cancer education in an urban African American community, *J Cancer Educ* 2010 Feb 10. [Epub ahead of print] PMID: 20146044.

Machtinger EL, et al: A visual medication schedule to improve anticoagulation control: a randomized, controlled trial, *Comm J Qual Patient Saf* 33:625–635, 2007.

MacLeod ML, Zimmer LV: Rethinking emancipation and empowerment in action research: lessons from small rural hospitals, *Can J Nurs Res* 37:78–84, 2005.

Makosky DC, et al: Assessing the scientific accuracy, readability, and cultural appropriateness of a culturally targeted smoking cessation program for American Indians, *Health Promot Pract* 10:386–393, 2009.

Mancuso JM: Assessment and measurement of health literacy: an integrative review of the literature, *Nurs Health Sci* 11:77–89, 2009.

Marks R: Ethics and patient education: health literacy and cultural dilemmas, *Health Promot Pract* 10:328–332, 2009.

Martinez D, et al: Development of a cancer camp for adult Spanish-speaking survivors: lessons learned from Camp Alegria, *J Cancer Educ* 23(1):4–9, 2008.

Martyn KK, et al: Mexican adolescents' alcohol use, family intimacy, and parent-adolescent communication, *J Fam Nurs* 15:152–170, 2009.

McKinlay JB: Epidemiological and political determinants of social policies regarding the public health, *Soc Sci Med* 13A:541–558, 1979.

Meade CD: Producing videotapes for cancer education: methods and examples, *Oncol Nurs Forum* 23:837–846, 1996.

Meade CD: Improving understanding of the informed consent process and document, *Semin Oncol Nurs* 15:124–137, 1999.

Meade CD: *Creating educational tools: from concept to product,* Montreal, Canada, 2009, Society for Behavioral Medicine (abstract).

Meade CD, Byrd JC: Patient literacy and the readability of smoking education literature, *Am J Public Health* 79:204–206, 1989.

Meade CD, Calvo A: Developing community-academic partnerships to enhance breast health among rural and Hispanic migrant and seasonal farmworkers, *Oncol Nurs Forum* 28:1577–1584, 2001.

Meade CD, Menard J, Luque J, Martinez-Tyson D, Gwede CK: Creating community-academic partnerships for cancer disparities research and health promotion. health promotion practice, *Health Promotion Practice* 2009 Oct 12 [Epub ahead of print] PMID: 19822724.

Meade CD, et al: Impact of culturally, linguistically and literacy relevant videotaped cancer information among Hispanic farmworker women, *J Cancer Educ* 17:50–54, 2002a.

Meade CD, et al: Screening and community outreach programs for priority populations: considerations for oncology managers, *J Oncol Manag* 11(5):14–22, 2002b.

Meade CD, et al: Focus groups in the design of prostate cancer screening information for Hispanic farmworkers and African American men, *Oncol Nurs Forum* 30:967–975, 2003.

Meade CD, et al: Impacting health disparities through community outreach: utilizing the CLEAN look (Culture, Literacy, Education, Assessment, Networking), *Cancer Control* 14:70–77, 2007.

Meade CD, et al: Addressing cancer disparities through community engagement: improving breast health among Haitian women, *Oncol Nurs Forum* 36:716–722, 2009.

Meade CD, McKinney WP, Barnas G: Educating patients with limited literacy skills: the effectiveness of printed and videotaped materials about colon cancer, *Am J Public Health* 84:119–121, 1994.

Meade CD, Smith CF: Readability formulas: cautions and criteria, *Patient Educ Couns* 17:153–158, 1991.

Meleis AI: Culturally competent care, *J Transcult Nurs* 10:12, 1999.

Melvin CL, et al: Recommended cessation counseling for pregnant women who smoke: a review of the evidence, *Tob Control* 9 (Suppl 3):iii80–iii84, 2000.

Minkler M: Community-based research partnerships: challenges and opportunities, *J Urban Health* 82(2 Suppl 2):ii3–ii12, 2005.

Minkler M, Wallerstein N, editors: *Community-based participatory research for health: from process to outcomes*, ed 2, San Francisco, 2008, Jossey-Bass.

Minkler M, Wallerstein N, Wilson N: Improving health through community organization and community building. In Glanz K, Rimer BK, Visnawath K, editors: *Health behavior and education: theory, research, and practice*, ed 4, San Francisco, 2008, Jossey-Bass, pp 288–312.

Mohrmann CC, et al: An analysis of printed breast cancer information for African American women, *J Cancer Educ* 15:23–27, 2000.

Morris NS, et al: Single item literacy screener: evaluation of a brief instrument to identify limited reading ability, *BMC Fam Pract* 21, 2006.

Murphy-Knoll L: Low health literacy puts patients at risk: The Joint Commission proposes solutions to national problem, *J Nurs Care Qual* 22:205–209, 2007.

The National Literacy Act of 1991: PL 102–173, 1991.

National Adult Literacy Survey: *Technical report and data file user's manual for 2003 National Assessment of Adult Literacy*, NCES 2009476. Published online August 11, 2009: nces.ed.gov/pubsearch/pubsinfo.asp?pubid=2009476.

Nielsen-Bohlman L, et al: *Health literacy: a prescription to end confusion*, Institute of Medicine report, Washington, DC, 2004, National Academies Press.

Nightingale F: *Notes on nursing*, New York, 1859, Appleton-Century-Crofts.

Nutbeam D: Health literacy as a public health goal: a challenge for contemporary health education and communication strategies into the 21st century, *Health Promot Int* 15:259–267, 2000.

Nutbeam D: The evolving concept of health literacy, *Soc Sci Med* 67:2072–2078, 2008.

Nutbeam D: Defining and measuring health literacy: what can we learn from literacy studies? *Int J Public Health* 54(5):303–305, 2009.

Nyswander DB: Education for health: some principles and their application, *Health Educ Mono* 14:65–70, 1956.

Office of Minority Health (OMH): *Assuring cultural competence in health care: recommendations for national standards and an outcomes-focused research agenda*, Rockville, MD, 1999, The Author, www.omhrc.gov/clas/cultural1a.htm.

Olshansky E, et al: Participatory action research to understand and reduce health disparities, *Nurs Outlook* 53:121–126, 2005.

Osborn CY, et al: Measuring adult literacy in health care: performance of the newest vital sign, *Am J Health Behav* 31(Suppl 1):S36–S46, 2007.

Paasche-Orlow MK, et al: The prevalence of limited literacy, *J Gen Intern Med* 20:175–184, 2005.

Paasche-Orlow MK, Wolf MS: The causal pathways linking health literacy to health outcomes, *Am J Health Behav* 31(Suppl):S19–S26, 2007.

Padilla GV, Bulcavage LM: Theories used in patient/health education, *Semin Oncol Nurs* 7:87–96, 1991.

Pandit AU, et al: Education, literacy, and health: mediating effects on hypertension knowledge and control, *Patient Educ Couns* 75:381–385, 2009.

Parker EA, et al: Community action against asthma: examining the partnership process of a community-based participatory research project, *J Gen Intern Med* 18:558–567, 2003.

Parker RM, et al: The test of functional health literacy in adults: a new instrument for measuring patients' literacy skills, *J Gen Intern Med* 10:537–541, 1995.

Paul CL, et al: Direct telemarketing of smoking cessation interventions: will smokers take the call? *Addiction* 99:907–913, 2004.

Peerson A, Saunders M: Health literacy revisited: what do we mean and why does it matter? *Health Promot Int* 24:285–296, 2009.

Pender NJ, Murdaugh CL, Parsons MA: *Health promotion in nursing practice*, ed 5, Englewood Cliffs, NJ, 2005, Prentice Hall.

Petersen R, et al: Moving beyond disclosure: women's perspectives on barriers and motivators to seeking assistance for intimate partner violence, *Women Health* 40:63–76, 2004.

Pollard RQ, et al: Adapting health education material for deaf audiences, *Rehabil Psychol* 54:232–238, 2009.

Powe BD, et al: Testicular cancer among African American college men: knowledge, perceived risk, and perceptions of cancer fatalism, *Am J Mens Health* 1:73–80, 2007.

Prochaska JO, DiClemente CC: Stages and processes of self-change of smoking: toward an integrative model of change, *J Consult Clin Psychol* 51(3):390–395, 1983.

Quinn G, et al: Adapting smoking relapse-prevention materials for pregnant and postpartum women: formative research, *Matern Child Health J* 10:235–245, 2006.

Quinn GP, et al: Evaluation of educational materials from a social marketing campaign to promote folic acid use among Hispanic women: insight from Cuban and Puerto Rican ethnic subgroups, *J Immigr Minor Health* 11(5):406–414, 2009. Epub 2008 Jun 17.

Rankin SH, Stallings KD: *Patient education: principles and practices*, ed 4, New York, 2000, Lippincott Williams & Wilkins.

Rawl SM, et al: The impact of age and race on mammography practices, *Health Care Women Int* 21:583–597, 2000.

Redman BK: *The practice of patient education*, ed 10, St. Louis, 2006, Elsevier.

Roberts NJ, et al: The development and comprehensibility of a pictorial asthma action plan, *Patient Educ Couns* 74:12–18, 2009.

Ronis DL, Hong O, Lusk SL: Comparison of the original and revised structures of the Health Promotion Model in predicting construction workers' use of hearing protection, *Res Nurs Health* 29:3–17, 2006.

Rosenstock I: Why people use health services, *Milbank Mem Fund Q* 44:94–127, 1966.

Rosenstock IM, Strecher VJ, Becker MH: Social learning theory and the health belief model, *Health Educ Q* 15(2):175–183, 1988.

Rubin A, et al: Automated telephone screening for problem drinking, *J Stud Alcohol* 67:454–457, 2006.

Rue CB: *The public health nurse in the community*, Philadelphia, 1944, Saunders.

Schapira MM, Meade C, Nattinger AB: Enhanced decision-making: the use of a videotape decision-aid for patients with prostate cancer, *Patient Educ Couns* 30:119–127, 1997.

Schillinger D, et al: Does literacy mediate the relationship between education and health outcomes? A study of a low-income population with diabetes, *Public Health Rep* 121:245–254, 2006.

Schillinger D, et al: Effects of self-management support on structure, process, and outcomes among vulnerable patients with diabetes: a three-arm practical clinical trial, *Diabetes Care* 32:559–566, 2009.

Sepulveda AR, et al: Feasibility and acceptability of DVD and telephone coaching-based skills training for carers of people with an eating disorder, *Int J Eat Disord* 41:318–325, 2008.

Sheehan CA: A brief educational video about prostate cancer screening: a community intervention, *Urol Nurs* 29:103–111, 117, 2009.

Shin Y, et al: Test of the health promotion model as a causal model of commitment to a plan for exercise among Korean adults with chronic disease, *Res Nurs Health* 28:117–125, 2005.

Simon MA, et al: Heeding our words: complexities of research among low-literacy populations, *J Clin Oncol* 27:1938–1940, 2009.

Smedley BD, et al, editors: *Unequal treatment: confronting racial and ethnic disparities in health care*, Washington, DC, 2003, National Academies Press.

Stallings KD, Rankin SH: *Patient education in health and illness*, ed 5, 2005, Lippincott Williams & Wilkins.

Steuart GW, Kark SO: *A practice of social medicine: a South African team's experiences in different African communities*, Edinburgh, 1962, Livingstone.

Strecher VJ, et al: The role of self-efficacy in achieving health behavior change, *Health Educ Q* 13:73–92, 1986.

Strickland J, et al: Health promotion in cervical cancer prevention among the Yakama Indian women of the Wa'Shat Longhouse, *J Transcult Nurs* 10:190–196, 1999.

Sudore RL, et al: Unraveling the relationship between literacy, language proficiency, and patient-physician communication, *Patient Educ Couns* 75:398–402, 2009.

US Department of Health and Human Services: *Making health communication programs work*, NIH Pub No 05-5145, Bethesda, MD, 2005, Office of Cancer Communications, National Cancer Institute.

US Department of Health and Human Services, Centers for Disease Control and Prevention, National Center for Chronic Disease Prevention and Health Promotion: *The health consequences of smoking: A report of the Surgeon General*, Atlanta, 2004, Office on Smoking and Health.

US Department of Health and Human Services, Public Health Services: *Healthy People 2010*, ed 2, vol 1: Understanding and improving health; vol 2: Objectives for improving health, Washington DC, 2000, US Government Printing Office.

Van Wyk NC: Health education as education of the oppressed, *Curationis* 22:29–34, 1999.

Villarruel AM, et al: Predicting condom use among sexually experienced Latino adolescents, *West J Nurs Res* 29:724–738, 2007.

Waite KR, et al: Literacy, social stigma, and HIV medication adherence, *J Gen Intern Med* 23:1367–1372, 2008.

Wallace LS, et al: Brief report: screening items to identify patients with limited health literacy skills, *J Gen Intern Med* 21:874–877, 2006.

Wallerstein N, Bernstein E: Empowerment education: Freire's ideas adapted to health education, *Health Educ Q* 15:379–394, 1988.

Wallerstein NB, Duran B: Using community-based participatory research to address health disparities, *Health Promot Pract* 73:12–23, 2006.

Watters EK: Literacy for health: an interdisciplinary model, *J Transcult Nurs* 14:48–54, 2003.

Weiss BD, et al: Quick assessment of literacy in primary care: the newest vital sign, *Ann Fam Med* 3:514–522, 2005.

Werle GD: The lived experience of violence: using storytelling as a teaching tool with middle school students, *J Sch Nurs* 20(2): 81–87, 2004.

Wells KJ, et al: Patient navigation: state of the art or is it science? *Cancer* 113:1999–2010, 2008.

Wilkinson GS, Robertson GJ: *Wide Range Achievement Test 4 professional manual*, Lutz, FL, 2006, Psychological Assessment Resources.

Wilson FL, et al: Using the teach-back and Orem's self-care deficit nursing theory to increase childhood immunization communication among low-income mothers, *Issues Compr Pediatr Nurs* 31:7–22, 2008.

Wilson N, et al: Getting to social action: the Youth Empowerment Strategies (YES!) project, *Health Promot Pract* 9:395–403, 2008.

Wolf MS, et al: Patients' shame and attitudes toward discussing the results of literacy screening, *J Health Commun* 12:721–732, 2007.

Woolfe SH, et al: Promoting informed decision choice: transforming health care to dispense knowledge for decision making, *Ann Intern Med* 143:293–300, 2005.

World Health Organization: *Health promotion and community action in developing countries*, Geneva, 1994, The Author.

World Health Organization: *Health promotion glossary*. Prepared by D. Nutbeam, WHO/HPR/HEP/98.1 (definition of health literacy), www.who.int/hpr/NPH/docs/hp_glossary_en.pdf, p. 10.

World Health Organization Commission on the Social Determinants of Health: *Achieving health equity: from root causes to fair outcomes*, Geneva, 2007, World Health Organization.

Yost KJ, et al: Bilingual health literacy assessment using the Talking Touchscreen/laPantalla Parlanchina: development and pilot testing, *Patient Educ Couns* 75:295–301, 2009.

Case Management

Jean Cozad Lyon, Karyn Leavitt Grow

Additional Material for Study, Review, and Further Exploration

evolve WEBSITE

http://evolve.elsevier.com/Nies
- Quiz
- Case Studies
- Glossary
- WebLinks

OBJECTIVES

Upon completion of this chapter, the reader will be able to do the following:
1. Define case management and care management, and compare the differences.
2. Discuss the purpose of providing case management services.
3. Identify the origin and purpose of case management.
4. Distinguish between case management and care management.
5. Discuss trends that influence the development of case management programs.
6. Incorporate case management concepts into clinical practice settings.
7. Identify educational preparation and skills recommended for case managers.

KEY TERMS

care management
case management
client-centered case management

continuum of care
discharge planning
system-centered case management

utilization review

OUTLINE

Overview of Case Management
    Care Management
Origins of Case Management
    Public Health
    Case Management in Mental Health
    Case Management and the Elderly
    Disease-Specific Case Management
Purpose of Case Management
Utilization Review and Managed Care
Trends That Influence Case Management
Case Manager Education Preparation
    Nurse Case Managers
Case Manager Services
Case Manager Roles and Characteristics

Case Identification
The Referral Process
Case Management Models
    Hospital-Based Case Management
    Case Management Models Across the Health Care
      Continuum
    Community Case Management Models
Application of Case Management in
  Community Health
    Public Health Clinic Settings
    Occupational Health Settings
    High-Risk Clinic Settings
Research in Case Management
International Case Management

OVERVIEW OF CASE MANAGEMENT

Case management is a term that describes a wide variety of patient care coordination programs in acute hospital and community settings. The term *case management* applies to community health settings, which include public and mental health settings and population groups of all ages.

Since the late 1980s and the 1990s, a variety of case management programs have emerged (Huber, 2002). From 1990 to 2005, case management evolved rapidly in response to changes in the health care environment and increased managed care programs. Client service use reflects a greater emphasis on health care costs; therefore third-party payers evaluate the appropriate use of health care resources such as diagnostic tests, laboratory tests, length of hospital visits, and duration of home health care services. Managed care organizations (MCOs) may deny reimbursement to health care providers that exceed the expected costs. Health care providers must closely monitor their use of resources; therefore they introduced various forms of case management programs.

The development of case management models in acute hospital and community settings created confusion over what programs and services compose case management and how case management differs from other services such as social services and discharge planning. A single definition of case management does not exist. The Case Management Society of America (CMSA) (2002) offers the following definition of case management:

Case management is a collaborative process of assessment, planning, facilitation and advocacy for options and services to meet an individual's health needs through communication and available resources to promote quality cost-effective outcomes. (p. 5)

The philosophy statement published by CMSA (2005) states:

The philosophy of case management is that all individuals, particularly those experiencing catastrophic and high chronicity injuries or illnesses, should be evaluated for case management services. The key philosophical components of case management address care that is holistic and client-centered, with mutual goals, allowing stewardship of resources for the client and the healthcare system. (p. 6)

According to the American Nurses Association, nursing case management is "a health care delivery process whose goals are to provide quality health care, decrease fragmentation, enhance the client's quality of life, and contain costs" (1992).

Many labels describe case management within a profession. In addition to case management, other titles include case coordination, care management, geriatric care management (GCM), integrated care management, continuing care coordination, continuity coordination, and service coordination. Multiple case management labels cause further confusion among health care professionals and health care consumers.

Case management takes on many forms depending on the level, discipline, organization, situation, and basic client care needs that are addressed (White and Hall, 2006).

Some hospitals, health maintenance organizations (HMOs), and other insurance companies inaccurately use the term *case management* to describe "utilization management," "managed care," or the method of monitoring and controlling service use within a system or care episode to control cost. Many of these providers have case management programs that transcend use control and monitor the patient following hospital discharge. Some of the programs provide continued services to high-risk clients for an indefinite time, regardless of the client's location (Box 9-1).

Case management programs aim to provide a service delivery approach to ensure the following: cost-effective care, alternatives to institutionalization, access to care, coordinated services, and patient's improved functional capacity (Lyon, 1993). These goals apply to community health and acute care settings.

Care Management

Care management consists of programs that apply systems, science, incentives, and information to improve medical practice and to allow clients and their support systems to participate in a collaborative process with a goal of improving medical, social, and mental health conditions more effectively. The overall goal of care management is to improve the coordination of services provided to clients who are enrolled in a care management program and to minimize or eliminate duplication (Center for Health Care Strategies [CHSC], 2007).

The framework used in care management includes the identification of clients or groups of people at high risk for poor health care outcomes who have potential for improvements in the outcomes if their care is coordinated. The care coordination is designed to meet the needs of the individual clients and the client's right as a consumer to be a decision maker in the care planning process and, at the same time, minimize or eliminate the duplication of the services provided (CHSC, 2007).

Examples of groups of people who may be served by care management services include the elderly, children from low-income families who receive Medicaid services, and groups of people with chronic illnesses (see Box 9-2).

BOX 9-1 POSSIBLE CASE MANAGEMENT FUNCTIONS

- Identifying the target population
- Determining screening and eligibility
- Arranging services
- Monitoring and follow-up
- Assessing
- Planning care
- Reassessing
- Assisting clients through a complex, fragmented health care system
- Care coordination and continuity

ORIGINS OF CASE MANAGEMENT

Case management has a long history with the mentally ill, elderly patients, and the community setting (Steinberg and Carter, 1983). Public health, mental health, and long-term care settings have implemented and studied case management services and have reported them in their literature for many years (Mahn and Spross, 1996; Weil and Karls, 1985).

Public Health

Community service coordination, which was a forerunner of case management, appeared in public health programs in the early 1900s. During this time, health care providers reported these community service and case management programs in the nursing literature. Programs focused on community education in sanitation, nutrition, and disease prevention became prevalent. Lillian Wald conducted many of these programs at the Henry Street Settlement House in New York City. The Metropolitan Life Insurance Company later expanded nursing services for individuals, families, and the community (Conger, 1999) to include disease prevention and health promotion.

The concept of continuum of care originated following World War II to describe the long-term services required for discharged psychiatric patients (Grau, 1984). Service coordination evolved into case management; this term first appeared in social welfare literature during the early 1970s.

Case Management in Mental Health

During the late 1960s and early 1970s, mental health care emphasized moving patients from mental health institutions back into the community (Crosby, 1987; Pittman, 1989). The Community Mental Health Center Act of 1963 placed federal approbation on deinstitutionalization, which emphasized the importance of community mental health services. Mental health providers began to move patients from large state institutions to the community.

Several problems resulted from the deinstitutionalization of mentally ill patients. In 1977, Congress acknowledged that many disabled people were deinstitutionalized without basic needs, proper follow-up, or health care monitoring. Congress further recognized that a systematic approach to service delivery could have prevented many state hospital readmissions. Case management in community mental health helped avoid client service fragmentation (Pittman, 1989).

Case Management and the Elderly

Specific elderly services recognized that age-generic programs do not adequately assist older people. Many older people have special, population-specific health care needs. Thus, case management services frequently target the elderly population, specifically homebound individuals, or those with complex problems. However, not all older people who subscribe to multiple services require a case manager. Older adults may not need a case manager if they possess adequate functional status and can coordinate and access services for themselves, if they have family support, or if they have formal or informal caregivers who provide these functions for them. These individuals require information about options, available services, and follow-up assistance (Lyon et al., 1995).

Disease-Specific Case Management

Case management services are often provided for individuals who are identified as having medical conditions that are high-cost or high-volume acute and chronic illnesses. Examples of these illnesses include chronic obstructive pulmonary disease and chronic cardiac conditions such as congestive heart failure. The goal of disease-specific case management is to keep these individuals as healthy as possible and stable in their home environment. One particular goal is to decrease the frequency and length of hospital stays and consequently decrease health care costs.

PURPOSE OF CASE MANAGEMENT

Case management is client centered and system centered. Client-centered case management assists the client or patient through a complex, fragmented, and often confusing health care delivery system and achieves specific client-centered goals. System-centered case management recognizes that health care resources are finite. The upward spiral in health care costs causes third-party payers such as Medicare, MCOs, and insurance companies to demand cost-effective health care. Client consumers insist on cost-effective, quality care. This demand forces health care providers to reevaluate the way they administer care, to emphasize quality improvement, and to focus on decreasing cost. Health care resources then become allocated to those populations with the greatest needs.

Case management is used to promote and integrate the coordination of clinical services, linking patients to community services and agencies. Case managers monitor resources used by clients, support collaborative practice and continuity of care, and enhance patient satisfaction (Yamamoto and Lucey, 2005).

For hospitalized patients, health care service coordination begins either upon the patient's admission or shortly thereafter and continues following the patient's discharge for an unspecified time. The patient's physical and psychosocial status and the plan's success will determine the length of the case manager's evaluation and intervention (Lyon, 1993; Lyon et al., 1995).

ETHICAL INSIGHTS

Ethical Issues in Case Management

There are several ethical issues that a case manager should take into consideration when working with populations. Some of these include:

1. Right to privacy. Confidentiality of clients served must be maintained. Communicating patient information to others who are involved with the client's care must be done only with the client's knowledge and permission.
2. Health care resources are expensive and limited. The case manager must use appropriate, reliable, and accessible resources for individual clients or groups of clients with the same identified needs.
3. Respect for the client's right to be informed about his or her care and services and that the client has a right to choose to receive services or not.
4. Clients have the right to know what resources are available to them and have the right to select providers of the resources.

UTILIZATION REVIEW AND MANAGED CARE

Equity and cost-effectiveness require management and allocation of available resources in a hospital, community, city, state, or particular health care client population. System-centered case management rations and sets priorities for those in a larger group or population who could benefit from specific services.

Case management programs are often motivated by the need to evaluate, use, and allocate health care resources. Many case management programs evolved from utilization review departments. These departments showed that monitoring service use alone is insufficient for managing patient populations with diverse resource needs. Over time, the utilization review nurses assumed the additional case manager responsibilities.

TRENDS THAT INFLUENCE CASE MANAGEMENT

Numerous trends influenced case management programs. During the 1970s, hospitals billed Medicare, Medicaid, and other third-party payers for client services and received reimbursement. Health care costs skyrocketed and rapidly became the basis for discussion and concern throughout the health care industry and the country. In 1983, PL 98-21 of the Social Security Amendments introduced the prospective payment system (PPS) in the acute care setting. Under the PPS, health care providers receive a fixed amount of money based on the relative cost of resources they use to treat Medicare patients within each diagnosis-related group. Other third-party payers followed this example and negotiated reimbursement schedules through preferred provider programs or managed care contracts (U.S. Department of Commerce, 1990).

Health care costs continue to escalate, the population is aging, and the elderly population is increasing. Many elderly suffer from chronic illness and require health care resources.

These issues influenced, and still influence, the introduction of case management services to control costs and distribute health care resources in a variety of settings.

CASE MANAGER EDUCATION PREPARATION

It is essential to determine what classification of health care provider is best qualified to provide case management services. Traditionally, case managers were social workers (SWs) who assumed the role of discharge planner. Client health care needs have become more complex, the need for ongoing patient assessment has emerged, and available resources have become more numerous and diverse; therefore nurses have become case managers. Several health care organizations exclusively employ SWs in case manager roles, others exclusively employ nurses in case management, and others use a combination of SWs and nurses, depending on the client population's needs. Combining the strength and knowledge of the nurse's clinical background with the SW's community service background is a combination that can efficiently move a client through the complex health care system (Lyon et al., 1995).

Nurse Case Managers

Although both nurses and SWs have proved themselves to be excellent case managers, this chapter focuses on the nurse case manager in discussing educational requirements. A nurse case manager's optimum education level is debatable. Basic nursing education for case managers required by employers can vary. Some may require a baccalaureate degree, and others may not. In some settings, a master's degree may be required. Some programs are more interested in prior experience, continuing education, and case management certification than the entry-level nursing degree. Education and experience requirements may vary depending on the program's geographic location, specific client needs, and available staff.

Nurses with master's degrees and a focus in case management are readily available in urban settings. This gives facilities the opportunity to hire case managers who are academically prepared in theory and clinical experience. Rural areas that do not have master's-level academic programs are at a great disadvantage in recruiting and hiring qualified nurses. To fill the case manager role, rural facilities promote nurses to case management positions, provide them with continuing education programs, and offer them necessary job-related experience. Although this is not the ideal solution, it is often the only option for smaller facilities and those in more remote parts of the United States.

Regardless of the educational requirements in the individual case management program, case managers need a minimum skill level to ensure success in the role. These skills include sound knowledge of reimbursement structures; knowledge of available resources within the institution, organization, or community; working knowledge of the identification and evaluation of quality outcomes; the ability to perform cost-benefit ratios; and an understanding of financial strategies. In addition to the required knowledge, the nurse case manager needs the following characteristics: flexibility, creativity, excellent communication skills, and the ability to work autonomously.

Case Manager Certification Options

There are two options for case managers to become certified as case managers. The certifications are offered by the Case Management Society of America (CMSA) and by the American Nurses Credentialing Center (ANCC).

Case Management Society of America (CMSA). Certification as a case manager through the CMSA is offered through Certified Case Manager Certification (CCMC). The certification granted is the Certified Case Manager (CCM) credential. The following are the requirements of the applicant:

- Possess a good moral character
- Meet acceptable standards of practice
- Provide a job description for each case management position held
- Meet the continuum of care requirement
- Hold an acceptable license or certification based on a postsecondary degree program in a field that promotes the psychosocial or vocational well-being of the persons being served
- Ensure that the license or certification grants the ability to practice without the supervision of another licensed professional
- Perform the following essential activities of case management:
  1. Assessment
  2. Coordination
  3. Planning
  4. Monitoring
  5. Implementation
  6. Evaluation
  7. Outcomes
  8. General (Commission for Case Manager Certification, 2009)

American Nurses Credentialing Center (ANCC). The ANCC offers certification in nursing case management. Eligibility to take the certification examination includes the following:

- Hold a current, active registered nurse (RN) license within a state or territory of the United States or the professional, legally recognized equivalent in another country
- Have practiced the equivalent of 2 years full time as an RN
- Have a minimum of 2000 hours of clinical practice in case management nursing within the last 3 years
- Have completed 30 hours of continuing education in case management nursing within the last 3 years

Several other certifications in specialty case management are available. A few of these include disability management, health care quality, utilization management, managed care, and case management administrator certification. Case management professionals who are interested in obtaining certification should carefully research the options available for certification and select the credentialing program that fits their work performed, education, and future career goals (CMSA, 2005).

CASE MANAGER SERVICES

Although case management programs differ in structure and design, case managers provide some services regardless of the program's location. There appears to be a consensus in the literature that there are six core functions or activities that delineate case management: assessment, coordination, planning, monitoring, implementation, and evaluation in multiple environments. The focus of each of these functions varies depending on the case management model (CMSA, 2005).

Examples of care coordination include assisting the client or family member with medical appointments, equipment acquisition, home meal delivery, home follow-up services (e.g., home health or public health nursing), appointment transportation, and medical insurance or Medicare form completion. The types of services differ depending on the location of the case management program, the population of clients, and the scope of case management services. Some case managers in managed care environments monitor whether the patient keeps medical appointments and follows the prescribed course of treatment.

The coordination of health care services for hospitalized patients begins at admission or shortly thereafter and continues after discharge for an unspecified time (Ethridge and Lamb, 1989; Lyon, 1991). Depending on the setting, community case management services continue for varying lengths of time. Some programs continue service coordination indefinitely for populations such as the high-risk elderly or the chronically ill. Other programs move patients' case management status from active to inactive when the patient no longer requires services. However, these clients become active again if their condition changes. Case management services continue in the home health care setting until the client is discharged from the program. It is widely recognized that early intervention on the part of a case manager and appropriate referrals prevent costly complications and can result in better health outcomes (Thurkettle and Noji, 2003).

CASE MANAGER ROLES AND CHARACTERISTICS

The individual case manager's role will vary depending on the specific program's services. The role functions of case managers are defined by the CMSA as including assessment, planning, facilitation, and advocacy, achieved through collaboration with the client and others involved in the client's care (CMSA, 2002).

The ANCC describes the practice of a nurse case manager as follows:

Nurse case managers actively participate with their clients to identify and facilitate options and services, providing and coordinating comprehensive care to meet patient/client health needs, with the goal of decreasing fragmentation and duplication of care, and enhancing quality, cost-effective clinical outcomes. Nursing case management is a dynamic and systematic collaborative approach to provide and coordinate health care services to a defined population. Nurse case managers continually evaluate each individual's health plan and specific challenges and then seek to overcome obstacles that affect outcomes. A nurse case manager uses a framework that includes interaction, assessment, planning, implementation, and evaluation. Outcomes are evaluated to determine if additional actions such as reassessment or revision to a plan of care are required to meet clients' health needs. To facilitate patient outcomes, the nurse case manager may fulfill the roles of advocate, collaborator, facilitator, risk manager, educator, mentor, liaison, negotiator, consultant, coordinator, evaluator, and/ or researcher (ANCC, 2009, www.nursingworld.org).

Nurse case managers must be flexible. The health care environment experiences rapid change, and new regulations and reimbursement schedules frequently emerge. The health care provider must respond to these changes rapidly to remain competitive. It is an ideal job for the self-directed nurse who enjoys being involved in a larger health care team within the organization and in the larger community.

CASE IDENTIFICATION

Identification of case management clients occurs in many ways, and each program should determine the criteria for eligibility for case management services. These criteria depend on the services provided, the service's location, the population served, and whether the service is in an acute care or community setting. Some programs are diagnosis based and use many community health care resources; for example, clients with chronic obstructive pulmonary disease often require numerous hospitalizations. Programs may focus on a particular population (e.g., the elderly) and establish criteria to identify which clients to target for services (e.g., the high-risk elderly who are chronically ill or frail and would benefit from case management services).

All clients referred for case management must undergo screening to determine their appropriateness for inclusion in the program. Not all referred clients need the services of a nurse case manager. Often, a nurse can arrange community services or instruct the client and family in the most appropriate follow-up based on client need and program design. The screening instrument must be comprehensive enough to determine which clients meet the program's criteria and user friendly enough to allow the screener to evaluate the clients rapidly to determine their appropriateness for the program. The screener should refer clients to more suitable services within the community if they are not appropriate candidates for a particular case management program. For example, a nurse may refer a human immunodeficiency virus (HIV)–positive client to a case management program for high-risk clients in the community, but the program may not accept clients with HIV and acquired immunodeficiency syndrome (AIDS) because the community already has a program for HIV-positive clients. Instead, the nurse should refer the client to a case management program that focuses exclusively on comprehensive service coordination for clients with HIV and AIDS.

THE REFERRAL PROCESS

The nurse may perform program referrals in a variety of ways. In the acute care hospital setting, referrals are usually based on patient diagnosis or other criteria that trigger a nurse case manager referral (e.g., patient rehospitalization). Internal mechanisms alert the case manager of the patient's admission (e.g., a computerized list).

A variety of tools are used to identify people who would benefit from case management services. These tools include health-risk screening tools, evidence-based criteria, risk stratification through data management, and referrals from hospitals, health care providers, and families. Information is collected by the case manager and analyzed to determine whether the individual being referred is a candidate for case management services (CMSA, 2005).

In community settings, referrals originate from a variety of sources such as a client's family, a primary care provider, or a hospital case manager. These referrals may be written or verbal. Staff in community agencies can also make service referrals; for example, the American Heart Association or American Cancer Society may receive calls from clients and families requesting information and assistance.

CASE MANAGEMENT MODELS

The literature has reported a variety of case management models. These models may be hospital based or community based, and some provide client services across the health care continuum. Further, case management models are designed for a variety of populations.

Hospital-Based Case Management

The acute care setting uses the following essential models of case management: the New England model, the discharge planner and arbitrator model, and the geriatric specialist model. In these models, the case manager provides patient services during hospitalization and performs short-term or limited intervention after discharge.

New England Model

The New England model of case management is a primary nursing care delivery system operated within the hospital (Bower, 1992; Zander, 1988, 1990). In this client-centered model, an RN provides primary nursing care to one patient group and case management to another patient group. The nurse may or may not provide primary nursing care to the case management group. In the case management role, the nurse is responsible for clinical nursing care and the financial outcome of each managed care patient. The nurse measures the financial outcome through critical paths and aims to discharge each patient within the allotted number of hospital days under the PPS (Bower, 1992; Zander, 1988, 1990).

The New England model resembles a modified primary nursing model with additional managed care responsibilities more closely than case management because the primary nurse provides direct patient care and financial managed care responsibilities. An essential part of the nurse's responsibilities includes use of critical paths to determine the patient's progress and monitor consumed resources (a utilization review or managed care function). The nurse performs a limited telephone follow-up after discharge and may make a single home visit. Using staff nurses for patient follow-up after discharge can create problems. Administration must find replacements for staff nurses in the acute-care setting when staff performs phone calls or home visits. It must also consider the education and experience level of the staff nurse acting in the community health nursing role.

Discharge Planner and Arbitrator Case Management Model

In this model, the RN patient care provider is the discharge planner and the manager of utilization review strategies and quality assurance activities. A multidisciplinary utilization review team also maximizes resource use and discharge planning services. The program's quality assurance component incorporates an evaluation process of patient outcomes that results from the community service discharge referrals from all discharge planning sources (Bair, Griswold, and Head, 1989).

Geriatric Clinical Nurse Specialist Model

The case managers in this model are master's-prepared geriatric clinical nurse specialists who augment the staff nurses' basic care. The case managers use a comprehensive discharge planning protocol for hospitalized elderly patients, whom the staff nurses follow (Naylor, 1990; Neidlinger, Scroggins, and Kennedy, 1987). This protocol includes a comprehensive patient assessment and a comprehensive discharge plan for posthospital care. The protocol may include assessment of the patient's health status, orientation level, skill level, motivation level, sociodemographic data, health status knowledge, and perception levels. The discharge plan is based on patient assessment. Case managers often monitor patients on a short-term basis through telephone or home visits for at least 2 weeks following discharge.

Another model is that of the geriatric care manager. An RN or a master's-level social worker provides comprehensive care through in-home visits, telephone contact with clients, ongoing coordination, monitoring, and follow-up for 8 months on average (Enguidanos et al., 2003).

Case Management Models Across the Health Care Continuum

Some models provide patient discharge services from the acute hospital setting and continue with long-term case management services in the community setting after discharge. The Arizona model is one example of this case management model.

Arizona Model

In this case management model, nurse administrators, educators, researchers, and clinicians are case managers. They are responsible for patients during hospitalization and refer patients to appropriate community services following discharge (Ethridge, 1991; Ethridge and Johnson, 1996; Ethridge and Lamb, 1989). For several months or years, nurse case

managers may work with chronically ill individuals who have frequent exacerbations or are entering terminal phases of their disease (Bower, 1992).

Private Pay Care Management

Private pay care management is another type of service offered in many communities. In this program, a care manager offers case management services on a contract basis or in conjunction with an existing program. If the client does not meet the criteria for an existing care management program or if an existing program's services expire before the client is satisfied, the client or family must pay for the case manager's services. Families who need service coordination assistance often request this service. The length of time the care manager provides these services depends on the client's needs.

Pharmacy Model of Case Management

Pharmacy case management has a focus on medication management for clients with chronic illness who take multiple medications (Huber, 2002). The goal of pharmacy case management is to manage the client's polypharmacy to ensure the correct medications are taken by clients in the correct doses and frequency.

The Medication Interest Model (MIM) is dedicated to the topic of how to improve medication adherence across all medication classes (Shea, 2006). The MIM consists of a set of interview techniques that can be applied by clinicians in a variety of settings. New interviewing techniques are used along with well-established techniques that include task-specific interview questions. It is a model that can be used for research, training, and communication for improving medication adherence (Shea, 2008).

Community Case Management Models

Some case managers provide services exclusively in the community setting after discharge. Proponents argue that discharge planning and case management should be two separate and distinct functions with separate staff, procedures, and accountability. Supporters of this model believe case management's purpose is much broader than discharge planning and includes alternative planning to institutionalization, which ensures cost-effective care, access to comprehensive care, coordinating services, and improved client functional capacity (Simmons and White, 1988). The Denver model and the Indianapolis model are two exclusively community-based case management models.

Clinical Example: Denver Case Management Model

In 1989, the Denver Regional Council of Governments evaluated counselor-facilitated hospital discharges in five metro-area Colorado hospitals. The sample included 1040 people aged 75 years or older and continued for 8 weeks after discharge. The counselor intervention system resulted in fewer deaths, a 21% decrease in the number of discharged individuals in nursing homes, and an increase in those released into their homes rather than institutions. The research supported the trend toward case management services and services in the home for high-risk, high-cost cases in particular (Denver Regional Council of Governments, 1989).

APPLICATION OF CASE MANAGEMENT IN COMMUNITY HEALTH

Case management can be used in all community health settings, with interventions at the primary, secondary, and tertiary levels of prevention, based on the community program and population served. Nurses working as case managers in the community setting will have diverse roles and responsibilities.

Public Health Clinic Settings

Depending on the services provided in the public health setting, the nurse has an opportunity to provide education, screening, and referrals as needed to the clients served. Examples of primary prevention can include an antepartum clinic, where the nurse interacts with women and can teach about pregnancy, diet, and exercise during pregnancy.

Working with parents in pediatric settings, the nurse case manager can teach nutrition, growth, and development and provide anticipatory guidance (primary level of prevention). The nurse can also screen children for growth and development and make referrals as needed to the Women, Infants, and Children (WIC) program, and other specialty programs available in the area for the clients' needs (secondary prevention).

Nurses can also serve as case managers working with elderly, providing nutrition education (primary prevention), screening for hypertension (secondary prevention), and even assisting with medication management and care of chronic diseases (tertiary prevention). The opportunities for community health nurses to provide case management services are vast, depending upon the location, populations served, and resources available in the community.

Occupational Health Settings

More employers are providing health screening and education to their employees to keep their work force healthy. Community health nurses who work in occupational health settings are in a position to provide primary prevention in health education classes designed for the needs of the employees. These classes can be designed on the basis of the health

status of workers, to prevent the types of injuries to which they are prone. The nurse in this setting can also provide primary prevention by offering flu shots and other immunizations to keep the employees healthy.

Secondary prevention can be provided to employees through screening clinics for hypertension and other potential chronic illnesses or health problems to which the employees may be more susceptible because of the nature of work performed. Referrals can be made as needed for follow-up with these employees. The occupational health nurse would continue to follow these employees and case manage any health issues that could impact the employees' ability to perform the duties of their jobs.

Case management for tertiary prevention can include keeping in touch with injured employees and monitoring their recovery, therapy, or other services that are provided to the employees in the process of returning to health and their jobs. The occupational health nurse who provides case management services to these employees offers them education, referrals as needed, and assistance in their recovery process.

High-Risk Clinic Settings

There are many examples of health care settings that provide services to high-risk clients in which the nurse serves as case manager. A few examples include HIV clinics, settings that provide health care services to high-risk perinatal clients, clients who have received transplants, dialysis settings, oncology clinics, and infusion centers. The case management services offered by the nurse are determined by the specific needs of the clients seen in these settings. The models of case management are also developed for the needs of the clients.

Clients with Chronic Diseases

The community health nurse who interacts with clients with chronic diseases can be instrumental in monitoring the client in the community, monitoring medication management, assessing clients to identify problems early, and intervening with the physician to modify therapy (see Box 9-2). With patients with chronic obstructive pulmonary disease, hypertension, or congestive heart failure, early intervention on the part of the nurse can decrease the need for hospitalization and, if the patient is hospitalized, ensure early hospitalization with a shorter length of stay.

Home Health and Hospice Settings

The community health nurses working in home health or hospice services are often assigned a case load of clients for whom they provide case management services. In both of these settings, the nurse case manager provides primary, secondary, and tertiary prevention to clients. These services are designed on the basis of the individual needs of clients and their families. Coordination of care, referrals, assessment, medication management, patient and family education, and the development of plans of care are just a few of the nursing functions that are provided through a case management model.

RESEARCH IN CASE MANAGEMENT

Results of case management research are scarce in the literature; the documented studies describe the implemented programs and evaluate the program outcomes. An example is given in the Research Highlights box.

RESEARCH HIGHLIGHTS

Geriatric Care Management for Low-Income Seniors: A Randomized Controlled Trial

Counsell et al. (2007) conducted a randomized clinical control study of 951 adults 65 years or older with annual incomes less than 200% of the federal poverty level whose primary care physicians were randomly assigned to the intervention group (474 patients) or usual care (477 patients) in community-based health centers. The intervention consisted of 2 years of home-based care management by a nurse practitioner and social worker who collaborated with the primary care physician and a geriatrics interdisciplinary team and were guided by twelve care protocols for common geriatric conditions. Results of the study showed that integrated and home-based geriatric care management resulted in improved quality of care and reduced acute care utilization among a high-risk group. Improvements in health-related quality of life issues were mixed, and physical function outcomes did not differ between groups.

Case management programs in all settings require further study. Terms used in case management programs should be defined for comparison across clinical sites. Programs with similar organizational structures and services can then be compared across settings. Critical to the success of case management programs is the inclusion of costs and cost savings. The researcher or case manager must report the program's description, and the case manager's role and professional background. Well-defined patient and program outcomes are essential to the evaluation of case management programs. With the implementation of well designed research with measurable outcomes, management in health care settings across the continuum of care can identify the most cost-effective programs for specific populations served.

INTERNATIONAL CASE MANAGEMENT

As more Americans are traveling outside of the United States in search of affordable health care, a new need for case management has emerged. There is a now a need for international case management with great potential and new opportunities. New challenges are emerging in the need for ongoing consumer-relevant quality in the international case management arena (The PCM Editorial Review Board, 2008).

▍ S U M M A R Y

Case management programs will continue to emerge in all health care settings. These programs will change as the needs of the population change. A common need among all programs is to collect data on the efficacy of programs, measuring client and program outcomes to ensure that the services that are offered are meeting targeted goals.

Staff who work as case managers should consider obtaining certification to develop common knowledge and skills among case management providers and better validate the services provided.

CASE STUDY APPLICATION OF THE NURSING PROCESS

The following case study is an example of a comprehensive case management program. Case management programs and the served populations are diverse; this is only one example of case management implementation.

Judy, the case manager at an HIV early intervention program, received a call from Don, a white man aged 29 years. Don had just moved from a neighboring state, where he recently discovered he was HIV positive. A clinic administered his HIV test, and he did not receive any health services. He found the HIV clinic's phone number in the phone book and did not have a local health care provider. He was a construction worker before he moved, but the company laid him off. He moved to Reno to find work because new building and growth abounded in the area. He moved into a local motel and paid rent for the following 2 weeks. He did not have health insurance, but he was eligible for continued health insurance coverage through the Consolidated Omnibus Budget Reconciliation Act (COBRA). Unfortunately, he could not afford to pay the COBRA premium because he was unemployed. He felt desperate, alone, isolated, and depressed, and he needed help.

Judy performed an intake screening and assisted Don in receiving needed services. She scheduled appointments with the clinic's health care providers and met with him to identify the services he needed. Judy completed her assessment after Don attended the clinical appointment and met with her for case management.

Assessment

Don was HIV positive, but he did not have any symptoms of AIDS. He took medication, ate well, maintained good physical condition and dentition, and owned a car. Although he had limited finances, he paid his rent for 2 weeks. He did not have health insurance and could not afford medications or laboratory tests. Judy developed the following plan:

Individual

Judy used Ryan White grant funds to finance Don's services through the clinic. She applied for housing assistance and scheduled an appointment with the clinic's SW to discuss his financial situation and job prospects. The pharmacist provided his medications, which were funded by the clinic; explained the drugs in detail; and offered to answer questions.

Family

Don was estranged from his family. His mother, who lived 2000 miles away, was aged 65 years, widowed, and retired. Don had not visited his two siblings in 10 years and chose not to have family contact. Although Don had friends at his last job, he had not made friends in Reno. Before moving, he was in a relationship with a woman for 2 years. After the relationship ended, he did not know where she lived.

CASE STUDY   APPLICATION OF THE NURSING PROCESS—cont'd

Community

Judy knew Don could access a solid network of community services. Don was new in the community, and he did not have social support; therefore Judy identified that he needed to contact job placement services and attend an HIV support group.

Diagnosis

Judy developed the following nursing diagnoses for Don:

Individual

- Deficient knowledge related to HIV, including knowledge of the disease, medications, and available resources
- Inadequate income from unemployment

Family

- Lack of family and social support
- Poor family communication patterns

Community

- Adequate services through the HIV clinic
- Coordination of services through case management

Planning

Judy made the following plan, which is open for modification, and established goals with Don.

Individual
Short-Term Goals

- Don will find employment within 2 months. If his employer does not provide health care benefits, the clinic program will continue to provide them.
- If Don does not find work and cannot pay rent, local HIV funding will be used to provide housing assistance.

Long-Term Goal

- The clinic will provide health care services, medications, laboratory tests, and other outpatient services.

Family
Short-Term Goal

- Don was not interested in communicating with his family. Judy respected his wishes and did not pursue the issue in the short term.

Long-Term Goal

- Judy will ask Don again if he is interested in having contact with his family. Judy will offer Don the opportunity of family counseling to explore his feelings regarding his family and allow Don to determine whether he wants to communicate with any of his family members.

Community
Short-Term Goal

- Judy will collect information on available community resources to share with Don.

Long-Term Goal

- Judy will evaluate Don's involvement in using community resources. As needed, Judy will offer Don more options of resources that are available and that are appropriate.

Intervention
Individual

Acting as his case manager, Judy connected Don with job opportunities, housing, and community support groups. Judy explained the available programs and allowed Don to choose his services.

Don had to attend his scheduled clinic appointments, take his medication, and contact his case manager regularly.

Family

Judy knows that Don is estranged from his family. As appropriate, Judy will continue to approach Don about exploring his feelings about his family with a professional counselor. If Don is interested in making contact with any of his family members, Judy will assist in the coordination of this process.

Community

The plan supplemented the services that Don could not afford. The plan focused on Don's individual needs in health care, employment, housing, and support groups. Judy will provide Don with available services in the community. As new programs become available, Judy will contact Don to explain the services and make referrals to services that both she and Don believe are appropriate.

Evaluation
Individual

Judy evaluated the results of Don's comprehensive case management plan on a continuing basis. If Don obtained employment in construction, he could support himself adequately and would require financial assistance primarily with his medications. If he did not find a job, or if his health status changed and he was unable to work in construction, then Judy would need to modify the plan.

Family

Judy evaluated Don's interest in getting in touch with his family. She will assist him in getting referred for family therapy. When and if Don wishes to contact any of his family, Judy will assist him in making arrangements.

Community

Judy will need to connect Don with community support groups to establish friendships and gain social support.

LEARNING ACTIVITIES

1. Contact case management programs in the community and acute care setting.
2. Interview case management program directors. Ask them about their program's structure and process, the program's acceptance criteria, and their referral sources.
3. Ask the directors what data they collect on their clients and what is reported to their administration.
4. Ask the directors about their program's required education and experience levels for case managers.
5. Spend a day with a case manager, and ask about his or her various roles and services.
6. Participate in a client/family interview.

REFERENCES

American Nurses Association: *Case management by nurses*, Washington, DC, 1992, The Association. www.nursingworld.org.

American Nurses Credentialing Center: *Case management nursing*, 2009, www.nursingworld.org.

Bair NL, Griswold JT, Head JL: Clinical RN involvement in bedside-centered case management, *Nurs Econ* 7(3):150–154, 1989.

Bower KA: *Case management by nurses*, Washington, DC, 1992, American Nurses Publishing.

Case Management Society of America: *Standards of practice for case management*, Little Rock, AR, 2002, The Author.

Case Management Society of America: *Philosophy of case management*, 2005, The Author. www.cmsa.org/ABOUTUS/DefinitionofCaseManagement/tabid/104/Default.aspx.

Center for Health Care Strategies, Inc.: *Care management definition and framework*, Hamilton, NJ, 2007, Fact Sheets.

Commission for Case Manager Certification: *Certified Case Manager (CCM) certification requirement*, 2009, www.ccmcertification.org.

Conger MM: Nursing case management: a managed care organizational strategy. In Conger MM, editor: *Managed care: practice strategies for nursing*, Thousand Oaks, CA, 1999, Sage Publications.

Counsell SR, Callahan CM, Clark DO, et al: Geriatric care management for low-income seniors, *JAMA* 298:2623–2633, 2007.

Crosby RL: Community care of the chronically mentally ill, *Journal of Psychosocial Nursing* 25(1):33–37, 1987.

Denver Regional Council of Governments: *DRCOG study may trigger new national policy*, Denver, 1989, The Author.

Enguidanos SM, Gibbs NE, Simmons WJ, et al: Kaiser Permanente Community Partners Project: improving geriatric care management practices, *J Am Geriatr Soc* 51:710–714, 2003.

Ethridge PA: Nursing HMO: Carondelet St. Mary's experience, *Nurs Manage* 22(7):22–27, 1991.

Ethridge PA, Johnson S: The influence of reimbursement on nurse case management practice: Carondelet's experience. In Cohen EL, editor: *Nurse case management in the 21st century*, St. Louis, 1996, Mosby.

Ethridge PA, Lamb GS: Professional nursing case management improves quality, access, and costs, *Nurs Manage* 20(3):30–35, 1989.

Grau L: Case management and the nurse, *Geriatr Nurs* 5(8):372–375, 1984.

Huber DL: The diversity of case management models, *Lippincotts Case Manag* 7(6):212–220, 2002.

Lyon JC: *Descriptive study of models of discharge planning and case management in California*, Ann Arbor, MI, 1991, University of California, San Francisco, University Microfilms International (doctoral dissertation).

Lyon JC: Models of nursing care delivery and case management: clarification of terms, *Nurs Econ* 11(3):163–169, 1993.

Lyon JC, et al: In *Case management for high risk elderly*, Paper presented at the 123rd annual meeting of the American Public Health Association, San Diego, 1995.

Mahn VA, Spross JA: Nursing case management as an advanced practice role. In Hamric AB, Spross JA, Hanson CM, editors: *Advanced nursing practice: an integrative approach*, Philadelphia, 1996, Saunders.

Naylor MD: Comprehensive discharge planning for hospitalized elderly: a pilot study, *Nurs Res* 39(3):156–161, 1990.

Neidlinger SH, Scroggins K, Kennedy LM: Cost evaluation of discharge planning for hospitalized elderly, *Nurs Econ* 5(5):225–230, 1987.

Pittman DC: Nursing case management: holistic care for the deinstitutionalized mentally ill, *J Psychosoc Nurs* 27(11):23–27, 1989.

Shea SC: *Improving medication adherence: how to talk with patients about their medications*, Philadelphia, 2006, Lippincott Williams & Wilkins.

Shea SC: The "Medication Interest Model." An integrative clinical interviewing approach for improving medication adherence—part I: clinical applications, *Prof Case Manag* 6(13):305–315, 2008.

Simmons WJ, White M: Case management and discharge planning: two different worlds. In Volland P, editor: *Discharge planning: an interdisciplinary approach to continuity of care*, Owings Mills, MD, 1988, National Health Publication.

Steinberg RM, Carter GW: *Case management and the elderly*, Lexington, MA, 1983, Lexington Books, DC Health.

The PCM Editorial Review Board: The PCM journal "think tank" on case management predictions for 2009, *Prof Case Manag* 13:299–301, 2008.

Thurkettle MA, Noji A: Shifting the healthcare paradigm: the case manager's opportunity and responsibility, *Lippincotts Case Manag* 8(4):160–165, 2003.

US Department of Commerce/International Trade Administration: *Health and medical services: US industrial outlook*, Washington, DC, 1990, The Author, US Document.

Weil M, Karls J: *Case management in human service practice*, San Francisco, 1985, Jossey-Bass.

Weinberger M, et al: The cost-effectiveness of intensive post discharge care: a randomized trial, *Med Care* 26(11):1092–1101, 1988.

White P, Hall ME: Mapping the literature of case management nursing, *J Med Libr Assoc* 94(2 Suppl):E99–E106, 2006.

Yamamoto L, Lucey C: Case management "within the walls" a glimpse into the future, *Crit Care Nurs Q* 28(2):162–178, 2005.

Zander KS: Nursing case management: strategic management of cost and quality outcomes, *J Nurs Adm* 18(5):23–30, 1988.

Zander KS: Managed care and nursing case management. In Mayer GG, Madden MJ, Lawrenz E, editors: *Patient care delivery models*, Gaithersburg, MD, 1990, Aspen.

Health Care System

Anita W. Finkelman

OBJECTIVES

Upon completion of this chapter, the reader will be able to do the following:

1. Analyze landmark health care legislation and its influence on the delivery system.
2. Describe the organization of the public health care subsystem at the federal, state, and local levels.
3. Compare and contrast the scope of the private health care subsystem and the public health care subsystem.
4. Describe the roles of the members of the health care team.
5. Discuss the relationship of critical health care issues to the health care organization and health care providers.
6. Discuss future concerns for the health care delivery system.

KEY TERMS

accreditation
alternative therapies
client rights
community health center
health care reform

managed care
managed care organizations
  (MCOs)
Medicaid
Medicare

outcomes measures
public health
quality care
telehealth

OUTLINE

Major Legislative Actions and the Health Care System
  Federal Legislation
  State Legislative Role
  Legislation Influencing Managed Care
Components of the Health Care System
  Private Health Care Subsystem
  Public Health Subsystem
  Federal Level Subsystem
  State Level Subsystem
  Local Health Department Subsystems
  Health Care Providers

Critical Issues in Health Care Delivery
  Managed Care
  Quality Care
  Fraud and Abuse
  Information Technology
  Consumerism, Advocacy, and Client Rights
  Coordination and Access to Health Care
  Disparity in Health Care Delivery
  Health Care Reform
**Future of Public Health and the Health
  Care System**

The health care system of the United States is dynamic, multifaceted, and not comparable with any other health care system in the world. It is regularly praised for its technological breakthroughs, frequently criticized for its high costs, and often difficult to access by those most in need. This chapter describes landmark health care legislation, the components of the health care system, critical health care organization and provider issues, and the role of government in public health and health care reform and presents a futuristic perspective.

MAJOR LEGISLATIVE ACTIONS AND THE HEALTH CARE SYSTEM

An examination of the major legislative actions that federal and state governments have taken and recognition of their influence on health and health care delivery are critical to understand the evolution of the health care system in the United States. Throughout the twentieth century, the U.S. Congress enacted bills that had a major influence on the private and public health care subsystems. Legislation pertaining to health increased in scope in each decade of the twentieth century, with the goal of improving the health of populations and coping with changing health care needs. During the last two decades, concerns about an increase in health care costs and the growth of managed care stimulated even more legislation. Indeed, health care reform/health insurance reform were major issues during the 2008 presidential election. Further, throughout much of 2009, Congress debated numerous bills and amendments proposed to help reduce costs, increase access, and improve quality.

Federal Legislation

The following discussion describes some of the landmark federal laws that have influenced health services and health care professionals. These are summarized in Table 10-1.

- *Pure Food and Drugs Act of 1906:* This act established a program to supervise and control the manufacture, labeling, and sale of food. Subsequent legislation included meat and dairy products, pharmaceuticals, cosmetics, toys, and household products. Since 1927, the Food and Drug Administration (FDA) has administered elements of this act.
- *Children's Bureau Act of 1912:* The Children's Bureau was founded to protect children from the unhealthy child labor practices of the time and to enact programs that had a positive effect on children's health. In 1921, the Sheppard-Towner Act extended children's health care programs by providing funds for the health and welfare of infants.
- *Social Security Act of 1935 and its amendments (1965, 1972):* The Social Security Act and its subsequent amendments have had a far-reaching effect on health care for many groups. The Social Security Administration (SSA) provides welfare for high-risk mothers and children. Benefits were later expanded to include health care provisions for older adults and the handicapped. This major governmental action was the enactment of legislation for Medicare and Medicaid.
- *Medicare, Title XVIII Social Security Amendment (1965):* This federal program, administered by the Centers for Medicare and Medicaid Services (formerly Health Care Financing Administration [HCFA]), pays specified health care services for all people 65 years of age and older who are eligible to receive Social Security benefits. People with permanent disabilities and those with end-stage renal disease are also covered. The objective of Medicare is to protect older adults and the disabled against large medical outlays. The program is funded through a payroll tax of most working citizens.

TABLE 10-1	CRITICAL FEDERAL LEGISLATION RELATED TO HEALTH CARE
DATE	**LEGISLATION**
1906	Pure Food and Drugs Act
1912	Children's Bureau Act
1921	Sheppard-Towner Act
1935	Social Security Act
1944	Public Health Act
1945	McCarren-Ferguson Act
1946	Hill-Burton Act
1953	Department of Health, Education and Welfare as a cabinet-status agency; in 1979 divided into U.S. Department of Education and DHHS
1956	Health Amendments Act
1964	Nurse Training Act
1965	Social Security Act amendments: Title XVIII Medicare; Title XIX Medicaid
1970	Occupational Safety and Health Act
1972	Social Security Act amendments: Professional Standards Review Organization; further benefits under Medicare and Medicaid, including dialysis
1973	Health Maintenance Act
1974	National Health Planning Resources Act
1981, 1987, 1989, 1990	Omnibus Budget Reconciliation Acts
1982	Tax Equity and Fiscal Responsibility Act
1985	Consolidated Omnibus Budget Reconciliation Act
1988	Family Support Act
1990	Health Objectives Planning Act
1996	Health Insurance Portability and Accountability Act
1996	Welfare Act
2004	Nurse Reinvestment Act
2003	Medicare Reinvestment Act
2008	Mental Health Parity and Addictions Equity
2010	Patient Protection and Affordable Care Act

Individuals or providers may submit payment requests for health care services and are paid according to Medicare regulations. See Chapter 11 for more information on Medicare.

- *Medicaid, Title XIX Social Security Amendment (1965):* This combined federal and state program provides access to care for the poor and medically needy of all ages. Each state is allocated federal dollars on a matching basis (i.e., 50% of costs are paid with federal dollars). Each state has the responsibility and right to determine services to be provided and the dollar amount allocated to the program. Basic services (i.e., ambulatory and inpatient hospital care, physical therapy, laboratory, radiography, skilled nursing, and home health care) are required to be eligible for matching federal dollars. States may choose from a wide range of optional services including drugs, eyeglasses, intermediate care, inpatient psychiatric care, and dental care. Limits are placed on the amount and duration of service. Unlike Medicare, Medicaid provides long-term care services (e.g., nursing home and home health) and personal care services (e.g., chores and homemaking). In addition, Medicaid has eligibility criteria based on level of income.

TABLE 10-2 2009 USDHHS POVERTY GUIDELINES

PERSONS IN FAMILY OR HOUSEHOLD	48 CONTIGUOUS STATES AND D.C.	ALASKA	HAWAII
1	$10,830	$13,540	$12,460
2	$14,570	$18,220	$16,760
3	$18,310	$22,890	$21,060
4	$22,050	$27,570	$25,360
5	$25,790	$32,240	$29,660
6	$29,530	$36,920	$33,960
7	$33,270	$41,590	$38,260
8	$37,010	$46,270	$42,570
For each additional person, add	$3,740	$4,680	$4,300

From U.S. Department of Health and Human Services: *Computations for the 2009 annual update of the HHS Poverty Guidelines for the 48 contiguous states and the District of Columbia, 2009:* aspe.hhs.gov/poverty/09poverty.shtml.

Table 10-2 provides the U.S. Department of Health and Human Services (USDHHS) poverty guidelines for 2009. The Medicaid population has complex needs, and managed care organizations may not be able to provide optimum services to these beneficiaries. See Chapter 11 for more information on Medicaid.

- *Public Health Act of 1944:* The Public Health Act consolidated all existing public health legislation into one law. Since then, many new pieces of legislation have become amendments. Examples of some of its provisions, either in the original law or in amendments, provided for or established the following:
  - Health services for migratory workers
  - Family planning services
  - Health research facilities
  - National Institutes of Health (NIH)
  - Nurse training acts
  - Traineeships for graduate students in public health
  - Home health services for people with Alzheimer's disease
  - Prevention and primary care services
  - Rural health clinics
  - Communicable disease control
- *McCarren-Ferguson Act of 1945:* The McCarren-Ferguson Act has had a major influence on the insurance industry by giving states the exclusive right to regulate health insurance plans (Knight, 1998). No federal government agency is solely responsible for monitoring insurance. Some federal agencies are involved in insurance reimbursement; however, the structure of the benefit program for federal employees and military personnel, Medicare, and Medicaid allows Congress to pass laws that can override state laws if the laws meet certain criteria.
- *Hill-Burton Act of 1946:* The Hill-Burton Act authorized federal assistance in the construction of hospitals and health centers with stipulations about services for the uninsured. As a result, hospitals with obligations to care for the uninsured were built in towns and cities across

the United States. Through these measures, hospital care became more accessible, but, by the late 1990s, the high cost of health care, combined with decreasing lengths of stay and increasing use of primary care, forced the closure of many of the hospitals built with Hill-Burton funds.

- *Health Amendments Act of 1956:* The Health Amendments Act, Title II, authorizes funds to aid registered nurses (RNs) in full-time study of administration, supervision, or teaching. In 1963, the Surgeon General's Consultant Group on Nursing noted that there were still too few nursing schools, nursing personnel were not put to good use, and there was limited nursing research. As a result, in 1964, the Nurse Training Act provided funds for loans and scholarships for full-time study for nurses and funds for construction of nursing schools.
- *Occupational Safety and Health Act of 1970:* The Occupational Safety and Health Act focuses on the health needs and risks in the workplace and environment. It continues to provide critical programs important to the workplace and the community. See Chapter 30 for more information on both the Occupational Safety and Health Act and the Occupational Safety and Health Administration.
- *Health Maintenance Organization Act of 1973:* The HMO Act provides grants for HMO development. The act requires that employers offer federally qualified HMOs as a health care coverage option to employees and established that states were responsible for the oversight of HMOs. Although initially it was not successful in stimulating HMO growth, this legislation has had a long-term effect on the growth of managed care.
- *National Health Planning and Resources Act of 1974:* The National Health Planning and Resources Act assigned health planning responsibility to the states and local health systems agencies. In addition, it requires health care facilities to obtain prior approval from the state for expansion in the form of a certificate of need (CON).
- *Omnibus Budget Reconciliation Acts (1981, 1987, 1989, and 1990):* The Omnibus Budget Reconciliation Acts were each enacted in response to the huge federal deficit. They have influenced funding for nursing homes, home health agencies, and hospitals and set up guidelines and regulations about several issues, including a move from process to outcome evaluation, use of restraints, and prescription drugs for Medicaid recipients.
- *Tax Equity and Fiscal Responsibility Act of 1982:* The Tax Equity and Fiscal Responsibility Act was a major amendment to the Social Security Act of 1935, establishing the prospective payment system (PPS) for Medicare, the diagnosis-related group (DRG) system. This law changed health care radically by introducing a new reimbursement method. See Chapter 11 for more information on DRGs.
- *Consolidated Omnibus Budget Reconciliation Act of 1985:* COBRA is a federal law that affects health care delivery and reimbursement. It requires all hospitals with emergency services that participate in Medicare to treat any client in their emergency services, whether or not that client is covered by Medicare or has the ability to

pay. This legislation includes requirements for Medicaid services for prenatal and postnatal care to low-income women in two-parent families in which the primary spouse is unemployed. Another important requirement of COBRA focuses on the problem of the loss of insurance when a person loses his or her job. With the growing number of unemployed, COBRA is even more important. Employers who terminate an employee must continue benefits for the employee and dependents for a specified period of time if the employee had health benefits before the termination. COBRA is an example of how a federal law can affect state health care practices. The federal government must determine who receives federal Medicare funds; therefore COBRA provides the opportunity for the federal government to legislate health care delivery at the state level.

- *Family Support Act of 1988:* The Family Support Act expanded coverage for poor women and children and required states to extend Medicaid coverage for 12 months to families who have increased earnings but are no longer receiving cash assistance. This act also required states to expand Aid to Families With Dependent Children (AFDC) coverage to two-parent families when the principal wage earner is unemployed.

- *Health Objectives Planning Act of 1990:* The Health Objectives Planning Act was initiated in response to the 1979 report *Healthy People: The Surgeon General's Report on Health Promotion and Disease Prevention.* After that report, the federal government began to take a directive approach in identifying and monitoring national health care goals. *Healthy People 2000, Healthy People 2010,* and *Healthy People 2020* are also results of the Health Objectives Planning Act.

- *Health Insurance Portability and Accountability Act of 1996:* The Health Insurance Portability and Accountability Act (HIPAA) addressed several insurance issues. Critical issues were the portability of coverage and preexisting conditions. This law established that insurers cannot set limits on coverage of longer than 12 months. This is a complex law, but it is important for consumers with preexisting conditions.

- *Welfare Reform Act of 1996:* The Welfare Reform Act placed restrictions on eligibility for AFDC, Medicaid, and other federally funded welfare programs. This law decreased the number of people on welfare and forced many individuals to take low-paying jobs, many of which do not offer health insurance. Between 1994 and March 1999, welfare rolls dropped 47% (DeParle, 1999). Many individuals, particularly underserved women and children, subsequently lost Medicaid coverage.

- *The State Child Health Improvement Act (SCHIP) of 1997:* This has been a critical law providing insurance for children and families who cannot afford health insurance. This law has been very important to children's health. The law was extended several times and then it was not renewed by the Bush administration. In January 2009 the law was renewed again by the Obama administration.

- *Medicare Modernization Act of 2003:* The Medicare Modernization Act was the most significant law in 40 years for senior health care. After being implemented in January 2006, the law provided seniors and people living with disabilities with some prescription drug benefit coverage, more choices, and better benefits.

- *Nurse Reinvestment Act of 2003:* The Nurse Reinvestment Act is significant because it is a response to the critical nursing shortage that is present across the country. Funding is provided to increase enrollments and number of practicing nurses.

- *Mental Health Parity and Addictions Equity Act of 2008:* A similar act was passed in the 1990s, but it was not an effective law. Improving over the earlier law, this act mandates that if a group health plan includes medical/surgical benefits and mental health benefits and/or substance use disorder benefits, the financial requirements (e.g., deductibles and copayments) and treatment limitations (e.g., number of visits or days of coverage) that apply to mental health benefits must be no more restrictive than the predominant financial requirements or treatment limitations that apply to substantially all medical/surgical benefits.

- *Patient Protection and Affordable Care Act of 2010:* The Health Care Reform Act is an extremely complex and comprehensive piece of legislation. One of the primary intents of the act is to reduce the number of uninsured Americans, and a number of provisions directly address this intent. For example, it requires all U.S. citizens and legal residents to have qualifying health coverage, either provided through employers, individually purchased, or provided by federal plans (i.e., Medicare, Medicaid, CHIPS). It also dramatically changes eligibility requirements for Medicaid, allowing coverage of childless adults with incomes up to 133% of the federal poverty line and expands CHIPS. Further, it subsidizes premiums for lower and middle income families, and requires coverage of dependent adult children up to age 26 for those with group policies (Kaiser Family Foundation, 2010).

The Health Care Reform Act includes significant insurance reforms. For example, it will: (1) establish high-risk pools to provide health coverage to individuals with preexisting conditions; (2) prohibit insurers from placing lifetime limits on the dollar value of coverage; (3) prohibit insurers from disallowing coverage for some individuals because of pre-existing health conditions and dropping policyholders when they get sick; and (4) require health plans to provide some types of preventive care and screenings without consumer cost-sharing (i.e., copayments or coinsurance). The act will also create programs to foster nonprofit, member-run health insurance companies that can offer health insurance, create state-based health insurance exchanges through which individuals and small businesses can buy coverage, and permit states to form compacts that will allow insurers to sell policies in any participating state.

There is considerable confusion and debate on how the act will be implemented and funded. Indeed, most of the provisions will not be in place for at least four years (2014) and some will not be implemented for several years beyond that. Funds for government-financed elements (i.e., Medicare, Medicaid, CHIPS) will be through a combination of new fees and taxes and variety of cost-saving measures. For example, there will be taxes on indoor tanning and new Medicare taxes for those in high-income brackets. The act requires fees for pharmaceutical companies and medical devices, as well as penalties for those who do not obtain health insurance. To cut costs there will be significant cuts to the Medicare Advantage program and modifications and reductions in Medicare spending. It also enhances efforts to reduce administrative costs, streamline care, and reduce fraud and abuse.

Until passage of the Health Care Reform Act in 2010, the thrust of federal legislation has been on either prevention of illness through influencing the environment (e.g., Occupational Safety and Health Act of 1970) or provision of funding to support programs that influence health care (e.g., Social Security Act of 1935). Beginning with the Sheppard-Towner Act of 1921 and continuing to the present, federal grants have increased the involvement of state and local governments in health care. The involvement of the federal government through fiscal allocations to state and local governments provided money for programs not previously available to state and local areas. Similar services became available in all states. Funds supporting these services were accompanied by regulations that applied to all recipients. Many state and local government programs were developed on the basis of availability of federal funds. The involvement of the federal government through funding has served to standardize the public health policy in the United States (Pickett and Hanlon, 1990).

The rising number of uninsured and underinsured strongly influenced passage of the Health Reform Act of 2010, and although it is anticipated that about 32 million additional citizens will have insurance, universal coverage continues to be a concern. As mentioned, it will take a number of years to fully implement the act and the long-term effects will not be known for at least a decade. Further, legal and legislative challenges to some provisions are anticipated.

State Legislative Role

State governments are also directly involved in health care policy, legislation, and regulation. State governments focus particularly on financing and delivery of services and oversight of insurance. The latter has become important as managed care has grown. The Institute of Medicine (IOM) (1988) report *Future of Public Health* noted that it is the state's responsibility to see that functions and services necessary to address the mission of public health are in place throughout the state. The IOM framed the public health enterprise in terms of three functions: assessment, policy development, and assurance. The Association of State and Territorial Health Officials (ASTHO) (2007) described the "public health duties of states" and expanded on the three core functions of public health as the basis. The state health care functions are as follows (p. 7):

- Assessment of health needs based on statewide data collection
- Assurance of an adequate statutory base for health activities in the state

- Establishment of statewide health objectives, delegating power to localities as appropriate and holding them accountable
- Assurance of appropriate organized statewide effort to develop and maintain essential personal, educational, and environmental health services; provision of access to necessary services; and solution of problems inimical to health
- Guarantee of a minimum set of essential health services
- Support of local service capacity, especially when disparities in local ability to raise revenue and/or administer programs require subsidies, technical assistance, or direct action by the state to achieve adequate service levels

Legislation Influencing Managed Care

Prior to passage of the Health Care Reform Act in 2010, much of the recent legislation (i.e., usually state level) influencing managed care organizations (MCOs) is in response to consumers' concerns about MCOs' efforts to control costs. Considerable variability exists across states in MCO legislation, and usually these acts are in response to consumer calls for reform (Levy, 2002). The following examples describe a growing number of legislative acts that provide more control over managed care:

- *Provider protection initiatives (PPIs):* The need for the removal of "gag rules" has been one area of concern for providers and clients. MCOs use gag rules to control what their providers discuss with clients about all treatment options. Additionally, many MCOs provide financial incentives to providers to control costs. These incentives are paid to providers based on their performance data (e.g., number of hospital admissions, length of stay, types of treatment, and types and number of prescriptions ordered).
- *Any willing provider initiatives:* Provider panels are the lists of providers that are approved by an MCO for reimbursement. These initiatives require that MCOs accept any provider on their provider panels who meets plan requirements and is willing to agree to the contract.
- *Direct access legislation:* Client freedom-of-choice legislation is rapidly growing as clients become more concerned about their lack of provider choice and want direct access to providers without obtaining prior approval.
- *Mandated benefits requirement:* This legislation mandates specific minimum health care benefits. Examples of these are the designation of specific basic services, emergency care without prior approval, coverage for experimental treatments, mental health parity, diabetes management, prostate screening, chiropractic treatment, and hospice services.
- *Consumer rights:* Consumers are demanding more rights than just provider choice. Examples include coverage for specific benefits, such as emergency services without prior approval; longer lengths of stay (e.g., obstetric and mastectomy); detailed disclosure of benefits and plan procedures; provider choice; and impartial mechanism for grievances. Efforts have been made to pass a national patients' rights bill, but this has not occurred even though many states passed this type of legislation.

COMPONENTS OF THE HEALTH CARE SYSTEM

The current health care system consists of private and public health care subsystems (Figure 10-1). The private health care subsystem includes personal care services from various sources, both nonprofit and profit, and numerous voluntary agencies. The major focus of the public health subsystem is prevention of disease and illness. These subsystems are not always mutually exclusive, and their functions sometimes overlap.

With the rapid growth of technology and increased demands on the private and public health care subsystems, health care costs have become prohibitive. Cost-effectiveness and cost containment have become a critical driving force as health care delivery system changes are made, and cost-effectiveness often conflicts with the provision of quality care.

Community health nursing requires an understanding of the mission, organization, and role of the private and the public health care subsystems and the contexts within which they function to effectively collaborate with health care organizations to reach community health goals. An organizational framework in which private and voluntary organizations and the government work collaboratively to prevent disease and promote health is essential. Public health and community health nurses are in a unique position to provide leadership and facilitate change in the health care system.

Private Health Care Subsystem

Most personal health care services are provided in the private sector. Services in the private subsystem include health promotion, prevention and early detection of disease, diagnosis and treatment of disease with a focus on cure, rehabilitative-restorative care, and custodial care. These services are provided in clinics, physicians' offices, hospitals, hospital ambulatory centers, skilled care facilities, and homes. Increasingly, these private sector services are available through MCOs.

Private health care services in the United States began with a simple model. Physicians provided care in their offices and made home visits. Clients were admitted to hospitals for general care if they experienced serious complications during the course of their illness. Currently, a variety of highly skilled health care professionals provide comprehensive, preventive, restorative, rehabilitative, and palliative care. A broad array of services is available, which range from general to highly specialized with multidelivery configurations.

Personal care provided by physicians is delivered under the following five basic models:

1. The solo practice of a physician in an office continues to be present in some communities.
2. The single specialty group model consists of physicians in the same specialty, who pool expenses, income, and offices.
3. Multispecialty group practice provides for interaction across specialty areas.
4. The integrated health maintenance model has prepaid multispecialty physicians.
5. The community health center, developed through federal funds in the 1960s, addresses broader inputs into health such as education and housing.

Managed care has become the dominant paradigm in health care, affecting many aspects of health care delivery. Managed care involves capitated payments for care rather than fee-for-service. Health care providers, including physicians, hospitals, community clinics, and home care providers, are integrated in a system such as an HMO. See Chapter 11 for a more detailed discussion of managed care and reimbursement.

Voluntary Agencies

Voluntary or nonofficial agencies are a part of the private health care system of the United States and developed at the same time that the government was assuming responsibility for public health. In the United States during the 1700s and early 1800s, voluntary efforts to improve health were virtually nonexistent because early settlers from Western Europe were not accustomed to participating in organized charity. Immigration expanded to include slaves from Africa and people from Eastern Europe, and their well-being received little attention.

Toward the end of the nineteenth century, new immigrants brought a heritage of social protest and reform. Wealthy businesspeople, such as the Rockefellers, Carnegies, and Mellons, responded to the needs and set up foundations that provided health and welfare money for charitable endeavors. District nurses, such as Lillian Wald, established nursing practices in the large cities for the poor and destitute. Services did not focus just on illness but also on work conditions, health, communicable diseases, living conditions, and language skills.

Voluntary agencies can be classified into the following categories (Hanlon and Pickett, 1990):

1. Specific diseases, such as the American Diabetes Association, American Cancer Society, and National Multiple Sclerosis Society
2. Organ or body structures, such as the National Kidney Foundation or the American Heart Association

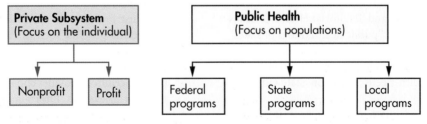

FIGURE 10-1 U.S. health care system.

3. Health and welfare of special groups, such as the National Council on Aging or the March of Dimes
4. Particular phases of health, such as the Planned Parenthood Federation of America

Philanthropic groups also support research and programs. Many professional organizations, such as the American Medical Association and the American Nurses Association, have a significant role in advocacy and in providing professional expertise.

Voluntary organizations provide major sources of help in prevention of disease, promotion of health, treatment of illness, advocacy, consumer education, and research. For example, private and voluntary organizations currently support clients with acquired immunodeficiency syndrome (AIDS). In many cities, the Chicken Soup Brigade provides meals for clients with AIDS who are unable to cook for themselves, and AIDS support groups exist in most larger communities.

Overlap of services often occurs among the numerous private, voluntary, and public agencies. The private and public agencies provide a wide array of services, but sometimes duplication causes them not to be cost-effective. Without voluntary and official agencies, the array of services would be less than what is currently available.

The future is somewhat uncertain for voluntary agencies because major changes are occurring in health care. In the mid-1990s, the Pew Health Professions Commission projected that the emerging health care system would be an amalgam of different public and private forces that would work together to provide integrated, resource-conscious, population-based services (O'Neil and Pew Health Professions Commission, 1998). It was projected that the system would also be more innovative and diverse in how it responded to health needs and more concerned with disease prevention and promotion of health. The Pew Health Professions Commission's projection has not yet been fully realized.

Public Health Subsystem

The U.S. Constitution mandates that the federal government "promote the general welfare of its citizens." The public health subsystem is required by law to address the health of populations. Activities are covered by legal provisions at the local, state, and federal levels of government. At the federal level, Congress enacts laws and writes rules and regulations. The various departments of the executive branch implement and administer them. Interpretations of, and amendments to, the Constitution and Supreme Court decisions over time have changed and increased the role of the federal government in health activities.

Federal policies and practices have had an increasing influence on local and state governments in meeting health and social problems, and many laws have been enacted to respond to changing health needs. Coordination of federal services under several agencies culminated in the establishment of the Department of Health, Education, and Welfare under President Eisenhower in 1953. In 1979, this department was separated into the Department of Education and the DHHS. The DHHS is currently the second largest department of the federal government; only the Department of Defense is larger.

Public health refers to the efforts organized by society to protect, promote, and restore the people's health. Public health programs, services, and institutions emphasize the prevention of disease and address the health needs of the population as a whole. Public health activities typically respond to changing technology and social values, but the goals remain the same (i.e., to reduce the amount of disease, premature death, and disease-produced discomfort and disability).

The public health subsystem is concerned with the health of the population and a healthy environment. The scope of public health is broad and encompasses activities that promote good health. The public health subsystem is organized into multiple levels (i.e., federal, state, and local) to more effectively provide services to those who are unable to obtain health care without assistance and to establish laws, rules, and regulations to protect the public.

Federal Level Subsystem

Most health-related activities at the federal level are implemented and administered by the DHHS. This department is directed by the Secretary of the DHHS, numerous undersecretaries, and assistant secretaries. The Surgeon General is the principal deputy to the assistant secretary of the DHHS. The DHHS has 11 major agencies (Box 10-1).

Other federal agencies perform activities related to health. For example, the Department of Education is involved with health education and school health. The Department of Agriculture administers the inspection of meat and milk and provides funds for the Women, Infants, and Children program (supplemental nutrition), the food stamp program, and the school-based nutrition program.

Scope of Health Services of the Federal Level Subsystem

The federal government targets the following major health areas: the general population, special populations, and international health. For the general population, federal activities include protection against hazards, maintenance of vital and health statistics, advancement of scientific knowledge through research, and provision of disaster relief. In recent years, public health efforts have been directed toward changing behaviors by fostering healthy eating habits, exercise, and preventing tobacco, drug, and alcohol use. Other programs have provided nutritional food and food stamps to individuals and families to ensure adequate food intake.

Services for special populations include protection of workers against hazardous occupations and work conditions and health care for veterans, Native Americans, Alaska natives, federal prisoners, and members of the armed services. In addition, the federal government provides special services for children, older adults, the mentally ill, and the vocationally handicapped.

In the international arena, the federal government works with other countries and international health organizations (e.g., the World Health Organization and the Red Cross) to promote various health programs throughout the world.

BOX 10-1 STRUCTURE OF THE U.S. DEPARTMENT OF HEALTH AND HUMAN SERVICES

The USDHHS is composed of several agencies that provide different services related to U.S. health care. Among them are the following:

- The **Administration on Aging** is the agency responsible for coordinating home and community-based services for older persons and their caregivers.
- The **Centers for Medicare and Medicaid Services** administers those programs.
- The **Administration for Children and Families** provides family assistance (welfare), child support, Head Start, and other programs to strengthen the family unit.
- The **Centers for Disease Control and Prevention (CDC)** conducts and supports programs directed to prevent and control infectious diseases; they assist states during epidemics. In addition, they provide services related to health promotion and education and professional development and training.
- The **Food and Drug Administration** provides surveillance over the safety and efficacy of foods, pharmaceuticals, and other consumer goods.
- The **Health Resources and Services Administration** is concerned with the development of health services programs and

facilities. The Division of Nursing is in this unit. A major focus of this agency is funding grants for nursing education and training. The **Indian Health Service** is also in this unit, providing health services for Native Americans and Alaska Natives.

- The **National Institutes of Health (NIH)** perform and support research programs. The focus of their efforts is to develop and extend the scientific knowledge base related to their respective areas. The National Institute for Nursing Research is part of NIH, and it focuses on nursing research.
- The **Substance Abuse and Mental Health Services Administration** awards grants and funds research related to problems with substance abuse and mental health.
- The **Agency for Healthcare Quality and Research** works to improve quality, safety, efficiency, and effectiveness of health care services for all Americans.
- The **Agency for Toxic Substances and Disease Registry** serves the public by using the best science, taking responsive public health actions, and providing trusted health information to prevent harmful exposures and diseases related to toxic substances.

The IOM report *HHS in the 21st Century: Charting a New Course for a Healthier America* (IOM, 2008) does not recommend major reorganization of the DHHS but rather an approach that would transform it. The recommendations center on five key areas:

1. Define a twenty-first century vision.
2. Foster adaptability and alignment.
3. Increase effectiveness and efficiency of the U.S. health care system.
4. Strengthen the DHHS and public health and the health care workforce.
5. Improve accountability and decision making.

It is anticipated that the DHHS will play a major role in any health care reform initiatives because it accounts for a very large segment of the country's health care dollar.

State Level Subsystem

States are responsible for the health of their citizens and are the central authorities in the public health care system. The organization and activities of public health services vary widely among the states. Most state agencies are directed by a health commissioner or secretary of health who is typically appointed by the governor. Each state also has a health officer, who is usually a physician with a degree and experience in public health. In some states, the health officer directs the health department. Many states have boards of health, which determine policies and priorities for allocation of funds. Staffing of the state agency varies among states; however, compared with other state programs, state health programs usually have a large staff.

The state health department, however, does not stand alone. It is highly dependent on the federal level for resources and guidance. For example, funds that the federal government contributes to Medicaid, which is jointly funded by the federal government and states, have been reduced. This has had a major impact on services that states can provide to their most vulnerable citizens. Cooperation between the state

and federal levels has also been brought to the forefront with efforts to plan for bioterrorism, an event that would necessitate cooperation and sharing. The United States requires an integrated system so that both federal and state levels work to the benefit of all citizens.

Scope of Health Services of the State Level Subsystem

Each state is responsible for its own public health laws; therefore state policy is widely varied. Factors that affect the level of state services include state-legislated or mandated services, political factors related to division of power between state and local health departments (LHDs), and competition among officials, providers, and the business community.

As discussed in previous chapters, the three core functions of public health are assessment, policy development, and assurance (IOM, 1988). Assessment activities include the collection of data pertaining to vital statistics, health facilities, and human resources; epidemiological activities, such as communicable disease control, health screening, and laboratory analyses; and participation in research projects. In the area of policy development, states formulate goals, develop health plans, and set standards for local health agencies. Assurance activities involve inspection in a variety of areas, licensing, health education, environmental safety, personal health services, and resource development.

Nurses represent the largest group of professionals providing health services. State legislatures determine licensure requirements and enact nurse practice acts. State boards of nursing are the administrative arm for implementation of these laws and regulations.

Local Health Department Subsystems

Several provisions of the 2010 Health Care Reform Act address improvement of quality and access to care. For example, it promotes establishment of local consortiums of health care providers to coordinate health care services for low-income uninsured and underinsured populations. It also substantially increases funds for community health centers and finances newly developed school-based health centers and nurse-managed health clinics.

LHDs are generally responsible for the direct delivery of public health services and protection of the health of citizens though not all communities/counties have LHDs. State and local governments (i.e., city and county) delegate the authority to conduct these activities. The organization of LHDs varies widely depending on community size, economics, partnerships with the private health care system, health care facilities, business support, health care needs, transportation, and the number of citizens requiring public health care. Some LHDs function as district offices of the state health department; others are responsible to local government and the state; and still others are autonomous, particularly those in large cities. LHDs may be a separate agency or a division within an agency, such as the DHHS.

A health officer or administrator appointed by local government directs the LHDs. At least half of the states require that the health officer of an LHD have a medical degree. An interdisciplinary team carries out the activities of the department. Public health nurses and health inspectors represent the two largest groups of professional staff members. Other professional staff members include dentists, social workers, epidemiologists, nutritionists, and health educators.

Scope of Services of the LHD Subsystem

LHDs are responsible for determining the health status and needs of their constituents. This involves identifying unmet needs and taking actions to meet these needs. Most services to groups and individuals are provided at the local level. These services fall into the following four major categories:

1. *Community health services* include control of communicable disease (i.e., surveillance and immunizations), maternal-child health programs, nutrition services, and education. Health promotion education is directed toward changing behavior; individuals are encouraged to eat healthy foods, increase their amount of exercise, and decrease their use of tobacco, drugs, and alcohol. Other programs provide nutritious food and food stamps to individuals and families. Preventive screening for potential problems throughout the lifespan is a major activity of LHDs.
2. *Environmental health services* include food hygiene (e.g., inspection of food-producing and food-processing plants and restaurants); protection from hazardous substances; control of waste, air, noise, and water pollution; and occupational health. The objective of these activities is to provide a safe environment.
3. *Personal health services* provide care to individuals and families in clinics, schools, and prisons. In many areas, home health care services are provided through the LHD.
4. *Mental health services* are provided through the LHDs in many communities. These services are supported by funds offered by local and regional mental health and mental retardation facilities and programs. See Chapter 24 for more information on community-based mental health care.

In the preceding description of the three government levels that provide public health services (i.e., local, state, and federal), distinctive and overlapping roles have been discussed. The federal government has been assuming a larger role in the protection of the population through regulation and funding. It finances specific programs (e.g., Medicare and categorical programs for mothers and infants) and provides direct care to special populations (e.g., veterans). States establish health codes, regulate the insurance industry, and license health care facilities and personnel. States also provide funds for services offered through Medicaid. Direct care activities funded by state health departments may include care in mental hospitals, state medical schools, and associated hospitals. LHDs are the primary agencies that provide direct services to communities, families, and individuals.

LHDs establish local health codes, fund public hospitals (i.e., city-county), and provide services to populations and individuals at risk who often lack health insurance. Programs and services for state health departments and LHDs vary across jurisdictions. The services provided reflect the values of the residents and officials, available resources, and perceived needs of their respective populations within their state and local area. Although the goals of the public health subsystem do not change, the programs and services change to meet the changing needs of the public.

Health Care Providers

Providers of health care are individuals, groups, and organizations that deliver or support health care services. This section describes health care providers, including provider organizations, health care professionals, and nontraditional providers.

Provider Organizations

The following are examples of health care provider organizations:

- Hospital
- Clinic
- Physician practice
- Ambulatory care center
- Home health agency
- Long-term care facility
- Skilled nursing facility
- Rehabilitation center
- Hospice service
- Public health department
- School health clinic
- Birthing center
- Ambulatory surgical center
- Occupational health clinic
- Crisis clinic
- Community health center
- Any other type of organization that provides health care to the community

Health care provider organizations are undergoing tremendous changes. This is particularly true of hospitals, which are merging, consolidating, and closing. As discussed previously, the Hill-Burton Act provided funds to increase hospital beds and accomplished this goal. However, currently there are too many beds. With the increasing shift to ambulatory and primary care, hospital stays have shortened, and the patients who are admitted to the hospital are more acutely ill and require more intensive care (Box 10-2). Consequently, decreased hospital stays result in more home care admissions or more discharges to long-term care facilities for short-term recovery and rehabilitation. Figure 10-2 provides data about length of hospital stays.

⚖ ETHICAL INSIGHTS

Universal Health Care

Universal health care has been a topic of interest in the United States for some time. The United States is the only developed country that does not have some form of universal health care. Although the Health Care Reform Act of 2010 should significantly reduce the number of uninsured individuals, it is estimated that following full implementation in 2017, there will still be about 13 million people without any health care coverage and many with inadequate coverage. Thus, the question of universal health coverage remains important. Clients without health coverage have a direct impact on communities, and we should consider the following questions: How do we deal with this question? What additional reforms will be necessary to resolve this question? Is health care a right of all citizens? These are difficult questions particularly in light of a growing problem in health care disparities in the United States.

Health Care Professionals

The health care team has been growing and changing over the last few years with new types of health care professionals added and other members of the team taking on new responsibilities. The following is a brief review of the major types of professional and nonprofessional members of the health care team:

- *Registered nurse (RN):* This appears to be a simple designation that should be familiar to the reader. However, different educational routes exist to obtain a license to practice nursing, including diploma, associate degree, and baccalaureate degree. In addition, many nurses now obtain master's degrees and doctorates. These advanced degrees provide them with the opportunity to do more independent practice, teach, and conduct research. RNs practice in all types of health settings.
- *Nurse practitioner (NP):* This is a nurse who has obtained education beyond a baccalaureate degree and has studied content related to primary care. An NP specializes in such areas as adult health, pediatrics, neonatology, gerontology, and psychiatric nursing. NPs may work in clinics, the community, a private practice, the home, the hospital, and long-term care facilities (i.e., any setting in which health care is provided).
- *Clinical nurse leader (CNL):* This is a new position and requires a master's degree. The CNL is a provider and manager of care at the point of care for individuals and cohorts and does not have a clinical specialty in the master's program. The types of positions that CNLs are taking are variable, though many are in acute care settings.
- *Clinical nurse specialist (CNS):* This nurse has a master's degree in a specialty area and provides acute care and guides other nursing staff in providing care.
- *Nurse-midwife (NM):* This is a nurse who has completed an additional educational program focused on midwifery. NMs work in all types of settings in which women's health and obstetrical services are provided.
- *Licensed practical nurse or licensed vocational nurse (LPN or LVN):* LPNs and LVNs perform some specific nursing functions and play a critical role in providing direct client care. They have high school degrees and additional training (usually 1 year) and work in all types of settings, typically under the direct supervision of an RN or a physician.
- *Physician (MD or DO):* A physician has a medical degree; most specialize in a specific area of practice (e.g., internal medicine, surgery, pediatrics, and gynecology).
- *Physician assistant (PA):* The PA is a "physician extender" who provides medical services under the supervision of a licensed physician. The role was developed in the 1960s in response to a shortage of primary care physicians in certain areas. PAs generally work in primary care.
- *Registered dietitian (RD):* This health care professional assesses the client's nutritional status and needs. RDs work in hospitals, long-term care facilities, clinics, community health, and homes.

BOX 10-2   PRIMARY CARE AND PRIMARY PREVENTION

Primary health care is essential health care based on practical, scientifically sound, and socially acceptable methods and technology made universally accessible to individuals and families in the community through their full participation and at a cost that the community and country can afford to maintain at every stage of their development in the spirit of self-reliance and self-determination.... It is the first level of contact of individuals, the family, and the community with the national health system bringing health care as close as possible to where people live and work (World Health Organization [WHO], www.who.org, 2009).

Primary care is usually provided by a physician, nurse practitioner, or physician's assistant. Generally, the primary care provider's practice is in family medicine, internal medicine, or pediatrics. The primary care provider is responsible for health maintenance and for treatment of common illnesses and may refer clients to specialists as needed.

Primary prevention is a type of intervention that promotes health and prevents disease. Primary prevention includes immunizations and contraception, as well as promotion of good nutrition, exercise, and healthy lifestyle choices (e.g., avoidance of tobacco, limitation of alcohol).

How do these definitions compare? The WHO definition and the definition of primary care that is usually used in the United States are similar. Primary prevention is an intervention that is used in primary care services.

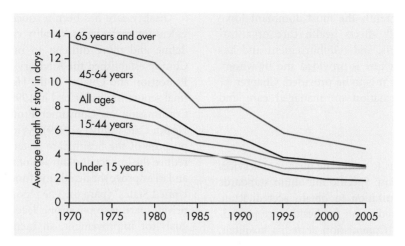

FIGURE 10-2 Discharge and length of stay for all payers. (From U.S. National Center for Health Statistics: *Vital and health statistics, series 13,* Washington, DC, The Author.)

- *Social worker (SW):* SWs assist clients and their families with problems related to reimbursement, access to care, housing, care in the home, transportation, and social problems. They have been used as discharge planners, particularly in acute care facilities or hospitals, often as case managers; however, they work in all types of settings. SWs may also have additional education to specialize in counseling.
- *Occupational therapist (OT):* OTs assist clients with impaired functions or disabilities to reach the clients' maximum level of physical and psychosocial independence. They work in all types of settings.
- *Speech-language pathologist:* Speech-language pathologists assist clients who need rehabilitative services related to speech and hearing. They work in all types of settings.
- *Physical therapist (PT):* PTs assist clients who are experiencing musculoskeletal problems. PTs focus on maximizing physical functioning and work in all types of settings (e.g. hospitals, long-term care/rehabilitation, home health).
- *Pharmacist:* Pharmacists prepare and dispense medications. Pharmacists have become much more involved in client education about medications and in monitoring and evaluating the effects of medications. They work in all types of settings, including the local drug store, where they play a critical role in ensuring safe prescriptions and providing consumer education.
- *Respiratory therapist (RT):* RTs provide care to clients with respiratory illnesses. They use oxygen therapy, intermittent positive pressure respirators, artificial mechanical ventilators, and inhalation therapy. Most RTs work in hospitals and long-term care, but they are becoming more common in home health care.
- *Chiropractor:* Chiropractors are concerned with improving the function of the clients' nervous system with various treatment modalities (e.g., spinal manipulation, diet, exercise, and massage). Visits to chiropractors have increased as the consumer has become more interested in nontraditional medical interventions. Chiropractors are mostly community based.

- *Paramedical technologists:* Paramedical technologists work in various medical technology areas (e.g., radiology, nuclear medicine, and other laboratories).
- *Unlicensed assistive personnel (UAP):* This member of the health care team has caused some controversy in last few years; however, the UAP is a critical member of the team. UAPs provide more direct client care, supervised by RNs. The amount of education and training of UAPs is highly variable.

Nontraditional Health Care Providers

Nontraditional health care providers deliver alternative or complementary therapies. During the last two decades, consumers have become more interested in this type of care and have demanded that it be available.

Although many large medical centers are now developing programs and centers that offer complementary therapies, reimbursement for these services is lagging. The NIH agreed to conduct research focused on a wide array of alternative therapies and their effects on health and disease. As a result, in 1998, the NIH established the National Center for Complementary and Alternative Medicine to meet the need. This represents a major change in the scientific and medical communities.

Alternative therapies, provided by a variety of health care providers, include massage therapy, herbal therapy, healing touch, energetic healing, acupuncture, and acupressure. Ethnic healers, such as *curanderos,* and folk healers are also found in some communities. Training and licensure requirements vary but will probably become more standard as their care becomes more accepted in established medical practice. Many nurses have incorporated alternative therapies in their practice and are seeking continuing education on this topic.

CRITICAL ISSUES IN HEALTH CARE DELIVERY

Managed Care

Managed care refers to any method of health care delivery designed to reduce unnecessary use of services, increase cost containment or cost-effectiveness, and ensure high-quality care. Managed care is currently the most dominant force in health care delivery. It affects health care organizations, health care providers, and reimbursement and has a direct influence on what care is provided and by whom, where, when, and whether it is to be provided. Chapter 11 provides additional information on managed care and reimbursement.

Quality Care

Accreditation is one means to assess the quality of services and care of the organization. Specific minimum standards must be met by an organization to obtain accreditation. Many groups provide accreditation for health care providers and MCOs. The Joint Commission accredits hospitals, home care agencies, long-term care facilities, ambulatory care centers, and MCOs. The National Committee for Quality Assurance (NCQA) accredits MCOs and uses the Health Plan Effectiveness Data and Information Set (HEDIS) to collect data about more than 90% of health care plans to measure performance and consumer satisfaction. Medicare also uses HEDIS. The American Healthcare Commission also accredits MCOs (NCQA, 2009).

Purchasers of care (insurers and MCOs) are also concerned about the accreditation status of MCOs when they negotiate MCO contracts. Insurers and MCOs are concerned about the accreditation status of health care provider organizations, as are nursing schools that use clinical sites for educational purposes. Health care providers should also be concerned about the accreditation status of their employers. The Consumer Assessment of Healthcare Providers and Systems (CAHPS) is a survey and reporting tool administered by the Agency for Healthcare Research and Quality (AHRQ). CAHPS collects data and reports on consumer experience with specific aspects of their health plans. This type of survey provides data that help purchasers of plans compare and contrast plans (AHRQ, 2009).

Currently, quality care monitoring focuses on improvement. With the improvement approach, outcomes measures have moved to the forefront. Accrediting organizations require outcomes data and use them to assess overall performance. Practitioners use outcomes to identify the treatment goals with the client. Report cards are used to compare and contrast health care organizations and health care plans. These report cards are available to the consumer, providers, and insurers. Quality data are no longer hidden and will continue to be available as new methods are developed to assess improvement based on outcomes (Beyers, 2003; McCarthy, 2002).

The IOM developed frameworks to monitor health care quality and health care disparities. AHRQ now collects data using the framework and publishes the report annually on the Internet (access the report at www.ahrq.gov). Despite all these efforts to evaluate and accredit to ensure quality care, the United States has not really been all that successful. There is still discussion about what constitutes quality care and how to best assess quality. The number of errors continues to be high, and clients continue to be dissatisfied.

Quality care has been a concern of consumers and providers for many years. Quality care is a difficult concept to define and more difficult to measure. In 1996, President Clinton established the Advisory Commission on Consumer Protection and Quality in the Health Care Industry, and its final report was published in 1999 (The President's Advisory Commission on Consumer Protection and Quality in the Health Care Industry, 1999). As identified in this report, "the purpose of the health care system must be to continuously reduce the impact and burden of illness, injury, and disability and to improve the health and functioning of the people of the United States" (para 6). The report strongly supports public-private partnerships, strong leadership with clearly defined goals for improvement, an increase in consumer strength and rights, a focus on vulnerable populations, promotion of accountability, reduction in errors and an increase in health care safety, fostering of evidence-based practice, adaptation of organizations for change, an increase in health care workforce involvement, and investment in information systems.

The report from the President's Advisory Commission on Consumer Protection and Quality in the Health Care Industry (1999) had a major impact in that it stimulated a series of more in-depth explorations of the health care delivery system, which resulted in a series of reports developed by the IOM *Quality Chasm* series. The IOM defines quality as "the degree to which health services for individuals and populations increase the likelihood of desired health outcomes and are consistent with current professional knowledge" (Chassin and Galvin, 1998, p. 1000). The following is a brief description of the content of some of these important reports that are changing health care delivery.

To Err Is Human: Building a Safer Health System

The first report, *To Err Is Human: Building a Safer Health System* (Kohn, Corrigan, and Donaldson, 1999), focused on safety within the health care delivery system. Data indicated that there have been, and continue to be, serious safety problems. Examples include the following:

- When data from one study were extrapolated, the findings indicated that at least 44,000 Americans die each year as a result of a medication error, and another study indicated the number could be as high as 98,000 (American Hospital Association, 1999; as cited in Kohn et al., 1999).
- In a given year more people die as a result of medical errors than because of motor vehicle accidents (43,664), breast cancer (41,491), or AIDS (12,113) (Centers for Disease Control and Prevention [CDC], 2009).

There are clear problems, and, to date, the focus has only been on hospital errors. This, however, does not negate the presence of medical errors in community, home care, long-term care, ambulatory care, or primary care areas and other health care settings. These are settings that require further exploration.

The report on safety clearly states that there is no one answer to solving this problem. This report defines safety as "freedom from accidental injury" and defines error as "the failure of a planned action to be completed as intended or the use of a wrong plan to achieve an aim" (Kohn et al., 1999, p. 3). Errors are directly related to outcomes, which is a significant concern in quality improvement efforts. Patient safety is a critical component of quality.

This initiative represents a collaborative effort from a health care professional organization, an accrediting organization, and consumers. Getting the patient involved is a very important strategy; however, the critical next step is listening to the patient. The four key messages from this report are, first, the magnitude of harm that results from medical errors is great; second, errors result largely from systems' failures, not individual failures; third, voluntary and mandatory reporting programs are needed now to improve patient safety; and, fourth, the IOM committee and others call on health care systems to focus on error reduction as an important part of their operations and to embrace organizational change needed to reorient error-ridden systems and process (Maddox, Wakefield, and Bull, 2001).

Crossing the Quality Chasm

The second major report, *Crossing the Quality Chasm* (IOM, 2001), focused on developing a new health care system for the twenty-first century, one that improves care. The first conclusion from the report is that the system is in need of fundamental improvement. The report emphasizes the impact of the rapid change in the health care system: new medical science, new technology, rapid availability of information, and so on. Health care providers cannot keep up, and "performance of the health care system varies considerably" (IOM, 2001, p. 3). As was noted in *To Err Is Human*, the system is fragmented, is poorly organized, and does not make the best use of its resources.

Another conclusion from the report is the impact that the increase of chronic conditions has had on the system. With people living longer, mostly because of the advances in medical science and technology, more are living with chronic conditions. Many of these patients also have comorbid conditions—complicated problems that require collaborative treatment efforts. The health care system is ineffective in dealing with these problems. To address these multiple concerns, the report supports changes that were identified by Wagner, Austin, and Von Korff (1996):

1. Need for evidence-based, planned care
2. Reorganization of practices to meet the needs of patients who require more time, a broad array of resources, and closer follow-up
3. Systematic attention to patients' need for information and behavioral change
4. Ready access to necessary clinical expertise
5. Supportive information systems

The report recommendations for an agenda for crossing the quality chasm, which are directly related to nursing, include the following:

- All health care constituents, including policy makers, purchasers, regulators, health professionals, health care trustees and management, and consumers, commit to a national statement of purpose for the health care systems as a whole and to a shared agenda.
- Clinicians and patients and the health care organizations that support care delivery adopt a new set of principles to guide the redesign of care processes.
- Health care organizations design and implement more effective organizational support processes to make change in the delivery of care possible.
- Purchasers, regulators, health professions, educational institutions, and the DHHS create an environment that fosters and rewards improvement by (1) creating an infrastructure to support evidence-based practice, (2) facilitating the use of information technology, (3) aligning payment incentives, and (4) preparing the workforce to better serve patients in a world of expanding knowledge and rapid change (IOM, 2001, p. 5).

Leadership by Example

Leadership by Example was a report requested by Congress that examined the federal government's quality enhancement processes (Corrigan, Eden, and Smith, 2003). It focused on six government programs: Medicare, Medicaid, the State Children's Health Insurance Program, the Department of Defense TRICARE and TRICARE for Life programs, the Veterans Administration program, and the Indian Health Services program. Approximately 100 million people are covered by these programs. The report concluded that improvement was needed in several areas. Among the findings:

1. There is a lack of consistent performance measurement across and within programs.
2. The usefulness of quality information has been questioned.
3. There is a lack of a conceptual framework to guide the evaluation.
4. There is a lack of computerized clinical data.
5. There is a lack of commitment to guide decisions.
6. There is a lack of a systematic approach for assessing the quality enhancement activities.

The report noted that federal leadership is needed because the federal government is in a unique position to assume a lead role in developing a national health care quality improvement initiative. The federal government is the largest purchaser of care and has a major impact on many people. It provides direct care to many: military personnel and their families, Native Americans, and veterans. Through these programs, the federal government can establish models to improve care. Further, as a regulator, federal leadership can affect many health care providers who are not in the federal system; for example, health care organizations that accept Medicare or Medicaid funds must comply with federal regulations (Hurtado, Swift, and Corrigan, 2001). Sponsorship of research, education, and training are other areas in which the federal government has a major impact. The report's conclusions recommend that the federal government lead by example and coordinate government roles in improving health care quality.

Who Will Keep the Public Healthy?

This report brought public health into the forefront by focusing on issues including globalization, rapid travel, scientific and technological advances, and demographic changes. It provided an in-depth exploration of the educational needs for improved public health. To address current and future public health problems, it was pointed out that there is a great need for appropriately prepared public health professionals. Eight content areas were identified in this report aimed at public health professionals: informatics, genomics, communication, cultural competence, community-based participatory research, global health, policy and law, and public health ethics. These areas are in addition to the long-held core components of public health: epidemiology, biostatistics, environmental health, health services administration, and social and behavioral science (Gebbie, Rosenstock, and Hernandez, 2003).

Health Professions Education

In the report *Health Professions Education* (Greiner and Knebel, 2003) the education of health professionals is viewed as a bridge to quality care. This discussion included the need to have qualified, competent staff in order to improve health care. The report indicated that health professions education must change to meet the growing demands of the health care system today. It identified five core competencies that all apply to all health care professions: (1) provide patient-centered care, (2) work in interdisciplinary teams, (3) employ evidence-based practice, (4) apply quality improvement, and (5) utilize informatics. The authors noted that all health professionals "should be educated to deliver patient-centered care as members of an interdisciplinary team, emphasizing evidence-based practice, quality improvement approaches, and informatics" (Greiner and Knebel, 2003, p. 3).

Priority Areas for National Action: Transforming Health Care Quality

In *Priority Areas for National Action* Adams and Corrigan (2003) identified nineteen priority areas that should be addressed to improve quality. Obesity was listed as an "emerging area." These priority areas were identified to promote care coordination and self-management/health literacy and enhance the continuum of care across the lifespan. The nineteen areas that they identified are:

1. Care coordination
2. Self-management/health literacy
3. Asthma—appropriate treatment for persons with mild/ moderate persistent asthma
4. Cancer screening that is evidence based—focus on colorectal and cervical cancer
5. Children with special health care needs (are at increased risk for chronic physical, developmental, behavioral condition)
6. Diabetes—focus on appropriate management of early disease
7. End-of-life with advanced organ system failure—focus on congestive heart failure and chronic obstructive pulmonary disease
8. Frailty associated with old age—preventing falls and pressure ulcers, maximizing function, and developing advance care plans
9. Hypertension—focus on appropriate treatment of early disease
10. Immunization—children and adult
11. Ischemic heart disease—prevention, reduction of recurring events, and optimization of functional capacity
12. Major depression—screening and treatment
13. Medical management—preventing medication errors and overuse of antibiotics
14. Nosocomial infections—prevention and surveillance
15. Pain control in advanced cancer
16. Pregnancy and childbirth—appropriate prenatal and intrapartum care
17. Severe and persistent mental illness—focus on treatment in the public sector
18. Stroke—early treatment in the public sector
19. Tobacco dependence treatment in adults

These areas should be used as a guide by health care providers. Further, communities can use this list to develop their community health focus and thus improve the quality of life and care of populations in the community.

Keeping Patients Safe: Transforming the Work Environment of Nurses

The IOM report *Keeping Patients Safe: Transforming the Work Environment* is an important report for nurses in all types of settings (Page, 2004). This report addressed critical quality and safety issues with a particular focus on nursing care and nurses and examined these issues from the perspective of the work environment. It presented methods for designing the work environment so that nurses may provide safer patient care and described concerns related to the nursing shortage, health care errors, patient safety risk factors, the central role of the nurse in patient safety, and work environment threats to patient safety.

Fraud and Abuse

Health care fraud has been an ongoing problem. The billions of dollars spent on health care and struggles for control between providers, consumers, and MCOs have provided an arena that lends itself to fraud and abuse. Officials estimate that up to 10% of the total health care expenditures in 2003, or about $170 billion, was lost to fraud and abuse (National Health Care Anti-Fraud Association [NHCAA], 2007). To address this problem, a number of actions have been taken. Among them are the False Claims Act Amendments (1986), which allow private citizens to collect a percentage of recovered funds if they report fraudulent Medicare claims and monies are recovered as a result (Stanton, 2001). HIPAA contains a set of provisions that address fraud, including a Fraud and Abuse Control Program, the Medicare Integrity Program, and the Health Care Fraud and Abuse Data Collection Program. Each of these programs is designed to address concerns over health care fraud. In addition, HIPAA dramatically increased funding for fraud enforcement activities (Michael, 2003).

Major health care fraud and abuse incidents have influenced the most vulnerable of the population (i.e., the mentally ill and older adults). In recent years, overbilling and unnecessary visits in home health care were reported across the United States, which resulted in widespread reforms to Medicare reimbursement for home health services (Infante and McAnaney, 2004). President Obama's Health Reform Act focuses attention on enhanced efforts to reduce fraud and abuse in public programs. It encourages screening of providers, and enhanced oversight for initial claims for durable medical equipment suppliers. The act requires Medicare and Medicaid program providers and suppliers to establish compliance programs and develops a database to share fraud and abuse information across federal and state programs. Finally, it increases penalties for submitting false claims and increases funding for anti-fraud activities (Kaiser Family Foundation, 2010).

Information Technology

The development of information technology over the last decade has been phenomenal. Clinical staff members use computers in all health care settings. Telehealth is growing, which means that clients can receive care via technology, such as computer, video, or interactive television. The Internet has opened doors for consumers and providers, and health information has exploded. Although information availability has been enhanced to millions of people, which resulted in an explosion of knowledge regarding health and health issues, the quality of this information is sometimes questionable. Providers must address the source and content of Internet information. There is a drive now to move the health care system to electronic medical records (EMRs), though it will take funding and effort to make this a reality across the health care delivery system.

Consumerism, Advocacy, and Client Rights

The growth of managed care has increased the strength of consumerism. Over the past decade, the baby boom generation has been subsidizing the health care system and paying more in premiums than it has taken out in claims. However, growing concern exists that, as this generation ages, it will demand more care than previous generations. Consumers are now critical of the health care system and demanding changes as they encounter problems. MCOs and providers are recognizing the importance of the consumer voice and the need for explanations. Client- or customer-centered health care is a term that has become commonly used in health care, and more effort has been made to provide the consumer with information.

Client rights are now an important health care issue that individual states and the federal government have been addressing through legislation. In 1999, the House and Senate passed bills that focused on client rights in the managed care environment, but more needs to be done to improve client rights. Client rights issues that are vitally important are information disclosure, physician and provider choice, direct access to specialists, reimbursement for emergency care, and reimbursement denial. As has been discussed, there is still no national patients' bill of rights.

Coordination and Access to Health Care

The social justice foundation of public health is yet to be realized because many inequalities in access to health care still exist. The United States has more than 47 million uninsured individuals (Cover the Uninsured, 2009). Characteristics of uninsured people reflect a wide range of incomes, races, and occupations, although children, minorities, the poor, and those with less education are overrepresented.

Health care providers often function in isolation from one another and provide fragmented services. Although multiple services are available for the wellness–serious illness continuum, coordination is lacking. Services range from office-clinic, home care, adult day care, acute care institutions, and specialized institutions to skilled nursing facilities. The services provided by one agency or one provider do not help the individual transit, or move, across boundary lines and receive services offered by others. Handoffs are a time of increased risk for errors reducing the quality of care. In addition, the services tend to be geographically separated, and each agency has different criteria for access. The focus of services has not kept pace with the changing needs of individuals and populations. Millions of Americans lack access to health care services, and inadequate financial resources are a deterrent to available health services.

The current health care system is pluralistic and competitive, and it provides fragmented and uncoordinated care. Private care agencies and institutions are in competition with one another for clients, health professionals, and resources. Even with recent reforms, two hospitals in the same geographic area may be competing for the same clients while other communities may not have a hospital at all, have only minimal services, or lack essential services such as obstetrics. Hospital home care programs are in direct competition with private home care agencies. Hospitals diversify services to become economically viable; therefore, they compete with HMOs for the ambulatory market. Public health services can be viewed as indirectly competing for resources. This fragmentation and duplication must be overcome to provide coordinated, collaborative, and accessible service to all citizens.

Disparity in Health Care Delivery

Disparity in health care delivery is certainly related to the number of uninsured and underinsured, but it is also more than this. The IOM (2002) report *Unequal Treatment: Confronting Racial and Ethnic Disparities in Health Care* addressed potential causes of disparities in health care. The report observed that bias and stereotyping on the part of health care providers might contribute to differences in care. Disparities in care were particularly found in cancer, cardiovascular disease, HIV/AIDS, diabetes, and mental illness. To address this problem, there needs to be more cross-cultural education for health care professionals, including nurses, to improve awareness of cultural and social factors and their impact on health care.

Health Care Reform

The United States appeared to be ready for health care reform when the Clinton administration took office (Skocpol, 1994). By 1990, support for reform had reached a 40-year high in the polls, and the election of Bill Clinton in 1992 brought the health care debate onto the national agenda. Believing reform of the health care system to be part of his election mandate, the new president assembled an ambitious plan to produce legislation for national reform of the health care system. The process was initially supported by diverse sectors of the system, but some participants began to distance themselves and ultimately opposed reform. This was true in the case of many major power constituents (i.e., businesses, physicians, and insurance companies). Ultimately, the bills failed.

With the Obama administration, a great deal of effort has been made at the federal level to achieve major health care reform. As discussed, when fully implemented, the Patient Protection and Affordable Care Act will dramatically influence virtually all components of the Health Care System. Significant reforms will be seen in private health insurance, per se, in addition to changes in Medicare and Medicaid. Additionally, it is anticipated that about 75% of the uninsured will obtain health coverage. How exactly these changes will influence health, health care economics, and health care delivery, however, remains to be seen.

⚖ ETHICAL INSIGHTS

Limited Health Care for Some

The health care system in the United States is complex, with social policies that favor pluralism, free choice, and free enterprise. The private sector personal care subsystem provides the majority of care to individuals. The private sector includes nonprofit agencies, for-profit agencies, and voluntary organizations. The public health subsystem provides limited personal care services for socially marginalized populations but, for the most part, subsidizes the private sector through Medicare and Medicaid reimbursement to provide these services.

FUTURE OF PUBLIC HEALTH AND THE HEALTH CARE SYSTEM

Changes in the health care system are coming. With implementation of the Health Care Reform Act, the health care system will be required to set limits on the care provided; identify criteria for use of technology; and determine which conditions will be treated, which interventions are effective, and who should receive the care. With implementation of health care reforms, the debate will continue. Questions include:

- What health care services should be provided?
- Who should have access to health care services?
- Who should pay for health care services?
- How should health care be delivered?
- What is the role of the government?

The importance of health promotion, disease prevention, and a population-based approach to health care is becoming increasingly recognized. The IOM reports indicate a need for improvement in all sectors of the health care delivery system. There is recognition of the need for an electronic medical record, which, to be effective, would have to incorporate care provided in the community. The growing concern over bioterrorism and roles of health care organizations, practitioners, and the government must address the community health components of the system. Local, state, and national political leaders must begin to grapple with the health of the population and the need to reduce the levels of health care expenditures in a voluntary environment.

Futurists rarely identify the public health subsystem as a component of the health care system, but this is changing. Indeed, the history of the public health subsystem's involvement with the poor and disenfranchised is a major influence in inattention to their problems. Furthermore, focus on environmental influences on the population is critical for the future health of any nation.

Predicting future trends in human values is more difficult than predicting scientific discoveries or the patterns of disease. However, Koop (1989) stated that the ultimate test of the public health subsystem is whether it effectively serves the people by their measurements, not those of the public health profession. The past two decades have brought a significant shift in thinking about the future of the health care system. Consumer rights and further efforts to control or limit health care costs while improving access will be critical issues to be resolved in the future. How these decisions and implementation of health care reform law, will affect public health is unclear.

▋ SUMMARY

The health care system is complex and changes quickly. Federal, state, and local legislation and policies affect the system, and understanding the legislation and its effect on the health care delivery system is critical for any nurse. In addition, the development of managed care has demonstrated how important it is for health care providers to understand the reimbursement system and to learn how to advocate for their clients.

The many different types of health care organizations and health care providers also affect the health care system. Interdisciplinary care will be necessary for success in the system and to ensure that the client receives cost-effective, quality care. There are many concerns about health care, including cost, access, the number of uninsured, quality, and health care fraud and abuse. Resolving these problems will not be an easy task, but it must be done. Understanding the system helps as health care providers learn to function in the rapidly changing system.

▋ LEARNING ACTIVITIES

1. Describe the organization of the state and local health departments.
2. Visit the LHD, and learn what services are provided. How do these services relate to *Healthy People 2020* objectives?
3. Identify regional and state health services.

4. Visit a voluntary agency. Determine the services it offers and how the agency collaborates with the local public health agency. Does the agency have a website? If so, visit it and find out what information is available to consumers and professionals.

5. Discuss how critical health care issues (e.g., managed care, quality care, fraud and abuse, diversity and disparity) affect health care organizations in the community.

6. Cite examples of health care consumerism in the local community. What are their histories?

7. Give a personal reaction to health care fraud and abuse. How should the principles found in the Code for Nurses apply in practice?

8. Visit the website for the AHRQ (www.ahrq.gov), and search for practice guidelines related to community health. Select one and review it. How might the guideline apply to a community health nurse?

9. Review the current national health care quality report and the national disparities report on the Internet. They can be accessed at www.ahrq.gov. What are the frameworks or matrices used to structure the report? What is the status of health care and disparities?

REFERENCES

Adams K, Corrigan J, editors: *Priority areas for national action: transforming health care quality*, Washington, DC, 2003, National Academies Press.

Agency for Healthcare Research and Quality: *Consumer assessment of health plans*, Washington, DC, AHRQ. www.ahrq.gov. Accessed January 10, 2009.

American Hospital Association: *Hospital statistics*, Chicago, 1999, The Author.

Association of State and Territorial Health Officials: Public health: an essential component of a healthy America, www.astho.org/Programs/Health-Reform/Health-Reform-Essential-Components/2007.

Beyers M: Viewpoint: report cards are here to stay, *Patient Care Manag* 19(1):10–11, 2003.

Centers for Disease Control and Prevention, National Center for Health Statistics: Deaths: final data for 2006, *Natl Vital Stat Rep* 57(14):2009. www.cdc.gov/nchs/data/nvsr/nvsr57/nvsr57_14.pdf.

Chassin M, Galvin R: The urgent need to improve health care quality, *JAMA* 280(2):1000–1005, 1998.

Corrigan J, Eden J, Smith B, editors: *Leadership by example*, Washington, DC, 2003, National Academies Press.

Cover the Uninsured. Fact sheets, www.covertheuninsured.org/Factsheets. Accessed January 10, 2009.

DeParle J: States struggle to use windfall born of shifts in welfare law, *New York Times* August 29, 1999.

Gebbie K, Rosenstock L, Hernandez L, editors: *Who will keep the public healthy?* Washington, DC, 2003, National Academies Press.

Greiner A, Knebel E, editors: *Health professions education*, Washington, DC, 2003, National Academies Press.

Hanlon G, Pickett J: *Public health administration and practice*, ed 9, St. Louis, 1990, Mosby.

Hurtado M, Swift E, Corrigan J, editors: *Envisioning the national health care quality report*, Washington, DC, 2001, National Academies Press.

Infante M, McAnaney K: Home health agencies can avoid fraud charges with compliance plans, *Hosp Home Health* 21(5):49–51, 2004.

Institute of Medicine: *The future of public health*, Washington, DC, 1988, National Academies Press.

Institute of Medicine: *Crossing the quality chasm*, Washington, DC, 2001, National Academies Press.

Institute of Medicine: *Unequal treatment: confronting racial and ethnic disparities in health*, Washington, DC, 2002, National Academies Press.

Institute of Medicine: *HHS in the 21st century: charting a new course for a healthier America*, Washington, DC, 2008, National Academies Press.

Kaiser Family Foundation: Focus on health reform 2010. www.kff.org/healthreform/upload/8061.pdf 2010b.

Knight W: *Managed care: what it is and how it works*, Gaithersburg, MD, 1998, Aspen.

Kohn L, Corrigan J, Donaldson M, editors: *To err is human: building a safer health system*, Washington, DC, 1999, National Academies Press.

Koop CE: An agenda for public health, *J Public Health Policy* 10:7, 1989.

Levy D, editor: *2002 State by state guide to managed care law*, Gaithersburg, MD, 2002, Aspen.

Maddox P, Wakefield M, Bull J: Patient safety and the need for professional and educational change, *Nurs Outlook* 49(1):8–13, 2001.

McCarthy M: U.S. government releases nursing home report cards, *Lancet* 360:1670, 2002.

Michael JE: What home healthcare nurses should know about fraud and abuse, *Home Healthc Nurse* 21(8):523–530, 2003.

National Committee for Quality Assurance: Accreditation 2009, www.ncqa.org/tabid/66/Default.aspx.

National Health Care Anti-Fraud Association: Health care fraud: a serious and costly reality for all Americans, http://www.nhcaa.org/eweb/docs/nhcaa/PDFs/aboutnhcaafinal.pdf. 2007.

O'Neil E: *Pew Health Professions Commission: Recreating health professional practice for a new century*, San Francisco, 1998, Pew Health Professions Commission.

Page A, editor: *Keeping patients safe: transforming the work environment of nurses*, Washington, DC, 2004, Institute of Medicine of the National Academies Press.

Pickett G, Hanlon JJ: *Public health administration and practice*, ed 9, St. Louis, 1990, Mosby.

Skocpol T: From social security to health security? *J Health Polit Policy Law* 19:239, 1994.

Stanton TH: Fraud and abuse enforcement in Medicare: finding middle ground, *Health Aff* 20(4):28–38, 2001.

The President's Advisory Commission on Consumer Protection and Quality in the Health Care Industry: Quality First: Better health care for all Americans, Washington, DC. 1999, U.S. Government Printing Office.

U.S. Department of Health and Human Services: *Healthy People 2010*, Washington, DC, 2000, US Government Printing Office.

U.S. Department of Health and Human Services: *Computations for the 2009 annual update of the HHS Poverty Guidelines for the 48 contiguous states and the District of Columbia*, 2009, aspe.hhs.gov/poverty/09poverty.shtml.

Wagner E, Austin B, Von Korff M: Organizing care for patients with chronic illness, *Milbank Q* 74(4):511–542, 1996.

11

Economics of Health Care

Carrie Morgan, Melanie McEwen

Additional Material for Study, Review, and Further Exploration

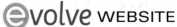 WEBSITE

http://evolve.elsevier.com/Nies
- Quiz
- Case Studies
- Glossary
- WebLinks

OBJECTIVES

Upon completion of this chapter, the reader will be able to do the following:

1. Discuss factors that influence the cost of health care.
2. Identify terms used in the financing of health care.
3. Discuss public financing of health care.
4. Discuss private financing of health care.
5. Discuss health insurance plans.
6. Describe trends in health care financing.
7. Describe the effects of economics on health care access.
8. Identify the future of health care economics.

KEY TERMS

access
actuarial classifications
adverse selection
ambulatory care
capitated reimbursement
carrier
carve-out service
coinsurance
co-payment
cost containment
cost shifting
current procedural terminology
    (CPT) codes

deductible
diagnosis-related group
    (DRG)
effectiveness
flexible spending account
gatekeepers
health care providers
health insurance plans
health maintenance organization
    (HMO)
indemnity plan
managed care groups
managed care plans

mandates
Medicaid
Medicare
medigap insurance
outcomes
out-of-pocket expenses
preferred provider organization
    (PPO)
premiums
primary care provider
prospective payment system (PPS)

OUTLINE

Factors Influencing Health Care Costs
    Historical Perspective
    Use of Health Care
    Lack of Preventive Care
    Lifestyle and Health Behaviors
    Societal Beliefs
    Technological Advances
    Aging of Society
    Pharmaceuticals
    Shift to For-Profit

Public Financing of Health Care
    Medicare
    Medicaid
    Governmental Grants
Philanthropic Financing of Health Care
Health Insurance Plans
    Historical Perspective
    Types of Health Care Plans
    Reimbursement Mechanisms of Insurance Plans
    Covered Services

Economics represents the science of allocation of resources. Resources are commonly known as goods or services, for example, health care services. Economics affects all aspects of health care. Nurses have traditionally avoided the arena of health care economics, preferring to focus on the actual, direct care of the client. So strong is the feeling of social justice that some nurses express a reluctance to be informed of the individual client's health care financing source for fear that this knowledge will influence their care. Community health nurses who deal with the medically underserved have had more experience in this area. However, even these nurses may have only rudimentary knowledge.

Health care costs continue to rise and consume a greater percentage of our nation's resources. Nursing can no longer ignore the intricacies of health care financing. The health of individuals, families, and aggregates is influenced by economics. Economically disadvantaged individuals who have difficulty obtaining the basics, such as food and shelter, are less likely to have access to health care. Passage of the Patient Protection and Affordable Care Act (PL 111-148), however, should dramatically influence health care access. Indeed, when fully implemented, almost all citizens will have health insurance, either provided by their employers, through private purchase, or, for those from low income groups, through state and federal government sources (ie Medicare, Medicaid, CHIPs).

This chapter focuses on the economics of health care. It specifically discusses factors that influence health care costs, terminology of health care financing, and trends in health care economics. This chapter also addresses the future of health care financing. Box 11-1 presents terms and definitions that are important to the discussion of these topics.

FACTORS INFLUENCING HEALTH CARE COSTS

Historical Perspective

Until the 1930s, the predominant method of individual health care financing in the United States was self-payment. Health care providers charged a fee for the services they rendered, and the patient paid these out-of-pocket expenses. The price of the service was under the control of the provider and generally represented the cost of providing that service. A certain amount of "charity" services was expected. The assumption was that those who could pay would pay and those who could not pay should receive care and pay what they could.

The concept of public financing of health care for a specific aggreagate was restricted and varied from geographic area to area until the term *public health* came into common use.

The following types of hospitals existed:

1. Public hospitals, which received public funds and served the health care needs of the entire population regardless of ability to pay
2. Private hospitals, which cared mainly for those whose ability to pay was greater than that of the general population
3. For-profit hospitals, which were limited in number, received funds from investors, and cared for those who could definitely pay

This system worked well as long as the number of those who could pay outnumbered those who could not. During the Great Depression, with more than 25% of the population out of work, the number of those capable of paying for health care was greatly reduced. Because public financing of health care was limited, hospitals, physicians, and other providers of health care went bankrupt.

In 1929, schoolteachers in Dallas, Texas negotiated a prepaid health provision contract with Baylor Hospital. The teachers paid a sum of money each month, which guaranteed them access to health care through Baylor Hospital. The concept of insurance for health care proved extremely successful for Baylor Hospital. By 1939, this insurance plan had grown to include other groups and hospitals and became Blue Cross-Blue Shield (Koch, 2008).

Health insurance, or the idea of paying a small fee for guaranteed health care, appealed to the public. Societal concerns were mainly focused on sick care and acquisitions of curative therapies whenever needed. A public view that health insurance would provide freedom from fear that illness would impoverish them developed and prevails today. Health care providers envisioned guaranteed payment for their services (Higgins, 1997). During World War II, faced with a limited workforce and governmental restrictions on wages, employers began to see health insurance as a means of supplying workers' benefits without granting a wage increase.

To extend this same "insurance" to the general population, the Social Security Act of 1935 was amended in 1965 to create Medicare and Medicaid. Medicare provided indemnity

BOX 11-1   TERMINOLOGY USED IN HEALTH CARE FINANCING

The financing of health care has given rise to new terminology. Nurses, as providers of care and consumers of services, need to be knowledgeable about these terms to increase their understanding of health care financing.

Terms Pertaining to Consumers

Access: Ability to obtain health care services in a timely manner, at a reasonable cost, by a qualified practitioner, and at an accessible location.

Carve-out service: A service (i.e., mental health care) provided within a standard benefit package, but delivered exclusively by a designated provider or group.

Charges: The posted prices of provider services.

Coinsurance: Cost sharing required by a health plan whereby the individual is responsible for a set percentage of the charge for each service.

Co-payment: Cost sharing required by the health plan whereby the individual must pay a fixed dollar amount for each service.

Deductible: Cost sharing whereby the individual pays a specified amount before the health plan pays for covered services.

Fee schedule: List of predetermined payment rates for medical services.

Flexible spending account (FSA): A mechanism by which an employee may pay for uncovered health care expenses through payroll deductions.

Gatekeeper: Person in an MCO who decides whether a patient will be referred for specialty care. Doctors, nurses, nurse practitioners, and physician assistants function as gatekeepers.

Health care provider: An individual or institution that provides medical services (e.g., physicians, hospitals, or laboratories).

Health maintenance organization (HMO): A managed care plan that acts as an insurer and sometimes a provider for a fixed prepaid premium. HMOs usually employ physicians.

Health plan: A health insurance plan that pays a predetermined amount for covered services.

Indemnity plan: A health plan that pays covered services on a fee-for-service basis.

Managed care plan: A health plan that uses financial incentives to encourage enrollees to use selected providers who have contracted with the plan.

Medicaid: Joint federal- and state-funded programs that provide health care services for low- income people.

Medicare: A health insurance program for people over 65 years of age, those who are disabled, and those with end-stage renal disease.

Medicare Advantage: Medicare recipients may choose to enroll in a coordinated care plan, private fee-for-service, or medical savings account plan created by the Balanced Budget Act of 1997.

Medigap insurance: Privately purchased individual or group health insurance plan designed to supplement Medicare coverage.

Out-of-pocket expenses: Payment made by the individual for medical services.

Point of service (POS): A managed care plan that combines prepaid and fee-for-service plans. Enrollees may choose to use the services of an uncontracted provider by paying an increased copayment.

Portability: An individual changing jobs is guaranteed coverage with the new employer without a waiting period or having to meet additional deductible requirements.

Preferred provider organization (PPO): A health plan that contracts with providers to furnish services to the enrollees of the plan. Usually no insurance copayment is required.

Premium: Amount paid periodically to purchase health insurance benefits.

Primary care provider: A generalist physician, typically a family physician, internist, gynecologist, or pediatrician, who provides comprehensive medical services.

Terms Pertaining to Providers

Ambulatory care: Medical services provided on an outpatient basis in a hospital or clinic setting.

Capitation: Payment mechanism that pays health care providers a fixed amount per enrollee to cover a defined set of services over a specified time period regardless of actual services provided.

Care management: Process used to improve quality of care by analyzing variations in and outcomes for current practice in the care of specific health conditions.

Cost containment: Reduction of inefficiencies in the consumption, allocation, or production of health care services.

Customary charge: Physician payment based on a median charge for a given service within a 12-month period.

Diagnosis-related group (DRG): A system of payment classification for inpatient hospital services based on the principal diagnosis, procedure, age and gender of the patient, and complications.

Effectiveness: Net health benefit provided by a medical service or technology for a typical patient in community practice.

Fully capitated: A stipulated dollar amount established to cover the cost of all health care services delivered for a person.

Maximum allowable costs: Specified cost level established by the health plan.

Outcome: The consequences of a medical intervention in a patient.

Physician's current procedural terminology (CPT) codes: A list of codes for medical services and procedures performed by physicians and other health care providers that has become the health care industry's standard for reporting physician procedures and services.

Practice guidelines: An explicit statement of what is known and believed about the benefits, risks, and costs of particular courses of medical action intended to assist decisions made by practitioners, patients, and others about appropriate health care for specific and clinical conditions.

Utilization review: A formal prospective, concurrent, or retrospective assessment of the medical necessity, efficiency, and appropriateness of health care services.

Terms Pertaining to Third-Party Payers

Actuarial classification: Classification of enrollees that is determined by use of the mathematics of insurance, including probabilities to ensure adequacy of the premium to provide future payment.

Administrative costs: Costs that the insurer incurs for utilization review, marketing, medical underwriting, agents' commissions, premium collection, claims processing, insurer profit, quality assurance activities, medical libraries, and risk management.

Adverse selection: Larger proportion of people with poorer health status enroll in specific plans or options. Plans that enroll a subpopulation with lower-than-average costs are favorably selected.

Capital cost: Depreciation, interest, leases and rentals, taxes, and insurance on tangible assets.

Carrier: An organization that contracts with the CMMS to administer claims processing and make Medicare payments to health care providers.

Cost contract: Arrangement between a managed health care plan and the CMMS for reimbursement of the costs of services provided.

Cost shifting: The cost of uncompensated care is passed on to the insured, resulting in higher costs for those with insurance coverage.

Mandate: A state or federal statute or regulation that requires coverage for certain health services.

Risk assessment: Statistical method used to estimate claims costs of enrollees.

insurance to those over the age of 65 years, and Medicaid, a state-administered health plan, provided a source for financing health care for the poor and the disabled.

As a result of these health care resources, the majority of the population was protected by indemnity health care insurance from various sources. The indemnity plans lacked an incentive for limitation of use and few or no provisions for health promotion. The emphasis was placed on illness care, providers received a fee only when a service was rendered, and all costs of services were reimbursed. Insulated from rising health care costs, health care consumers demanded complex and technologically advanced services whenever illness struck. These demands for costly services represented the major driving force in rising health care costs.

By the 1980s, the first efforts to curtail health care costs were made by the federal government. With institution of the prospective payment system (PPS), hospital reimbursement for Medicare patients was based on a classification system that identified costs according to diagnosis and client characteristics. The PPS prompted an evolution towards managed care, dramatically altering health care financing through the end of the twentieth century, and into the first decade of the 21st century. Despite containment efforts, however, costs of health care have continued to rise.

The spiraling health care costs starting from the mid 1960s and persisting into the 21st century were fueled by the presence of technologic advances, society's sense of entitlement to these therapies, a guaranteed payer, and the prevailing medical orientation toward curative measures. Prior to implementation of Medicare and Medicaid, national health expenditures represented less than 5% of the GDP. Forty years later, however, costs have risen exponentially, and now comprise about 17% of the GDP (CMS, 2010a).

Use of Health Care

According to economic principles, use is influenced by the existence of a desirable product, the demand for the product, and the availability of financial funding for a product. Health care is the product, and the demand for this product increases when funding is available. In an attempt to reduce unnecessary utilization, insurance plans began to limit coverage for certain services and people; thus the move toward 'managed care'. Restrictions on use of health care, such as the establishment of a "gatekeeper," requirement of preauthorization for some services, limited coverage for preexisting illnesses, and exclusion of those participants whose use was deemed exorbitant, have been instituted. These restrictions have had only limited success in curbing health care costs. In 2004, spending for health care in the U.S. was more than double that of other developed countries (i.e. those in the Organization for Economic Cooperation and Development [OCED]). Indeed, average per capita spending in that year was $2560 (8.9% of GDP) for OCED countries, compared with $6102 (15.3% of GDP) in the U.S. (Congressional Research Service, 2007).

Expenses for health care vary according to types of care and sources of funding (Table 11-1). In 1960, out-of-pocket expenditure for physicians' fees was 61.6% compared with 7.2% governmental expenditure for these fees. By 2007, the out-of-pocket expenditure for physicians' fees was only 10.4%, and governmental expenditure proportion had risen to 33.7%. Similar patterns are evident for other health costs as a percentage of government financing has increased across all sectors. For example, by 2007, 55% of hospital costs and more than 62% of nursing home costs were paid by governmental sources (CMS, 2010a).

Lack of Preventive Care

Until recently, little to no incentive has existed to prevent illness or promote health. Curative measures have traditionally been the focus of health care. Soaring health care costs and an improved knowledge of health have heightened the public's awareness of their obligation to assume responsibility for their health by amending many unhealthy behaviors. As a result, more people are demanding preventive health care from the provider and their health care contractors. Public financing of health care has increased funding for such preventive care as screening tests, periodic examinations, and immunizations. Use of these preventive health services has increased, but disparities persist relating to ethnic background and economic status (National Center for Health Statistics [NCHS], 2009). There continues to be a gap between the amount of funding available for preventive treatment modalities and funding for curative treatments.

Lifestyle and Health Behaviors

A healthy lifestyle does not ensure good health but has been shown to contribute to longevity and productivity (Harvard Men's Health Watch, 2009). The five leading causes of death and illness can be positively affected by changes in lifestyle. Recent studies have found that a low-fat diet, exercise, maintaining a optimal weight, smoking cessation, and stress reduction can modify or even prevent most chronic illnesses. Smoking cessation reduces the incidence of lung cancer. Seat belt use reduces the severity of injuries incurred during moving vehicle accidents. Effective treatment of illness must be coupled with a change in lifestyle. In the near future, access to expensive and unique medical treatment will probably be influenced less by the patient's ability to pay and more by the person's commitment to compulsory lifestyle changes. For example, legislation has levied "sin taxes" on products whose use has been associated with chronic illnesses. The Commonwealth of Kentucky has the highest rate of adult smoking in the country. To offset the cost of Medicaid care, the legislature has levied a $0.30 per package cigarette tax. This income will be utilized to fund care for, prevention of, and research on chronic illness (Commonwealth of Kentucky Department of Revenue, 2005).

Old movies dramatize the change in lifestyle that has taken place in the past 30 years. The current "smoke-free" environment appears shocking when contrasted to the nonchalant attitude toward smoking that was pervasive 40 years ago. The advent of the Health Belief Model and Pender's Health Prevention Model has given rise to numerous studies into methods of achieving lifestyle changes. The total effects of

TABLE 11-1   PERSONAL HEALTH CARE EXPENDITURES, ACCORDING TO TYPE OF EXPENDITURE AND SOURCE OF FUNDS: UNITED STATES, SELECTED YEARS 1990-2007

TYPE OF PERSONAL HEALTH CARE EXPENDITURES AND SOURCE OF FUNDS	1990	2000	2001	2002	2003	2004	2005	2006	2007
Amount per capita	$2,398	$4,049	$4,352	$4,695	$4,979	$5,281	$5,588	$5,902	$6,219
Amount in Billions									
All personal health care expenditures	$609.4	$1,135.3	$1,231.4	$1,340.2	$1,447.5	$1,550.2	$1,655.6	$1,765.5	$1,878.3
Percent Distribution									
All sources of funds	100.0	100.0	100.0	100.0	100.0	100.0	100.0	100.0	100.0
Out-of-pocket payments	22.5	17.0	16.3	15.9	15.5	15.2	14.9	14.4	14.3
Private health insurance	33.4	35.1	35.5	35.8	36.0	36.2	36.2	36.1	36.2
Other private funds	5.0	4.8	4.4	4.2	4.4	4.2	4.2	4.2	4.2
Government	39.0	43.1	43.8	44.2	44.0	44.5	44.7	45.2	45.3
Federal	28.6	32.8	33.5	33.6	33.6	34.0	34.0	35.2	35.3
State and local	10.5	10.4	10.4	10.6	10.4	10.5	10.7	10.1	10.0
Amount in Billions									
Hospital care expenditures	$253.9	$413.2	$444.3	$486.5	$527.4	$566.8	$601.5	$649.3	$686.3
Percent Distribution									
All sources of funds	100.0	100.0	100.0	100.0	100.0	100.0	100.0	100.0	100.0
Out-of-pocket payments	4.4	3.1	2.9	3.0	3.3	3.3	3.3	3.3	3.3
Private health insurance	38.3	33.3	33.6	33.9	35.6	35.8	35.5	36.4	36.9
Other private funds	4.1	4.9	4.3	4.2	4.7	4.5	4.5	4.6	4.6
Government	53.2	58.8	59.1	58.9	56.4	56.5	56.8	55.7	55.2
Medicaid	15.9	16.9	17.1	17.3	17.1	17.1	17.3	17.0	17.2
Medicare	31.2	30.9	30.7	29.1	29.1	29.2	29.6	28.9	28.2
Amount in Billions									
Physician services expenditures	$157.5	$290.3	$315.1	$339.5	$366.7	$393.6	$422.2	$449.7	$478.8
Percent Distribution									
All sources of funds	100.0	100.0	100.0	100.0	100.0	100.0	100.0	100.0	100.0
Out-of-pocket payments	19.3	11.1	10.5	10.1	10.2	10.2	10.5	10.3	10.4
Private health insurance	43.0	48.5	48.7	49.1	48.4	48.5	49.0	49.3	49.4
Other private funds	7.2	7.3	7.1	6.9	7.1	6.7	6.5	6.5	6.5
Government	30.6	33.1	33.8	33.8	34.2	34.6	34.2	33.9	33.7
Medicaid	4.5	6.6	6.9	7.2	6.9	7.1	7.0	6.9	6.9
Medicare	19.0	20.6	20.3	19.9	20.1	20.0	20.5	20.4	20.1
Amount in Billions									
Nursing home expenditures	$52.7	$93.8	$99.1	$103.2	$110.5	$115.2	$120.6	$125.4	$131.3
Percent Distribution									
All sources of funds	100.0	100.0	100.0	100.0	100.0	100.0	100.0	100.0	100.0
Out-of-pocket payments	37.5	27.9	26.9	25.1	27.6	26.9	26.1	26.1	26.9
Private health insurance	5.8	7.8	7.7	7.5	7.8	7.5	7.3	7.4	7.5
Other private funds	7.5	4.4	3.8	3.4	3.8	3.7	3.6	3.6	3.5
Government	49.2	59.8	61.7	64.0	60.7	61.9	62.9	62.9	62.1
Medicaid	47.5	47.3	49.3	44.6	45.0	44.7	44.6	43.5	41.7
Medicare	9.3	12.1	12.5	13.1	13.3	14.7	15.8	16.8	17.7
Amount in Billions									
Prescription drug expenditures	$40.3	$121.5	$140.8	$162.4	$174.2	$188.8	$199.7	$216.8	$227.5
Out-of-pocket payments	$59.1	$31.5	$30.2	$29.9	$44.1	$46.2	$48.7	$46.7	$47.6
Private health insurance	$24.4	$46.5	$47.5	$47.8	$83.4	$90.0	$95.8	$96.2	$99.1
Government	$16.6	$21.9	$22.4	$22.3	$46.6	$52.6	$55.2	$73.9	$80.8
Local	$12.6	$17.1	$17.5	$17.5	$18.9	$21.2	$22.5	$15.1	$14.3
Federal	$0.5	$1.9	$1.7	$1.6	$27.8	$31.4	$32.7	$58.7	$80.8

Data are compiled from various sources by the Centers for Medicare and Medicaid Services. From Centers for Medicare and Medicaid Services, Office of the Actuary: *National health accounts, national health expenditures,* Baltimore, 2009, The Author: www.cms.hhs.gov/statistics/nhe.

these changes are just now being seen. Meanwhile, the health care system must continue to contend with the results of years of unhealthy lifestyles.

Health care funding has changed to provide funding for preventive services. Some insurance plans provide monetary incentives, such as reduction in insurance premiums, for those who participate in behavioral changes toward a healthier lifestyle. Medicare will pay for many screening procedures performed for specific persons at specified times (CMS, 2010b). Funding for behavioral changes, however, is often limited, inadequate, or unavailable. Weight loss programs, support groups for smoking cessation, or participation in relaxation programs are not considered reimbursable treatment regimens, but more expensive pharmaceutical interventions are reimbursable.

Societal Beliefs

With the advent of such wonders as penicillin, society began to believe that the eradication of disease was just a few years away. More and more resources were dedicated to this elusive search. Armed with the belief that disease would soon be eliminated, societal interest in preventive care was limited. The general belief was that more money available for health care meant better health care and the greater likelihood that illness would be cured. Society views insurance as an economic shield protecting against all disease and illness. The belief in cure rather than prevention, combined with this financial safety net, encouraged society to become a passive participant in health care. The feeling "I don't have to worry, I have insurance" became the pervasive societal thought (Sloan, 2004).

Health care professionals also were slow to embrace preventive care. Most efforts were directed toward curing illness. With what seemed to be an unending source of financing for curative care, illness prevention seemed counterproductive.

As health care costs accelerated at an alarming rate and technological advances did not keep up with the increase in illnesses, the health of society had to become a collaborative effort between society itself and the health care industry. Although the United States spends more money on health care than any other industrialized country, it ranks significantly behind many other countries in health status indicators (NCHS, 2009; OECD, 2008). People still expect the health care industry to cure them when they are ill, but there is an increase in preventive care interest. Interest in health education, health promotion, and behavioral changes has increased. Research into barriers and facilitators to lifestyle changes has increased but is not funded at the same level as curative measures (OECD, 2008).

Technological Advances

Modern society has come to expect miraculous technological advances. In response to this demand, and supplied with funding from various sources, technological advances have become too numerous to mention. The United States leads the world in laboratory and clinical research. People come from all over the world for education and to train in leading American centers for excellence (Weintraub and Shine, 2004). The United States exceeds other industrialized countries in the availability and use of these technological advances. For example, in 2006, France reported 5.3 magnetic resonance imaging (MRI) scanners for every 1 million population compared with the 26.5 MRI scanners available in the United States. For the same year, the United Kingdom performed angioplasties at a rate of 54.2 per 100,000 population and the United States performed 250.2 per 100,000 population (OECD, 2008). Technological advances can save the lives of people who would otherwise die. These advances, although remarkable, are expensive and result in 20% of the population consuming 80% of the health care resources. As the health care dollar shrinks, these advances raise ethical questions involving health care access and rationing. Restriction on technology can result in significantly reduced cost of health care, but the delays, inconvenience, and limitations to care with rationing will be strongly resisted by most Americans.

Aging of Society

Health care expenditures increase with age. According to the most recent population projections, individuals older than 65 years constituted about 13% of the total population in 2010. This population is expected to increase to almost 21.5% by the year 2050 (U.S. Census Bureau, 2008). Further, the percentage of those older than 85 years will increase from the present level of 1.9% of the total population to about 4.4% of the total population. This is concerning because health care costs increase dramatically as individuals age. For example, the average health care expenditures for Americans aged 65 to 75 years was $10,800 in 2004, compared with $25,700 for those 85 years and older (NCHS, 2009). The number of persons aged 20 to 64 years will decrease from 58.1% to 53.4% during the next 40 years (Figure 11-1). This means that the number of those consuming the greatest amount of health care resources will increase more rapidly than those who provide the monetary support for these resources. It has been estimated that nearly one third of expenditures for health care are incurred during middle age; half will be incurred during the senior years; and for those older than 85 years, one third will be incurred during the last year of life (Alemayehu and Warner, 2004).

Pharmaceuticals

A relatively new phenomenon that has influenced health care economics is the utilization of drugs, both over-the-counter and prescription drugs. New drugs are improving health outcomes and quality of life. These new drugs and new uses for older drugs are curing some illnesses, preventing or delaying other chronic diseases, and hastening recovery from other illnesses. As a result, during the last several decades, costs of prescription drugs have risen dramatically and have become a very significant part of health expenditures. Seniors in particular were hugely affected, as many have chronic illnesses that require daily medications.

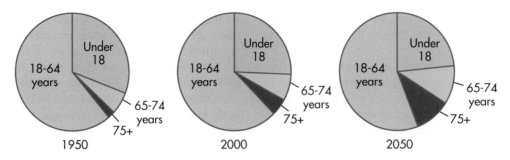

FIGURE 11-1 Percentage of population in four age-groups: United States, 1950, 2000, and 2050. Sources: U.S. Census Bureau, 1980 Census of Population, General Population Characteristics, United States Summary (PC80-1-B1) [data for 1950]; Table 1 NA-EST2002-ASRO-03-National Population Estimates-Characteristics, eire.census.gov/popest/data/national/tables/asro/NA-EST2002-ASRO-03.php accessed on March 18, 2004; Special tabulation of U.S. Interim Projections by Age, Sex, Race, and Hispanic Origin, www.census.gov/ipc/www/usinterimproj/accessed on March 18, 2004.

To help alleviate the costs of prescriptions for seniors, in 2003, Medicare added a pharmaceutical benefit for enrollees. With implementation of the the Medicare Prescription Drug and Modernization Act, all Medicare recipients were eligible to purchase insurance coverage to offset the costs of prescription drugs. As with other health care services, once a funding source has been established, utilization and costs increase. For 2006, the United States expenditure for pharmaceuticals was 1.5 times that of other industrialized countries (OCD, 2008). As shown in Figure 11-2, many Americans routinely use prescription medications and related costs have risen from less than 5% of total health care expenditures in 1980 to more than 10% of expenditures in 2007 (NCHS, 2009).

Shift to For-Profit

The final contributor to the increase in health care costs is a national shift from nonprofit health care to for-profit health care. This has given rise to the new phrase "health care industry." More and more large-profit organizations are taking over smaller community organizations. As the emphasis is on profit, mechanisms of achieving higher reimbursement have been developed.

The prospective reimbursement rates are based on diagnoses and patient characteristics. These are represented by codes, following the *International Classification of Diseases*, 10th edition, or ICD-10 (CDC, 2010). Physician services are coded according to current procedural terminology (CPT) codes. Coding of the patient's illness can result in an increase in reimbursement. Specialists in coding, as well as computer programs, are employed by both third-party payers and service providers. Third-party payers' code specialists scrutinize the claims for the appropriated data to support the code. Service provider code specialists are paid to ensure that the code is as accurate as possible to obtain the higher reimbursement. The appropriateness of services is based on the diagnosis code. For example, spirometry is appropriate (reimbursable) when the patient's diagnosis code indicates a variety of pulmonary and nonpulmonary conditions. Specialists in coding can quickly identify these codes, thus increasing payment for services. Physician visits, or CPT codes, are reimbursed on the basis of the documentation of the degree of "medical decision making" and time spent with the patient. Computerized medical record programs almost ensure that the visit can be reimbursed at the highest rate possible. This has changed health care practices to the utilization of services that are low in costs and higher in reimbursement. High-cost services are limited or not offered. Figure 11-3 illustrates how the nation's health care dollar was spent in 2007.

Fraudulent claims are another source of health care cost increase. Medicare and Medicaid fraud is estimated to cost these programs billions of dollars each year and curtailing this abuse is one of the major sources of cost savings attributed to the new health reform act. Consumers and providers are asked to help identify fraud by closely scrutinizing their health care bills for charges for services not delivered (Box 11-2).

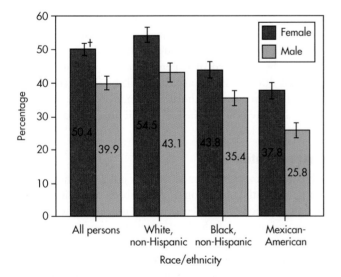

FIGURE 11-2 Percentage of persons reporting use of at least one prescription drug during the preceding month, by sex and race/ethnicity—United States, 1999-2002. (From National Center for Health Statistics: *Health, United States, 2005. Table 91.* Hyattsville, Md, 2005. National Center for Health Statistics.)

PUBLIC FINANCING OF HEALTH CARE

As the popularity and benefits of employer-provided insurance plans were recognized, it became evident that the health care of some segments of society was being neglected. The

The Nation's Health Dollar, Calendar Year 2007: Where it Went

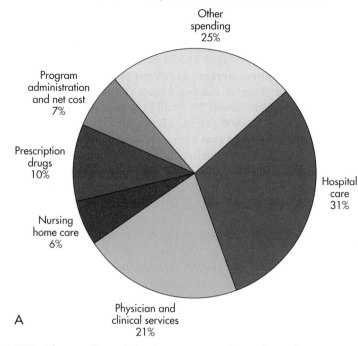

A

NOTE: Other spending includes dentist services, other professional services, home health, durable medical products, over-the-counter medicines and sundries, public health, other personal health care, research and structures and equipment.

The Nation's Health Dollar, Calendar Year 2007: Where it Came From

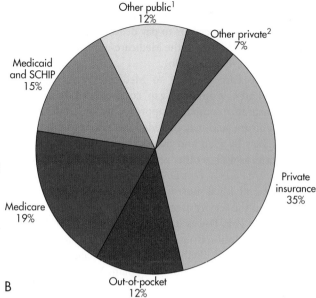

B

[1]Other public includes programs such as workers' compensation, public health activity, Department of Defense, Department of Veterans Affairs, Indian Health Service, State and local hospital subsidies and school health.

[2]Other private includes industrial in-plant, privately funded construction, and non-patient revenues, including philanthropy.

NOTE: Numbers shown may not add to 100.0 because of rounding.

FIGURE 11-3 The nation's health care dollar, calendar year 2007. (From Centers for Medicare and Medicaid Services, Office of the Actuary, National Health Statistics Group, 2007.)

BOX 11-2 MEDICARE FRAUD

What is fraud?
- Billing Medicare for services not received
- Billing Medicare for services other than those received
- Use of another's Medicare card to obtain services

Be suspicious if providers tell you:
- Medicare wants you to have this service.
- They know how to get Medicare to pay for service.
- The more services provided, the cheaper they are.

Be suspicious if providers:
- Change co-payment of Medicare-approved services
- Advertise "free" consultations to those with Medicare
- Claim they represent Medicare
- Use pressure to persuade you of need for high-priced services
- Use telemarketing as a marketing tool

Whenever you receive a Medicare payment notice, review it for errors. Make sure Medicare was not billed for services not received.

Modified from Centers for Medicare and Medicaid Services: *Medicare fraud: detection and prevention tips,* Baltimore, no date, The Author: www.medicare.gov/FraudAbuse/Tips.asp.

1960s, with a pervasive thrust for social justice in the public and political arenas, presented the ideal opportunity for governmental participation in health care financing. In 1965, the federal government enacted the first movement toward universal health care coverage. Titles XVIII and XIX of the Social Security Act created Medicare and Medicaid, respectively.

Medicare

Medicare is a federal entitlement program, which is intended to help cover the costs of health care for people 65 years of age and older and people who are disabled or have end-stage renal disease. Medicare is divided into Part A, Part B, Part C, and Part D. Medicare Part A is basically hospital insurance. Services covered by Medicare Part A include inpatient care in hospitals and skilled nursing facilities (not unskilled or long-term care). It also covers hospice care and some home health care. Most U.S. residents are eligible for premium-free Medicare Part A benefits when they reach age 65, based on their own or their spouse's employment. Although Medicare Part A is an entitlement program, the enrollee must pay a deductible for health services. The deductible paid by the beneficiary when admitted as a hospital inpatient was $1,100 in 2010. The Part A deductible is the beneficiary's only cost for up to 60 days of Medicare-covered inpatient hospital care in a benefit period. Beneficiaries had to pay an additional $275 per day for days 61 through 90 in 2010, and $550 per day for hospital stays beyond the ninetieth day in a benefit period (CMS, 2010b).

Those individuals who are eligible for Medicare Part A may purchase Medicare Part B for a monthly fee. Medicare Part B is medical insurance and helps pay for physician services, hospital outpatient care, durable medical equipment, and other services, including some home health care. The monthly premium paid by beneficiaries enrolled in Medicare Part B averaged $96.40 in 2010. In addition to the monthly premium, Part B requires subscribers to pay deductibles ($155 in 2010) and coinsurance (20% of the Medicare-approved amount for most services) (CMS, 2010b).

Medicare Part C refers to Medicare Advantage Plans. Medicare Part C is optional "gap" coverage and is provided by private insurance companies approved by, and under contract with, Medicare, and may include HMOs and PPOs. Covered services vary by plan and may include vision, hearing, and dental care, as well as other services and supplies not covered by Medicare Parts A, B or D. Costs vary by plan, and to be eligible, the individual must have Medicare Parts A and B and must live in the service area of the plan (CMS, 2010b).

Medicare Part D was initiated in 2006 to help defray the costs of prescription drugs. Like Parts B and C, Medicare Part D is optional, and eligible Medicare recipients must enroll in an approved prescription drug plan. Most participants in Medicare Part D pay a monthly premium (average $32), a yearly deductible and co-payments, with out-of-pocket costs based on the plan selected and drugs used. In addition to the costs above, the enrollee is responsible for 100% of the costs between $2830 and 4550; this is termed the "coverage gap" or "donut hole." Once out of pocket costs for drugs reaches $4550, Medicare will pay 95% of the costs of prescription drugs for covered individuals (CMS, 2010b).

Medicaid

Medicaid was initiated in 1965 by Title XIX of the Social Security Act. Medicaid is a public welfare assistance program that finances health care coverage for the indigent and children. Eligibility for this program, a joint state and federal venture, is dependent on the size and income of the family, and priority participation is given to children, pregnant women, and the disabled.

The federal government sets baseline eligibility requirements for Medicaid. State governments that wish to provide care to more citizens through this program can lower the eligibility requirements. For example, the federal government may set 100% of poverty as an eligibility requirement, but Kentucky may set the requirement as 110% of poverty. This means that a family living in Kentucky can have an income slightly above the federal standard and still qualify for Medicaid.

The federal government mandates covered services, but state governments may provide more services. Mandated services covered by Medicaid for eligible recipients include inpatient and outpatient hospital cae, pregnancy-related care, vaccines for children, family planning services, rural health clinic services, home health care, laboratory and x-ray services and Early and Periodic Screening, Diagnosis, and Treatment (EPSDT) services for children under age 21. Optional services that states may elect to provide include: optometrist services and glasses, intermediate care facilities for the mentally disabled, rehabilitation, physical therapy, and hospice (Kaiser Family Foundation, 2009a).

Four out of ten financially disadvantaged persons under the age of 65 years are covered by Medicaid (see Table 11-1).

In 2006, the average expenditure per eligible recipient of Medicaid was about $4700, but there was very wide variation based on the population and services provided. For example, Medicaid payments for children (52% of all Medicaid beneficiaries) averaged $1,750 per child, and adults (24% of beneficiaries) averaged $2,500 per person. Medicaid payments for those in nursing homes (long-term care facilities), however, - about 3% of all beneficiaries - averaged an astounding $26,600 per individual (CMS, 2009a). Indeed, it should be noted that almost 43% of all Medicaid funds go to pay for long-term health care. Medicaid payments per enrollee also vary dramatically from state to state. In 2005, the average payment was $4,662 per enrollee; California had the lowest expenditure ($2,700) and New York had the highest ($7,730) (Kaiser Family Foundation, 2009a).

Aside from Medicaid, many children under the age of 18 years are eligible for the Children's Health Insurance Program (CHIP). Established in 1997 and reauthorized in 2009, CHIP is a program that provides insurance for children of low socio-economic families who do not qualify for Medicaid. Like Medicaid, the program is administered by the states with the cost being shared with the national government. President Obama's health care reform plan requires expansion of Medicaid and CHIP to cover many of those who were previously uninsured.

Governmental Grants

Unlike individual health care services, governmental grants are directed toward funding large populations and multitudes of aggregates. Historically, the bulk of health promotion and disease preventive measures have been limited to this arena of public health care. The main funding for these foundation public health services is provided from the government on different levels. On the national level the U.S. Department of Health and Human Services (DHHS) administers this funding.

A variety of funding grants are available through the DHHS (USDHHS, 2007). These health grants are administered through the public health department at each governmental level or community. A large part of the federal government funding provided to the states is through "block grants." These are "blocks" of funds provided to the states to impact the health of the public as a whole. There are specific restrictions as to how these monies can be spent including limitations in the populace that receive the services and what types of programs are to be funded. The states use these monies to provide for the care of the public within these restrictions. Depending on the health needs of the state, these monies may be spent to provide direct aggregate care but most often are used for health promotion activities that are directed at a larger percentage of the population. Each level of government may make funds available for a specific health need of the members of the community.

To ensure that the needs of the community are being addressed, health care providers and programs may be required to compete for these funds. Submission of proposals, grant applications, or requests must be submitted, reviewed, and prioritized. Allocation of funds is provided on the basis of need and program merit. This type of funding is directed toward the populace in general and not to specific individuals. When the funding is no longer provided, the programs cease, which can result in lack of continuity of care.

Currently, the funding priorities are closely related to the achievement of the *Healthy People 2020* objectives. Limitations on the amounts provided are related to governmental resources.

PHILANTHROPIC FINANCING OF HEALTH CARE

A limited amount of the nation's estimated $1.5 trillion health care bill is paid by philanthropic sources whose priorities are usually capricious and research or disease oriented. Eligibility for services through these associations is generally limited to the specific disease or population of interest, as with the American Heart Association. Few direct services are rendered, and these are awarded on individual case consideration. Ancillary health care needs such as transportation, parental housing, or wigs may be addressed. Informational and research activities constitute the majority of services provided by these types of organizations. The organizations fund many educational programs that increase awareness of specific diseases, screening procedures, and preventive measures.

Exceptions do exist, and national organizations such as the Shriners operate health care institutions designed to provide specialty care for a specific population group. These services and all costs related to this care, including transportation, are often provided to the eligible person free of charge. The only requirement for this care is sponsorship by a member of the supporting organization.

HEALTH INSURANCE PLANS

Historical Perspective

During the 1930s, in an effort to provide care and avoid bankruptcy, health care providers began to establish health insurance plans. One of the most recognizable of these plans is Blue Cross and Blue Shield. Those enrolled in the plan, called *enrollees,* paid a monthly fee for a guarantee of health care. Providers delivered services to the enrollees and collected payment from the health insurance plan. The insurance plan paid fees plus its administrative costs from money collected from the enrollees.

During World War II when prices and wages were frozen, industries began to offer health insurance as a fringe benefit. In 1953, as a further incentive to obtain health care coverage, money spent on health insurance was declared tax exempt. Over the years, workers' union groups began to negotiate for these benefits. With more available financial resources, the health care expenditures increased. Reimbursement based on operational costs represented a strong incentive for expansion (Higgins, 1997). By 2008, 65% of those under the age of 65 years were covered by insurance, 95% of which was obtained through the workplace. Reasons for being uninsured were costs, change in employment, change in marital status, and death of spouse or parent (NCHS, 2008).

Types of Health Care Plans

This early Blue Cross and Blue Shield was an example of an indemnity plan. This plan paid all of the costs of covered services provided to the enrollee. The enrollee enjoyed free choice of the provider and services. Indemnity plans preserve the enrollee's right of choice and allow the person to manage his or her own health care. These plans lack incentives for cost containment. Although indemnity plans are still available, the monthly cost of enrollment has increased to exorbitant amounts, making these plans cost prohibitive. In an effort to infuse these incentives while preserving freedom of choice, mechanisms of cost sharing were introduced. These cost-sharing methods include co-payment, deductible amounts, and coinsurance. All of these represented efforts to have the enrollee share in the cost of medical care (Table 11-2).

As health care costs escalated, variations in health care insurance plans were developed. Industries, the major providers of insurance coverage, began to look for a more economical means of providing health care to their employees. Large industrial giants, such as Kaiser Permanente, decided

TABLE 11-2	**CONSUMER ADVANTAGES AND DISADVANTAGES OF INSURANCE REIMBURSEMENT PLANS**	
TYPE	**ADVANTAGES**	**DISADVANTAGES**
Indemnity	No gatekeeper	High premiums
Fee for service	Unlimited choice of providers	Potential for overuse
	Full access to all services	No incentive for cost containment
Managed care	"Credentialed" providers promote quality assurance	
HMO	Comprehensive care	Restricted to plan provider
	Lower premium	Potential for lower quality care to maximize costs
	No deductibles or co-payment	
PPO	Greater selection of providers than with HMO	Gatekeeper
	Expedited provider reimbursement	Additional cost for out-of-plan provider
	Lower premiums	Potential for lower quality care to maximized costs
POS	More flexibility	Deductible
	Comprehensive services with plan	20%-50% co-payment for out-of-plan services
		Primary care provider referral needed for specialized care

HMO, Health maintenance organization; *POS,* point of service; *PPO,* preferred provider organization.

to assemble their own health care program. They built hospitals, hired physicians, and provided health care services to their employees. In an effort to market this concept, Dr. Paul Elwood coined the phrase "health maintenance organization" (HMO) (Higgins, 1997). HMOs were designed to provide more comprehensive care, but this type of program lacks enrollee freedom of choice. Preventive care is covered and encouraged, but care is somewhat restricted, and care providers are encouraged to reduce costs by providing only the most necessary services. This loss of choice led to a decrease in popularity of HMOs. In the U.S., the number of HMO plans peaked in the mid 1990s when about 31% of the populations were enrolled in them. By 2009, however, only 20% of the U.S. population were enrolled in HMOs (Kaiser Family Foundation, 2009b).

In an effort to compete with the HMO, physicians and hospitals organized the independent practice model (IPM). The IPM was a separate entity that provided services to enrollees of one insurance company. This model evolved into the preferred provider organization (PPO). These types of insurance plans negotiated with health care providers for services at a reduced rate in exchange for a guaranteed increase in consumers. A negotiated reimbursement rate allows the cost of the plan to be somewhat controlled. Plan enrollees are offered cost incentives for choosing health care from within the plan's network of health care providers. As they receive a specific amount of reimbursement, regardless of the rendered services, providers have an incentive to be cost-conscious in the services provided (Ginsburg, 2004). PPOs are more flexible than HMOs, but to receive full benefits, the covered individual must use network providers. PPOs are the most common type of insurance plan in the U.S., and in 2009, about 60% of insured workers were enrolled in them (Kaiser Family Foundation, 2009b).

Point of service (POS) plans combine elements of the HMO and the PPO. In POS plans, the covered individual designates an in-network physician as the primary health care provider (PCP). If the individual goes outside of the network for care, they will be responsible for most of the costs unless referred by the PCP. POS plans were common during the early years of the centruy, but in 2009 accounted for only about 10% of all health insurance plans (Kaiser Family Foundation, 2009b).

Costs of private health insurance are staggering, and often prohibitively high. In 2009, the average annual costs of insurance provided to through employers was $4,800 for an individual and $13,400 for a family. Surprisingly, that year there was very little variation based on plan type; costs for an HMO were $4,900/single ($13,500/family); costs for a PPO were $4,900/single ($13,900/family) and POS plans were $4,800/single ($13,000/family) (Kaiser Family Foundation, 2009b). The similarity in costs have no doubt contributed to the relative increase in the proportion choosing a PPO over the more restrictive POS and HMO plans.

Multistate networks or alliances are health insurance–purchasing cooperatives that establish purchasing pools responsible for negotiating health insurance arrangements for employers, employees, and state Medicaid recipients. These alliances use the volume of health consumers that they represent as leverage to negotiate contracts for health care coverage. Provider membership into the alliance is voluntary but exclusive. If the provider is located in an area in which the alliance is the predominant insurance plan, the provider is financially forced to join and accept the negotiated reimbursement.

Another means of providing the enrollee with choice, but at the same time allowing the plan to control prices, is a "cafeteria plan." Insurance providers may offer the enrollee or consumer a wide variety of choices. Employers may specify the amount of money that will be contributed toward health care. The consumers may then customize their health care coverage, depending on their needs and willingness to pay. By choosing the types of services they want covered and the provider of these services, consumers have some control over their own health care costs. Consumers assume financial responsibility for any costs that exceed the employer's contributing amount (Clark, 2003).

Reimbursement Mechanisms of Insurance Plans

When insurance plans were initially offered, the customary method of reimbursement was a fee for the service rendered, or retrospective reimbursement. Calculation of the fee was based on the cost of providing the service. Included in this "umbrella" of costs were such things as salaries, supplies, equipment, building depreciation, utilities, and taxes. Cost-based reimbursement encouraged inflated prices and fraud. Physicians were encouraged to overtreat patients, and participants were encouraged to overuse the health care system.

Prospective reimbursement (i.e. the PPS), a concept derived from the HMO method of payment, seemed to be an effective financial alternative to cost-based reimbursement. Prospective reimbursement meant that care, no matter what the provider's cost, would be reimbursed according to a predetermined amount. The government introduced this method of reimbursement for Medicare in 1983, and an immediate savings was noted. For determination of the prospective amount, Medicare depended on the diagnosis-related group (DRG) to calculate the reimbursement. The amount to be paid to the provider was determined according to the client's primary and secondary diagnoses, age, gender, and complications. This amount was deemed sufficient cost for health care ascertained to be adequate for treatment. If the provider, at first limited to hospitals, could provide the treatment for less than this amount, a profit was made. If the required services cost more than this amount, then the provider took a loss (Rozzini, Sabatini, and Trabucchi, 2005).

Implementation of the PPS led to a reduction in Medicare costs but did not result in overall health care cost savings as intended. Hospitals developed cost shifting as a means of supplementing the loss of Medicare funding. Private insurance's reimbursement continued to be cost based. Therefore hospitals could include the loss from caring for Medicare patients in their cost. Private insurance companies were paying for the cost of providing care to their enrollees and Medicare patients.

Only a few years after implementation of the PPS by Medicare, private health care plans followed the government's lead. In an effort to ensure appropriate reimbursement, more sophisticated methods of calculating the relative cost of health care were developed. Actuarial classifications ensured that adequate premiums were charged for the projected health care needs of those enrolled, and other means of cost control began to emerge. Managed care groups negotiated with health care providers to render care for a specified amount of reimbursement based on community ratings modified by group-specific demographics (Turner, 1999). Prospective reimbursement created incentives to control costs but also led to instances of undertreatment and underuse of the system (see Table 11-2).

Covered Services

Insurance plans have always designated the types of services for which the plan would be financially responsible. When first developed, health insurance was meant to be a means of protecting an individual or family from economic catastrophe should a serious illness occur. Once an employee's fringe benefit included health insurance coverage, expanded benefit packages were developed. The scope of covered services began to increase to such things as physician's office visits, medication, and dental costs. Unions began to negotiate for these expanded covered medical services in lieu of additional wages.

When health care costs increased, the price of enrollment into the insurance plans increased. Industries began to balk at paying these higher premium rates. Workers became disgruntled when their employers passed the cost of increased rates to them. To curtail the escalating premium price, insurance companies began to limit the covered services and dictate the conditions under which these services would be covered. Sites of care delivery changed. Many treatments were required to be delivered outside the hospital, or in ambulatory care centers. The patient was held financially responsible for "uncovered" services. Providers were pressured to comply with these requirements. Providers began to modify the delivery of health care to accommodate for these changes. Following implementation of the PPS and various managed care options, the rate of hospitalization declined dramatically, and the number of outpatient services increased. As a result, for example, in 2007 63% of all surgical procedures were performed on an outpatient basis compared with 16% in 1980 (NCHS, 2009).

All of these changes resulted in conflicts among providers, patients, employers, and the insurance plans, particularly when services deemed necessary by the consumer and provider were denied insurance coverage. Employers looked to the insurance companies to provide health care services at a reasonable price. Insurance companies searched for ways to control costs, and providers searched for ways to deliver needed care within the confines of the health care policy.

COST CONTAINMENT

Limiting health care costs is an imperative. All recent presidents including Clinton, Bush, and Obama have recognized that spiraling health care costs have eroded an already suffering economy. In 1960, health care expenditures represented 5.15% of the GNP; by 1995, health care expenses had risen to 13.4% of the GNP, and in 2007, health expenditures represented about 16% of the GNP, with no indication of a slowdown (ODEC, 2008).

Early in his presidency, President Obama stated that "one of the greatest threats not just to the well-being of our families and the prosperity of our businesses, but to the very foundation of our economy…is the exploding cost of health care in America today" (White House Forum on Health Reform, 2009). Costs have to be controlled to meet the public's demand for unlimited health care. This is known as cost containment. Numerous attempts to control costs have been made over the years, but none has been more than marginally successful.

Historical Perspective of Cost Containment

In addition to implementation of the PPS, in the mid 1980s, health insurers and governmental sources attempted to curtail unnecessary proliferation of medical technology by requiring a certificate of need (CON) for additions to current health care buildings or services. To further reduce use, hospital records were reviewed for the appropriateness of care provided. Admission and treatment of those hospitalized were reviewed by peer standard review organizations. Physicians and other medical personnel reviewed the hospital records and counseled the attending physician about unnecessary or excessively lengthy stays in the hospital, as well as unwarranted services.

⚖ ETHICAL INSIGHTS

Cost Containment: Whom Will You Deny?

You are the gatekeeper, meeting with others in your organization to determine what services to provide to clients. You have $400,000 to divide among four clients. Who will receive the required treatment? Who will not?

1. Child with broken leg needs physical therapy (estimated cost: $10,000)
2. 55-year-old man requiring knee replacement surgery and physical therapy (estimated cost: $40,000)
3. 76-year-old requiring hip replacement (estimated cost: $40,000)
4. 32-year-old woman with leukemia, requiring a bone marrow transplant (estimated cost: $350,000)

What factors should be considered in the decision?
How much does the cost of treatment affect the decision?
How much does the age of the patient affect the decision?
Is social justice a factor in the decision?

The cost reduction, as a result of prospective payment and other efforts, gave rise to the managed care revolution. Unable to shift costs to another entity, and with a predetermined reimbursement rate, providers searched for the most cost-effective mechanism of care provision. Greater ability to predict the cost of care enabled health care plans to negotiate the best value for their premiums.

RESEARCH HIGHLIGHTS

Hospital Readmissions From Home Health Care Before and After Prospective Payment

In an effort to control the Medicare home health expenditure, home health reimbursement was changed from fee for service to a prospective payment system (PPS). This changed the reimbursement from a per-visit fee to episodes of care. Each episode of care begins on the first billable day and proceeds for a period of 60 days. Reimbursement is based on the diagnosis and type and level of care predicted to be required.

Utilizing a comprehensive evaluative tool, the OASIS, a client is placed in a home health resource group (HHRG). Payment for services is based on the HHRG. Another important factor is that payment is received in two parts: 60% at the start of care and 40% after the episode of care is completed. Adjustment in final payment results from changes in the client's condition and may result in more or less than anticipated.

Unplanned hospital readmissions are an aspect of adverse change in patient condition or outcome chosen to be studied by these investigators. This study was designed to compare characteristics of clients rehospitalized during home health care before PPS and after PPS.

The sample size of 76 clients was chosen from a Midwestern U.S., not-for-profit, Medicare-certified, hospital-affiliated, home health care agency. This agency served approximately 280 to 300 clients daily. Characteristics of the clients at time of rehospitalization were determined utilizing a Hospital Readmission Inventory. This instrument has an interrater reliability of 96%. Closed-case medical records were reviewed.

The sample was matched for characteristics such as age, sex, marital status, referral sources, and length of stay in home health care. The primary diagnosis at hospital discharge and readmission before PPS was chronic obstructive pulmonary disease and congestive heart failure. Post-PPS hospital discharge and readmission diagnosis was circulatory associated. Pre-PPS length of stay was 13 days compared with 9.01 for post-PPS clients.

From this study it is difficult to conclude whether PPS has any negative effect on home health care patient outcomes. The data set does confirm that during the first 2 weeks after discharge, there was an increase in the number of different nurses caring for the client compared to a care provided by the same nurse providing care to the home health client. Post-PPS clients were judged to be sicker at the time of rehospitalization and were almost twice as likely to be readmitted for another diagnosis. It is concluded that, since the institution of PPS in 2000, the hospital length of stay has decreased, resulting in clients being sicker at time of discharge.

The study shows that the first 2 weeks following hospital discharge are the most critical. Payments for home health services are suspended at the time of readmission pending a client's return to home health care after rehospitalization. If the client does not return to home health care and the agency has completed five visits, 60% of the payment will awarded. If the agency has not completed the five visits, only 11% of the amount will be awarded. This might serve as an incentive for agencies to increase the number of visits after the initial hospital discharge but not for clients discharged the second time.

From Anderson MA, Clarke MM, Helms LB, Foreman MD: Hospital readmission from home health care before and after prospective payment, *J Nurs Scholarsh* 37(1):73-79, 2005.

Current Trends in Cost Containment

The managed care form of health care financing changed economic incentives and forced health care providers to rethink health management decisions. Treatment recommendations may be tied more to "Can you afford this?" rather than "This is best for you." Costs of the service rendered, rather than enhancement of revenue through service provision, must be considered. These economic or cost-containment incentives can be divided into the following broad categories: capitated reimbursement, access limitation, and rationing.

Capitated Reimbursement

The increasing visibility of managed care models and their associated success in cost containment through the use of prospective reimbursement to influence provider practice gave rise to various arrangements that link health care financing to service delivery or managed care. Managed care organizations create partnerships with health care providers using financial incentives to prevent overuse. Statistical norms, practice parameters, and population data determine the capitated, or maximum, payment for services. This is the maximum reimbursement amount that the health care provider will receive for the provision of care. The actual cost of provision of care does not affect the reimbursement. Health care providers must provide appropriate medical care while being cognizant of health care costs. As a reward for conservative practices, health care providers may receive a specified amount of money or a percentage of the agreed reimbursement if services are delivered below the limit

set by the third-party payer. Providers whose services are inadequate or exceed this limit may be excluded from the network.

Cost Containment Through Access Limitation

All third-party payers, or insurance plans, control access to health care through designation of covered services. Managed care organizations designate the type of covered services and specify the conditions under which the service is covered. Some services may only be accessed upon approval or referral from physicians who are used as gatekeepers. The enrollee must choose a primary care provider and consult this provider for a referral before seeking specialty services. Without this referral, the enrollee is financially responsible for the service. Even with the referral, choices may be limited to the providers who have contracted with the managed care plan.

Managed care plans may require that less costly health care modalities or medications be used. Exceptions to these modalities require justification. More technologically advanced and expensive treatments may be accessed under the most stringent conditions. Preauthorization requirements determine the medical necessity of the service. The process is so complex that the client may not be aware that the service is not covered until the reimbursement for the service is denied.

Cost Containment Through Rationing

Rationing is best described as determining the most appropriate use of health care or directing the health care where it can do the most good. The following case dramatizes the problem.

Clinical Example

A middle-aged woman had ovarian cancer diagnosed. After conventional and high-dose chemotherapy failed, her physician recommended an autologous bone marrow transplantation, which was considered experimental at the time. The procedure was approved and performed. Medical costs exceeded $200,000, but the patient died 2 months later.

Was this a wise use of medical resources? Health care is not an exact science; too many variables exist. What appears to be the best course of action for one is not the best course of action for another. Making accurate treatment decisions is difficult, and the ramifications of a mistake are great. Health care providers and third-party payers, including the federal government, are currently investigating the outcomes of health care practices to determine what methods, if any, can be instituted to improve the accuracy of these choices. Research into the area of treatment outcomes has brought about such treatment changes as laparoscopic surgery, genetically determined cancer treatment, and gender-specific interventions.

TRENDS IN HEALTH FINANCING

The public's demand for affordable health care has created a new environment for health care financing. Competition among health care providers and third-party payers has led to new and innovative health care. Outpatient services, patient education packages, electronic health records, and telehealth are just a few of these innovations. Increased competition has required insurance plans to be sensitive to the needs of the employee organizations and their enrollees. Individualized plans of covered services can be created. Enrollees can choose the plan that provides them with the services they desire at a selected cost. Health care providers advertise to ensure that the consumer selects an insurance plan in which their services are included. Some providers, such as hospitals, campaign for provision into a plan.

Cost Sharing

Aware of the amount that the employer is willing to contribute for basic coverage, a third-party payer or insurance plan may propose several options, giving the employee freedom to choose services desired. Employees willing to pay may be able to increase the covered services not provided by the basic plan. Cost sharing may also require the consumer to pay an increased portion of the bill for covered services in return for lower premiums. Enrollees may opt to pay a higher premium for freedom to choose providers, or elimination of the gatekeeper. This can result in increased consumer control of health care.

Health Care Alliances

The creation of powerful regional or statewide insurance purchasing pools or health alliances is seen as one of the means of reform for the health care industry. The alliance would define basic benefits that all insurers would have to offer to everyone at the same price regardless of health status. These alliances would be chartered to not regulate insurance prices. Health alliances would collect premiums and help consumers choose among competing insurers and plans. The consumer's choice would be based on published, simple, standard information about benefits and outcomes of the different available plans. Plans would have to compete by offering better outcomes or less cost. Insurers would have to contract with providers that find ways of delivering cost-efficient care. Medicare is currently participating in health care alliances. Enrollees are given a choice between the traditional Medicare Parts A and B, or Medicare Advantage.

Self-Insurance

Some organizations have used health care information collected by insurance plans to self-insure their employees. This has enabled industries and other types of organizations to reduce the administrative cost of insurance, which has been estimated to represent 12.5% of the cost of insurance. Unlike the large industrial HMOs, self-insured status organizations administer their own health care plan but purchase health care services from an established insurance plan.

Flexible Spending Accounts

Another source of funding for uncovered services is the flexible spending account (FSA). The employee determines how much he or she will have to spend for uncovered services and has this amount deducted from his or her paycheck. When these services are incurred, the employee can secure payment for these services from this account. The employee continues to pay into the account until the estimated amount is reached. If the employee overestimates the cost, the remaining amount is forfeited. If the cost of the services exceeds the estimate, only the amount estimated will be paid.

Health Promotion and Disease Prevention

"We can agree that if we want to bring down skyrocketing costs, we'll need to modernize our system and invest in prevention," stated President Obama (White House Forum, 2009). Unfortunately, reimbursement for health promotion and disease prevention continues to be limited. Most health insurances, both private and public, pay for screening procedures. However, funding or reimbursement for treatment modalities such as support groups for smoking cessation, home safety evaluation, or relaxation techniques is not common. Obesity is one of this nation's most common health problems, yet weight loss programs are not reimbursed.

Research into barriers and facilitators to changes in lifestyle continues to be funded well below curative treatment research. Lifestyle change interventions are slow to be developed and even more difficult to implement and evaluate (Reid et al., 2009). For example, research into weight loss strategies found that documenting all food intake was effective in initial and sustained weight loss (Hollis et al., 2008). Until these types of interventions are directly financed, most likely they will not become widely implemented.

HEALTH CARE FINANCING REFORM

It has been estimated that more than 45 million Americans are uninsured or underinsured. In 2007, about 21% of Americans did not have health insurance at some point during the year. The rates were highest among those those between the ages of 18 and 24 years (35% are uninsured) and among Hispanics (36% are uninsured). Lack of insurance is the major factor associated with lack of access to medical care. Uninsured adults are more than 3 times as likely as insured adults to go without needed medical care (NCHS, 2009).

Access to Health Care

Access to health care is a complex situation that is defined by the circumstances of the individual. The primary concern is inadequate access to health care, which leads to unnecessary illness. Most Americans want to believe that the best possible health care will be available for themselves and their family members at any time regardless of their age, sex, race, or ability to pay. Anything that obstructs this pursuit can be considered a barrier to the access of health care.

Financial support for health care, through either private insurance coverage or participation in government programs is the mechanism that is largely responsible for access. Lack of a source for health care financing due to lack of insurance coverage, preexisting conditions, unapproved care, or nonparticipating physicians represent the most frequent factors attributed to difficulty in obtaining care. According to the National Health Interview Survey in 2007, 16% of the American population lacked health insurance; as a result, millions reported that they delayed seeking health care or did not received health care because of cost (NCHS, 2009). Other impediments to health care access are physical barriers, including structural inaccessibility, lack of appropriate equipment, or inability to communicate.

Inequality in the distribution of health care services represents another type of physical barrier. Even those with insurance coverage may be unable to locate "participating" health care providers. Transportation difficulty, conflict with work hours, and failure to provide services exemplify these types of physical barriers. Opportunities to seek health care, especially preventive health care, during work hours is often discouraged by employers. Rural areas and inner cities have been recognized as medically underserved for many years. Government incentives for increasing available medical services in these areas have not solved the problem.

Sociological barriers to health care access exist among poor and ethnic Americans. Poor outpatient diagnosis and treatment, increased use of emergency departments for primary care, and reluctance to hospitalize were possible explanations. Language and fear of reprisals have become important sociological barriers. Many of the poor and uninsured are illegal aliens, and seeking medical attention, even during illnesses, may result in severe repercussions.

Historical Perspective

National health insurance is not a new concept. European countries began a social model of health insurance in the early 1900s. In 1916, President Theodore Roosevelt advocated enactment of a form of national medical coverage. President Franklin Roosevelt wanted national health insurance to be part of the Social Security Act of 1935 but that provision did not pass (Higgins, 1997). During the administration of President Lyndon Johnson, however, a modified form of national health insurance, Medicare and Medicaid, was instituted.

Before the 1930s, most Americans were uninsured. Most health care providers considered it their duty to donate time and services to charity. Hospitals and clinics maintained charity wards. Society believed that those who could, and those who could not, should help themselves. The enactment of governmental entitlement programs, coupled with the availability of health care insurance as a benefit of occupation, helped change this belief. Quickly, the pervasive societal view was that those who could not help themselves should get government assistance, or go to work (Higgins, 1997).

As discussed earlier, in the 1960s, Medicare and Medicaid brought about national health insurance coverage for older adults, the disabled, and those, especially children, living below the poverty level. Expansion of Medicaid with CHIPS in the 1990s, expanded care coverage for children of the "working poor", or those whose parent's employers did not provide insurance.

During the 1992 presidential campaign, Bill Clinton promised to reform America's health care system, ensure universal coverage, and reduce medical care costs without damaging the economy. At that time, it was thought that basic health care coverage for all individuals could be achieved over several years. After a year of debate and numerous proposals, the Clinton plan eventually failed to reach a consensus because of wide-spread opposition from various health care provider groups and organizations as well as lack of support of the public.

Societal Perceptions

Social justice, in the form of equal health care for all, is a concept that most Americans support. Most people state that health care should be one of those necessities available to all without consideration of what it costs. Despite this, efforts to provide universal coverage through increased governmental involvement in health care have failed because of a number of factors including rejection of much higher taxes, objection to paying for care for non-citizens, concerns over access and availability, and fears of rationing. Managed care has been somewhat successful in containing escalating health care costs by diminishing and limiting use, but the public is very aware of the spiraling costs and rapidly aging population.

The current dilemma is how to provide health care to all Americans that is acceptable and affordable. Other countries provide their citizens with universal health care, but there are aspects of this care that are unpopular with U.S. society. The most concerning or pressing problem relates to funding source as significant tax increases would be necessary to provide coverage for all. Waiting several months for nonemergent treatment, lack of choice of treatment, and inaccessible or unavailable diagnostic and treatment modalities are not acceptable to most Americans. Indeed, most Americans want assurance that all of the health care services that they and their families need, now and in the future, will be available no matter what the condition, age of the patient, job status or ability to pay.

Health Care Reform - 2010

During the 2008 presidential campaign, health care reform was a key issue. The election of President Obama and Democratic Party majorities in both houses of Congress helped pave the way for significant changes in health care financing. After hundreds of deliberations that were often contentious, and after more than a year of debate, Congress passed the Patient Protection and Affordable Care Act (PL111-148), which was signed into law March 23, 2010. Although the Act does not ensure 'universal coverage' per se, the Congressional Budget Office (CBO) estimated that when fully implemented, it will ensure that an additional 32 million people will have access to health insurance coverage (Kaiser Family Foundation, 2010).

The Health Care Reform Act is an extremely complex piece of legislation and the final version of the bill exceeded 2000 pages. There are many health-related provisions of the law. These include: mandating that all citizens obtain health insurance; expanding Medicaid eligibility; subsidizing insurance premiums for low income purchasers; prohibiting denial of coverage for pre-existing conditions; and establishing health insurance exchanges. Costs for expansion of coverage and subsidies will be offset by a combination of taxes and fees, reduction in payments for Medicare and Medicaid services and prescription drugs, and enhanced efforts to reduce Medicare fraud and abuse. Box 11-3 outlines some of the major provisions covered.

A few of the provisions of the Health Care Reform Act will be implemented in 2010, but most do not take effect until 2014, and it will not be fully implemented until 2018. Further, the Act remains very controversial, and legislative and legal challenges are anticipated. All health care providers and consumers should remain alert to both short and long-term changes in health care financing and health care delivery that will result.

ROLES OF THE COMMUNITY HEALTH NURSE IN THE ECONOMICS OF HEALTH CARE

Researcher

Nurses need to be engaged in research into provision of efficient, cost-effective health care. Nurses are in a pivotal role to investigate culturally sensitive treatment modalities, health education, disease prevention, and factors to change behaviors. Health promotion and disease prevention are more cost-effective than curative treatment modalities. Community health nurse researchers need to investigate, develop, and evaluate the effectiveness of health promotion and disease prevention. Research on health promotion intervention outcomes, program cost/benefit analysis, and health informatics are just a few of these areas.

Educator

Health education is the foundation of community health nursing practice. Community health nurses agree that knowledge empowers clients to actively participate in their health care. Funding for this education is provided primarily through public governmental plans. Educational plans for individuals are almost nonexistent. In the area of health care economics, the nurse needs to demonstrate the effectiveness and value of this education. Outcome measures for health education need

---

BOX 11-3   HIGHLIGHTS OF THE PATIENT PROTECTION AND AFFORDABLE CARE ACT (P.L. 111-148)

Individual Mandate – Requires U.S. citizens and legal residents to have qualifying health coverage.

Employer Requirements – Requires employers with more than 50 employees to offer coverage or vouchers for full-time employees; requires employers with more than 200 employees to enroll employees into health insurance plans offered by the employer.

Expansion of Medicaid – Expands Medicaid to all individuals under age 65 with incomes up to 133% of the federal poverty line.

Expansion of CHIP – Requires states to maintain current income eligibility levels for children enrolled in CHIP until 2019.

Premium and Cost-Sharing Subsidities to Individuals – Creates insurance exchanges to provide premium credits and subsidies to individuals and families with incomes between 133% and 400% of the federal poverty level.

Changes to Private Insurance – Establishes a temporary national high-risk pool to provide health coverage to individuals with pre-existing medication conditions; establishes a process for reviewing increases in health plan premiums and requires justification of increases; provides dependent coverage for children up to age 26 for all individual and group policies; prohibits health plans

from placing lifetime limits on the dollar value of coverage and from rescinding coverage; establishes a website to help residents identify health coverage options; permits states to form health care choice compacts and allow insurers to sell policies in any state participating in the compact.

Cost Containment Provisions – Requires rules to simplify health insurance administration by adopting a single set of rules for payment, verification and claims status; restructures payments to Medicare Advantage plans; reduces waste, fraud and abuse in public programs by allowing providers screening enhanced oversight periods for new providers and suppliers; increases penalties for submitting false claims.

Prevention and Wellness – improves prevention by covering preventive services and eliminating cost-sharing for preventive services in Medicare and Medicaid; requires qualified health plans to provide preventive services, recommended immunizations, preventive care for infants, children and adolescents and additional preventive care and screening for women; provides grants for small employers who establish wellness programs; requires chain restaurants and foods sold from vending machines to disclose the nutritional content of each item.

From **"Summary of New Health Reform Law"**, (#8061) The Henry J. Kaiser Family Foundation, April 2010. This information was reprinted with permission from the Henry J. Kaiser Family Foundation. The Kaiser Family Foundation is a non-profit private operating foundation, based in Menlo Park, California, dedicated to producing and comunicating the best possible analysis and information on health issues.

to be established. Measuring these outcomes will provide evidence of the value of this education ("Health Illiteracy Leads to Billions in Avoidable Costs," 2004).

Provider of Care

Any service delivered by the nurse needs to be appropriate, necessary, and cost-effective. Nurses, in all areas of practice, need to be cost conscious. Judicious application of the nursing process is imperative. An accurate assessment is the foundation for an appropriate nursing diagnosis. Goals for care, jointly established between members of the community and the community health nurse, will guide the choice of interventions. Evaluation, using previously developed outcome measures, will provide appropriate modifications to the plan.

Nurses can serve as program service providers, health education providers, and health program participants. Nurses need to participate in the grant proposal process, program design, and evaluation of these programs. They need to be familiar with and participate in the statistical information gathering process that serves as the basis for determining community health need.

Advocate

Nurses must become more involved in the economics of health care. Too often, nurses are cognizant of the effects of changes in health care economics but feel powerless to act. Increasing knowledge of health care funding and policy making will empower nurses to advocate for the type of funding that provides appropriate care to obtain the greatest good. The large number of nurses provides our occupation with political clout. Nurses need to utilize this political power to influence health care funding. Nurses need to advocate for increase in health promotion/disease prevention funding from both the public and the private sector. Nurses need to plan programs, seek funding, and evaluate program effectiveness through outcome measures. Nurses need to constantly seek sources of funding for health programs through any available sources.

SUMMARY

Health care economics is influencing health care practice at all levels. Nurses must become aware of the economics of health care to practice in this new era. Patient outcomes are quickly being seen as a measurement for health care financing. As the health care system evolves toward health promotion and disease prevention, nursing will play a pivotal role. Community health nurses, whose domain of practice has encompassed these areas, will be in the forefront of this change.

This chapter has presented the basics of health care economics. An understanding of these elements is essential for the practice of nursing. This is an ever-changing field with new innovations and changes coming every day. To be effective, the nurse must be attentive to these developments.

LEARNING ACTIVITIES

1. Create a health care system including services, eligible recipients, funding resources, and qualifying requirements for these services.
2. Evaluate a family's health care coverage. Investigate the type of coverage and the ability of this coverage type to meet the needs of the family. Is there another type of insurance coverage that would meet more of the family's needs? What prohibits their ability to obtain this coverage?
3. Investigate the Health Care Reform Act from the points of view of the consumer, health care provider, and third-party payer. How will it affect the concerns of each of these constituents?
4. Interview representatives from health care provider groups, insurance plans, and consumer groups regarding their suggestions for health care reform.
5. Interview public health nurses employed in a public health department regarding their perception of funding for health promotion/disease prevention.
6. Investigate political influences on health care reform. Interview governmental officials regarding what influences their health care policy decisions.

REFERENCES

Alemayehu B, Warner K: The lifetime distribution of health care costs, *Health Serv Res* 39: 627–642, 2004.

Centers for Disease Control and Prevention (CDC): *International Classificaiton of Diseases, Tenth Revision, clinical Modivicaiton (ICD-10-CM)*, 2010. http://www.cdc.gov/nchs/icd/icd10cm.htm#10update.

Centers for Medicare and Medicaid Services (CMS): *National health expenditure projections, 2009–2019*, Baltimore MD, 2010a, The Author. http://www.cms.gov/NationalHealthExpendData/downloads/proj2009.pdf.

Centers for Medicare and Medicaid Services: *Medicare fraud: detection and prevention tips*, Baltimore, no date, The Author. www.medicare.gov/FraudAbuse/Tips.asp.

Centers for Medicare and Medicaid Services (CMS): *Medicare and you. 2010*, 2010b. http://www.medicare.gov/Publications/Pubs/pdf/10050.pdf.

Clark K: Cost cure-all? Or unhealthy shift? Employers seek to pass on the workers more of the burden of soaring medical costs, *US News World Rep* 135(21):38–39, 2003.

Commonwealth of Kentucky Department of Revenue: *Tobacco taxes*, Frankfort, KY, 2005, The Author. revenue.ky.gov/business/tobaccotax.htm.

Congressional Research Service: *U.S. Health Care Spending – Comparison with other OCED countries*, 2007. http://digitalcommons.ilr.cornell.edu/cgi/viewcontent.cgi?article=1316&context=key_workplace.

Ginsburg P: Controlling health care costs, *N Engl J Med* 351:1591–1593, 2004.

Harvard Medical School Harvard's Men's Health Watch 13(8), 2009.

Health illiteracy leads to billions in avoidable costs, *Oncol News Int* 13(6):53, 2004.

Higgins W: How did we get this way? *Health Care Econ* 11:35, 1997.

Hollis J, Gullion C, Stevens V, et al: Weight loss during the intensive intervention phase of weight loss maintenance trial, *J Prevent Med* 35(2):118–126, 2008.

Kaiser Family Foundation: *Employer Medical Benefits*, 2009b. Annual Survey http://ehbs.kff.org/pdf/2009/7936.pdf.

Kaiser Family Foundation: *Medicaid: A primer*, 2009a. http://www.kff.org/medicaid/upload/7334-03.pdf.

Kaiser Family Foundation: *Focus on Health Reform*, 2010. http://www.kff.org/healthreform/upload/8061.pdf 2010b.

National Center for Health Statistics: *Health: United States, 2009*, Hyattsville, Md, 2010, The Author. http://www.cdc.gov/nchs/data/hus/hus09.pdf#126.

Organisation for Economic Co-operation and Development: *Health at a glance*, 2008. www.oecd.org/document/16/0,3343,en_2649_34631_2085200_1_1_1_1,00.html.

Reid G, van Teijlingen E, Douglas F, et al: The reality of partnership working when undertaking an evaluation of a national well men's service, *J Mens Health* 6(1):36–49, 2009.

Rozzini R, Sabatini T, Trabucchi M: Diagnosis related groups and hospital costs in elderly dependent patients, *J Am Geriatr Soc* 53:174–175, 2005.

Sloan T: Consumer-driven to nowhere: study throws cold water on recent efforts to beat health care cost inflation, *Mod Healthcare* 34(49):21, 2004.

Turner SO: *The nurse's guide to managed care*, Gaithersburg, Md, 1999, Aspen.

U.S. Census Bureau: *U.S. interim projections by age, group: 2010–2050*, 2008. http://www.census.gov/population/www/projections/summarytables.html.

US Department of Health and Human Services: *Grants and funding*, Hyattsville, Md, 2007, The Author. www.hhs.gov/grants/index.shtml.

Weintraub W, Shine K: Is a paradigm shift in US healthcare reimbursement inevitable? *Circulation* 109:1448–1455, 2004.

White House Forum on Health Reform: March 5, 2009, www.whitehouse.gov/assets/documents/White_House_Forum_on_Health_Reform_Report.pdf.

12

Policy, Politics, Legislation, and Community Health Nursing

*Linda Thompson Adams, Deborah M. Tierney**

Additional Material for Study, Review, and Further Exploration

evolve WEBSITE

http://evolve.elsevier.com/Nies
- Quiz
- Case Studies
- Content Updates
- Glossary
- WebLinks

OBJECTIVES

Upon completion of this chapter, the reader will be able to do the following:
1. Discuss the nurse's role in political activities.
2. Discuss the power of nursing to influence and change health policy.
3. Identify the social and political processes that influence health policy development.
4. Identify the legislative, judicial, and administrative (executive) processes involved in establishing federal, state, or local health policy.
5. Discuss current health policy issues, including restructuring of the health care system.
6. Discuss nursing's involvement in private health policy.

KEY TERMS

administrative agencies	Lillian Wald	policy analysis
Clara Barton	lobby	political action committees
coalition	lobbyist	politics
Florence Nightingale	Mary Wakefield	public health law
government	nursing policy	public policy
health policy	organizations	Ruth Watson Lubic
institutional policies	organizational policies	social policy
Lavinia Dock	policy	Sojourner Truth

OUTLINE

Introduction to Health Policy and the Political Process
  Definitions
  Healthy People 2020
Structure of the Government of the United States
  Balance of Powers
The Legislative Process
  How a Bill Becomes a Law

Overview of Health Policy
  Public Health Policy
  Health Policy and the Private Sector
Public Policy: Blueprint for Governance
  Policy Formulation: The Ideal
  Policy Formulation: The Reality
  Steps in Policy Formulation and Analysis

*The authors would like to acknowledge the contributions of Denise Snow and MaryAnne Laffin, who wrote this chapter for the previous edition.

INTRODUCTION TO HEALTH POLICY AND THE POLITICAL PROCESS

This chapter addresses the interrelationships of the processes through which health policies are determined and instituted. Politics and legislation are the routes through which public health policies are established. Policy, politics, and legislation are the forces that determine the direction of health programs at every level of government, as well as the private sector. These programs are crucial to the health and well-being of the nation, the state, the community, and the individual. Nurses influence the maintenance and improvement of the health of individuals, groups, and communities by contributing to policy and legislative advancement.

The health care delivery system, including nursing practice and research, is profoundly influenced by policies set by both government and private entities. Nurses who understand the system of health policy development and implementation can effectively interpret and influence policies that affect nursing practice and health of individuals, families, groups, and communities.

The more a nurse knows about the political process, the more he or she tends to become involved. Individual nurses may become politically active on a local, state, or national level. Nurses may work collectively within a group such as the National Student Nurses Association, the American Nurses Association (ANA), and state boards of nursing to lobby for health causes. The profession of nursing is about 3 million strong (ANA, 2009; HRSA, 2010), and together nurses can be patient advocates, change agents, and policy makers. Nurses are respected by lawmakers and act as consultants in both the legislative and executive branches. It is the hallmark of the U.S. system of government that citizens have the right to have an influential voice in the governance of the community. Nurses are able to communicate concerns about conditions and issues in health care, the health care needs of individuals and communities, as well as the profession of nursing. United, nurses can influence political leaders to make changes to the health care system that are beneficial to all. Experienced nurses in the political arena can mentor novice nurses. Many individual nurses in the past and present have been instrumental in working with legislation and politics. Information on a few exemplary nurse heroines who illustrate this point follows:

- Florence Nightingale was the first nurse to exert political pressure on a government (Hall-Long, 1995). She transformed military health and knew the value of data in influencing policy. She was a leader who knew how to use the support of followers, colleagues, and policy makers.
- Sojourner Truth became an ardent and eloquent advocate for abolishing slavery and supporting women's rights. Her work helped transform the racist and sexist policies that limited the health and well-being of African Americans and women. She fought for human rights and lobbied for federal funds to train nurses and physicians (Mason, Leavitt, and Chaffee, 2007).
- Clara Barton was responsible for organizing relief efforts during the U.S. Civil War. In 1882, she successfully persuaded Congress to ratify the Treaty of Geneva, which allowed the Red Cross to perform humanitarian efforts in times of peace. This organization has had a lasting influence on national and international policies (Hall-Long, 1995; Kalisch and Kalisch, 2004).
- Lavinia Dock was a prolific writer and political activist. She waged a campaign for legislation to allow nurses to control the nursing profession instead of physicians. In 1893, with the assistance of Isabel Hampton Robb and Mary Adelaide Nutting, she founded the politically active American Society of Superintendents of Training School for Nurses, which later became the National League for Nursing (Kalisch and Kalisch, 2004). She was also active in the suffrage movement, advocating that nurses support the woman's right to vote (Lewinson, 2007).
- Lillian Wald's political activism and vision were shaped by feminist values. Working in the early 1900s, she recognized the connections between health and social conditions. She was a driving force behind the federal government's development of the Children's Bureau in 1912. Wald appeared frequently at the White House to participate in the development of national and international policy (Mason et al., 2007).
- Dr. Ruth Watson Lubic is a nurse-midwife who crusaded for freestanding birth centers in this country. After realizing the birth center model through the Maternity Center Association in New York City, Dr. Lubic expanded the model to Washington, DC, where the infant mortality rate was twice the national average. In 1993, Lubic was awarded the MacArthur Fellowship Grant and, in 2001, the Institute of Medicine's Lienhard Award (Institute of Medicine, 2001; Lyttle, 2000).

Definitions

Policy denotes a course of action to be followed by a government, business, or institution to obtain a desired effect. The Merriam-Webster definition is "a definite course or method of action selected from among alternatives and in light of given conditions to guide and determine present and future decisions." Policy encompasses the choices that a society, segment of society, or organization makes regarding its goals and priorities and the ways it allocates its resources to attain those goals. Policy choices reflect the values, beliefs, and attitudes of those designing the policy (Mason et al., 2007).

Public policy denotes precepts and standards formed by governmental bodies that are of fundamental concern to the state and the whole of the general public. The field of public policy involves the study of specific policy problems and governmental responses to them. Political scientists involved in the study of public policy attempt to devise solutions for problems of public concern. They study issues such as health care, pollution, and the economy. Public policy overlaps comparative politics in the study of comparative public policy, with international relations in the study of foreign policy and national security policy, and with political theory in considering ethics in policy making. See the example in Table 12-1.

Health policy is a statement of a decision regarding a goal in health care and a plan for achieving that goal. For example, to prevent an epidemic, a program for inoculating a population is developed and implemented, and priorities and values underlying health resource allocation are determined.

Nursing policy specifies nursing leadership that influences and shapes health policy and nursing practice. Nursing, and therefore nursing leadership, is shaped dramatically by the impact of politics and policy. Effective nursing leadership is a vehicle through which both nursing practice and health policy can be influenced and shaped.

Institutional policies are rules that govern work sites and identify the institution's goals, operation, and treatment of employees.

Organizational policies are rules that govern organizations and their positions on issues with which the organization is concerned (Mason et al., 2007).

Social policy is policy associated with individuals and communities. In very general terms, social policy can be defined as the branch of public policy that advances social welfare and enhances participation in society. Social safety nets, however, often contribute to social exclusion, especially in urban settings, instead of being universally accessible. In most Western societies, social protection usually depends on contributory social insurance schemes to which only regular job holders have access (either in their own right or as dependents). In the United States, this is particularly evident with respect to the way the health care system and Social Security retirement benefits work.

Social justice argues that all individuals and groups receive fair treatment in society, as well as impartially sharing in the benefits of that society (Almgren, 2007).

Administrative agencies are departments of the executive branch with the authority to implement or administer particular legislation.

Laws are rules of conduct or procedure; they result from a *combination* of legislation, judicial decisions, constitutional decisions, and administrative actions.

Public health law focuses on legal issues in public health practice and on the public health effects of legal practice. Public health law typically has three major areas of practice: police power, disease and injury prevention, and the law of populations. Statute, ordinance, or code prescribes sanitary standards and regulation for the purpose of promoting and preserving the community's health. Public health law consists of legislation, regulations, and court decisions enacted by government at the federal, state, and local levels to protect the public's health. This includes case law and treaties.

Statutes are any laws passed by a legislative body at the federal, state, or local level.

Organizations are associations that set and enforce standards in a particular area; a group of individuals who voluntarily enter into an agreement to accomplish a purpose.

A professional association (also called a professional body, professional organization, or professional society) is a nonprofit organization seeking to further a particular profession, the interests of individuals engaged in that profession, and the public interest. It is a volunteer group that seeks to join large numbers of individuals who have a significant wealth of knowledge and experience in a particular field. There are also pooled funds for lobbying purposes (Thomas, 1997). The roles of these professional organizations are viewed as maintaining the control and oversight of the professional occupation, as well as safeguarding the public trust. There is an

TABLE 12-1	TERMINOLOGY EXAMPLE
TOPIC	**EXAMPLE**
Public policy	A local or regional effort to prevent the sale of tobacco or alcohol to minors. Public policy directs that the right to health of the majority must be preserved over individual freedoms and corporate interests.
Public health law	New York State Public Health Law §2164: "Every person in parental (statute) relation to a child in this state shall have administered to such child an adequate dose of an immunizing agent against poliomyelitis, mumps, measles, diphtheria, rubella, varicella, *Haemophilus influenza* type B, and hepatitis B…"
Common law	The Supreme Court decision in *Roe v. Wade*, making first-trimester abortion legal, is an example of how common law becomes enforceable.
Regulation	Reporting communicable diseases to the state and local health departments, which then report them to the CDC.
Treaty	Multilateral treaty: Treaty to eliminate all forms of discrimination against women

element of protecting the interests of the professional practitioners, similar to a cartel or labor union. Inherent in these organizations is the promotion of general standards for the performance of its members and the expectation of continued professional development.

Many professional bodies are involved in the development and monitoring of professional educational programs and the updating of skills, and thus perform professional certification to indicate that a person possesses qualifications in the subject area. Sometimes membership of a professional body is synonymous with certification, though not always. Membership of a professional body, as a legal requirement, can in some professions form the primary formal basis for gaining entry to and setting up practice within the profession. Professional bodies also act as learned societies for the academic disciplines underlying their professions.

Nongovernmental organizations are international organizations that use donations and grants to assist communities in need, with minimal support from, or influence of, a particular nation.

Healthy People 2020

The publication of *Healthy People 2000* by U.S. Surgeon General C. Everett Koop in 1990 led to a resurgence of interest by the federal government in the health and welfare of Americans. However, fiscal resources for public health interventions declined, and only marginal progress was made in meeting the goals. In early 2000, *Healthy People 2010* (U.S. Department of Health and Human Services [USDHHS], 2009) marked the beginning of the new millennium and an enhanced focus on population-based health promotion strategies. Many *Healthy People 2010* objectives directly or indirectly involved health policy. The most recent update, *Healthy People 2020* (USDHHS, 2009) enhances the focus on the social determinents of health and adds even greater emphasis on health policy (*Healthy People 2020* box).

♥ HEALTHY PEOPLE 2020

Selected Objectives Related to Public Policy

OBJECTIVE	BASELINE	GOAL
DSC -4: Eliminate disparities in employment rates between working-aged adults with and without disabilities		
ECBP -4: Increase the proportion of the nation's elementary, middle, and senior high schools that have a nurse-to-student ratio of at least 1:750		
EH – 1: Increase the proportion of persons served by community water systems who receive a supply of drinking water that meets the resignations of the Safe Drinking Water Act.		
EH – 10: Reduce air toxic emissions to decrease the risk of adverse health effects caused by airborne toxins		
FS – 9: Increase the number of states that have prohibited sale or distribution of unpasteurized dairy products		
IID – 21: Increase the proportion of children under age 6 years who participate in fully operational population-based immunization registries		
IVP 10: Increase the number of States and the District of Columbia with laws requiring bicycle helmets for bicycle riders		
IVP 15: Increase age-appropriate vehicle restraint system use in children		
IVP 16: Increase the number of States with strong graduated driver licensing laws		
MCH 22: Ensure appropriate newborn blood-spot screening and follow-up testing		
NWS 18: Increase the number of States that have State-level policies that incentivize food retail outlets to provide foods that are encouraged by the dietary guidelines.		
NWS – 19: Increase the number of states with nutrition standards for foods and beverages provided to preschool-aged children in childcare		
OH – 2: Increase the proportion of the U.S. population served by community water systems with optimally fluoridated water		
TU-3: Reduce the illegal sales rate to minors through enforcement of laws prohibiting the sale of tobacco products to minors		
TU-13: Establish laws in States, District of Columbia, Territories, and Tribes on smoke-free indoor air that prohibit smoking in public places and worksites		
T-16: Increase the State tax on tobacco products		
28-11: Increase the proportion of newborns who are screened for hearing loss by one month of age, have audiologist evaluation by three months of age, and are enrolled in appropriate intervention services by six months of age	93% to 97% 12 states	95% 50 states and DC

From U.S. Department of Health and Human Services: *Healthy People 2020*, 2009 Draft Objectives.

Virtually all of the areas of *Healthy People 2020* have multiple policy-related objectives, and the *Healthy People* box lists only a few of them. Building on previous iterations, the updated draft version has four "over-arching goals" for 2020: attain high quality, longer lives free of preventable disease, disability, injury, and premature death; achieve health equity, eliminate disparities, and improve the health of all age groups; create social and physical environments that promote good health for all; and promote quality of life, health development, and health behaviors across all life stages. Another forward-looking recommendation is making *Healthy People 2020* into a Web-accessible database that is searchable and interactive and will allow users to tailor the document to the public's needs. The intent is that enhanced focus on social determinants represents a "deliberate shift away from the perception that access to health care services will ever solve all of our health care problems" (USDHHS, 2009).

STRUCTURE OF THE GOVERNMENT OF THE UNITED STATES

Government is the structure of principles and rules determining how a state, country, or organization is regulated. Among its purposes are regulation of conditions beyond individual control and provision of individual protection through a population-wide focus. These tasks are accomplished through passage and enforcement of laws. Requirements of childhood immunizations for school attendance, vector control, and sewage treatment are examples of regulations to protect the health of the population.

Government can also be viewed as the sovereign power vested in a nation or state. Sovereign power is the independent and supreme authority of the nation or state. Historical documents describe the government's responsibility for health in the United States and the subsequent authority to enact laws (including health laws). These documents reflect the values of the country's founders. They give the government the authority to enact laws, but they also limit that power. The earliest of these statements was the Mayflower Compact, through which the Pilgrims committed themselves to making "just and equal laws" for the general good. The Declaration of Independence later established the doctrine of inalienable rights, life, liberty, and the pursuit of happiness. However, it was not until the Constitution of the United States was signed by the representatives of the individual states that the federal government realized its sovereign power. At the same time that power was realized, a limit to that power was placed on the federal government. The drafters of the Constitution sought to balance the need to empower the new federal government to "establish Justice, insure domestic Tranquility, provide for the common defence, promote the general Welfare, and secure the Blessings of Liberty" for its people but with limits on that power. That balance is achieved in several important ways.

The federal government is a government of limited powers, which means that for a federal action to be legitimate, it must be authorized. Only those actions that are within the scope of the Constitution, the supreme law of the land, are authorized. The Constitution separates governmental powers among the branches of government (Table 12-2).

Some examples of the separation of powers doctrine that are written into the U.S. Constitution include the following:

- The legislature is prohibited from interfering with the courts' final judgments.
- The Supreme Court cannot decide a "political question"; it must be an actual case or controversy.
- Congress must present a bill to the President before it can become law (Box 12-1).
- The President needs consent of the Senate to appoint Supreme Court Justices or to make treaties.

TABLE 12-2	GOVERNMENT BRANCHES
BRANCH OF GOVERNMENT	**INCLUDES**
Executive branch	The president, the vice president, and the administrative agencies
Legislative branch	The Senate and the House of Representatives (Congress)
Judicial branch	At the federal level: district courts, circuit courts, and the Supreme Court
	At the state level: state and county courts

BOX 12-1   **AN EXAMPLE OF THE PRESIDENT'S RESPONSE TO A HOUSE BILL (A PRESIDENT MAY OR MAY NOT RESPOND TO A BILL)**

State Children's Health Insurance Program or SCHIP

H.R. 2 (and related bills H.R. 57, H.R. 72, and S. 275) became Public Law 111-3, The Children's Health Insurance Reauthorization Act of 2009. This was signed into law by President Barack Obama on February 4, 2009. It went into effect on April 1, 2009.

- Allows certain state plans under Titles XIX (Medicaid) or XXI (State Children's Health Insurance Program) (SCHIP, referred to in this Act as CHIP) of the Social Security Act (SSA) that require state legislation to meet additional requirements imposed by this Act additional time to make required plan changes.
- Provides for coordination of CHIP funding for the 2009 fiscal year.
- Amends SSA Title XXI to reauthorize the CHIP program through FY2013 at increased levels.
  See www.thomas.gov for more information.

- The President and members of Congress are elected; the Judiciary is appointed.

The Constitution not only set forth the responsibilities of the federal government, but it also provided for the individual citizen's rights and freedoms. These are contained in the ten amendments, which were added after the original Articles of the Constitution were ratified in 1787. These ten amendments, added in 1791, are known as the Bill of Rights. The rights guaranteed in the Bill of Rights, such as the rights of free speech and freedom of religion, only applied to the laws and actions of the *federal* government. It would take another 72 years for these rights to be guaranteed within the states. "Liberty interests" and "privacy rights" have been found to exist by determinations by the Supreme Court and have become guiding principles in setting policy and enacting legislation. Note that these rights are only applicable to state or federal government's interaction with people. Violations of restrictions on rights such as free speech do not apply to nongovernmental entities, unless a specific law states otherwise.

Balance of Powers

Federalism is the relationship and distribution of power between the national and the state governments. This balance flows directly from the text of the Constitution: "The powers not delegated to the United States by the Constitution, nor prohibited by it to the States, are reserved to the States respectively, or to the *people*."

States retain powers not delegated to the federal government; therefore much of public health law is under state jurisdiction and, as a result, varies considerably from state to state. These powers to enact laws for the public welfare are referred to as the states' "police powers." Additionally, states may delegate these powers to local governments. In the United States, legislative activities of the three levels of government (federal, state, and local) may vary greatly in their expectations, actions, and results. The state legislatures, for the most part, are directly involved in health care, yet the federal government influences health policy, directly and indirectly, through the financing of health care for many groups (e.g., Medicare), regulation activities (e.g., approval of drugs), and setting of standards (e.g., air quality).

ADMINISTRATIVE AGENCIES

One of the most dramatic changes in American government since the ratification of the Constitution is the growth of administrative agencies. Federal administrative agencies have broad power. They exercise all of the powers of government: executive, legislative, and judicial.

The Food and Drug Administration is one such administrative agency. Its power is in regulating the pharmaceutical industry, as well as the food industry.

Decisions affecting the public's health are made not only at every level of government but also in each branch of government. The separation and balance of powers, referred to as checks and balances, is as important to health as it is to the economic or military status of the country.

The legislative branch (i.e., Congress at the federal level; legislature, general assembly, or general court at the state level) enacts the statutory laws that are the basis for governance. The executive branch administers and enforces the laws, which are broad in scope, through regulatory agencies. These agencies, in turn, define more specific implementation of the statutes through rules and regulations (i.e., regulatory or administrative law). The judiciary body provides protection against oppressive governance and against professional malpractice, fraud, and abuse. Its function, through the courts, both state and federal, is to determine the constitutionality of laws, interpret them, and decide on their legitimacy when they are challenged. Decisions of the U.S. Supreme Court are binding law for the nation. Decisions of the individual state's highest court are binding law within that state alone. The courts also have jurisdiction over specific infractions of laws and regulations.

THE LEGISLATIVE PROCESS

How a Bill Becomes a Law

As stated in the previous section, there is a balance of powers within the government at both state and federal levels. The three branches of government, executive, judicial, and legislative, form a three-legged stool that is in equilibrium.

Along with a separation of powers of the three branches of government, there is an additional mechanism that balances the power of the Congress: bicameralism. Bicameralism ensures that the power to enact laws is shared between the House of Representatives and the Senate. The procedure through which legislation must pass to eventually become law is similar for all U.S. legislative bodies. Once a concept has been drafted into legislative language, it becomes a bill, is given a number, and moves through a series of steps. The bill's passage is sometimes smooth, but, more often than not, the bill is extensively altered through amendments or even killed.

In Congress and in the 49 states that have a two-house legislature, a bill must succeed through the two legislative bodies, that is, the House of Representatives and the Senate (Figure 12-1). Nebraska, which has a single-house legislature, is the exception. A bill that has moved successfully through the legislative process has one final hurdle, which is the chief executive's approval. The approval may be a clear endorsement, in which case the governor or president signs it. If the executive neither signs nor vetoes it, the bill may become law by default. An explicit veto conclusively kills the bill, which then can be revived only by a substantial vote of the legislature to override the veto. This is another example of the checks and balances of the government process.

Issues that find their way into the legislative arena are commonly controversial, and proponents and opponents quickly align themselves. Defeating a bill is much easier than getting one passed; therefore the opposition always has the advantage. Health legislation, which usually requires preventive action (e.g., toxic waste management) or creates a new service (e.g., nursing center organizations for Medicare recipients), is at a disadvantage from several standpoints.

Few elected officials are knowledgeable about the health care field. Although health is readily recognized as a national resource, it is not easily quantified into the economic terms that make the issue easy to grasp. Other disadvantages are the backgrounds, biases, and ambitions of each legislator. Despite these obstacles, good health laws can be passed when concerned nurses and other health care workers understand the legislative process and use it effectively. Nurses should educate their elected officials and be expert tutors for them. In addition, this is yet another mode of intervention on behalf of clients for nurses. Legislation passed to reduce or prevent abuse for all children is as important as physical and emotional care of the abused child.

OVERVIEW OF HEALTH POLICY

Public Health Policy

To review, *public policy* refers to decisions made by legislative, executive, or judicial branches of one of the three levels of government (local, state, or federal). These decisions are intended to direct or influence actions, behaviors, or decisions of others. Public health policies influence health care through the monitoring, production, provision, and financing of health care services.

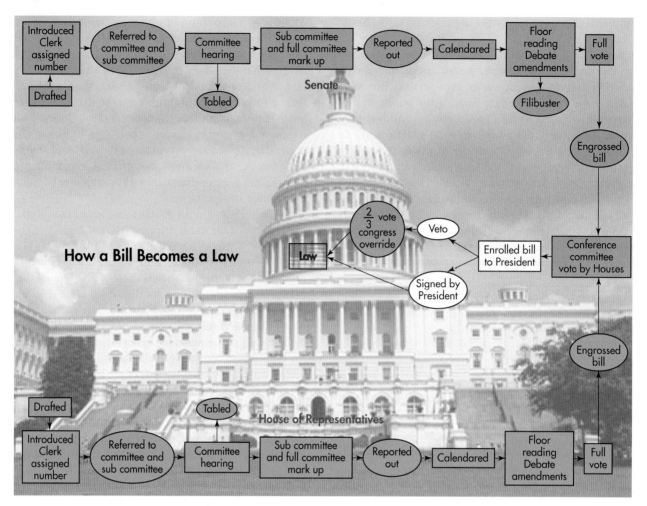

FIGURE 12-1 How a bill becomes a law at the federal level. (Retrieved October 19, 2009, from publicdomainclip-art.blogspot.com/2007_09_01_archive.html.)

Everyone, from health care providers to consumers, is affected by health policies. Likewise, health policy influences corporations, employers, insurers, colleges of nursing, hospitals, clinics, producers and retailers of medical technology and equipment, as well as senior care facilities.

The authority for the protection of the public's health is largely vested with the states, and most state constitutions specifically delineate their responsibility. Municipal subdivisions of states, such as counties, cities, or towns, generally have the power of local control of the services conferred by the state legislature. The responsibility of local, state, and federal governments for health services under varying circumstance sometimes complicates attempts to determine the locus of political decision making. The supremacy of the state prevails in most instances; therefore the state is a critical arena for political action. An example is the state's authority to license health professionals and health care institutions.

Each state establishes policies or standards for goods or services that impact the health of its citizens. However, if the federal government or the local government imposes a higher standard than the state requires, the lower standard is negated by the higher standard. An example would be standardization of pasteurized milk. A state may hold to one standard whereas interstate commerce of the federal jurisdiction may dictate a higher standard that must be met by that state.

The federal government has a strong influence on the health services available in each state. Constitutionally, this authority is derived from the federal role in interstate commerce and through broad interpretation of the "general welfare" clause (e.g., Medicare and Medicaid). States vary considerably in resources allocated to provide health programs; therefore significant de facto authority derives from the promise of revenues or threats to remove funding (e.g., funds for interstate highway repair are often tied to air quality requirements). Federal funds typically fully or partially fund most health care programs.

Compliance by states with federal program standards is voluntary, but the advantage of the revenue, which is withheld from the states that fail to comply, is seldom ignored. Programs such as a statistical reporting system of sexually transmitted infections and control are standardized across the country in response to the indirect but marked effect of federal funding.

Health Policy and the Private Sector

In addition to the public policy making sector, health policies can also be made through the private sector. For example, an insurance company or an employer will determine what illnesses and preventative care will be covered by the insurance program, what drugs are included in the formulary, and how much to charge for an insurance policy. The private sector includes employers, professional organizations (e.g., American Hospital Association), nonprofit health care organizations (American Heart Association), and for-profit corporations that deliver, insure, or fund health care services outside of government control. In particular, health insurance companies and managed care organizations (MCOs) are increasingly setting policies that impact a large number of individuals.

In the private sector, health policy evolves differently than in the public sector. One difference is that private health policy is largely influenced by theories of economics and business management as compared with the social and political theories that predominate in the public sector. In the private sector economics is central, whereas in the public sector economics is but one of many factors. In the private sector decisions can be swift and are often proactive, whereas in the public sector decisions are slow and deliberate, and more reactive. Private sector needs are determined by consumerism, market trends, and economics. Public sector needs are determined by voting shifts, electoral realignment, and term limits (Pulcini et al., 2000). Box 12-2 provides the history of government-funded health care.

PUBLIC POLICY: BLUEPRINT FOR GOVERNANCE

Policy is directed by values. It articulates the guiding principles of collective endeavors, establishes direction, and sets goals. It influences and, in turn, is influenced by politics. Policy directives may become realized or obstructed at any stage in the political process.

Policy Formulation: The Ideal

In ideal circumstances, authorized authoritative bodies (e.g., state health departments, the DHHS, the Centers for Medicare and Medicaid Services) rationally determine actions to create, amend, implement, or rescind health care policy. These groups decide what is right, or best, and then develop the political strategies to effect the desired outcomes. The question of whether a particular policy is advocated or adopted depends on the degree that a group or society as a whole may benefit without harm or detriment to subgroups. Of all the seemingly endless limitless factors that may influence policy formation, group need and group demand should be the strongest determinants. The premises supporting the goals of health policy should be equitable distribution of services and the guarantee that the appropriate care is given to the right people, at the right time, and at a reasonable cost.

Policy Formulation: The Reality

In the real world, policy for health care exemplifies both conflict and social change theories. Health policy is the product of continuous interactive processes in which interested professionals, citizens, institutions, industries, and other interested groups compete with one another for health care dollars and policy initiatives. They also compete with one another for the attention of various branches of government. The most obvious and prominent among these is the legislative branch, although policy is also made through regulatory mechanisms and court decisions. Health policy may also issue from the recommendations of fact-finding commissions established by the legislative or executive branch (Box 12- 3).

BOX 12-2   HISTORY OF GOVERNMENT-FUNDED HEALTH CARE

1965: The Social Security Act established both Medicare and Medicaid. Medicare was a responsibility of the Social Security Administration (SSA), whereas federal assistance to the state Medicaid programs was administered by the Social and Rehabilitation Service (SRS). SSA and SRS were agencies in the Department of Health, Education, and Welfare (HEW).

1977: The Health Care Financing Administration (HCFA) was created under HEW to effectively coordinate Medicare and Medicaid.

1980: HEW was divided into the Department of Education and the Department of Health and Human Services (HHS).

2001: HCFA was renamed the Centers for Medicare and Medicaid Services (CMS). CMS is the federal agency that administers the Medicare and Medicaid program.

2010: Patient Protection and Affordable Care Act was a very comprehensive attempt to improve access to care by providing health insurance to most nation's uninsured.

BOX 12-3   BALANCING THE RESPONSIBILITIES OF THE GOVERNMENT WITH INDIVIDUAL RIGHTS

Example of Statutory and Common Law

Jacobson v. Commonwealth of Massachusetts (1905)

- Massachusetts passes a statute requiring everyone to be vaccinated for smallpox.
- Jacobson refuses to be vaccinated, claiming the requirement of vaccination violated his liberty interests of bodily integrity and decisional privacy.
- The U.S. Supreme Court ruled that "a community has the right to protect itself against an epidemic of disease which threatens the safety of its members." Also, that individual liberty "does not import an absolute right in each person to be, at all times and in all circumstances, wholly freed from restraints. There are manifold restraints to which every person is necessarily subject for the common good."
- Result of the ruling: In this instance, the Supreme Court ruled that the Massachusetts law was constitutional. But when the Court rules against a statutory law, the Supreme Court's decision becomes the law.

From U.S. Supreme Court, *Jacobson v. Commonwealth of Massachusetts*, 197 U.S. 11 (1905).

Health policy is rarely created through discrete, momentous determinations in relation to single problems or issues. It often evolves slowly because changes in the social beliefs and values that underlie established policy develop within the context of actual service delivery. Once a direct health care service is offered, especially an official tax-funded service, it is often difficult to discontinue it. Existing programs create tradition by establishing vested interest and a sense of entitlement on the part of the public. An example is the annual updating of the Centers for Disease Control and Prevention (CDC) recommended childhood and adolescent vaccination schedule. This is also an example of professional organizations working with government agencies to promote the well-being of individuals and communities (Box 12-4).

Steps in Policy Formulation and Analysis

The tangible formulation of public policy begins with the most critical step, which is defining the issue and placing it in the agenda. The next step is the commitment of resources, most often through the passage of legislation. A regulatory schedule for the implementation of the law into program is formulated. Then, an evaluation process is designed that satisfies regulatory and legislative remedies should they be needed. Analysis of health policy is an objective process that identifies the sources and consequences of policy decisions in the context of the factors that influence them. Health policy analysis determines those who benefit and those who experience a loss as the result of a policy. These considerations are critical in order to develop health policies that are fair to all who are affected.

A MAJOR PARADIGM SHIFT

Policy is based on values, and the first step in forming policy is identification of the issue. Therefore, it would seem rational to define "health" as the starting point for any policy annexed to health care issues. Historically, health was defined in the context of infectious diseases. Current definitions encompass prevention and management of chronic conditions. The World Health Organization (WHO) considers health to be the state of complete physical, mental, and social well-being and not merely the absence of disease or infirmity. Despite this broad definition, it is only in the most recent decades that WHO is refocusing on its initial definition as it attempts to deal with environmental issues of nuclear contamination and industrial toxins in industrialized nations and the exploration of carcinogenic commercial products such as tobacco products. On a global level, WHO is working to eliminate antibiotic-resistant bacteria and find a way to solve the human immunodeficiency virus (HIV) pandemic. The emergence of HIV has changed the global health paradigm from the traditional notions of containment and treatment to a more comprehensive approach of social intervention. Thus there is a realization that health is a basic human right and that health problems are linked to government actions, and hence affect human rights.

Human rights violations occur when governments fail to provide their people with the infrastructure, services, and information necessary to promote health, reduce risk, and control disease. For example, for every year of education a woman has, infant mortality is decreased by 10%; yet education of women is not a global reality.

On a national level, the CDC is committed to achieving true improvements in people's lives by accelerating health impact and reducing health disparities. All people, and especially those at greater risk of health disparities, will achieve their optimal lifespan with the best possible quality of health in every stage of life. However, a shift in the paradigm of health concepts would necessitate a substantial reallocation of resources because the vast majority of health spending is directed at medical care and biomedical research and, as such, reflects a viewpoint of health care as a commodity. Considering that more than 47 million have no health insurance and 11.7% of children are uninsured, it becomes clear that the health and human rights relationship is not yet reflected in our health policies.

The Effective Use of Nurses

The Health Resources and Services Administration (HRSA) provides general resources and information to the public and for use in the development of policy by the government. The nursing workforce development programs administered by the HRSA through Title VIII funding provide federal support for nurse workforce development. Title VIII provides the largest source of federal funding for nursing education at the undergraduate and graduate levels and favors institutions that educate nurses for practice in rural and medically underserved communities. In 2007, these programs provided loans, scholarships, traineeships, and programmatic support to more than 70,000 nursing students and nurses.

An issue that is vital to effective health care delivery relates to nurse staffing. The current nursing shortage has been a topic of concern of nurses for many years and is now a health care crisis. Compounding the problem is the fact that nursing colleges and universities across the nation are struggling to expand enrollment to meet the rising demand for nursing care. A shortage of nursing faculty and changing demographics contribute to the projection that all fifty states will experience a shortage of nurses by 2015. The Nurse Education, Expansion, and Development Act of 2009 was introduced to amend Title VIII to authorize capitation grants for nursing schools to increase the number of faculty and students.

NURSES' ROLES IN POLITICAL ACTIVITIES

The Power of One and Many

There are about 3 million registered nurses in the United States (ANA, 2010). Registered nurses are the largest health care professional group. One in 44 women voters is a registered nurse. Why are nurses not more politically active? In 1997, Winter and Lockhart found that there are many factors contributing to the political activism of nurses. Factors identified that facilitate political involvement include being raised in a family that was politically active and having positive role models who exemplified the importance of involvement in health policy, social issues, etc. Hindrances to political action included lack of resources, the slow nature of the political process, time constraints, perceived lack of support from peers and society, gender issues, administrative structure, negative experiences, frustration, burnout, and apathy. More effort needs to be given to educate nurses about the importance of being informed on health policy issues and to encourage them to be politically active. Exposure to positive role models is particularly important. Nurses must obtain the tools to overcome factors that impede involvement. Nurses most often identify positive role models as the major influence that assisted them to become politically active in the profession. Therefore, mentorship at the student level up to expert level is important. Box 12-5 shows responses to a survey about what helped in developing awareness in the profession, policy, and politics.

Nurses as Change Agents

The public, as well as the government, recognizes the nursing profession as indispensible, necessary, and a valuable national resource. In their advocacy role, nurses are seen as professionals whose knowledge, skills, and caring concern are used to promote both the individual's and the community's well-being. Nurses have a unique status in caring for patients; they are interpreters of the health care system to the public, and their professional activites are influenced by

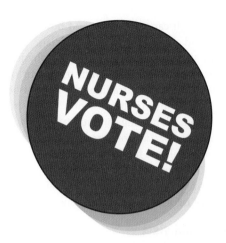

BOX 12-5	RESPONSES TO POLICY ACTIVISM SURVEY

Positive Influences and the Importance of Mentorship

"I became involved in politics through a relationship with a professor who felt strongly about an issue."

"I have found communication among peers to be informative and often inspiring. That has motivated my involvement in health care issues."

"I became aware of the potential role nurses could play related to policy as an undergrad. I had a few dynamic professors that were very inspiring by their involvement and passion related to various issues. At that point I didn't consider myself as someone to get involved but I think it ignited a spark for some day...."

"My exposure to professors that were actually involved in different 'causes' and not just teaching the course made a huge difference in my perspective of getting involved. The continual role model/mentor is also a huge inspiration."

"...nurses who take an interest in current events and enjoy discussing their opinions regarding public policies."

"I think if you don't get exposed to that 'spark' throughout your career it goes out. An inspiring speaker at a professional meeting will get me every time!"

"I was inspired by my professor who was past president for New York State Nurses Association."

"It would be great if one of the clinical nurse specialists at my hospital asked some nurses in a unit what they thought about something and how we could try to change or fix it. We just need that little nudge and some guidance to kindle that passion."

Negative Experiences Influencing Awareness

"I became more aware of the policies from my institution, from preceptors, and when I had a problem. I was more aware as a novice because I was scared to do something that was going to get me into trouble."

"I became more involved at the institutional level after being 'wronged' by administration in regard to a policy, procedure, or benefit."

"I was usually unaware of a policy until it affected me directly; therefore the need to know became paramount."

government-funded programs. The private business sector is also involved. Therefore, public health nurses must know how to participate in the political process. To do this effectively, they need a sound knowledge of the community, state, and national government organization and function and a clear understanding of how these bodies collectively interact to influence policy. Nurses must know how to influence the creation of health care legislation and how to contribute to the election and appointment of key officials.

Although there are more nurses than physicians, hospital administrators, insurance administrators, or other health care professionals, nursing traditionally has not been seen as a major political influence because of a lack of public policy consensus within the nursing community. Unity within professional organizations, coalitions, and lobby efforts is changing this perception. Policy is fundamental to governance; therefore nurses need to know about the formation of public policy and the acts of government and its agencies. Tables 12-3 and 12-4 give sources of information on these issues.

Nurses as Lobbyists

A lobbyist is a person who, voluntarily or for a fee, represents himself or herself, another individual, an organization, or an entity before the legislature. A lobbyist typically represents special interest groups. The term derives from the fact that lobbyists usually stay in the areas (lobbies) next to the Senate and House chambers, seeking to speak with legislators and their aides as they walk to and from the chambers, or as they await legislative action that might affect their interests.

To lobby is to try to influence legislators; it is an art of persuasion. Influencing lawmakers to pass effective health legislation requires the participation of individual nurses and nursing organizations. There are currently more than 100 national nursing organizations. Many also have state chapters. Professional organizations make advocacy easier for members through the use of the Internet. Policy action centers are now part of many organizations' websites. E-mail alerts can be sent instantly to members residing in targeted districts to contact their legislator on a particular bill or issue. By entering one's postal zip code and with a push of a button, a template letter can be signed and sent to one's legislator.

TABLE 12-3   SOURCES FOR LEGISLATIVE INFORMATION

GOVERNMENT LEVEL	INFORMATION AVAILABLE	LOCATION
Federal	Background of members of Congress Committee assignments	Congressional Directory
	Terms of service	Government documents section of selected public or university libraries
	Congressional news	*Congressional Quarterly Weekly Report*
	Vote tabulations	Government documents section of selected public or university libraries
	Bills in process or legislated (bill number needed)	U.S representative or senator (may have local office)
	Health and nursing issues in U.S. Congress	ANA
	ANA-PAC *(The American Nurse)*	600 Maryland Ave SW Suite 100 Washington, DC 20024 (202) 554-4444
	Public health issues in U.S. Congress *(The Nation's Health)*	APHA 1015 15th St NW Washington, DC 20005 (202) 789-5600
State	Bills in process or legislated (bill number needed)	State representative or senator (may have local office)
	Health and nursing issues in state legislature, state PACs for nursing	SNA (for location, see April directory issue of the *American Journal of Nursing*) National League for Nursing

ANA, American Nurses Association; *APHA,* American Public Health Association; *PAC,* political action committee; *SNA,* state nurses association.

TABLE 12-4   SOURCES FOR ELECTORAL INFORMATION

GOVERNMENT LEVEL	INFORMATION AVAILABLE	LOCATION
State	State government operations	Secretary of State (state capitol)
	Political subdivisions	Office of Lieutenant Governor (state capitol)
	Legislative information telephone number	
	State election laws and procedures	
	Campaign finance reports	
County or municipal	Similar to state as appropriate to local government	County clerk (county courthouse)
	Political jurisdictions for each household address	City clerk (city hall)
General	Government information	
	Political jurisdictions for each household address	League of Women Voters
	Names of current office holders in local jurisdictions	1730 M Street NW Washington, DC 20036 (202) 429-1965 Telephone directory (major cities)

The goal of the first contact with an official is to establish that the nurse is a concerned constituent, as well as a credible source of information on health issues. The image of nurses caring for people is a definite advantage at this point. Nurses are considered the most ethical of all health care providers and are considered to be trustworthy. In communities in which nurses have already established strong political credentials, their colleagues will be more readily accepted. An individual who establishes a reputation as a reliable and accurate resource as a lobbyist has substantial influence.

Legislators rely heavily on lobbyists to educate them on issues, and they usually want to hear from all sides before taking a position on an issue. The official must trust the lobbyists to give accurate, though predictably biased information. Information needs to be timely and up-to-date.

Each official represents a constituency with varied needs and interests, and each vote must be weighted within this context. The positions taken by legislators will not always be to an individual or organization's liking. Evaluation of their performance should be based on their overall voting pattern, not just on individual votes. Many organizations regularly tally and publish the records of each federal legislator on all issues related to nursing and health. This information can be helpful in evaluating elected officials. Collective action by nursing and health care organizations is critical to meeting their goals. Professional associations monitor legislative activity related to relevant health issues and link the process to their membership. This continual surveillance of the legislative environment is critical because even seemingly minor amendments can have profound effects on health issues. Thorough legislative surveillance requires the participation of people who are knowledgeable about nursing, health care, and the political intricacies of the legislative process. The ANA, The American Academy of Nursing (AAN), and the National League for Nursing have full-time staff lobbyists who work with Congress. State associations also work with state legislators. State legislative contacts become the eyes, ears, and voices of their professional organizations. These associations can then provide testimony and comment on relevant state and federal issues. However, regardless of the effectiveness of association lobbyists in promoting the interests of nurses and society, they always need grassroots cooperation to truly influence decisions. In the final analysis, a sufficiently high number of communications from individual constituents, via e-mail messages, telephone calls, and letters has the greatest influence. Lobbying is an ongoing activity for health policy issues influencing nursing and health care delivery. Lobby basics (Box 12-6) provide an overview of the lobbying process.

Nurses and Political Action Committees

Political action committees (PACs) have been important sources of collective political influence since the 1970s. These nonpartisan entities promote the election of candidates believed to be sympathetic to their interests. PACs are established by professional associations, businesses, and labor organizations and are highly regulated by federal and state laws that stipulate how they may contribute financially to campaigns. The advantage of a PAC is that small donations

---

BOX 12-6   ABCs OF LOBBYING ON A STATE LEVEL

Before the Meeting
- Appointments will have been made with your legislator(s) for the Lobby Day. Tell the staff that you are a constituent and what issue(s) you would like to discuss with your representative. If your legislator is unavailable, you may have a scheduled appointment with a member of the legislative staff.
- If possible, put together a delegation of nurses to attend the meeting. A number of individuals from the legislator's district who are concerned about the same issue will make a big impression. Take along students from their districts, as the legislators are impressed with their participation.

Preparing for the Meeting
- Establish your agenda and goals. For example, focus on educating the legislators on the profession of nurse midwifery, the legislation that this group would like them to sponsor, the concerns about the malpractice insurance crisis and the benefit to women's and children's health. Nurse practitioners would focus on the cost-benefit of NP's as primary care providers in all settings, including health care homes.
- Research your legislator's stance prior to the meeting. It is important that you know your official's position so that you can present your stance more effectively and have an intelligent discussion.
- Meet with the midwifery delegation that will participate in the lobbying. It is important that you review what each person will say during the meeting. Select someone as the group leader and make a list of points to be made and questions to be asked by each individual.

- Prepare materials. Review the packet of information you will leave with your legislator. It is important to include your name and phone number in the packet so that your legislator will have a contact person for more information. Leaving a business card would be appropriate.

During the Meeting
- Be on time for your meeting.
- Be concise and diplomatic. Keep your presentation short and to the point.
- Be a good listener. Look for indications of your legislator's views and watch for opportunities to provide useful information in order to strengthen or counter particular views.
- Stress why the issues concern you and others in your district.
- Don't be intimated. Your legislator is in office to serve you. It is important to have a general knowledge of the issues, but you don't have to know every little detail. If he/she asks a question that you do not know the answer to, simply say that you do not know but are willing to find out. Find out the best way to get the information to him/her (fax, e-mail, or a follow-up phone call).

After the Meeting
- Write a follow-up letter. After your visit, write a letter thanking your legislator for his/her time. Cards are included in your folder for you to mail prior to leaving the legislative building.
- Stay in contact with your legislator. Remember your goal is to strengthen midwifery relationships with your legislators.

From New York State Association of Licensed Midwives (NYSALM): *The Voice of Midwives* letter.

from many members add up to a significant donation to a campaign fund in the name of the organization. This gains the attention of the candidate and earns good will for the group.

Valid concern exists about the correlation of major PAC contributions and legislators' votes on special interest legislation. However, as long as PACs are a reality of political life, nurses need to recognize their power and support those that are committed to electing candidates sympathetic to health care issues.

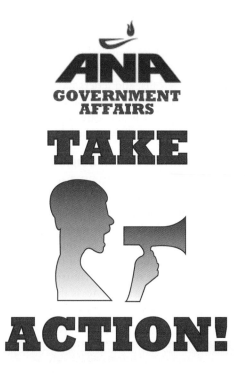

Most national associations of health care providers have PACs. Among the more powerful are those representing hospitals, nursing homes, health insurers, home health agencies, and pharmaceutical companies. A PAC that makes major political contributions is the American Medical Political Action Committee, sponsored by the American Medical Association. State medical associations also have strong PACs. This means that organized medicine has a powerful influence on national and state elections and on health care legislation at both levels.

Nurses in Public Office

President Barack Obama named Mary Wakefield, PhD, RN, administrator of the HRSA on February 20, 2009. HRSA is an agency of the DHHS.

HRSA works to fill in the health care gaps for people who live outside the economic and medical mainstream. The agency uses its $7 billion annual budget (FY 2008) to expand access to quality health care in partnership with health care providers and health professions training programs.

"As a nurse, a PhD, and a leading rural health care advocate, Mary Wakefield brings expertise that will be instrumental in expanding and improving services for those who are currently

uninsured or underserved," President Obama said in announcing her appointment. "Under her leadership, we will be able to expand and improve the care provided at the community health centers, which serve millions of uninsured Americans and address severe provider shortages across the country."

She has served on the Medicare Payment Advisory Commission, as chair of the National Advisory Council for the Agency for Healthcare Research and Quality, as a member of President Clinton's Advisory Commission on Consumer Protection and Quality in the Health Care Industry, and as a member of the National Advisory Committee to HRSA's Office of Rural Health Policy (HRSA, 2010).

There are currently three nurses in the 111th Congress. They are Lois Capps of California, Eddie Johnson of Texas, and Carolyn McCarthy of New York.

Other women who have been active in the federal government are Carolyne Davis, who, in 2001, served as the administrator of the Health Care Financing Administration (renamed the Centers for Medicare and Medicaid Services), Shirley Chater, was Commissioner of the Social Service Administration, and Patricia Montoya was Commissioner for Children, Youth, and Families. Virginia Trotter Betts, who served as the President of the ANA, was also the Senior Advisor on Nursing and Policy to the Secretary of HHS in Washington, DC. Likewise, Dr. Beverly Malone resigned as President of the ANA in 1999 to assume the position of Deputy Assistant Secretary of the HHS. In this capacity, she advised the Assistant Secretary for the HHS, Dr. David Satcher, in program and political matters, policy and program development, and setting of legislative priorities. Janet Heinrich is Associate Administrator of the Bureau of Health Professionals and Michele Richardson is Director of the Division of Nursing.

In the future, more nurses need to run for public office at all three levels of government. Whether serving as political appointees or career bureaucrats, nurses have much to offer. Young and beginning nurses should accept the challenge of helping to advance the nursing practice and the nation's health.

Shift in CDC Policy

The existence of awareness of the health and human rights relationship is also seen nationally. In its 2004 annual report, the CDC describes health broadly and in terms similar to those used by WHO (CDC, 2004). The CDC's commitment to protecting health is reinforced and guided by a set of four overarching Health Protection Goals that focus on better health for all people by accelerating health impact and achieving health equity. An example goal is that all people, and especially those at greater risk of health disparities, will achieve their optimal lifespan with the best possible quality of health in every stage (CDC, 2008). Box 12-7 illustrates the shifts in CDC philosophy.

Nursing's Involvement in Private Health Policy

Nursing should incorporate private health policy into its policy agenda. Nurses can influence private health care organizations from internal and external positions. From an internal

BOX 12-7	SHIFTS IN PHILOSOPHY AT THE CDC
FROM	**TO**
Disease orientation	Health protection focus
Designing and implementing sponsored programs	Informing and guiding health system actors
Allocating agency resources	Leveraging resources to steer larger health system
Emphasis on clinical prevention	Focus on prevention and health protection
Transaction-based relationships	Partnerships and strategic alliances
Program requirements	Incentives for participation/cooperation
Collecting and analyzing health data	Creating integrated health information systems
Issuing advisories and guidelines	Building decision-support system

From Centers for Disease Control and Prevention: *State of the CDC: fiscal year 2008*, The Author.

perspective, nurses can hold important management positions in MCOs. This would allow direct involvement in policy setting. Nurses can also support and use nursing research that demonstrates positive clinical and economic outcomes. This would serve to validate the importance of nursing within the health system (Pulcini et al., 2000).

External strategies that nurses can use to influence private health policy include participation in discussions regarding quality and managed care (Pulcini et al., 2000). Nurses should monitor the quality ratings of MCOs and suggest changes in providers accordingly. Nurses can also build entrepreneurial practices to provide lower-cost services for underserved groups and can encourage clients to call and write their managed care plan organization to request that nursing services be reimbursable. Nurses should work cooperatively with other health professions to influence MCOs to improve quality of care.

Restructuring of the Health Care Industry

Health care reform was a major topic of discussion during the 2008 presidential election. With the election of President Obama and significant Democratic majorities in both the Senate and the House, it appeared that health care reform would pass easily. After the failed attempt at comprehensive reform, during the early years of the Clinton presidency, politicians recognized some of the major concerns and issues and addressed them proactively. For example, strong opposition from many health care provider groups (i.e., physicians) and the health care industry groups (i.e., insurers, pharmaceutical companies, hospitals) led to failure of the Clinton plan. In 2009, Congressional leaders early on sought ways to attract leaders of these groups and convince them to support reform measures.

A great deal of debate on what should be included in reform was evident throughout 2009. Major items of contention included whether to require all Americans to purchase coverage (i.e., a health insurance mandate), whether there

would be a "government option" whereby people could elect to be covered by an extension of Medicare (or another, similar government-sponsored and funded program), whether government funds will pay for abortions, and how all of the changes and mandates would eventually be financed. After much public and private debate, in March 2010, the House of Representatives rather reluctantly passed the bill which the Senate had approved in late 2009, and President Obama signed it into law on March 23, 2010.

Although the 2010 Patient Protection and Affordable Care Act is extremely controversial, and the long-term effects of its implementation are unclear, health care reform is a nursing issue, and few nurses will argue with the statement that reform is needed in the health system in the United States. In virtually every practice arena, nurses see the inequalities and inadequacies that diminish the nation's level of wellness. Recognition of these problems is important to discussions of reform, and changing policies and targeting popular beliefs that create barriers to reform are essential in correcting the inequalities and inadequacies.

The economic structure of the United States is a market economy. There is a strong and prevailing political and popular belief in market-driven systems. Competition, which includes increasing quality and lowering costs, drives the market economy, thereby theoretically creating an even more robust economy with better goods and services. In the health care arena, efforts to lower costs have been aimed at decreasing payments to providers, hospitals, and pharmaceutical companies. Providers, in turn, avoid unprofitable patients. Competition between insurers exists less by increasing quality or lowering costs than by shifting costs. The business of health care generates huge administrative costs that, along with profits, divert resources from providing care to the demands of business.

These are some of the areas targeted by the Health Reform Act. For example, insurers will no longer be able to drop coverage for those who are seriously ill as the act prohibits health insurance plans for placing lifetime limits on coverage and prohibits insurers from rescinding coverage for those who are diagnosed with chronic or life-threatening conditions. Additionally, mechanisms to reduce administrative costs are encouraged (Kaiser Family Foundation, 2010).

Popular sentiments about governmental control over health care have mirrored attitudes concerning the governmental role in general; this was very evident during the debates over reform. The politically viable range of cost-control measures available to public programs has been limited to cutbacks in payments to providers rather than limits on the demand for clinical services or limits on individual choice.

In addition to overall health care reform, one of the issues that is vital to effective health care delivery relates to nurse staffing. Staffing has been a topic of concern of nurses for many years because inadequate and inappropriate staffing can threaten patients' safety, the nurses' health, and commitment to the profession. Inappropriate staffing also contributes to pressure experienced by nurses because of increasing patient intensity, increasing complexity of care, and fatigue.

The Registered Nurse Safe Staffing Act of 2005 (S. 71/H.R. 1372) was introduced in Congress to address these concerns. See Box 12-8 for highlights of the Bill. It was later referred to committees in both the Senate and the House of Representatives.

RESEARCH HIGHLIGHTS

National Sample of Registered Nurses

The Division of Nursing, a component of the HRSA, helps direct policy through the National Sample Survey of Registered Nurses. This survey has been conducted nine times since 1977 and was done most recently in March 2008 and preliminary findings were released in 2010 (HRSA, 2010). The national survey looks at trends in demographics, employment, education, and compensation among registered nurses (RNs).

- Number of licensed RNs in the United States grew by almost 5.3% between 2004 and 2008 to a new hight of slightly more than 3 million.
- Average age of RNs climbed to 47.0 years, the highest average age since the first comparable report was published in 1980.
- Average annual earning for RNs were $66,973.
- Real earnings (comparable dollars over time) have grown almost 16% since 2004.
- The share of RNs whose initial nursing education was a bachelor's degree in nursing rose from 31% to 33.7% between 2004 and 2008.
- Employment in nursing rose to almost 85% of RNs with active licenses, the highest since 1980.
- RNs with master's or doctorate degrees rose to more than 400,000, an increase of 32% from 2000.

Data from Health Resources and Services Administration: The registered nurse population: Initial findings from the 2008 national sample survey of registered nurses, Washington, DC, 2010. The Author.

Chief Nurse Executive

In 2002, then Michigan Governor Jennifer Granholm appointed the nation's first state chief nurse executive. The position focuses on policy and legislation related to Michigan's nursing workforce, as well as nursing's unique expertise in addressing the health care needs of the state (Michigan Department of Community Health, 2002).

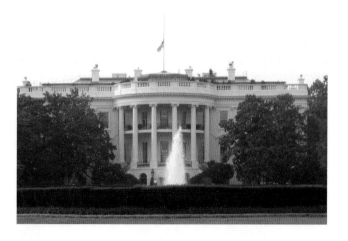

BOX 12-8   **THE REGISTERED NURSE SAFE STAFFING ACT OF 2007 (H.R. 4138/S.73)**

The Registered Nurse Safe Staffing Act of 2007 amends part D (Miscellaneous) of title XVIII (Medicare) of the Social Security Act (SSA) to: (1) require each participating hospital to adopt and implement a staffing system that ensures a number of registered nurses on each shift and in each unit of the hospital to ensure appropriate staffing levels for patient care; (2) provide for the public reporting of certain staffing information, including a daily posting for each shift in the hospital of the current number of licensed and unlicensed nursing staff directly responsible for patient care; (3) prescribe recordkeeping, data collection, and evaluation requirements for participating hospitals; (4) specify civil monetary penalties for violations of such requirements; and (5) provide whistleblower protections.

From H.R. 4138—110th Congress: Registered Nurse Safe Staffing Act of 2007. (2007). In GovTrack.us (database of federal legislation). Retrieved January 12, 2010, from www.govtrack.us/congress/bill.xpd?bill=h110-4138&tab=summary.

A State Organization: NYSALM

In New York State, more than 1000 licensed midwives recognized a need for organized advocacy on the state level. The American College of Nurse-Midwives, which represents nearly 10,000 certified nurse-midwives and certified midwives nationally, did not have a mechanism in its structure (bylaws) to develop state organizations. In 1999, the midwives of New York State formed the New York State Association of Licensed Midwives (NYSALM). NYSALM's organizational objectives include effecting legislation and regulations for its members. Each year, NYSALM brings midwives of the state together for a lobby day in the state capitol. In a few short years, their lobbying efforts have been successful in advancing their profession. NYSALM reaches out to student midwives, encouraging their participation as advocates early in their professional career. Box 12-9 lists priorities supported by the ANA.

Nurses and Coalitions

When two or more groups join to maximize resources, increasing their influence and improving their chances of success in achieving a common goal, it is called a coalition. Coalitions of health care providers often work together on issues such as family violence and fluoridation of water supplies. An outstanding example of such cooperative action is the establishment of rehabilitation programs for health professionals whose practice has been impaired by substance abuse or mental health problems.

Nursing and consumer groups often form coalitions to advance their shared interests in health promotion. The ANA joined 16 other organizations (e.g., American College of Nurse Practitioners, American Red Cross, Department of Veterans Affairs, and Sigma Theta Tau) to form a coalition called Nurses for a Healthier Tomorrow. Responding to concerns about a potentially dangerous shortage of nurses, this coalition hopes to raise funds for a national advertising

From American Nurses Association: *Federal issues* www.nursingworld.org/
MainMenuCategories/ANAPoliticalPower/Federal/Issues.aspx. Accessed April
29, 2010.

BOX 12-9 FEDERAL ISSUES AND REGULATORY PRIORITIES OF THE ANA

Nursing Shortage
Fiscal year 2009 Omnibus Appropriations Act
Funding for workplace development
Immigration and the nurse workforce

Appropriate Staffing
Adequate nursing facility staffing
Nurse Reinvestment Act
Mandatory overtime

Workplace Rights
Barriers to practice for advanced practice registered nurses
Advanced practice nursing Medicaid reimbursement
Healthcare Truth and Transparency Act

Workplace Health and Safety
Health care worker safety
Safe patient handling and movement

Patient Safety/Advocacy
American Recovery and Reinvestment Act
Association health plans
Medicaid cost containment and Medicaid cuts in funding

BOX 12-10 PROFESSIONAL ORGANIZATIONS JOINING FORCES: AMERICANS FOR NURSING SHORTAGE RELIEF ALLIANCE (ANSRA)

ANSRA is a coalition of thirty-seven nursing organizations that was founded in the early 2000s to influence policy and funding decisions related to nursing shortages. It does this through

- Media attention to the nation's growing nursing shortage
- Advocacy for legislation that will reverse the nursing shortage
- Working with Congress to increase funding through the Nurse Reinvestment Act
- Promoting nursing education, retention, and faculty development
- Developing funding initiatives for nursing education loans and scholarships
- Researching into nursing workforce, staffing issues

In September 2004, ANSRA presented a briefing to Congress, titled "The Nursing Faculty Shortage: A National Perspective." In early 2005, ANSRA held a reception for members of Congress and their health legislative assistants to bring the nursing faculty shortage to the attention of federal policy makers.

campaign designed to recruit new nurses and encourage existing ones to remain in the profession (Box 12-10). The coalition hopes to attract major health insurers, managed care companies, pharmaceutical firms, health care providers, nursing schools, and hospitals to support the campaign. The campaign focuses on the message that nurses are essential to the health care team and that they save health care dollars.

The campaign shows that an increased demand exists for nurses, both in specialty areas and outside the hospital (ANA, 1999).

Nurses and Health Policy Development

As the role of nurses in changing health care policy increases in importance, more nurses are needed who are equipped for this challenge. A strong cadre of nursing leaders who have the vision for change is essential to promoting nursing's policy agenda. National fellowships and internships are available for nurses who are interested in taking leadership roles (Sharp, 1999).

The Robert Wood Johnson Health Policy Fellowship is a 1-year career development program for midcareer health professionals. The goal of this program is to help nurses gain an understanding of the health policy process and contribute to the formulation of new policies and programs. Robert Wood Johnson Health Policy fellows are selected from academic faculties from diverse disciplines, including medicine, dentistry, nursing, public health, health services administration, economics, and social services. After an extensive orientation on the legislative and executive branches of government, the fellows work with a member of Congress or on a congressional health committee (Sharp, 1999).

The President's Commission on White House Fellowships offers 20 fellowships each year to nurses early in their careers; the average age is 33 years. The White House fellows participate in an education program that involves working with government officials, scholars, journalists, and private-sector leaders to explore U.S. policy in action. Nurses who have been White House fellows may work at the Centers for Medicare and Medicaid Services and the Office of Science and Technology Policy, among others (Sharp, 1999). These fellowship programs are competitive, but strong leaders are desperately needed.

Nurses and Campaigning

Helping someone win an election is a sure way of gaining influence. All candidates are grateful for campaign assistance and usually remember to thank those who have helped. Although campaign contributions are commonly thought of as financial, they can also take the form of participation in campaign activities. Nurses are frequently unable to contribute much money; therefore, they can provide these invaluable services. For the novice, veteran campaigners are eager to help him or her learn the necessary skills. Initially, a volunteer can address or stuff envelopes for mailings. The volunteer can also invite friends and neighbors for a social gathering to meet the candidate, thereby providing an opportunity to discuss issues of concern with constituents.

Telephone banks help a candidate identify supporters, opponents, and the critical undecided voter. These latter voters can make a difference on election day and are courted by all candidates. The telephone interviews are highly structured and easily handled by inexperienced campaign workers. Direct contact with potential voters may occur later in the form of house-to-house block walks or poll work on election day. The confidence that this requires comes with experience and a strong commitment to the candidate and the cause. Hosting a social function to allow nurse colleagues to meet the candidate is a welcome contribution to the campaign. Nurses are substantial in number, and their voting record is humanistic; therefore they are valued as a political force.

Government employees may be restricted by policies that limit or disallow political activism. Nurses employed at any level of government should be aware of such prohibitions.

Nurses and Voting Strength

With around 3 million members, nurses make up the largest profession in health care (ANA, 2010; HRSA, 2010). It is estimated that one in forty-five voters is a registered nurse (Hadley, 1996). Therefore if every registered nurse voted, the influence of registered nurses on health policy would be tremendous. If the nursing profession is to meet the challenges of the twenty-first century and work as a profession to positively influence the health of populations, political action is necessary, and an understanding of the factors that motivate or impede political action is needed (Winter and Lockhart, 1997).

INTERNET AND POLITICAL PROCESS

A 30-day window of opportunity is typical for public input into the development of regulations. Written comments about a political issue are made part of the public record. To facilitate correspondence, websites have been set up to promote contacting agencies, governmental organizations, and political figures. Nurses need to be aware of some of the important websites. Furthermore, many legislators may have their own web pages so that the nurse can easily access their offices. Numerous websites related to health policy issues may be accessed through the WebLinks section of this book's website at http://evolve.elsevier.com/Nies/.

The Internet can provide almost unlimited access to information. However, access to information does not ensure the quality or credibility of the information. The user is responsible for evaluation of the information and separation of quality information from misinformation. Nurses need to be information and communication technology literate. Technology literacy is the ability of an individual, working independently and with others, to responsibly, appropriately, and effectively use technology tools to access, manage, integrate, evaluate, create, and communicate information. Technology fluency builds upon technology literacy and is demonstrated when nurses: apply technology to real-world experiences, adapt to changing technologies, modify current as well as create new technologies, and personalize technology to meet personal needs, interests, and learning style.

Twitter is a free social networking and microblogging service that enables its users to send and read each other's updates, known as *tweets*. Tweets are text-based posts of up to 140 characters, displayed on the author's profile page and delivered to other users—known as followers—who have subscribed to them. Senders can restrict delivery to those in their circle of friends or, by default, allow open access.

Users can send and receive tweets via the Twitter website, Short Message Service (SMS), or external applications. The service is free over the Internet, but using SMS may incur phone service provider fees. Facebook is a free-access social networking website that is operated and privately owned by Facebook, Inc. According to its website, users can join as individuals or join networks organized by location, work interests, profession, school, or hobbies. People and groups add others to their network and can share personal and professional information. YouTube provides a means of sharing user-generated video and audio media. It is a subsidiary of Google, Inc. The 44th president of the United States, Barack Obama, has included YouTube video on the White House website and also links to Twitter, Facebook, and Flickr.

■ SUMMARY

Historically, nurses have been able to make significant differences in the quality of life experienced by the members of the communities in which they serve. By understanding how government works, how bills become laws, and how legislators make decisions, nurses can influence policy decisions through individual efforts such as electronic letter writing, social networking, participation in political campaigns, and selection of candidates who support policies conducive to improving the health and welfare of all citizens. When organized in lobbying groups, coalitions, and PACs, or when holding office, nurses can be a powerful force that brings about change in the delivery and quality of the health care of aggregates.

■ LEARNING ACTIVITIES

1. Develop an "insight" bulletin board, with each class member contributing cartoons, anecdotes, and clippings about issues affecting public health or nursing.
2. Look at a current public health issue that affects your community, including an understanding of the causes, effect on the public, and possible solutions. Influence its resolution through any of the following activities:
   a. Write a succinct letter to the editor of a local newspaper.
   b. Write a position paper and submit it to the "opinion page" of a local newspaper.
   c. Write to elected or appointed officials whose jurisdiction may be influential on the issue.
   d. Meet with an elected or appointed official to discuss the issue in groups of two or three. Write a one-page summary of your "talking points" to leave with the official.
   e. Call in to a radio talk show about the issue.
   f. Volunteer to speak on the issue to appropriate consumer or professional groups.
3. With a group of two or three, meet with an elected official for a 15-minute appointment to ask about the official's concerns and priorities. Remember to refer to the "ABCs of Lobbying" prior to meeting with the official.
4. Invite an elected official who is sympathetic to nurses to speak to the local chapter of the National Student Nurses Association to discuss the political process and health policy.

5. Invite an elected official to spend a day engaging in appropriate activities with a public health nurse or nursing student. Take black-and-white photos for press use.
6. Invite a medical reporter from the press, radio, or television to observe public health nursing activities that would appeal to the public.
7. Participate in a group organized around a public health issue (e.g., disposable diapers, toxic waste, or fluoride).
8. Serve as a volunteer in a campaign for a candidate who is supportive or potentially supportive of public health or nursing issues.
9. Serve as a volunteer for a political party.

REFERENCES

Almgren G: *Health care, politics, policy and services*, New York, 2007, Springer.

American Nurses Association: ANA advises on health care reform, *Capital Update* 11(8):1, 1993.

American Nurses Association (ANA): 2009. www.nursingworld.org/Function/menucategory/aboutANA.aspx, accessed March 1, 2010.

Centers for Disease Control and Prevention: Annual report, 2004: www.cdc.gov.

Centers for Disease Control and Prevention: State of the CDC: fiscal year: 2008,The Author: www.cdc.gov/about/stateofcdc/FY08/cd/SOCDC/SOCDC2008.pdf.

de Vries C, Vanderbilt M: Nurses gain ground during reform debate, *Am Nurse* 26(10):2–3, 1994.

Hadley EH: Nursing in the political and economic marketplace: challenges for the 21st century, *Nurs Outlook* 44(1):6–10, 1996.

Hall-Long BA: Nursing's past, present, and future political experiences, *Nurs Health Care Perspect* 16(1):24–28, 1995.

Health Resources and Services Administration: *The registered nurse population: Initial findings from the national 2008 sample survey of registered nurses*, Washington, DC, 2010, The Author.

Healthy People 2020: Secretary's Advisory Committee on National Health Promotion and Disease Prevention for 2020: *U.S. Department of Health and Human Services*,

2009: www.healthypeople.gov/HP2020/advisory/PhaseI/PhaseI.pdf. Accessed May 20, 2008.

Institute of Medicine: Biographical information: *2001 Lienhard Award Recipient Ruth Watson Lubic*, 2001, The Author: www.iom.edu/subpage.asp?id=5046.

Kaiser Family Foundation: Focus on health reform 2010. www.kff.org/healthreform/upload/8061.pdf 2010b.

Kalisch PA, Kalisch BJ: *American nursing: a history*, ed 4, Philadelphia, 2004, Lippincott Williams & Wilkins.

Lewinson SB: A historical perspective on policy, politics and nursing. In Mason DJ, Leavitt JK, Chaffee MW, editors: *Policy and politics in nursing and health care*, ed 5, Philadelphia, 2007, Saunders.

Litman T: *Health, politics and policy*, ed 3, Albany, NY, 1997, Delmar.

Lyttle B: Humanizing childbirth, *Am J Nurs* 100(10):52–53, 2000.

Mason DJ, Leavitt JK, Chaffee MW: Policy and politics: a framework for action. In Mason DJ, Leavitt JK, Chaffee MW, editors: *Policy and politics in nursing and health care*, ed 4, Philadelphia, 2002, Saunders.

Mason DJ, Leavitt JK, Chaffee MW: Policy and politics: a framework for action. In Mason DJ, Leavitt JK, Chaffee MW, editors: *Policy and politics in nursing and health care*, ed 5, St. Louis, 2007, Saunders.

Michigan Department of Community Health: 2002, www.Michigan.gov.mdch/0,1607,7=132-3150=40178-135921--,00,html. Accessed March 1, 1010.

Pulcini J, et al: Health policy and the private sector: new vistas for nursing, *Nurs Health Care Perspect* 21(1):22–28, 2000.

Sharp N: Wanted: nurse leaders to craft health policy, *Nurse Pract* 24(10):85–86, 89, 1999.

Thomas J: *Introduction—the role of professional associations, Library Trends, Fall 1997*, findarticles.com/p/articles/mi_m1387/is_n2_v46/ai_20365179. Accessed July 18, 2009.

US Department of Health and Human Services: *Healthy People 2010*, Conference ed, Washington, DC, 2000, The Author.

US Department of Health and Human Services, Centers for Medicare and Medicaid Services: FY 2005 budget in brief, 2004: www.dhhs.gov/budget/05budget/centersformed.html#med.

US Department of Health and Human Services, Office of Disease Prevention and Health Promotion, *Healthy People 2020*: The Road Ahead, Nov 3, 2009. Accessed March 1, 2010.

US Department of Health and Human Services, Health Resources and Services Administration: Accessed March 1, 2010.

Winter MK, Lockhart JS: From motivation to action: understanding nurses' political involvement, *Nurs Health Care Perspect* 18(5):244–250, 1997.

Cultural Diversity and Community Health Nursing

*Carrie L. Abele**

Additional Material for Study, Review, and Further Exploration

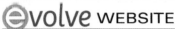 WEBSITE

http://evolve.elsevier.com/Nies
- Quiz
- Case Studies
- Glossary
- WebLinks

OBJECTIVES

Upon completion of this chapter, the reader will be able to do the following:

1. Critically analyze racial and cultural diversity in the United States.
2. Analyze the influence of sociocultural, political, economic, ethical, and religious factors that influence

the health of culturally diverse individuals, groups, and communities.

3. Identify the cultural aspects of nursing care for culturally diverse individuals, groups, and communities.
4. Apply the principles of transcultural nursing to community health nursing practice.

KEY TERMS

biomedical
cultural imposition
cultural negotiation
cultural stereotyping
culture
culture shock
culture specific
culture universal
culture-bound syndrome

culturological assessment
dominant value orientation
ethnocentrism
Leininger's theory of culture care
   diversity and universality
magicoreligious
naturalistic
norms
poverty

religion
socioeconomic status (SES)
spirituality
subculture
transcultural nursing
value
yin-yang theory

OUTLINE

---

*The author would like to acknowledge the contribution of Margaret M. Andrews, who wrote this chapter for the previous edition.

CULTURAL DIVERSITY

Cultural diversity is a multifaceted and complex concept that refers to the differences among people, especially those related to values, attitudes, beliefs, norms, behaviors, customs, and ways of living. It is essential that all nurses understand how cultural groups view life processes, how cultural groups define health and illness, how healers cure and care for members of their respective cultural groups, and how the cultural background of the nurse influences the way in which care is delivered. Nurses in community health settings also need to understand the diversity or differences that occur in families, groups, neighborhoods, communities, and public and community health care organizations.

TRANSCULTURAL PERSPECTIVES ON COMMUNITY HEALTH NURSING

Nurses' knowledge of culture and cultural concepts improves the health of the community by enhancing their ability to provide culturally competent care. Culturally competent community health nursing requires that nurses understand the lifestyle, value system, and health and illness behaviors of diverse individuals, families, groups, and communities. Nurses also should understand the culture of institutions that influence the health and well-being of communities. Nurses who have knowledge of, and an ability to work with, diverse cultures are able to devise effective interventions to reduce risks in a manner that is culturally congruent with community, group, and individual values.

In the United States, metaphors such as *melting pot, mosaic,* and *salad bowl* describe the cultural diversity that characterizes the population. Although there is a tendency to identify the federally defined racial and ethnic minority groups when referring to the cultural aspects of community

health nursing, all individuals, families, groups, communities, and institutions, including nurses and the nursing profession, have cultural characteristics that influence community health. When planning and implementing health care, community health nurses need to balance cultural diversity with the universal human experience and common needs of all people.

POPULATION TRENDS

The population of the United States is becoming increasingly diverse. In recent years, the populations within the federally defined minority groups have grown faster than the population as a whole. In 1970, minority groups accounted for 16% of the population. By 1999, this share increased to 30%. Assuming that current trends continue, the U.S. Census Bureau (2009) projects that, by 2025, more than half of all children will be minorities and that, by 2050 minorities will account for 54% of the total population. For the first time in U.S. history, minorities will make up a majority of the total population.

Furthermore, the numbers of certain minority groups, such as Hispanics, are growing considerably faster than those of whites and other groups. If current demographic trends continue, the United States will have the following population composition by the year 2050: white, 44%; Hispanic, 30%; black, 15%; Asian, 9%; and American Indians and Alaska Natives, 2% (U.S. Census Bureau, 2009).

Although the nursing profession has representatives from diverse groups, minorities are generally underrepresented. Currently about 81.8% of registered nurses (RNs) in the United States are white/non-Hispanic. Estimates for each minority group are as follows: black, 4.2%; Hispanic, 1.7%; Asian and Pacific Islander, 3.1%; and Native American and Alaska Native,

0.3% (Health Resources and Services Administration [HRSA], 2009). Additionally, each minority group is distributed differently around the country. Black nurses are more likely to be found in the South, Hispanics in the West or South (i.e., especially states bordering Mexico), and Asian and Pacific Islanders in the West or Northeast. Native American and Alaska Native nurses are predominantly in states with reservations.

The United States has grown and achieved its success largely through immigration. Since 1991, more than 13 million legal immigrants have come to United States (U.S. Department of Homeland Security, 2006). In 2003, the U.S. population included 33.5 million foreign-born individuals, or 11.7% of the total population. Among those foreign born, 53.3% were born in Latin America, 25% in Asia, 13.7% in Europe, and the remaining 8% in other regions of the world (U.S. Census Bureau, 2004). The number of immigrants and refugees in the United States is projected to continue to increase.

In addition, people from other countries will continue to seek treatment in U.S. hospitals, particularly for cardiovascular, neurological, and cancer care, and U.S. nurses will have the opportunity to travel abroad to work in a variety of health care settings in the international marketplace. In the course of a nursing career, it is possible to encounter foreign visitors, international university faculty members, international high school and university students, family members of foreign diplomats, immigrants, refugees, as well as members of more than 130 different ethnic groups, and Native Americans from more than 557 federally recognized tribes. A serious conceptual problem exists within nursing in that nurses are expected to know, understand, and meet the health needs of these culturally diverse individuals, groups, and communities.

Members of some cultural groups desire culturally relevant health care that incorporates their specific beliefs and practices. An increasing expectation exists among members of certain cultural groups that health care providers will respect their "cultural health rights," an expectation that frequently conflicts with the unicultural, Western biomedical worldview taught in most U.S. educational programs that prepare nurses and other health care providers.

Given the multicultural composition of the United States and the projected increase in the number of individuals from diverse cultural backgrounds, concern for cultural beliefs and practices of people in community health nursing is becoming increasingly important. Nursing is inherently a transcultural phenomenon, in that the context and process of helping people involves at least two people who often have different cultural orientations or intracultural lifestyles.

CULTURAL PERSPECTIVES AND *HEALTHY PEOPLE 2020*

Healthy People 2020, the new proposed prevention agenda for the nation, identifies priority areas and objectives. By developing a set of national health targets, which includes eliminating racial and ethnic disparities in health, U.S. health officials, together with state and local officials and members of the private sector, set goals to increase the quality and years of healthy life for all Americans (U.S. Department of Health and Human Services [USDHHS], 2009).

The *Healthy People 2020* proposed objectives embrace and focus on ways to close the gaps in health outcomes. Particularly targeted are racial and ethnic disparities in areas including diabetes, acquired immunodeficiency syndrome (AIDS), heart disease, infant mortality rates, cancer screening and management, and immunizations. The objectives bring focus on disparities among racial and ethnic minorities, women, youth, older adults, people of low income and

---

♥ HEALTHY PEOPLE 2020

Selected Proposed Objectives Related to Cultural Health

OBJECTIVE

PHI–11: Increase the proportion of all degrees awarded to members of underrepresented racial and ethnic groups among the health professions, allied and associated health profession fields, the nursing field, and the public health field

BDBS–2: Reduce hospitalizations for sickle cell disease among children age 9 years and under

C–Reduce the overall cancer death rate

CKD–1: Reduce the rate of new cases of end-stage renal disease (ESRD)

D–4: Reduce the rate of lower extremity amputations in persons with diabetes

FP–8: Reduce pregnancy rates among adolescent females

HDS–1: Reduce coronary heart disease deaths

HDS–3: Reduce stroke deaths

HIV–17: Reduce HIV incidence among adults and adolescents

IID–18: Achieve and maintain effective vaccination coverage levels for universally recommended vaccines among young children

IVP–Reduce firearm-related deaths

MICH–7: Reduce low birth weight (LBW) and very low birth weight (VLBW)

NWS–2: Reduce the proportion of adults who are obese

SA–6: Reduce past-month use of illicit substances

From US Department of Health and Human Services: *Healthy People 2020*: 2009 draft objectives. Accessed from www.healthypeople.gov/HP2020/Objectives/TopicAreas.aspx.

SIDS, Sudden infant death syndrome, *NA*, not available.

education, and people with disabilities (USDHHS, 2000). The *Healthy People 2020* box lists selected objectives from *Healthy People 2020* specific to cultural health issues.

The aims of *Healthy People 2020* are the promotion of healthy behaviors, promotion of healthy and safe communities, improvement of systems for personal and public health, and prevention and reduction of diseases and disorders. The initiative is a tool for monitoring and tracking health status, health risks, and use of health services.

Addressing Racial and Ethnic Disparities in Health Care

As in many nations, people in the United States who come from various racial, ethnic, cultural, and socioeconomic backgrounds often experience marked disparities in health care. The occurrence of many diseases, injuries, and other public health problems is disproportionately higher in some groups; access to health care may be more restricted, and the overall quality of health care is deemed inferior, for people from certain racial, ethnic, and cultural populations. Although the overall health of the U.S. population has improved during the past several decades, research reveals that all people have not shared equally in those improvements. For example, 17% of Hispanic adults and 16% of black adults report that they are in fair or poor health, compared with 10% of non-Hispanic whites (Agency for Healthcare Research and Quality, 2005).

Primary care provides the foundation for the health care system, and research indicates that having a usual source of care increases the chance that people will receive adequate preventive care and other important health services. Data from the Agency for Healthcare Research and Quality (2005) reveal the following facts:

- Cancer mortality rates are 35% higher in black Americans than in whites.
- Black Americans who have diabetes are seven times more likely to have amputations and renal failure than are whites with diabetes.
- Thirty percent of Hispanics and 20% of black Americans lack a usual source of health care (compared with fewer than 16% of whites).
- Hispanic children are nearly three times as likely as non-Hispanic white children to have no usual source of health care.
- Black Americans (16%) and Hispanic Americans (13%) are more likely to rely on hospitals or clinics for health care than are whites (8%).

During the past two decades, health disparities have become the focus of numerous federal, state, and local government studies, and one of the major goals of *Healthy People 2020* is to achieve health equity, eliminate disparities, and improve the health of all groups (USDHHS, 2009). Therefore, it is essential to look at how to overcome these and other identified factors that contribute to poorer health among members of some minority groups. A recent study by the Commonwealth Fund (2007) found that disparities in health care can be reduced or even eliminated when adults have health care insurance and a medical home, which is defined as "a health care setting that provides patients with timely, well-organized care and enhanced access to providers." According to the survey, when adults have insurance and a medical home, "their access to needed care, receipt of routine preventive screenings, and management of chronic conditions improve substantially."

TRANSCULTURAL NURSING

In 1959, Madeleine Leininger, a nurse-anthropologist, used the term transcultural nursing to define the philosophical and theoretical similarities between nursing and anthropology. In 1968, Leininger proposed her theory-generated model, and, in 1970, she wrote the first book on transcultural nursing, *Nursing and Anthropology: Two Worlds to Blend* (Leininger, 1970). According to Leininger (1978), transcultural nursing is "a formal area of study and practice focused on a comparative analysis of different cultures and subcultures in the world with respect to cultural care, health and illness beliefs, values, and practices with the goal of using this knowledge to provide culture-specific and culture-universal nursing care to people" (p. 493). Culture specific refers to the "particularistic values, beliefs, and patterning of behavior that tend to be special, 'local,' or unique to a designated culture and which do not tend to be shared with members of other cultures" (Leininger, 1991, p. 491), whereas culture universal refers to the "commonalties of values, norms of behavior, and life patterns that are similarly held among cultures about human behavior and lifestyles and form the bases for formulating theories for developing cross-cultural laws of human behavior" (Leininger, 1991, p. 491).

Although many nurse-scholars have developed theories of nursing, Leininger's theory of culture care diversity and universality is the only one that gives precedence to understanding the cultural dimensions of human care and caring. Leininger's theory is concerned with describing, explaining, and projecting nursing similarities and differences focused primarily on human care and caring in human cultures. Leininger used worldview, social structure, language, ethnohistory, environmental context, and the generic or folk and professional systems to provide a comprehensive and holistic view of influences in cultural care and well-being. The following three models of nursing decisions and actions may be useful in providing culturally congruent and competent care (Andrews and Boyle, 2008; Leininger, 1978, 1991, 1995; Leininger and McFarland, 2002):

1. Culture care preservation and maintenance
2. Culture care accommodation and negotiation
3. Culture care repatterning and restructuring

Among the strengths of Leininger's theory is its flexibility for use with individuals, families, groups, communities, and institutions in diverse health systems. Leininger's Sunrise Model (Figure 13-1) depicts the theory of cultural care diversity and universality and provides a visual representation of the key components of the theory and the interrelationships among its components.

The term *cross-cultural nursing* is sometimes used synonymously with *transcultural nursing*. The terms *intercultural*

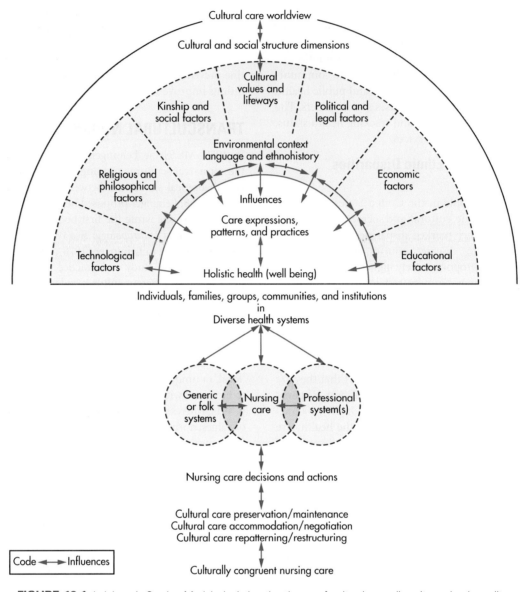

FIGURE 13-1 Leininger's Sunrise Model, depicting the theory of cultural care diversity and universality. (From Leininger MM: *Culture, care, diversity, and universality: a theory of nursing,* New York, 1991, National League for Nursing Press.)

nursing and *multicultural nursing* and the phrase "ethnic people of color" are also used. Since Leininger's early work, many nurses have contributed significantly to the advancement of nursing care of culturally diverse clients, groups, and communities, and some of their contributions are mentioned in this chapter.

One of the major challenges that community health nurses face in working with clients from culturally diverse backgrounds is overcoming individual ethnocentrism, which is a person's tendency to view his or her own way of life as the most desirable, acceptable, or best and tendency to act in a superior manner toward individuals from another culture. Nurses also must beware of cultural imposition, which is a person's tendency to impose his or her own beliefs, values, and patterns of behavior on individuals from another culture. When clients' cultural values and expressions of care differ

from those of the nurse, the nurse must exercise caution to ensure that mutual goals have been established.

OVERVIEW OF CULTURE

In 1871, the English anthropologist Sir Edward Tylor was the first to define the term *culture*. According to Tylor (1871), culture refers to the complex whole, including knowledge, beliefs, art, morals, law, customs, and any other capabilities and habits acquired by virtue of the fact that one is a member of a particular society. Culture represents a person's way of perceiving, evaluating, and behaving within his or her world, and it provides the blueprint for determining his or her values, beliefs, and practices. Culture has four basic characteristics:

1. It is learned from birth through the processes of language acquisition and socialization.

2. It is shared by members of the same cultural group.
3. It is adapted to specific conditions related to environmental and technical factors and to the availability of natural resources.
4. It is dynamic.

Culture is an all-pervasive and universal phenomenon. However, the culture that develops in any given society is always specific and distinctive, encompassing the knowledge, beliefs, customs, and skills acquired by members of that society. Within cultures, groups of individuals share beliefs, values, and attitudes that are different from those of other groups within the same culture. Ethnicity, religion, education, occupation, age, sex, and individual preferences and variations bring differences. When such groups function within a large culture, they are termed *subcultural groups.*

The term subculture is used for fairly large aggregates of people who share characteristics that are not common to all members of the culture and that enable them to be a distinguishable subgroup. Ethnicity, religion, occupation, health-related characteristics, age, sex, and geographic location are frequently used to identify subcultural groups. Examples of U.S. subcultures based on ethnicity (e.g., subcultures with common traits such as physical characteristics, language, or ancestry) include blacks, Hispanics, Native Americans, and Chinese Americans. Subcultures based on religion include members of the more than 1200 recognized religions, such as Catholics, Jews, Mormons, Muslims, and Buddhists. Those based on occupation include health care professionals (e.g., nurses and physicians), career military personnel, and farmers. Those based on health-related characteristics include the blind, hearing impaired, and mentally challenged. Subcultures based on age include adolescents and older adults, and those based on sex or sexual preference include women, men, lesbians, and gay men. Those based on geographic location include Appalachians, Southerners, and New Yorkers.

Culture and the Formation of Values

According to Leininger (1995), value refers to a desirable or undesirable state of affairs. Values are a universal feature of all cultures, although the types and expressions of values differ widely. Norms are the rules by which human behavior is governed and result from the cultural values held by the group. All societies have rules or norms that specify appropriate and inappropriate behavior. Individuals are rewarded or punished as they conform to, or deviate from, the established norms. Values and norms, along with the acceptable and unacceptable behaviors associated with them, are learned in childhood.

Every society has a dominant value orientation, a basic value orientation that is shared by the majority of its members as a result of early common experiences. In the United States, the dominant value orientation is reflected in the dominant cultural group, which is made up of white, middle-class Protestants, typically those who came to the United States at least two generations ago from northern Europe. Many members of the dominant cultural group are of Anglo-Saxon descent; thus, they are sometimes referred to as white Anglo-Saxon Protestants (WASPs). In the United States, the dominant cultural group places emphasis on educational achievement, science, technology, individual expression, democracy, experimentation, and informality.

Although an assumption is sometimes made that the term *white* refers to a homogeneous group of Americans, a rich diversity of ethnic variation exists among the many groups that constitute the dominant majority. Countries of origin include those of eastern and western Europe (e.g., Ireland, Poland, Italy, France, Sweden, and Russia). The origins of people in Canada, Australia, New Zealand, and South Africa can ultimately be traced to western Europe. Appalachians, the Amish, Cajuns, and other subgroups are also examples of whites who have cultural roots that are recognizably different from those of the dominant cultural group.

Values and norms vary, sometimes significantly, among various cultural groups. According to Kluckhohn and Strodtbeck (1961), several basic human problems exist for which all people must find a solution. They identified the following five common human problems related to values and norms:

1. What is the character of innate human nature (human nature orientation)?
2. What is the relationship of the human to nature (person-nature orientation)?
3. What is the temporal focus (i.e., time sense) of human life (time orientation)?
4. What is the mode of human activity (activity orientation)?
5. What is the mode of human relationships (social orientation)?

Human Nature Orientation

Innate human nature may be good, evil, or a combination of good and evil. Some believe that life is a struggle to overcome a basically evil nature; they consider human nature to be unalterable or able to be perfected only through great discipline and effort. For others, human nature is perceived as fundamentally good, unalterable, and difficult or impossible to corrupt.

According to Kohls (1984), the dominant U.S. cultural group chooses to believe the best about a person until that person proves otherwise. Concern in the United States for prison reform, social rehabilitation, and the plight of less fortunate people around the world is a reflective perception of the belief in the fundamental goodness of human nature. Recent scientific advances, such as the advent of stem cell research and genome studies, have necessitated consideration of ethical quandaries regarding human nature. Questions emerge as to whether science can or should pursue activities that could alter the basic human orientation.

Person-Nature Orientation

The following three perspectives examine the ways in which the person-nature relationship is perceived:

1. Destiny, in which people are subjugated to nature in a fatalistic, inevitable manner
2. Harmony, in which people and nature exist together as a single entity
3. Mastery, in which people are intended to overcome natural forces and put them to use for the benefit of humankind

Most Americans consider humans and nature clearly separated; this is an incomprehensible perspective for many individuals of Asian heritage. The idea that a person can control his or her own destiny is alien to many individuals of culturally diverse backgrounds. Many cultures believe that people are driven and controlled by fate and can do very little, if anything, to influence it. Americans, by contrast, have an insatiable drive to subdue, dominate, and control their natural environment.

For example, the reader should consider three individuals in whom hypertension has been diagnosed, where each embraces one of the values orientations described. The person whose values orientation is destiny may say, "Why should I bother watching my diet, taking medication, and getting regular blood pressure checks? High blood pressure is part of my genetic destiny and there is nothing I can do to change the outcome. There is no need to waste money on prescription drugs and health checkups." The person whose values orientation embraces harmony may say, "If I follow the diet described and use medication to lower my blood pressure, I can restore the balance and harmony that were upset by this illness. The emotional stress I've been feeling indicates an inner lack of harmony that needs to be balanced." The person whose values orientation leads to belief in active mastery may say, "I will overcome this hypertension no matter what. By eating the right foods, working toward stress reduction, and conquering the disease with medication, I will take charge of the situation and influence the course of my disease."

Time Orientation

People can perceive time in the following three ways:

1. *The focus may be on the past, with traditions and ancestors playing an important role in the client's life.* For example, many Asians, Native Americans, East Indians, and Africans hold particular beliefs about ancestors and tend to value long-standing traditions. In times of crisis, such as illness, individuals with a values orientation emphasizing the past may consult with ancestors or ask for their guidance or protection during the illness.
2. *The focus may be on the present, with little attention paid to the past or the future.* These individuals are concerned with the current situation, and they perceive the future as vague or unpredictable. Nurses may have difficulty encouraging these individuals to prepare for the future (e.g., to participate in primary prevention measures).
3. *The focus may be on the future, with progress and change highly valued.* These individuals may express discontent with the past and present. In terms of health care, these individuals may inquire about the "latest treatment" and the most advanced equipment available for a particular problem.

The dominant U.S. cultural group is characterized by a belief in progress and a future orientation. This implies a strong task or goal focus. This group has an optimistic faith in what the future will bring. Change is often equated with improvement, and a rapid rate of change is usually normal.

Activity Orientation

This values orientation concerns activity. Philosophers have suggested the following three perspectives:

1. *Being,* in which a spontaneous expression of impulses and desires is largely nondevelopmental in nature
2. *Growing,* in which the person is self-contained and has inner control, including the ability to self-actualize
3. *Doing,* in which the person actively strives to achieve and accomplish something that is regarded highly

The person often directs the doing toward achievement of an externally applied standard, such as a code of behavior from a religious or ethical perspective. The Ten Commandments, Pillars of Islam, Hippocratic oath, and Nightingale pledge are examples of externally applied standards.

The dominant cultural value is action oriented, with an emphasis on productivity and being busy. As a result of this action orientation, Americans have become proficient at problem solving and decision making. Even during leisure time and vacations, many Americans value activity.

Social Orientation

Variations in cultural values orientation are also related to the relationships that exist with others. Relationships may be categorized in the following three ways:

1. *Lineal relationships:* These exist by virtue of heredity and kinship ties. These relationships follow an ordered succession and have continuity through time.
2. *Collateral relationships:* The focus is primarily on group goals, and family orientation is important. For example, many Asian clients describe family honor and the importance of working together toward an achievement of the group versus a personal goal.
3. *Individual relationships:* These refer to personal autonomy and independence. Individual goals dominate, and group goals become secondary.

The social orientation among the dominant U.S. cultural group is toward the importance of the individual and the equality of all people. Friendly, informal, outgoing, and extroverted members of the dominant cultural group tend to scorn rank and authority. For example, nursing students may call faculty members by their first names, clients may call nurses by their first names, and employees may fraternize with their employers.

Members of the dominant culture have a strong sense of individuality. However, family ties are relatively weak, as demonstrated by the high rate of separation and divorce in the United States, as well as the frequently widespread geographic separation of extended families. In many U.S. households, the family has been reduced to its smallest unit: the single-parent family.

When making health-related decisions, clients from culturally diverse backgrounds rely on relationships with others in various ways. If the cultural values orientation is lineal, the client may seek assistance from other members of the family and allow a relative (e.g., parent, grandparent, or elder brother) to make decisions about important health-related matters. If collateral relationships are valued, decisions about the client may be interrelated with the influence of illness on the entire family or group. For example, among the Amish, the entire community is affected by the illness of a member because the community pays for health care from a common fund. Members join together to meet the needs of the client and family for the duration of the illness, and the roles of many in the community are likely to be affected by the illness of a single member.

In another example, there are approximately 10.3 million undocumented residents living in the United States (Passel, 2005). These individuals often create their own social groups in which they seek to protect themselves from being discovered by immigration authorities. These groups fear that attempting to access the health care system may lead to deportation, and they often have "underground" or private access to home remedies and pharmaceuticals for their health care. As a result, they often enter the formal health care system via emergency departments when their health status has declined considerably.

A values orientation that emphasizes the individual is predominant among the dominant cultural majority in the United States. Decision making about health and illness is often an individual matter, with the client being responsible, although members of the nuclear family may participate to varying degrees.

Culture and the Family

The family remains the basic social unit in the United States. Although various ways exist to categorize families, the following are commonly recognized types of constellations in which people live together in society:

- Nuclear (i.e., husband, wife, and child or children)
- Nuclear dyad (i.e., husband and wife alone, either childless or with no children living at home)
- Single parent (i.e., either mother or father and at least one child)
- Blended (i.e., husband, wife, and children from previous relationships)
- Extended (i.e., nuclear plus other blood relatives)
- Communal (i.e., group of men and women with or without children)
- Cohabitation (i.e., unmarried man and woman sharing a household with or without children)
- Gay (i.e., same-gender couples with or without children)

In addition to structural differences in families cross-culturally, accompanying functional diversity may exist. For example, among extended families, kin residence sharing has long been recognized as a viable alternative to managing scarce resources, meeting child care needs, and caring for a handicapped or older family member. Sometimes the shared household is an adaptation for survival and protection. In general, families with a culturally diverse heritage include a large number of adults and a larger number of children.

The family constellations associated with teen parenting are unique and provide a special socialization context for infants. For example, Hispanic teen mothers receive more child care help from grandmothers and peers than do white teen mothers. Among blacks and Puerto Ricans, the presence of the maternal grandmother ameliorates the negative consequences of adolescent childbirth on the infant. In addition, grandmothers are more responsive and less punitive in their

interactions with the infant than their daughters (Andrews and Boyle, 2008). Three-generational households can have an influence on the infant's development: by influencing the mother's knowledge about development and providing other more responsive social interactions with infants.

Families from diverse backgrounds are often characterized as being more conservative in terms of sex roles and parenting values and practices than white families. For example, traditional Japanese-American and Mexican-American families are family centered, enforce strict gender and age roles, and emphasize children's compliance with authority figures. Children of culturally diverse backgrounds are involved in family interactions that differ from those of children from the dominant U.S. cultural group. The values of children of immigrants typically evolve, depending on how far removed they are from the country of origin. These children may detach from their cultural traditions, becoming more individually focused or autonomous—often to the dismay of the elders in the family. Often the language of the ancestors is forgotten, or in certain subcultures, forbidden to be spoken, so that the children may assimilate to the dominant culture.

Relationships that may seem apparent sometimes warrant further exploration by nurses interacting with clients from culturally diverse backgrounds. For example, the dominant cultural group defines siblings as two people with the same mother, the same father, the same mother and father, or the same adoptive parents. In some Asian cultures, a sibling relationship is defined as involving infants who are breastfed by the same woman. In other cultures, certain kinship patterns, such as maternal first cousins, are sibling relationships. In some African cultures, anyone from the same village or town may be called "brother" or "sister."

Certain subcultures, such as Roman Catholics, who may be further subdivided by ethnicity into those who are Italian, Polish, Spanish, Mexican, and so on, recognize relationships such as "godmother" and "godfather." The godmother/godfather is an individual who is not the biological parent but promises to assist with the moral and spiritual development of an infant and agrees to care for the child in the event of parental death. The godparent makes these promises during the religious ceremony of baptism.

When providing care for infants and children, the nurse must identify the primary provider of care because this individual may or may not be the biological parent. For example, among some Hispanic groups, female members of the nuclear or extended family (e.g., sisters or aunts) are sometimes the primary providers of care. In some black families, the grandmother may be the decision maker and primary caregiver of the children.

CULTURE AND SOCIOECONOMIC FACTORS

No single indicator can adequately capture all facets of economic status for entire populations, but measures such as median or average annual income, employment rate, poverty rate, and net worth are most often used. The economic status of most individuals, especially children, is better reflected by the pooled resources of family or household members than by their individual earnings or incomes. Socioeconomic status (SES) is a composite of the economic status of a family or unrelated individuals based on income, wealth, occupation, educational attainment, and power. It is a means of measuring inequalities based on economic differences and the manner in which families live as a result of their economic well-being. Most families with racially or ethnically diverse backgrounds have a lower SES than the population at large, with a few exceptions (e.g., Cuban Americans and subgroups of Asian Americans).

Poverty is another factor that dramatically influences health and well-being. National poverty data are calculated using the official U.S. Census Bureau definition of poverty, which has remained standard since its initial introduction in the mid-1960s. Under this definition, poverty is determined by comparing pretax cash income with the poverty threshold, which adjusts for family size and composition. Table 13-1 provides an overview of the poverty thresholds according to size of family and number of related children under age 18 years residing in the home. The poverty guidelines are issued each year by the USDHHS. The guidelines are a simplification of the poverty threshold for administrative purposes, such as determining financial eligibility for federal programs (e.g., Head Start, National School Lunch, Medicaid, Aid to Families with Dependent Children) (U.S. Census Bureau, 2007).

According to the U.S. Census Bureau (2008), the poverty rate in 2007 was 12.5%. The distribution of the poor varies considerably on the basis of certain factors such as age, race or ethnicity, and marital status. For example, 24.5% of the black population, 10.2% of the Asian population, and 21.5% of the Hispanic population live in poverty. In addition, children under 6 years of age are particularly vulnerable to poverty, with 20.8% of all U.S. children in this age-group being poor.

Distribution of Resources

Status, power, and wealth in the United States are not distributed equally throughout society. Rather, a small percentage of the population enjoys most of the nation's resources, primarily through ownership of multibillion-dollar corporations, large pieces of real estate in prime locations, and similar assets. The U.S. population has traditionally been divided into the following three social classes: upper, middle, and lower. SES may be calculated by considering a variety of factors, but it is customarily determined by examining factors such as total family income, occupation, and educational level. In a less formalized examination of SES, factors such as age, sex, material possessions, health status, family name, location of residence, family composition, amount of land owned, religion, race, and ethnicity may also be considered.

A disproportionate number of individuals from the racially and ethnically diverse subgroups are members of the lower socioeconomic class, whereas a larger percentage of members of the dominant cultural group (i.e., WASPs) belong to the upper and middle socioeconomic classes. The United States has socioeconomic stratification; therefore, the idealization of America as the land of opportunity often applies more to members of the upper and middle classes than to those of the lower class. The outcome of social stratification is social inequality. For example, school systems, grocery stores, and recreational facilities vary significantly between the inner city, which has a high percentage of minority residents, and the suburbs, which are overwhelmingly WASP.

For many years, health care settings have been the subject of study and concern regarding distribution of resources, with members of racial and ethnic minority groups compellingly pointing out the inequalities. Because financing of health care in the United States largely relies on a combination of federally funded insurance (i.e., Medicare) and employer-provided health insurance, those from the highest SES and elders tend

TABLE 13-1	POVERTY THRESHOLDS FOR 2009 BY SIZE OF FAMILY AND NUMBER OF RELATED CHILDREN UNDER 18 YEARS								
	RELATED CHILDREN UNDER 18 YEARS								
SIZE OF FAMILY UNIT	NONE	ONE	TWO	THREE	FOUR	FIVE	SIX	SEVEN	EIGHT OR MORE
One person (unrelated individual)									
Under 65 years	11,161								
65 years and over	10,289								
Two people									
Householder under 65 years	14,366	14,787							
Householder 65 years and over	12,968	14,731							
Three people	16,781	17,268	17,285						
Four people	22,128	22,490	21,756	21,832					
Five people	26,686	27,074	26,245	25,603	25,211				
Six people	30,693	30,815	30,180	29,571	28,666	28,130			
Seven people	35,316	35,537	34,777	34,247	33,260	32,108	30,845		
Eight people	39,498	39,847	39,130	38,501	37,610	36,478	35,300	35,000	
Nine people or more	47,514	47,744	47,109	46,576	45,701	44,497	43,408	43,138	41,476

Note: The poverty thresholds are updated each year using the change in the average annual Consumer Price Index for All Urban Consumers (CPI-U). Since the average annual CPI-U for 2009 was lower than the average annual CPI-U for 2008, poverty thresholds for 2009 are slightly lower than the corresponding thresholds for 2008.
Source: U.S. Census Bureau. http://www.census.gov/hhes/www/poverty/threshold/threshold09.html

to receive the best health care. In contrast, those from low SES groups (i.e., those without health insurance or with Medicaid) tend to receive less health care. Thus, in the United States, SES largely determines acess to health care, as well as the quality of care received.

Education

One of the components considered in determining SES is educational level. Educational attainment is perhaps the single most important factor. In recent years, there has been an improvement in the level of education among those who have historically been less educated (e.g., elders, women, minorities). For example, women have a higher rate of high school completion than men. Also, dropout rates for both blacks and Hispanics are steadily declining (National Center for Educational Statistics, 2008).

Research suggests that differences between white and Mexican-American children's home educational development can be accounted for by differences in levels of formal schooling rather than by cultural differences or economic indices. According to a study by Garcia Coll (1990), mothers who had received more years of formal education inquired and praised their children more often than did mothers with less education. In contrast, the lower the mother's level of formal education, the more often she used modeling as a teaching strategy. Compared with white mothers, Hispanic mothers inquired and praised less often and used modeling, visual cues, directives, and negative physical control more often. However, these differences disappeared entirely when the mother's or father's educational level was controlled statistically. This study contributes to an understanding of the ways in which educational level attained by people from culturally diverse backgrounds affects the didactic aspects of the child-rearing environment.

CULTURE AND NUTRITION

Long after assimilation into U.S. culture has occurred, many members of various ethnic groups will continue to follow culturally based dietary practices and eat ethnic foods. When a new group of immigrants arrives in the United States, neighborhood food markets and ethnic restaurants are often established soon after arrival. The ethnic restaurant is often a place for members of the cultural group to meet and mingle, and customers from the dominant cultural group may be of secondary interest. Food is an integral part of cultural identity that extends beyond dietary preferences.

Nutrition Assessment of Culturally Diverse Groups

Factors that must be considered in a nutrition assessment include the cultural definition of food, frequency and number of meals eaten away from home, form and content of ceremonial meals, amount and types of food eaten, and regularity of food consumption. Twenty-four-hour dietary recalls or 3-day food records traditionally used for assessment may be inadequate when dealing with clients from culturally diverse

backgrounds. Standard dietary handbooks may fail to provide culture-specific diet information because nutritional content and exchange tables are usually based on Western diets. Another source of error may originate from the cultural patterns of eating. For example, among low-income urban black families, elaborate weekend meals are frequent, whereas weekday dietary patterns are markedly more moderate.

Although community health nurses may assume that food is a culture-universal term, they may need to clarify its meaning with the client. For example, certain Latin-American groups do not consider greens, an important source of vitamins, to be food and fail to list intake of these vegetables on daily records. Among Vietnamese refugees, dietary intake of calcium may appear inadequate because low consumption rates of dairy products are common among members of this group. However, they commonly consume pork bones and shells, providing adequate quantities of calcium to meet daily requirements.

Food is only one part of eating. In some cultures, social contacts during meals are restricted to members of the immediate or extended family. For example, in some Middle Eastern cultures, men and women eat meals separately, or women are permitted to eat with their husbands but not with other males. Among some Hispanic groups, the male breadwinner is served first, then the women and children eat. Etiquette during meals, use of hands, type of eating utensils (e.g., chopsticks or special flatware), and protocols governing the order in which food is consumed during a meal all vary cross-culturally.

Dietary Practices of Selected Cultural Groups

Cultural stereotyping is the tendency to view individuals of common cultural backgrounds similarly and according to a preconceived notion of how they behave. However, not all Chinese like rice, not all Italians like spaghetti, and not all Mexicans like tortillas. Nevertheless, aggregate dietary preferences among people from certain cultural groups can be described (e.g., characteristic ethnic dishes and methods of food preparation, including use of cooking oils); the reader is referred to nutrition texts on the topic for detailed information about culture-specific diets and the nutritional value of ethnic foods.

Religion and Diet

Cultural food preferences are often interrelated with religious dietary beliefs and practices. As indicated in Table 13-2, many religions have proscriptive dietary practices and some use food as symbols in celebrations and rituals. Knowing the client's religious practice as it relates to food makes it possible to suggest improvements or modifications that will not conflict with religious dietary laws.

Fasting and other religious observations may limit a person's food or liquid intake during specified times. For example, many Catholics fast or abstain from meat on Ash Wednesday and each Friday of Lent, Muslims refrain from eating during the daytime hours for the month of Ramadan but are permitted to eat after sunset, and Mormons refrain from ingesting all solid foods and liquids on the first Sunday of each month.

TABLE 13-2	DIETARY PRACTICES OF SELECTED RELIGIOUS GROUPS
RELIGION	**DIETARY PRACTICE**
Hinduism	All meats are prohibited.
Islam	Pork and intoxicating beverages are prohibited.
Judaism	Pork, predatory fowl, shellfish, other water creatures (fish with scales are permissible), and blood by ingestion (e.g., blood sausage and raw meat) are prohibited. Blood by transfusion is acceptable. Foods should be kosher (meaning "properly preserved"). All animals must be ritually slaughtered by a shochet (i.e., quickly with the least pain possible) to be kosher. Mixing dairy and meat dishes at the same meal is prohibited.
Mormonism (Church of Jesus Christ of Latter-day Saints)	Alcohol, tobacco, and beverages containing caffeine (e.g., coffee, tea, colas, and select carbonated soft drinks) are prohibited.
Seventh-Day Adventism	Pork, certain seafood (including shellfish), and fermented beverages are prohibited. A vegetarian diet is encouraged.

CULTURE AND RELIGION

According to the *Yearbook of American and Canadian Churches* (National Council of Churches, 2005), in North America, more than 226 million people are affiliated with organized religion. A recent Gallup Poll (Gallup, 2008) found that 78% of Americans report that they believe in God. Further, about 66% note that they are members of a church, synagogue, or mosque. The largest religious groups are Protestant, 48%; Catholic, 23%; Jewish, 2%; Mormon, 2%; and other, 12%. The largest specific Protestant denominations are, in order, Baptist (other than Southern Baptist), Methodist, Southern Baptist, Lutheran, and Presbyterian.

Although the nurse cannot be an expert on each of the estimated 1200 religions practiced in the United States, knowledge of health-related beliefs and practices and general information about religious observances are important in providing culturally competent nursing care. For example, when planning home visits or scheduling clinic visits for members of a specific religious group, the nurse should consult the group's religious calendar and work around designated holy days. The nurse should also know the customary days of religious worship observed by members of the religion. Most Protestants worship on Sundays, whereas Muslims' holy day of worship extends from sunset on Thursday to sunset on Friday, and Jews and Seventh-Day Adventists' holy day extends from sunset on Friday to sunset on Saturday. Roman Catholics may worship in the late afternoon or evening of Saturday or all day Sunday. Some religions may meet more than once weekly.

In addition to regularly scheduled weekly religious services, most major religions also recognize special days of observance

or celebration that last from 1 day (e.g., Christmas, Easter, Rosh Hashanah, and Janmashtami) to 1 month (e.g., Ramadan). Some days of commemoration or observation are based on a lunar calendar and some have rotating dates; the nurse may consult official information sources, such as religious leaders or religious calendars, to verify exact dates. The nurse should also ask clients what religious practices they follow, because individual activity within the religious organization may vary widely.

As an integral component of the individual's culture, religious beliefs may influence the client's explanation of the cause of illness, perception of its severity, and choice of healer. In times of crisis, such as serious illness and impending death, religion may be a source of consolation for the client and family and may influence the course of action believed to be appropriate.

Religion and Spirituality

Religious concerns evolve from, and respond to, the mysteries of life and death, good and evil, and pain and suffering. Nurses frequently encounter clients who find themselves searching for a spiritual meaning to help explain illness or disability. Some nurses find spiritual assessment difficult because the topic is abstract and personal, whereas others feel comfortable discussing spiritual matters. Comfort with personal spiritual beliefs is the foundation for effective assessment of spiritual needs in clients.

Although religions offer various interpretations of many of life's mysteries, most people seek a personal understanding and interpretation at some time in their lives. Ultimately, this personal search becomes a pursuit to discover a supreme being (e.g., Allah, God, Yahweh, or Jehovah) or some unifying truth that will render meaning, purpose, and integrity to existence.

An important distinction must be made between religion and spirituality. Religion refers to an organized system of beliefs concerning the cause, nature, and purpose of the universe, especially belief in or the worship of a god or gods. More than 1200 religions are practiced in the United States. Spirituality, in contrast, is born out of the individual's unique life experience and personal effort to find purpose and meaning in life. Box 13-1 provides suggested guidelines for assessing the spiritual needs of culturally diverse clients.

SHARED BELIEFS AMONG VARIOUS RELIGIONS: THE "GOLDEN RULE"

Buddhism: "Hurt not others in ways that you yourself would find hurtful." (Udana-varga 5:18)

Christianity: "Whatsoever you would that men should do to you, do you even so to them." (Matthew 7:12)

Confucianism: "Do not do to others what you do not want them to do to you." (Analects 15:23)

Hinduism: "One should not behave towards others in a way which is disagreeable to oneself." (Mahabharata 5:1517; Mencius Vii.A.4)

Islam: "Not one of you is a believer until he loves for his brother what he loves for himself." (Number 13 of Al-Nawawi's Forty Hadiths)

Judaism: "Thou shalt love thy neighbor as thyself." (Leviticus 19:18)

Taoism: "Regard your neighbor's gain as your own gain and your neighbor's loss as your own loss." (T'ai Shang Kan Ying P'ien)

BOX 13-1 METHODS OF ASSESSING SPIRITUAL NEEDS IN CULTURALLY DIVERSE CLIENTS

Environment
- Does the client have religious objects in the environment?
- Does the client wear outer garments or undergarments that have religious significance?
- Are get-well greeting cards religious in nature or from a representative of the client's church?
- Does the client receive flowers or bulletins from a church or other religious institution?

Behavior
- Does the client appear to pray at certain times of the day or before meals?
- Does the client make special dietary requests (e.g., kosher diet; vegetarian diet; or diet free from caffeine, pork, shellfish, or other specific food items)?
- Does the client read religious magazines or books?

Verbalization
- Does the client mention a Supreme Being (e.g., God, Allah, Buddha, or Yahweh), prayer, faith, church, or religious topics?
- Does the client request a visit by a clergy member or other religious representative?
- Does the client express anxiety or fear about pain, suffering, or death?

Interpersonal Relationships
- Who visits the client? How does the client respond to visitors?
- Does a church representative visit?
- How does the client relate to nursing staff and roommates?
- Does the client prefer to interact with others or remain alone?

Data from Andrews MM, Boyle JS, editors: *Transcultural concepts in nursing care,* ed 5, Philadelphia, 2008, Lippincott Williams & Wilkins.

Religion may influence decisions regarding prolongation of life, euthanasia, autopsy, donation of a body for research, disposal of a body and body parts including fetus, and type of burial. The nurse should use discretion in asking clients and their families about these issues and gather data only when the clinical situation necessitates that the information be obtained. The nurse should encourage clients and families to discuss these issues with their religious representative when necessary. Before dealing with potentially sensitive issues, the nurse should establish rapport with the client and family by gaining their trust and confidence in less-sensitive areas.

Childhood and Spirituality

Serious illness during childhood is especially difficult. Children have spiritual needs that vary according to the child's developmental level and the religious climate that exists in the family. Parental perceptions about the illness of their child may be partially influenced by religious beliefs. For example, some parents may believe that a transgression against a religious law is responsible for a congenital anomaly in their offspring. Other parents may delay seeking medical care because they believe that prayer should be tried first. Certain types of treatment (e.g., administration of blood or medications

containing caffeine or other prohibited substances and selected procedures) may be perceived as cultural taboos, which are to be avoided by children and adults.

CULTURE AND AGING

Values held by the dominant U.S. culture, such as emphasis on independence, self-reliance, and productivity, influence aging members of society. Americans define people 65 years and older as "old" and limit their work. In some other cultures, people are first recognized as being unable to work and then identified as being old. In some cultures the wisdom, not the productivity, of the older adult is valued; the diminishment of one's activity level and reduction of physical stamina associated with growing old are accepted more readily without loss of status among culture members. Retirement is also culturally defined, with some older adults working as long as physical health continues and others continuing to be active but assuming less physically demanding jobs.

The main task of older adults in the dominant culture is to achieve a sense of integrity in accepting responsibility for their own lives and having a sense of accomplishment. Individuals who achieve integrity consider aging a positive experience, make adjustments in their personal space and social relationships, maintain a sense of usefulness, and begin closure and life review. Not all cultures value accepting responsibility for an individual's own life. For example, among Hispanics, Asians, Arabs, and other groups, older adults are often cared for by family members who welcome them into their homes when they are no longer able to live alone. The concept of placing an older family member in an institutional setting to be cared for by strangers is perceived as an uncaring, impersonal, and culturally unacceptable practice by many cultural groups.

Older adults may develop their own means of coping with illness through self-care, assistance from family members, and social group support systems. Some cultures have developed attitudes and specific behaviors for older adults that include humanistic care and identification of family members as care providers. Older adults may have special family responsibilities (e.g., the older Amish adults provide hospitality to visitors, and older Filipino adults spend considerable time teaching the youth skills learned during a lifetime of experience).

Older adult immigrants who have made major lifestyle adjustments in the move from their homeland to the United States or from a rural to an urban area, or vice versa, may need information about health care alternatives, preventive programs, health care benefits, and screening programs for which they are eligible. These individuals may also be in various stages of culture shock, the state of disorientation or inability to respond to the behavior of a different cultural group because it holds sudden strangeness, unfamiliarity, and incompatibility to the newcomer's perceptions and expectations (Leininger and McFarland, 2002).

Several examples of how being an elderly immigrant influences health can be found in the nursing literature. Wilmoth and Chen (2003), for example, studied living arrangements and symptoms of depression among middle-aged and older immigrants and concluded that immigrants had significantly more depressive symptoms than nonimmigrants. Further, immigrants who lived alone or with family had more depressive symptoms than those who lived with a spouse. In another example, Becker (2002) found that many older Cambodians wanted to return to their homeland to die.

CROSS-CULTURAL COMMUNICATION

Verbal and nonverbal communication are important in community health nursing and are influenced by the cultural background of the nurse and client. Cross-cultural, or intercultural, communication refers to the communication process between a nurse and a client with different cultural backgrounds as each attempts to understand the other's point of view from a cultural perspective.

Nurse-Client Relationship

From the introduction of the nurse to the client through termination of the relationship, communication is a continuous process for the community health nurse. First impressions are important in all human relationships; therefore cross-cultural considerations concerning introductions warrant a few brief remarks. To ensure a mutually respectful relationship, the nurse should introduce himself or herself and indicate how the client should refer to the nurse (i.e., by first name, last name, or title). Having done so, the nurse should ask the client to do the same. This enables the nurse to address the client in a manner that is culturally appropriate, thereby avoiding potential embarrassment. For example, some Asian and European cultures write the last name first; confusion can be avoided in an area of sensitivity (i.e., the client's name).

Space, Distance, and Intimacy

Sense of spatial distance is significant because culturally appropriate distance zones vary widely. For example, nurses may back away from clients of Hispanic, East Indian, or Middle Eastern origin who invade personal space with regularity in an attempt to bring the nurse closer into the space that is comfortable to them. Although nurses are uncomfortable with clients' close physical proximity, clients are perplexed by the nurse's distancing behaviors and may perceive the community health nurse as aloof and unfriendly. Table 13-3 summarizes the four distance zones identified for the functional use of space that are embraced by the dominant cultural group, including most nurses.

Interactions between clients and nurses may also depend on the client's desired degree of intimacy, which may range from formal interactions to close personal relationships. For example, some Southeast Asian clients expect those in authority (e.g., nurses) to be authoritarian, directive, and detached.

In contrast, Appalachian clients traditionally have close family interaction patterns that often lead them to expect close personal relationships with health care providers. The Appalachian client may evaluate the nurse's effectiveness on

TABLE 13-3	FUNCTIONAL USE OF SPACE
ZONE	**REMARKS**
Intimate zone (0 to 1.5 feet)	Visual distortion occurs. Best for assessing breath and other body odors.
Personal distance	Perceived as an extension of the self, similar (1.5 to 4 feet) to a "bubble." Voice is moderate. Body odors are inapparent. Visual distortion does not occur. Much of the physical assessment will occur at this distance.
Social distance (4 to 12 feet)	Used for impersonal business transactions. Perceptual information is much less detailed. Much of the interview will occur at this distance.
Public distance (>12 feet)	Interaction with others is impersonal. Speaker's voice must be projected. Subtle facial expressions are imperceptible.

Data from Hall E: Proxemics: the study of man's spatial relations. In Galdston I, editor: *Man's image in medicine and anthropology*, New York, 1963, International Universities Press.

the basis of interpersonal skills rather than professional competency. Appalachian clients are likely to be uncomfortable with the impersonal, bureaucratic orientation of most health care institutions. Likewise, clients of Arab, Latin-American, or Mediterranean origin often expect an even higher degree of intimacy and may attempt to involve the nurse in their family system by expecting participation in personal activities and social functions. These individuals may come to expect personal favors that extend beyond the scope of professional nursing practice and may believe it is their privilege to contact the nurse at home at any time of the day or night for care.

Overcoming Communication Barriers

Nurses tend to have stereotypical expectations of the client's behavior. In general, nurses expect behavior to consist of undemanding compliance, an attitude of respect for the health care provider, and cooperation with requested behavior throughout the examination. Although clients may ask a few questions for clarification, slight deference to recognized authority figures (e.g., health care providers) is expected. However, individuals from culturally diverse backgrounds may have significantly different perceptions about the appropriate role of the individual and family when seeking health care. If nurses find themselves becoming annoyed that a client is asking too many questions, assuming a defensive posture, or otherwise feeling uncomfortable, they may pause for a moment to examine the source of the conflict from a cross-cultural perspective.

During illness, culturally acceptable "sick-role" behavior may range from aggressive, demanding behavior to silent passivity (Cockerham, 2009). Complaining, demanding behavior during illness is often rewarded with attention among Jewish and Italian-American clients, whereas Asian and Native-American clients are likely to be quiet and compliant during illness. Furthermore, during an interview, Asian clients may provide the nurse with the answers they think the nurse wants to hear, which is behavior consistent within their cultural value for harmonious relationships with others. The nurse should attempt to phrase questions or statements in a neutral manner that avoids foreshadowing an expected response. Appalachian clients may reject a community health nurse whom they perceive as prying or nosy because a cultural ethic of neutrality mandates that people mind their own business and avoid assertive or argumentative behavior.

Nonverbal Communication

Unless the nurse makes an effort to understand the client's nonverbal behavior, he or she may overlook important information such as that which is conveyed by facial expressions, silence, eye contact, touch, and other body language. Communication patterns vary widely cross-culturally, even for seemingly "innocent" behaviors such as smiling and handshaking. For example, among many Hispanic clients, smiling and handshaking are considered an integral part of sincere interaction and essential to establishing trust, whereas a Russian client may perceive the same behavior by the nurse as insolent and frivolous.

Gender issues also become significant. For example, among some groups of Middle Eastern origin, men and women do not shake hands or touch each other in any manner outside of the marital relationship. However, if the nurse and client are both female, a handshake is usually acceptable.

Wide cultural variation exists when interpreting silence. Some individuals find silence extremely uncomfortable and make every effort to fill conversational lags with words. In contrast, Native Americans consider silence essential to understanding and respecting the other person. A pause after a question signifies that what the speaker has asked is important enough to be given thoughtful consideration. In traditional Chinese and Japanese cultures, silence may mean that the speaker wishes the listener to consider the content of what has been said before continuing. The English and Arabs may use silence out of respect for another person's privacy, whereas the French, Spanish, and Russians may interpret it as a sign of agreement. Asian cultures often use silence to demonstrate respect for elders.

Eye contact is among the most culturally variable nonverbal behaviors. Although most nurses have been taught to maintain eye contact while talking with clients, individuals from culturally diverse backgrounds may misconstrue this behavior. Asian, Native-American, Indochinese, Arab, and Appalachian clients may consider direct eye contact impolite or aggressive, and they may avert their own eyes during the conversation. Native-American clients often stare at the floor when the nurse is talking. This culturally appropriate behavior indicates that the listener is paying close attention to the speaker.

In some cultures, including Arab, Hispanic, and some black groups, modesty for women is interrelated with eye contact. For Muslim women, modesty is achieved in part by avoiding eye contact with men, except for their husband, and keeping the eyes downcast when encountering members of

the opposite sex in public situations. In many cultures, the only women who smile and establish eye contact with men in public are prostitutes. Hasidic Jewish men also have culturally based norms concerning eye contact with women. The male may avoid direct eye contact and turn his head in the opposite direction when walking past or speaking to a woman. The preceding examples are intended to be illustrative and are not exhaustive; nor do they represent values, actions, and beliefs of all members of the cultural groups described.

Language

To assess non–English-speaking clients, the nurse may need the help of an interpreter. Interviewing a non–English-speaking person requires a bilingual interpreter for full communication. Even the person from another culture or country who has a basic command of English may need an interpreter when faced with the anxiety-provoking situation of becoming ill, encountering a strange symptom, or discussing sensitive topics, such as birth control, gynecological concerns, or urological problems. The nurse may be tempted to ask a relative or friend of another client to interpret because this person is readily available and is anxious to help. However, this is disadvantageous because it violates confidentiality for the client, who may not want personal information shared with another. Furthermore, the friend or relative, although fluent in ordinary language, is likely to be unfamiliar with medical terminology, clinical procedures, and medical ethics.

Whenever possible, the nurse should use a bilingual team member or trained medical interpreter. This person knows interpreting techniques, has a health care background, and understands clients' rights. The trained interpreter is also knowledgeable about cultural beliefs and health practices, can help bridge the cultural gap, and can provide advice concerning the cultural appropriateness of recommendations.

Although the nurse is in charge of the client-nurse interaction, the interpreter is an important member of the health care team. Whenever feasible, the nurse should ask the interpreter to meet the client before the visit to establish rapport and learn about the client's age, occupation, educational level, and attitude toward health care. This enables the interpreter to communicate on the client's level.

The nurse should allow more time for visits with culturally diverse clients who require an interpreter. With the third person repeating everything, it can take considerably longer than interviewing English-speaking clients. The nurse will need to focus on the major points and prioritize data.

Line-by-line and summarization are interpretation styles. Translation of line-by-line ensures accuracy, but it takes more time. The nurse and client should speak only a sentence or two and then allow the interpreter time to interpret. The nurse should use simple language, not medical jargon that the interpreter must simplify before translating. Summary translation is faster and useful for teaching relatively simple health techniques with which the interpreter is already familiar. The nurse should be alert for nonverbal cues as the client talks because they can give valuable data. A good interpreter will also note nonverbal messages and communicate those to the

- Before locating an interpreter, the nurse should know what language the client speaks at home because it may be different from the language spoken publicly (e.g., French is sometimes spoken by aristocratic or well-educated people from certain Asian or Middle Eastern cultures).
- The nurse should avoid interpreters from a rival tribe, state, region, or nation (e.g., a Palestinian who knows Hebrew may not be the best interpreter for a Jewish client).
- The nurse should be aware of the gender difference between the interpreter and client to avoid violation of cultural mores related to modesty.
- The nurse should be aware of the age difference between the interpreter and client.
- The nurse should be aware of socioeconomic differences between the interpreter and client.
- The nurse should ask the interpreter to translate as closely to verbatim as possible.
- An interpreter who is not a relative may seek compensation for services rendered.

community health nurse. Box 13-2 summarizes suggestions for the selection and use of an interpreter.

Although use of an interpreter is ideal, the nurse may find himself or herself in a situation with a non–English-speaking client when no interpreter is available. Box 13-3 provides some suggestions for overcoming language barriers when an interpreter is not available.

Touch

Touching the client is a necessary component of a comprehensive assessment. Although benefits exist in establishing rapport with clients through touch, including the promotion of healing through therapeutic touch, physical contact with clients conveys various meanings cross-culturally. In many cultures (e.g., Arab and Hispanic), male health care providers may be prohibited from touching or examining all or certain parts of the female body. During pregnancy, the client may prefer female health care providers and may refuse to be examined by a man. The nurse should be aware that the client's significant other also might exert pressure on health care providers by enforcing these culturally meaningful norms in the health care setting.

Touching children may also have variable meanings cross-culturally. For example, Hispanic clients may believe in *mal ojo* (evil eye), in which an individual becomes ill as a result of excessive admiration by another. Many Asians believe that personal strength resides in the head and that touching the head is considered disrespectful. The nurse should approach palpation of the fontanelle of an infant of Southeast Asian descent with sensitivity. The nurse may need to rely on alternative sources of information (e.g., assessing for clinical manifestations of increased intracranial pressure or signs of premature fontanelle closure). Although it is the least desirable option, the nurse may need to omit this part of the assessment.

Gender

Violating norms related to appropriate male-female relationships among various cultures may jeopardize the therapeutic nurse-client relationship. Among Arab Americans, a man is never alone with a woman, except his wife, and is usually accompanied by one or more other men when interacting with women. This behavior is culturally significant, and failure to adhere to the cultural code (i.e., set of rules or norms of behavior used by a cultural group to guide their behavior and interpret situations) is viewed as a serious transgression, often

- The nurse should be polite and formal.
- The nurse should greet the client using his or her last or complete name. The nurse should gesture to himself or herself and say his or her name. The nurse should offer a handshake or nod and smile.
- The nurse should proceed in an unhurried manner. The nurse should pay attention to efforts by the client or family to communicate.
- The nurse should speak in a low, moderate voice. The nurse should remember that he or she may have a tendency to raise the volume and pitch of his or her voice when the listener appears not to understand and the listener may perceive that the nurse is shouting or angry.
- The nurse should use words that he or she may know in the client's language. This indicates that the nurse is aware of and respects the client's culture.
- The nurse should use simple words, such as "pain" instead of "discomfort." The nurse should avoid medical jargon, idioms, and slang. He or she should avoid using contractions such as "don't," "can't," and "won't." The nurse should use nouns repeatedly instead of pronouns. For example, the nurse should say, "Do you take medicine?" instead of "You have been taking your medicine, haven't you?"

- The nurse should pantomime words and simple actions while verbalizing them.
- The nurse should give instructions in the proper sequence. For example, he or she should say, "First, wash the bottle. Second, rinse the bottle," instead of "Before you rinse the bottle, sterilize it."
- The nurse should discuss one topic at a time. He or she should avoid use of conjunctions. For example, the nurse should say, "Are you cold [while pantomiming]?" and "Are you in pain?" instead of, "Are you cold and in pain?"
- The nurse should determine whether the client understands by having the client repeat instructions, demonstrate the procedure, or act out the meaning.
- The nurse should write out several short sentences in English and determine the client's ability to read them.
- The nurse should try a third language. Many Indo-Chinese speak French. Europeans often know three or four languages. The nurse should try Latin words or phrases.
- The nurse should ask who among the client's family and friends could serve as an interpreter.
- The nurse should obtain phrase books from a library or bookstore, make or purchase flash cards, contact hospitals for a list of interpreters, and use both formal and informal networking to locate a suitable interpreter.

one in which the lone male will be accused of sexual impropriety. The best way to ensure that cultural variables have been considered is to ask the client about culturally relevant aspects of male-female relationships, preferably at the beginning of the interaction before an opportunity arises to violate culturally based practices.

HEALTH-RELATED BELIEFS AND PRACTICES

One of the major aspects of a comprehensive cultural assessment concerns the collection of data related to culturally based beliefs and practices about health and illness. Before determining whether cultural practices are helpful, harmful, or neutral, the nurse must first understand the logic of the belief system underlying the practice and then be sure to grasp fully the nature and meaning of the practice from the client's cultural perspective.

Health and Culture

The first step in understanding the health care needs of clients is to understand personal culturally based values, beliefs, attitudes, and practices. Sometimes this requires considerable introspection and may necessitate that the nurse confront his or her own biases, preconceptions, and prejudices about specific racial, ethnic, religious, sexual, or socioeconomic groups. The next step is to identify the meaning of health to the client, remembering that concepts are derived, in part, from the way in which members of their cultural group define health.

Considerable research has been conducted on the various definitions of health that may be held by various groups. For example, Jamaicans define health as having a good appetite, feeling strong and energetic, performing activities of daily living without difficulty, and being sexually active and fertile. For traditional Italian women, health means the ability to interact socially and perform routine tasks such as cooking, cleaning, and caring for oneself and others. On the other hand, some individuals of Hispanic origin believe that coughing, sweating, and diarrhea are a normal part of living rather than symptoms of ill health, because the frequency of these problems in the clients' country of origin is high. Individuals may define themselves or others in their group as healthy even though the nurse identifies symptoms of disease.

Cross-Cultural Perspectives on Causes of Illness

For clients, symptom labeling and diagnosis depend on the degree of difference between the individual's behaviors and those the group define as normal. Other issues that the nurse should consider include the client's beliefs about the causation of illness, level of stigma attached to a particular set of symptoms, prevalence of the disease, and meaning of the illness to the individual and family.

Throughout history, humankind has attempted to understand the cause of illness and disease. Theories of causation have been formulated on the basis of religious beliefs, social circumstances, philosophical perspectives, and level of knowledge. Disease causation may be viewed from the following three major perspectives: biomedical (i.e., sometimes used synonymously with the term *scientific*), naturalistic (i.e., sometimes used synonymously with the term *holistic*), and magicoreligious.

Biomedical Perspective

The biomedical (i.e., scientific) theory of illness causation is based on the following:
1. All events in life have a cause and effect.
2. The human body functions more or less mechanically (i.e., the functioning of the human body is analogous to the functioning of an automobile).
3. All life can be reduced or divided into smaller parts (e.g., the human person can be reduced into body, mind, and spirit).
4. All of reality can be observed and measured (e.g., with intelligence tests and psychometric measures of behavior).

Among the biomedical explanations for disease is the germ theory, which posits that microscopic organisms such as bacteria and viruses are responsible for many specific disease conditions. Most educational programs for nurses and other health care providers embrace biomedical, or scientific, theories that explain the causes of physical and psychological illnesses.

Naturalistic Perspective

Another way in which clients may explain the cause of illness is from the naturalistic (i.e., holistic) perspective. This viewpoint is found most frequently among Native Americans, Asians, and others who believe that human life is only one aspect of nature and a part of the general order of the cosmos. Individuals from these groups believe that the forces of nature must be kept in natural balance or harmony to maintain health and well-being.

Many Asians subscribe to the yin-yang theory, in which health is believed to exist when all aspects of the person are in perfect balance. Rooted in the ancient Chinese philosophy of Tao, the yin-yang theory states that all organisms and objects in the universe consist of yin or yang energy forces. The origin of the energy forces is within the autonomic nervous system, where balance between the opposing forces is maintained during health. Yin energy represents the female and negative forces (e.g., emptiness, darkness, and cold), whereas yang forces are male and positive, emitting warmth and fullness. Foods are classified as hot and cold in this theory and are transformed into yin and yang energy when metabolized by the body. Yin foods are cold, and yang foods are hot. Cold foods are eaten when one has a hot illness, and hot foods are eaten when one has a cold illness. The yin-yang theory is the basis for Eastern or Chinese medicine.

The naturalistic perspective posits that the laws of nature create imbalance, chaos, and disease. Individuals embracing the naturalistic view use metaphors such as the healing power of nature, and they may call the earth "Mother." For example, from the perspective of the Chinese, illness is not seen as an intruding agent but rather as a part of life's rhythmic course and an outward sign of the disharmony that exists within.

Many Hispanic, Arab, black, and Asian groups embrace a hot-cold theory of health and illness, an explanatory model with its origin in the ancient Greek humoral theory. Blood, phlegm, black bile, and yellow bile, the four humors of the body, regulate basic bodily functions and are described in terms of temperature, dryness, and moisture. The treatment of disease consists of adding or subtracting cold, heat, dryness, or wetness to restore the balance of the humors.

Beverages, foods, herbs, medicines, and diseases are classified as hot or cold according to their perceived effects on the body, not on their physical characteristics. Illnesses believed to be caused by cold entering the body include earache, chest cramps, paralysis, gastrointestinal discomfort, rheumatism, and tuberculosis. Illnesses believed to be caused by overheating include abscessed teeth, sore throats, rashes, and kidney disorders.

According to the hot-cold theory, the individual as a whole, rather than a specific ailment, is significant. Those who embrace the hot-cold theory maintain that health consists of a positive state of total well-being, including physical, psychological, spiritual, and social aspects of the person. Paradoxically, the language used to describe this artificial dissection of the body into parts is a reflection of the biomedical-scientific perspective, not a naturalistic or holistic one.

Magicoreligious Perspective

Another way in which people explain the causation of illness is from a magicoreligious perspective. The basic premise of this explanatory model is that the world is seen as an arena in which supernatural forces dominate. The fate of the world and those in it depends on the action of supernatural forces for good or evil. Examples of magical causes of illness include the belief in voodoo or witchcraft among some blacks and others from circum-Caribbean countries. Faith healing is based on religious beliefs and is most prevalent among selected Christian religions, including Christian Scientists. Various healing rituals may be found in many religions, such as Roman Catholicism, Mormonism (i.e., Church of Jesus Christ of Latter-day Saints), and others (Andrews, 2008).

A combination of worldviews is possible, and many clients are likely to offer more than one explanation for the cause of their illness. As a profession, nursing largely embraces the biomedical-scientific worldview, but some aspects of holism have begun to gain popularity. These include a wide variety of techniques for management of chronic pain (e.g., hypnosis, therapeutic touch, and biofeedback). Many nurses hold a belief in spiritual power and readily credit supernatural forces with various unexplained phenomena related to clients' health and illness states.

Folk Healers

All cultures have their own recognized symptoms of ill health, acceptable sick-role behavior, and treatments. In addition to seeking help from the nurse as a biomedical-scientific health care provider, clients from many groups may also seek help from folk or religious healers.

Numerous types of folk healers exist, each with a unique scope of practice. Hispanic clients may turn to a *curandero* (male folk healer) or *curandera* (female folk healer), spiritualist, *yerbo* (herbalist), or *sabador* (healer who manipulates muscles and bones). In many instances, people from diverse cultures will combine folk healing and biomedicine. Among the main reasons for seeking care from folk healers is the perception that biomedical practitioners (e.g., physicians and nurses) fail to provide holistic care and use medicines that are not natural.

Some black clients may mention having received assistance from a *hougan* (voodoo priest or priestess), spiritualist, or "old lady" (an older woman who has successfully raised a family and specializes in child care and folk remedies). Likewise, Native-American clients may seek assistance from a shaman or a medicine man or woman. Clients of Asian descent may mention that they have visited herbalists, acupuncturists, or bone setters.

Each culture has its own healers, most of whom speak the native tongue of the client, make house calls, and cost significantly less than healers practicing in the biomedical-scientific health care system. In addition to relying on folk healers, many cultures rely on lay midwives (e.g., *parteras* for Hispanic women) or other health care providers to meet the needs of pregnant women.

In some religions, spiritual healers may be found among the ranks of the ordained or official religious hierarchy ranks and are called priest, bishop, elder, deacon, rabbi, brother, or sister. Other religions have a separate category of healer (e.g., Christian Science "nurses" [not licensed by states] or practitioners) (Andrews, 2008).

A comprehensive discussion of the variety of healing beliefs and practices used by the numerous cultural groups is beyond the scope of this chapter. However, the nurse should be aware of alternative practices and folk healers that are used by the groups for which they care. The nurse should also be aware that most indigenous healing practices are innocuous, regardless of whether they are effective.

Cultural Expressions of Illness

A wide cultural variation exists in the manner in which certain symptoms and disease conditions are perceived, diagnosed, labeled, and treated. The disease that is grounds for social ostracism in one culture may be reason for increased status in another. For example, epilepsy is contagious and untreatable among Ugandans, a cause for family shame among Greeks, a reflection of a physical imbalance among Mexican Americans, and a sign of having gained favor by enduring a trial by God among the Hutterites.

Bodily symptoms are also perceived and reported in a variety of ways. For example, individuals of Mediterranean descent tend to report common physical symptoms more often than people of northern European or Asian heritage. The Chinese do not have a translation for the English word *sadness,* yet all people experience the feeling of sadness at some time in their life. To express emotion, Chinese clients sometimes somaticize their symptoms. For example, a client may complain of cardiac symptoms because the center of emotion in the Chinese culture is the heart. If the client has experienced a loss through death or divorce and is grieving, he or she may describe the loss in terms of a pain in the heart. Although some biomedical-scientific clinicians may refer to this as a psychosomatic illness, others will recognize it as a culturally acceptable somatic expression of emotional disharmony.

Cultural Expression of Pain

To illustrate the manner in which symptom expression may reflect the client's cultural background, pain, an extensively studied symptom, is used. Pain is a universally recognized phenomenon and an important aspect of assessment for clients of various ages. Pain is a private, subjective experience that is greatly influenced by cultural heritage. Expectations, manifestations, and pain management are all embedded in a cultural context. The definition of pain, like that of health or illness, is culturally determined.

The term *pain* is derived from the Greek word for penalty, which helps explain the long association between pain and punishment in Judeo-Christian thought. The meaning of painful stimuli for individuals, the way people define their situation, and the influence of personal experience combine to determine the experience of pain.

Much cross-cultural research has been conducted on pain (Ludwig-Beymer, 2008; Zborowski, 1969). Pain has been found to be a highly personal experience that depends on cultural learning, the meaning of the situation, and other factors unique to the individual. Health care professionals have identified silent suffering as the most valued response to pain. The majority of nurses have been socialized to believe that, in virtually any situation, self-control is better than open displays of strong feelings.

Studies of nurses' attitudes toward pain reveal that the ethnic background of clients is relevant to the nurses' assessment of physical and psychological pain. Nurses view Jewish and Spanish clients as experiencing suffering the most and Anglo-Saxon Germanic clients as experiencing suffering the least. In addition, nurses who infer relatively greater client pain tended to report their own experiences as more painful. In general, nurses with an eastern or southern European or African background tend to infer greater suffering than do nurses of northern European background. Years of experience, current position, and area of clinical practice are unrelated to inferences of suffering (Ludwig-Beymer, 2008).

In addition to expecting variations in pain perception and tolerance, a nurse should expect variations in the expression of pain. Individuals turn to their social environments for validation and comparison. A first important comparison group is the family, which transmits cultural norms to its children.

Culture-Bound Syndromes

Clients may have a condition that is culturally defined, known as a culture-bound syndrome. Some of these conditions have no equal from a biomedical or scientific perspective, but others, such as anorexia nervosa and bulimia, are examples of health problems found primarily among members of the dominant U.S. cultural group. Table 13-4 presents selected examples from among more than 150 culture-bound syndromes that have been documented by medical anthropologists.

MANAGEMENT OF HEALTH PROBLEMS: A CULTURAL PERSPECTIVE

After a symptom is identified, the first effort at treatment is often self-care. In the United States, an estimated 70% to 90% of all illness episodes are treated first, or exclusively, through self-care, often with significant success. The availability of over-the-counter medications, a relatively high literacy level, and influence of the mass media in communicating health-related information to the general population have contributed to the high percentage of self-treatment. Home treatments are attractive because they are accessible compared with the inconvenience associated with traveling to a physician, nurse practitioner, and pharmacist, particularly for clients from rural or sparsely populated areas. Furthermore, home treatment may mobilize the client's social support network and provide the sick individual with a caring environment in which to convalesce.

However, the nurse should be aware that not all home remedies are inexpensive. For example, urban black populations in the Southeast sometimes use medicinal potions that cost much more than an equivalent treatment with a biomedical intervention.

Various nontraditional interventions are gaining the recognition of health care professionals in the biomedical-scientific health care system. Acupuncture, acupressure, therapeutic touch, massage, biofeedback, relaxation techniques, meditation, hypnosis, distraction, imagery, and herbal remedies are interventions that clients may use alone or in combination with other treatments.

Cultural Negotiation

Cultural negotiation refers to the process in which messages, instructions, and belief systems are manipulated, linked, or processed between the professional and lay models of health problems and preferred treatment. In each act, the nurse gives attention to eliciting the client's views regarding a health-related experience (e.g., pregnancy, complications of pregnancy, or illness of an infant).

Katon and Kleinman (1981) describe negotiation as a bilateral arrangement in which two principal parties attempt to work out a solution. The goal of negotiation is to reduce conflict in a way that promotes cooperation. Cultural negotiation is used when conceptual differences exist between the client and the nurse, a situation that may occur for one or more of the following reasons:

- The nurse and client may be using the same words but applying different meanings to them.
- The nurse and client may apply the same term to the same phenomenon but have different notions of its causation.
- The nurse and client may have different memories or emotions associated with the term and its use.

TABLE 13-4	SELECTED CULTURE-BOUND SYNDROMES	
GROUP	**DISORDER**	**REMARKS**
Whites	Anorexia nervosa	Excessive preoccupation with thinness, self-imposed starvation
	Bulimia	Gross overeating, then vomiting or fasting
Blacks	Blackout	Collapse, dizziness, or inability to move
	Low blood	Not enough blood or weakness of the blood that is often treated with diet
	High blood	Blood that is too rich in certain components from ingesting too much red meat or rich foods
	Thin blood	In women, children, and the elderly; renders the individual more susceptible to illness in general
	Diseases of hex, witchcraft, or conjuring	Sense of being doomed by a spell, part of voodoo beliefs
Chinese or Southeast Asians	Koro	Intense anxiety that the penis is retracting into the body
Greeks	Hysteria	Bizarre complaints and behavior because the uterus leaves the pelvis and goes to another part of the body
Hispanics	Empacho	Food forms into a ball and clings to the stomach or intestines, causing pain and cramping
	Fatigue	Asthma-like symptoms
	Mal ojo (evil eye)	Fitful sleep, crying, and diarrhea in children caused by a stranger's attention; sudden onset
	Pasmo	Paralysis-like symptoms of face or limbs; prevented or relieved by massage
	Susto	Anxiety, trembling, and phobias from sudden fright
Native Americans	Ghost	Terror, hallucinations, and sense of danger
Japanese	Wagamama	Apathetic childish behavior with emotional outbursts

In cultural negotiation, the nurse provides scientific information while acknowledging that the client may hold different views. If the client's perspective indicates that behaviors would be helpful, positive, adaptive, or neutral in effect, the nurse should include these in the plan of care. However, if the client's perspective would result in behaviors that may be harmful, negative, or nonadaptive, the nurse should attempt to shift the client's perspective to that of the practitioner (Spector, 2008).

Pregnancy and childbirth are social, cultural, and physiological experiences; therefore, an approach to culturally sensitive nursing care of childbearing women and their families must focus on the interaction between cultural meaning and biological functions. Childbirth is a time of transition and social celebration that is of central importance in any society; it signals realignment of existing cultural roles and responsibilities, psychological and biological states, and social relationships. Child rearing is also a period during which culturally bound values, attitudes, beliefs, and practices permeate virtually all aspects of life for the parents and child (Andrews and Boyle, 2008). Careful assessment and attention to culturally based practices are particularly important during these occasions.

MANAGEMENT OF HEALTH PROBLEMS IN CULTURALLY DIVERSE POPULATIONS

The factors responsible for the health disparity between minority and white populations are complex and defy simplistic solutions. Health status is influenced by the interaction of physiological, cultural, psychological, and societal factors that are poorly understood for the general population and even less so for minorities. Despite the shared characteristic of economic disadvantage among minorities,

common approaches for improving health are not possible. Rather, solving problems among minorities necessitates activities, programs, and data collection that are tailored to meet the unique health care needs of many different subgroups. Solutions to health care problems among culturally diverse populations include the following:
- Providing health information and education
- Delivering and financing health services
- Developing health professionals from minority groups
- Enhancing cooperative efforts with the nonfederal sector
- Improving methods of data development
- Promoting a research agenda on minority health issues

Providing Health Information and Education

Minority populations tend to be less knowledgeable or less aware of some specific health problems than whites. This is demonstrated by the following (American Cancer Society, 2008; USDHHS, 2000):
- Blacks have the highest mortality rate and shortest survival rate for many cancers.
- Blacks receive less information about cancer and heart disease than nonminority groups.
- Blacks tend to underestimate the prevalence of cancer, give less credence to the warning signs, obtain fewer screening tests, and receive a diagnosis at later stages of cancer than whites.
- Many professionals and lay people, both minority and white, do not know that heart disease is as common in black men as in white men and that black women die of coronary heart disease at a higher rate than white women.
- Among Mexican Americans, cultural attitudes regarding obesity and diet are often barriers to achieving weight control.

Programs to increase public awareness about health problems have been well received in several areas. For example, the Healthy Mothers, Healthy Babies Coalition, which provides an education program in both English and Spanish, has contributed to increased awareness of measures to improve the health status of mothers and infants. In addition, increased knowledge among blacks of hypertension as a serious health problem is one of the accomplishments of the National High Blood Pressure Education program. The success of these efforts indicates that carefully planned programs have a beneficial effect, but efforts must continue and expand to reach even more of the target population and focus on additional health problems.

Planning Health Information Campaigns

Sensitivity to cultural factors is often lacking in the health care of minorities. Key concepts for the nurse to consider in designing a health information campaign include meeting the language and cultural needs of each identified minority group, using minority-specific community resources to tailor educational approaches, and developing materials and methods of presentation that are commensurate with the educational level of the target population. Furthermore, the powerful influences of cultural factors over a lifetime in shaping people's attitudes, values, beliefs, and practices concerning health require health information programs to be sustained over a long period. The following are examples of ways in which the nurse can interweave these concepts into health promotion efforts:

- The nurse should involve local community leaders who are members of the targeted cultural group to promote acceptance and reinforcement of the central themes of health promotion messages.
- Health messages are more readily accepted if they do not conflict with existing cultural beliefs and practices. Where appropriate, messages should acknowledge existing cultural beliefs.
- The nurse should involve families, churches, employers, and community organizations as a support system to facilitate and sustain behavioral change to a more healthful lifestyle. For example, although hypertension control in blacks depends on appropriate treatment (e.g., medication), blood pressure can be improved and maintained by family and community support of activities such as proper diet and exercise.
- Language barriers, cultural differences, and lack of adequate information on access to care complicate prenatal care for Hispanic and Asian women who have recently arrived in the United States. By using lay volunteers to organize community support networks, programs have been developed to disseminate culturally appropriate health information.

Health Education

Although printed materials and other audiovisual aids contribute to the educational process, client education is inherently interpersonal. The success of educational efforts is often determined by the credibility of the source and is highly dependent on the skill and sensitivity of the nurse in communicating information in a culturally appropriate manner. Education

programs are particularly critical and necessary for several health problems with the greatest influence on minority health, such as hypertension, obesity, and diabetes. For example, if patients with diabetes could improve their self-management skills through education, a significant number of complications (e.g., ketoacidosis, blindness, and amputations) could be avoided, saving human misery and health care dollars.

Delivering and Financing Health Services

Innovative models for delivering and financing health services for minority populations are needed. According to community health experts, models should increase flexibility of health care delivery, facilitate minorities' access to services, and improve efficiency of service and payment systems. One of the most commonly used indicators of adequacy of health services for a population is distribution of health care providers; however, this is an inadequate measurement. The following observations exemplify the problems associated with health services for minorities:

- The disparities in death rates between minorities and whites remain despite overall increases in health care access and use.
- Language problems hinder refugees and immigrants when they seek health care.
- Blacks with cancer postpone seeking diagnosis of their symptoms longer than whites and delay initiation of treatment once diagnosed (American Cancer Society, 2008).
- A smaller proportion of black women than white women begin prenatal care in the first trimester of pregnancy (USDHHS, 2000).

Models of Health Promotion

In most health models, SES is assumed to affect health status through environmental or behavioral factors. These models posit that poor families may not have the economic, social, or community resources needed to remain in good health. For example, poverty is thought to affect children's well-being by impacting health and nutrition, the home environment, caregiver interactions with children, caregiver mental health, and neighborhood conditions. The deficits associated with poverty may lead to an inadequate diet, which results in poor growth and delayed development. Likewise, poor housing results in increased risk for exposure that leads to other environmental hazards; overcrowding results in increased risk for infectious diseases such as tuberculosis, meningitis, influenza, and related conditions; and community violence threatens the safety and well-being of children. The combined effect of these stressors is thought to provide the foundation for a cycle of hopelessness and depression among family members, who, in turn, may engage in risky health behaviors (e.g., smoking, substance abuse, and poor dietary habits resulting in obesity and high cholesterol levels) and unfavorable family interactions.

Although many Latino children live in poverty, they enjoy relatively good health compared with children in other low socioeconomic groups. This has been called an epidemiological paradox. It is believed that strong family-community support fosters optimum family health behaviors. The assumption is that if the family promotes beneficial health behaviors among its members, these behaviors will become integrated into the culture. Healthy lifestyle behaviors become an integral component of the family identity, traditions, and history.

Continuity of Care

Continuity of care is associated with improved health outcomes and is presumably greater when a client is able to establish an ongoing relationship with a care provider. Many of the leading causes of death among minorities (e.g., cancer, cardiovascular disease, and diabetes) are chronic rather than acute problems; therefore they require extended treatment regimens. Consider the following:

- Refugees are eligible for special refugee medical assistance during their first 18 months in the United States. However, after this period, refugees who cannot afford private health insurance and are ineligible for Medicaid or state medical assistance may become medically indigent.
- Many Native Americans and Alaska Natives live in areas where the availability of health care providers is half the national average.

Health Care Financing Problems

As mentioned previously, problems associated with financing health care tend to be more common in minority groups than in the dominant cultural group. Consider the following (National Center for Health Statistics, 2008):

- Economic inequalities cause members of minority groups to disproportionately rely on Medicaid for their health care needs.
- Older minority people are less likely than whites to supplement Medicare with additional private insurance.
- Proportionately, three times as many Native Americans, blacks, Hispanics, and certain Asian and Pacific Islander groups as whites live in poverty.
- In 2008, 30.4% of Hispanics lacked insurance coverage, compared with 17% of blacks and 9.9% of whites.

To better manage health problems and reduce the disparity in health indicators, these issues of financing must be addressed. Failure to do so will result not only in continued inequity in access to services but also in continued poor health among minority groups.

Developing Health Professionals from Minority Groups

The need to increase the number of health professionals from minority groups has been recognized for decades. With few exceptions, minorities are underrepresented as students and practitioners of the health professions. Although the number of minority nursing students has been steadily increasing, there still are proportionately more white nursing students.

Differences in the availability of health personnel resources in minority communities are apparent, regardless of the minority group being considered. Communities located in urban-metropolitan areas have significantly more professional resources. Among the factors that contribute to the imbalances in minority representation in health professions are the size of a minority population, number of cultural subgroups, and

demographic features. Efforts to encourage more students from minority groups are ongoing, and government and private foundations offer grants, scholarships, and low-cost loans to recruit and retain students from underserved minority groups in nursing and other health care professions. Minority and nonminority health professional organizations, academic institutions, state governments, health departments, and other organizations from the public and private sectors should work together to develop strategies to improve the availability and accessibility of health care professionals to minority communities (Sullivan Commission, 2004).

Enhancing Cooperative Efforts with the Nonfederal Sector

Activities to improve minority health should involve participation of organizations at all levels (i.e., community, municipal, state, and national). Community involvement in developing health promotion activities can contribute to their success by providing credibility and visibility to the activities and facilitating their acceptance. Changes in health behavior frequently depend on personal initiative and are most likely to be triggered by efforts from locally based sources.

However, not all minority communities have the ability to identify their own health problems and initiate activities to address them. Support from the state and federal governments and private sector assistance is needed to assist with identifying and solving health-related problems afflicting the minority community. Assistance may be provided to minority communities in the following ways:

1. The use of technical assistance to identify high-risk groups
2. Assistance with planning, implementing, and evaluating programs to address identified needs
3. Specialized community services (e.g., federally funded projects for infants and frail older adults)
4. Programs supported by businesses and industries (e.g., health promotion programs organized by unions)

The private sector can also serve as an effective channel for programs targeted to minority health projects. National organizations concerned with minorities, such as the National Urban League and the National Alliance for Hispanic Health include health-related issues in their national agendas and are actively seeking effective ways to improve the health of minorities. Organizations such as these have a powerful potential for effecting change among their constituencies because they have strong community-level grassroots support.

Promoting a Research Agenda on Minority Health Issues

The National Center on Minority Health and Health Disparities (NCMHD) (http://ncmhd.nih.gov/) was developed in 2000 to assist in the investigation of factors affecting minority health. Its mission is to promote minority health and to ultimately eliminate health disparities. The NCMHD conducts and supports research that examines risk factor prevalence and treatment services. It also reviews health education interventions, preventive services interventions, and sociocultural factors that influence health and outcomes of care.

For further information on current research related to culture and community health nursing, the reader should search library databases for reports of completed studies. Electronic bulletin boards also may be valuable when searching for research in progress and for communicating with researchers studying a particular phenomenon of interest. An example of recent nursing research related to culturally competent care is discussed in Research Highlights.

RESEARCH HIGHLIGHTS

Nutritional Patterns of Recent Immigrants

Edmonds (2005) examined the nutritional patterns of 23 recently immigrated women from Honduras to assist in understanding health-related nutritional issues in this Hispanic subgroup. She determined that the Honduran women had made both positive and negative changes in their diets since coming to the United States. Rice, beans, natural fruit juices, tortillas, bananas, beef, and eggs were reported as the typical foods eaten every day in Honduras. Positive changes in diets included eating a greater variety of fruits and vegetables, cooking with less grease, baking more frequently than frying, and using vegetable oil rather than lard. They also ate more meat and dairy products. Negative changes noted were more skipped meals and eating foods high in fat and calories (e.g., fast foods). Research suggests that classes be taught in Women, Infants, and Children (WIC) programs and other venues that would support the Hondurans' traditional diet and focus on how to eat nutritionally in fast-food restaurants, eat a balanced diet, plan meals and cook ahead, and read food labels.

From Edmonds VM: The nutritional patterns of recently immigrated Honduran women, *J Transcult Nurs* 16(3):226-235, 2005.

ROLE OF THE COMMUNITY HEALTH NURSE IN IMPROVING HEALTH FOR CULTURALLY DIVERSE PEOPLE

This chapter provides data detailing the health care problems of culturally diverse individuals, families, groups, and communities. Given the complexity of the problems and the wide variation in incidence and distribution of these problems within specific subgroups, no simple method exists for providing culturally sensitive community health nursing care to all clients. However, the following strategies may assist the community health nurse when working with culturally diverse clients:

- Conduct a "culturological" assessment.
- Conduct a cultural self-assessment.
- Seek knowledge about local cultures.
- Recognize the political issues of culturally diverse groups.
- Provide culturally competent care.
- Recognize culturally based health problems.

Culturological Assessment

All nursing care is based on a systematic, comprehensive assessment of the client; therefore the community health nurse must gather cultural data on clients from racially and ethnically diverse backgrounds. A culturological assessment refers to a systematic appraisal or examination of individuals, groups, and communities regarding their cultural beliefs, values, and practices to determine explicit nursing needs and intervention practices

within the cultural context of the people being evaluated (Leininger, 1995). The term culturological is a descriptive reference to cultural phenomena in their broadest sense.

Culturological assessments are as vital as physical and psychological assessments. Culturological assessments tend to be broad and comprehensive because they deal with cultural values, belief systems, and ways of living now and in the recent past. In conducting a culturological assessment, the community health nurse should be involved in determining and appraising the traits, characteristics, or smallest units of cultural behavior as a guide to nursing care. The following section summarizes major data categories pertaining to the culture of clients and offers suggested questions that the nurse may ask to elicit needed information.

Brief History of Ethnic and Racial Origins of the Cultural Group with Which the Client Identifies

- With what ethnic group or groups does the client report affiliation (e.g., Hispanic, Polish, Navajo, or a combination)? To what degree does the client identify with the cultural group (e.g., "we" concept of solidarity or a fringe member)?
- What is the client's reported racial affiliation (e.g., black, Native American, or Asian)?
- Where was the client born?
- Where has the client lived (i.e., country and city) and when (i.e., during what years)? If the client has recently relocated to the United States, knowledge of prevalent diseases in the country of origin may be helpful.

Values Orientation

- What are the client's attitudes, values, and beliefs about birth, death, health, illness, and health care providers?
- Does culture influence the manner in which the client relates to body image change resulting from illness or surgery (e.g., importance of appearance, beauty, strength, and roles in cultural group)?
- How does the client view work, leisure, and education?
- How does the client perceive change?
- How does the client value privacy, courtesy, touch, and relationships with individuals of different ages, of different social class, or caste, and of the opposite sex?
- How does the client view biomedical-scientific health care (e.g., suspiciously, fearfully, or accepting)? How does the client relate to people in a different cultural group (e.g., withdrawal, verbal or nonverbal expression, or negative or positive attitude)?

Cultural Sanctions and Restrictions

- How does the client's cultural group regard expression of emotion and feelings, spirituality, and religious beliefs? How are dying, death, and grieving expressed in a culturally appropriate manner?
- How is modesty expressed by men and women in the client's cultural group? Does the client's cultural group have culturally defined expectations about male-female relationships, including the nurse-client relationship?

- Does the client have restrictions related to sexuality, exposure of body parts, or certain types of surgery (e.g., amputation, vasectomy, or hysterectomy)?
- Does the client have restrictions against discussion of dead relatives or fears related to the unknown?

Communication

- What language does the client speak at home? What other language does the client speak or read? In what language would the client prefer to communicate with you?
- What is the written and spoken English fluency level of the client? Remember that the stress of illness may cause clients to use a more familiar language and temporarily forget some English.
- Does the client need an interpreter? If so, is a relative or friend available whom the client would like to have interpret? Is anyone available with whom the client would prefer not to interpret (e.g., member of the opposite sex, a person younger or older than the client, or a member of a rival tribe or nation)?
- What are the rules (i.e., linguistics) and modes (i.e., style) of communication?
- Is it necessary to vary the technique of communication during the interview and examination to accommodate the client's cultural background (e.g., tempo of conversation, eye contact, sensitivity to topical taboos, norms of confidentiality, and style of explanation)?
- How does the client's nonverbal communication compare with that of individuals from other cultural backgrounds? How does it affect the client's relationship with the nurse and with other members of the health care team?
- How does the client feel about health care providers who are not of the same cultural background (e.g., black, middle-class nurse, or Hispanic of a different social class)? Does the client prefer to receive care from a nurse of the same cultural background, sex, or age?
- What are the overall cultural characteristics of the client's language and communication processes?
- With which language or dialect is the client most comfortable?

⚖ ETHICAL INSIGHTS
Disclosure of HIV/AIDS Status

Ortiz (2005) examined the experiences of 19 Latinas who disclosed they were living with HIV/AIDS. She described how the women decided to disclose their HIV status to partners, family members, friends, and employers. Four categories emerged: timing of the disclosure, the need to disclose, controlling disclosure, and supportive disclosing. These factors were influenced by the Latinas' relationship with others, the perceived risks to the women and others, the need to disclose, the wish to give support to themselves or others, and the desire to control who should know and when. It was concluded that nurses should be knowledgeable of the realities of Latinas' lives and to be able to incorporate that knowledge into comprehensive care plans that will help them maximize the utilization of appropriate resources.

Ortiz CE: Disclosing concerns of Latinas living with HIV/AIDS, *J Transcult Nurs* 16(3):210-217, 2005.

Health-Related Beliefs and Practices

- To what cause(s) does the client attribute illness and disease (e.g., divine wrath, imbalance in hot-cold or yin-yang, punishment for moral transgressions, hex, or soul loss)?
- What does the client believe promotes health (e.g., eating certain foods, wearing amulets to bring good luck, exercise, prayer, ancestors, saints, or intermediate deities)?
- What is the client's religious affiliation (e.g., Judaism, Islam, Pentecostalism, West African voodooism, Seventh-Day Adventism, Catholicism, or Mormonism)?
- Does the client rely on cultural healers (e.g., curandero, shaman, spiritualist, priest, minister, or monk)? Who determines when the client is sick and when the client is healthy? Who determines the type of healer and treatment that should be sought?
- In what types of cultural healing practices does the client engage (e.g., herbal remedies, potions, massage, wearing talismans or charms to discourage evil spirits, healing rituals, incantations, or prayers)?
- How does the client perceive biomedical-scientific health care providers? How do the client and family perceive nurses? What are the expectations of nurses and nursing care?
- What comprises appropriate "sick-role" behavior? Who determines what symptoms constitute disease and illness? Who decides when the client is no longer sick? Who cares for the client at home?
- How does the client's cultural group view mental disorders? Do they show differences in acceptable behaviors for physical versus psychological illnesses?

Nutrition

- What nutritional factors are influenced by the client's cultural background?
- What meanings does the client attach to food and eating? With whom does the client usually eat? What types of foods does the client usually eat? What does the client define as food? What does the client believe comprises a "healthy" versus an "unhealthy" diet?
- How does the client prepare foods at home (e.g., type of food preparation; cooking oils used; length of time foods, especially vegetables, are cooked; amount and type of seasoning added to various foods during preparation)?
- Do religious beliefs and practices influence the client's diet (e.g., amount, type, preparation, or delineation of acceptable food combinations, such as kosher diets)? Does the client abstain from certain foods at regular intervals, on specific dates determined by the religious calendar, or at other times?
- If the client's religion mandates or encourages fasting, what does the term *fast* mean to the client (e.g., refraining from certain types or quantities of foods, eating only during certain times of the day)? For what period of time is the client expected to fast?

- During fasting, does the client refrain from liquids or beverages? Does the religion allow exemption from fasting during illness, and, if so, is the client believed to have an exemption?

Socioeconomic Considerations

- Who constitutes the client's social network (i.e., family, peers, and healers)? How do they influence the client's health or illness status?
- How do members of the client's social support network define caring (e.g., being continuously present, doing things for the client, or looking after the client's family)? What are the roles of various family members during health and illness?
- How does the client's family participate in the client's nursing care (e.g., bathing, feeding, touching, and being present)?
- Does the cultural family structure influence the client's response to health or illness (e.g., beliefs, strengths, weaknesses, and social class)? Does a key family member have a role that is significant in health-related decisions (e.g., grandmother in many black families or eldest adult son in Asian families)?
- Who is the principal wage earner in the client's family? What is the total annual income? This is a potentially sensitive question that should be asked only if necessary. Does the family have more than one wage earner? Does the family have other sources of financial support (e.g., extended family or investments)?
- What influence does economic status have on lifestyle, place of residence, living conditions, ability to obtain health care, and discharge planning?

Organizations Providing Cultural Support

- What influence do ethnic and cultural organizations have on the client's receiving health care (e.g., National Association for the Advancement of Colored People, Black Political Caucus, churches, schools, Urban League, and community-based health care programs and clinics)?

Educational Background

- What is the client's highest educational level obtained? Does the client's educational background affect the client's knowledge level concerning the health care delivery system, how to obtain the care needed, teaching and learning skills, and written material that is distributed in the health care setting (e.g., insurance forms, educational literature, information about diagnostic procedures and laboratory tests, and admissions forms)?
- Can the client read and write English, or does he or she prefer another language? If English is the client's second language, are materials available in the client's primary language?
- What learning style is most comfortable or familiar? Does the client prefer to learn through written materials, oral explanation, or demonstration?

Religious Affiliation

- How does the client's religious affiliation influence health and illness (e.g., death, chronic illness, body image alteration, and cause and effect of illness)?
- What is the role of the client's religious beliefs and practices during health and illness?
- Does the client believe in healing rituals or practices that can promote well-being or hasten recovery from illness? If so, who performs these?
- What is the role of significant religious representatives during health and illness? Does the client have recognized religious healers (e.g., Islamic imams, Christian Scientist practitioners or nurses, Catholic priests, Mormon elders, and Buddhist monks)?

Cultural Aspects of Disease Incidence

- Does the client have specific genetic or acquired conditions that are more prevalent in a specific cultural group (e.g., hypertension, sickle cell anemia, Tay-Sachs disease, or lactose intolerance)?
- Are any socioenvironmental diseases more prevalent among the client's specific cultural group (e.g., lead poisoning, alcoholism, AIDS, drug abuse, or ear infections)?
- Do diseases exist against which the client has an increased resistance (e.g., skin cancer in darkly pigmented individuals)?

Biocultural Variations

- Does the client have distinctive physical features that are characteristic of a particular racial group (e.g., skin color or hair texture)? Does the client have variations in anatomy that are characteristic of a particular racial or ethnic group (e.g., body structure, height, weight, facial shape and structure [nose, eye shape, and facial contour], or upper and lower extremity shape)?
- How do anatomical and racial variations affect the assessment?

Developmental Considerations

- Does the client have distinct growth and development characteristics that vary with his or her cultural background (e.g., bone density, psychomotor patterns of development, or fat folds)?
- What factors are significant in assessing children from the newborn period through adolescence (e.g., expected growth on standard grid, culturally acceptable age for toilet training, introduction of various types of foods, sex differences, discipline, and socialization to adult roles)?
- What is the cultural perception of aging (e.g., is youthfulness or the wisdom of old age more highly valued)?
- How are older people handled culturally (e.g., cared for in the home of adult children or placed in institutions for care)? What are culturally acceptable roles for older adults?
- Does the older adult expect family members to provide care, including nurturance and other humanistic aspects of care?

- Is the older adult isolated from culturally relevant supportive people or enmeshed in a caring network of relatives and friends?
- Has a culturally appropriate network replaced family members in performing some caring functions for older adults?

Cultural Self-Assessment

Community health nurses can engage in a cultural self-assessment. Through identification of health-related attitudes, values, beliefs, and practices that are part of the personal cultural meaning brought to the nurse-client interaction, the nurse can better understand the cultural aspects of health care from the perspective of the client, family, group, or community. Everyone has ethnocentric tendencies that must be brought to a level of conscious awareness so that efforts can be made to temper ethnocentrism and view reality from the perspective of the client.

Knowledge About Local Cultures

Community health nurses can learn about the cultural diversity characteristics of the subgroup or subgroups that are most prevalent within their communities. The nurse cannot know about all health-related beliefs and practices of the diverse groups served, but he or she can study select ones. The nurse can accomplish this cultural study by a review of nursing, anthropology, sociology, and related literature on culturally diverse groups; in-service programs held at community health agencies, educational institutions in the community, or organizations serving minority groups; enrollment in courses on transcultural or cross-cultural nursing and medical anthropology; and interviews with key members of the subgroups of interest, such as clergy members, nurses, physicians, and others, to obtain information about the influence of culture on health-related beliefs and practices.

Recognition of Political Issues of Culturally Diverse Groups

Awareness of the political aspects of health care for culturally diverse groups and communities can help community health nurses influence legislation and funding priorities aimed at improving health care for specific populations. Recognized for their leadership role in community health matters involving culturally diverse groups, community health nurses may be invited by political leaders to participate in political decision making affecting the health of a targeted subgroup. Community health nurses should also be active politically, both individually and collectively, to influence legislation affecting culturally diverse individuals, groups, and communities, and they should offer to serve on key community committees, boards, and advisory councils that impact the health of culturally diverse groups.

Providing Culturally Competent Care

When caring for individuals and families from culturally diverse backgrounds, the community health nurse can assess, diagnose, implement, and evaluate nursing care in a manner that is culturally congruent, competent, relevant, and appropriate. To provide this culturally appropriate nursing care, the nurse must create a relationship of mutual respect by becoming aware of the cultural similarities and differences between herself or himself and the client. A guideline for gathering cultural data has been presented, and the nurse may use this guideline or a similar one for identifying significant areas in which the nurse and client differ. Knowledge about biocultural variations in health and illness is particularly important when conducting cultural assessments.

Recognition of Culturally Based Health Practices

As discussed previously, the community health nurse should attempt to understand the nature and meaning of culturally based health practices of clients, groups, and communities. Once the practices are understood, the nurse can make a determination regarding their appropriateness in a particular context. Generally, the nurse should decide whether a cultural practice is useful, neutral, or harmful to the client, group, or community. The nurse should encourage or "tolerate" helpful and neutral practices, whereas he or she should discourage harmful practices.

The classification of some cultural healing practices is not so easily determined. For example, many Southeast Asians practice coining, which is the rubbing of a coin over body surfaces to expel "bad winds" that are believed to cause illness. Coining leaves abrasions on the skin. Community health nurses are faced with an ethical dilemma when coining is practiced on young children, because this practice may be construed by some members of the dominant cultural group as child abuse. This practice is not useful, so the nurse must make the decision whether it is neutral or harmful. An argument for the practice being neutral is based on the facts that the abrasions usually heal quickly, no harm is done to the child as a result of the practice, and the practice is meaningful to parents who have much confidence in the healing powers associated with coining.

The argument can also be made that the practice is harmful. The red marks and skin abrasions caused by the coining place the child at increased risk for skin infection. Given that the child may require antibiotics or other medication for a respiratory disorder, encouragement of coining may prevent the child from receiving needed medical intervention and delay treatment.

As a solution, the community health nurse may suggest that parents combine traditional treatment with Western biomedicine (i.e., they can use coining in conjunction with a biomedical intervention). Therefore the healing will occur in a manner that has involved the use of both folk and professional health care systems.

RESOURCES FOR MINORITY HEALTH

Community health nurses will find federal resources for improving the health care of the federally defined minority populations through the USDHHS. Within the USDHHS, the Office of Minority Health (OMH) and the Indian Health

Service (IHS) divisions relate to health promotion, disease prevention, service delivery, and research on minority groups.

Office of Minority Health

The OMH coordinates federal efforts to improve the health status of racial and ethnic minority populations (i.e., blacks, Hispanics, Native Americans and Alaska Natives, and Asians and Pacific Islanders). The OMH is directed by the deputy assistant secretary for minority health and was established by the Disadvantaged Minority Health Improvement Act of 1990 (PL 101-527), which was signed by President George H. W. Bush on November 6, 1990. Under the directives of the act, the OMH has the following responsibilities:

- Establish short- and long-range goals and objectives relating to disease prevention, health promotion, service delivery, and research on the health of minority people.
- Promote increased participation of disadvantaged people, including minorities, in health service and health promotion programs.
- Create a national minority health resource center.
- Support research, demonstrations, and evaluations of new and innovative models that increase understanding of disease risk factors and support better information dissemination, education, prevention, and service delivery to minority communities.
- Promote minority health–related activities in the corporate and voluntary sectors.
- Develop minority-focused health information and health promotion materials and teaching programs.
- Assist providers of primary care and preventive services in obtaining assistance of bilingual health professionals when appropriate.

As the focal point for minority health efforts, the OMH plays a key role in major initiatives launched by the USDHHS secretary. Table 13-5 lists some of the initiatives.

Indian Health Service

The Indian Health Service (IHS) is responsible for providing federal health services to Native Americans and Alaska Natives. Federal Indian health services are based on the laws that Congress has passed pursuant to its authority to regulate commerce with the Indian Nations as specified in the Constitution and other documents.

The primary responsibility of the IHS is to elevate the health status of Native Americans and Alaska Natives to the highest level possible. The mission is to ensure quality, availability, and accessibility of a comprehensive, high-quality health care delivery system, providing maximum involvement of Native Americans and Alaska Natives in defining their health needs, setting health priorities for their local areas, and managing and controlling their health programs.

The IHS also acts as the principal federal health advocate for Native Americans by ensuring that they have knowledge of, and access to, all federal, state, and local health programs to which they are entitled as American citizens. The IHS also works with these programs so Native Americans will be cognizant of their entitlements.

The IHS carried out its responsibilities through development and operation of a health services delivery system designed to provide a broad-spectrum program of preventive, curative, rehabilitative, and environmental services. This system integrates health services delivered directly through IHS facilities and staff with those purchased by IHS through contractual arrangements. Tribes are also actively involved in program implementation.

The 1975 Indian Self-Determination Act (PL 93-638), as amended, builds on IHS policy by giving tribes the option of staffing and managing IHS programs in their communities and provides funding for improvement of tribal capability to contract under the act. The 1976 Indian Health Care Improvement Act (PL 94-437), as amended, was intended to elevate the health care status of Native Americans and Alaska Natives to a level equal to that of the general population

TABLE 13-5 FEDERALLY SPONSORED INITIATIVES TO IMPROVE THE HEALTH OF MINORITY GROUPS

INITIATIVE	DESCRIPTION
Health Resources and Services Administration Health Disparity Collaboratives (HDC)	HDC is a broad, multiyear plan to improve the health status of underserved populations. It seeks to ensure that clients receive evidence-based care, and it encourages clients to be active participants in their own care.
Racial and Ethnic Approaches to Community Health (REACH 2010)	This program was launched in 1999 to eliminate health disparities in six priority areas: cardiovascular diseases, immunizations, breast and cervical cancer screening and management, diabetes, HIV/AIDS, and infant mortality. REACH 2010 supports community coalitions in designing, implementing, and evaluating community-driven strategies to eliminate health disparities.
National Breast and Cervical Cancer Early Detection Program (NBCCEDP)	NBCCEDP provides breast and cervical cancer screening, diagnosis, and treatment to low-income, medically underserved, and uninsured women (emphasizing recruitment of minority women).
Ryan White Comprehensive AIDS Resources Emergency (CARE) Act B	Ryan White CARE Act provides services to persons living with HIV disease, primarily racial and ethnic minorities.
National Center on Minority Health and Health Disparities (NCMHD)	NCMHD leads, coordinates, supports, and assesses the NIH research efforts to reduce and ultimately eliminate health disparities.

HIV, Human immunodeficiency virus; *NIH*, National Institutes of Health.

through a program of authorized, higher resource levels in the IHS budget. Appropriated resources were used to expand health services, build and renovate medical facilities, and step up the construction of safe drinking water and sanitary disposal facilities. It also establishes programs designed to increase the number of Native-American health professionals for Native-American needs and to improve health care access for Native Americans living in urban areas.

The operation of the IHS health care delivery system is managed through local administrative units called service units. A service unit is the basic health organization for a geographic area served by the IHS program, just as a county or city health department is the basic health organization in a state health department. These are defined areas usually centered around a single federal reservation in the continental United States or a population concentration in Alaska.

The IHS serves approximately 50% of the total Native-American and Alaska Native population in the United States, primarily those residing on reservations.

SUMMARY

To provide community health nursing for individuals, groups, and communities representing the hundreds of different cultures and subcultures found in the United States, the nurse should include cultural considerations in nursing care. Guidelines for gathering data from clients of culturally diverse backgrounds have been suggested in this chapter and are interwoven throughout the text. Knowledge about culture-specific and culture-universal nursing care is foundational and is an integral component of community health nursing.

CASE STUDY   APPLICATION OF THE NURSING PROCESS

Community health nurse Maria Gonzales visited the home of 5-year-old Nguyen Van Nghi, who was discharged from the hospital on the previous day. The pediatrician had diagnosed pneumonia and "suspected failure to thrive" in the child because the child's growth fell below the third percentile on a standard growth chart for height and weight, and he performed poorly on a screening test used to identify developmental delays for a 5-year-old child.

Residing in the home were the child's parents, four siblings, grandmother, aunt, uncle, and three cousins. Although the child's father and uncle spoke some English, other members of the household communicated in a language unfamiliar to Maria, which "sounded like Chinese." When Maria approached the child, he did not look at her or speak to her, even when she called him Nguyen (pronounced "we'en").

Assessment

In a brief survey of the Nguyens' home, Maria noted that the home and furnishings were modest but very clean. The pantry held a considerable amount of food, including rice and dried noodles. The small refrigerator smelled of fish and contained some vegetables that Maria did not recognize. She did not see any green vegetables, milk, or other dairy products.

During her initial assessment of Nghi, Maria observed multiple tender, ecchymotic areas with petechiae between the ribs on the front and back of the body, resembling strap marks. Suspecting child abuse, Maria told the family that she would return later in the day with an interpreter. She located an interpreter who spoke Mandarin Chinese and briefed him about her concerns with child abuse. When Maria and the interpreter returned to the client's home, she instructed the interpreter to ask the parents for an explanation of the bruises. The interpreter told Maria that the family was Vietnamese and could not understand his Chinese dialect. Both the interpreter and the child's father knew a little French and awkwardly managed to communicate.

The interpreter advised the nurse that, in the Vietnamese culture, the person's family name is given first, followed by the middle name and then the first name. Only a few different family names exist among the Vietnamese; therefore it is common practice to call people by their given first name. At this point, Maria also learned that the child was actually 4 years old, because the Vietnamese consider a newborn to be 1 year old at birth.

The interpreter explained that a Vietnamese healer performed *cao gio,* or coining, to exude the "bad wind" from Nghi. *Cao gio* is

performed by applying a special menthol oil to the painful or symptomatic part of the body and then rubbing a coin over the area with firm, downward strokes. When Nghi's condition seemed to worsen after his hospital discharge, his grandmother convinced his parents that Western biomedicine had failed and that their son required the stronger power of folk healing.

Diagnosis
- Maria must set priorities and focus on selected cultural data categories because they seem most relevant for the Nguyen family at present.

Individual
- High risk for Nghi's pneumonia to worsen
- Potential for child abuse/neglect
- Possible physical and/or developmental delay (low weight/height for age)

Family
- Increased risk for poor health outcomes related to distrust of Western health care practices
- Increased risk for nutritional deficits

Community
- Potential for poor health of area Vietnamese immigrants related to knowledge deficit of good nutritional practices and general health promotion

Planning
Individual
Short-Term Goals
- Nghi's pneumonia will resolve.
- Nghi will show no more evidence of practice of "coining."

Long-Term Goal
- Nghi's height and weight will increase proportionally to at least 50th percentile for age.

Family
Short-Term Goals
- Family members will cease practice of "coining."
- Caregivers will recognize the importance of completing the antibiotics as prescribed.

CASE STUDY   APPLICATION OF THE NURSING PROCESS—cont'd

Long-Term Goal
- A family nutritional assessment will be completed, and adjustments will be made to their diet to provide needed nutrients.

Community
Long-Term Goal
- Leaders of the area's Vietnamese community will work with area health care providers to promote good nutritional practices.

Intervention
Individual
Through the interpreter, Maria was able to communicate with the Nguyen family that it was vital for Nghi to complete the prescribed antibiotics. She also attempted to convey the potentially harmful effect of the practice of coining and suggested that that procedure be stopped. She set a follow-up appointment for the following day.

Family
Maria was able to bring a Vietnamese interpreter for the follow-up appointment. So, in addition to reiteration of the importance of taking the medications, she was able to teach about basic nutritional principles and perform additional nutritional assessments. Although Nghi was not as small as initially thought, he was still below the 50th percentile for his age. Maria gave nutritional pamphlets written in Vietnamese to the parents and provided them with information on where to find low-cost foods in the neighborhood.

Community
Working with the health department's social worker and the Vietnamese interpreter, Maria visited several area markets to gather information on diet and nutritional practices of Vietnamese immigrants. They decided that they would seek a small grant to develop more teaching materials on nutrition for this population.

Evaluation
Individual
By the third follow-up visit, Maria determined that, although Nghi still had a residual cough, his chest was clearing. In addition, there was no evidence of coining. Further, Maria was shown that the family's refrigerator now contained whole milk and some leafy green vegetables. It was decided that she would return in 6 weeks for a follow-up visit to weigh and measure Nghi.

Family
The presence of the interpreter who spoke Vietnamese and who was familiar with the culture was vital. And, by the third visit, most of the family members appeared to be at ease with Maria. Mrs. Nguyen asked a number of questions about nutrition and other health issues and requested that Maria monitor the heights and weights of the other children.

Community
The health department's social worker was able to identify a small grant to develop and purchase teaching materials for the Vietnamese population. They applied for the funds and are eagerly waiting to hear the outcomes.

Levels of Prevention
The following are examples of three levels of prevention as applied to the case study.

Primary Prevention
- Nutritional education for the Nguyen family
- Health education targeted to developing comfort with the U.S. health care system and Western medicine
- Education related to potentially harmful practices (e.g., coining)

Secondary Prevention
Monitoring the height and weight of Nghi and his siblings

Tertiary Prevention
- Evaluation of resolution of pneumonia

■ LEARNING ACTIVITIES

1. Examine the vital statistics of a community, and compare differences in morbidity and mortality rates for whites and racial and ethnic subgroups. What data are available according to racial and ethnic heritage? What data are missing?
2. Visit an inner-city grocery store and compare quality, prices, customer services, and variety of products with those of a suburban grocery store.
3. Select a client from a racially or ethnically diverse background, and conduct a cultural assessment.
4. Interview someone from a racial or ethnic background different from your own to determine beliefs about illness causation, use of the lay and professional health care delivery systems, and culturally based treatments.
5. Dine at an ethnic restaurant. While dining, notice the type of cultural heritage in restaurant decor and information about the culture available from the menu, placemats, or elsewhere in the restaurant. Ask the owner or manager about the history of the restaurant.
6. Attend religious services at a church, temple, synagogue, or place of worship for a religion unfamiliar to you.
7. Interview an official representative (e.g., priest, elder, monk, or bishop) of a religion unfamiliar to you. Ask about health-related beliefs and practices, healing rituals, support network for the sick, and dietary practices.
8. Watch prime-time television and note the racial and ethnic diversity that is present during the commercials. During the program, note the role played by racially and ethnically diverse characters. Are they heroes or heroines or the "bad guys"? What are their occupations, SES, religions, and lifestyles?
9. Skim a popular magazine for references to racially and ethnically diverse subgroups. What is being written? Is the nature of the article favorable or unfavorable?

REFERENCES

Agency for Healthcare Research and Quality: *Addressing racial and ethnic disparities in health care: fact sheet, AHRQ 00-P041*, Rockville, MD, 2005, The Author.

American Cancer Society: *Cancer facts & figures for African Americans: 2007-2008*, 2008: www.cancer.org/downloads/STT/CAFF2007AAacspdf2007.pdf.

Andrews MM: Religion, culture and nursing. In Andrews MM, Boyle JS, editors: *Transcultural concepts in nursing care*, ed 5, Philadelphia, 2008, Lippincott Williams & Wilkins.

Andrews MM, Boyle JS, editors: *Transcultural concepts in nursing care*, ed 5, Philadelphia, 2008, Lippincott Williams & Wilkins.

Becker G: Dying away from home: quandaries of migration for elders in two ethnic groups, *J Gerontol B Psychol Sci Soc Sci* 57B(2):S79–S95, 2002.

Cockerham WC: *Medical sociology*, ed 11, Upper Saddle River, NJ, 2009, Prentice Hall.

The Commonwealth Fund: *Closing the divide: how medical homes promote equity in health care: results from the Commonwealth Fund 2006 healthcare quality survey*, 2007. www.commonwealthfund.org/Content/Publications/Fund-Reports/2007/Jun/Closing-the-Divide--How-Medical-Homes-Promote-Equity-in-Health-Care--Results-From-The-Commonwealth-F.aspx.

Edmonds VM: The nutritional patterns of recently immigrated Honduran women, *J Transcult Nurs* 16(3):226–235, 2005.

Gallup Poll: *Religion*, 2008. www.gallup.com/poll/1690/Religion.aspx.

Garcia Coll CT: Developmental outcome of minority infants: a process-oriented look into our beginnings, *Child Dev* 61:270, 1990.

Health Resources and Services Administration: *The registered nurse population: findings from the 2004 national sample survey of registered nurses*, 2009. bhpr.hrsa.gov/healthworkforce/rnsurvey04/2.htm.

Katon W, Kleinman A: Doctor-patient negotiation and other social science strategies in patient care. In Eisenberg L, Kleinman A, editors: *The relevance of social science for medicine*, Boston, 1981, D. Reidel.

Kluckhohn F, Strodtbeck F: *Variations in value orientations*, Evanston, IL, 1961, Row, Peterson.

Kohls LR: *Survival kit for overseas living*, Yarmouth, ME, 1984, Intercultural Press.

Leininger MM: *Nursing and anthropology: two worlds to blend*, New York, 1970, Wiley.

Leininger MM: *Transcultural nursing: concepts, theories, and practice*, New York, 1978, Wiley.

Leininger MM: *Culture, care, diversity, and universality: a theory of nursing*, New York, 1991, National League for Nursing Press.

Leininger MM: *Transcultural nursing: concepts, theories, research and practice*, ed 2, New York, 1995, McGraw-Hill.

Leininger MM, McFarland MR: *Transcultural nursing: concepts, theories, research and practice*, ed 3, New York, 2002, McGraw-Hill.

Ludwig-Beymer PA: Transcultural aspects of pain. In Andrews M, Boyle JS, editors: *Transcultural concepts in nursing care*, ed 5 Philadelphia, 2008, Lippincott Williams & Wilkins.

National Center for Educational Statistics: Fast facts: status dropout rate: 2008. nces.ed.gov/fastfacts/display.asp?id=16.

National Center for Health Statistics: People without health insurance coverage by race and ethnicity: 2008. www.cdc.gov/Features/dsHealthInsurance/.

National Council of Churches: *Yearbook of American and Canadian churches*, New York, 2005, Office of Minority Health.

Ortiz CE: Disclosing concerns of Latinas living with HIV/AIDS, *J Transcult Nurs* 16(3): 210–217, 2005.

Passel JS: Estimates of the size and characteristics of the undocumented population: Pew Hispanic Center/Pew Research Center, Washington, DC, 2005, http://pewhispanic.org/files/reports/44.pdf.

Spector R: *Cultural diversity in health and illness*, ed 7, Upper Saddle River, NJ, 2008, Prentice Hall.

Sullivan Commission: Missing persons: minorities in the health professions: *Report of the Sullivan Commission on diversity in the healthcare workforce*, 2004. admissions.duhs.duke.edu/sullivancommission/documents/Sullivan_Final_Report.pdf.

Tylor EB: *Primitive culture*, London, 1871, Murray.

US Census Bureau: Foreign-born populations in the United States: 2003. Washington, DC, 2004, The Author. www.census.gov/prod/2004pubs/p20-551.pdf.

US Census Bureau: Income, poverty, and health insurance coverage in the United States: 2007: Washington, DC, 2008, The Author. www.census.gov/prod/2008pubs/p60-235.pdf.

US Census Bureau: An older and more diverse nation by mid-century (press release): 2009. www.census.gov/Press-Release/www/releases/archives/population/012496.html.

US Department of Health and Human Services: *Healthy People 2020: 2009 Draft Objectives*, Washington, DC, 2009, htt://pewhispanic.org/files/reports/44.pdf.

US Department of Homeland Security: *Yearbook of immigration statistics, 2004*, Washington DC, 2006, US Department of Homeland Security, Office of Immigration Statistics.

Wilmoth JM, Chen PC: Immigrant status, living arrangements, and depressive symptoms among middle-aged and older adults, *J Gerontol B Psychol Sci Soc Sci* 58B(5):S305–S313, 2003.

Zborowski M: *People in pain*, San Francisco, 1969, Jossey-Bass.

Environmental Health

*Bridgette Crotwell Pullis**

Additional Material for Study, Review, and Further Exploration

evolve WEBSITE

http://evolve.elsevier.com/Nies
- Quiz
- Case Studies
- Glossary
- WebLinks

OBJECTIVES

Upon completion of this chapter, the reader will be able to do the following:

1. Describe the broad areas of environmental health about which community health nurses must be informed, and name environmental hazards in each area.
2. Recognize potential social, cultural, economic, and political factors affecting environmental health.
3. Apply the basic concepts of critical theory to environmental health nursing problems.
4. Identify aggregates at risk for particular environmental health problems.
5. Distinguish between environmental health approaches that focus on altering individual behaviors and those that aim to change health-damaging environments.
6. Formulate critical questions about environmental conditions that limit the survival and well-being of communities.
7. Understand the skills needed to facilitate community participation and partnership in identifying and solving environmental health problems.
8. Propose collective strategies in which community health nurses can participate to address the environmental health concerns of specific aggregates.

KEY TERMS

aggregate
atmospheric quality
critical theory
environment
environmental health
environmental justice

environmental racism
food quality
housing
living patterns
participatory action research
Precautionary Principle

radiation risks
sick building syndrome
waste control
water quality
work risks

OUTLINE

A Critical Theory Approach to Environmental Health
  Adults
  Children (Parents or Guardian)
Areas of Environmental Health
  Living Patterns
  Work Risks
  Atmospheric Quality

Water Quality
Housing
Food Quality
Waste Control
Radiation Risks
Effects of Environmental Hazards
Efforts to Control Environmental Health Problems

*The author would like to acknowledge the contributions of Joanne M. Hall, Carolyn H. Robinson, and Tonya J. Broyles, who wrote this chapter for the previous edition.

The U.S. Department of Health and Human Services (USDHHS) (2000) defines environmental health as

...those aspects of human health, disease, and injury that are determined or influenced by factors in the environment. This includes the study of both direct pathological effects of various chemical, physical, and biological agents, as well as the effects on health of the broad physical and social environment, which includes housing, urban development, land-use and transportation, industry and agriculture. (p. 8-3) (Figure 14-1)

Environmental health is vitally important to community health nursing practice. Accumulated evidence shows that the environmental changes of the past few decades have profoundly influenced the status of public health. The safety, beauty, and life-sustaining capacity of the physical environment are unquestionably of global consequence. The ecological approach of the 1960s and 1970s tended to focus on clean water, clean air, and protected natural resources in specific locales. Since the beginning of the twenty-first century, it has become apparent that the world must address urgent environmental difficulties, including extinction of some species,

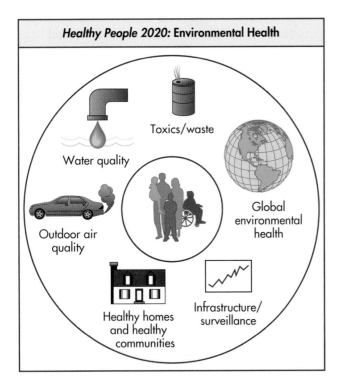

FIGURE 14-1 *Healthy People 2020:* elements of environmental health. (From US Department of Health and Human Services: *Healthy People 2010*, ed 2, Washington, DC, 2000, US Government Printing Office.)

diminishment of tropical rain forests, proliferation of toxic waste dumps, progressive destruction of the ozone layer, shortage of landfill sites, consequences of climate change, threats of terrorism, development of deadly chemical and ballistic weapons, adulteration of food by pesticides and herbicides, oceanic contamination through toxic dumping and petroleum spills, overcrowding of urban areas, and traffic congestion.

This chapter uses critical theory to explore the health of communities in relation to the environment. Critical theory is particularly useful in examining environmental health, as it offers a framework for discussion and a basis for describing community health nursing practice (Bent, 2003; Clark, Barton, and Brown, 2002; Stevens and Hall, 1992). Applying critical theory is a way of thinking upstream (Chapter 3). Critical theory is an approach that raises questions about oppressive situations, involves community members in the definition and solution of problems, and facilitates interventions that reduce health-damaging effects of environments. By applying the nursing process in a critical fashion, nurses can be dynamically involved in the design of interventions that alter the precursors of poor health.

Recognition of the gravity and pervasiveness of environmental hazards can be overwhelming. Looking beyond the individual to recognize the environmental determinants of illness and wellness can be complicated and alarming. Intervening to improve the quality of air, water, housing, food, and waste disposal and reducing the risks of occupational injury and radiation require basic social, economic, and political changes. Nurses must be aware of their ability to bring about changes in health-damaging environments. Nurses are becoming increasingly active in efforts to reduce medical waste and to increase awareness of the effects of the environment on human beings.

Any nurse, those new to environmental health, as well as experienced practitioners, may need guidance for his or her efforts. One often-cited environmental principle is the Wingspread Statement on the Precautionary Principle, developed in 1998. The statement says that "when an activity raises threats of harm to human health or the environment, precautionary measures should be taken even if some cause-and-effect relationships are not fully established scientifically" (Wingspread Conference, Global Development Research Center, 1998). "This document can be accessed at www.gdrc.org/u-gov/precaution-3.html." The Precautionary Principle originated from concern that the use and release of hazardous substances into the environment have had negative consequences and that the public must become involved in calling attention to these activities.

Throughout this chapter, clinical examples illustrate how environmental health problems affect the everyday lives of aggregates. The term aggregate refers to a group that shares a common aspect, such as age, gender, race, economic status, cultural perspective, chronic illness, or area of residence. Aggregates may be a community in which the members know and interact with each other, such as a barrio neighborhood or a labor union. Aggregates may also be "theoretically defined" categories of individuals who may or may not interact regularly with others in the defined group, such as "crack cocaine users," "women with physical disabilities," or "men over the age of 65."

Two other terms used frequently throughout this chapter are *environment* and *community's health*. Environment is the accumulation of physical, social, cultural, economic, and political conditions that influence the lives of communities. The community's health depends on the integrity of the physical environment, the humaneness of the social relations in the environment, the availability of resources necessary to sustain life and manage illness, the equitable distribution of health risks, attainable employment and education, cultural preservation and tolerance of diversity among subgroups, access to historical heritage, and a sense of empowerment and hope.

A CRITICAL THEORY APPROACH TO ENVIRONMENTAL HEALTH

Critical theory suggests that community health nurses must be aware of environmental threats or factors that might detrimentally affect the safety and well-being of particular aggregates or deprive them of access to resources necessary in the pursuit for health. This may include recognizing, supporting, and maintaining positive environmental influences. Public buildings, schools, workplaces, and mass transportation systems are environmental structures that are vital to people's everyday functioning. Ordinarily, society takes these systems and structures for granted, ignoring or overlooking potentially harmful environmental situations.

For example, the experiences of agricultural workers exposed to pesticides bring into question what society takes for granted about the environment. A recent study determined that farm workers and pesticide applicators who accumulate agricultural chemicals on their skin and clothing take these substances home with them, increasing their children's exposure to toxicants (Thompson et al., 2008). Nurses must provide answers to farm workers who ask questions such as "What do I do if I'm exposed to a pesticide? How long should I wait until after a pesticide application to go back into the field? How do I find out how toxic a certain pesticide is? Where can I get information on a specific pesticide?" In addition, nurses must advocate for pesticide legislation that will help protect the health of agricultural workers, as well as the safety of the food chain.

According to *Healthy People 2010* (USDHHS, 2000), of the worldwide preventable illnesses, 25% are caused by poor environmental quality. Indeed, it is estimated that air pollution contributes to 50,000 premature deaths annually in the United States. The data suggest nurses need to ask critical questions about their clients' work and home environments to help discern the contributions of specific hazards to their health. This can be accomplished by taking an environmental health history. An environmental health history can benefit the client in the following ways:

- Increase awareness of environmental/occupational factors
- Improve timelines and accuracy of diagnosis
- Prevent disease and aggravation of conditions
- Identify potential work-related environmental hazards, and/or environmental hazards in and around clients' homes

Environmental health histories should be obtained for both adults and children, although the relationship between the environment and children's health is frequently overlooked (National Environmental Education Foundation [NEEF], 2008). Also, although frequently overlooked, a parent's occupational exposures may put the child at risk for particular health problems.

The following are some suggestions for environmental health screenings (NEEF, 2008).

Adults

- What kind of work do you do? How long on the job? Types of work exposures?
- Do you notice health problems you are having while you are at work? At home? In the community? In a specific location?
- What is the age of your home? Characteristics of heating and ventilation? Do you live near an industrial site or landfill?
- Have you recently used pesticides, solvents, insecticides, or weed killers?
- What kinds of hobbies do you have?
- Has your workplace been treated recently for insects, weeds, or other pest problems?

Children (Parents or Guardian)

- Where does your child go to school, day care, playgrounds?
- Have any of these places been treated recently (e.g., sprayed) for insects, weeds, or other pest problems?
- Does your child help with gardening activities?
- What are sources of food, water (e.g., well water)? Is someone in the household breastfeeding an infant?
- Do parents have any occupational exposure to potential health threats (e.g., lead, pesticides, x-rays)?

According to Bent (2003), when looking at the community through a critical lens, nurses have the opportunity to promote "community-based" and "community-focused health" (p. 224). In identifying environmental sources of health problems, nurses must be involved with the affected communities. Rather than impose their views of the problem, nurses should share their ideas and dialogue with community members. For example, nurses should listen to what the community believes is problematic, help raise consciousness about environmental dangers, and help bring about change (Bent, 2003; Clark et al., 2002). If nurses become involved in conducting community assessments and analyses, they can learn how the community members perceive themselves, their health, and their environmental influences.

The ultimate goal of the critical practice of community health nursing is liberating people from health-damaging environmental conditions (Bent, 2003). From a critical standpoint, helping communities become more aware of the environmental effects on health and helping them make needed changes in their environment are legitimate nursing actions. Collective actions have been instrumental in accomplishing positive environmental changes since the 1980s. Some of the mechanisms have included strategic organization, litigation, public hearing testimony, letter-writing campaigns, legislative lobbying, and mass demonstrations. Currently, organizing, informing, and fund-raising for environmental causes are also done via the Internet. The immediate online donations from private individuals in the United States and elsewhere in response to the January 2010 earthquake in Haiti and the December 2004 Southeast Asia tsunami facilitated rapid availability of resources for minimizing loss of life and restoring basic necessities, such as clean water and shelter. Public response to "acute" environmental disasters needs to be extended to an ongoing, consistent pressure to ensure day-to-day environmental integrity; hence, "chronic" environmental problems need to be addressed more effectively.

A critical perspective can help nurses plan and implement aggregate-level interventions because it emphasizes collective strategies for change. Acting collectively can empower nurses to impact environmental health. Assessing environmental health problems, planning and implementing interventions, and evaluating the effectiveness of community-based actions need to be based on a wide lens. Community health nurses should be familiar with physical surroundings and their mutual interaction with cultural realities, social relations, economic circumstances, and political conditions of communities, applying a critical perspective to community health.

AREAS OF ENVIRONMENTAL HEALTH

Environmental health hazards are ubiquitous in communities across the United States and place adults and children at risk for disease or injury. This chapter divides the vast field of environmental health into the following subcategories: living patterns, work risks, atmospheric quality, water quality, housing, food quality, waste control, and radiation risks (Table 14-1). The brief discussions of these areas are only introductions to environmental health and, as such, focus on basic problems and strategies to address them. The following sections define these eight areas of environmental health, provide clinical examples of problems relevant to each category, and describe the community health nursing responses to the environmental health concerns. Table 14-2 provides examples of health problems within each area.

It should be noted that a critical perspective does not separate the idea of a safe social environment from a safe physical environment. For example, interpersonal violence is a significant and growing risk, with consequences ranging from bodily injury to psychiatric aftereffects that may last for decades in some individuals. There are intergenerational patterns of abuse, hate crimes toward marginalized groups, sexual predators, and hazards of combat that might be considered from an environmental health perspective. There are also occupational hazards of sexual harassment, racial discrimination, and workplace distresses that have resulted in shooting sprees. Issues of violence are discussed in more depth in Chapter 27.

Finally, we must be prepared for the public health effects of terrorism. Terrorism is a word that evokes many images

TABLE 14-1	AREAS OF ENVIRONMENTAL HEALTH
AREA	**DEFINITION**
Living patterns	Living patterns are the relationships among people, communities, and their surrounding environments that depend on habits, interpersonal ties, cultural values, and customs.
Work risks	Work risks include the quality of the employment environment and the potential for injury or illness posed by working conditions.
Atmospheric quality	Atmospheric quality refers to the protectiveness of the atmospheric layers, the risks of severe weather, and the purity of the air for breathing purposes.
Water quality	Water quality refers to the availability and volume of the water supply and the mineral content levels, pollution by toxic chemicals, and the presence of pathogenic microorganisms. Water quality consists of the balance between water contaminants and existing capabilities to purify water for human use and plant and wildlife sustenance.
Housing	Housing is an environmental health concern and refers to the availability, safety, structural strength, cleanliness, and location of shelter, including public facilities and family dwellings.
Food quality	Food quality refers to the availability, relative costs, variety, and safety of foods, and the health of animal and plant food sources.
Waste control	Waste control is the management of waste materials resulting from industrial and municipal processes, human consumption, and efforts to minimize waste production.
Radiation risks	Radiation risks are health dangers posed by the various forms of ionizing radiation relative to barriers preventing exposure of humans and other life forms.
Violence risks	The environmental risks of violence include the potential for victimization through the violence of particular individuals and the general level of aggression in psychosocial climates.

TABLE 14-2 EXAMPLES OF ENVIRONMENTAL HEALTH PROBLEMS

AREA	PROBLEMS
Living patterns	Drunk driving
	Secondhand smoke
	Noise exposure
	Urban crowding
	Technological hazards
Work risks	Occupational toxic poisoning
	Machine-operating hazards
	Sexual harassment
	Repetitive motion injuries
	Carcinogenic worksites
Atmospheric quality	Gaseous pollutants
	Greenhouse effect
	Destruction of the ozone layer
	Aerial spraying of herbicides and pesticides
	Acid rain
Water quality	Contamination of drinking supply by human waste
	Oil spills in the world's waterways
	Pesticide or herbicide in filtration of groundwater
	Aquifer contamination by industrial pollutants
	Heavy metal poisoning of fish
Housing	Homelessness
	Rodent and insect infestation
	Poisoning from lead-based paint
	Sick building syndrome
	Unsafe neighborhoods
Food quality	Malnutrition
	Bacterial food poisoning
	Food adulteration
	Disrupted food chains by ecosystem destruction
	Carcinogenic chemical food additives
Waste control	Use of nonbiodegradable plastics
	Poorly designed solid-waste dumps
	Inadequate sewage systems
	Transport and storage of hazardous waste
	Illegal industrial dumping
Radiation risks	Nuclear facility emissions
	Radioactive hazardous wastes
	Radon gas seepage in homes and schools
	Nuclear testing
	Excessive exposure to x-rays

and a range of reactions from rage to grief and loss. Acts of terrorism have drawn the public and political focus to establishing environmental security. Bioterrorism and homeland security are new areas where nurses will have an impact. A critical perspective is needed now more than ever, as security issues are linked to religious imperatives, moral stances, values, profit motives, health care systems and information, and cultural differences. These issues are also clearly in the scope of community health nursing and are discussed in more detail in Chapter 28.

Living Patterns

Living patterns are the relationships among people, communities, and their surrounding environments that depend on habits, interpersonal ties, cultural values, and customs. Most people live within areas that require almost daily contact with potential health risks and threats. These include intoxicated or impaired drivers, secondhand smoke, urban crowding, noise exposure, unabated traffic, and the stress of increased mechanization (Environmental Protection Agency [EPA], 2002; Frumkin, 2002).

Urban sprawl is an emerging issue and an example of a living pattern that is of increasing concern. Urban sprawl has been defined as the conversion of land to nonagricultural or nonnatural uses at a faster rate than the population growth (EPA, 2002). The sprawling development often occurs more rapidly than the expansion of the infrastructure (e.g., schools, sewer systems, water lines) needed for support. Typically, the desire to own one's vehicle, coupled with inadequate public mass transportation systems, contributes to a greater dependence on the automobile. This results in high volumes of traffic and a constant need to build more highways. Consequences of sprawl include air and water pollution, floods, infrastructure expenses, and a decrease in natural areas and forests (EPA, 2002; Frumkin, 2002) (see photos on page 251 depicting urban sprawl). The health implications of urban sprawl are found in Table 14-3.

Living patterns reflect an individual's lifestyle choices (e.g., tobacco use, eating a diet rich in saturated fats, leading a sedentary lifestyle, becoming emotionally distressed while living with a substance abuser). Living patterns also contribute to population exposure to environmental conditions affected by mass culture, media, social policy, ethnic customs, and technology.

Clinical Example

In an urban Chinese-American community, the economic aftershocks of a major earthquake caused the closure of a number of businesses. Some of these family businesses moved to parts of the city less characterized by the use of Chinese languages. These moves caused many elderly, non–English-speaking family members to experience depression, characterized by loss of appetite.

The community health nurses in the area began visiting these elders and brought interpreters with them. In their assessments, the nurses focused on psychiatric symptoms and suggested ventilation of emotions. They encouraged the Chinese elders to attend a local senior center staffed and attended mostly by European Americans. In some cases, they recommended psychiatric evaluations. In almost every instance, the elderly Chinese resisted these interventions.

The nurses failed to establish an alliance with the very strong Chinese family organizations before imposing their solutions. They also neglected to investigate Chinese cultural patterns before attempting to assist them with the life pattern ramifications of the earthquake. Generally, Chinese people do not readily talk about feelings with outsiders, and they do not conceptualize distress in psychiatric terms. They interpret the presence of fatigue and disturbances in eating and sleeping patterns as physical illness. They expect health care personnel to recognize and help them with these physical symptoms. The suggestion that socializing in centers populated by English speakers would cure their illness seemed quite incredulous to the families.

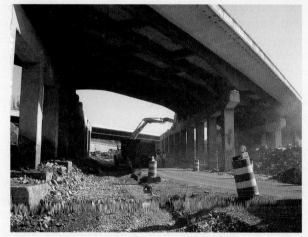

Construction of new interstate bypass to relieve traffic congestion due to urban sprawl.

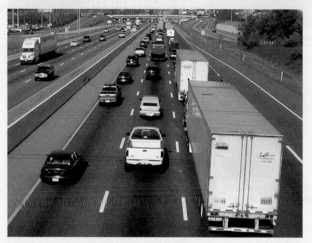

Motor vehicle emissions (primary mobile source of air pollutants).

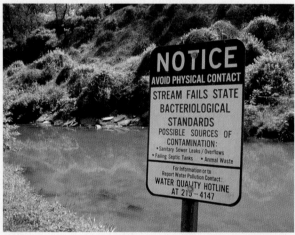

Polluted creek within 25 feet of children's urban playground in Knoxville, Tennessee.

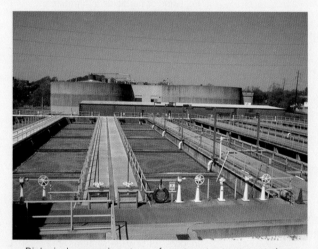

Biological processing stage of wastewater treatment plant.

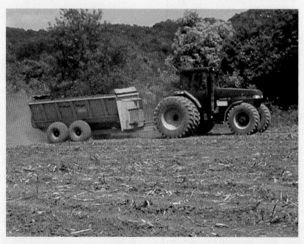

Land application of biosolids as part of a "sustainable" waste management program.

TABLE 14-3 MAJOR AIR POLLUTANTS

POLLUTANT	SOURCES	EFFECTS
Ozone: A colorless gas that is the major constituent of smog at the earth's surface	Ozone is formed in the lower atmosphere as the result of chemical reactions between oxygen, volatile organic compounds, and nitrogen oxides in the presence of sunlight, particularly during hot weather. Sources of this harmful pollutant include vehicles, factories, landfills, lawn equipment, farm equipment, and industrial solvents.	Ozone can irritate the respiratory tract, produce impaired lung function, and cause throat irritation, chest pain, cough, and susceptibility to lung infection. Individuals with asthma and other existing respiratory conditions are particularly vulnerable. Ozone can also reduce agricultural yields and injure forests and other vegetation.
Carbon monoxide: A colorless and odorless gas that is emitted in the exhaust of motor vehicles and other kinds of engines during combustion of fossil fuels	Carbon monoxide is emitted from cars, buses, trucks, and other small engines and from some industrial processes. High concentrations can be found in confined spaces (e.g., parking garages, poorly ventilated tunnels, or along roadsides during periods of heavy traffic).	Carbon monoxide reduces the ability of the blood to deliver oxygen to vital tissues, affecting primarily the cardiovascular and nervous systems. Lower concentrations have been shown to adversely affect individuals with heart disease and to affect exercise performance. Higher concentrations can cause symptoms such as dizziness, headaches, and fatigue.
Nitrogen dioxide: A light brown gas at lower concentrations; in higher concentrations, a significant component of brown urban haze	Nitrogen dioxide forms from the burning of fuels in utilities, industrial boilers, cars, and trucks.	Nitrogen dioxide is a major component of smog and acid rain. When concentrations are high, it can cause increased respiratory illnesses (e.g., chest colds and coughing) in children. For asthmatics, it may cause increased breathing difficulty.
Sulfur dioxide: A colorless gas, odorless at low concentrations but pungent at very high concentrations	Sulfur dioxide is emitted from industrial, institutional, utility, and apartment-house furnaces and boilers, as well as petroleum refineries, smelters, paper mills, and chemical plants.	Sulfur dioxide is one of the major components of smog. At high concentrations, it can harm humans; asthmatics are particularly vulnerable. It can also harm vegetation and metals and acidify lakes and streams.
Particulate matter: Droplets from smoke, dust, ash, and condensing vapors that can be suspended in the air for long periods of time	Particulates are emitted from industrial processes, vehicles, wood smoke, dust from paved and unpaved roads, construction, and agriculture.	Particulates can affect breathing and elicit respiratory symptoms, causing increased respiratory disease and lung damage. Children, elders, and people with heart or lung disease are especially at risk. They can also damage paint, soil, and clothing and reduce visibility.
Lead: A metal found in nature as well as a by-product of industry; can contaminate substances (e.g., soil, dust) that can be directly inhaled	Metals processing is the major source of lead emissions into the air today. Lead is generally found near lead smelters, waste incinerators, utilities, and lead-acid battery manufacturers.	Lead can adversely affect mental development and performance, kidney function, and blood chemistry. Young children are particularly at risk to its effects.

From Environmental Protection Agency: *What are the six common air pollutants?* April 7, 2006: www.epa.gov/air/urbanair/6poll.html.

One unfortunately common problem associated with living patterns relates to residing near hazardous facilities (e.g., waste incinerators, sewage treatment plants, landfills, refineries, and some correctional facilities). Discriminatory land use ensures that many impoverished and marginalized groups, especially people of color, live in close proximity to industrial contamination. This is called environmental racism (Chakraborty and Zandbergen, 2007; Northridge et al., 2003; Norton et al., 2007). People who live near such environmental hazards are in danger of becoming victims of illness and injury related to violence, poisonings and exposures, fires, and malignant and nonmalignant disease.

Many communities lack sufficient resources to respond when urban development and technological advances jeopardize the health and well-being of families in affected areas. The environmental movement of the 1960s and 1970s succeeded in building political power capable of passing monumental environmental reforms; however, charges that poor and minority communities are dumping grounds for environmental hazards have been substantiated by governmental agencies (EPA, 2008a; Shavers and Shavers, 2006).

Difficulties in alerting state and federal officials about environmental health dangers and difficulties in obtaining compensation for environmental toxin–causing disease and death often result in resident revictimization. Tightly knit social structures in the affected community and a lack of low-cost housing in other neighborhoods may hinder residents from leaving an area that poses potentially severe health risks from exposure to hazards. Residents may be unwilling to disrupt family ties and cultural roots to start over elsewhere, or they may be unable to afford a move. These residents may live with uncertainty and conflict. Long-term, community-wide effects of division, animosity, distrust, cynicism, and despair can abound in these situations.

In the 1990s, the central issues of equity and justice emerged in environmental health policy. In 1994, President

Year	Legislation
1970	Clean Air Act
	Poison Prevention Packaging Act
	Occupational Health and Safety Act
	Hazardous Materials Transportation Control
	National Environmental Policy Act
1971	Lead-Based Paint Poisoning Prevention Act
1972	Federal Water Pollution Control Act Amendments
	Noise Control Act
1976	Resource Conservation and Recovery Act
	Toxic Substances Control Act
1977	Clean Water Act
1980	Low Level Radiation Waste Policy Act
	Comprehensive Environmental Response, Compensation, and Liability Act (i.e., Superfund)

Clinton signed Executive Order 12898, which required all federal agencies to develop comprehensive strategies for achieving environmental justice. This legislation has served to increase public participation and access to information, as well as provision of education about multiple risks and cumulative exposures (EPA, 2005) (Box 14-1). Much remains to be done, however, to attain environmental justice in the United States.

Work Risks

Work risks include poor employment environments and potential injury or illness due to working conditions. Environmental health problems posed by work risks include such issues as sexual harassment, occupational toxic poisoning, machine-operation hazards (e.g., falls, crushing injuries, burns), electrical hazards, repetitive motion injuries, carcinogenic particulate inhalation (e.g., of asbestos, coal dust), and heavy metal poisoning (Centers for Disease Control and Prevention [CDC], 2005c; Krieger et al., 2008; Le Moual, Kennedy, and Kauffmann, 2004). Prevention of work-related health problems requires integrated action to improve job safety and the working environment.

Worldwide, it is estimated that job-related accidents and illnesses claim more than 2 million lives annually, and this number appears to be rising because of industrialization in developing countries (World Health Organization [WHO], 2005). In 2007, there were 4,002,700 recorded cases of non-fatal illnesses and injuries in the United States. In that year, there were approximately 5488 occupational fatalities; fishing, mining, construction, and agriculture have the highest rates of work-related deaths (U.S. Department of Labor, Bureau of Labor Statistics, 2008).

These statistics do not reflect unreported health problems. For example, a clerical worker leaves the office every day with back strain and a headache because of ventilation problems in the building. After 5 years on a repetitive hand-movement job task, an employee develops carpal tunnel syndrome. An operating room nurse has a miscarriage and recalls that

many of her coworkers have also been unable to carry their babies to term. A dry cleaner often leaves work feeling light-headed and dizzy from inhaling solvents at the shop, and one day she has a car accident on her way home. As a result, collective problems related to employment or occupation are often perceived as individualized injuries, and no one "connects the dots."

Clinical Example

Sanitation workers in an urban area experienced an increasing incidence of puncture injuries while transporting hazardous wastes from the public medical center; these puncture injuries caused several hepatitis cases. When the story became public, members of the city health commission contacted community health nurses and instructed them to politically support the interests of the city and the medical center "at all costs." Subsequently, the sanitation workers' union contacted the community health nursing office and requested information about procedures for safely packaging medical wastes. They also requested that a nurse speak to their membership about immediate measures for preventing further injuries on the job.

The nurses met to resolve the conflict. Most agreed that the sanitation workers had pressing needs for education and support. Despite the city's demand for loyalty, they decided to "choose sides" with the workers and respond to their requests. They collectively drafted a letter to the city health commission and arranged a meeting with the commissioners to discuss their plan to assist the sanitation workers. The health commission held a press conference, which depicted the nurses' actions as mediational efforts that benefited the union and the city. Eventually, the nurses and the commission developed a new medical waste disposal plan, and injured workers received reasonable compensation through an out-of-court settlement.

Atmospheric Quality

Atmospheric quality refers to the amount of protection in the atmospheric layers, the risks of severe weather, and the purity of the air. Environmental dangers related to atmospheric quality include nitrogen dioxide, lead, particulate matter, and sulfur dioxide emitted from power plants, as well as motor vehicle emissions, by-products of industrial processes, and waste incinerators (see Table 14-3). Tornadoes, electrical storms, smog, gaseous pollutants (e.g., carbon monoxide), excessive hydrocarbon levels, aerial herbicide spraying, and acid rain all contribute to air pollution. In addition, mercury, a potent neurotoxin released into the air from coal-fired power plants and waste incinerators, has resulted in fish consumption advisories in 48 states (EPA, 2007a).

Two significant issues related to atmospheric quality are of global concern. First, the amount of protection in the atmospheric layers is diminishing (EPA, 2008e). Chemicals such as chlorofluorocarbons, halons, and carbon tetrachloride, which have been in widespread use for refrigeration, air conditioning, and aerosol propellants, remain in the atmosphere. These molecules cause depletion of the atmosphere's protective ozone layer. The resulting "holes" in the ozone layer allow excess ultraviolet radiation to penetrate, which causes harmful effects on many organisms. Long-term problems include increases in skin cancer and cataracts, suppression of immune response, and environmental damage.

Second, there is a disruption in the key processes that break down atmospheric carbon dioxide. The ongoing devegetation of the earth's surface, especially cutting the tropical rain forests, not only releases the carbon stored in the biomass, but it also eliminates sources of photosynthesis (i.e., the process by which plants absorb carbon and release oxygen) (U.S. Department of Commerce, 2006). The loss of carbon dioxide–consuming resources increases carbon dioxide and traps part of the heat reemitted by the earth. As a result, the earth's surface temperature is increasing (i.e., the "greenhouse effect"), causing potentially catastrophic ecological consequences. Scientists predict that within a few decades, significant regional climate changes will have occurred, causing sea levels to rise and, in turn, causing serious coastal wetland loss.

Severe weather conditions, another aspect of atmospheric quality that affects the public's health, can have dramatic results in the form of injury and loss of life, destruction of plants and wildlife, and property damage (Burns, 2002; Ivers and Ryan, 2006). Climatic changes associated with global warming may contribute to increasing the frequency and severity of the earth's weather extremes. Climatic disruption may be implicated in global geophysical destabilization, exemplified by earthquakes and tsunami effects.

Ground-level ozone, the primary component of smog, is the most common outdoor air pollutant in the United States. Ozone is formed when nitrogen oxides (created by the burning of fossil fuels in power plants, automobiles, and industry) react with oxygen and sunlight (EPA, 2008e). Ozone, along with other hazardous atmospheric pollutants, causes and/or contributes to asthma, allergic reactions, bronchitis, lung cancer, chronic respiratory disease, and death and harms animal and plant species (Ciencewicki, Trivedi, and Kleeberger, 2008; National Toxic Inhalation Study Group, 1998). Further, sulfur dioxide, a by-product of burning coal and other fossil fuels, contributes to acid rain, which affects terrestrial ecosystems by increasing soil acidity, reducing nutrient availability, mobilizing toxic metals, leaching soil chemicals, and altering species composition (EPA, 2007b).

Clinical Example

During a recent summer, a sudden increase occurred in the number of emergency calls from residents of a particular urban neighborhood to a medical hotline. These calls often involved elderly women who collapsed in their homes. In one case, an asthmatic child had severe dyspnea.

The emergency calls continued, and two community health nurses noted that respiratory difficulties were often implicated. These nurses decided to visit the neighborhood and investigate. It was near rush hour, and within minutes the traffic on the nearby freeway slowed to a crawl, apparently from road construction. Through their direct observations and critical assessment, these nurses determined that heavy car exhaust fumes seemed to stagnate around several residential buildings in the area. The nurses notified the Environmental Protection Agency and the city transportation department and recommended further investigation and resolution of the problem.

One week later, the nurses returned to the neighborhood and observed that the traffic moved more efficiently, although road construction continued. Within several weeks, the number of emergency medical calls decreased.

Water Quality

Water quality refers to the water supply's availability, volume, mineral content levels, toxic chemical pollution, and pathogenic microorganism levels. Water quality consists of the balance between water contaminants and the existing capabilities to purify water for human use and plant and wildlife sustenance. Water quality problems include experiencing droughts, dousing reservoirs with chemicals to reduce algae, contaminating aquifers with pesticides and fertilizers, leaching lead from water pipes, and oil spilling from transport tankers or leaking offshore wells. Other sources of water pollution are microbial contamination from poorly managed or maintained septic or sewage systems and animal feedlot wastes (Hamilton, Miller, and Myers, 2004; EPA, 2008b). Water pollution can be from point sources (a well-defined source, e.g., factory wastewater discharge) or nonpoint sources (urban runoff, domestic lawn care, and air-to-water transfer).

Advances in water treatment technologies in industrialized countries have controlled many water-related diseases such as cholera, typhoid, dysentery, and hepatitis A. Despite this, disease outbreaks resulting from contamination by untreated groundwater and inadequate chlorination are increasing in both urban and rural areas. In addition, more than 42 million Americans obtain their drinking water from private water supplies (e.g., wells) that have no treatment or monitoring guidelines (CDC, 2008). Other potential water contaminants include accelerated soil erosion caused by construction, agriculture, and deforestation; these can contribute to high sediment levels in drinking water supplies. This necessitates higher levels of water treatment to remove heavy metals and chemicals. Heavy metal and toxic chemical pollution may also occur during the water treatment process or in the drinking water distribution system. The EPA monitors drinking water for more than 80 organic and inorganic pollutants that have potential health effects in humans, including those who are most vulnerable, such as children and those with weakened immune systems (EPA, 2007c). Pesticides, herbicides, and carcinogenic industrial waste infiltrate an increasing amount of groundwater, the underground source of half the U.S. population's drinking water (U.S. Geological Survey, 2005). This is particularly tragic because groundwater is uniquely susceptible to long-term contamination. Unlike river or lake water, once groundwater becomes contaminated, it is impossible to cleanse.

Clinical Example

In a Midwestern farm community, there is growing concern about agricultural pesticide and herbicide seepage into groundwater. Families obtain water from their own wells rather than a central municipal source. The families recognized the potential long-term carcinogenic effects of the chemicals involved. Although family farmers decreased their use of these chemicals, the large-scale agribusiness companies continued to use excessive amounts of these chemicals.

County community health nurses lobbied local officials to begin a comprehensive program to monitor groundwater pollutants and enforce standards for herbicide and pesticide use; however, the powerful agribusiness companies pressured these officials to stand back. Together, some county farmers and nurses organized grass-roots information and support groups among rural families. The families and nurses, in coalition with environmental activist groups in the state, established several participatory action research projects. These projects included collecting and testing samples from each family well, forming a local umbrella organization called "Water Watch" to coordinate actions and communications, and involving a research project with a federal health agency to track the health problems of local residents who used these water sources on a long-term basis. The organization also disseminated an emergency plan for drinking-water distribution if wells were found to have toxic levels of pesticides, herbicides, or other pollutants.

Housing

Housing is an environmental health concern, and it refers to the availability, safety, cleanliness, and location of shelter, including public facilities and individual or family dwellings. According to *Healthy People 2010*, four of the major environmental health problems related to housing are elevated indoor allergen levels, radon poisoning, lead-based paint poisoning, and exposure to tobacco smoke (USDHHS, 2000).

Other environmental health problems related to housing include fire hazards; lack of access for disabled people; illnesses caused by overcrowding, dampness, and rodent or insect infestation; psychological effects of architectural design (e.g., low-cost, high-rise housing projects); injuries sustained from collapsed building structures; and exposure deaths from inadequate indoor heating or cooling.

Poor housing conditions can contribute to the spread of infectious disease (EPA, 2008d), as well as cardiovascular and respiratory disorders, cancers, allergies, and mental illnesses (Barton et al., 2007; Rauh, Landrigan, and Claudio, 2008). The term sick building syndrome describes a phenomenon in which public structures and homes cause occupants to experience a variety of symptoms, such as headache, fatigue, and exacerbation of allergies. This typically results from poor ventilation and building operations, hazardous building materials, furniture and carpeting substances, and cleaning agents (EPA, 2008d).

Other problems may arise related to building structures, composition, and settings. For example, commercial buildings with offices near underground parking garages may cause workers to have carbon monoxide intoxication. Formaldehyde, asbestos, and volatile organic compounds—which are common components of thermal insulation, cement, flooring, furnishings, and household consumer products—have carcinogenic properties. Additionally, "toxic mold" arising from chronically damp wood and improperly sealed areas in homes and offices has recently been recognized as contributing to respiratory irritation, allergies, and infections in susceptible individuals (EPA, 2008d).

Much controversy surrounds the economic hardship that industry, government, business, and multidwelling owners would face if they were forced to reduce concentrations

of such toxic elements. Enforcement of mandatory toxic abatement, however, will ensure a safer future and exemplify community-level response to environmental health risks.

Clinical Example

In a large, northeastern U.S. city, an economic recession led to massive unemployment, rising housing costs, and drastically reduced housing subsidies. Simultaneously, funding was cut for several public health and mental health facilities. The result left approximately 4000 people "houseless." The local shelters housed a total of 500 people each night, but none of these shelters accepted women. More than a dozen people died of exposure to the elements during the winter.

Community health nurses met with local church groups who started a shelter for women. This coalition acquired a building in an area where many shelterless people congregated. They offered accommodations for 75 women. After 3 months, the city took over the women's shelter because the churches experienced difficulties filling the beds and maintaining the project's financial solvency. The city changed the shelter to a dwelling for 50 men and 25 women because women did not use it sufficiently.

In their evaluation, the nurses consulted with several shelterless women and workers from a popular soup kitchen. The answer was relatively simple. The women did not feel safe going to the shelter because the area had a high-crime reputation and lacked street lighting. Eventually, a new coalition formed, composed of community health nurses, several women who were or had been shelterless, a representative from the police force, and the church groups. A new women's shelter opened in a safer, well-lit neighborhood close to public transit lines.

Food Quality

Food quality refers to availability and relative cost of food, variety and safety of food, and the health of animal and plant food sources. Food quality problems include malnutrition, bacterial food poisoning, carcinogenic chemical additives (e.g., nitrites, dyes, and cyclamate), improper or fraudulent meat inspection or food labeling, microbial epidemics among livestock (e.g., *Escherichia coli*), food products from diseased animal sources, and disruption of vital natural food chains by ecosystem destruction. Further, increased mobility and globalized trade means that contaminants may rapidly be carried to distant destinations, through marketing, importing, and air travel.

Potential microbial contaminants of foods include bacteria (e.g., *Shigella salmonella*, *E. coli*, *Campylobacter*), parasites (e.g., *Balantidium coli*, *Cryptosporidium parvum*, *Entamoeba histolytica*), and viruses (e.g., calicivirus, rotavirus, hepatitis A virus, enterovirus) (CDC, 2005b). After increasing throughout the 1990s, the rates of food-borne illnesses are now declining. The biggest decline has been seen in *E. coli 0157*, most frequently identified in uncooked hamburger. The United States currently depends on the Foodborne Diseases Active Surveillance Network (FoodNet) of CDC's Emerging Infections Program to collect data on diseases caused by enteric pathogens transmitted through food.

Agrichemicals, such as pesticides and fertilizers; materials from mechanical handling devices; detergents; and organic packaging materials can also contaminate food. Toxic chemicals from farming and ranching may be introduced into the food chain, increasing risk of reproductive and mutagenic effects in humans (Driehuis et al., 2008; EPA, 2008c; Knobeloch et al., 2009). For instance, farmers spray dioxin-containing weed killers on rangeland. Beef cattle graze on the land, herbicide accumulates in their fatty tissue, and the contaminated meat is sold in markets. The complexity of transfer of these contaminants makes for difficulty in establishing causality and tracing accountability for these health risks.

Unsuitable handling, storage, processing, and transport techniques can damage food and make it unsuitable for consumption. Further, additives are often used to improve food properties. For example, vitamins and minerals are used to enhance nutritional content; salt, sugars, and monosodium glutamate are used to improve flavor; dyes are used to enhance color; leavening agents, gums, or thickening agents are used to improve consistency; and various preservatives are used to increase shelf life. Many of these additives are not nutritious, and some may be harmful. Additionally, residues from the overuse of antibiotics in animal husbandry remain in meat and milk products, causing consumers to develop resistance, thus rendering these antibiotics ineffective in treating human infections (Hurd and Malladi, 2008). Another potential threat related to food quality involves "genetically modified" (GM) or genetically engineered foods. GM foods have been in existence since the early 1970s and are created by a process in which scientists splice plant or animal genes with particular traits into the DNA of other organisms (Whitney, Maltby, and Carr, 2004). This technology has contributed to crops and livestock that grow faster, are more resistant to disease and insects, and produce higher yields and greater nutritive value; often GM crops require less water and fertilizer (Davies, 2003).

There is concern that genetic alteration of food is growing despite the fact that the long-term health effects of eating GM food are unknown. Some believe that allergies and other immunity problems may proliferate as unique antigens are present on GM proteins, and GM foods have unpredictable metabolic processes in animals, humans, and plants (Whitney et al., 2004). Although the U.S. Department of Agriculture and the U.S. Food and Drug Administration set policy for foods produced from new plant varieties and breeding, a number of groups and organizations have called for increased public awareness on the potential risks of genetically engineered foods and are working to require more stringent testing of them.

Clinical Example

A southern U.S. town with a population of 10,000 has a large population of black farm workers and a smaller, but significant, number of white residents who are textile workers. Located well off the interstate arteries, the town experienced very high food costs from shipping difficulties. Many families tapered their diets and ate mostly bread, rice, beans, and eggs. Health assessments of school-age children and toddlers indicated deficiencies of vitamins contained in fresh fruits and vegetables.

Local physicians, county health nurses, and the Parent-Teacher Association joined forces to improve the nutritional situation. The most popular proposed solution involved a community garden project. The groups leased land from the county, and the project began. Conflict arose when black community leaders realized that the mostly white textile workers formed their own garden project and competed with the original garden project for the town's support.

The nurses and parents originally involved in planning the project met to avert a crisis. They decided to focus on reaching church leaders and women in both black and white sectors of the town in the hope of supporting a dialogue and a equitable solution to the problem. Parents and church leaders spread the word in their respective communities. A community meeting was held at a convenient time for women in the town and at a neutral place that was acceptable to both groups.

Although tensions were strong enough to prevent the formation of a joint garden, the solution reached in the meeting caused each group to feel successful. On a per-capita basis, town funds were allocated to two gardening projects. The groups agreed that they would share vegetable and fruit yields, depending on the yield from each site. In addition, the cooperative plan increased the total garden space allotted by 50% and began a gardening "tool library" so neither group had to purchase new tools.

Waste Control

Waste control is the management of waste materials resulting from industrial and municipal processes, human consumption, and efforts to minimize waste production. Environmental health problems related to waste control include nonbiodegradable plastics, inefficient recycling programs, unlicensed waste dumps, inadequate sewage systems for increasing populations, unsafe dumping of industrial toxins, exportation of radioactive medical wastes, illicit dumping, and nonenforcement of environmental regulations.

American consumers' increasing trash production and the improper treatment, storage, transport, and disposal of waste are a significant concern. Routinely, commercial and institutional wastes are dumped with household waste in the same municipal incinerator, landfill, or sewer system. These commercial enterprises are generally exempt from the strict waste regulation applied to industry, although they often generate the same hazardous materials. Small businesses such as dry cleaners, photography laboratories, pesticide formulators, construction sites, and car repair shops discard a variety of substances that can cause serious public health problems.

Traditionally, U.S. economic development has produced optimal wealth with the assumption that the environmental health consequences would be minor. This notion of sustainable development has proved inadequate, and cumulative hazardous episodes necessitate tough pollution control technologies. The sustainability paradigm has led to a shift from disposing to recycling of wastes reclaimed from sewage, called biosolids. Biosolids refer to sewage sludge that has been treated for pathogens to meet the regulatory requirements for land application. This has been a cost-effective practice, but more study needs to be conducted on human health risks of biosolid distribution in the ecosystem (see photo on page 251 depicting waste disposal).

There are a number of potential health problems associated with waste management. For example, solid waste landfills accumulate methane gas, a by-product of decomposing organic wastes. Without proper venting, this volatile gas can move through soil and cause fires and explosions in nearby areas. Waste incineration is not the best solution because it causes particulate air pollution and is ineffective in the combustion of many materials. Improper design, operation, or waste site location causes hazardous substances to spread through air, soil, and water to poison humans, animals, and plant life. Alarmingly, only a percentage of hazardous waste actually reaches the designated waste sites; much is disposed of in open pits and in bodies of water, with dangerously uncertain long-term effects. New methods are only now being developed to estimate long-term rates of leaching of materials in various types of waste sites, based on probability principles (Sanchez and Kosson, 2005).

In 1980, Congress passed the Environmental Response Compensation and Liability Act, which established a revolving fund called the Superfund, to clean up several hundred of the worst abandoned chemical waste disposal sites. One of the most notorious sites is the Love Canal in Niagara Falls, New York. For 40 years before the 1960s, more than 80 different types of chemicals including benzene, dioxin, trichloroethylene, toluene, and chloroform were dumped in an abandoned canal. Afterward, the covered area became the site for a school and several hundred homes. In the winters of 1976 and 1977, heavy snowfall and rain caused toxic wastes to reach the surface. Subsequently, the inhabitants experienced elevated miscarriage rates, blood and liver abnormalities, birth defects, and chromosome damage.

Clinical Example

In a city on the Mississippi River, an outbreak of shigellosis was traced to a group of high school students who had been swimming in a particular area of the river. The local meatpacking plant was releasing waste material, including human and animal feces, directly into the river.

After intervening to contain the *Shigella* outbreak, the local community health nurses began to assess the situation. Their research indicated that the meatpacking facility had been in violation of waste control laws for some time. City officials imposed fines, which the company paid, but the dumping continued. A sign at the riverside prohibited swimming. Frustrated by their attempts to negotiate with the city and the plant, the nurses wrote a letter to the state capital newspaper, which had a large state readership, and the local newspaper. In the letter, they voiced concern about the community's health and the river's ecological integrity. Both papers published their informative letter as a commentary, which prompted responses from two local environmental groups, several activist groups located downriver, and a national organization concerned with clean water. These groups provided legal support and brought a collective suit against the meatpacking company. Subsequently, the company improved its waste treatment process to avoid paying a large award in the civil suit.

Radiation Risks

Radiation risks are health dangers posed by various forms of ionizing radiation relative to barriers that prevent human exposure and other life form exposure. Radiation risks include nuclear power emissions, radioactive hazardous wastes, medical and dental radiographs, and wartime nuclear weapon dangers. According to WHO (2009c), the three primary sources and distribution of radiation exposure to the world's population are radon (43%), medical exposure (20%), and other nonnatural sources (19%).

Manufactured sources of radiation contribute to humans' continuous exposure to ionizing radiation. Potential environmental radioactive pollution results from nuclear weapons testing, nuclear waste disposal, accidents at nuclear power plants, and the transportation, storage, loss, and misuse of radioactive sources (WHO, 2009c).

There is considerable disagreement regarding the safety of nuclear industries. Although some studies have found an increased risk of health problems among people and animals living near nuclear facilities such as power plants and waste storage sites (Harrison, Gustafson, and Dixon, 2003), other studies have found that there is no increased risk (Slama et al., 2008; Brownless, 2008; Harris and Miller, 2008). In addition, nuclear wastes remain dangerously radioactive for thousands of years; a safe way to dispose of them does not exist. Interim collection centers currently stockpile much of the waste. There is a quandary not only about how, where, and when to dispose of newly generated nuclear wastes, but also about how to manage improperly disposed radioactive materials.

Millions of Americans are exposed to dangerous levels of radiation in the form of radon gas in their homes, schools, and workplaces. Radon contamination is the second leading cause of lung cancer mortality in the United States, contributing to an estimated 15,000 to 20,000 deaths of this disease each year (EPA, 2008f). Radon is a radioactive radium decay product that occurs naturally in certain kinds of phosphate- and uranium-containing rock, such as granite and black shale, and is associated with an increased risk of cancer. Radon may be present in building materials, drinking water, and soil. Radon gas diffuses into dwellings, mostly through soil, and is prevalent where uranium-bearing land is common. Radon seeps through basement walls, pipes, and cracks in the foundation and is trapped in buildings with inadequate ventilation.

Cumulative exposure to excessive or ill-performed radiographs can also cause radiation damage in the body (Martin, 2008; Hampton, 2006). People who work with medical sources of radiation, such as radium or radioactive iodine, are at increased risk for development of cancers and for having children with birth defects. Older x-ray machines may emit excessive levels of radioactivity; all such equipment should undergo regular testing for leakage.

Ammunition (bombs and bullets) made with depleted uranium was used in wars in Europe and Asia and also contributes to health hazards from radiation (Salbu et al., 2005; Milacic, 2008). The long-term health consequences are purported to include teratogenic, immunological, and cancerous conditions, posing danger to both local populations and military personnel. Continued investigation is needed to identify long-term consequences of this practice.

Clinical Example

During wartime, federal standards related to radioactive environmental contamination and the public's "right to know" are suspended for military projects. In the middle of the Persian Gulf War, information "leaked" about a military installation in the southwestern desert near Deserttown. The installation planned test explosions of several new nuclear bombs, which they called nuclear "devices."

Local townspeople expressed concern, but the military did not confirm or deny these plans. The possible dates for the tests were also unknown. Residents began to panic, and several families moved. Others built makeshift shelters and began stockpiling food. There was an increase in psychiatric hospitalization rates. The town reached a crisis when a spate of three related adolescent suicides occurred in 2 months. The entire community appeared disorganized, helpless, and hopeless.

Town officials organized town meetings. Public health nurses offered community education about the health effects of ionizing radiation and answered questions, but this did not raise resident morale. The nurses decided to contact other communities that faced similar threats to determine how they dealt with them.

When these communities received word about Deserttown, they organized a letter-writing campaign and a support demonstration. They converged on Deserttown for a weekend rally and celebration of solidarity. The youth of Deserttown extended this demonstration by performing weekly vigils at the military site. One year later, the community was more united and less depressed, and the adolescent suicide rate had decreased significantly. The nuclear threat remained.

EFFECTS OF ENVIRONMENTAL HAZARDS

Environmental hazards are ubiquitous, and their effect on the public's health is complex and generally interconnected (Smith, 2008). Nurses must understand the multiple and complex sequences leading to health disorders. For example, nuclear power plant emissions may contaminate water and air supplies, affecting water quality, atmospheric quality, and radiation risk. Overcrowded housing may exacerbate problems in managing human waste, which may taint foodstuffs and contribute to the spread of communicable disease.

Certain environmental exposures have been found to have a direct relationship to the development of some cancers, chronic diseases, and other health-related problems (Boyd and Genuis, 2008). Furthermore, oppressive environments may affect health directly. In one case, an American company dumped dangerous waste material in Mexico rather than pay for proper disposal (Schrieberg, 1991). Poor children who lived nearby and scavenged for food in the dump picked up and played with the shiny, brightly colored radioactive medical waste. The severe burns they suffered and the wine-colored spots on their skin were direct effects of the illegally dumped toxic waste.

Effects of environmental risks may also be indirect, such as in the case of global warming (Akhtar et al., 2009; Pan and Kao, 2009). It has been hypothesized that the sea level will eventually rise from the melting polar ice caps. The resulting coastal inundation and flooding will threaten large areas of low-lying agricultural land and food supplies in many regions of the world. Rising global temperatures may enhance the quantity and distribution of parasites, insects, and other disease vectors, potentially increasing the prevalence of a variety of infectious diseases.

Effects of environmental hazards may be general or specific. For example, the ramifications of high unemployment, drought, and extensive smog cover affect the public generally, whereas the particular housing needs of elderly people who use walkers or canes, the occupational risks of electrical line repair workers, and the mentally incapacitating effects of elevated blood lead levels in children affect the public more specifically.

Environmental health effects can be immediate, long term, or transgenerational. Burns, gunshot wounds, hurricane damage, and outbreaks of gastrointestinal distress among cafeteria customers are examples of immediate effects from health-damaging environments. Examples of long-term health effects include gradual occupational hearing loss, "black lung" in coal miners, and increased rates of thyroid cancer among young victims of the Chernobyl accident (Ron, 2007). Transgenerational effects occur with female factory workers exposed to radiation at plutonium-processing plants. The radiation causes chromosomal anomalies, which result in birth defects.

ETHICAL INSIGHTS

Agent Orange

The controversial legacy of the Agent Orange defoliant (which contained dioxin) that was sprayed by the U.S. Army during the Vietnam War has caused pain for numerous citizens (past, present, and future). This toxic chemical killed many people in Vietnam, including civilians.

Environmental exposures after the World Trade Center attack resulted in significant adverse health effects. The dust produced bronchial hyperactivity, persistent cough, and increased risk for asthma. Pregnant women who were inside or near the World Trade Center on September 11, 2001, bore small-for-gestational-age babies, possibly related to exposures to polycyclic aromatic hydrocarbons and particulates. Further, scientists hypothesize that the future risk of chronic respiratory disease may be increased, because of occupational exposure to inhaled particulate matter (Lorber et al., 2007).

Some negative environmental health effects may be reversible. Smokers who have quit demonstrate regeneration of cilia in the lungs after months to years, for example. Radiation damage to human cells and silicosis damage to lung capacity, however, are irreversible. Conversely, heavy metal exposure from many environmental hazards causes cumulative effects. Lead slowly collects in the long bones, and the lead can re-release into the body. This release may cause acute poisoning and additional damage over time (Meyer, Brown, and Falk, 2008).

EFFORTS TO CONTROL ENVIRONMENTAL HEALTH PROBLEMS

The 1970s were the decade of environmental concern. Cynicism toward institutions grew during the years of U.S. involvement in Vietnam, and legislative activism for environmental preservation exploded (Burger, 1989). During the 1970s, Congress created new agencies to regulate environmental conditions on a national level, including the EPA, Occupational Safety and Health Administration, and the Nuclear Regulatory Commission. The EPA has enormous responsibilities for protecting the environment and minimizing risks to human health. Among its roles are health surveillance and monitoring; setting standards for air and water quality; evaluating environmental risks; acquiring information; screening new chemicals; performing basic research and training; and establishing, evaluating, and enforcing regulatory efforts.

The legislative activism of the 1970s was aimed toward a comprehensive national environmental policy. For example, stricter automobile fuel and emissions standards created improvements in air quality, which caused lead levels in urban air to decrease dramatically over the next decade (Bingham and Meader, 1990). The momentum to control environmental pollution in the United States slowed in the 1980s and 1990s with several policy reversals and the defunding of regulatory mechanisms.

This trend has continued into the twenty-first century. For example, one piece of recent legislation regulating mercury pollution from power plants drew criticism from environmental advocates who noted that the rule was too weak. The Clean Air Mercury Rule is aimed at coal-fired power plants, which is the nation's largest remaining source of mercury emissions. According to the EPA, the rule will decrease mercury in two phases, eventually capping national mercury emissions at 15 tons by 2018 (down from about 48 tons). Environmental advocates argue that the EPA's mercury rule violates the 1900 Clean Air Act, ignores the science on mercury hazards, and allows industry to pollute beyond the 2018 deadline.

Other laws and regulatory structures are weak or nonexistent with regard to environmental health problems. For example, federal mandates for recycling do not exist, although local communities have made great strides in this area. Comprehensive groundwater legislation, similar to adopted measures to preserve marine and surface waters, also does not exist. Additionally, the EPA tends to set priorities for the reduction of environmental problems but does not allocate the resources necessary to accomplish these goals.

Most of the U.S. environmental health efforts have aimed for short-term results rather than anticipating future issues and problems. A crucial need exists in the development of human resources in the area of environmental health. Nurses in all areas of practice should be aware of the implications the environment has for their clients and their health. It is for this reason that nurses need to take and record an environmental health history on every client. The means of taking an environmental health history is discussed later in this chapter.

GLOBAL ENVIRONMENTAL HEALTH

Environmental health addresses all of the physical, chemical, and biological factors external to a person, and all the related factors impacting behaviours. It encompasses the assessment and control of those environmental factors that can potentially affect health. (WHO, 2009a)

The WHO goes on to say that the target of environmental health is disease prevention and the creation of environments that support health.

Globalization and industrialization in the developing world have increased the number of health problems related to the environment. Urbanization has made it difficult to maintain clean air, clean water, and good sanitation practices. Consequently, humans are now exposed to serious amounts of environmental hazards (CDC, 2005c).

Large-scale hazards related to global environmental conditions include climate change, stratospheric ozone depletion, loss of biodiversity, degradation, stresses on food-producing systems, and changes in the hydrological systems and freshwater supplies. As corporations become global entities, many escape U.S. standards by moving operations to unregulated areas of the world. Global environmental health hazards cannot be fully outlined here, but it is incumbent on nursing as a profession to take a strong stance on global health at the international level.

EMERGING ILLNESSES RELATED TO THE ENVIRONMENT

The new science focusing on identifying and treating emerging illnesses recognizes the relationship between environmental change, human activities, disease, and public health. Emerging illness refers to newly identified diseases, as well as diseases that are establishing new niches in parts of the world where they previously were nonexistent. Urban areas are susceptible to this phenomenon because they are densely populated and permit rapid entrance of microbes and contaminants from other countries due to the large number of seaports and airports (Center for Children's Health and the Environment, 2002).

For example, global climate change, along with international commerce and travel, contributed to the entry and propagation of the West Nile virus in the United States (Epstein, 2001). Increased air and water temperatures facilitate the spread of vector-borne diseases transmitted by mosquitoes (e.g., West Nile virus). As a result, in 2003, there were 9862 reported cases of, and 264 related deaths because of, West Nile virus in the United States (CDC, 2005a).

Similarly, severe acute respiratory syndrome (SARS) and H1N1 virus (swine flu) were recently added to the list of environmental challenges for health professionals throughout the world. SARS swept through China and Southeast Asia before spreading to many parts of the world, including Canada and

RESEARCH HIGHLIGHTS

I PREPARE: Development and Clinical Utility of an Environmental Exposure History Mnemonic

The I PREPARE environmental exposure history mnemonic is a quick reference tool created for primary care providers. A total of 159 health care providers, both students and professionals, were asked to evaluate a prototype mnemonic, to suggest new health history questions, and to propose the deletion of less-relevant questions. The prototype was formatted as a pocket guide. The goal of this evaluation was to create a practical and clinically relevant mnemonic, rather than to obtain quantitative estimates of validity. This mnemonic serves as a mental cue to facilitate the collection and documentation of health information in a systematic manner.

I—Investigate Potential Exposures
P—Present Work
R—Residence
E—Environmental Concerns
P—Past Work

A—Activities
R—Referrals and Resources
E—Educate

Questions to ask are presented for each letter in the mnemonic, except for Referrals and Resources, which provides sources of additional information. A checklist of strategies to prevent or minimize exposures can be used by the health care provider to help clients identify potential exposures. The sequence of I PREPARE makes intuitive sense by cueing the provider to ask specific questions and provide educational materials to the client. The final version was reprinted on heavy laminated material. The I PREPARE mnemonic increases the repertoire of tools clinicians have available to elicit an appropriate health history. The national improvements in the quality of environmental exposure history are predicated, in part, on the creation of simple and convenient tools for use in clinical practice.

From Paranzino GK, et al: I PREPARE: Development and clinical utility of an environmental exposure history mnemonic, *AAOHN J* 53(1):37-42, 2005.

the United States, during the winter of 2002-2003 (WHO, 2009d). Likewise, the H1N1 influenza pandemic apparently started in central Mexico in the spring of 2009 before spreading to more than 74 countries by mid-June of that year (CDC, 2009; WHO, 2009b). International travel greatly contributed to the rapid spread of SARS, which epidemiologists have now identified as a global health threat.

Other Emerging Threats

It is a misconception that the United States is exempt from the environmental health hazards that less-developed nations must endure. Within the past decade, we are beginning to recognize that our environmental public health infrastructure is quite weak and that the United States is susceptible to many of the same problems that burden the rest of the world. For example, the illegal use of pesticides, medical waste incineration, and the increased incidence of asthma related to air pollution are just a few of the challenges facing the United States today. The manufacturing of methamphetamine in home-based laboratories has risen dramatically in the past 5 years, and the "cooking process" emits dangerous levels of toxic chemicals into the air. Similarly, the abandoned labs also pose a threat.

Since September 11, 2001, U.S. citizens realize that our country is not safe from terrorist attacks. Terrorist attacks can take many forms, some of which could include biological or chemical warfare or nuclear retaliation. Ongoing reports of actual attacks (e.g., the hotel attacks in India in 2008) and threats of attacks promote recognition of personal vulnerability and the need to be aware and prepared.

There is also the threat of natural disasters that can disrupt and oftentimes overwhelm private and public health systems. Natural disasters, such as the tsunami that struck the coast of Indonesia in December 2004, Hurricane Katrina in August 2005, and the devastating earthquake in the Sichuan Province of China in 2008, and in Haiti in 2010, require mobilization of disaster relief units that offer substantial assistance and expertise. Natural disasters such as hurricanes, tornados, and earthquakes frequently receive notable publicity, but other, more insidious disasters such as droughts, floods, heat waves, and extreme cold also pose major public health concerns. The aforementioned threats can cause significant mortality and morbidity and, therefore, have the potential to burden the health care delivery system.

Nursing Actions

Nurses must work with the public to promote more stringent and actively enforced environmental legislation and regulations. In the twenty-first century, actions must include not only national but also worldwide environmental policies. Ozone depletion, global warming, fossil fuel burning, marine dumping, active land mine abandonment in war-torn areas, mass relocation of refugees across national borders, and destruction of tropical rain forests are among key global environmental health concerns.

In an era of globalization, nurses must support actions for biodiversity, including pushing back the deserts, replanting the forests, stabilizing the climate, and seeking alternative development pathways that do not destroy plant and animal species. The development of state-of-the-art methods for removing pollutants from the biosphere, managing ecosystems, handling hazardous wastes, and preserving oceans depends on the integration of scientific knowledge, complex sociopolitical processes, and values. In recognition of threats to the biosphere and exploitation of the world's ecosystems, environmental integrity will require international assistance, ameliorative actions, and an environmentally educated global public.

Environmental concerns for clean air, clean water, and freedom from noxious chemicals must become global nursing concerns. Community health nurses can be catalysts to neighborhood efforts to produce safe living environments.

Community health nursing must expand its theory and practice to incorporate the fact that individual and community health ultimately depends on global environmental integrity. Many organizations work to preserve and protect the environment and could benefit from the active involvement and support of nurses. Box 14-2 lists some of these organizations. Nursing must broaden its borders to include a global perspective. Global sustainability will be achieved through commitment to strong ethical principles and social justice and with initiatives for environmental responsibility in daily personal activity.

BOX 14-2   ENVIRONMENTAL ORGANIZATIONS

- American Farmland Trust
- Animal Preservation League
- Citizens for a Better Environment
- Clean Water Action
- Earth Regeneration Society
- Forests Forever
- Greenpeace
- International Rivers Network
- National Environmental Law Center
- National Toxics Campaign
- Natural Resources Defense Council
- Ocean Alliance
- Pesticide Action Network
- Radioactive Wastes Campaign
- Rainforest Action Network
- Sierra Club
- Toxics Coordinating Project
- Trust for Public Land
- U.S. Public Interest Research Group
- Wilderness Society

Websites for these organizations can be accessed through the WebLinks section of the book's website at http://evolve.elsevier.com/Nies.

For further information, see the report by the Institute of Medicine Committee on Enhancing Environmental Health Content in Nursing Practice: *Nursing, health, and the environment*, Washington, DC, 1995, National Academies Press.

APPROACHING ENVIRONMENTAL HEALTH AT THE AGGREGATE LEVEL

In the United States, personal independence and individual responsibility for success and failure are valued. These values can lead nurses to overlook environmental hazards and instead blame individual clients for their health problems. By placing responsibility for the cause and cure of health problems exclusively on the individual, the belief is reinforced that all individuals are free to exert meaningful control over the quality and length of their lives. Such a perspective absolves society, government, industry, and business from accountability.

Research suggests that changing individual behaviors does not lead to significant reductions in overall morbidity and mortality in the absence of basic social, economic, and political changes (Bhatia and Wernham, 2008). Emphasizing only interventions that address deleterious personal habits through exercise programs, weight-loss regimens, smoking-cessation classes, and stress-reduction tactics fails to take into account the broader environmental origins of disease, injury, and ecological degradation. An attempt to approach health at the aggregate level is the *Healthy People 2020* initiative (USDHHS, 2009). It focuses on health promotion and disease prevention in specific areas, such as environmental health. The *Healthy People* box lists selected *Healthy People 2020* environmental health objectives.

Nursing is not alone in its focus on individual health-promoting interventions. Most health agencies, health care institutions, and corporate workplaces, however, have principally addressed the idea of "controllable risk" in the individual, with much less effort directed toward reducing risks in the environment. In addition, the government has also reduced its overall focus on environmental health. The effectiveness and power of agencies such as the EPA and the National Institute for Occupational Safety and Health have declined over the past 25 years. Therefore fewer studies of environmental health risks and enforcement regulatory policies have been conducted.

 HEALTHY PEOPLE 2020

Selected Objectives for Environmental Health

OBJECTIVE
EH–1 Increase the proportion of persons served by community water systems who receive a supply that meets the regulations of the Safe Drinking Water Act
EH–2 Reduce waterborne disease outbreaks arising from water intended for drinking among persons served by community water systems.
EH–4 Increase recycling of municipal solid waste
EH–9 Increase use of alternative modes of transportation for work commutes to reduce motor vehicle emissions and improve the nation's air quality
EH–10 Reduce air toxic emissions to decrease the risk of adverse health effects caused by airborne toxins
EH–13 Eliminate elevated blood lead levels in children
EH–17 Increase the proportion of persons living in homes at risk that have an operating radon mitigation system

From U.S. Department of Health and Human Services: *Healthy People 2010*, ed 2, Washington, D.C, 2000, US Government Printing Office.
US Department of Health and Human Services: *Healthy People* 2020–2009 Draft Objectives. Wasington DC. http://www.healthypeople.gov/hp2020/Objectives/TopicAreas.aspx

Protecting Vulnerable Aggregates

Community health nurses have a mandate to assist vulnerable aggregates who have fewer options in protecting themselves from pollution, inadequate housing, toxic poisoning, unsafe products, and other hazards. Non–English-speaking individuals, children, very-low-income women and families, undocumented manual laborers, and people from racial and ethnic minorities are just some of the groups in the United States who hold minimal influence with industry, government, business, and other large institutions for environmental changes and compensations for harm from environmental hazards.

Interventions designed for individuals may overlook unhealthy environments. Further, although environmental hazards can be serious, the implication persists that little can alter the impact of technological and industrial growth. Therefore individuals are compelled to adjust to environments that might cause illness and injury.

Community health nurses who base their practices on theory are better prepared to respond to collective challenges. These nurses can facilitate community participation in identifying and solving environmental health problems and bring about changes that improve environments and eliminate hazards.

CRITICAL COMMUNITY HEALTH NURSING PRACTICE

Community health nurses who approach environmental health critically are action oriented (Ortner, 2004; Stevens and Hall, 1992). Several clinical examples throughout the chapter illustrate how nurses can focus their efforts by organizing groups of people, taking a stand, and acting as advocates for change. The nurses ask critical questions, stay engaged with the communities they serve, form coalitions, and use various collective strategies. In the interest of educating future practitioners about the critical practice of environmental community health nursing, the following sections discuss each of these interventions.

Taking a Stand: Advocating for Change

An old labor union folk song asks, "Whose side are you on?" Although a nurse may acknowledge that there are multiple sides to health and environmental issues, nurses cannot ultimately avoid taking a stand. Nurses must make individual and collective decisions about which interests they want to serve with their specialized knowledge and skills. To say that all must be served is certainly an ideal; however, people often experience consequences of hazardous environments inequitably. Vulnerable groups are exposed to more health-damaging effects than less-vulnerable groups (Chakraborty and Zandbergen, 2007; EPA, 2008a; Northridge et al., 2003; Norton et al., 2007). Nurses have the potential to increase or decrease these inequities through the decisions they make about the positions they accept and the interventions they undertake.

Environmental problems are clearly intertwined with social, political, and economic policies, resource barriers, and the interests of those in positions of control. Nurses need to connect the immediate and long-term health problems experienced by particular communities to this larger sphere of influence.

Asking Critical Questions

Community health nurses must also consider the relationships between nonhealth policies and health policies. They should ask how policies concerning ecological preservation, energy, housing, immigration, civil rights, crime, nutrition, minimum wage, occupational safety, and defense might affect the well-being of people. Addressing critical questions such as who has access to resources in this country, and whose interests are served in the existing system, provides a way to include social, political, and economic factors in environmental nursing assessments. Box 14-3 provides a sample set of questions that are useful in this endeavor. Nurses can ask these critical questions when approaching environmental health problems.

Dialogue resulting from critical questioning can frame the problem and assist in building collective strategies. Ideally, those directly affected by the problem should explore these questions collectively. However, even one individual involved in the situation can begin to explore a problem from this perspective and define an initial basis for action.

Facilitating Community Involvement

Approaching community health from a critical perspective requires working to improve health conditions and creating the context in which people can identify health-damaging

---

BOX 14-3   CRITICAL QUESTIONS ABOUT ENVIRONMENTAL HEALTH PROBLEMS

- What is the problem?
- Who is defining the problem?
- In what terms is the problem described?
- How are others in the situation viewing the problem?
- What is the history of the problem?
- How did things get the way they are?
- What other situations does this problem directly affect?
- Who does the problem affect?
- Whose health is damaged because things are this way?
- Who benefits from the way things are?
- Whose interests do current solutions serve?
- What are the economic inequities in the situation?
- Who has political power in the situation?
- Who knows about the problem?
- Who needs to know more about the problem?
- How effective are current programs, strategies, and policies?
- What are the barriers to solving the problem?
- What strategies may alleviate the problem?
- How successful have these strategies been?
- What existing groups might deal with this problem?
- What resources are needed to solve the problem?
- How accessible are the resources?
- How can nurses evaluate potential solutions?

problems in their environments. One important nursing goal is to help people learn from their own experiences and analyze the world with an intention to change it. It is essential that the affected people participate in the process of identifying and working to solve environmental problems. To foster active participation, nurses must be prepared to take leadership positions and join in mutual exchanges with community members that consider each person's experience. The nurse's role changes from presenting solutions and directing lifestyle changes to asking critical questions and helping groups reflect on the problematic environmental realities of their lives.

A second nursing role is to provide support, information, and expertise to groups to assist them in meeting the goals they set for environmental change. Rather than trying to compel people to behave in certain ways, nurses should assist aggregates in their collective search for effective change strategies. Actions dictated from those outside the situation are often culturally inappropriate and will most likely fail. Lasting rapport with aggregates depends on honesty, fairness, and mutuality in interactions over extended periods of time.

Using critical questions, community health nurses can help community members look beyond immediate environmental problems and explore social, cultural, economic, and political circumstances that contribute to them. Nurses can share their knowledge about the scientific basis for health problems, their insights about the historical origins of particular environmental hazards, their technical skills, and their expertise in communicating and organizing. Nursing expertise is not used to dominate a group but rather to develop a mutual plan of action to deal with the problems a group has collectively identified. By addressing people's everyday concerns and targeting the problems they identify, nurses situate their efforts in community struggles.

Forming Coalitions

Another very important nursing task that arises from approaching environmental health from a critical perspective involves forming coalitions to produce social change. By initiating dialogue and building a strong base of collective support, nurses join with communities to eliminate hazards and improve public health. Nurses can approach existing community organizations, churches, and family and friendship networks to help mobilize aggregate members who have not previously socialized or acted together. Nurses can then expose hazards, assess needs, plan actions, report abuses, and secure appropriate resources, personnel, funding, and legislative changes.

The environmental justice movement is an excellent example of coalition building wherein members of racial and ethnic minority groups have organized grassroots groups to address lead contamination, pesticide use, water and air pollution, native self-government, nuclear testing, and workplace safety. These groups focus on the disproportionate environmental challenges they face. Drawing insights from the civil rights movement and the environmental movement, environmental justice groups have forged alliances with many conventional environmental and civil rights organizations to mount formal responses to environmental threats (EPA, 2009).

For example, the Mothers of East Los Angeles, one grassroots organization fighting for environmental justice, acquired the support of Greenpeace, Natural Resources Defense Council, Environmental Policy Institute, Citizens' Clearinghouse on Hazardous Waste, National Toxics Campaign, and Western Center on Law and Poverty to bring a lawsuit against state and federal agencies that granted a private corporation permission to build and operate a toxic waste incinerator in their urban neighborhood. Coalition allies provided the Mothers of East Los Angeles with valuable technical advice, expert testimony, lobbying, research, and legal assistance. The grassroots group spearheaded efforts in which hundreds of East Los Angeles residents placed intense political pressure on the state and federal agencies by attending every public hearing about the incinerator project. In the ensuing state supreme court battle, the decision prevented construction of the proposed facility.

Nurses can be instrumental in these efforts by helping community groups make connections with larger, more powerful organizations. Nurses can organize forums whereby community groups meet with scientific experts who can help them gather evidence about health threats, with business managers whose actions impinge on the economic life of the community, with industry leaders whose companies create ecological hazards, and with legislators who can bring community concerns to lawmaking bodies. Using available institutional resources, skills, and knowledge, nurses can also explore what is happening elsewhere. Making connections with groups in other locales who are struggling for similar environmental changes can enhance collective strength and solidarity. Press releases, media events, interviews, television spots, speeches, newsletters, and leaflets are important means of calling attention to a situation and raising awareness among communities.

It is important to recognize that when nurses work to build coalitions for improving environmental conditions, each issue or problem requires appropriate strategic action based on its own merits. Allies in a current struggle may have been adversaries in a previous struggle. For example, although a bank refused to help farm families by granting farm loan extensions last month, it may be an ally this month when a superhighway development project threatens its location and an adjacent poor neighborhood. An ally need not be in complete agreement with the core group's philosophy, political agenda, or moral beliefs. It is a good idea to brainstorm about all the possible groups in a locale that may have a stake in the outcome of an issue. A good coalition-building strategy is to consider the future and contemplate how one struggle, or one set of allies, can extend its network and subsequently form new coalitions for emerging issues.

Using Collective Strategies

Nurses can use a variety of strategies to intervene at the aggregate level and facilitate improvement in a community's health. Nurses can organize people to change health-damaging environments through combinations of strategies including coalition building; consciousness-raising groups; educational forums in neighborhoods, workplaces, schools, churches, and social clubs; seminars for health care providers, city officials, teachers, and employers; community needs assessments; dissemination of clinical research and policy analyses; use of mass media; canvassing; litigation; legislative lobbying; testimony at public hearings; demonstrations; and participatory research.

One collective strategy that is an effective aggregate-level community health nursing intervention is participatory action research. Participatory action research calls for nurses, community members, and other resource people to work together in identifying environmental health problems, designing the studies, collecting and analyzing the data, disseminating the results, and posing solutions to the problems (Gershon et al., 2008; Kelly, 2005). With the assistance of community health nurses, community members gather information on suspected environmental hazards, document their effects on health, educate their communities, persuade corporations to clean up, and lobby local, state, and federal governments for stricter regulations and improved enforcement. The goal of the research process is not merely the production of knowledge, but rather the generation of open discussion and debate that intensifies a community's consciousness of health-impairing environmental constraints. Box 14-4 presents an abstract of an article about illustrating a type of participatory action research related to environmental health.

Although nurses have not traditionally used all of these collective strategies to intervene in community health matters, environmental hazards are multiplying geometrically, pushing nurses to expand their skills repertoire. Pioneers such as Hollie Shaner, RN, have embraced that concept and are blazing the path to environmental awareness (Sattler, 2003). In the 1990s, Shaner frequently left her home where she avidly separated and recycled, and arrived at the Vermont hospital where she worked, where none of the waste was recycled. Shaner was not comfortable throwing everything into a "red bag" and decided that there must be a way to change the environmental unfriendliness of her place of employment. She began voluntarily recycling the hospitals' cardboard and then began to recycle the newspapers, glass, and plastics. In addition, she received a grant from the state of Vermont to maximize her efforts in medical waste reduction. The efforts and savings did not go unnoticed by the hospital, as Shaner

| BOX 14-4 | PARTICIPATORY ACTION RESEARCH |

Rates of overweight children and adolescents have nearly tripled over the past 30 years. Many barriers exist to healthy eating and physical activity for children and adolescents, including factors in the school and community environment. The Nutrition Friendly Schools and Communities (NFSC) model was developed to address these modifiable school environment factors with the intent of preventing the development of obesity among children and adolescents. The NFSC model was built upon the Coordinated School Health Program, the Baby Friendly Hospital Initiative, participatory research, and empowerment evaluation. The purpose of the NFSC environmental intervention is to actively engage the school community to prevent overweight in students through a multilevel, participative intervention that facilitates coordinated changes in the school environment in the following areas: health education, physical education, health services, food services, school policy, staff wellness, psychosocial services, and family/community involvement. The NFSC model is the basis by which school communities develop a plan and evaluation that lead to a healthy school environment and prevent the development of overweight in children.

From Vecchiarelli S, et al: Using participatory action research to develop a school-based environmental intervention to support healthy eating and physical activity, *Am J Health Educ* 36(1):35-42, 2005.

received a new job title of clinical waste reduction coordinator in which she saves the hospital $175,000 per year.

Shaner also authored a book for the American Hospital Association on medical waste management. She quickly realized the negative impact the health care industry was having on the environmental health of the communities served. Mercury was being released into the streams from medical waste, and dioxins were being released into the air from medical waste incineration. From this realization, in 1996, Shaner and a small group of other health professionals launched a campaign to lead the health care industry toward environmental stewardship. This campaign, supported by the American Nurses Association, was named Health Care Without Harm. "The goal of the campaign was to reduce the environmental health risks that were being created by the health care industry" (Sattler, 2003, p. 8). The campaign still exists and is building momentum; today there are 433 participating organizations in 52 different countries (Health Care Without Harm, 2005).

If nurses do not possess these types of organizational skills, they can learn from experts in the community who have experience with conducting mass media campaigns, organizing demonstrations, canvassing neighborhoods, participating in class-action litigation, and testifying at public hearings. Nurses can also consult many available books about political action.

CASE STUDY   APPLICATION OF THE NURSING PROCESS

In July 2001, the *Metro Pulse* newspaper reported an extensive air pollution problem in the city of Knoxville, Tennessee (Tarr, 2001). The American Lung Association had recently named Knoxville as the ninth most polluted city in the country, based on the ozone contamination in the air. The following case study expands on some of the reported facts of the situation to construct hypothetical nursing interventions.

Knoxville's community health nurses and the public health department have long been involved with city residents and have been aware of high rates of asthma in particular neighborhoods. In the wake of alarming newspaper and research articles about the dangerous incidence of air pollution and related asthma, the nurses decided to make the health issues a priority. The community health nurses and several nursing students assigned to their department researched the topics and uncovered the following information.

Asthma has long been recognized as a condition in which an acute respiratory response may follow inhalation of a material to which a person is sensitized. Only recently, though, have scientists focused on agents that cause nonspecific generalized inflammation, such as air pollution (Thurston and Bates, 2003).

A study conducted by the University of Southern California and funded by the California Environmental Protection Agency's Air Resources Board provides strong evidence that ozone can *cause*, as well as exacerbate, asthma (McConnell et al., 2002). The study found that days with higher ozone concentration resulted in significantly higher school absences due to respiratory illness, and children living in high-ozone communities who actively participated in several sports were more likely to develop asthma than children in communities not participating in sports.

Indeed, the nation's leading group of pediatricians, the American Academy of Pediatrics (AAP) (2004) revised its policy statement on outdoor air pollution and the health hazards to children. The AAP's Committee on Environmental Health strengthened its warning of the dangers that air pollution poses to children because of the recent studies correlating air pollution with asthma and negative lung growth and function. Estimates are that more than 20 million Americans have asthma (Asthma and Allergy Foundation, 2004).

An economically depressed neighborhood in Knoxville, hypothetically called Trent Park, is situated near numerous railways, freeways, and industrial yards. High numbers of African-American, Latino, and Southeast Asian residents live in the older homes that line the streets of Trent Park. Isolated by language and economic circumstances, many Trent Park residents do not know they are exposed to these environmental health hazards.

Assessment

Elena Garcia, an 8-year-old girl who lives in Trent Park, presented at the pediatric primary clinic at the health department at 8 AM on an early November morning, accompanied by her mother. Elena had had asthma diagnosed 2 months previously and was now in mild respiratory distress. Elena explained to the nurse that she had gone trick-or-treating the night before in her neighborhood. It had turned cold that weekend, and she had also played outside in her neighborhood with friends the day before. In addition, Mrs. Garcia explained that Elena had contracted a respiratory virus a few days ago. The nurse realized that Elena and her mother both mentioned several factors such as her playing outside on a cold afternoon/evening in a polluted neighborhood with a respiratory virus that could have exacerbated her asthma.

At the clinic visit, the nurse assessed the following:

- Elena's heart rate and cardiovascular status
- Elena's pattern of breathing, which includes rate, rhythm, and effort
- Elena's asthma medication history
- Evidence of diaphoresis, papillary dilation, and fear, which are all features of the adrenergic response to hypoxia
- Elena's global central nervous system function, such as alertness, cooperation, and motor activity
- Elena's stress level and coping skills
- Mrs. Garcia's stress level and coping skills

Diagnosis
Individual

- Ineffective airway clearance related to environmental exposure to air pollution
- Deficient knowledge related to precipitating factors that can cause/worsen an asthma attack
- Anxiety related to ongoing fear of daughter's illness

Family

- Risk for family crisis related to instability caused by the illness
- Deficient knowledge related to precipitating factors that can cause/worsen an asthma attack

Community

- Risk for increased incidence of asthma due to air pollution
- Inadequate programs for asthma screening

Planning

A plan of care is developed at the individual, family, and community levels. Mutual goal setting and contracting are essential if the outcome is to be optimal.

Individual
Long-Term Goals

- Client will not exercise outdoors on a day with high pollution levels.
- Client will reduce exposure to allergy triggers.
- Client will avoid tobacco smoke.
- Client will keep pets out of the bedroom.
- Client will experience successful maintenance of asthma.

Short-Term Goals

- Client will begin to keep an asthma diary and identify which allergy triggers are problematic.
- Client will remain free of acute asthma attacks.

Family
Long-Term Goals

- Family will follow the city's daily air quality index.
- Family will encourage child to stay indoors on days with high pollution levels.
- Family will remove as many allergy triggers from home as possible.
- Family will enforce the pets-out-of-the-bedroom policy.
- Family will cope effectively with daughter's asthma.

Short-Term Goals

- Family will provide encouragement for client to keep asthma diary to identify which allergy triggers are problematic.
- Family will express emotions regarding daughter's acute asthma attack.

Community
Long-Term Goals

- Citizens will be involved in decision-making process about proposed activities that could pose an environmental hazard.
- Citizens will encourage utility companies, government, and industries to reduce air pollution.
- Citizens will be encouraged to use mass transit and carpools to reduce vehicle emissions.
- Citizens will encourage officials to build new schools away from polluted areas.

Short-Term Goals

- Citizens will be alerted about the air pollution problem in the area.
- Citizens will be educated about the air quality index and its implications for outdoor activity.

Intervention

The actions of the community health nurses in coalition with community members comprise interventions at the individual, family, and aggregate levels.

Continued

CASE STUDY   APPLICATION OF THE NURSING PROCESS—cont'd

Individual

- Identify Trent Park children in whom asthma is diagnosed and treated and plan follow-up home visits to provide education on basic pathophysiology, symptoms of distress, and environmental controls needed for successful asthma management.
- Redesign the community health agency's child health assessment protocol, adding several observations designed to detect symptoms of asthma and several questions that establish whether there are specific triggers for asthma in the home.
- Coordinate with school nurses to ensure they incorporate similar changes in their health assessment protocols.
- Establish an agreement with the state's TennCare Child Health Program that ensures it will screen for asthma if physicians, school nurses, or community health nurses recommend it.
- Prepare an educational pamphlet with members of Trent Park that details Trent Park residents' air pollution and asthma risks. The community health nurses mail the pamphlet to individual physicians and nurses who provide services to children in Trent Park.
- Prepare translations of the pamphlet in languages and reading levels appropriate for Trent Park residents and mail it to individual households.

Family

- Initiate a family-to-family program in which a core group of Trent Park community members attend educational meetings with the community health nurses. In these meetings, they share information about the environmental origins of air pollution and asthma and its prevention, diagnosis, and treatment. These specially trained community members then take charge of the program, sharing their knowledge with extended family members and neighboring families.
- Coordinate with school nurses to establish a health education program in Trent Park schools in which school-aged children learn about air pollution and asthma. Encourage these children to take their knowledge home and teach younger preschool-aged siblings about staying indoors on hot, sunny days when the ozone levels are apt to be the highest.
- Investigate how community health nurses might better assist Trent Park families by helping them apply for and obtain nutritional resources such as food stamps, food bank supplements, and school lunch programs. With improved nutritional status and immune system, symptoms of asthma may decrease.
- Facilitate the formation of a support group for families with children who have had asthma. The community health nurses volunteer their offices for evening meeting space and provide information about health care, social services, and government disability assistance.

Community

- Provide pamphlets with announcements about community health nurses' willingness to offer asthma education programs at churches, schools, hospitals, workplaces, medical association meetings, and nursing association meetings.
- Involve members of the Trent Park community at planning meetings and include African-American, Latino, and Southeast Asian community members.
- Contact neighborhood leaders, church leaders, ethnic clubs, the local Parent-Teacher Association, a senior citizen organization in the neighborhood, the Black Women's Health Project, and a local Latino women's political organization and organize planning meetings.

- Start multicultural grassroots effort by Citizens United to Combat Air Pollution (CUTCAP) that travels door to door educating Trent Park residents about the dangers of air pollution as it relates to asthma.
- Establish ties with local physicians, nurses, and health care institutions who allocate adequate funds and personnel to accomplish the coalition's goals.
- Establish a timeframe for evaluating the Trent Park project.
- Encourage nursing students and community health nursing faculty from the local university and college programs to participate in the interventions.
- Lobby state legislatures, municipal officials, local medical associations, local hospitals, and city clinics regarding plan implementation.
- Form broader coalitions with Knoxville churches, local nurses association, several preschool and day care centers, and the Knoxville School Board to design a comprehensive, nonduplicative, cost-effective asthma screening program that will test all children in Knoxville on a regular basis.
- Contact researchers at a local university's environmental sciences program and request that they work with the coalition to conduct a house-to-house study of asthma triggers sources.
- Designate a CUTCAP committee to do daily reviews of the Environmental Protection Agency (EPA) index for air quality, and provide monthly reports to Trent Park and surrounding communities.
- Contact state environmental groups for advice on local efforts and join in their fight for stricter regulation of air pollutants and toxic wastes.
- Contact local media (e.g., television, radio, and newspaper) about running a series of stories about Knoxville air pollutants and related asthma risks; supply information and contacts for interviews and photographs.

Evaluation

Individual

- Evaluate the child and mother's understanding of asthma treatments at follow-up home visits.
- Facilitate the evaluation of ongoing interventions.
- Track the number of asthma screening tests Trent Park children receive and the rates of asthma to determine the effectiveness of their efforts in these areas.
- Keep close contact with the school nurses and organize an after-school educational and screening program at schools that are understaffed.
- Ask school nurses to report on the educational sessions' success.

Family

- Document participation levels at educational programs and family training sessions.
- Document ongoing participation in referrals and support groups.

Community

Although local officials supported their plan, CUTCAP's efforts at pushing for a comprehensive asthma screening program met a great deal of opposition from the state legislature. When repeated negotiations continued to fail, CUTCAP decided to align with environmental and civil rights groups who were suing the state of Tennessee for failure to provide federally mandated asthma screening tests for low-income children. The CUTCAP coalition became plaintiffs in the class-action suit. The community health nurses from Trent Park gave expert testimony in the case.

The court case proceeded, and some members of the state legislature began to show more interest in an asthma screening program; another vote was scheduled. The Trent Park Coalition participated in an Air Pollution and Asthma Awareness Day at the state capitol the week before the vote. They were active in the demonstration and gave speeches about their local experiences. They visited the offices of individual legislators, informing them of Trent Park's situation. Citing the tentative results from the environmental scientists' house-to-house research study and the community health nurses' asthma screening statistics proved very useful. This evidence strengthened the coalition members' arguments about the need for a comprehensive asthma screening program in the state. The coalition also shared these data with the national environmental groups with whom they worked. These groups used the data in testimony before federal legislators to secure federal funding

for a new program to reduce emissions from automobiles and trucks by implementing an annual mandatory emissions test for all vehicles in the state.

Levels of Prevention
Primary Prevention
Educating the community regarding air pollution and its relationship to asthma.

Secondary Prevention
Screening at-risk populations for asthma and testing blood levels for air pollutants.

Tertiary Prevention
Follow-up treatment for people with asthma and reducing air pollutants from the community environment.

SUMMARY

This chapter provided a glimpse into the complex world of environmental health from a critical community health nursing perspective. The case study and clinical examples illustrate that nurses must evaluate the broader picture in assessing the environmental health status of communities and the vulnerable aggregates within communities. In preventing, minimizing, and resolving environmental health problems, nurses must recognize patterns, detect subtle changes, identify underlying issues, and work collaboratively with a variety of individuals and groups. In the past, environmental threats to health were usually suspected only when other possible causes of illness were ruled out. Nurses can expect this pattern to change dramatically in the twenty-first century as environmental health moves increasingly to the forefront of the public health agenda.

LEARNING ACTIVITIES

1. Identify a health-related problem associated with some aspect of the environment. It may be a problem in a nearby community, a problem publicized in the media, or a difficulty experienced by a family. Examine the problem using the sample series of critical questions listed in Box 14-3. Without sharing the results, present the problem to the group and ask them to discuss it by responding to the same questions. Were there differences or similarities in the initial results and the group's answers? On what points did everyone agree? Why? What questions caused the most disagreement? Why? Now repeat the entire activity by involving people other than nursing students in the group discussion. How did this discussion compare with the previous discussion and responses?

2. Attend meetings that hold environmental hazard discussions. If meetings or public forums are not available in the vicinity, write for information about the state's actions to

fight environmental hazards. The reference librarians at colleges or public libraries can suggest ways of contacting sources and will supply addresses. Organizations that are likely to sponsor forums and provide information include those listed in Box 14-2, the EPA, the National Institute for Occupational Safety and Health, state and municipal agencies for environmental protection and occupational health, environmental caucuses of political parties, the American Public Health Association, the local public health department, farmers' organizations, and labor unions.

3. This chapter described how to use participatory research as an intervention in dealing with ecological hazards. In a group, brainstorm about possibilities for participatory action research projects in the area. Try to identify examples from a variety of environmental health areas. Be creative in planning. How might a nurse mobilize community support and participation in the research? What groups would be approachable? What critical questions might facilitate dialogue about the problem? What kinds of data could be collected, and how could they be used? How could research results be publicized? What ramifications could the completed study have for community members, other communities in the state, and community health nurses in other locales?

4. Nurses may have to supplement their knowledge of collective strategies by reading books about political action and by learning from community members who are experienced in political organizing. Visit a college or public library to investigate books and journal articles outside the nursing literature. Compile a list of references related to one of these political strategies (e.g., grassroots organizing, legislative lobbying, community education, policy analysis, use of the media, coalition building, citizen surveys, public protest, letter-writing campaigns, or consciousness-raising groups). Exchange reference lists with peers to benefit from their efforts. Then choose one or two books of interest and read them.

REFERENCES

Akhtar AZ, Greger M, Ferdowsian H, et al: Health professionals' roles in animal agriculture, climate change, and human health, *Am J Prev Med* 36(2):182–187, 2009.

American Academy of Pediatrics: *Air pollution: children more at risk than adults*, www.aap.org/advocacy/releases/decpollution.htm (press release), 2004.

Asthma and Allergy Foundation: *Asthma facts and figures*, www.aafa.org/display.cfm?id=8&sub=42, 2004.

Barton A, Basham M, Foy C, et al: The Watcombe housing study: the short term effect of improving housing conditions on the health of residents, *J Epidemiol Community Health* 61:771–777, 2007.

Bent KN: Perspectives on critical and feminist theory in developing nursing praxis, *J Prof Nurs* 9(5):296–303, 2003.

Bhatia R, Wernham A: Integrating human health into environmental impact assessment: an unrealized opportunity for environmental health and justice, *Environ Health Perspect* 116(8):991–1000, 2008.

Bingham E, Meader WV: Governmental regulation of environmental hazards in the 1990s, *Annu Rev Public Health* 11:419–434, 1990.

Boyd DR, Genuis SJ: The environmental burden of disease in Canada: respiratory disease, cardiovascular disease, cancer and congenital affliction, *Environ Res* 106(2):240–249, 2008.

Brownless GP: Does protecting humans protect the environment? A crude examination for UK nuclear power plants and the marine environment using information in the public domain, *J Radiol Prot* 28(4):525–538, 2008.

Burger EJ: Human health: a surrogate for the environment: the evolution of environmental legislation and regulation during the 1970s, *Regul Toxicol Pharmacol* 9:196–206, 1989.

Burns WG: Climate change and human health: the critical policy agenda, *JAMA* 287(17):2287, 2002.

Center for Children's Health and the Environment: *Emerging illnesses in urban environments*, www.childenvironment.org/factsheets/emerging_illnesses.htm, 2002.

Centers for Disease Control and Prevention: *2003 West Nile virus activity in the United States*, www.cdc.gov/ncidod/dvbid/westnile/surv&controlCaseCount03_detailed.htm, 2005a.

Centers for Disease Control and Prevention: Preliminary FoodNet data on the incident of infection with pathogens transmitted commonly through food: 10 sites—United States, 2004, *MMWR Surveill Summ* 54(14):352–356, 2005b.

Centers for Disease Control and Prevention: *Worker health chartbook 2004, NIOSH 2004–146*, www2a.cdc.gov/NIOSH-Chartbook/, 2005c.

Centers for Disease Control and Prevention: *Drinking water*, www.cdc.gov/ncidod/dpd/healthywater/privatewell.htm, 2008.

Centers for Disease Control and Prevention: Novel influenza A (H1N1) virus infection—Mexico, March-May 2009, *MMWR Morb Mortal Wkly Rep* 58(21):585–589, 2009.

Chakraborty C, Zandbergen PA: Children at risk: racial/ethnic disparities in potential exposure to air pollution at school and home, *J Epidemiol Community Health* 61:1074–1079, 2007.

Ciencewicki J, Trivedi S, Kleeberger SJ: Oxidants and the pathogenesis of lung disease, *J Allergy and Clin Immunol* 3(122):456–468, 2008.

Clark L, Barton JA, Brown NJ: Assessment of community contamination: a critical approach, *Public Health Nurs* 19(5):354–365, 2002.

Davies WP: An historical perspective from the green revolution to the gene revolution, *Nutr Rev* 61(6):S124–S134, 2003.

Driehuis F, Spanjer MC, Scholten JM, et al: Occurrence of mycotoxins in feedstuffs of dairy cows and estimation of total dietary intakes, *J Dairy Sci* 91(11):4261–4271, 2008.

Environmental Protection Agency: *Urban sprawl modeling, air quality monitoring and risk communication: The Northeast Ohio Project, EPA/625/R-02/016*, Washington, DC, 2002, The Author.

Environmental Protection Agency: *Ensuring risk reduction in communities with multiple stressors: environmental justice and cumulative risks/impacts*, Washington, DC, 2004, The Author.

Environmental Protection Agency: *Highlighting success: the region 9 environmental justice small grant program, fiscal years 1994–99, EPA 909-R99–002*, Washington, DC, 2005, The Author.

Environmental Protection Agency: *What are the six common air pollutants?* April 7, 2006, www.epa.gov/air/urbanair/6poll.html.

Environmental Protection Agency: *2005/2006 National listing of fish advisories*, www.epa.gov/waterscience/fish/advisories/2006/tech.pdf, 2007a.

Environmental Protection Agency: *The effects of acid rain*, www.epa.gov/acidrain/effects/index.html, 2007b.

Environmental Protection Agency: *What are the health effects of contaminants in drinking water?* www.epa.gov/safewater/dwh/health.html, September 2007c.

Environmental Protection Agency: *About environmental justice*, Washington, DC, 2008a, The Author.

Environmental Protection Agency: *Drinking water contaminants*, www.epa.gov/safewater/contaminants/index.html#ucmr, 2008b.

Environmental Protection Agency: *Food safety*, www.epa.gov/agriculture/tfsy.html#pesticideinfood, October 2008c.

Environmental Protection Agency: *Indoors air facts No. 4 (revised): Sick building syndrome (SBS)*, www.epa.gov/iaq/pubs/sbs.html, February 2008d.

Environmental Protection Agency: *Ozone layer depletion*, www.epa.gov/ozone/basicinfo.html, September 2008e.

Environmental Protection Agency: *Radon*, www.epa.gov/radon/healthrisks.html, 2008f.

Epstein PR: West Nile virus and the climate, *J Urban Health* 78:367–371, 2001.

Frumkin H: Urban sprawl and public health, *Public Health Rep* 117:201–212, 2002.

Gershon RM, Rubin MS, Qureshi KA, et al: Participatory action research methodology in disaster research: results from the World Trade Center evacuation study, *Disaster Med Public Health Preparedness* 2(3):142–149, 2008.

Global Development Research Center: *Wingspread statement on the precautionary principle*, Wingspread Conference, Kobe, Japan, 1998, Global Development Research Center. www.gdrc.org/u-gov/precaution-3.html.

Hamilton PA, Miller TL, Myers DN: *Water quality in the nation's streams and aquifers: Overview of selected findings, 1991–2001, US Geological Survey circular 1265*, Reston, VA, 2004, US Geological Survey.

Hampton T: Researchers examine long-term risks of exposure to medical radiation, *JAMA* 296(6):638–640, 2006.

Harris JT, Miller DW: Radiological effluents released by US commercial nuclear power plants from 1995–2005, *Health Phys* 95(6):734–743, 2008.

Harrison TW, Gustafson EM, Dixon JK: Radiologic emergency: protecting schoolchildren and the public, *Am J Nurs* 103(5):41–49, 2003.

Health Care Without Harm: About us www.noharm.org/aboutUs/HCWHStory, 2005.

Hurd HS, Malladi S: A stochastic assessment of the public health risks of the use of macrolide antibiotics in food animals, *Risk Anal* 28(3):695–710, 2008.

Institute of Medicine Committee on Enhancing Environmental Health Content in Nursing Practice: *Nursing, health, and the environment*, Washington, DC, 1995, National Academies Press.

Ivers LC, Ryan ET: Infectious diseases of severe weather-related and flood-related natural disasters, *Curr Opin Infect Dis* 19:408–414, 2006.

Kelly PJ: Practical suggestions for community interventions using participatory action research, *Public Health Nurs* 22(1):65–73, 2005.

Knobeloch L, Turyk M, Imm P, et al: Temporal changes in PCB and DDE levels among a cohort of frequent and infrequent consumers of Great Lakes sportfish, *Environ Res* 109:66–72, 2009.

Krieger N, Chen JT, Waterman PD, et al: The inverse hazard law: blood pressure, sexual harassment, racial discrimination, workplace abuse and occupational exposures in US low-income black, white, and Latino workers, *Soc Sci Med* 67:1970–1981, 2008.

Le Moual N, Kennedy SM, Kauffmann F: Occupational exposures and asthma in 14,000 adults from the general population, *Am J Epidemiol* 160(11):1108–1116, 2004.

Lorber M, Gibb H, Grant L, et al: Assessment of inhalation exposures and potential health risks to the general population that resulted from the collapse of the World Trade Center towers, *Risk Analysis* 27(5):1203–1221, 2007.

Martin CJ: Radiation dosimetry for diagnostic medical exposures, *Radiat Prot Dosimetry* 128(4):389–412, 2008.

McConnell R, et al: Asthma in exercising children exposed to ozone: a cohort study, *Lancet* 359:386–391, 2002.

Meyer PA, Brown MJ, Falk H: Global approach to reducing lead exposures and poisoning, *Mutat Res* 659(1–2):166–175, 2008.

Milacic S: Health investigations of depleted uranium clean-up workers, *Med Lav* 99(5):366–370, 2008.

National Environmental Education Foundation: *Pediatric environmental history initiative*, dev. neefusa.org/, 2008.

National Toxic Inhalation Study Group: Environmental pulmonary edema: an update, *Rev Environ Health* 13(1–2):27–58, 1998.

Northridge ME, et al: Environmental equity and health: understanding completely and moving forward, *Am J Public Health* 93(2):209–213, 2003.

Norton JM, Wing S, Lipscomb HJ, et al: Race, wealth, and solid waste facilities in North Carolina, *Environ Health Perspect* 115:1344–1350, 2007.

Ortner P: The nurse as change agent: an approach to environmental health advocacy, *Policy Polit Nurs Pract* 5(2):125–130, 2004.

Pan TC, Kao JJ: Inter-generational equity index for assessing environmental sustainability: an example of global warming, *Ecol Indic* 9(4):725–1721, 2009.

Rauh VA, Landrigan PJ, Claudio L: Housing and health: intersection of poverty and environmental exposures, *Ann NY Acad Sci* 1136:276–288, 2008.

Ron E: Thyroid cancer incidence among people living in areas contaminated by radiation from the Chernobyl accident, *Health Phys* 93(5):502–511, 2007.

Salbu C, et al: Oxidation states of uranium in depleted uranium particles from Kuwait, *J Environ Radioact* 78(2):125–135, 2005.

Sanchez F, Kosson DS: Probabilistic approach for estimating the release of contaminants under field management scenarios, *Waste Manag* 25(4):463–472, 2005.

Sattler B: The greening of health care: environmental policy and advocacy in the health care industry, *Policy Polit Nurs Pract* 4(1):6–13, 2003.

Schrieberg D: Death from a healing machine: radioactive waste goes on Mexican odyssey after sale of medical device, *San Francisco Examiner* 1:12, 1991.

Shavers VS, Shavers BS: Racism and health inequity among Americans, *JAMA* 98(3):386–396, 2006.

Slama R, Boutou O, Ducot B, et al: Reproductive life events in the population living in the vicinity of a nuclear waste processing plant, *J Epidemiol Community Health* 62(6):513–521, 2008.

Smith KR: Comparative environmental health assessments: a brief introduction and application in China, *Ann NY Acad Sci* 1140:31–39, 2008.

Stevens PE, Hall JM: Applying critical theories to nursing in communities, *Public Health Nurs* 9:2–9, 1992.

Tarr J: Knoxville's pollution rivals that of Los Angeles, Houston and Atlanta, but Green Power might help clear the air, *Metro Pulse* 11(18):2001.

Thompson B, et al: *Para Ninos Saludables:* a community intervention trial to reduce organophosphate pesticide exposure in children of farmworkers, *Environ Health Perspect* 116(5):687–694, 2008.

Thurston GD, Bates DV: Air pollution as an underappreciated cause of asthma symptoms, *JAMA* 290:1915–1917, 2003.

U.S. Department of Commerce, National Oceanic and Atmospheric Administration: *Scientific assessment of ozone depletion*, www.esrl.noaa.gov/csd/assessments/2006/, 2006.

U.S. Department of Health and Human Services: *Healthy People 2020*. 2009 Draft Objectives. Washington DC. http://www.healthypeople.gov/hp2020/Objectives/TopicAreas.aspx.

U.S. Department of Health and Human Services: *Healthy People 2010*, ed 2, Washington, DC, 2000, US Government Printing Office.

U.S. Department of Labor, Bureau of Labor Statistics: *Current injury, illness, and fatality data*, www.bls.gov/iif/, 2008.

U.S. Geological Survey: *How does water get into the ground?* September pubs.usgs.gov/of/1993/ofr93–643/, 2005.

Whitney SL, Maltby HJ, Carr JM: This food may contain…." What nurses should know about genetically engineered foods, *Nurs Outlook* 52:262–266, 2004.

World Health Organization: *World day for safety and health at work 2005: a background paper*, Geneva, 2005, International Labour Office.

World Health Organization: *Environmental health*, www.who.int/topics/environmental_health/en/, 2009a.

World Health Organization: *Influenza A (H1N1) update 46*, www.who.int/csr/don/2009_06_10a/en/index.html, 2009b.

World Health Organization: *Ionizing radiation in our environment*, www.who.int/ionizing_radiation/env/en/, 2009c.

World Health Organization: *SARS*, www.who.int/csr/sars/guidelines/en/index.html, 2009d.

Globalization and International Health

Julie Cowan Novak

Additional Material for Study, Review, and Further Exploration

evolve WEBSITE

http://evolve.elsevier.com/Nies
- Quiz
- Case Studies
- Glossary
- WebLinks

OBJECTIVES

Upon completion of this chapter, the reader will be able to do the following:

1. Describe globalization and international patterns of health and disease.
2. Discuss the World Health Organization (WHO) concepts of "health for all" and primary health care.
3. Identify international health care organizations and how they collaborate to improve global nursing and health care.
4. Describe the role of the community or public health nurse in international health.
5. Discuss key elements and effective models for successful international service learning community health projects including ICAM and FURCO.

KEY TERMS

Bill and Melinda Gates Foundation
Carter Center
Centers for Disease Control and Prevention (CDC)
Declaration of Alma-Ata
globalization
health for all by the year 2000

International Council of Nurses (ICN)
Millennium Development Goals
nongovernmental organizations (NGOs)
Pan American Health Organization (PAHO)
primary care
primary health care

United Nations
United Nations International Children's Emergency Fund (UNICEF)
World Bank
World Health Organization (WHO)

OUTLINE

Population Characteristics
Environmental Factors
Patterns of Health and Disease
International Agencies and Organizations

International Health Care Delivery Systems
   The Role of the Community Health Nurse in International Health Care
Research in International Health

Health care and health care reform are sources of critical debate throughout the world. Human health and its influence on every aspect of life are central to the global agenda. Nurses, as first responders, expert care providers, and leaders in international health care assessment, planning, evaluation, and policy development, promote and restore health to individuals, families, and communities across settings and geographic boundaries. Nurses must study models of health promotion, community assessment, community empowerment, and service learning to improve health care access and efficient and effective delivery. Community public health nurses must also be aware of forces that threaten health in the global community.

Our global society, the worldwide Internet, and reduction in travel time provide access that was unimaginable a decade ago. Globalization, the process of increasing social and economic dependence and integration as capital, goods, persons, concepts, images, ideas, and values cross state boundaries, is inextricably linked to the benefits and challenges of our time.

This chapter highlights population characteristics; international patterns of health and disease; social, cultural, and economic factors; international health care agencies and organizations; health care providers; health care delivery systems; and the community public health nurse's role as a leader in the global community. The chapter presents an International Community Assessment Model (ICAM) and the FURCO service learning framework (Furco, 2002) for faculty and student discovery, learning, reflection, engagement, policy, and system design.

Population characteristics, including patterns of growth, demographics, and pandemics, are among the many health issues that merit attention and study because they have global effects that threaten human life. This chapter explores these issues and other environmental factors, including identified stressors and patterns of health and disease.

POPULATION CHARACTERISTICS

More than 1 billion people entered the twenty-first century without benefiting from the health care revolution. Enormous population growth presents a threat to the health and the economy of many nations. The exponential nature of world population growth is evident. In 1804, after 2 to 5 million years of human existence, the world population exceeded 1 billion. Between 1804 and 1927, the population reached 2 billion and, between 1927 and 1960, 3 billion. The population soared to 4 billion between 1960 and 1974 and 5 billion between 1974 and 1987. In 1999, the world population grew to 6 billion and, in 2006, 6.6 billion. The population is projected to reach 8 billion by 2025 and 10 to 12 billion by midcentury (United Nations Population Division, 2008). Ninety-nine percent of the growth is expected to occur in resource-poor countries (Population Reference Bureau [PRB], 2006).

In any society, large populations create pressure. For example, feeding a population becomes problematic in developing countries when famine, international trade problems, and war occur. Malnutrition, disease, or death may be the outcome. Pressures from population growth are also felt in industrialized nations. Although food may be plentiful, overcrowding leads to pollution, stress, disease, and violence. Each of these challenges represents a major barrier to economic growth. The poor suffer this burden of excess mortality and morbidity disproportionately. Thus, improving quality of life (QOL) through health promotion, effective health care delivery systems, and the enhancement of the environmental infrastructure will address the origins of poverty and ultimately increase productivity and improve QOL.

World population distribution is uneven. More than 50% of the population lives in China (1.3 billion), India (1.1 billion), the United States (299 million), and Indonesia (225 million) (PRB, 2006). In 2007, 30% of the world population consisted of children. 8% were over 60 (WHO, 2009). In developed countries life expectancy is increasing; however, in countries severely affected by the human immunodeficiency virus/acquired immunodeficiency syndrome (HIV/AIDS) epidemic, life expectancy has dropped to 35 to 40 years. In these countries the working age population has dwindled while the birth rate has risen. At today's age-specific mortality rates, a girl born in Zambia can expect to live 43 years whereas a girl born in Japan can expect to live 86 years. Malcolm Potts, a world-renowned population theorist, predicted that "by the twenty-first century the world may end up divided not into political or economic groups but by demographic structure," where countries will be classified into slow-growth or fast-growth countries instead of rich or poor countries. This will eventually further divide the rich and poor (Potts, 1994).

As the world population grows, a global trend toward urbanization occurs; people live closer together and migrate to urban areas for employment. For example, in 1975, 38.5% of the world's population lived in urban areas. By 1994, the proportion of urban dwellers swelled to 45%; this proportion is expected to reach 50% by 2015 (United Nations Population Division, 2008). With increasingly dense living arrangements and global travel, the health of the general population is threatened by environmental factors and disease, for example, the H1N1 influenza pandemic.

> *Others say the human population level is OK and can continue to increase because science will meet our needs with new sources of energy and things like that. But even if we sustain 10 billion people, then as it goes, it will be 15 billion, then 20 billion. Impossible! (Dalai Lama University of Virginia Nobel Laureates Conference 1998 [speech])*

ENVIRONMENTAL FACTORS

The relationship between humans and their environment is an important component of individual, family, and global health. The field of environmental health and sustainable development has exploded since 1990. Environmental stressors are categorized into five types. First, stressors such as lead poisoning and air pollution directly assault human health. Second, stressors such as the effects of air pollution on products and structures damage society's goods and services. Third, stressors such as noise and litter affect QOL. Fourth, stressors such as global warming interfere with the ecological balance. Finally, natural disasters, terrorism, and war affect all of the above.

Air, water, and land pollution are among the consequences of environmental stressors. For example, 50% of the worldwide air pollution problem is attributable to the chemical pollutant carbon monoxide. Other primary pollutants, such as nitrogen monoxide, sulfur oxides, particulate matter, and hydrocarbons, combine with carbon monoxide to create 90% of the world's pollution. In developing countries, only 75% of the urban population and 50% of the rural population have sanitation facilities, which is a significant contributing factor to water pollution.

Agricultural, industrial, residential, and commercial wastes increase land pollution. For example, chemical fertilizers have displaced natural fertilizers; synthetic pesticides have displaced natural means of pest control; and petrochemical products, such as detergents, synthetic fiber, and plastics, have replaced soap, cotton, and paper. Disposable goods have replaced reusable goods, resulting in increased waste. Production technologies are contributing to worldwide environmental and ecological stress.

PATTERNS OF HEALTH AND DISEASE

Lifestyles, health and cultural beliefs, infrastructure, economics, and politics affect existing illnesses and society's commitment to prevention. Disease patterns vary throughout the world; therefore primary causes of mortality differ in developed and developing countries. Racial, ethnic, and access disparities exist within and between countries. Of 57 million deaths worldwide in 1 year, 33 million are from noncommunicable disease, 18 million are from communicable disease, and 5 million are from injuries and violence (Marmot, 2008).

Cardiovascular disease (CVD), cancer, respiratory disease, stroke, violence, and traumatic injury are the primary causes of mortality in *developed countries*. Infections, malnutrition, and violence are the primary causes of mortality in *developing countries*; however, CVDs are becoming more prevalent. Once plagued with high rates of infectious disease, developed countries significantly reduced high mortality rates from these diseases through improved sanitation, nutrition, immunization, and improved health care. Most developed countries have a more stable economy and a wide range of industrial and technological development. These countries experience an epidemiological transition. For example, the morbidity and mortality profile of a country changes from a lesser developed country profile to a developed country profile. Many developed countries experienced an epidemiological transition from having an infectious disease profile to having a chronic disease profile and are now plagued by chronic diseases such as CVD, respiratory disease, and cancer, secondary to air pollution and the tobacco use pandemic. This altered profile has created a demographic transition from traditional societies, where almost everyone is young, to societies with rapidly increasing numbers of middle-aged and elderly people.

Among the infectious diseases that contribute to high rates of mortality in developing countries are AIDS, tuberculosis (TB), endemic malaria, hepatitis B, rheumatic heart disease, parasitic infection, and dengue fever. These diseases claim the lives of millions, yet it is estimated that these diseases could be reduced by up to 50% through effective public health interventions. Many of these diseases will join smallpox as a disease known only to history through the development and implementation of immunization programs or to the twenty-first century threats of bioterrorism. Immunization is the most powerful and cost-effective strategy at our disposal for many infectious diseases (Centers for Disease Control and Prevention [CDC], 2005). TB recommendations included in the "Commission for Africa" report were presented to world leaders attending the G8 summit in Scotland in 2005. The paper calls for wealthy nations to double their aid to Africa in order to rebuild systems to deliver public health services, provide staff training, develop new medicines, and provide better sexual and reproductive health services. The WHO "two diseases, one patient" strategy should be supported to provide integrated TB and HIV care; 70% of the 14 million people worldwide who have both HIV and TB are in Africa (WHO, 2005b). The bacille Calmette-Guérin (BCG) vaccine series induces active immunity, but it does not reduce the transmission of infectious types of TB. At least one third of the world's population harbors the TB pathogen, *Mycobacterium tuberculosis*. The WHO programs "Roll Back Malaria," "Stop TB," "HIV/AIDS Control," "Tobacco Free Initiative (TFI)," "Avian Influenza Pandemic Preparedness," and more recently the H1N1 pandemic target key infectious and chronic disease issues of the twenty-first century.

AIDS continues to be a grave global concern. The WHO "3 by 5 Initiative" (WHO, 2005c) proposed treating 3 million people living with HIV/AIDS by the end of 2005. In 2004, more than 28.5 million adults and children were estimated to be living with AIDS in sub-Saharan Africa, and 40 million adults and children worldwide were living with this disease. The total number of AIDS deaths from 1981 to 2008 exceeds 25 million (UNAIDS, 2009). The worldwide number of people living with HIV is 33.4 million (UNAIDS, 2009). Newly infected HIV cases totaled 2.7 million, and AIDS deaths were 2.0 million in 2008 (UNAIDS, 2009).

Although AIDS is a global epidemic, it varies demographically in different parts of the world. For example, the estimated male-female ratio of HIV infections in North America is 5:2, whereas in Africa the ratio is 1:1 (WHO, 2007a). Urbanization and within-country migration play a role in the spread of AIDS. For instance, in Rwanda the HIV seroprevalence is 14 to 20 times higher in urban areas versus rural areas. Annually, HIV threatens more lives as more people migrate to the world's largest cities. In 2010, 50% of the developing world lived in cities. This is an increase from 25% in 1970.

Substantial reductions in HIV seroprevalence occurred after several countries deployed "ABC" (Abstinence, Be faithful, Condom use) strategies. In 1985, 35% of those infected with HIV were women. By 2004, 50% of infected people worldwide were women (Dworkin and Ehrhardt, 2007).

Malaria is a life-threatening parasitic disease transmitted by mosquitoes. Today approximately 40% of the world's population is at risk for malaria. Malaria is found throughout the tropical and subtropical regions of the world and causes more than 300 million acute illnesses and at least 1 million deaths annually. Malaria kills an African child every 30 seconds. Effective low-cost strategies are available for its prevention, treatment, and control, including insecticide-treated nets and new generation medications, including artemisinin-based combination therapies (WHO, 2005a). Efforts are ongoing to develop a malarial vaccine.

With 4.9 million deaths annually worldwide, tobacco control is a critical component of the international health care agenda. By 2020, an estimated one in seven deaths will be tobacco related. Since 1990, tobacco control and secondhand smoke policies have been implemented at various political levels in the United States and abroad. The magnitude and consequences of the tobacco pandemic were unexpected. Smoking prevention and cessation programs, state and federal mandates, tobacco taxation, the tobacco settlement, antitobacco media campaigns, strict licensing of tobacco retailers, the elimination of tobacco vending machines and point-of-sale advertising, and the elimination of tobacco sales by pharmacies have made an impact on tobacco sales in the United States. Because of health concerns and cost, many countries from Ireland to New Zealand have developed tobacco-free policies. Although American adults have enrolled in cessation programs, the tobacco industry has targeted youth and dramatically increased international exports. A global commitment to tobacco control can avert millions of premature deaths in the next half century.

In 2003 the first global public health treaty was adopted at the World Framework Convention on Tobacco Control. The treaty was designed to reduce tobacco-related deaths and diseases around the world (WHO, 2007a). In 2005, the WHO Tobacco Free Initiative (TFI) group, in furthering the aims and objectives of the WHO Framework Convention on Tobacco Control (tobacco product regulation provisions) and on the recommendation of the WHO Study Group on Tobacco Product Regulation, five meetings have been convened by the WHO Tobacco Laboratory Network most recently in Rio de Janeiro.

Proposed activities included:
- Assess capabilities of each member, and make an inventory.
- Conduct collaborative study on smokeless tobacco.
- Initiate a quality management program that will lead to accreditation in the future.
- Develop and initiate training programs and capacity building.
- Establish a communication channel for network members, including a website and an expert panel for assistance.
- Develop a compendium of global testing methods for tobacco product emissions and contents.
- Participate in international research and standardization activities.
- Define periodic meetings for scientific research and exchange of information and to identify research priorities and agendas.
- Exchange information with policy makers and regulators (WHO, 2009).

The global approach to tobacco control can guide the development of effective interventions based upon best evidence and best practice. Countering potential threats to health resulting from economic crises, unhealthful environments, or risky behavior is critical. Promotion of a healthy lifestyle underpins a proactive strategy for risk reduction, tobacco use prevention and cessation, immunization provision, cleaner air and water, adequate sanitation, healthful diets, fitness and exercise programs, and safe transportation.

INTERNATIONAL AGENCIES AND ORGANIZATIONS

Promoting worldwide health is humankind's greatest challenge. Several global agencies, such as the WHO, the Pan American Health Organization (PAHO), the United Nations, the United Nations International Children's Emergency Fund (UNICEF), the World Bank, the CDC, and nongovernmental organizations play important roles in improving the health of all nations. Founded in 1948, the World Health Organization (WHO) is an international health agency of the United Nations. With six regional offices in the United States, Congo, Denmark, Egypt, India, and the Philippines, the WHO directs and coordinates international health efforts, producing and disseminating global health standards and guidelines, helping countries to address public health issues, and supporting health research (WHO, 2007a). The WHO goal of "health for all by the year 2000" was framed at the Alma-Ata conference in the former USSR in 1978. The conference defined "health for all" as "the attainment by all citizens of the world by the year 2000 of a level of health that will permit them to lead a socially and economically productive life" (WHO, 1999, p. 65). The target year for achievement was extended to 2010, once again without attainment.

The Alma-Ata conference on primary health care expressed the need for urgent action by all governments. The WHO statement of beliefs, goals, and objectives is outlined in the Declaration of Alma-Ata, which is presented in Box 15-1. The concept of primary health care stresses health as a fundamental human right for individuals, families, and communities; the unacceptability of the gross inequalities and disparities in health status; the importance of community involvement; and

---

BOX 15-1   DECLARATION OF ALMA-ATA

The International Conference on Primary Health Care, meeting in Alma-Ata this twelfth day of September in the year Nineteen hundred and seventy-eight, expressing the need for urgent action by all governments, all health and development workers, and the world community to protect and promote the health of all the people of the world, hereby makes the following Declaration:

I. The Conference strongly reaffirms that health, which is a state of complete physical, mental, and social well-being and not merely the absence of disease or infirmity, is a fundamental human right and that the attainment of the highest possible level of health is a most important worldwide social goal, whose realization requires the action of many other social and economic sectors in addition to the health sector.

II. The existing gross inequality in the health status of the people, particularly between developed and developing countries and within countries, is politically, socially, and economically unacceptable and is therefore of common concern to all countries.

III. Economic and social development, based on a New International Economic Order, is of basic importance to the fullest attainment of health for all and to the reduction of the gap between the health status of developing and developed countries. The promotion and protection of the health of the people are essential to sustained economic and social development and contribute to a better quality of life and to world peace.

IV. The people have the right and duty to participate individually and collectively in the planning and implementation of their health care.

V. Governments have a responsibility for the health of their people which can be fulfilled only by the provision of adequate health and social measures. In the coming decades, a main social target of governments, international organizations, and

Continued

BOX 15-1   DECLARATION OF ALMA-ATA—cont'd

the whole world community should be the attainment by all peoples of the world by the year 2000 of a level of health that will permit them to lead a socially and economically productive life. Primary health care is the key to attaining this target as part of development in the spirit of social justice.

VI. Primary health care is essential health care based on practical, scientifically sound, and socially acceptable methods and technology made universally accessible to individuals and families in the community through their full participation and at a cost that the community and country can afford to maintain at every stage of their development in the spirit of self-reliance and self-determination. It forms an integral part both of the country's health system, of which primary health care is the central function and main focus, and of the overall social and economic development of the community. It is the first level of contact for individuals, the family, and the community with the national health system bringing health care as close as possible to where people live and work and it constitutes the first element of a continuing health care process.

VII. Primary health care:

1. reflects and evolves from the economic conditions and sociocultural and political characteristics of the country and its communities and is based on the application of the relevant results of social, biomedical, and health services research and public health experience;

2. addresses the main health problems in the community, providing promotive, preventive, curative, and rehabilitative services accordingly;

3. includes at least: education concerning prevailing health problems and the methods of preventing and controlling them; promotion of food supply and proper nutrition; an adequate supply of safe water and basic sanitation; maternal and child health care, including family planning; immunization against the major infectious diseases; prevention and control of locally endemic diseases; appropriate treatment of common diseases and injuries; and provision of essential drugs;

4. involves, in addition to health sector, all related sectors and aspects of national and community development, in particular agriculture, animal husbandry, food industry, education, housing, public works, communication, and other sectors; and demands the coordinated efforts of all those sectors;

5. requires and promotes maximum community and individual self-reliance and participation in the planning, organization, operation, and control of primary health care making fullest use of local, national, and other available resources; and to this end, develops through appropriate education the ability of communities to participate;

6. should be sustained by integrated, functional, and mutually supportive referral levels, on health workers, including physicians, nurses, midwives, auxiliaries, and community workers, as applicable, and on traditional practitioners as needed, suitably trained socially and technically to work as a health team and to respond to the expressed health needs of the community; and

7. relies, at local and referral levels, on health workers, including physicians, nurses, midwives, auxiliaries, and community workers, as applicable, and on traditional practitioners as needed, suitably trained socially and technically to work as a health team and to respond to the expressed health needs of the community.

VIII. All governments should formulate national policies, strategies, and plans of action to launch and sustain primary health care as part of a comprehensive national health system and in coordination with other sectors. To this end, it will be necessary to exercise political will, to mobilize the country's resources, and to use available external resources rationally.

IX. All countries should cooperate in a spirit of partnership and service to ensure primary health care for all people because the attainment of health by people in any one country directly concerns and benefits every other country. In this context the joint WHO-UNICEF report on primary health care constitutes a solid basis for the further development and operation of primary health care through the world.

X. An acceptable level of health for all the people of the world by the year 2000 can be attained through a fuller and better use of the world's resources, a considerable part of which is now spent on armaments and military conflicts. A genuine policy of independence, peace, détente, and disarmament could and should release additional resources that could well be devoted to peaceful aims and in particular to the acceleration of social and economic development of which primary health care, as an essential part, should be allotted its proper share.

The International Conference on Primary Health Care calls for urgent and effective national and international action to develop and implement primary health care throughout the world and particularly in developing countries in a spirit of technical cooperation and in keeping with a New International Economic Order. It urges governments, WHO and UNICEF, and other international organizations, and multilateral and bilateral agencies, nongovernmental organizations, funding agencies, all health workers and the whole world community to support national and international commitment to primary health care and to channel increased technical and financial support to it, particularly in developing countries. The Conference calls on all the aforementioned to collaborate in introducing, developing and maintaining primary health care in accordance with the spirit and content of this Declaration.

Reprinted, by permission, from *Alma-Ata: Primary health care, report of the international conference on primary health care,* "Health for All" Series, 1:2-6, Geneva, September 6-12, 1978, World Health Organization.

the active role of all sectors. Primary health care seeks to obtain the highest level of health care for all people. The program promotes seven elements of primary health care, including health education regarding disease prevention and cure, proper food supply and nutrition, adequate supply of safe drinking water and sanitation, maternal and child health care, immunizations, control of endemic diseases, and the provision of essential drugs.

A primary health care system should provide the entire population with universal coverage; relevant, acceptable, affordable, and effective services; a spectrum of comprehensive services that provide for primary, secondary, and tertiary

care and prevention; active community involvement in the planning and delivery of services; and integration of health services with development activities to ensure that complete nutritional, educational, occupational, environmental, and safe housing needs are met. In 2004, the WHO Global Strategy on Diet, Physical Activity, and Health was adopted (WHO, 2007a).

The Pan American Health Organization (PAHO) is an international public health agency with nearly a century of experience in working to improve the health and living standards of the Americas. It serves as the regional office of WHO and is recognized as part of the United Nations system.

Founded in 1945 after World War II, the United Nations (UN) now comprises 192 nations committed to world peace and security through international cooperation. The UN provides the means to resolve global conflicts and formulates policies that affect all nations. Regardless of size, wealth, or political system, all member nations have an equal vote in the decision-making process. UN decisions reflect world opinion and the moral authority of the community of nations (United Nations, 2008). In 2000, the Millennium Development Goals were developed to coordinate and strengthen global efforts to meet the needs of the poorest of the poor. Governments throughout the world and leading global development agencies agreed on a target date of 2015 for meeting the following goals:

1. Eradicate extreme hunger and poverty.
2. Achieve universal primary education.
3. Promote gender equality, and empower women.
4. Reduce child mortality.
5. Improve maternal health.
6. Combat HIV/AIDS, malaria, and other infectious diseases.
7. Ensure environmental sustainability.
8. Develop global partnerships. (United Nations, 2000, 2006)

Collaborating with the UN are nongovernmental organizations (NGOs) such as the Carter Center and the Bill and Melinda Gates Foundation. Founded in 1982, the Carter Center is a nonprofit NGO founded by former President and First Lady, Jimmy and Rosalynn Carter, and based in Atlanta, Georgia. The Carter Center has three objectives: (1) to prevent and resolve conflicts, (2) to enhance freedom and democracy, and (3) to improve health.

The bond of our common humanity is stronger than the divisiveness of our fears and prejudices. God gives us the capacity for choice. We can choose to alleviate suffering. We can choose to work together for peace. We can make these changes—and we must. (Former U.S. President Jimmy Carter, Carter Center, 2008)

Founded in 2000, the Bill and Melinda Gates Foundation has local, national, and global objectives. Globally, the foundation focuses on reducing extreme poverty, improving health, and increasing public library access. Within Africa, the foundation has had a profound effect on improving access to antiviral medications and prevention and treatment for HIV/AIDS, TB, and malaria.

Created in 1946, the United Nations International Children's Emergency Fund (UNICEF) was founded to assist millions of sick and hungry children in war-ravaged Europe and China. In 1950, the UNICEF mandate was expanded to address needs of children and women throughout the world. UNICEF works for children's survival, development, and protection by developing and implementing community-based programs with well-documented achievements in child health, nutrition, education, water, sanitation, and women's rights. In 1953 the name was shortened to the UN Children's Fund; however, the UNICEF acronym was retained (WHO, 2007a).

Within a dramatically changing world economy, the major goal of the World Bank is to improve the health status of individuals living in areas that lack economic development.

Since 1970, the World Bank has become more focused on health-related initiatives to promote sustainable economic growth (Ruger, 2005). Projects range from alleviating poverty to safe water to effective sanitation to affordable housing. Financial assistance for the education of health care providers, the improvement of internal infrastructures, and funding for projects related to health status and disease prevention and control has been provided. The five largest shareholder countries include France, Germany, Japan, the United Kingdom, and the United States (World Bank, 2007a). Since 1963, the World Bank has provided $31 billion in loans and credits, currently funds 158 educational projects in 83 countries, and commits, on average, $1 billion for health, nutrition, and population projects in new lending annually (World Bank, 2007b).

The Centers for Disease Control and Prevention (CDC), located in Atlanta, Georgia, is one of the thirteen major operating components of the U.S. Department of Health and Human Services (USDHHS). The principal agency in the U.S. government for protecting the health and safety of all Americans and for providing essential human services, the CDC was founded in 1946 to help control malaria. The CDC has remained at the forefront of public health efforts to prevent and control infectious and chronic diseases, injuries, workplace hazards, disabilities, and environmental health threats. Today, the CDC is globally recognized for conducting research and investigations and for its action-oriented approach. The CDC applies research and findings to improve people's daily lives and responds to health emergencies—something that distinguishes the CDC from many of its peer agencies. The CDC is committed to achieving evidence-based health improvements. The agency is defining specific health impact goals to prioritize and focus its work and investments, to measure progress, and to work toward attainment of the CDC National Public Health Performance Standards and accreditation of U.S. public health departments.

Representing 12 million nurses in 129 countries, the International Council of Nurses (ICN) has addressed nursing and health care needs for more than a century. Nursing research, advanced practice nursing, doctoral education, first responder, disaster preparedness, mass casualty, policy, and advocacy have received increased emphasis over the past two decades in ICN and other nursing organizations worldwide. The ICN has five core values including visionary leadership, inclusiveness, flexibility, partnership, and achievement. The ICN Code for Nurses is the foundation for ethical nursing practice throughout the world (ICN, 2008). ICN and WHO are attempting to address the global shortage of nurses and other health care providers.

INTERNATIONAL HEALTH CARE DELIVERY SYSTEMS

When comparing health care systems, developed and developing countries can learn much from one another. Although transferring specialized medical technologies from developed to developing countries may not always be appropriate, developing countries are currently learning from health care reform policies and the technological revolution in developed countries. Likewise, developed countries have much to learn about low-technology initiatives such as oral rehydration therapy for the treatment of diarrhea and the delivery of primary health care as defined by the WHO. Participatory approaches to health care delivery, such as community involvement in health and education, are also essential. This exchange is important given the state of the current health care policy in developed countries. Many developed countries have made health care inaccessible to portions of their general public.

Even in countries with socialized medicine, medical costs increase annually and citizens are faced with paying supplemental medical fees or co-payment. There is a need to expand the knowledge base that made the twentieth-century health care revolution possible. In the twenty-first century, it is critical to provide research and development that are relevant to infectious diseases that overwhelmingly affect the poor. In addition, it is necessary to systematically generate an information base that countries can use to shape the future of their health care system (WHO, 2010).

The Lalonde Report (1974) proposed the "health field concept" as a useful way to consider the determinants of health such as biology, lifestyle, environment, and health services. This report emphasized lifestyle and environment as determinants of health outside the traditional medical sphere. It became the basis for rethinking new paradigms for health care delivery. The report signified the early beginnings of a health care paradigm shift from the traditional medical model to a more holistic system–environment perspective (Boothroyd and Eberle, 1990, p. 2). In the 1980s and 1990s, the rising costs of health care were a major catalyst for change, focusing attention on the need to provide alternative models of care. Over the past three decades, population-based approaches to health promotion and disease prevention have been developed to address system access, cost, efficiency, and effectiveness (Wall, Novak, and Wilkerson, 2005). Day surgery and outpatient services, nurse-managed clinics, ambulatory care, and home care provide alternatives to hospital-based care. In each of these areas, the nurse plays a prominent role and has the potential to bring a needed dimension of health promotion and disease prevention as individuals, families, and communities attempt to navigate a complex health care system.

Nurses must think more broadly about potential collaborators in solving the problems of the health care delivery system. Disciplines such as industrial engineering have much to offer nursing and other health care professionals, as engineering principles are applied to information technology, system design, patient safety, medication administration and reconciliation, simulation, chronic disease management, and hospital and clinic development, design, and renovation. The doctor of nursing practice (DNP) was developed by nursing leaders and endorsed by the American Association of Colleges of Nursing in order to reengineer health care (Wall, Novak, and Wilkerson, 2005). More than 100 programs have admitted DNP students with 200 programs in the developmental phase.

In 2010, U.S. expenditures for health care are projected to be 18% of the gross domestic product (GDP) (Centers for Medicaid and Medicare Services, 2008) while 49.4 million Americans are uninsured (Urban Institute, 2010). A market-based developed country such as the United States treats health care as a market commodity; therefore it focuses on curative medicine rather than preventive medicine because it creates more capital. A market-based health care system could lead to a goal opposite that of health for all. Theoretically, the advent of the managed care system in the United States proposed a capitated model to cut health care costs. Few managed care models, however, propose universal access or the comprehensive primary health care that WHO, U.S. President Barack Obama, and the late Senator Edward Kennedy advocate.

Given the two basic health care systems, market based and population based, and the fact that countries at different levels of development need to learn from each other, it is evident that a single model of health care delivery is not appropriate for every country. For example, in 1985, Cuba was recognized for reaching WHO's goal of "health for all." Cuba began to demonstrate to the world that health care could be provided as a basic human right rather than a privilege. In addition, Canada developed a universal health care system and Canadian community health nurses (CHNs) created innovative models for practice. Canada's Achieving Health for All provided a health promotion framework that includes fostering public participation in decisions that affect health, strengthening community health service networks with the disadvantaged communities they serve, and coordinating public health policy efforts (Epp, 1996).

The pressure for change provides the opportunity for reform, and the broad goal of health for all should guide this reform. Effective health care delivery systems must increase access and efficiency; improve health status through health promotion and disease prevention; eliminate health disparities; and protect individuals and families from financial loss due to catastrophic illness. One lesson learned from Canada's experience is that a narrow focus on individual responsibility and biology, with acute interventions does not ensure the overall health of a country. Thirty years after the start of the "Health for All" programs, inequity in health is still linked to socioeconomic rank. This suggests that a collective responsibility or population-based focus must be established with less emphasis on the individual. Collective mandates such as required physical education classes in elementary and middle schools will be instrumental in changing the social and economic environments in which people live. Preventative health programs are the first line in reducing disease by providing education on healthy living choices (Low, 2008). McKinlay, as cited in Low (2008), argues that treatment of disease is akin to standing downstream and pulling people out of the river after they have fallen in. In contrast, health promotion stresses preventative health care, taking into account how social structure produces ill health and the economic framework of a society, shape lifestyle choices. They are thus analogous to upstream activities where people are prevented from falling into the river in the first place (Low, 2008).

The Role of the Community Health Nurse in International Health Care

In a rapidly changing health care environment, the nursing role is becoming less traditional and much more diverse. The traditional structure of provider roles is challenged as professional disciplines are recruited to provide expanded and diverse health care services. The nursing role is reciprocal, and it is interdependent with clients and families, physicians, and other health care professionals. The nurse's role expectations and societal expectations influence the formation of behavior patterns specific to the professional nursing role. These expectations provide the basis for the role of the community and public health nurse in international health care.

Florence Nightingale was the first nurse to establish international linkages and networks that became vastly important to her own country and to nursing throughout the world. As the first woman and nurse inducted into the Royal Statistics Society, she recognized the importance of evidence-based nursing and health care. Every obstacle to health and wellness confronted her. She overcame obstacles systematically, developing the foundation and legacy for modern nursing and community and public health nursing. Nightingale channeled her energies into all aspects of health from the care of wounded soldiers at Scutari in the Crimea to the broad public policies that affected health in her time.

CHNs seek to ensure the attainment of health for all in a cost-effective, efficient, accessible health care system. They must be involved in research, community assessment, planning, implementation, management, evaluation, health services delivery, disaster preparedness and emergency response, health policy, advocacy, and legislation. Nurses in all countries coordinate their work with other health care personnel, as well as local and global community leaders. Health for all requires attitudes, levels of competence, knowledge, and skills that differ substantially from those required in traditional nursing. The changes in the health environment, such as technological advancements, changes in the morbidity and mortality patterns of the population, and social and political changes, all form the basis for the nursing role.

With the development of the nurse practitioner (NP) role over the past 40 years in the United States and over the past 20 years abroad, nurses with advanced degrees and areas of specialization have strengthened the community-based health care system. The development of the DNP degree in the United States and PhDs in nursing in a variety of countries further elevates the knowledge and skill base for nursing's role in reengineering health care (Wall et al., 2005).

As primary health care and primary care may be practiced differently in other countries, the NP and the CHN face multiple challenges. Primary health care refers to essential services that support a healthy life. It involves access, availability, service delivery, community participation, and the citizen's right to health care. In contrast, primary care refers to first-line or point-of-access medical and nursing care controlled by providers and focused on the individual. Primary care may not be the norm, particularly in communities in developing or lesser-developed countries that have overwhelming needs for basic necessities such as safe drinking water and sanitation. The needs of the group outweigh the needs of the individual.

Nurses can make a difference in helping solve the existing and emerging health problems in countries throughout the world. The advent of technology has enhanced global communication and facilitated travel. It is important that nurses throughout the world understand each other and learn from one another. Nurses are the most valuable assets of any health care system. Community public health nursing can improve access to care for the most vulnerable and hard-to-reach groups in any country. In its many forms, nursing is relevant and will further expand in the future. The future demands evidence-based learning, engagement, service and growth in information technology, and local and global health policy. Population-based nursing experts are critical to solving the challenges of the fragmented, mismanaged, expensive, ineffective, inefficient health care delivery system that exists in many parts of our global community.

RESEARCH IN INTERNATIONAL HEALTH

Since 1990, international nursing research has focused predominantly on the following three areas: (1) student and faculty educational exchange programs, (2) diverse clinical experiences, and (3) the international development of home care or transition from hospital to home.

WHO collaborating centers in nursing provide a framework for research, education, and service delivery partnerships. Purdue University and the University of Virginia, both affiliates of Case Western Reserve University and the University of Mexico WHO Collaborating Centers, contributed to a partnership for educational programming, clinical practice, and research for graduate students in primary health care nursing and community health. Team Reach Out South Africa is presented in the case study.

Crigger and colleagues (2004) focus on ethical issues related to introducing antibiotic resistance into the second- and third-world community assessment and clinic development in Honduras, while Altman (2009) immerses her "Spanish for Health Care Professionals" nursing students in orphanages and clinics in Nicaragua.

U.S. models of home health care are developing in many countries. These models provide a variety of services to bridge the gap between the hospital and community-based care. Sources of home care include home visits by nurses from official government public health agencies, nonprofit voluntary agencies, and for-profit home care agencies. Examples of home care services include assistance with activities of daily living, treatment, rehabilitation, transportation, and respite for caregivers. Home care service providers in the United States and abroad face many challenges. Estimating financial implications and calculating potential caseloads are complex factors in the design of effective delivery systems.

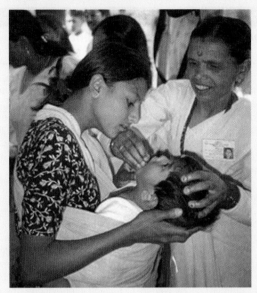

Nepalese child receives vitamin A supplement. Over 3 million Nepali children are now receiving twice-yearly vitamin A supplements in a program instituted by the U.S. Agency for International Development (USAID). Approximately 15,000 child deaths are averted each year in Nepal as a result of this program. (From U.S. Agency for International Development, Washington, DC [www.usaid.gov.])

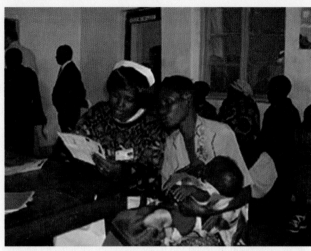

Malaria is the number one killer among children in Tanzania. A child health nurse consults with a mother at a maternal-child health clinic in Iringa, Tanzania. (From U.S. Agency for International Development, Washington, DC [www.usaid.gov.] John Dunlop.)

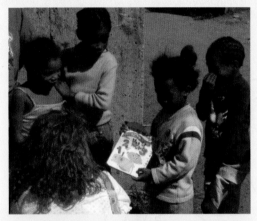

Community home health visits, Cape Town South Africa. (Julie Cowan Novak)

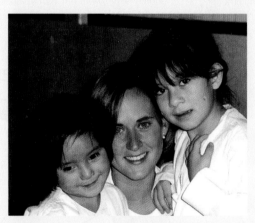

Nurse-managed clinics San Luis, Xochimilco and Mexico City. (Julie Cowan Novak)

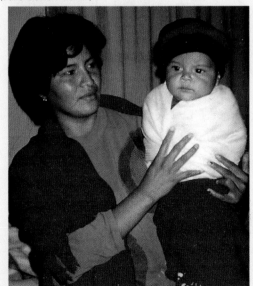

Nurse-managed public health clinic, Universidad Nacional Autonomo de Mexico, San Luis, Xochimilco, Mexico. (Julie Cowan Novak)

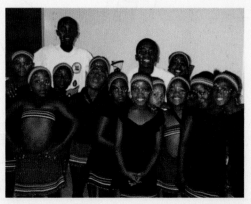

Cape Town, South Africa school inauguration and health fair. (Julie Cowan Novak)

CASE STUDY   APPLICATION OF INTERNATIONAL COMMUNITY ASSESSMENT

International Community Assessment Model (ICAM): A Collaborative Model for Community Assessment, Education, and Health Care Delivery

In Mexico and South Africa the provision of equitable health care services to a population that is geographically and educationally disparate is both economically and logistically challenging. Both countries are further challenged by a lack of infrastructure necessary for health promotion, protection, and maintenance. South Africa is challenged by extreme poverty and staggering rates of HIV/AIDS and TB. In planning interventions, nurses need a globally diverse assessment tool and methodology to empower communities in developing countries to achieve health care goals and reduce health care costs. U.S. nursing students gaining international health care experience in a community in rural Mexico and urban South Africa can implement the International Community Assessment Model (ICAM) (Figure 15-1) before planning targeted programs with local community leaders. The ICAM, tested in rural Mexico and as a component of Team Reach Out South Africa, is part of an ongoing project. U.S. nursing students compare and contrast practices in various countries using the ICAM and FURCO Service Learning Model (Figure 15-2). Service learning is discipline specific, experiential, and embedded in course objectives and relies heavily on reflection and journaling.

Community Empowerment

Nurses can collaborate with health and environmental experts in implementing a community empowerment framework (Novak and Novak in Richards, et al 1998). In community empowerment, the community identifies its problems and a plan of action, and environmental experts and nurses remain consultants and team members to assist community members (May, Mendelson, and Ferketich, 1995). This process aids the community in developing interventions that are culturally acceptable, breaking down cultural barriers. In developing countries, health-promotion programs that do not involve community participation and education often fail after the experts leave the community.

Assessment

During the assessment phase, the nurse identifies key influential community members and leaders and encourages them to join a board of community partners with the goal of assessing community health. The community partners may choose to use the ICAM for the purpose of providing a globally diverse assessment framework and for data gathering. Assessment of community culture helps identify potential cultural barriers to nursing interventions. The center of the model assesses the heart of the community's culture by identifying individual, family, and community characteristics, including their history, demographics, values, beliefs, rituals, and the effect of these characteristics on social and economic conditions.

The ICAM assesses the following:

• *Recreation:* Community cardiovascular fitness; stress management; energy renewal; and relaxation through sports, hobbies, and games.

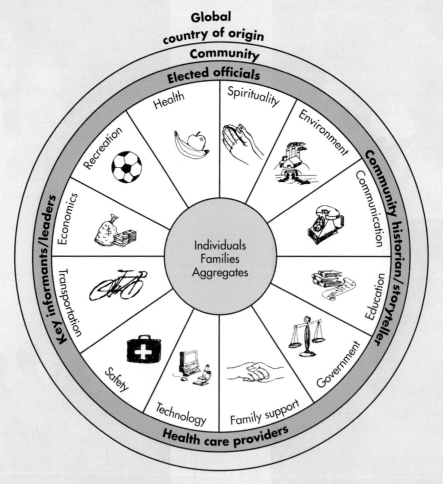

FIGURE 15-1 International Community Assessment Model.

Continued

International Community Assessment Model (ICAM): A Collaborative Model for Community Assessment, Education, and Health Care Delivery

- *Perceptions:* Community perceptions of health, including community members' physical, social, and mental balance and lifestyle choices.
- *Spirituality:* The community's religious beliefs and practices.
- *Support systems:* Family support systems, including parental support of children and adult children, adult children's support of their parents, and support among extended family members. (Family is defined as a group of individuals who share common experiences and goals and are often linked together by genetics, marriage, living situation, or a common emotional bond.)

The physical environment encompasses the community's infrastructure, including homes, water sources, waste disposal sites, roadways, buildings for businesses and shops, factories, power lines, and considerations related to occupational health (e.g., nurses must seek new collaborators in solving the complex problems of the health care delivery system). Industrial and biomedical engineering have much to offer nursing and the other health care disciplines, as engineering principles are applied to system design, information technology, patient safety and quality, simulation, and hospital and clinic development, design, and renovation. Throughout the United States advanced practice nursing is evolving to the DNP. This innovation in nursing will revolutionize health care and improve public health safety and quality. (Wall, Novak, and Wilkerson, 2005). More than 100 programs have admitted DNP students with 200 programs in developmental phase.

The ICAM also assesses the following:

- *Education:* The concept of education reflects the community's knowledge, skills, level of schooling or training, and literacy rate.
- *Transportation:* Transportation is defined as how community members travel from point A to point B.
- *Safety:* Evaluation of the community's safety includes examining potential dangers in the community that could lead to injury or death and examining safety measures and plans developed by the community to prevent these problems.
- *Government and politics:* How the community is governed or ruled is examined.
- *Economy:* The efficacy of economic resources is analyzed in terms of production, dispersal, and expenditure of resources.
- *Communication:* Communication is evaluated by examining face-to-face and community-wide information exchange through speech, body language, writing, and drawings. Key components of the community's communication are native languages and forms of communication, such as letters, telephone, computer networks, electronic health records, the Internet, fax machines, television, billboards, signs, magazines, newspapers, and telegrams.
- *Access:* Electricity, public sanitation, public water systems, radio, television, technology, computers, the Internet, fax machines, libraries, industrial machinery, and agricultural practices must be examined.

The ICAM will allow the board to examine all the public health threats to the community and additional barriers to an effective cultural awareness, sensitivity, proficiency, and humility.

The ICAM also reflects the importance of assessing the country of origin and global effects on the community. When assessing a community, the nurse must consider the external factors affecting the community. For example, the economy depends on vendors and international purchasing of their main exports.

After the community assessment, the collaborative team should develop an educational program that identifies potential challenges to an educational program or intervention. This program should motivate community partners to identify these problems and then search for effective solutions. As partners become further aware of the health care barriers or health hazards, resources should be provided that will aid in their response.

Next, partners should be assisted in completing a survey and offering focus groups related to needs assessment and attitudes.

The nursing team, local experts, key community informants, and partners need to establish the root cause of problems in a collaborative manner in order to develop effective interventions.

Planning and Intervention

The board and community identify central issues, challenges and barriers. The board then enters the planning phase of the intervention campaign. Community board members can collaborate with environmental experts and the nurse to identify individual, family, and community educational and service learning goals, strategies, and interventions based on best evidence and practice.

The collaborative team will subsequently analyze possible interventions. This body of knowledge will allow the community partners to determine which, if any, of the proposed interventions would be relevant and appropriate for their community. In addition, they may be able to apply these ideas in creating their own interventions. When the community partners have selected or developed an intervention for their project, they can be encouraged to create strategies to educate the community.

Implementation

Before the project is implemented, the outcome of the community needs assessment must be clarified. The community must be given the opportunity to provide feedback to all collaborators regarding proposed interventions. The partners should be willing to compromise to meet the community's needs. After the community-wide education has occurred and necessary consensus and compromise have been achieved, the project can be implemented. At this point, the community members are trained to maintain the project. Once the implementation is completed, evaluation of the project can begin to ensure that the goals and objectives of the board are met.

Evaluation

The collaborative team should evaluate the project in a formative and summative manner. In addition, the nurse should conduct community surveys to determine whether members continue to recognize the need to maintain the project and to provide feedback related to progress. The ICAM was tested in rural Mexico and is being tested in South Africa as part of the ongoing Team Reach Out project. The targeted communities have a high incidence of poverty. As a result, 80% of the communities reside in crowded living conditions. Many factors in the community pose serious health threats including infectious disease, chronic conditions, tobacco use, secondhand smoke, farm chemicals, and air pollution.

Field workers are often powerless and have minimal recourse when exposed to unhealthy environmental contaminants causing increased morbidity and mortality.

In rural Mexico, the top three causes of mortality in the communities are cardiac disorders, diabetes, automobile accidents, and dramatic increases in violence, particularly in urban Mexico and border communities. The leading causes of morbidity are respiratory infections, diabetes, hypertension, and gastrointestinal illnesses. The community's high rate of gastrointestinal illness is related to poor access to potable water. The community historians, community political leaders, key employers, full-time staff at nurse-run clinics, local community health faculty, and the *pasantes* (nursing graduates who have completed 1 year of community service at nurse-run clinics and public health agencies) are critical to the success of the project.

International Community Assessment Model (ICAM): A Collaborative Model for Community Assessment, Education, and Health Care Delivery

Evaluation—cont'd

A multidisciplinary team of key influential community members, environmental experts, and nurses will further assess the community using the ICAM model. The goal of this assessment is to assist the community members in further diagnosing the community's health care needs and other issues as they are identified. Nurses collaborate with community partners to develop culturally proficient interventions. After the interventions are developed, the local partners, clinic staff, and *pasantes* continue to evaluate the effectiveness of these interventions, promoting a sense of ownership of the project in the community and helping to ensure improvements in health care long after the multidisciplinary team leaves the community (see Case Study: Team Reach Out South Africa).

CASE STUDY   **TEAM REACH OUT SOUTH AFRICA**

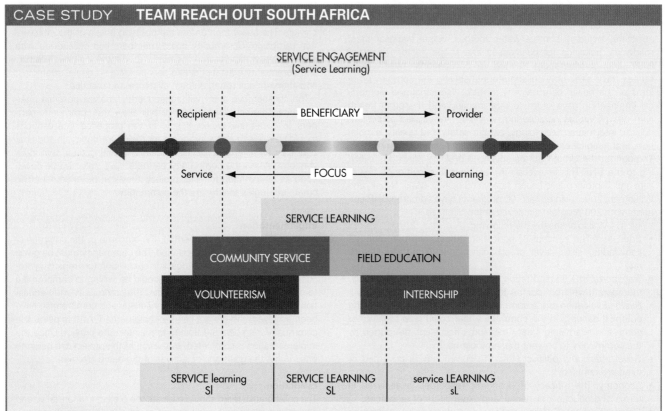

FIGURE 15-2 FURCO Service Learning Model.

Team Reach Out started as a student-initiated service-learning project with the goal of providing ongoing assistance to the victims of Hurricane Katrina. Four years after Hurricane Katrina, Team Reach Out refocused efforts to Cape Town, South Africa. In 2009, four senior nursing students and one science student integrated their leadership skills with the application of public health knowledge, compassion, and concern as they worked in partnership with several international health agencies. This case reviews the service-learning framework (Furco, 1996, 2002), course planning, implementation, and evaluation.

Service learning is a reciprocal partnership that bridges the gap between professional education and society. It is a powerful teaching and learning strategy that engages students in learning while helping communities to help themselves (Poirrier, 2001). Service learning provides an experiential, collaborative, discipline-based relationship between students and community members for a reciprocal service learning experience and allows an opportunity for reflection. Service learning sets the stage for a lifelong commitment to the development of civic duty, social awareness, and engagement while providing unique learning experiences that focus on building citizenship, cultural diversity, community partnerships, knowledge of community resources, critical thinking skills, and respect for humankind.

Both students and the community benefit from service learning. Students benefit from the exposure to real-life dilemmas and first-hand experience of joint team efforts. Communities benefit from the knowledge and creativity available from academia (Richards, Novak, and Davis, 2009).

The faculty team leader/advisor completed an exploratory trip to Johannesburg and Cape Town, South Africa, in March 2008, meeting with prospective community partners. Each of the local health care leaders invited the development of a collaboration. Due to the richness of each setting and the overwhelming need for human and financial resources, the choice was extremely difficult. Cape Town was selected as the city site through a comprehensive assessment using the International Community Assessment Model (ICAM) (Novak and Novak, 2001, 2007, 2009, 2010). Health care and educational partners within the city were selected in collaboration

Continued

with the Christel House Academy school nurse, faculty, and staff. Subsequently, students from the School of Nursing and College of Science were invited to apply through notification in their respective student newsletters. Selection was based on the clarity of the student's goals and understanding of cultural humility and service learning. After selection, each student wrote an additional travel grant application to the university's Office of Engagement. Below is a description of the partners involved in this project and the experiences each provided.

Partners

Christel House International is a 501(c)(3) public charity that operates learning centers in impoverished neighborhoods with the goal of creating sustainable social and educational impact. Between 1999 and 2002, Christel House opened five learning centers in Mexico, India, South Africa, Venezuela, and the United States. Currently, Christel House serves more than 3000 students, their families, and communities. Christel House K-12 Academy in Cape Town helps children around the world break the cycle of poverty, realize their hopes and dreams, and become self-sufficient, contributing members of society (Christel House, 2009). The Academy invited the students to participate in the inaugural celebration of a new school facility and campus. Weekend cultural experiences included a trip to Robben Island, an ecological and historical heritage site where Nelson Mandela was imprisoned from 1963 to 1990; Table Mountain, a protected natural habitat with 1500 plant species; and a game and nature preserve.

The Themba Care Orphanage provides a safe and compassionate environment for approximately twenty children who are HIV positive. In the majority of cases the parents had died of AIDS; however, some children were placed in the setting by their parents to avoid stigma within their respective communities. The orphanage is run by an executive director, two registered nurses/"sisters," a teacher, a staff of five nursing assistants, and local volunteers. Team Reach Out worked with volunteers from three different U.S. universities on site. In addition to one older child, 95% of the children at the orphanage ranged in age from 18 months to 4 years. Students were able to complete Denver Developmental Screenings and health assessments and to work with the sisters in medication dispensation and reconciliation. The majority of the children demonstrated global developmental delay on the screenings. Students played with, fed, and cared for the children in this warm, caring, inviting preschool environment. The students reflected their difficulty in saying goodbye to the children.

The Gatesville Medical Center is a multispecialty large private Indian hospital located in Cape Town. Team Reach Out students were able to care for pediatric patients and effectively compare and contrast this South African state-of-the-art private hospital with other health care settings. Diagnoses included respiratory syncytial virus, pneumonia, asthma, gastroenteritis/dehydration, and meningitis.

The Tafelsig Community Health Center provides care to approximately 9000 low-income patients each month. In addition to health promotion visits across the lifespan, upper and lower respiratory tract infections, gastroenteritis, and urinary tract infections were common diagnoses. A minor emergency/urgent care clinic is on site. Tafelsig also has one of the largest TB and HIV/AIDS patient populations in Cape Town. Students were able to complete health assessments and immunize patients under the supervision of South African registered nurse specialty clinic coordinators and their faculty advisor.

The students' week of clinical experiences culminated with a presentation of a health fair at the academy. This health fair focused on school and family health promotion and included the following stations: prenatal and newborn care and parenting; prevention of TB, HIV/AIDS, and malaria; health care careers; science experiments (with premed students); and health screenings including height, weight, blood pressure, glucose, and cholesterol. The academy ran special bus routes from the school to and from area shanty towns to bring parents and other community members to the school health fair. The students worked with the World Health Organization, the Centers for Disease Control and Prevention, Johnson & Johnson, and local Cape Town universities to ensure culturally appropriate materials for the health fair. The Christel House Academy Health Fair was attended by 600 children and 200 parents.

Student Responses

Team Reach Out South Africa students provided poignant and insightful reflections regarding their experiences. Community partners indicated that the students were very professional and were able to provide much-needed support. Phase three of the project was implemented in March 2010 in collaboration with local South African community partners.

Summary

Students felt strongly that service learning enhanced their community public health experience while building relationships with community service organizations. Students reported encountering minimal barriers to the implementation of this project and also were not reluctant to participate in these activities. Students also agreed that they would continue to participate in service-learning activities in the near future. Table 15-1 includes more student reflections on their experiences. Table 15-2 and Box 15-2 highlight students' feelings about service learning in general (Richards and Novak, 2010).

TABLE 15-1 STUDENT REFLECTIONS ON TEAM REACH OUT PROJECTS

Team Reach Out Biloxi Student Reflections

"It was a wonderful experience to be able to meet so many interesting people and use our knowledge of health care to provide support to this community."

"Every victim was thinking about their neighbor in terms of their needs."

"Everyone expressed appreciation and hope."

"My most meaningful memory is the incredible impression each Mississippian made on me. It was amazing to me that through all of the tragedy, devastation, and loss, their southern hospitality and gentleness was still very much alive."

Team Reach Out South Africa Student Reflections

"We were so fortunate to see the health care extremes, from the poorest of the poor clinics to the private hospitals. It was such a diverse spectrum to work in."

"Traveling to South Africa was an eye-opening experience in so many ways. I'll never forget the striking beauty of the country contrasted with the devastating poverty that runs rampant; I was both impressed and surprised by the resourcefulness of their healthcare system."

"The trip was incredible. So much poverty and beauty and riches in the same area. The people touched my life and I hope that I did the same for some of them."

CASE STUDY   **TEAM REACH OUT SOUTH AFRICA—cont'd**

TABLE 15-2   STUDENT AND PROVIDER RESPONSES OF SERVICE-LEARNING QUESTIONNAIRE

PURDUE UNIVERSITY SCHOOL OF NURSING SERVICE-LEARNING QUESTIONNAIRE STRONGLY AGREE (5), AGREE (4), UNDECIDED (3), DISAGREE (2), STRONGLY DISAGREE (1)	STUDENT AVERAGE (N = 5)
1. Service learning at Purdue University School of Nursing may be a catalyst for	
a. Assisting societal needs	4.75
b. Student learning	4.8
c. Building relationships with community service organizations	4.6
d. Engagement opportunities	4.8
2. I encountered significant barriers to completing this service-learning activity.	1.8
3. Service learning should only be integrated into senior course leadership.	2.4
4. Service learning enables a positive change through leadership.	4.4
5. I was reluctant to participate in community and civic service-learning activities.	1.2
6. Service learning is a community-building and democracy-building activity.	4
7. I plan to continue service-learning activities in the immediate future.	4.2
8. This experience embraced the concepts of reciprocity between learning and the community being served.	4.2
9. This experience allowed students to engage in activities that addressed community needs	4.8

(Richards and Novak, 2010.)

BOX 15-2   STUDENT RESPONSES: WHAT IS THE DEFINITION OF SERVICE LEARNING?

Providing services to those in need while at the same time learning in your field of interest and having the ability to work with those less fortunate. It is a hand-on learning experience that, for me, was life changing and eye opening.

It is volunteering with doing something that you are in the field of doing or obtaining a degree in.

Service learning is a unique way of learning in and about a community and providing services for the betterment of a community. Service projects provide communities with people who are able to use their time, resources, and expertise in order to improve or help the community in which they are serving. At the same time, the people involved in the service project are learning from their experiences with the project.

Service learning is a volunteering project that is done to help the community in some positive way while the volunteer has the opportunity to broaden their own horizons by learning something new.

Utilizing skills and knowledge acquired in the classroom as a means to enhance the community (Richards and Novak, 2010).

REFERENCES

Christel House International: 2009, www.christelhouse.org. Accessed July 6, 2009.

Poirrier G: *Service learning: curricular applications in nursing*, New York, 2001, National League for Nursing.

Richards E, Novak J, Davis L: Disaster response after Hurricane Katrina: a model for an academic-community partnership in Mississippi, *J Community Health Nurs* 26(3):114–120, 2009.

Richards E, Novak J: From Biloxi to Cape Town: Curricular integration of service learning, *J Community Health Nurs* 27(1):46–50, 2010.

SUMMARY

Community public health nurses face many exciting challenges in health care reform and designing effective systems of health care delivery. These include being responsive to emerging needs and health issues in the population, developing multidisciplinary practice models that adhere to the principles of primary health care in the context of a reengineered health care system, and mobilizing research dissemination and practice implementation strategies to ensure evidence-based practice as the norm rather than the exception. Using evidence-based models as a framework for local to global community public health partnerships and projects should be tested and evaluated. There is still much to be done to meet the challenge of

WHO's goal of "health for all." Studying the progress achieved in other countries is critical; however, success will ultimately depend on societal commitment to addressing complex issues of poverty, disparity, and health care inaccessibility.

LEARNING ACTIVITIES

1. Discuss population characteristics and the threat of population growth to health and health care systems.
2. Compare and contrast the incidence and treatment of people living with AIDS, TB, and malaria. Discuss methods of prevention.

3. Explain the incidence of death from AIDS in Africa, Mexico, and the United States. What might account for the differences?
4. Compare population-focused nursing in a developing country with community health nursing in the community. How are they the same, and how do they differ?
5. Conduct research and compare the rates of life expectancy and infant mortality in Africa, Mexico, and the United States. What factors might account for the similarities and differences in rates between the developing and the developed countries?

6. Describe the key elements of an effective health care delivery system. Will the focus of future health care services reflect downstream thinking, or will the orientation uphold models of prevention and promotion that deal with root causes of health problems?
7. Test the International Community Assessment Model (ICAM) in a community. Evaluate its effectiveness.
8. Describe the FURCO Service Learning Model and its potential application in local to global projects in your university.

REFERENCES

Altman MI: Culture and healthcare delivery in Nicaragua: crossing a cultural divide, *Purdue Nurse* January: 12, 2009.

Boothroyd P, Eberle M: *Healthy communities: what they are, how they're made, CHS Research Bulletin, UBC Centre for Human Settlements*, Vancouver, 1990, University of British Columbia.

Carter Center: About the center, 2008, www.cartercenter.org/about/index.html.

Centers for Disease Control and Prevention: 2005, www.cdc.org.

Center for Medicare and Medicaid Services: Table 1: National health expenditures aggregate, 2008, www.cms.gov/nationalhealthExpendData/downloads/tables.pdf.

Crigger N, et al: A model of antibiotic use in a lay Honduran population, *Int J Nurs Stud* 41(7):745–753, 2004.

Dworkin SL, Ehrhardt AA: Going beyond "ABC" to include "GEM": critical reflections on progress in the HIV/AIDS epidemic, *Am J Public Health* 97(1):128–134, 2007.

Epp J: *Achieving health for all: a framework for health promotion*, Ottawa, 1996, Health and Welfare Canada.

Furco A: Service learning: A balanced approach to experiential education. In Taylor B, editor: *Expanding boundaries: Serving and learning*, Washington, DC, 1996, Corporation for National Service.

Garrett B, Buettgens M, Doan L, Headen I, Holahan J: Urban Institute (2010). Without healthcare reform, number of unanswered could increase significantly over next decade. The Cost of Failure to Enact Health Reform: 2010–2020. http://rwjf.org/files/research/57449.pdf.

International Council of Nurses: About ICN, 2008, www.icn.ch/abouticn.htm.

Lalonde M: *A new perspective on the health of Canadians*, Ottawa, 1974, Minister of Supply and Services.

Low J, Theriault L: Health promotion policy in Canada: Lessons forgotten, lessons still to learn, *Health Promot Int* 23(2):200–206, 2008.

Marmot M: *The social determinants of global health and resolving tensions: Readings in global health*, Washington, DC, 2008, American Public Health Association, p. 3.

May KM, Mendelson C, Ferketich S: Community empowerment in rural healthcare, *Public Health Nurs* 12(1):25–30, 1995.

Population Reference Bureau: *World population data sheet*, 2006, www.prb.org.

Potts M: Common sense prevailing at population conference, *Lancet* 344:809, 1994.

Querreno R, et al: *Key issues in health development: poverty and ill-health, Division of Intensified Cooperation with Countries and People in Greatest Need*, 1998, www.who.int/ico/key.htm.

Reiff FM, et al: Low cost safe water for the world, a practical interim solution, *J Public Health Policy* 17(4):389–408, 1996.

Rosenkoetter MM: A framework for international healthcare consultations, *Nurs Outlook* 45(4):182–187, 1997.

Ruger JP: The changing role of the World Bank in global health, *Am J Public Health* 95(1):60–70, 2005.

UNAIDS 2009, November *AIDS Epidemic Update*, www.unaids.org/en/knowledgecenter/HIV Data/2009.

United Nations: *Resolution adopted by the General Assembly: United Nations Millennium Declaration*, New York, 2000, The Author.

United Nations: *The Millennium Development Goals report*, New York, 2006, The Author.

United Nations: The UN in brief, 2008, un.org/Overview/uninbrief/.

Wall B, Novak J, Wilkerson S: The doctor of nursing practice: reengineering healthcare, *J Nurs Educ* 44(9):396–403, 2005.

Williams AB: Nursing, health, and human rights: a framework for international collaboration, *J Assoc Nurses AIDS Care* 15(3):75–77, 2004.

World Bank: About us, 2007a, www.worldbank.org.

World Bank: *Ten things you never knew about the World Bank*, Washington, DC, 2007b, The Author.

World Health Organization: *Tobacco Free Initiative*, (2009), www.who.int/tobacco/global_interaction/en.

World Health Organization: *Roll back malaria info sheet*, Geneva, 2005a, The Author. www.who.int/malaria/docs/Basicfacts.pdf.

World Health Organization: *TB recommendations included in the "Commission for Africa" report*, 2005b, www.who.int/tb/commission_for_africa/en/print.html.

World Health Organization: *The 3 by 5 initiative*, 2005c, www.who.int/3by5/about/initiative/en/index.html.

World Health Organization: *Working for health: an introduction to the World Health Organization*, Geneva, 2007a, WHO Press.

World Health Organization: *About WHO*, 2007b, www.who.int/about/en/.

World Health Organization: *Global summary of the AIDS epidemic*, December 2007, 2008, www.who.int/hiv/data/2008_global_summary_AIDS_ep.png.

World Health Organization (WHO): *Global health atlas database*, 2010, Author.

16

Child and Adolescent Health

Susan Rumsey Givens, Mary Brecht Carpenter

Additional Material for Study, Review, and Further Exploration

evolve WEBSITE

http://evolve.elsevier.com/Nies
- Quiz
- Case Studies
- Glossary
- WebLinks

OBJECTIVES

Upon completion of this chapter, the reader will be able to do the following:

1. Identify major indicators of child and adolescent health status.
2. Describe how socioeconomic circumstances influence child and adolescent health.
3. Discuss the individual and societal costs of poor child health status.
4. Discuss public programs and prevention strategies targeted to children's health.
5. Apply knowledge of child and adolescent health needs in planning appropriate, comprehensive care at the individual, family, and community levels.

KEY TERMS

adolescent pregnancy
child maltreatment
childhood immunization
Children's Health Insurance Program (CHIP)
cultural competence
Early and Periodic Screening, Diagnosis, and Treatment (EPSDT)
fetal alcohol spectrum disorders (FASD)
infant mortality
lead poisoning
Medicaid
preconceptional counseling
prenatal care
preterm birth
Special Supplemental Nutrition Program for Women, Infants, and Children (WIC)

OUTLINE

Issues of Pregnancy and Infancy
    Infant Mortality
    Preterm Birth and Low Birth Weight
    Preconceptional Health
    Prenatal Care
    Prenatal Substance Use
Childhood Health Issues
    Accidental Injuries
    Obesity
    Immunization
    Lead Poisoning
    Child Maltreatment
    Children with Special Health Care Needs
Adolescent Health Issues
    Adolescent Pregnancy and Childbearing
    Violence

Sexually Transmitted Infections
Tobacco, Alcohol, and Drug Use
Factors Affecting Child and Adolescent Health
    Poverty
    Racial Disparities
    Single Parenting
    Parents' Educational Status
    Health Care Use
Strategies to Improve Child and Adolescent Health
    Monitoring and Tracking
    Healthy People 2020: Child and Adolescent Health
    Health Promotion and Disease Prevention
Public Health Programs Targeted to Children and Adolescents
    Health Care Coverage Programs
    Direct Health Care Delivery Programs

Sharing Responsibility for Improving Child and Adolescent Health
  Parents' Role
  Community's Role
  Employer's Role

Government's Role
Community Health Nurse's Role
Legal and Ethical Issues in Child and Adolescent Health
  Ethical Issues

A nation's destiny lies with the health, education, and well-being of its children. The United States has made tremendous progress over the past century toward improving children's lives. Improvements in public health measures—such as sanitation, infectious disease control, environmental regulation, health screening, and education—and remarkable strides in medical care have all contributed to the good health status that most children enjoy. However, these improvements have not equally benefited children of all races and ethnic groups, children at all income levels, or children in all geographic areas of the country. For example, significant disparities persist in the health status of white children versus children of color. Children living in suburban areas and most outer urban areas experience superior access to health care services compared with children living in rural areas and inner cities, especially if they are poor.

Although most of the nation's children are healthy and succeed in school, many are not enjoying optimal health and well-being and are not reaching their full potential as contributing members of society. Despite improvements, the mortality and morbidity rates for U.S. children in all age groups are unacceptably high. Consider:

- More than 28,000 infants die every year before reaching their first birthday.
- More than half a million babies are born prematurely. Many of these children will suffer long-term effects, including cerebral palsy, respiratory and vision problems, physical disabilities, and learning difficulties.
- Eighteen percent of children aged 0 to 18 years live in poverty.
- Every year, nearly 800,000 children are documented victims of child maltreatment; most are under the age of 4 years.
- More than 140,000 girls aged 15 to 17 years give birth each year.
- Seventy-five percent of students have consumed alcohol by the end of high school; nearly one quarter are cigarette smokers.
- Violence is the second leading cause of death among adolescents (National Center for Health Statistics, 2009).

The health of a child has long-term implications. The health habits adopted by children and youth will profoundly influence their potential to lead healthy, productive lives. The physical and emotional health experienced by a child plays a pivotal role in his or her overall development and the well-being of the entire family. Children who go to school sick or hungry, who cannot see the chalkboard or hear the teacher, who have learning disabilities, who are troubled by abusive parents or disruptive living circumstances, or who fear for their safety at home or in school often do not perform on the level of their counterparts who are healthy, well nourished, well cared for at home, and safe and secure in their world. From fetal life onward, the health and well-being of individuals has a substantial impact on their futures.

In 2007, there were about 73.9 million children in the United States under age 18 years, forming about 25% of the country's population. The number of children is expected to increase to 80 million by the year 2020, but the proportion of children as compared with adults has been decreasing since the mid-1960's baby boom (Federal Interagency Forum on Child and Family Statistics, 2008). The demographic composition of the nation is important to planners and policy makers because it influences how resources will be allocated. For example, a growing child population necessitates more resources for schools, child care, and health care.

The ethnic and racial composition of the United States' child and adolescent population is also changing. The percentage of children living in the United States with at least one foreign-born parent rose from 15% in 1994 to 22% in 2007. About 20% of school-age children speak a language other than English at home.

In 2007, 57% of children living in the United States were white, non-Hispanic; 21% were Hispanic; 15% were black; 4% were Asian; and 4% were of all other races (Figure 16-1). The percentage of children who are Hispanic has increased

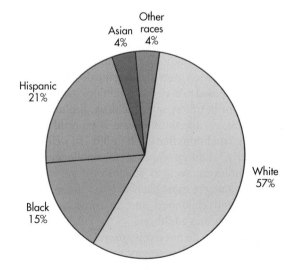

FIGURE 16-1 Percentage distribution of U.S. children by race/ethnicity, 2008. (From Federal Interagency Forum on Child and Family Statistics: *America's children in brief: key national indicators of well-being, 2008:* www.childstats.gov/americaschildren/demo.asp. Accessed May 1, 2009.)

faster than that of any other racial or ethnic group, growing from 9% of the child population in 1980 to 21% in 2007. By 2020, it is projected that nearly one in four children in the United States will be of Hispanic origin (Federal Interagency Forum on Child and Family Statistics, 2008).

Children are a dependent population and rely primarily on parents or other adults to protect and promote their health and well-being. Community health nurses can learn more about this important population group and the positive and negative factors that influence their health. Nurses can use this information to help improve the chances that children will grow up to be healthy, both physically and emotionally.

This chapter focuses on the health status of children and adolescents and the medical, socioeconomic, environmental, educational, safety, and public health factors that community health nurses must address to improve child and adolescent health. This chapter also discusses indicators of child and adolescent health status, the individual and societal costs of poor child health, public programs targeted to children's health, and strategies to improve child and adolescent health at the individual, family, and community levels.

ISSUES OF PREGNANCY AND INFANCY

The health of the mother before, during, and after pregnancy has a direct impact on the health of her children. Predictors of healthy child development include genetic endowment, maternal health, environmental stresses, and health behaviors throughout her life. The conditions that surround a child's fetal development and early years shape his or her life. Protection and promotion of maternal and child health can help ensure a healthy future for the child.

- Women who are not in optimal health before becoming pregnant are at increased risk for poor pregnancy outcomes.
- Children whose mothers have late or no prenatal care, or who smoked or used illegal drugs during pregnancy, are more likely to be born with low birth weights and serious health conditions (e.g., birth defects, learning disabilities, and vision and hearing deficits).
- A fetus exposed to maternal conditions such as hypertension; poor nutrition; maternal drug, alcohol, or tobacco exposure; or infectious disease is more likely to have chronic conditions that affect health and well-being.
- Similarly, children exposed to unsafe environmental conditions, such as secondhand smoke or lead-based paint, are more likely to have chronic conditions throughout childhood and, in some cases, through adolescence and adulthood.
- Children who do not receive preventive health care and do not obtain all necessary immunizations are more likely to have preventable diseases or chronic conditions that could have been prevented or minimized and controlled.

The first year of life is the most hazardous until the age of 65 years. Therefore, it is particularly important for women to be as healthy as possible before becoming pregnant, to receive prenatal care and adopt healthy lifestyle choices, and for infants to receive primary health care to maintain health and prevent or minimize serious, long-lasting health problems.

Infant Mortality

Infant mortality, the death of an infant during the first year of life, is a critical gauge of children's health status. It is an important marker because it is related to several factors, including maternal health, medical care quality and access, socioeconomic conditions, and public health practices. Infant mortality reflects the health and welfare of an entire community and is used as a broad indicator of health care and health status. Box 16-1 lists some terms and definitions associated with infant health and mortality.

Surprisingly, the United States ranks a dismal twenty-ninth in infant mortality behind most other industrialized nations, including Japan, Sweden, Spain, Hong Kong, Italy, France, and Canada (Table 16-1). Fifty years ago, the United States ranked twelfth. The gap in infant mortality between the United States and other nations has occurred despite the United States' comparatively high per capita spending on health care and technological advancements.

Despite a poor ranking among other nations in the world, in the past century, the infant mortality rate in the United States declined substantially (Figure 16-2). The 2006 infant death rate of 6.71 deaths per 1000 live births (MacDorman and Mathews, 2008) was the lowest infant mortality rate ever recorded in this country. The incidence of infant mortality has decreased largely because of public health measures and improved standard of living (e.g., improved sanitation, a clean milk supply, immunizations against deadly childhood diseases, the increased availability of nutritious food, and enhanced access to maternal health care). Technological advances in neonatal care, for example, the introduction of synthetic lung surfactant, have also contributed to reductions in infant mortality. However, declines in infant mortality have stagnated during the past decade.

The three leading causes of infant death in the United States are congenital malformations, deformities, and chromosomal abnormalities; disorders relating to short gestation and low birth weight; and sudden infant death syndrome

---

BOX 16-1   INFANT HEALTH DEFINITIONS

Infant death: Death of an infant before his or her first birthday.
Infant mortality rate: Number of infant deaths per 1000 live births.
Preterm birth: Birth before 37 completed weeks of gestation.
Very preterm birth: Birth before 32 completed weeks of gestation.
Late preterm birth: Birth from 34 to 36 completed weeks of gestation.
Term birth: Birth from 37 to 41 completed weeks of gestation.

From MacDorman MF, Mathews TJ: *Recent trends in infant mortality in the United States,* NCHS data brief 9, Hyattsville, MD, 2008, National Center for Health Statistics.

TABLE 16-1	INTERNATIONAL COMPARISONS OF INFANT MORTALITY RATES* FOR SELECTED COUNTRIES AND TERRITORIES (2004)	
RANK	**COUNTRY**	**RATE**
1	Singapore	2.0
2	Hong Kong	2.5
3	Japan	2.8
4	Sweden	3.1
5	Norway	3.2
6	Finland	3.3
7	Spain	3.5
8	Czech Republic	3.7
9	France	3.9
10	Portugal	4.0
11	Germany	4.1
11	Greece	4.1
11	Italy	4.1
11	Netherlands	4.1
15	Switzerland	4.2
16	Belgium	4.3
17	Denmark	4.4
18	Austria	4.5
18	Israel	4.5
20	Australia	4.7
21	Ireland	4.9
21	Scotland	4.9
23	England/Wales	5.0
24	Canada	5.3
25	No. Ireland	5.5
26	New Zealand	5.7
27	Cuba	5.8
28	Hungary	6.6
29	Poland	6.8
29	Slovakia	6.8
29	**United States**	**6.8**
32	Puerto Rico	8.1
33	Chile	8.4
34	Costa Rica	9.0
35	Russian Federation	11.5
36	Bulgaria	11.7
37	Romania	16.8

From Centers for Disease Control and Prevention: *Health United States, 2007,* 2007: www.cdc.gov/nchs/data/hus/hus07.pdf#025. Accessed May 13, 2009.
*Infant mortality rate represents infant deaths per 1000 live births.

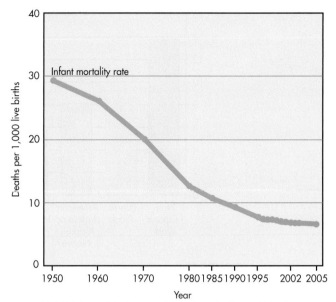

NOTES: Infant is defined as under 1 year of age. See Data Table for data points graphed and additional notes.

SOURCE: Centers for Disease Control and Prevention, National Center for Health Statistics, National Vital Statistics System.

FIGURE 16-2 Infant mortality rates by decade from 1950 to 2005. (From MacDorman MF, Mathews TJ: *Recent trends in infant mortality in the United States,* NCHS Data Brief, No. 9, Hyattsville, MD, 2008, National Center for Health Statistics.)

BOX 16-2	"BACK TO SLEEP" CAMPAIGN

The "Back to Sleep" campaign is named for its recommendation to place infants on their back during sleep to prevent sudden infant death syndrome (SIDS). This campaign is sponsored by the Eunice Kennedy Shriver National Institute of Child Health and Human Development, the Maternal and Child Health Bureau, the American Academy of Pediatrics, the SIDS Alliance, and the Association of SIDS and Infant Mortality Programs.

Since the initiation of "Back to Sleep" in 1994, the rate of SIDS has dropped more than 50% (Eunice Kennedy Shriver National Institute of Child Health and Human Development, 2008). The public education campaign encourages caretakers of healthy infants, born at term, to place them on their backs for sleep and to learn other ways to prevent SIDS, including eliminating soft sleeping surfaces and loose bedding, overheating, and exposure to secondhand smoke.

Despite dramatic reductions in the SIDS rate, there are still significant differences in the SIDS rates among racial and ethnic minorities. SIDS rates for non-Hispanic black and Native-American babies is over twice as high as for non-Hispanic white babies (MacDorman and Mathews, 2008). Reductions in the occurrence of SIDS, particularly among minority groups, would greatly lessen the overall infant mortality rate.

(SIDS) (Kung et al., 2007) (Box 16-2). Prematurity is a key risk factor for infant death. Socioeconomic factors also play an important role in infant mortality. Out-of-wedlock births pose greater risks for infant mortality, for example. In 2007, 40% of all babies were born to unmarried women, a rapidly increasing trend, particularly among Latino women (Martin et al., 2009). Infant mortality rates are also higher for children whose mothers receive late or no prenatal care, who are adolescents, who did not complete high school, who are unmarried, or who smoke during pregnancy.

Troubling disparities in infant mortality persist between racial and ethnic populations. For example, black infants continue to die at more than twice the rate of white infants (Figure 16-3) (MacDorman and Mathews, 2008). Identifying and remedying the causes of higher infant mortality rates among certain population subgroups remains a vexing societal problem (Box 16-3).

Preterm Birth and Low Birth Weight

Birth weight and length of gestation are the most important predictors of infant health. One reason infant mortality has declined so slowly in recent years is that the

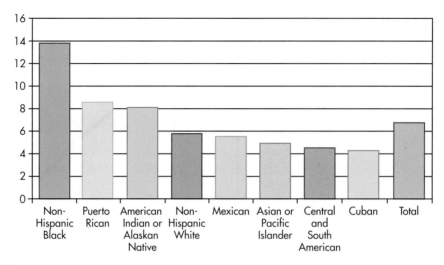

FIGURE 16-3 Infant mortality rates by race and ethnicity of mother, 2005. (From MacDorman MF, Mathews TJ: *Recent trends in infant mortality in the United States,* NCHS Data Brief, No. 9, Hyattsville, MD, 2008, National Center for Health Statistics.)

BOX 16-3	**SOURCES OF VITAL STATISTICS DATA FOR CHILDREN**

Information concerning an infant's birth, including the mother's total prenatal care visits, the mother's name and father's name, and the infant's weight and birth date, appears on a baby's birth certificate.

Information concerning an infant's death, such as the cause(s), date, and other details, appears on the death certificate. In each state, the vital statistics office in the state health department stores these certificates. This agency collects and regularly reports the aggregated data and forwards it to the National Center for Health Statistics.

The National Center for Health Statistics collects, analyzes, and publishes numerous reports on the health and well-being of the nation's infants. These data sources are very important in tracking the health of infants and the health of other population groups; they help determine necessary interventions from various perspectives (e.g., clinical, public health, public policy, and environmental).

---

preterm rate (birth before 37 completed weeks of gestation) has risen so quickly over the past two decades. About 13% of babies in the United States are born prematurely. A portion of this increase is due to increases in multiple births, but prematurity among single births has also risen (Martin et al., 2007). The greatest rise in preterm births has occurred in babies who are born between 34 and 36 6/7 completed weeks of gestation (late preterm). Indeed, 70% of babies born prematurely are born late preterm (Hamilton et al., 2009).

Infants born preterm or at a low birth weight have a far greater risk of death and physical and mental disabilities such as blindness, deafness, cerebral palsy, learning disabilities, and mental retardation than infants born at term with normal weight. Even babies born late preterm carry a risk for developmental delay that is 36% higher than for babies born at term (Morse et al., 2009).

Prematurity and low birth weight overlap. About half of preterm infants are born at low birth weight, but only two thirds of low-birth-weight babies are born prematurely. Babies born at term but at low birth weight are considered "growth restricted." Non-Hispanic black infants are disproportionately affected by preterm birth and low birth weight; indeed, they are nearly twice as likely as white infants to be born at low birth weight (Hamilton et al., 2009). Factors associated with preterm birth and low birth weight include the following:

- Minority status
- Maternal age of less than 17 years and more than 35 years
- Chronic health problems such as diabetes mellitus and hypertension
- Lack of prenatal care
- Induced labor and elective cesarean birth
- Multiple births
- Low socioeconomic status
- Unhealthy maternal habits (e.g., poor nutrition, obesity, alcohol and drug use, and cigarette smoking)

The development of advanced life-support technologies for small infants has significantly improved the survival rate of low-birth-weight babies. Success stories of tiny survivors are sensationalized in the news, but the long-term consequences of babies born even a few weeks early are not well publicized. Medical management of high-risk pregnancy and increasing numbers of labor inductions and elective cesarean births have helped to push the rate of late preterm birth upward. Consequences of late preterm birth can be long lasting and costly (Petrini et al., 2009; Morse et al., 2009; Bettegowda et al., 2008; Adams-Chapman, 2006; Institute of Medicine, Section IV, 2006). Because late preterm births account for the majority of preterm births, it is imperative that all possible measures are taken to decrease elective births before 39 weeks of gestation (Oshiro et al., 2009).

Preventing the occurrence of prematurity and low birth weight is a high priority for clinical and public health research and policy. Nurses can play important roles in preventing prematurity, through the provision of evidence-based primary care, research, screening, counseling, education, advocacy, referral, and implementation of interventions to reduce risk among target population groups.

Preconceptional Health

The good health of a woman before becoming pregnant is imperative to the health of her baby. Adapting healthy lifestyles and obtaining regular medical care before becoming pregnant can help to ensure a healthy pregnancy. Tiny developing fetal organ systems are highly vulnerable to the effects of maternal nutrition, drugs, alcohol, tobacco, chronic maternal diseases, environmental toxins, and other exposures. The fetus can suffer damage very early in pregnancy, even before a woman knows she is pregnant. This is important because approximately half of the pregnancies in the United States are unintended (Finer and Henshaw, 2006). Because of the likelihood that a woman may become pregnant, all women of childbearing age should adapt healthy lifestyles. Measures known to help ensure fetal health such as consuming 0.4 mg of the B vitamin folic acid every day, even before conception, will decrease the likelihood of defects of the brain and spine, known as neural tube defects (Wolff et al., 2009). The Centers for Disease Control and Prevention (CDC) estimates that 50% to 70% of neural tube defects could be prevented if this recommendation were followed before and during early pregnancy, yet fewer than one third of women get the recommended amount of folic acid (CDC, 2008). For women planning to become pregnant, preconceptional counseling is a prevention strategy that helps to identify potential risks to a fetus before pregnancy. Preconception assessment encourages health and lifestyle modifications that can lead to healthier babies.

Prenatal Care

Obtaining early and regular prenatal care greatly enhances a woman's chance of delivering a healthy, term baby. Prenatal care includes client education, risk identification, and monitoring and treatment of symptoms. It also includes referral to health, nutrition, and social service programs that can help a woman optimize her chances for a healthy pregnancy. In the past two decades, the Medicaid program was expanded to cover health care for increasing numbers of low-income pregnant women and infants. Still, fewer than 70% of women receive prenatal care beginning in the first trimester. Large disparities by race persist in the receipt of prenatal care. Non-Hispanic black and Hispanic women are more than twice as likely as non-Hispanic white women to receive late or no care (Martin et al., 2009). Examples of population groups that are less likely to receive early prenatal care include the following:
- Poor women who are under age 20 years and unmarried
- African-American, Hispanic, or Native-American women

- Women who live in isolated rural areas or medically underserved urban areas
- Women with less than 12 years of education

RESEARCH HIGHLIGHTS
Domestic Abuse and Infant Birth Weight

Medical records of almost 2000 women were reviewed to determine whether domestic abuse and other factors during pregnancy affected infant birth weight. The researcher concluded that physical or psychological abuse had a small but significant effect on birth weight. Single marital status, smoking, less than 12 years of education, and low weight gain were also significantly associated with low birth weight of infants.

From Kearney MH, Munro B, Ursula K, et al: Health behaviors as mediators for the effect of partner abuse on infant birth weight, *Nurs Res* 53(1):36-45, 2004.

Timely and comprehensive prenatal care increases the identification of specific and treatable causes of infant morbidity and mortality, such as maternal anemia, diabetes, hypertension, urinary tract infections, sexually transmitted infections, and poor nutrition. Comprehensive prenatal care is particularly important for low-income women. It can help them obtain other services such as the Special Supplemental Nutrition Program for Women, Infants, and Children (WIC) program, food stamps, smoking cessation, housing, child care, job training, substance abuse treatment, and domestic violence counseling.

Health education and counseling also are a part of comprehensive prenatal care and can provide women with the information they need to make lifestyle changes to help ensure a healthy pregnancy. Ideally, such counseling and treatment of chronic health conditions should begin before a woman becomes pregnant. Optimal health across her lifespan including treatment of chronic health conditions and the adaptation of a healthy lifestyle will have far more of an impact on healthy pregnancy than prenatal care alone.

Prenatal Substance Use

Tobacco, alcohol, and illicit drug use are social factors that affect health. During pregnancy, substance use profoundly affects the neurological and physical development of the fetus. The use of these substances, in any combination, worsens infant health and development outcomes.

Smoking

The adverse health effects of tobacco use during pregnancy are well documented and include low birth weight, prematurity, stillbirth, intrauterine growth retardation, preterm premature rupture of membranes, placenta previa, placental abruption, neurodevelopmental impairment, and SIDS (CDC, 2007b). Cigarette smoke contains more than 2500 chemicals. The fetal effects of most of these chemicals are unknown. However, what is known is when a pregnant woman inhales cigarette smoke, the oxygen supply to her fetus is disrupted by nicotine and carbon monoxide. Nicotine crosses the placenta and becomes concentrated in fetal blood and amniotic fluid. Nicotine concentrations in the fetus of a smoking woman can be as much as 15% higher than maternal levels. Secondhand smoke exposure also is dangerous to the fetus and newborn. It is linked to SIDS, decreased respiratory functioning, and childhood asthma. Pregnant women who are exposed to secondhand smoke have 20% higher odds of giving birth to a low-birth-weight baby than women who are not exposed to secondhand smoke during pregnancy (Leonardi-Bee et al., 2008; CDC, 2007b).

About 13% of women reported smoking during the last three months of pregnancy. Teenagers and young women have the highest rates of maternal smoking (CDC, 2007b). The elimination of tobacco use among pregnant women would significantly reduce the percentage of low-birth-weight infants, preterm delivery, intrauterine growth restriction, and infant mortality. Quitting is best. Merely reducing cigarette use during pregnancy may not be enough to benefit the fetus because women who cut back tend to inhale more deeply or take more puffs to get an equivalent amount of nicotine.

The need for widespread implementation of smoking cessation programs for women in the childbearing years is clear. Many smoking cessation programs have been developed and implemented by national, state, and local governments and organizations. Because pregnant women who have received even brief smoking cessation counseling are more likely to quit smoking, nurses should offer effective smoking cessation interventions to pregnant smokers at the first prenatal visit and throughout the pregnancy (Tong et al., 2008).

Alcohol and Illicit Drug Use

The use of alcohol and illicit drugs is a major risk factor for poor infant outcomes. No level of alcohol intake has been determined to be safe during pregnancy, but binge drinking (five or more drinks on the same occasion) is especially harmful to fetal development. Women who are pregnant or who may become pregnant should abstain from alcohol, yet an estimated 12% of pregnant women use alcohol during pregnancy and 2% of pregnant women report binge drinking (CDC, 2009a). Alcohol use during pregnancy can lead to spontaneous abortion, low birth weight, and a cluster of congenital defects, including the nervous system dysfunction called fetal alcohol spectrum disorders (FASDs). FASDs range from mild, subtle learning disabilities to severe learning disabilities. Children with FASD are at risk for psychiatric problems, criminal behavior, unemployment, and incomplete education. Many children with FASD also have physical abnormalities, growth deficiencies, and central nervous system disorders (Substance Abuse and Mental Health Services Administration, 2007).

Like alcohol, illicit drugs can also cause permanent harm to an unborn baby. Nearly 4% of pregnant women report using drugs such as marijuana, cocaine, ecstasy and other stimulants, and heroin. Risks to the baby include prematurity, low birth weight, birth defects, newborn withdrawal symptoms, and learning and behavioral problems. Further, illicit drug use often goes hand in hand with other maternal risks including tobacco and alcohol use, poor nutrition, and risk of sexually transmitted infections (Substance Abuse and Mental Health Administration, 2006).

Substance use is often a sign of more complex psychosocial problems such as depression, poverty, abuse, and violence. Because of serious potential risks to the developing fetus, women who are pregnant, or who could become pregnant, should be counseled to abstain from alcohol and the use of illicit drugs. For those women who already use alcohol and drugs, a comprehensive and long-lasting approach to treatment is required.

CHILDHOOD HEALTH ISSUES

At all ages, appropriate and timely medical care plays an important role in children's health status. However, other factors, including parental influences, nutrition, environmental hazards, community safety, and the overall quality of home life, exert even stronger influences over a child's well-being. Childhood is generally a healthy time of life, as evidenced by the improvement in many indicators of child health status over the past century. For example, the incidence of childhood disease has decreased because the majority of children receive a full complement of immunizations during infancy and toddlerhood.

The causes of childhood death vary with age. Parents and the community have important responsibilities in promoting healthy lifestyles, creating safe environments, and ensuring access to medical care. They must take steps to protect children from the leading threats to children's health (i.e., accidental injury and exposure to environmental toxins, abuse, and violence). Box 16-4 discusses screening newborns for genetic disorders.

BOX 16-4   NEWBORN SCREENING

Every infant born in the United States is screened shortly after birth for a number of genetic disorders. Often babies with genetic disorders appear healthy at birth; thus all babies are tested for select conditions that can lead to serious illness, mental retardation, or death if they are not identified and treated early.

Screening is conducted by collecting a few drops of blood from the newborn's heel. This sample is tested at a screening laboratory, and parents are notified of abnormalities.

Screening is state based so the number of conditions that babies are screened for varies from state to state. A movement is underway to standardize guidelines nationally and to make comprehensive screening available to all babies. All U.S. states and territories currently test for phenylketonuria, galactosemia, congenital hypothyroidism, and sickle cell disease. The March of Dimes recommends that babies are tested for 29 conditions including hearing loss.

From March of Dimes: *Newborn screening tests*, 2008: www.marchofdimes.com/professionals/14332_1200.asp. Accessed May 1, 2009.

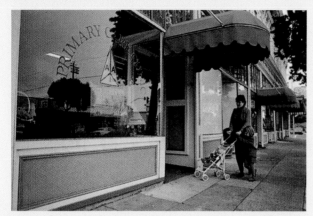

This clinic provides services through the Early and Periodic Screening, Diagnosis, and Treatment (EPSDT) Program, which was developed to provide health care for children in low-income families on Medicaid.

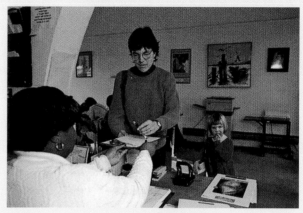

Unfortunately, clinic schedules are often crowded and clients may not be able to get appointments for several weeks.

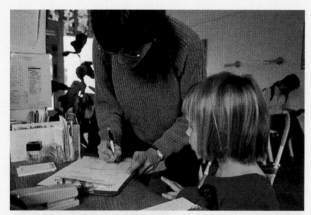

The nurse has an opportunity to observe the client and the family as they register and wait for their appointment. The parent registers the 5-year-old daughter for a school entry health physical. Medicaid insurance is verified for the physical examination.

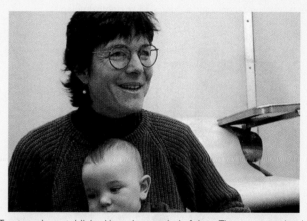

Trust can be established in a short period of time. The nurse can begin by explaining the steps in the clinic process so that the client knows what is expected. Always listen to the client attentively, and allow enough time for the client to reflect and respond to questions.

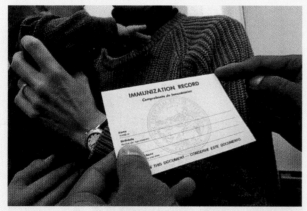

Reviewing immunization records is an important primary prevention role for the community health nurse. This is a teachable opportunity for the nurse to stress the importance of maintaining immunizations for the child. In California parents are provided with a yellow state immunization record for the child, which they should use for recording all immunizations and showing proof of immunizations when needed.

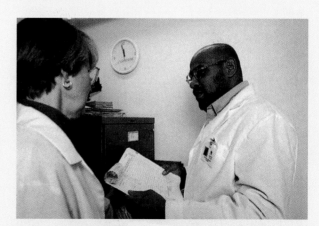

The nurse discusses any concerns about the client with the practitioner before the examination.

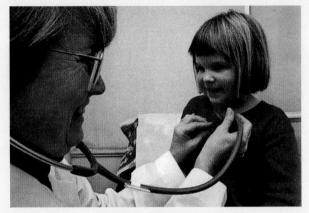

The practitioner performs the physical examination of the child with the help of the parent. The practitioner discusses the result of the vision test with the parent and the need for a follow-up appointment with an ophthalmologist. The child has not had a lead level done and requires booster immunizations. The practitioner orders laboratory tests, immunizations, and a referral to an ophthalmologist.

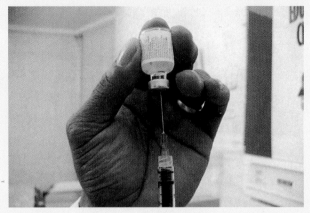

The clinic staff perform the laboratory work: hematocrit, urinary analysis, and lead level. The immunization consent forms have been signed by the parent. The nurse administers the immunizations and takes this opportunity to reinforce the importance of immunizations for both children.

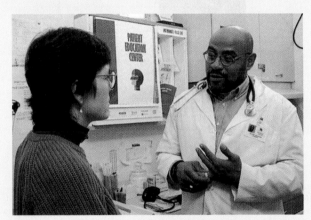

The nurse also offers suggestions to relieve the common side effects of immunizations.

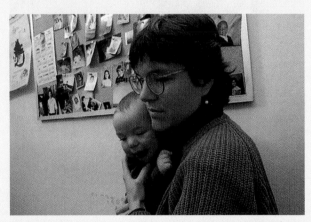

The parent asks about an ophthalmologist who takes Medicaid and about day care facilities in the area for the younger child. The parent also asks about family planning services in the community.

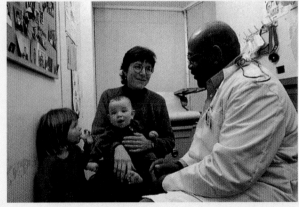

The family agrees to maintain immunizations for the children and to follow up with appointments with an ophthalmologist and a family planning clinic. The nurse returns the immunization record to the parent documenting today's immunization, as well as when the next immunizations are due. The nurse will call with a referral for an ophthalmologist, a family planning clinic, and a day care facility.

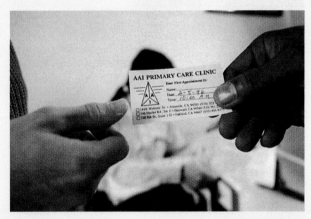

The nurse gives the parent a business card with the nurse's name and agency's address and phone number. The community health nurse advises the parent to call the nurse if there is anything else that the family may need.

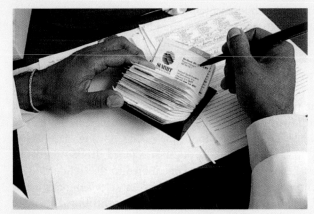

The nurse searches for resources for an ophthalmologist and a family planning clinic that accept Medicaid and a resource for day care providers. The nurse obtains phone numbers for a couple of ophthalmologists, a family planning clinic, and a day care consortium service.

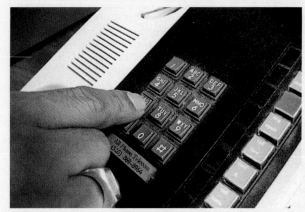

The nurse calls the day care consortium and finds out that there is a list of day care providers available.

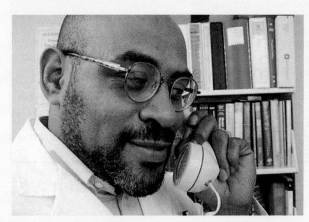

The nurse calls the family with the referrals for an ophthalmologist and a phone number to obtain a list of day care providers.

Story by Leonard Kaku, RN, MSN.
Photography by George Draper.

Accidental Injuries

Infants and young children are at great risk for accidental injuries. They are curious and eager to explore their environments, but they often lack the coordination and cognitive abilities to keep themselves safe from harm. Their small size and developing bones and muscles make them especially susceptible to injury. The leading cause of injury death for children under the age of 1 year is accidental suffocation due to choking or strangulation (CDC, 2008).

Motor vehicle injuries are the leading cause of death for children over the age of 1 year in the United States (CDC, 2008). Many injuries occur because adults fail to secure children in car seats in the back seat of the vehicle or to insist that older children buckle up. The most important step that a parent can take to ensure children's safety in a motor vehicle is to correctly secure them into car seats, or seat belts when they are older, for each ride. The National Highway Traffic Safety Administration recommends booster seats for children until they are at least 8 years of age or 4 feet 9 inches tall (U.S. Department of Transportation, 2009). The risk for motor vehicle accidents is highest for teens aged 16 to 19 years. Not wearing seat belts and drinking and driving contribute dramatically to this risk.

Traumatic brain injury is a leading cause of injury for adolescents, accounting for more than 240,000 emergency room visits, 36,000 hospitalizations, and more than 5700 deaths each year (CDC, 2008). High school sports–related concussions are an important contributor. Head injury from cycling and other wheeled sports, such as skateboarding, is a leading cause of child death and disability. Without proper head protection, a fall from as little as 2 feet can cause traumatic brain injury. The use of helmets and proper protective equipment can substantially reduce the risk of injuries. Other leading causes of accidental injury in children include pedestrian accidents, drowning, and burns. Box 16-5 discusses how toys can be another threat to small children.

Obesity

Obesity is a genuine health crisis in this country. With approximately 23 million children overweight or obese, this could be the first generation to lead sicker, shorter lives than their parents. (Levi et al., 2008)

Seventeen percent of children between the ages of 6 and 17 years are obese (Federal Interagency Forum on Child and Family Statistics, 2008). The percentage of obese children has nearly tripled since 1980. African-American children, particularly those living in the rural South, have the highest obesity levels. Minority groups, those with less income, and those with lower education levels are more likely to be overweight (Levi et al., 2008). The higher cost of healthy foods, food insecurity, and the lack of access to safe places to exercise contribute to obesity in lower-income communities (Widome et al., 2009).

Obesity in children is calculated on the basis of growth charts, physical development, gender, and age. Children at or above the 95th percentile are defined as *obese.* Those between the 85th and 95th percentile are *overweight.* Children at the 99th percentile or above are *severely obese.* Being overweight in childhood can lead to childhood type 2 diabetes and cardiovascular disease. The American Diabetes Association describes type 2 diabetes as a "new epidemic" among American children. Although there are a number of genetic risk factors associated with childhood type 2 diabetes, obesity is largely driving the trend toward this serious disease. In addition, overweight children often face social discrimination, which may lead to poor self-esteem and depression. Further, overweight adolescents are more likely to become obese adults. Obesity in adulthood can lead to a number of health problems, including hypertension, coronary disease, and diabetes.

A number of factors contribute to childhood obesity. The typical American diet, which is high in fat and calories and low in nutrients, has resulted in an increase in obesity. Widely available fast food, increasing portion sizes, vending machines in schools, sugar-sweetened drinks, and fewer meals eaten at home have contributed to the trend. Modern technologies such as electronic games, television, and readily accessible transportation have also contributed to more sedentary lifestyles.

Nurses can play a leading role in generating public awareness of factors that contribute to obesity, and focus on preventative measures is key. For example, breastfeeding provides some protection against later obesity. At least 60 minutes of moderately strenuous exercise is recommended for children most days of the week. Nurses can design and implement nutrition, healthy eating, and physical activities policies and standards in schools, and challenge policymakers and industry leaders such as fast-food restaurants to mobilize resources for good nutrition and fitness.

Immunization

Childhood immunization is a benchmark of child health. Maintaining appropriate immunization protects all members of the community, especially immunocompromised individuals and pregnant women who are particularly vulnerable to certain infectious diseases. Adequate immunization protects children against several diseases that kill or disable many children. Polio, a crippling disease of the past, has been eliminated in the United States thanks to the public health effort that made the polio vaccine accessible and affordable. Over the ensuing decades, new vaccines have been developed and children can now be protected from more than fourteen vaccine-preventable diseases. State laws requiring proof of vaccination before entry to school or child care have helped to ensure high vaccination levels.

Vaccine-preventable disease levels are at or near record lows, but many children and adolescents remain underimmunized. Widespread fears that childhood vaccines are linked to autism have prevented some parents from vaccinating their children. In 2009, however, the U.S. Court of Federal Claims ruled that childhood vaccines do not cause autism. This ruling is consistent with eighteen major scientific studies that have failed to show a link between vaccines and autism (U.S. Court of Federal Claims, 2009). Nurses can help to educate community members about the safety of vaccines and the consequences of undervaccination. The following vaccines are recommended for children and adolescents (CDC, 2009c):

- Diphtheria and tetanus toxoids and acellular pertussis vaccine
- Rotavirus vaccine (for selected populations)

- Measles, mumps, and rubella vaccine
- Hepatitis A vaccine
- Hepatitis B vaccine
- Varicella (chickenpox) vaccine
- *Haemophilus influenzae* type b conjugate vaccine (Hib)
- Influenza (yearly, for selected populations)
- Pneumococcal vaccine (for selected populations)
- Meningococcal vaccine (for selected populations)
- Human papilloma vaccine (for selected female adolescent populations)

Lead Poisoning

Lead poisoning is a preventable cause of childhood death, mental retardation, cognitive and behavioral problems, decreased growth, and neurological disabilities. The reduction of lead levels in both children and adults is among the greatest public health stories of the latter half of the twentieth century. Over the past three decades, lead has been removed from the manufacture of gasoline, household paint, food and drink cans, and plumbing systems. Public health, legislative, and commercial measures tremendously reduced the problem of lead poisoning in the United States, but, unfortunately, lead is still a threat. The neurotoxic properties of lead have been apparent for at least a century, but the nature and extent of subtle long-term effects were more recently realized. Often the signs of lead poisoning are difficult to recognize. Lead poisoning affects virtually every system in the body and rarely yields distinctive symptoms.

Before 1950, lead-based paint was quite common, but the 1972 Lead Paint Poisoning Prevention Act (CDC, 2009b) limited the manufacture of lead-based paint. However, many millions of housing units in the United States still contain lead-based paint. Most of these units are located in poor, inner-city neighborhoods. Contamination can result from contact with paint dust or chips (e.g., raising and lowering windows) and from exposure to contaminated soil. Lead can also be leached into water from lead pipes and fittings. Despite dramatic declines in blood lead levels for most U.S. populations, levels remain high among children in low-income families who live in older housing with lead-based paint. Black and Hispanic children are at greatest risk (Federal Interagency Forum on Child and Family Statistics, 2008).

Treatment for children with elevated lead levels is long and difficult and carries risks. Better prevention; eliminating risks in the environment, particularly in older housing units; more efficient tracking; and education of the public are essential to further reduce the menace of lead poisoning.

Child Maltreatment

Child maltreatment is another indicator of children's physical and emotional health status. In 2004, data collected from Child Protective Services agencies determined that approximately 900,000 children in the United States were victims of child maltreatment, and about 1500 children died because of abuse or neglect (U.S. Department of Health and Human Services, 2006). Because of the lack of identification and recognition and because of underreporting, the extent of child maltreatment is probably far greater than these statistics reveal.

Child abuse is defined as words or overt actions that cause harm, potential harm, or threat of harm to a child. Child abuse is deliberate and intentional; however, harm to a child may or may not be the intended consequence. For example a parent may hit a child causing a concussion. Hitting the child was intentional, but causing the concussion was not. Child abuse may be physical, sexual, or emotional. Child neglect is the failure to provide for a child's basic physical, medical, emotional, or educational needs or to protect a child from harm or potential harm. It may include failure to provide affection, warmth, understanding, and supervision adequate for healthy development (Leeb et al., 2008).

Child maltreatment affects children of all races, ages, and ethnicities. An estimated 14% of U.S. children are victims. Of these, 8% are victims of sexual abuse, 22% are victims of child neglect, 48% are victims of physical abuse, and 75% are victims of emotional abuse (Finkelhor et al., 2005). Girls are slightly more likely to be victimized than boys. Children from birth to age 3 years have the highest rate of victimization (U.S. Department of Health and Human Services, 2006).

There are many long-term effects of child abuse and neglect. The effects may be physical, such as brain damage in shaken baby syndrome; emotional, such as depression and low self-esteem; and behavioral, such as delinquency, promiscuity, eating disorders, poor academic achievement, and drug abuse.

Most often, the perpetrators of maltreatment are parents, victims themselves from a cycle of abuse. The two dominant characteristics of abusive parents include a history of substance abuse and abuse from their own parents. Often, caretakers do not intend to hurt their children. They may be stressed by poverty, illness, or disability, and they may lack social support systems or coping skills. Young and inexperienced parents may not understand the physical, emotional, and behavioral needs of their children.

Children are never responsible for the harm done to them by others, and yet they may feel guilty for causing it. Many professionals, including nurses, social service workers, and teachers, are required by law to report child abuse. Nurses in the community must understand their ethical and legal obligations to report child maltreatment. They can also help to create a climate that supports families and provides parents with alternatives to abusive behavior. Programs for parents can take many different forms. They may occur in parents' homes, in schools, in medical or mental health clinics, or in other community settings. Programs may involve one-on-one or group sessions. The ultimate goal is to prevent child maltreatment before it starts.

Children with Special Health Care Needs

Children and youth with special health care needs are those who have a chronic physical, developmental, behavioral, or emotional condition that necessitates health and related services beyond those required by children generally. All children receiving special education and all children with mental disorders are included in this group. An estimated 14% of the U.S. population of children and youth have special health care needs (U.S. Department of Health and Human Services, 2008b).

Children with special health care needs frequently have multiple service needs, including public health, physical and mental health care, specialized diagnostic services, social services, and educational, vocational, and sometimes corrective services. Families trying to obtain care for children with special needs face challenges in dealing with differing eligibility criteria, duplication and gaps in services, inflexible funding sources, geographic, cultural, and financial barriers, and poor coordination of care. Children with special needs can benefit from a coordinated, comprehensive, integrated system of care—often called a "medical home." A medical home is not a place, but rather an approach to providing care. Having a medical home strengthens the ability of children with multiple service needs to receive comprehensive care for complex conditions (Box 16-6).

BOX 16-6 THE PATIENT-CENTERED MEDICAL HOME

The American Academy of Family Physicians (AAFP), American Academy of Pediatrics (AAP), American College of Physicians (ACP), and the American Osteopathic Association have long endorsed the concept of a "medical home." This ideal suggests that every child, including special needs children, should have "accessible, continuous, comprehensive, family-centered, coordinated, culturally effective and compassionate" health care (AAFP et al., 2007).

A medical home should be within a community-based system with coordinated networks designed to promote the healthy development and well-being of children as they move from adolescence to adulthood. Such a system requires appropriate financing to support and sustain quality care, optimal outcomes, family satisfaction, and cost-efficiency.

ADOLESCENT HEALTH ISSUES

Adolescence is a time of generally good health. It is a period when preteens and teens form lifelong health habits, including dietary and exercise habits and emotional health skills such as problem-solving and coping strategies. Typically, adolescents do not use health services unless they have an underlying chronic condition or an acute illness. They rarely use preventive health services.

In their struggle to gain independence and with their sense of immortality, many adolescents engage in risk-taking behaviors, including alcohol and drug abuse, early and unprotected sexual activity, unsafe driving, and participation in delinquent and violent activities that threaten their health. Injury accounts for 80% of adolescent deaths (Federal Interagency Forum on Child and Family Statistics, 2008). The health threats that adolescents face at the beginning of the twenty-first century are very different from those that threatened the health of this age group only a generation or two ago. The community health nurse can help parents and communities understand the nonmedical, public health nature of these morbidities, and assist in developing community-wide strategies to effectively deal with them.

Adolescent Pregnancy and Childbearing

One of many risk-taking adolescent behaviors is sexual intercourse. Adolescent sexual activity is often unprotected and can result in pregnancy and sexually transmitted infections (STIs). Several factors predispose a child to engage in sexual activity in the teen years. Growing up in poverty, being a child of a teen mother, being the victim of sexual abuse or assault, lack of involvement with friends, family, school, and community, and dropping out of school are all factors that increase a girl's risk for pregnancy (Klein, 2005).

After many years of decline, the teen birth rate is once again on the rise. Adolescent pregnancy is a persistent and troubling problem (Figure 16-4). In 2007, the birth rate for teenagers 15 to 19 years was 42.5 per 1000 teens. Latinas and

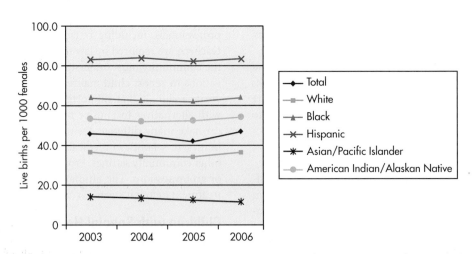

FIGURE 16-4 Adolescent births ages 15 to 19 years, by race and Hispanic origin of mother, 2003-2006. (From Martin JA, Hamilton BE, Sutton PD, et al: Births: final data for 2005, *Natl Vital Stat Rep* 56[6], 2007.)

black Americans have higher teen pregnancy rates than their white counterparts (Hamilton, Martin, and Ventura, 2009).

The consequences of early childbearing are significant. Teen childbearing poses serious health risks to the infant, including death, prematurity, low birth weight, and maltreatment. Researchers disagree on the causes of poor pregnancy outcomes among teenagers, but most agree on the importance of socioeconomic factors associated with young age, such as lack of education, low income, and inadequate prenatal care. Adolescent childbearing and parenting can have long-term, negative consequences for both child and mother. Children born to teenage parents are more likely to have poor health, are less likely to complete high school, and are more likely to end up on welfare (Annie E. Casey Foundation, 2000).

The causes and effects of teen pregnancy are complex, and the solutions are multifaceted. Primary prevention models are most successful when tailored to the community's individual needs. Components of such programs can include the following:

- Abstinence promotion
- Education about contraception and its availability
- Sexual education
- Character development
- Problem-solving skill development
- Peer counseling programs
- Strategies for ensuring teenagers' school success
- Job training

Such efforts are more likely to succeed when there are partnerships among parents, adolescents, and agencies for health, education, religion, social service, and government. Nurses working within such organizations can play leadership roles in developing community programs for adolescent pregnancy prevention.

Violence

Youth violence can be seen as a reflection of how well parents, schools, and the community are able to supervise and channel youth behavior in positive ways. A decline in the level of violence affecting adolescents in recent years is a positive public health trend. However, for too many of the nation's youth, violence is a way of life, a way of coping with challenging and difficult situations, and a significant public health problem.

Children aged 12 to 17 years are more than twice as likely as adults to be victims of serious crimes. Males are twice as likely as females to be victims (victimization rate of 14 per 1000 juveniles). Black males are the racial group most likely to be victimized (U.S. Department of Justice, 2009). Nearly all victims of juvenile violence know their offender (McCurley and Snyder, 2004).

Violence among youth is a multifaceted problem. Social factors, such as unemployment and poverty, strongly influence the risk of violent behavior exposure. Violence in the home, in the media, and in the community; gun ownership; and child abuse, violence, or severe corporal punishment may socialize youth to viewing violence as an expected and unavoidable part of life.

Handguns are readily accessible to America's youth. Federal law prohibits anyone under age 21 years from purchasing a handgun from a licensed dealer, but it does not prohibit anyone under age 21 years from purchasing a handgun from a non-licensed dealer. Teen violence does not have simple remedies. Solutions require community and neighborhood efforts to help young people diffuse anger and frustrations before they escalate; help parents, religious organizations, and schools assist their youth in managing anger and resolving conflicts; and work with children and teenagers to assure them that they are loved, appreciated, and accepted for who they are and that help is available. Reducing children's unsupervised exposure to guns, engaging communities in strengthening law enforcement, modifying the design of guns, and limiting the flow of illegal guns to youth are also strategies to reduce youth gun violence (Reich, 2002).

Sexually Transmitted Infections

STIs include human papillomavirus (HPV) infection, *Chlamydia*, herpes simplex virus type 2 (HSV-2), human immunodeficiency virus/acquired immunodeficiency syndrome (HIV/AIDS), hepatitis B, gonorrhea, syphilis, vaginal trichomoniasis, and certain other vaginal infections. A recent study by the CDC estimated that more than 26% of female adolescents are infected with at least one STI. The most common STI is cancer- and genital wart–associated HPV (18.3%), followed by *Chlamydia* (3.9%), trichomoniasis (2.5%), and HSV-2 (1.9%). Among the teenage girls who had an STI, 15% had more than one. About half of the teens in the study reported ever having sex. Forty percent of these had STIs (Forhan et al., 2008).

Compared with adults, teenagers are more likely to acquire STIs. For some infections, such as *Chlamydia trachomatis*, this may be due to a physiological susceptibility. Barriers to health care such as lack of transportation, concerns about confidentiality, and lack of access to preventive health services also contribute to a higher prevalence of STIs among teens. Although many STIs clear on their own, others can persist over time placing women at high risk for cervical cancer, pelvic inflammatory disease, ectopic pregnancy, and infertility. Young men infected with STIs do not suffer the same health consequences as women because male symptoms typically appear earlier and may be more apparent than female symptoms; thus men can obtain early treatment. Not only is a woman's health affected, especially if the infections go untreated, but infants born to women with STIs are at risk of infection and can suffer long-term consequences. Routine counseling and voluntary testing for sexually active teens and pregnant women is recommended. In addition, a vaccine against HPV types 16 and 18 (which are responsible for 70% of cervical cancer) and types 6 and 11 (responsible for nearly all genital warts) is now recommended routinely for 11- and 12-year-old girls.

Tobacco, Alcohol, and Drug Use

The use of tobacco, alcohol, and illicit drugs has serious and long-lasting consequences for adolescents and for society. The Youth Risk Surveillance System (CDC, 2007a) is a periodic, nationwide, school-based survey conducted by the CDC and state, territorial, tribal, and local education and health agencies. This survey monitors risky behaviors among youth and young adults. In 2007, the survey revealed:

- 20% of students had smoked cigarettes in the 30 days prior to the survey.
- 5.7% of students had smoked cigarettes on school property in the 30 days prior to the survey.
- 44.7% of students had at least one drink of alcohol in the 30 days prior to the survey.
- 26% of students had had five or more drinks of alcohol in a row (i.e., within a couple of hours) in the 30 days prior to the survey.
- 3.3% of students had used any form of cocaine (e.g., powder, crack, or freebase) one or more times in the 30 days prior to the survey.

The survey also found:

- 23.8% of students had drunk alcohol (other than a few sips) for the first time before age 13 years.
- 38.1% of students had used marijuana one or more times during their life.
- 13.3% of students had sniffed glue, breathed the contents of aerosol spray cans, or inhaled paints or sprays to get high one or more times during their life.

The Youth Risk Surveillance System provides a snapshot of trends. Among the findings of the most recent survey are that smoking rates among teens have declined since peaking in the mid-1990s. In contrast, illicit drug use by youths is constantly evolving as new drugs in new forms are introduced. Also, prescription drugs used outside of medical supervision, for example OxyContin and Ritalin, and nonprescription over-the-counter drugs such as cough and cold medicines have become more popular in recent years. According to the Monitoring the Future Project of the University of Michigan, rumors of the supposed benefits of using a drug usually spread much faster than information about the adverse consequences. It generally takes much longer for evidence of adverse consequences, such as death, disease, overdose, and addictive potential, to become widely known, thus contributing to the widespread use of both legal and illegal drugs (Johnston et al., 2009).

Participation in some community activities (e.g., team sports) is associated with a lower risk of illicit drug use (Office of Applied Studies, 2002). Likewise, participation in school-based, community-based, and church or faith-based activities lowers the risk of alcohol, tobacco, and illicit drug use (Office of Applied Studies, 2004).

FACTORS AFFECTING CHILD AND ADOLESCENT HEALTH

As in other age groups, social, nonmedical factors largely determine children's health. Children are dependent on their families or caregivers for their health and well-being; therefore the following factors significantly impact children's physical and mental health and overall well-being:

- Parents' or caregivers' income, education, and stability
- Security and safety of the home
- Nutritional and environmental issues
- Health care access and use

Poverty

Poverty is the greatest threat to child health. Child poverty in the United States is higher than in most other industrialized countries, including Canada and most western European countries (Children's Defense Fund, 2008). About 17% of the nation's children live below the poverty threshold (i.e., the federal poverty level), which was $18,310 for a family of three in 2009 (U.S. Department of Health and Human Services, 2009). Children are far more likely than adults to live in poverty, and young children are more likely than older children to live in low-income families.

Parental education plays a key role in child poverty. Eighty-two percent of children whose parents do not have a high school education live in low-income families. Even if parents have full-time employment, low education levels make their children susceptible to poverty (National Center for Children in Poverty, 2004).

Poverty by itself does not always place a child at risk; however, poor children face the following health and socioeconomic risks that can compound the burdensome influence of poverty (Federal Interagency Forum on Child and Family Statistics, 2008):

- Children in poverty have less access to nutritious food, shelter, and health care.
- Poor children are often deprived of advantages such as good schools, libraries, and other community resources.
- Deaths from unintended injuries, child maltreatment, homicide, STIs, and infectious diseases (including AIDS) are more common among poor children.
- Many poor children live in substandard housing, have stressful home lives, may live surrounded by drugs and crime, and lack positive and nurturing adult role models.
- Poor children may feel hopeless about the future.
- Poor children often suffer from low birth weight, asthma, dental decay, elevated blood lead levels, learning disabilities, and teenage unmarried childbearing.
- Poor children are more likely to move frequently. Residential instability and extreme living conditions of poor children who are homeless or migrants usually compound their health problems.

These social and economic burdens can be overwhelming to parents or caregivers and may cause them to neglect other matters, such as providing a nutritious breakfast before school, taking a child for a well-child appointment, or getting his or her immunizations completed on schedule. They can create a sense of despair and hopelessness among parents and children, which greatly hinders healthy behavior. These factors clearly increase a child's physical and emotional health risks.

Racial Disparities

Although children in the United States are healthier now than in any other time in our nation's history, overall improvements in health mask the poor health of some racial and ethnic subgroups. For example, as mentioned previously, the infant mortality rate has plunged over the past century, yet babies born to black mothers are twice as likely as babies born to white mothers to be born prematurely and to die in the first year of life. Native Americans and African Americans account for a disproportionate share of disabilities and deaths due to FASD. African-American and Hispanic mothers are less likely than white mothers to enter prenatal care early or to breast-feed their babies, and African-American youth are at higher risk for gun violence than white youth.

Eliminating health disparities is an important national health priority. *Healthy People 2020* targets persistent differences in health among children of varying racial and ethnic groups and calls for the elimination of disparities in health. Several factors appear to contribute to these disparities. These include systemic inequities in the health care system, such as lack of health insurance, limited access to quality care, poverty, and lack of education. One study showed, for example, that the race/ethnicity of children significantly influenced their wait time in emergency departments. Hispanic white children waited 18% longer than did non-Hispanic white children. Non-Hispanic black children waited 6% longer than non-Hispanic white children (James, Bourgeois, and Shannon, 2005).

Providing health care services that are culturally competent will help make care more acceptable to all races and cultures (Beach, Price, and Gary, 2005). Cultural competence requires that services and assistance are provided in a manner that demonstrates respect for individual dignity, personal preferences, and cultural differences. Community health nurses can develop the skills needed to provide culturally competent care by learning how to perform cultural assessments, cultural interpretation, culturally appropriate interventions, and cross-cultural communication.

Single Parenting

Family structure is associated with child well-being. Generally speaking, children living in households with two married parents fare better economically, socially, and academically. The number of children living in households headed by single parents has increased over the years. Approximately 32% of children do not live with two, married parents (Mills and Bhandari, 2003). Children in households headed by a single parent (usually the mother) are far more likely to live in poverty and thus have more health risks.

Parents' Educational Status

Children's health is also tied closely to their parents' education level. About 15% of U.S. children have a parent who has not received a high school diploma (Federal Interagency Forum on Child and Family Statistics, 2008). Low birth weight and infant mortality are more common in the children of less-educated mothers. Women with higher education are more likely to obtain prenatal care, delay childbearing until after adolescence, and breastfeed their babies. Women with less than 12 years of education are almost ten times more likely to smoke during pregnancy than mothers with 16 years of education.

Health Care Use

Children grow and develop rapidly between infancy and adolescence; therefore they are extremely vulnerable to the effects of illness and environmental factors that influence physical and emotional health. Preventive health and dental care offer children and parents a chance to periodically meet with a health care provider to do the following:

- Discuss the child's physical and emotional growth and development.
- Learn about good nutrition.
- Address safety issues, such as the use of car seats and seatbelts.
- Receive immunizations and vision and hearing screening.
- Learn about potential environmental threats to the child's health.
- Begin prompt treatment for a condition discovered during the examination.
- Ask other questions or obtain a referral if necessary.

Access to a regular health care source can facilitate prompt attention to acute medical problems, which can help prevent chronic, disabling conditions. For example, untreated ear infections can lead to hearing loss, which can lead to learning disabilities, school problems, and even school dropout. Resulting low self-esteem can increase the likelihood of depression, behavior problems, early sexual activity, STIs, and unplanned pregnancy. Comprehensive, regular health care helps all children achieve their potential.

STRATEGIES TO IMPROVE CHILD AND ADOLESCENT HEALTH

One of the most important ways to ensure the success and well-being of future generations is for each child to start life healthy and maintain his or her physical and emotional health status throughout childhood and adolescence. Since the beginning of the twentieth century, the nation has made remarkable progress in many areas of child and adolescent health, but the results are mixed. Fortunately, scientific, medical, environmental, parenting, and other knowledge can lessen or eliminate many of the problems. It is a matter of making these concerns a priority and taking the necessary steps to elicit change. Box 16-7 lists several resources for monitoring the health and well-being of children.

Monitoring and Tracking

The federal, state, and local governments and many national organizations collect and analyze data to track the well-being of children and adolescents. For example, the U.S. Department of Health and Human Services (2008a) generates a yearly report, Child Health USA, on more than fifty indicators of the well-being of America's children and youth. Such data are readily accessible online to citizens, health professionals, policymakers, and the media. A number of key indicators are tracked on a regular basis by the federal statistical system so that trends are revealed. State and local data also are used to track the well-being of children.

BOX 16-7 RESOURCES: MONITORING THE HEALTH AND WELL-BEING OF CHILDREN

Centers for Disease Control and Prevention (CDC). Monitors many health and disease prevention efforts, including the Youth Risk Behavior Surveillance System, which monitors youth tobacco, alcohol, and drug use; dietary behaviors; and sexual behaviors contributing to unintended pregnancy and sexually transmitted infections. www.cdc.gov.

Federal Interagency Forum on Child and Family Statistics. On an annual basis, produces *America's Children: Key National Indicators of Well-Being*, a report that includes detailed information on a set of key indicators of child well-being. www.childstats.gov.

National Center for Education Statistics (NCES). The primary federal agency for collecting and analyzing data related to education in the United States. www.nces.ed.gov.

National Center for Health Statistics (NCHS). Provides birth and death data, including birth certificate information. www.cdc.gov/nchs.

U.S. Bureau of Justice Statistics. Collects information about juvenile offenders. www.ojp.usdoj.gov/bjs.

U.S. Bureau of Labor Statistics. Provides a variety of employment data. www.bls.gov.

U.S. Census Bureau. Provides current census figures and analysis. www.census.gov.

U.S. Department of Health and Human Services (USDHHS). *Healthy People 2020* provides a framework of goals and objectives for the nation's health. www.healthypeople.gov.

U.S. Department of Health and Human Services (USDHHS). *Trends in the Well-Being of America's Children and Youth* monitors trends in the well-being of the nation's children on a yearly basis. http://aspe.hhs.gov/search/hsp/03trends.

Federal Interagency Forum on Child and Family Statistics Collects, monitors, and disseminates data on children and youth. http://www.childstats.gov/AMERICASCHILDREN/index.asp.

Healthy People 2020: Child and Adolescent Health

Many professions establish goals and set measurable objectives. Educators use these techniques to organize their teaching materials, measure their students' progress, and evaluate the effectiveness of their teaching strategies and plans. Health care professionals use them for similar purposes in client care. The individual community health nurse uses them in working with a family to ensure that the nurse and family are organized and guided by common purposes. Goals and objectives help the nurse and family evaluate progress and make necessary midcourse corrections.

These strategies are also important at the macro level and the programmatic level, where multiple players must collaborate to address complicated statewide or nationwide problems. In 1979, the Surgeon General of the United States embarked on an ambitious task of convening hundreds of public health experts, health care researchers, health professional organizations, and others to develop the first health goals and objectives for the nation. At each of the intervening decades, these groups have developed a new set of goals and objectives to help bring clear focus to the health concerns of the nation and to set measurable and attainable goals for different age-groups and issues across the country.

Healthy People 2020 (USDHHS, 2009) sets broad national health goals for the first decade of the twenty-first century. This initiative, like its predecessors, helps define the nation's health agenda and guides policy development. *Healthy People 2020* addresses many challenges facing the country and helps the public and private sectors understand the nation's leading

♥ HEALTHY PEOPLE 2020

Proposed Objectives for Child and Adolescent Health

OBJECTIVE

AHS HP2020–6b: Increase the proportion of persons (children and youth aged 17 years and under) who have a specific source of ongoing care.

AH HP2020–2: Increase the percentage of adolescents who participate in extracurricular and out-of-school activities.

EMC HP2020–1: Decrease the percentage of children who have poor quality of sleep.

EMC HP2020–3: Increase the proportion of elementary, middle, and senior high schools that require school health eduction.

EH HP2020–13: Eliminate elevated blood lead levels in children.

FP HP2020–8: Reduce pregnancy rates among adolescent females.

FP HP2020–9: Increase the proportion of adolescents aged 17 years and under who have never had sexual intercourse.

HIV HP2020: Reduce the number of new cases of perinatally acquired HIV/AIDS diagnosed each year and perinatally acquired AIDS.

IID HP2020–1: Reduce chronic hepatitis B virus infections in infants and young children (perinatal infections).

IID HP2020–14: Reduce or eliminate cases of vaccine-preventable disease.

IVP HP2020–16: Increase age-appropriate vehicle restraint system use in children.

IVP HP2020–28: Increase the proportion of public and private schools that require students to wear appropriate protective gear when engaged in school-sponsored physical activities.

MICH HP2020–1: Reduce the rate of child deaths.

MICH HP2020–5: Increase the proportion of pregnant women who receive early and adequate prenatal care.

MHMD–2: Reduce the rate of suicide attempts by adolescents.

Continued

HEALTHY PEOPLE 2020

Objectives for Child and Adolescent Health—cont'd

OBJECTIVE
NWMS Hp2020–5: Reduce the proportion of children and adolescents who are overweight or obese.
OH HP2020–4: Increase the proportion of low-income children and adolescents who received any preventive dental service during the past year.
PAF HP2020–2: Increase the proportion of the Nation's public and private schools that require daily physical eduction for all students.
PAF HP2020–8: Increase the proportion of children and adolescents that meet guidelines for television viewing and computer use.
SA HP2020–4: Reduce the proportion of adolescents who report that they rode, during the previous 30 days, with a driver who had been drinking alhocol.
TU HP2020–7: Reduce the initiation of tobacco use among children, adolescents, and young adults.

U.S. Department of Health and Human Services. Healthy People 2020 Draft Objectives 2009: http://www.healthypeople.gov/hp2020/Objectives/files/Draft2009Objectives.pdf

health problems, develops strategic plans for addressing them, and collaborates to reach common goals. The *Healthy People* table lists selected objectives from *Healthy People 2020* related to child and adolescent health.

Since the inception of the *Healthy People* initiative in 1979, child and adolescent health has improved. For instance, there have been improvements in infant, child, and adolescent mortality, use of prenatal care, adolescent smoking, pregnancy, and violence.

Health Promotion and Disease Prevention

Health promotion and disease prevention are more significant and cost-effective for children than for any other age group. Primary health care and early intervention for children and families can help prevent costly problems, suffering, and lost human potential. The following examples illustrate this point:

- The average medical cost for a healthy term newborn through the first year of life is $4,551. Medical costs for newborns with complications are twice that much, and the cost for low-birth-weight and premature babies is ten times that amount (March of Dimes, 2008). The costs do not end there. Infants who are born prematurely are more likely than healthy term infants to need specialized services for chronic conditions such as cerebral palsy, blindness, and learning disabilities.
- Preventing pregnancy among teenagers can reduce the dropout rate, welfare dependency, low birth weight, and infant mortality. It has been estimated that teen childbearing costs taxpayers at least $9.1 billion every year in expenses associated with health and foster care, criminal justice, and public assistance (Hoffman, 2006).

Health promotion and disease prevention strategies for improving child and adolescent health come in many forms and originate in research institutions, public agencies, private businesses, and community-based organizations. They can include the following:

- Clinical interventions
- Public health efforts that identify trends and develop population-based, community-wide, or individual strategies to affect these trends

- Philanthropic endeavors that fund initiatives at the community, state, and regional levels for the purpose of testing a strategy or establishing an initiative
- Public policy initiatives that create or improve public programs or provide incentives for nongovernmental entities to address identified problems

PUBLIC HEALTH PROGRAMS TARGETED TO CHILDREN AND ADOLESCENTS

A number of public programs address the health needs of children, and many target medically underserved or low-income individuals and families. In addition, local and state public health and social service agencies aim to protect the health of an entire community or state through programs such as water fluoridation, sanitation, and infectious disease control. Furthermore, broad-based strategies such as lead-based paint elimination, mandatory child safety seats in automobiles, bicycle helmet laws, teen pregnancy prevention programs, comprehensive school health clinics, and drug and violence prevention programs serve to improve the health of children through community-wide approaches.

Health Care Coverage Programs

Approximately 88% of American children under 18 years of age have some type of health insurance. Conversely, the number of children without any coverage is 12%, or 8.7 million children (Federal Interagency Forum on Child and Family Statistics, 2008). Hispanic children are far more likely than children of other races to be uninsured (Mills and Bhandari, 2003) (Figure 16-5). Those who do not have health insurance are more likely to lack a source of health care, to have unmet health needs, and to experience worse health outcomes than children with insurance (National Center for Health Statistics, 2006). Although most children are insured as dependents through their parent's workplace, an increasing number of children are losing this coverage. The cost of health insurance has risen over the years, and an increasing number of employers are no longer offering coverage for employees or their dependents. This is a more prevalent problem in small businesses and in businesses with mostly low-wage earners.

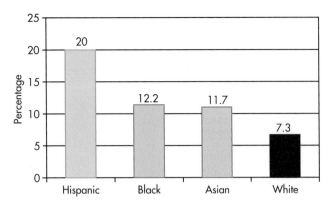

FIGURE 16-5 Children under 18 years of age lacking health insurance by race and Hispanic origin of mother, 2007. (From US Census Bureau: *Current population survey, 2008 annual social and economic supplement,* 2008: pubdb3.census.gov.macro/032008/health/h08_000.htm. Accessed May 12, 2009.)

Medicaid

The ability to pay for health care greatly influences whether a parent takes a child to see a health care provider. Medicaid (Title XIX of the Social Security Act) is a health insurance program for poor and low-income people. It is a federal/state entitlement program that plays an important role in providing health coverage for low-income women and children. Initiated in 1965, Medicaid is the largest source of funding for medical and health-related services for America's poor. In the late 1980s, Congress and states passed several pieces of legislation that expanded Medicaid eligibility for pregnant women, infants, and children in higher income groups in an effort to improve the nation's infant mortality rate and children's health status. Over the years, Medicaid has become a primary payer for prenatal care, deliveries, and child health. It now covers more than one in four children (U.S. Census Bureau, 2004).

Within broad national guidelines, each state establishes eligibility standards, determines the type and scope of services, and administers its own Medicaid program. States have some discretion in determining which population groups their program will cover. Thus, a pregnant woman or child who is eligible for the program in one state may not be eligible in another. Under federal guidelines, however, states must cover pregnancy-related services to pregnant women whose family income is at or below 133% of the federal poverty level and health coverage to children under the age of 6 years whose family income is at or below 133% of poverty. They also must cover children under age 19 years with family incomes under 100% of the federal poverty level. Several states go further than these minimum requirements.

Through the Early and Periodic Screening, Diagnosis, and Treatment (EPSDT) program, a child covered by Medicaid can receive a range of health and health-related services beginning in infancy. The program is designed to assure availability and accessibility of health care resources and to help Medicaid recipients and their parents effectively use these resources. The program's services far exceed those usually covered by private insurance and include the following:

- Health, developmental, and nutritional screening
- Physical examinations
- Immunizations
- Vision and hearing screening
- Certain laboratory tests
- Dental services

Children's Health Insurance Program (CHIP)

Medicaid does not cover all poor children, nor does it cover children in the "gap group," (i.e., children whose family income is above Medicaid limits but whose families do not receive health insurance through the parents' employment). This group is often called the working poor. These families may be able to qualify for the Children's Health Insurance Program (CHIP), a publicly subsidized health insurance program for children. CHIP was formed in 1997 to help close the gap between higher-income and lower-income families whose children need insurance. Each state sets its own guidelines regarding services and eligibility, and CHIP provides insurance to qualifying children up to the age of 19 years. Since reauthorization in 2009, about 7.4 million children are covered by CHIP (Centers for Medicare and Medicaid Services, 2009).

Expansions in public health care insurance programs have helped many children achieve insurance coverage, but many children still lack insurance or other health care coverage like Medicaid or CHIP for many reasons. Some of these include the following:

- Insurance is too expensive.
- Medicaid has a welfare stigma, and parents do not want to be associated with it.
- Medicaid application forms and processes can be complex and burdensome and can intrude on a family's privacy.
- Parents may be concerned that their illegal immigration status may be revealed.
- Parents may not consider the importance of health insurance.
- Parents may not know their child is eligible for programs such as Medicaid or CHIP.
- Applications and other information may not be available in the family's language.

Although insurance gives a child financial access to health care, some children may not obtain the health care they need for other reasons. Numerous health care or family barriers can still stand in the way. These may include the following:

- Lack of transportation
- Language barriers
- Misunderstanding or denial of the child's health problem
- Clinic or office hours that conflict with work or school schedules
- Overcrowded clinics with long delays in the waiting room (and parents often have more than one child in tow)

- Competing family or personal priorities that reduce the importance of obtaining care
- Some doctors' unwillingness to see Medicaid or low-income clients
- Parents' concerns that care providers are either unresponsive to their medical needs or interpersonally disrespectful
- Cost of deductibles or co-payments

To successfully meet the health needs of children and adolescents, especially those with known risk factors, the community health nurse must be cognizant of health care access issues, family and neighborhood influences, and other social concerns in a child's life. The nurse must be prepared to help the family solve problems, be their health care system advocate, and address the child's health needs in a culturally competent manner.

Direct Health Care Delivery Programs

Although Medicaid and SCHIP finance health care for their enrollees like private insurance, several other public programs deliver health care services directly to underserved populations. Most underserved aggregates live in inner cities or rural areas with few health care providers and facilities. Some have Medicaid, SCHIP, or insurance coverage, but many are uninsured.

Maternal and Child Health Block Grant

The Maternal and Child Health (MCH) Block Grant program (also called Title V, because it is the fifth section, or title, of the Social Security Act) allocates federal funds to the states, and the states must contribute their own funds for maternal and child health services. It is administered by the Maternal and Child Health Bureau as a part of the Health Resources and Services Administration, U.S. Department of Health and Human Services. Established in 1935, the Title V MCH Block Grant has provided health care services for mothers, children, and families over the years. In 2008, Title V received the highest rating possible from the White House in an assessment of effective federal programs. It has contributed to reductions in infant mortality, prevented disabling conditions in children, and improved the overall health of women and children (Alletto, 2009).

In most states, these federal and state resources are combined with local funding to help ensure the delivery of basic health care to pregnant women and children and help deliver additional services to children with special health care needs. Agencies in state health departments also monitor the health status of mothers and children throughout their respective states and work with other state agencies to develop programs to improve the health of this population.

Community and Migrant Health Centers Programs

The Community and Migrant Health Centers Programs began in 1965 and were two of the early programs of the U.S. Office of Economic Opportunity. Through a network of approximately 900 centers that operate more than 3600 service delivery sites, these health centers provide comprehensive primary and preventive health care to nearly 12.4 million low-income people, many of whom are uninsured or on Medicaid or CHIP (Health Resources and Services Administration, 2009). Health centers are located in medically underserved areas, which are mostly rural and inner-city areas. Health centers also obtain funds from sources such as local governments, foundations, corporations, and clients.

National Health Service Corps

The National Health Service Corps is another federal program that helps children and adolescents receive primary health care services. Currently, the National Health Service Corps supports more than 4000 physicians, nurses, and other health care providers who work in underserved areas of the country (National Health Service Corps, 2003). The program assists these professionals as students with medical, nursing, and other training through scholarships and loan repayment plans if they agree to provide a certain number of service years in a rural or urban underserved area.

School-Based and School-Linked Health Services

Adolescents are the least likely aggregate to use health care services, especially preventive services. Their adolescent health care needs are different from their childhood needs, and they may be uncomfortable seeing a pediatrician or their childhood provider. Furthermore, they may or may not be able to discuss sensitive topics such as puberty, contraception, and peer relationships with their parents. Some may not want their parents to know they have a health problem; therefore they may not want to see the family's health care provider out of concern for privacy and confidentiality. This can cause their health care needs to go unmet.

The school-based health movement began in the 1970s in a St. Paul, Minnesota, high school. Since then, school-based health clinics have grown to about 1700 centers serving 2 million adolescents in forty-four states (National Assembly on School-Based Health Care, 2007). Centers are more common in high schools, but some are located in elementary and middle schools. More conservative areas of the country are somewhat reluctant to allow adolescent health care at or near schools.

State dollars, mostly from general funds and the MCH Block Grant, are the primary sources of funding for school-based health care. An increasing number of health centers participate in the Medicaid and SCHIP programs, and some provide services within a managed care network.

Special Supplemental Nutrition Program for Women, Infants, and Children (WIC)

Although it is not a health program exclusively, the Special Supplemental Nutrition Program for Women, Infants, and Children (WIC) provides highly nutritious foods, nutrition education and counseling, and screening and referral to needed services for nearly 8.8 million low-income pregnant and breastfeeding mothers, their infants, and their children under 5 years of age each year (Food and Nutrition Service,

2007). About 75% of enrollees are infants and children. To be eligible, women and children must meet income guidelines established by each state, and a health professional must determine they are at "nutritional risk." Women and children who participate in Medicaid, the Food Stamp program, or the Temporary Assistance for Needy Families program are automatically income eligible for WIC.

WIC clinics operate in a number of sites including health clinics, hospitals, schools, public housing sites, and mobile clinics. Women participating in the program are encouraged to obtain prenatal care if they are pregnant. They also are encouraged to maintain healthy diets and obtain preventive health care for themselves and their children, including childhood immunizations. WIC participants receive checks or vouchers to purchase specific, nutritious foods. Most grocery stores and supermarkets participate in WIC and carry the foods designated by the program.

Established in 1972, WIC is one of the most successful, popular, and cost-effective public health programs. Some of the many benefits attributed to WIC include the following:

- Improved birth outcomes and health care cost savings
- Improved infant feeding practices, improved low-birth-weight rate, and more regular primary care
- Lower rates of childhood obesity

SHARING RESPONSIBILITY FOR IMPROVING CHILD AND ADOLESCENT HEALTH

Most children in the United States are born healthy and remain healthy throughout childhood. However, the protective factors operating in the lives of healthy children and the interventions they receive are not available to all children. Although public sector programs have attempted to provide a "safety net" for children, these interventions cannot address all needs of the children. For example, the health care system may provide emergency care to a 9-year-old child injured by gunfire in a drive-by shooting, but it cannot address the community conditions that perpetuate violence.

Child health is affected by many factors; therefore, the responsibility for improving children's health rests with the entire community. This responsibility begins with parents and includes health care professionals, community groups, businesses, and the public sector. When a child gets older, he or she can be responsible for practicing healthy behaviors and obtaining proper health care.

Parents' Role

Even before conception, a mother is responsible for ensuring the health of her fetus. Preconception care can help a woman learn about specific actions she can take to increase her chances for having a healthy baby, for example, achieving optimal weight and taking folic acid before she becomes pregnant (Stothard et al., 2009). During pregnancy, she should develop healthy behaviors, including proper nutrition and avoidance of tobacco, alcohol, drugs, and other behaviors that could harm her developing baby. This is particularly important in the early stages of gestation when fetal organ systems

| BOX 16-8 | BREASTFEEDING: THE FEEDING METHOD OF CHOICE |

Breastfeeding is uniquely superior for infant feeding. The practice imparts many health benefits for mothers and babies. Benefits for children include the following:
- Decreased incidence and severity of a wide range of infectious diseases
- Decreased infant mortality
- Decreased risk of SIDS
- Reduction in the incidence of diabetes, respiratory infections, and some cancers
- Lower risk of overweight and obesity
- Enhanced cognitive development

Benefits for mothers who breastfeed include the following:
- Decreased postpartum bleeding
- Earlier return to prepregnancy weight
- Decreased risk of breast and ovarian cancer

The American Academy of Pediatrics and many other health organizations recommend exclusive breastfeeding for the first 6 months of life (American Academy of Pediatrics, 2005).

are developing. It is also important for the mother to receive prenatal care early in pregnancy.

Starting with breastfeeding, parents must give their children nutritious food and ensure that they are immunized, receive needed health care services, and acquire healthful lifestyles. Breastfeeding provides many health benefits for mothers and their children (Box 16-8).

Another important task for parents is to ensure their children have a safe environment at home, in the neighborhood, and at school. They must protect their children from injury, violence, abuse, and neglect. Parents must learn how to nurture, guide, and protect their children effectively through the developmental stages of childhood and adolescence.

Community's Role

Families need support from their community and society to fulfill their roles and responsibilities. This is particularly true for families who live in poverty and for parents who are isolated and disenfranchised. Ensuring access to health care is an important community role, but communities also are responsible for promoting well-being, which goes far beyond the provision of traditional medical care.

Communities should work to create safe neighborhoods and support the development of community-based comprehensive health, education, and social service programs. Also, communities can promote community health education campaigns concerning prenatal care, smoking, nutrition, teenage pregnancy, drug and violence prevention, and other health topics. Communities and community organizations can sponsor health fairs, immunization drives, car safety seat checks, bicycle safety helmet campaigns, crime prevention and reduction programs, and other projects that help families develop healthy lifestyles and gain access to needed health services. Community health nurses can lead or contribute to any of these initiatives.

Communities are also well situated to facilitate the integration of health, education, and social services; to eliminate fragmentation and duplication of services; to provide culturally competent care; and to better organize more comprehensive and streamlined systems of care. Although many health and social service programs exist, they can be poorly coordinated with each other with little collaboration among the professional disciplines. Through public awareness campaigns, communities can facilitate the integration and coordination of services. For example, these initiatives can alert parents about the importance of immunizations, a safer environment, prenatal care, and other services and how and where to obtain these services.

The media are part of the community at large and should be involved in promoting child and adolescent health. The media significantly influence children's lives, their perceptions of the world, and their self-images. From developing informational campaigns about prenatal care and immunizations to discouraging violence and explicit sex in advertising and popular television programs, the media can have a profound effect on improving children's health and well-being.

Employer's Role

Business and industry have an enormous stake in the health of the nation's children. A strong, productive workforce is ensured only when the health, social, and educational needs of the next generation of workers are met. Furthermore, health risks cost employers in lost productivity and increased health care costs.

The private sector can play a role in improving the health of individual children or the community in general. An employer can make health care more accessible to families with children by offering affordable health insurance that covers employees and dependents. The provision of insurance plans that offers full pregnancy and well-child health care benefits is essential to employee health promotion.

Maintaining a workplace that allows flexible leave for prenatal and pediatric health care and allows time off to care for newborn and sick children can also contribute to child health improvements. In 1993, the Family and Medical Leave Act mandated that employers with 50 or more employees must allow a total of 12 work weeks of unpaid leave during any 12-month period for the birth, adoption, or foster care of a child or for the care of a seriously ill family member or the employee himself or herself (U.S. Department of Labor, 2009).

In addition, employers can sponsor education opportunities for employees about topics such as healthy diets, healthy pregnancies, substance abuse, and stress management. Businesses can also offer on-site child care and can work with community leaders and public officials to initiate community-wide health promotion projects targeted to children. Finally, employers can be catalysts in their communities for linking health, education, and social services for children.

Government's Role

In the United States, government's role in promoting or ensuring children's health is more limited than in many other countries. Other countries often have defined policies on children's health; the United States does not. Not only do such policies indicate that children are a priority of the citizenry, but they also help shape the operation of programs and their funding.

As discussed earlier, U.S. state and federal governments have several public health programs that provide assistance to children, especially to those at risk from poverty or other disadvantages. Monitoring the health of children is also a governmental role. Although these programs are not a substitute for a family's or caregiver's care and concern, they are important in protecting and promoting health and delivering services to those who would otherwise go without. Although programs with significant funding exist, many children with health problems do not receive the services they need for reasons previously discussed.

Managers and front-line workers (e.g., community health nurses, social workers, physicians, and caseworkers) in effective community programs should be encouraged to collaborate and thereby assist children with problems that adversely impact their health. "One-stop shopping" (i.e., user-friendly, accessible services for children and families) is an important concept for public and community programs to embrace to ensure that children easily receive needed services. Outreach and referral efforts should be an integral part of health initiatives to provide children with the services they require. Community health nurses are often an essential part of these efforts.

Community Health Nurse's Role

Public health nurses have always played pivotal roles in improving the health status of pregnant women, children, and adolescents. Within the community, the community health nurse is often most aware of children's health status, any barriers that prevent children from receiving necessary care, and other factors that may adversely affect their health. Armed with this information and knowledge about available health resources in the community, the community health nurse is as follows:

- An advocate for improved individual and community responses to children's needs
- A researcher for effective strategies to serve women and children
- A participant in publicly funded programs
- A promoter of social interventions that enhance the living situations of high-risk families
- A partner with other professionals to improve service collaboration and coordination

One important role of the community health nurse is to help link local health and social services with the school system. Children must be healthy to learn; however, children may come to school with vision, hearing, and other health problems that appropriate education, screening, and treatment could have prevented or alleviated. When children pass the preschool years, the school health nurse is sometimes their only connection to the health care system. School health nurses can be an important source of primary health care and health information for students and their families.

Community health nurses can alert the health professional community, business leaders, religious groups, and voluntary organizations to children's and adolescents' needs and the strategies that can improve their health. Community health nurses can influence the planning and implementation of necessary changes in the health care system to ensure improved children's health and to achieve the national health goals for the year 2020. Also, they can promote commitment within their own institutions for comprehensive, culturally competent care.

LEGAL AND ETHICAL ISSUES IN CHILD AND ADOLESCENT HEALTH

Every day, community health nurses are involved in making decisions. In each encounter with a client, the nurse's decisions or the family's choices have the potential to influence the health and well-being of the family or the community at large for better or for worse.

People often assume that health care professionals, particularly nurses, are by nature attuned to the ethical implications of their decisions. In addition, the community trusts that nurses are aware of the legal ramifications of their actions and decisions, of their client's decisions, and of the health care and legal systems' decisions. In reality, the ever-changing pressures of serving the community's health care needs leave little time to reflect on the ethical and moral implications of a given situation. In some cases, it may seem easier to avoid tough decisions. An ethical approach to decision making allows the community health nurse to evaluate a client's or a population's needs more honestly and completely and take appropriate action. Understanding the legal environment will help the nurse make informed decisions and effectively assist clients with their decision-making processes.

Ethical Issues

The complex nature of public health and health care delivery environments often sets the stage for conflicts of interest and values. Meanwhile, nurses and other health professionals must work within the system to improve child and adolescent health in a country of great differences. Such differences exist between races and cultures, and there are great dichotomies, such as the affluence of some and the poverty of many others. For the perinatal nurse, for example, ethical dilemmas may arise because she is an advocate for two clients: the pregnant woman and her fetus. The scope of ethical and legal dilemmas is broad. The Ethical Insights box includes specific ethical issues related to child and adolescent health.

These issues invariably involve value judgments and challenge a nurse's bounds of professional and personal duty. They also require the community health nurse to stay abreast of legislative changes at the local, state, and national levels and participate in professional activities that can help him or her stay current in these important matters. By recognizing the ethical implications of the care and advice they give

---

⚖ ETHICAL INSIGHTS

Ethical Issues Related to Child and Adolescent Health

- *Allocation decisions:* Given limited time and resources, what level of care should a nurse offer a child and his or her family?
- *Maternal-fetal conflict:* Sometimes there are opposing ethical concerns for the pregnant woman and her fetus, for example, whether the benefits of prolonging a pregnancy justify the risk of complications for a pregnant woman or whether court-ordered treatment for a substance-abusing pregnant woman overrides the right to autonomy for a pregnant woman.
- *Client autonomy:* In each specific case, who should make health care decisions for a young client, especially when opposing opinions arise? The client? The parents or guardian? The nurse or other health care professional? At what age does a child become mature enough to participate in such decision making? What laws does any given state have that affect adolescent client autonomy? What should the community health nurse do if he or she believes the client's or parent's decisions are not in the best interest of the client?
- *Privacy and confidentiality:* Is an intervention appropriate if the community health nurse identifies gross noncompliance, neglect, or abuse? Is it appropriate if the nurse must break confidentiality? When and how should the nurse take action?
- *"Gaming the system":* When the health care system's rules appear to impede the nurse's ability to serve the client's best interest, is it acceptable to circumvent the system? If so, what are the moral and legal costs?
- *Cultural competence:* The United States will continue to experience huge demographic changes and increased diversity; nurses will face different cultural definitions of what is and what is not acceptable or ethical. How should the community health nurse respond to a client or population group that does not share the same cultural outlook on health? What is the nurse's legal justification, if any, for responding in a certain way?
- *Health disparities and access to care:* What are the nurses' responsibilities in ensuring that women and children have access to health care? How can nurses influence policy decisions that impact community health care?
- *Prenatal diagnosis and newborn screening:* What are potential long-term consequences of identifying genetic conditions? Are parents fully informed of negative consequences of genetic diagnoses, including stigmatization, discrimination, and psychological consequences?

---

or the actions they take, nurses can embrace their duty to promote the health and well-being of individual clients and the community more completely, protect their clients from harm, and strive for health care fairness and justice for all clients.

Recognizing the value of engaging in a shared dialogue with colleagues regarding ethical decision-making issues and understanding the possible legal implications of their decisions are equally important. The choices can be complex; therefore receiving the guidance of an ethics board or gaining a second opinion can be critical to making the right choices. On a broader scale, a community health nurse's ethical perspective can enhance any discussion about individual client care and overall community health, and it also can affect the direction of the country's public health policy.

CASE STUDY APPLICATION OF THE NURSING PROCESS

By applying the principles of the nursing process to the individual, family, and community, the community health nurse can provide services to children and adolescents more systematically and effectively. Most communities offer a range of preventive services and other important programs that children need. The community health nurse must thoroughly understand the needs of the individual child and family and must be aware of available community resources to help meet the child's health needs.

Maria Martinez, a community health nurse working for the county health department, received a call from the high school nurse informing her that a 16-year-old high school student named Kaylah Mobando would come in that afternoon for a pregnancy test. Kaylah had already missed three menstrual periods and was afraid to talk about it with her family. She had a long discussion with the school nurse and asked her boyfriend to take her to the health department clinic after school for the pregnancy test.

Assessment

Kaylah's pregnancy test was positive, and she was an estimated 3 months pregnant. She was upset and would not speak with Maria at the health department. Maria arranged to make a home visit the next afternoon.

The school nurse told Maria that Kaylah wanted to keep her baby and that Kaylah's family struggled financially. Knowing that she needed to address a number of issues at the first home visit, Maria prepared by developing a list of possible assessment areas that covered individual, family, and community concerns. Her list included the following:

Individual
- Medical risk factors
- Emotional well-being, including concerns about domestic violence and sexual abuse
- Cultural beliefs and attitudes toward pregnancy and medical care
- Barriers to communication with providers, such as language, hearing, or sight
- Understanding and acceptance of pregnancy
- Health-promoting and risk-taking behaviors
- Understanding the importance of obtaining preventive care services
- Health insurance status
- Access to transportation

Family
- Adequacy of housing structure
- Safety of neighborhood
- Ability of family members to provide emotional support
- Ability of family to provide financial support

Community
- Availability of affordable and culturally sensitive prenatal and pediatric care
- Health and social services coordination
- Emotional guidance and counseling
- Educational opportunities for pregnant and parenting teenagers
- Job training
- Nutrition services such as WIC and food stamps
- Pregnancy and parenting education
- Child care availability

Assessment Data
Individual
- Kaylah was already in the early second trimester of pregnancy and had not received prenatal care. She also engaged in risk-taking behaviors (i.e., smoking, alcohol use, unprotected sex, and poor eating habits) potentially detrimental to her baby.
- During the interview, Kaylah seemed quiet and reserved. She said she was excited to have a baby, but she feared labor and delivery. Her boyfriend wanted her to keep the baby.
- She said she did not think about prenatal care much, but would probably visit a health clinic sometime before her delivery. Her family did not have health insurance, and she said they could not afford prenatal care.
- She wanted to keep the baby and remain in school, yet she did not have a realistic understanding of parental responsibilities.

Family
- When Kaylah told her parents she was pregnant, they expressed disappointment. Her mother voiced a willingness to provide emotional support, but her seemingly emotionally distant father expressed anger.
- Both parents expressed concern about how the family would manage financially.
- After a brief review of the family's financial situation, it appeared that Kaylah was eligible for Medicaid and WIC.

Community
- Maria determined that prenatal services were available, but only during school hours. Although the only clinic that accepted Medicaid clients was on the other side of town, a nearby obstetrical practice with a certified nurse-midwife on staff accepted clients with Medicaid coverage. However, their primary clientele was middle-class, married women.
- Applying for Medicaid and the WIC program required Kaylah to go to the welfare office and apply during school hours. However, the hospital outpatient department could make a preliminary Medicaid eligibility determination, which might be more convenient.
- Although Medicaid would pay for some prenatal classes, those nearby were geared to older, married couples.
- Kaylah's school encouraged her to remain in regular classes until her delivery date and participate in home study for a limited time thereafter.
- No parenting classes geared toward adolescents were available.
- Child care was not available at the high school, which made returning to school more difficult for Kaylah.
- Although the community has a lay home visitor program that matches mentors with pregnant and parenting teens and provides health information and encouragement, the project does not serve Kaylah's neighborhood.

Diagnosis
Individual
- Ineffective health maintenance related to the lack of prenatal care and the effect of poor nutrition, smoking, and alcohol use on fetal development
- Impaired parenting related to unrealistic expectations about parenting responsibilities
- Deficient knowledge of infant and child safety issues such as the use of child safety seats, prevention of lead poisoning, advantages of breastfeeding, and use of preventive health care, including immunizations

Family
- Interrupted family processes related to anger and disappointment over daughter's pregnancy
- Altered financial status resulting from the addition of another dependent to the family

Community

- Lack of coordinated, culturally sensitive, accessible prenatal and parenting services for adolescents
- Existing lay home visitor program not available

Planning

To ensure the action plan is complete, realistic, and successfully implemented, Maria must thoroughly identify the factors affecting Kaylah's health and well-being. In addition, Kaylah, her family, and Maria must set mutual goals.

Individual

Long-Term Goals

- Pregnancy outcome will be healthy for mother and infant.
- Kaylah will demonstrate successful parenting behaviors.
- Kaylah will complete high school.

Short-Term Goals

- Kaylah will obtain prenatal care.
- Kaylah will understand the reasons to change nutrition and substance use habits.
- Kaylah and the nurse will plan actions to change poor health habits.
- Kaylah will remain in school throughout her pregnancy and will use the home study program until she returns to school after her baby is born.
- Kaylah will enroll in parenting class. If classes are not available, she will use age-appropriate reading materials, films, videotapes, opportunities for group discussion with other teens, or visits with experienced parents.
- Kaylah will breastfeed her baby.
- Kaylah will speak with the community health educator to determine methods to protect the health and safety of her newborn.

Family

Long-Term Goal

- The family's ability to handle crises will improve with their ability to discuss problems and engage in mutual problem solving.

Short-Term Goal

- Kaylah's parents will display supportive behaviors, such as accompanying her to prenatal care appointments, helping her engage in healthy behaviors, and helping her arrange child care to remain in school.

Community

Long-Term Goal

- Accessible, comprehensive, culturally sensitive prenatal and other health care services will be established, including home visiting and parenting classes targeted to adolescents.

Short-Term Goals

- The health department clinic will extend evening hours to accommodate students and working families.
- A child care facility will open in or near the high school.

Intervention

The nurse, family, and individual must address their immediate, mutual goals to help Kaylah achieve a healthy birth outcome and begin successful parenting. Interdisciplinary planning between Kaylah's school health nurse, caseworker, community health nurse, primary pregnancy care provider, childbirth educator, and family planning nurse is critical. In addition, the nurse must be an advocate for community-wide change to ensure that the community is meeting individuals' needs.

Individual

Maria worked with the school nurse and other health professionals to help Kaylah obtain Medicaid and WIC; she was referred to an obstetrician who saw her regularly. Kaylah's pregnancy was also monitored by the school nurse who had her come to the clinic on a weekly basis to check her weight and blood pressure and to talk with her about pregnancy-related issues.

Working with the school nurse, Maria provided Kaylah with information on childbirth classes and nutrition, as well as booklets detailing how to promote a healthy pregnancy. She was counseled to avoid tobacco, alcohol, and all drugs. Near the end of the pregnancy, Kaylah was encouraged to attend parenting classes with her boyfriend.

Family

Maria and the social worker referred Kaylah's parents to other social service agencies that might be able to help financially. In particular, they focused on providers who could assist with utilities, job placement, and child care. The family was also referred to a family counselor who specialized in working with families with adolescent children.

Community

Maria worked with the Maternal Child Health Division of the County Health Department to help facilitate offering parenting classes at an area high school, targeting the learning needs of pregnant teens. She and the school nurse also met with school district officials and community leaders to stimulate dialogue about the consequences of dropping out of high school and facilitate action in policies such as child care for parenting teenagers to help them remain in school.

Evaluation

Evaluation strategies must involve both process and outcome measures on the individual, family, and community levels.

Individual

The school nurse was able to monitor Kaylah throughout her pregnancy and was aware that she finished classes for the term. Kaylah's pregnancy was unremarkable, and she delivered a healthy boy. Their health care expenses were covered by Medicaid, and the baby was determined to also be eligible for SCHIP. A home-based teacher was assigned to work with her for 1 month after delivery to ensure that she was able to keep up with her coursework. With the assistance of the social worker, Kaylah was able to place the baby in a subsidized day care facility, allowing her to finish school.

Family

Family counseling helped the family resolve some of their issues. Maria observed that Kaylah's parents were proud of their grandson and eager to help with his care.

Community

With the help of the school nurse and other interested parties, Maria was able to initiate a collaborative program in which health department nurses and developmental specialists offered parenting classes in high schools on a regular basis. They were also planning on writing for a Maternal Child Health Block Grant to implement a school-based clinic focusing on the needs of pregnant teens and their infants.

Continued

CASE STUDY   APPLICATION OF THE NURSING PROCESS—cont'd

Levels of Prevention
Primary
- Primary prevention depends largely on the child's age. For the youngest children, strategies include preconceptional counseling and the practice of healthy behaviors by mothers before pregnancy.
- Primary prevention also includes the prevention of unwanted pregnancy, which is especially important for adolescents.

Secondary
- Once pregnant, the woman must receive early and adequate prenatal care, practice healthy behaviors, obtain necessary social and supportive services, and prepare herself for becoming a parent.

- It is incumbent on the community to ensure that adequate preventive health services, such as prenatal care, nutrition and dietary counseling, pregnancy and parent education, and social services, are available.

Tertiary
- Initiate programs and services that prevent future unwanted pregnancy among teenagers and help the parenting teenager provide the best possible care to the child.
- Establish programs such as parenting classes; support services to help adolescents complete their education; coordination of health and social services for the mother and her child; and well-child care, immunizations, and nutrition services.

SUMMARY

Child and adolescent health status remains an important indicator of the nation's health. The health of a child sets the foundation for school readiness and future success. Child and adolescent health problems are a reflection of rapidly changing social conditions, not isolated events. Despite generally improving trends in health for most children, community health nurses must address discrepancies that exist between racial and ethnic groups. Poverty is the basis for many continuing health problems among children in this country, and nurses must recognize and treat it as such.

The best way to ensure the success and well-being of future generations is for each child to begin life healthy and maintain that health status throughout childhood. Any health problem (e.g., hunger and poor nutrition, increased lead blood levels, asthma, poor vision or hearing, anemia, dental caries, mental health problems, illicit drug use, or teen pregnancy) can interfere with school attendance, academic success, normal growth and development, learning ability, and life success.

The prevention of health problems is most significant and cost-effective for children. Each dollar spent on the prevention of physical and emotional problems in children is a sound investment. Primary health care and early intervention for children and families can help prevent costly problems, suffering, and lost human potential. Community health nurses can use their experience and "inside knowledge" of barriers to child health to educate others. Rather than limiting their approach to caring for the individual and family only, community health nurses can maximize their roles to collaborate and forge necessary alliances to solve children's health problems. Nurses are authority figures in the least expected places. Working on health care's front line is a powerful and very real position to members of Congress, state legislators, mayors, and other leaders. By creatively using this kind of power, community health nurses can contribute greatly to improving the health and well-being of all children.

LEARNING ACTIVITIES

1. Examine infant mortality statistics in the community and compare the rates with state and national averages. Is infant mortality higher for any particular racial or ethnic group within the community?
2. Determine how a non-English-speaking immigrant without finances or available transportation would obtain prenatal care.
3. Accompany a pregnant woman to a local department of social services and observe as she tries to establish Medicaid eligibility for herself and her unborn child.
4. Develop strategies to inform parents whose children are uninsured about the availability of SCHIP.
5. Spend a day with a school health nurse and analyze what could help prevent or address the health problems and issues he or she encountered throughout the day.
6. Survey businesses in the community to determine whether they offer maternity health insurance benefits, paid or unpaid maternity or paternity leave for new parents, and leave for prenatal care appointments. Is there a location within the worksite where women can pump breast milk? Use this information to develop a strategy to encourage family-friendly policies and practices in the business community.
7. If the community has a lay home visitor program, meet with a home visitor and, if possible, accompany him or her during home visits.
8. Communicate with those in policy-making positions by writing letters or holding meetings about children's needs.
9. Identify the public health and advocacy organizations in the community that are working to address children's health needs and identify their strategies for promoting child health within the community.

REFERENCES

Adams-Chapman I: Neurodevelopmental outcome of the late preterm infant, *Clin Perinatol* 33:947–964, 2006.
Alletto MM: *The power of prevention for mothers and children: the cost effectiveness of maternal and child health interventions*, Washington,

DC, 2009, Association of Maternal and Child Health Programs.
American Academy of Family Physicians, American Academy of Pediatrics, American College of Physicians, American Osteopathic Association: *Joint principles of the patient-*

centered medical home, March 2007. www.medicalhomeinfo.org/Joint%20Statement.pdf.
American Academy of Pediatrics: Breastfeeding and the use of human milk, *Pediatrics* 115(2):496–506, 2005.

Annie E. Casey Foundation: *When teens have sex: issues and trends*, 2000. www.aecf.org/kidscount/teen/index.htm.

Beach MC, Price EG, Gary TL: Cultural competence: a systemic review of health care provider educational interventions, *Med Care* 43(4):356–373, 2005.

Bettegowda VR, Dias T, Davidoff MJ, et al: The relationship between cesarean delivery and gestational age among U.S. singleton births, *Clin Perinatol* 35:309–323, 2008.

Centers for Disease Control and Prevention: *National youth risk behavior survey overview*, 2007a, www.cdc.gov/HealthyYouth/yrbs/pdf/yrbs07_us_overview.pdf.

Centers for Disease Control and Prevention: *Preventing smoking and exposure to secondhand smoke before, during, and after pregnancy*, 2007b, www.cdc.gov/NCCdphp/publications/factsheets/Prevention/smoking.htm.

Centers for Disease Control and Prevention: Alcohol use among pregnant and non-pregnant women of childbearing age—United States, 1991–2005, *MMWR Morb Mortal Wkly Rep* 58(19):529–532, 2009a, www.cdc.gov/mmwr/preview/mmwrhtml/mm5819a4.htm?s_cid=mm5819a4_e.

Centers for Disease Control and Prevention: *Lead poisoning prevention program*, 2009b, www.cdc.gov/nceh/lead/default.htm.

Centers for Disease Control and Prevention: *Vaccines and immunizations*, 2009c, www.cdc.gov/vaccines/default.htm.

Centers for Disease Control and Prevention, National Center for Injury Prevention and Control: *Web-based Injury Statistics Query and Reporting System* (WISQARS), May 5, 2008, www.cdc.gov/ncipc/wisqars.

Centers for Medicare and Medicaid Services: *National CHIP policy*, 2009, cms.hhs.gov/NationalCHIPPolicy/. Accessed May 12, 2009.

Children's Defense Fund: *State of America's children 2008*, Washington, DC, 2008, The Author.

Eunice Kennedy Shriver National Institute of Child Health and Human Development: *SIDS Back to Sleep Campaign*, 2008, www.nichd.nih.gov/sids.

Federal Interagency Forum on Child and Family Statistics: *America's children in brief: key indicators of wellbeing, 2008*, www.childstats.gov/americaschildren/index.asp. Accessed May 8, 2009.

Finer LB, Henshaw SK: Disparities in rates of unintended pregnancy in the United States, 1994 and 2001, *Perspect Sex Reprod Health* 38:90–96, 2006.

Finkelhor D, Ormrod RK, Turner HA, et al: The victimization of children and youth: a comprehensive national survey, *Child Maltreat* 10(1):5–25, 2005.

Food and Nutrition Service: *WIC participation and program characteristics 2006; summary*, 2007. fns.gov/oane/MENU/Published/WIC/FILES/PC2006/Summary.pdf. Accessed May 5, 2009.

Forhan SE, Gottlieb SL, Sternberg MR, et al: *Prevalence of sexually transmitted infections and bacterial vaginosis among female adolescents in the United States: data from the National Health and Nutritional Examination survey (NHANES) 2003–2004*, Poster Presentation, National STD Prevention Conference March 10–13, 2008, Division of STD Prevention, Centers for Disease Control and Prevention.

Hamilton BE, Martin JA, Ventura SJ: Births: preliminary data for 2007, *Natl Vital Stat Rep* 57(12):released March 18, 2009. www.cdc.gov/nchs/data/nvsr/nvsr57/nvsr57_12.pdf.

Health Resources and Services Administration: *The health center program: what is a health center?* 2009, bphc.hrsa.gov/about/. Accessed May 4, 2009.

Hoffman S: *By the numbers: the public costs of teen childbearing*, Washington, DC, 2006, National Campaign to Prevent Teen Pregnancy. www.thenationalcampaign.org/costs/pdf/report/BTN_National_Report.pdf.

Institute of Medicine, Section IV: Consequences of preterm birth. In Behrman RE, Butler AS, editors: *Preterm birth: causes, consequences, and prevention*, Washington, DC, 2006, National Humanities Press, pp. 311–345.

James CA, Bourgeois FT, Shannon MW: Association of race/ethnicity with emergency department wait times, *Pediatrics* 115(3):e310–e315, 2005.

Johnston LD, O'Malley PM, Bachman JG, et al: *Monitoring the future national results on adolescent drug use: overview of key findings, 2008*, (NIH Publication No. 09–7401), Bethesda, MD, 2009, National Institute on Drug Abuse.

Kaiser Family Foundation: *Children's health: why health insurance matters*, May 2002, www.kff.org/uninsured/loader.cfm?url=/commonspot/security/getfile.cfm&PageID=14132.

Klein JD: Committee on Adolescence: Adolescent pregnancy: current trends and issues, *Pediatrics* 116(4):281–286, 2005.

Kung HC, Hoyert DL, Xu JQ, et al: *E-stat deaths: preliminary data for 2005 health E-stats*, Hyattsville, MD, 2007, United States Department of Health and Human Services, Centers for Disease Control and Prevention. www.cdc.gov/nchs/products/pubs/pubd/hestats/prelimdeaths05/prelimdeaths05.htm.

Leeb RT, Paulozzi L, Melanson C, et al: *Child maltreatment surveillance: uniform definitions for public health and recommended data elements, version 1.0*, Atlanta, 2008, Centers for Disease Control and Prevention, National Center for Injury Prevention and Control.

Leonardi-Bee J, Smyth A, Britton J, et al: Environmental tobacco smoke and fetal health: systematic review and meta-analysis, *Arch Dis Child Fetal Neonatal Ed* 93:F351–F361, 2008.

Levi J, Vinter S, Laurent R St, et al: *F as in fat: how obesity policies are failing in America*, Washington, DC, 2008, Trust for America's Health, p. 143: healthyamericans.org/reports/obesity2008/.

MacDorman MF, Mathews TJ: *Recent trends in infant mortality in the United States*, NCHS data brief; 9, Hyattsville, MD, 2008, National Center for Health Statistics. www.cdc.gov/nchs/data/databriefs/db09.htm.

March of Dimes: *The cost of prematurity and complicated deliveries to U.S. employers*, report prepared by Thomson Reuters for the March of Dimes, October 29, 2008, marchofdimes.com/peristats/pdfdocs/cts/ThomsonAnalysis2008_SummaryDocument_final121208.pdf.

Martin JA, Hamilton BE, Sutton PD, et al: Births: final data for 2005, *Natl Vital Stat Rep* 56(6):2007. childstats.gov/americaschildren/tables.asp.

Martin JA, Hamilton BE, Sutton PD, et al: Births: final data for 2006, *Natl Vital Stat Rep* 57(7):2009.

McCurley C, Snyder HN: *Victims of violent juvenile crime*, U.S. Department of Justice, Office of Justice Programs, Juvenile Justice Bulletin, July 2004, www.ncjrs.gov/pdffiles1/ojjdp/201628.pdf.

Mills RJ, Bhandari S: Health insurance coverage in the United States, 2002, *Curr Popul Rep* 60–223, September 2003, U.S. Census Bureau: www.census.gov/prod/2003pubs/p60–223.pdf.

Morse SB, Zheng H, Tang Y, et al: Early school-age outcomes of late preterm infants, *Pediatrics* 123(4):e622–e629, 2009.

National Assembly on School-Based Health Care: *Capitol Hill briefing explains school-based health centers' role as first responders to students in crisis*, 2007, nasbhc.org/atf/cf/nationalrelease1.25.pdf. Accessed April 30, 2009.

National Center for Children in Poverty: *The effects of parental education on income*, New York, 2004, Columbia University, Mailman School of Public Health. www.nccp.org/pub_pei04.html.

National Center for Health Statistics: *Health, United States, 2006*, Hyattsville, MD, 2006, The Author.

National Center for Health Statistics: *Health, United States, 2008 with chartbook*, Hyattsville, MD, 2009, The Author. www.cdc.gov/nchs/data/hus/hus08.pdf#031.

National Governors' Association: *Maternal and child health update: states increase eligibility for children's health in 2007*, 2007, nga.org/Files/pdf/0811/MCHUPDATE.PDF. Accessed May 3, 2009.

National Health Service Corps: *About the NHSC*, 2003, nhsc.bhpr.hrsa.gov/about/. Accessed April 30, 2009.

Office of Applied Studies: *Team sports participation and substance use among youths*, National Survey on Drug Use and Health report, Rockville, MD, 2002, Substance Abuse and Mental Health Services Administration. www.oas.samhsa.gov/2k2/athletes/athletes_DrugUse.htm.

Office of Applied Studies: *Participation in youth activities and substance use among youths*, National Survey on Drug Use and Health Report, Rockville, MD, 2004, Substance Abuse and Mental Health Services Administration. www.oas.samhsa.gov/2k4/activities/activities.cfm.

Oshiro BT, Henry E, Wilson J, et al: Decreasing elective deliveries before 39 weeks of gestation in an integrated health care system, *Obstet Gynecol* 113:804–811, 2009.

Petrini JR, Dias T, McCormick MC, et al: Increased risk of adverse neurological development for late preterm infants, *J Pediatr* 154:169–176, 2009.

Reich K: editor: Children, youth, and gun violence, *Future Child* 12(2):2002, The David and Lucile Packard Foundation: www.futureofchildren.org/pubs-info2825/pubs-info_show.htm?doc_id=154414.

Safe Kids USA: *Preventing accidental injury*, 2009, usa.safekids.org. Accessed May 9, 2009.

Stothard KJ, Tennant PWG, Bell R, et al: Maternal overweight and obesity and the risk of congenital anomalies: a systematic review and meta-analysis, *JAMA* 301:636–650, 2009.

Substance Abuse and Mental Health Services Administration: *Results from the 2005 National Survey on Drug Use and Health: national findings*, Office of Applied Studies, NSDUH Series H-30, Publication No. SMA 06–4194, Rockville, MD, 2006, U.S. Department of Health and Human Services.

Substance Abuse and Mental Health Services. Administration: *Fetal alcohol spectrum disorders*, Rockville, MD, 2007, U.S. Department of Health and Human Services.

Tong VT, England LJ, Dietz PM, et al: Smoking patterns and use of cessation interventions during pregnancy, *Am J Prev Med* 35(4): 327–333, 2008.

U.S. Census Bureau: America's families and living arrangements: 2003, *Curr Popul Rep* 20–553, Annual Social and Economic Supplement: www.census.gov/prod/2004pubs/p20–553.pdf. 2004.

U.S. Court of Federal Claims: *Autism decisions and background information*, 2009, www.uscfc.uscourts.gov/node/5026.

U.S. Department of Health and Human Services: *Healthy People 2010*, conference ed, Washington, DC, 2000, U.S. Government Printing Office.

U.S. Department of Health and Human Services: 2009 poverty guidelines, *Fed Reg* 74(14): 4199–4201, 2009.

U.S. Department of Health and Human Services, Administration on Children, Youth, and Families: *Child maltreatment 2006*, [online], Washington, DC, 2006, Government Printing Office. www.acf.hhs.gov. Accessed February 20, 2008.

U.S. Department of Health and Human Services, Health Resources and Services Administration, Maternal and Child Health Bureau: *Child health USA 2007*, Rockville, MD, 2008a, U.S. Department of Health and Human Services. mchb.hrsa.gov/chusa07/index.html.

U.S. Department of Health and Human Services, Health Resources and Services Administration, Maternal and Child Health Bureau: *The National Survey of Children with Special Health Care Needs Chartbook 2005–2006*, Rockville, MD, 2008b, U.S. Department of Health and Human Services.

U.S. Department of Justice, Bureau of Justice Statistics: *Crime and victim statistics*, www.ojp.gov/bjs/cvict.htm. Accessed May 12, 2009.

U.S. Department of Labor: *Family and Medical Leave Act*, 2009, www.dol.gov/esa/whd/fmla. Accessed May 12, 2009.

U.S. Department of Transportation, National Highway Traffic Safety Administration: *Child passenger safety*, 2009, www.nhtsa.dot.gov. Accessed May 12, 2009.

Widome R, Neumark-Sztainer D, Hannan PJ, et al: Eating when there is not enough to eat: eating behaviors and perceptions of food among food-insecure youths, *Am J Public Health* 99:822–828, 2009.

Wolff T, Witkop CT, Miller T, et al: Folic acid supplementation for the prevention of neural tube defects: an update of the evidence for the United States Preventive Services Task Force, *Ann Intern Med* 150:632–639, 2009.

CHAPTER

17

Women's Health

Lori A. Glenn

Additional Material for Study, Review, and Further Exploration

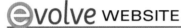 WEBSITE

http://evolve.elsevier.com/Nies
- Quiz
- Case Studies
- Glossary
- WebLinks

OBJECTIVES

Upon completion of this chapter, the reader will be able to do the following:

1. Identify the major indicators of women's health.
2. Examine prominent health problems among women of all age groups (i.e., from adolescence to old age).
3. Identify barriers to adequate health care for women.
4. Discuss issues related to reproductive health.
5. Explain the influence of public policy on women's health.
6. Discuss issues and needs for increased research efforts focused on women's health.
7. Apply the nursing process to women's health concerns across all levels of prevention.

KEY TERMS

breast cancer
cardiovascular disease
cesarean section
Civil Rights Act
domestic violence

ectopic pregnancy
Family and Medical Leave Act (FMLA)
family planning
hypertension
life expectancy

maternal mortality
multiple family configurations
osteoporosis
pelvic inflammatory disease (PID)
sexual harassment

OUTLINE

❤ HEALTHY PEOPLE 2020

Selected Proposed Objectives for Women's Health

OBJECTIVE

C HP2020–3: Reduce the female breast cancer death rate.

C HP2020–4: Reduce the death rate from cancer of the uterine cervix.

C HP2020–16: Increase the proportion of women aged 40 years and older who have received a breast cancer screening based on the most recent guidelines.

C HP2020–2: Increase the proportion of women with a family history of breast and/or ovarian cancer who receive genetic counseling.

MICH HP2020–3: Reduce maternal deaths.

MICH HP 2020–5: Increase the proportion of pregnant women who receive early and adequate prenatal care.

MICH HP2020–6b: Reduce cesarean births among low-risk (full term, singleton, vertex presentation) women; prior cesarean birth.

MICH HP2020–16: Increase the proportion of pregnant women who attend a series of prepared childbirth classes.

STD HP2020–1: Reduce the proportion of females aged 15-44 years who have ever required treatment for pelvic inflammatory disease (PID).

STD HP2020–7: Reduce the proportion of females with human papillomavirus (HPV) infection.

From U.S. Department of Health and Human Services. Healthy People 2020 Draft Objectives 2009. http://www.healthypeople.gov/hp2020/Objectives/files/Draft2009Objectives.pdf

To achieve "health for all" in the twenty-first century, health care services must be affordable and available to all. Although adequate health care for women is a key to realizing this goal, a significant number of women and their families face tremendous barriers in gaining access to health care. Additionally, knowledge deficits related to health promotion and disease prevention activities prevent women of all educational and socioeconomic levels from assuming responsibility for their own health and well-being.

Beginning in the 1970s, the women's movement called for the reform of systems affecting women's health. Women were encouraged to become involved as consumers of health services and as establishers of health policy. More women entered health professions in which they were previously underrepresented, and those in traditionally female-dominated professions, such as nursing and teaching, became more assertive in their demands to gain recognition for their contributions to society. Health care for women has evolved from the pelvic and breast focus to viewing the woman as a holistic being with specialized needs.

In "Preamble to a New Paradigm for Women's Health," Choi (1985) declared that collaboration and an interdisciplinary approach are necessary to meet the health care needs of women. She further stated that "essential to the development of health care for women are the concepts of health promotion, disease and accident prevention, education for self-care and responsibility, health risk identification and coordination for illness care when needed" (p. 14). To realize this paradigm, community health nurses must work with other health care professionals to formulate upstream strategies that modify the factors affecting women's health. Many *Healthy People 2020* objectives address health problems pertaining to women and include specific objectives and strategies to improve the health of this aggregate. The *Healthy People 2020* boxes in this chapter present a small selection of these objectives. This chapter examines the health of women from adolescence to old age. It explores the major indicators of health, including specific health problems and the socioeconomic, sociocultural, and health policy issues surrounding women's health. This chapter also discusses identification of current and future research aimed at improving the health of women. An understanding of these points will enable community health nurses to appropriately apply expertise in a community setting to help improve women's health.

MAJOR INDICATORS OF HEALTH

In the United States, data collected on major causes of death and illness appraise the health status of aggregates. These data are typically presented in terms of gender, age, or ethnicity and can help us interpret the levels of health in different groups. The primary indicators of health this chapter covers are life expectancy, mortality (i.e., death) rate, and morbidity (i.e., acute and chronic illness) rate.

There are 151.9 million women in the United States (Pleis, Lucas, and Ward, 2008). Of these women, 14% of those over the age of 18 years are considered in fair to poor health, while 18% have conditions that impair their daily functioning (Adams, Barnes, and Vickerie, 2007).

Many factors that lead to death and illness among women are preventable or avoidable. If certain conditions receive early detection and treatment, a significant positive influence on longevity and the quality of life could ensue. Recognition of patterns demonstrated by these indicators can address problems preventatively. This section presents an overview of these major indicators of health among women.

Life Expectancy

Except in a few countries, such as Bangladesh, Malawi, Niger, Pakistan, Qatar, and Zimbabwe, women typically experience greater longevity than their male counterparts (World Health

ANCHasjfка

Organization [WHO], 2004). For example, females born in the 1970s in the United States had an average life expectancy of 74.7 years, or 7.6 years longer than males born in the same year.

Life expectancy for Americans is at an all-time high, but the discrepancy between males and females remains. Males born in 2006 have a life expectancy of 76.5 years compared with 80.6 years for females. This suggests a trend toward narrowing the gap between male and female life expectancy (Heron et al., 2009). Ethnic/racial disparities in life expectancy unfortunately continued into the twenty-first century, as there is considerable variation between races. For example, black females gained an additional 7.1 years, rising from 69.4 years for those born in 1970 to 76.5 years in 2005. Although that is a significant gain, it falls behind the 80.8 years of life expectancy of white females born in that year (Heron et al., 2009).

Mortality Rate

Table 17-1 lists the six major causes of death among American women in 2004 by age group (CDC, 2007c). As age increases, the leading causes of death change. In the adolescent to early adulthood years, the leading cause is unintentional injuries (i.e., motor vehicle accidents, drug overdose). As middle age approaches, cancer takes over as the number one cause. Finally after the age of 65 years, the rates of cancer and cardiovascular disease even out as number one.

RESEARCH HIGHLIGHTS

Nurse Researchers Study the Inclusion of Women in Research

A group of nurse researchers examined more than 1000 articles published in nursing journals between 1995 and 2001 to determine whether women had been included in research studies focusing on the leading causes of mortality. They found that 87% of the studies did include women participants. They also noted that there appeared to be a slight increase in inclusion of women from the earlier years to the later years.

From Crane PB, et al: Inclusion of women in nursing research: 1995-2001, *Nurs Res* 53:237-242, 2004.

Cardiovascular Disease

About one in four Americans has one or more forms of cardiovascular disease (CVD) (e.g., high blood pressure, coronary heart disease, stroke, congenital defects, and rheumatic heart disease). CVD accounts for about 35.3% of all deaths in the United States, or about one out of every 2.8 deaths. One in ten women under age 60 years has some form of CVD; the ratio increases to one in three after age 65 years. Black women are more likely to die of CVDs than white women. In 2005, the CVD death rate among white females was 230.4 per 100,000, compared with 319.7 per 100,000 for black females. Black women are also more likely to die of stroke than white women (60.7 per 100,000 and 44 per 100,000, respectively) (American Heart Association [AHA], 2009a).

TABLE 17-1	FIVE LEADING CAUSES OF DEATH AMONG AMERICAN WOMEN FOR ALL RACES BY AGE GROUPS IN 2005
AGE GROUP (YR)	**CAUSE OF DEATH (IN RANK ORDER)**
15 to 19	Unintentional injury or accidents (51.7%) Suicide (8.8%) Homicide (7.5%) Cancer (7.3%) Heart disease (3.1%) Birth defects (2.8%)
20 to 24	Unintentional injury or accidents (40.5%) Homicide (8.4%) Cancer (8.0%) Suicide (7.6%) Heart disease (4.6%) Pregnancy complications (2.7%)
25 to 34	Unintentional injury or accidents (25.3%) Malignant neoplasm (15.1%) Heart disease (8.2%) Suicide (7.5%) Homicide (5.8%) HIV disease (4.4%)
35 to 44	Cancer (26.2%) Unintentional injuries (15.1%) Heart disease (12.4%) Suicide (5.0%) HIV disease (4.3%) Stroke (3.5%)
45 to 54	Cancer (36.2%) Heart disease (15.8%) Chronic obstructive pulmonary disease (5.4%) Unintentional injuries (7.4%) Cerebrovascular disease (4.2%) Diabetes mellitus (3.3%) Chronic liver disease (3.2%)
55 to 64	Cancer (41.5%) Heart disease (18.6%) Chronic lower respiratory disease (5.4%) Diabetes mellitus (4.3%) Cerebrovascular disease (4.2%) Unintentional injuries (2.9%)
65 to 74	Cancer (35.6%) Heart disease (22.1%) Chronic obstructive pulmonary disease (7.9%) Cerebrovascular disease (5.5%) Diabetes mellitus (4.3%) Kidney disease (1.9%)
75 to 84	Heart disease (27.5%) Cancer (22.6%) Cerebrovascular disease (8.3%) Chronic obstructive pulmonary disease (6.9%) Alzheimer's disease (4.0%) Diabetes mellitus (2.2%)
85+	Heart disease (27.2%) Cancer (22.0%) Cerebrovascular disease (7.5%) Chronic obstructive pulmonary disease (5.2%) Alzheimer's disease (3.9%) Diabetes mellitus (3.1%)

Modified from Centers for Disease Control and Prevention: *Leading cause of death in females, Women's health,* September 10, 2007a: www.cdc.gov/Women/lcod/04all.pdf. Accessed April 30, 2009.

Cardiovascular disease continues to be the number one overall killer of women. One out of every 2.4 deaths is from CVD, whereas one out of every 29 deaths is from breast cancer. In 2007, CVD caused more deaths among females (454,613, or 36.7%) than among males (409,867, or 34.2%) (AHA, 2009a). The overall number of deaths due to CVD decreased dramatically from 424.2 per 100,000 in 1950 to 273 per 100,000 in 2003.

Nevertheless, disparities continue related to prevention, diagnosis, and management of heart disease in women. After the age of 65 years, women are twice as likely to die because of heart disease as men (Vaccarino et al., 2003; American Heart Association, 2009b). Women have higher rates of complications after revascularization procedures (Jacobs, 2003) and higher rates of death after myocardial infarction (Wenger, 2004). This phenomenon exists because women display different symptoms of heart disease and are managed differently than men (Chang et al., 2003; Martin et al., 2004; Schulman et al., 1999). Physiologically, women have smaller arteries and higher rates of metabolic syndrome, diabetes, heart failure, and other comorbidities. They tend to be older at their first cardiovascular event, with more urgent and emergent presentations (Jacobs, 2003). These differences result in fewer preventative interventions, such as cholesterol screening, use of aspirin and other fibrinolytic therapy, and statin drugs to lower cholesterol (Downs, Clearfield, and Weis, 1998).

Rates of CVD among women can decline further when individuals become more aware of risk factors and accept responsibility for managing their own health and well-being (Kuehn, McMahon, and Creekmore, 1999). Concerned and motivated providers must encourage women to practice heart-healthy behaviors. In 2002, the American Heart Association launched the "Go Red" campaign for women and "The Heart Truth" program for health care providers designed to educate both about the unique features of women and heart disease.

Cancer

Cancer is the second leading cause of death in the United States. Of deaths in America in 2008, 23% were due to cancer. (American Cancer Society [ACS], 2009). Further, cancer is expected to become the overall leading cause of death in the next decade (Stewart, King, Thompson, Friedman, Wingo, 2004).

Cancer rates appear to be increasing for a number of reasons including lifestyle choices (smoking, diet, sun exposure), increasing exposure to environmental carcinogens, and, probably most important, age. To illustrate, death rates from cancer among women have increased from 136 per 100,000 women in 1960 to 167.3 per 100,000 women in 2000 (Stewart, et al., 2004). The ACS estimates that 296,000 deaths will occur among women as a result of cancer in 2009 (ACS, 2008).

In 1987, lung cancer surpassed breast cancer as the leading cause of cancer deaths in women, and death rates increased sharply until about 1990. Lung cancer deaths leveled off, and in 2005 26% of cancer deaths in American women were attributed to lung cancer. Breast cancer was the second most common cause and resulted in 15% of all cancer deaths (ACS,

2008). Colorectal cancer, the third most frequent cause of cancer deaths, accounts for 9% of all cancer deaths and claims the lives of some 28,000 women annually.

Other female-specific cancers include ovarian cancer (fifth most common cancer), uterine cancer (sixth most common cancer), and cervical cancer. Cervical cancer, in particular, has received considerable attention of late as it has been determined that 90% of women with cervical cancer have evidence of cervical infection with human papillomavirus (HPV) (ACS, 2009). In June 2006, the Food and Drug Administration (FDA) licensed Gardasil (Merck & Co., Inc.), the first vaccine to prevent HPV infection (CDC, 2007b; FDA, 2006). Since approval, more than 7 million doses have been given (CDC, 2007b). Gardasil has been shown to be highly effective in preventing the most common types of HPV infection and was approved for use in females between 9 and 26 years of age. For additional information consult the CDC's website (www.cdc.gov/vaccinesafety/Vaccines/HPV/gardasil.html).

The good news is that healthy lifestyle changes and early detection and intervention have contributed to the decrease in mortality rates from some cancers. For example, the death rate for colorectal cancer has been decreasing for the past 15 years because of early detection and treatment. Lung cancer deaths are beginning to show a slight decline that parallels a decreased incidence of smoking by women over the age of 18 years (ACS, 2009).

Five-year survival rates vary according to the type of cancer and stage at diagnosis. For instance, the 5-year survival rate for all clients with lung cancer is only 18%. For localized breast cancer, it is 98%, decreasing to 23% when diagnosed with distant metastases. Of cancers related to the reproductive tract, ovarian cancer has the lowest survival rate, as only around 46% of women survive for 5 years. When the cancer is diagnosed at an early stage, 5-year survival rate for women with colon cancer is 91% and for those with rectal cancer it is 89% (National Cancer Institute, 2009).

Early diagnosis and prompt treatment are major factors in surviving many types of cancer. According to the ACS (2008) this includes routine cervical cancer screening with Pap smear and HPV tests beginning 3 years after the onset of intercourse, and continuing annually. After age 30 years, women with three negative annual Pap tests can be screened every 3 years. Breast cancer screenings include regular self breast examination and annual clinical breast exam, with the addition of a mammogram after the age of 40 years or sooner with increased risk of hereditary breast cancer. Colorectal cancer screenings include annual fecal occult blood tests along with sigmoidoscopy every 5 years or colonoscopy every 10 years (ACS, 2008).

Certain health choices may reduce an individual's risk of cancer. All women need to avoid health-deteriorating practices and replace them with health-promoting behaviors. Women could reduce their risk for cancer by never smoking or by quitting if they already use tobacco products. Eating a nutritious, plant-focused, high-fiber diet, along with adopting a physically active lifestyle and maintaining a healthy body weight, protect against both heart disease and many cancers. Nutrition guidelines include avoiding salt-cured, smoked, nitrite-containing, and charred foods, high-fat food, and excessive alcohol (Rhodes, 2002; Vogel, 2003). Obesity has been associated with an increased risk for cancers such as colon and rectum, endometrium, and breast (ACS, 2008). Finally, the practice of safe sex has been shown to decrease the spread of cancer associated with sexually transmitted diseases such as HPV, hepatitis B and C, and human immunodeficiency virus (HIV).

Community health nurses must encourage all females (i.e., from childhood to old age) to adopt these healthy lifestyle choices and pursue early cancer detection. Community health nurses play a major role in providing cancer control services that should be culturally sensitive and appropriate to the targeted aggregate. If providers and clients applied everything known about cancer prevention, approximately two thirds of cancer cases would not occur.

Diabetes

In 2008, the number of patients with diabetes in the United States reached 24 million, or 8% of the population, with 25% of the population over 60 years of age being affected (CDC, 2008e). From 2003 to 2006, the number of patients with diagnosed diabetes had risen by 7.8%, especially among women (Cheung, Ong, and Cherny, 2009), although the number of men affected has exceeded women since 2006 (CDC, 2009a).

Diabetes mellitus is a chronic disease that causes premature death of many women and overall ranks sixth in mortality among that group, highest after the age of 45 years (CDC, 2007c). Diabetes ranks fourth as the cause of death among several aggregates, including Native American, black, and Asian, and is fifth among Hispanics (National Center for Health Statistics, 2004).

In addition to being a serious illness in itself, diabetes is a risk factor for the development of CVD; furthermore, it dramatically influences the severity and course of the CVD. In death certificates from 2004 where the cause of death was related to diabetes, 68% also listed CVD and 16% also listed stroke (CDC, 2008e). When comparing men and women with diabetes, of those who have myocardial infarction before age 65 years, women are more likely to have long-term health problems and to die (Norhammar et al., 2008). The good news is that the number of women hospitalized for diabetes has dropped, indicating that better management with tighter control of blood glucose has decreased complications (CDC, 2008c). The community health nurse is an important resource for supporting the tight control of diabetes to prevent its complications. An upstream approach to this problem includes helping women maintain a desirable weight throughout life in an effort to avoid nutrition-related causes of death, such as diabetes and CVD.

Maternal Mortality

According to the Safe Motherhood Organization (2005), complications of pregnancy and childbirth are the leading cause of disability and death among women between the ages of 14 and 49 years. In 2005, 536,000 women died,

mostly in developing countries. Forty percent of women have complications during pregnancy, childbirth, and the postpartum period; 15% are life-threatening problems.

Before 2003, maternal mortality was the death of a woman while pregnant or within 42 days after termination of pregnancy. The U.S. Standard Certificate of Death and the WHO's ICD-10 revised those guidelines in 2003 to include late causes of maternal death, defined as greater than 42 days but less than 1 year after the end of the pregnancy (Hoyert, 2007; WHO, 2007). The duration and the site of the pregnancy are irrelevant; causes are defined as related to or aggravated by the pregnancy or its management, but not from accidental or incidental causes.

It is important for community health nurses to be aware of the global situation surrounding maternal mortality. For each woman who dies in the developed world, 99 will die in the developing world (WHO, 2000), demonstrating that wide gaps continue to exist in the availability and quality of reproductive health care services globally.

The United States ranks seventeenth in maternal mortality among all nations. In 2005 the rate of maternal death was 12.1 per 100,000 pregnancies (Department of Reproductive Health and Research, 2005). Reduction of maternal mortality is one of the *Healthy People 2020* objectives for the United States.

Beginning in the 1950s, maternal mortality rates began to decline in the United States because of the use of blood transfusions, antimicrobial drugs, and the maintenance of fluid and electrolyte balance during serious complications of pregnancy and birth. The development of obstetric training programs and obstetric anesthesia programs was also important.

Racial discrepancy persists, however, in maternal mortality rates as in life expectancy. Table 17-2 illustrates how nonwhite women have a significantly higher incidence of death during pregnancy than whites. The gap in maternal mortality rates between black and white women has widened over the past several decades. Early in the twentieth century, black women were two times more likely to die of pregnancy-related complications than white women. Currently, black women are nearly four times more likely to die than white women (CDC, 2007c). Major risk factors for maternal death include lack

TABLE 17-2	MATERNAL MORTALITY RATE PER 100,000 LIVE BIRTHS—SELECTED YEARS			
YR	TOTAL	WHITES	BLACKS	OTHER (NONWHITE)
1985	7.8	5.2	20.4	18.1
1992	7.8	5.0	20.8	18.2
1995	7.1	4.2	22.1	18.5
2002	8.9	6.0	24.9	NA
2003*	12.1	8.7	30.5	NA

From Hoyert DL: Maternal mortality and related concepts, National Center for Health Statistics, *Vital Health Stat* 3(33), p 10, 2007.
*Includes the category of "late maternal deaths and sequelae of late maternal deaths" for the first time.
NA, Not available.

of antepartal care and family planning services, inadequate health education, and poor nutrition. An additional risk factor, regardless of race, is advancing age. Women aged 40 years and older have over three times the risk of dying of a pregnancy-related cause as women aged 30 to 39 years (National Center for Health Statistics, 2007). Intrinsic maternal factors, such as increasing frequency of hypertension and a greater likelihood of uterine hemorrhage, help explain this increase in the mortality rate among older mothers.

In 2005, maternal mortality was 15.1 per 100,000 live births, up from 12 per 100,000 in 2003 in the United States. Historically, the leading cause of maternal death is pulmonary embolism (17%), followed by pregnancy-induced hypertension, ectopic pregnancy, hemorrhage, stroke, and anesthesia (Cunningham et al., 2005). Of growing concern is the increasing cesarean section rate, incidence of maternal obesity, and increased age of mothers, which may be contributing to the rise in this rate (Kaiser, 2007). Death associated with legal surgical abortion is rare in the United States, with 33 reported in 2005 (Kung et al., 2008). Complications that result in death from legal abortion relate to the woman's age, the type of procedure, the gestational age of the fetus, and general health problems at the time of the abortion (Cates, Ellertson, and Stewart, 2004).

A medical, or induced, method of abortion using mifepristone (i.e., RU-486), an antiprogestin medication, together with prostaglandins has been used in the United States since September 2000. This method is as effective as surgical abortion and is considered a safe alternative to surgical abortion in pregnancies of less than 49 days (7 weeks). In 2005, 9.9% of the 820,151 legal abortions in the United States employed this method. Curettage as an abortion procedure is still the most widely used (Gamble et al., 2008).

Abortion is a controversial issue for providers and for the women in their care. Adequate access to affordable family planning services is key to decreasing the need for elective abortions. Consider this quote from Dr. Joycelyn Elders: "I never knew a woman who needed an abortion who wasn't already pregnant" (Elders, 2009). Nurses must continue to keep abreast of all available pregnancy prevention and termination options to provide the best counsel for women.

According to the CDC (2003), ectopic pregnancy is the leading cause of maternal death in the first trimester, accounting for 13% of maternal deaths. Since the 1980s, the incidence of ectopic pregnancy has increased fourfold to 11.3 per 1000 pregnancies among women 15 to 44 years of age. Racial discrepancy is evident and yields a rate of 14.7 per 1000 among nonwhites compared with 10.3 per 1000 among whites. This disparity continues to increase throughout the reproductive years of nonwhite women, possibly because sexually transmitted diseases (STDs) are more frequently diagnosed among nonwhite women, and these clients have less access to health care.

The most significant risk for ectopic pregnancy is previous pelvic inflammatory disease (PID) or salpingitis. Early diagnosis and treatment greatly reduce the mortality rate. Prevention interventions for women at risk for acquiring STDs are critical in reducing a woman's risk for an ectopic pregnancy. An important task of health care providers is to educate women and men on methods to reduce sexual health risk-taking behaviors. Additional risk factors for ectopic pregnancy include tubal pathology, previous ectopic pregnancy, tubal surgery, and the use of intrauterine contraceptive devices.

Morbidity Rate
Hospitalizations
The 2008 National Hospital Discharge Survey (CDC) reported that more women than men are hospitalized each year in the United States. Pneumonia resulted in an average hospital stay of 5.6 days, which occurred most frequently among women aged 65 years or older. Fractures accounted for an average of 5.8 days, malignant neoplasms for an average 6.7 days, and diseases of the heart for an average 4.7 days. The number one reason for hospitalization was childbirth, followed by circulatory, digestive, respiratory diseases, and finally injury or poisoning. The length of hospitalization after childbirth has increased along with the C-section rate since 1995 (DeFrances et al., 2006).

The prospective payment system for hospitalization resulted in an increased demand for skilled nursing services in the home. After hospitalization for several of these conditions, community health nurses may provide ongoing nursing care in the home by referral. Nurses practicing in home environments must be prepared to deliver high-tech and high-touch services. Chapter 33 discusses home health care in detail.

Chronic Conditions and Limitations
Women are more likely than men to be disabled from chronic conditions. Arthritis and rheumatism, hypertension, and impairment of the back or spine decrease women's activity level more often than they affect their male counterparts. In fact, twice as many women (24.3%) as men (11.5%) are limited in activity from arthritis and rheumatism. Women are more likely than men to have difficulty performing activities such as walking, bathing or showering, preparing meals, and doing housework (CDC, 2009d).

Functional limitations may require home health care that community health nurses supervise and deliver. Nurses plan and implement interventions based on functional assessments. The care plan facilitates optimal resumption of the individual's independence in personal care activities.

Surgery
Women are more likely than men to have surgery. Hysterectomy is the second most frequently performed major surgical procedure among women of reproductive age after C-section. Approximately 600,000 hysterectomies are performed each year (CDC, 2008g). Hysterectomy rates for women in the South are slightly higher than those in the Northeast (6.3 and 4.9 per 1000 women, respectively). Overall, rates of hysterectomy have decreased from 5.4 to 5.1 per 100 in the years 2000 to 2004 (Whiteman and Hillis, 2008).

The most common reason for hysterectomy is uterine fibroids or leiomyoma, which contributes to more than one third of all such surgeries, but considerably more for blacks (68%) than for whites (33%) (CDC, 2008g). White women more often have a diagnosis of endometriosis and uterine prolapse, which are the second and third most common reasons for hysterectomy. Hysterectomy rates are the highest in women aged 40 to 44 years (CDC, 2008g).

Optional procedures are becoming available to women. Myomectomy, or removing only the tumors with repair of the uterus, uterine artery ablation, and the use of a gonadotropin-releasing hormone to shrink the tumors can decrease the need for hysterectomy, but women may not know about these alternatives. Community health nurses function as advocates for women and can provide health education programs related to alternatives to hysterectomy, indications for hysterectomy and oophorectomy (i.e., removal of ovaries), and information regarding the type of surgical approach and the purpose of a second opinion. Second opinions and higher levels of education tend to decrease the rate of hysterectomies (Finkel and Finkel, 1990).

Birth by cesarean section is the most prevalent surgical procedure undergone by women in the United States and accounts for 32% of births. This rate has gone up more than 50% since 1996 (Hamilton, Martin, and Ventura, 2009). Several factors contribute to the high rates of C-section, including physician fear of malpractice suits, routine use of early induction of labor, and epidural anesthesia. The technology of fetal monitoring has been shown to increase the C-section rate without improving neonatal outcomes. Consumer demand has also played a part in this trend, as parents expect that the latest technological advances and advanced medical training can guarantee the "perfect baby" and report the procedure as attractive for its convenience and perceived safety. C-section is also thought of as a way to preserve the pelvic floor, despite no evidence to support this effect. C-section is a lifesaving procedure, yet should be performed judiciously for women and their babies who are at risk for life-threatening complications without the procedure. C-section involves the risks of any major surgery such as hemorrhage, infection, damage to adjacent structures, and those risks associated with anesthesia. Long-term sequelae for women include pelvic pain, along with formation of adhesions and placental abnormalities that lead to complications in subsequent pregnancies. Risks to the neonate include higher incidence of persistent pulmonary hypertension and respiratory diseases (Levine et al., 2001). Routine, high rates of C-section are not shown to improve outcomes for either mother or baby (American College of Nurse Midwives, 2005). Women should be made aware of the risks involved with interventions associated with birth and educated on how to best select their place of birth.

Mental Health

The most frequently occurring interruption in women's mental health relates to depression. Well-controlled epidemiological studies consistently demonstrate that women

BOX 17-1	*DSM-IV-TR* CRITERIA FOR MAJOR DEPRESSIVE DISORDER

- Depressed mood
- Significant decline in interest or pleasure
- Change in weight or appetite
- Insomnia or hypersomnia nearly every day
- Psychomotor agitation or retardation
- Fatigue or loss of energy nearly every day
- Feelings of worthlessness or excessive or inappropriate guilt
- Diminished ability to think or concentrate, or make decisions
- Recurrent thoughts of suicide or death
- Atypical symptoms of depression in women
- Increased appetite or weight gain
- Mood reactivity
- Leaden paralysis (heavy legs and arms)
- Sensitivity to personal rejection
- Absence of melancholia or catatonic features

From the American Psychological Association: *Diagnostic and statistical manual of mental disorders,* ed 4, Washington, DC, 2000, The Author.

experience depression at two to three times the rate of men (American Psychological Association, 2005). Symptoms of depression include depressed mood, apathy, anxiety, irritability, and thoughts of death and suicide (Evans et al., 1999). Unique to women are atypical symptoms including anxiety, increased appetite, weight gain, and somatic complaints along with increased rates of comorbid conditions. Women are more likely to attempt suicide but less likely to be successful (Urbanic, 2009). Women with socioeconomic barriers such as lower income and lower educational levels, racial/ethnic discrimination, unemployment, poor health, single parenthood, and high-stress jobs are at greater risk for depression than women with higher educational levels or higher economic status. Other risk factors include childhood negligence and abuse, parental death, negligence, and alcoholism (Urbanic, 2009).

Nurses practicing in community health settings should be aware of the signs and symptoms of depression and identify referral sources for professional help within the community. The nurse needs also to be aware of the impact a mother's depression may have on her child's development and family functioning. A woman experiencing depression may display some signs and symptoms listed in Box 17-1.

SOCIAL FACTORS AFFECTING WOMEN'S HEALTH

Health Care Access

In 2008, 14.7% of the U.S. population, or 43.1 million U.S. citizens, lacked health insurance coverage, with 19.7% (37.1 million) of persons between ages 18-64 reporting lack of health care insurance (CDC, 2009e). Owing to the nature of their employment, women frequently lack health insurance but may not be eligible for Medicaid benefits because their income is too high. Young adults (i.e., those between ages 16 and 24 years) make up approximately 50% of individuals without health insurance. Lacking economic means for meeting the costs of health care, these women are not likely to seek health care until they or a family member is in acute distress. Others may rely on home remedies, over-the-counter drugs, or folk healers for health care. Older adults, who are usually covered by Medicare, may also delay seeking health care. Older women on fixed incomes may have difficulty meeting co-payments required by Medicare and paying for prescription medications. Many senior citizens have paid hospitalization insurance premiums for policies that fail to meet the gap.

Education and Work

In the workplace, women traditionally predominate as secretaries, administrative assistants, registered nurses, teachers, cashiers, and retail sales people. However, in the 1980s, more women began to enter professions traditionally held by men (e.g., lawyers, physicians, and dentists), and in 2008, more than half (51%) of young professionals were women (U.S. Department of Labor, 2008). In 1970, 55.4% of all women aged 25 or older were high school graduates compared with 81.6% in 1995 and 85% in 2003. Of this same age group, 25.7% had completed college, which was more than three times the 1970 rate of 8.1% (U.S. Census Bureau, 2008a). An increasing number of women earned degrees in traditionally male-dominated professions. Table 17-3 reflects recent changes occurring in percentages of women receiving degrees in medicine, dentistry, law, and theology.

Employment and Wages

In 2008, 46.5% of the workforce were women. In addition, more than half (62%) of women with young children (younger than 6 years) were working outside the home (U.S. Department of Labor, 2005). In 1950, only 12% of women were combining these roles (Chadwick and Heaton, 1992).

TABLE 17-3 PERCENTAGES OF DEGREES RECEIVED BY WOMEN

DEGREE	1970	1980	1988	1996	2002	2007
Medicine (MD)	8.4	23.4	33.3	40.9	44.4	49.2
Dentistry (DDS or DMD)	0.9	13.3	26.7	35.8	38.5	44.5
Law (LLB or JD)	5.4	30.2	40.8	43.4	48.0	47.6
Theology (BD, MDiv, or MHL)	2.3	13.8	19.3	23.3	33.2	33.2

From US Department of Education: *Digest of education statistics,* Washington, DC, 2008, The Author.

Several questions concern women's health and well-being related to employment issues. A review of female-dominated versus male-dominated jobs discloses inequalities in wage and salary scales; despite the diminishing gap between women's and men's incomes, there is still much room for improvement. Table 17-4 depicts median annual earnings by type of household (U.S. Census Bureau, 2008b). Disparities in income based on sex are clear.

Women heads of households and their children are the poorest aggregate in the United States. This phenomenon is labeled "the feminization of poverty." In 2005, the poverty rate for single female heads of household was 36.9%, compared with 17.6% for men (Thibos, Lavin-Loucks, and Martin, 2007). The nurse working with impoverished families should be aware of social services, child care programs, emergency services, and other resources for families in need. The community health nurse often needs to act as case manager and advocate for families with social service agencies and other public entities.

Working Women and Home Life

Added to inequalities outside the home are inequalities within the home. A working woman is less likely to have a spouse or partner help with the home and children. Even when a spouse or partner is present, the burdens of housework and child care usually fall more heavily on women, regardless of ethnicity. Mothers generally spend more time than fathers preparing meals and training and disciplining their children. These multiple-role demands and conflicting expectations contribute to stress (American Academy of Pediatrics, 2005; Matthews and Power, 2002).

However, changes are occurring as younger and older men now report spending more time in family activities compared with middle-aged men. Blacks and Hispanics tend to spend a little more time working at family tasks than white men. Books and articles encourage wives and husbands to make their needs known, encouraging increased communication between partners. Marriage enrichment programs, often offered through churches and synagogues, teach couples how to communicate more effectively with each other, fostering equality between partners.

Family Configuration and Marital Status

Women are members of multiple family configurations (e.g., nuclear families, extended family units, single-parent units, families of group marriages, blended family units, adoptive

TABLE 17-4 MEDIAN ANNUAL EARNINGS (IN DOLLARS) BY TYPE OF HOUSEHOLD: 1969, 1979, 1989, 1999, 2003, AND 2007

HOUSEHOLD TYPE	1969	1979	1989	1999	2003	2007
Married couple with children	41,453	47,793	50,613	56,827	62,405	72,785
Female householder with children	16,327	18,468	17,651	26,164	29,307	33,370
Male householder with children	33,749	36,619	34,646	41,830	41,959	49,839

From DeNavas-Walt C, Proctor BD, Smith JC, US Census Bureau: Income, poverty, and health insurance coverage in the United States: 2007, *Curr Popul Rep Consum Income,* Washington, DC, 2008, US Government Printing Office: www.census.gov/prod/2008pubs/p60-235.pdf.

family units, nonlegal heterosexual unions, and lesbian family units). This diversity causes changes in women's roles within families. Whether or not they function in a traditional role, most women do whatever is necessary to maintain the integrity of their families. Early assessment of the strengths of family units by the community health nurse provides a database for positive nursing interventions established on upstream strategies to enhance each family's level of health and well-being.

Many women are delaying marriage, and an increasing number are not marrying. Overall, marriage rates have remained stable perhaps because the increasing number of remarriages balances the declining rate of first marriages. When a relationship ends in divorce or separation, more women than men have the responsibility of providing for themselves and their children. According to the U.S. Census Bureau (2007), single-parent households in 2006 represented 9% of all households with children, and one third of all children live with a single parent. Single mothers are most often the head of a single-parent family. Percentages of female single-parent households with children under the age of 18 years have been on the rise (U.S. Census Bureau, 2009) (Table 17-5). Even in the face of changing lifestyles, divorce, and increased mobility, which leads to long-distance relationships, most Americans report they remain connected to their extended families through parents, grandparents, siblings, aunts, and uncles.

One contemporary family configuration involves single women with one or more adopted children. Single-parent adoptions are legal, and an increasing number of single women are becoming adoptive parents. An often-ignored family structure is one headed by a lesbian parent. Lesbians who become parents have needs similar to those of all mothers. Many cities have lesbian-gay parent groups that provide support, anticipatory guidance, and strategies for coping in society. However, lesbian women often neglect their own health. This self-neglect may be traced to hostile and rejecting attitudes of health care providers (Zeidenstein, 2004). However, the parents or guardians must remain healthy to ensure the child's well-being.

TABLE 17-5	CHARACTERISTICS OF BLACK, WHITE, AND HISPANIC FEMALE-HEADED HOUSEHOLDS: 2007		
CHARACTERISTIC	BLACK	WHITE	HISPANIC
Never married (%)	51.5	27.4	39.7
Married and spouse absent (%)	12.1	11.3	17.8
Widowed (%)	11.1	16.9	9.6
Divorced (%)	21.7	40.6	26.4
No. of children per female-headed household	1.87	1.65	1.82

Modified from US Census Bureau *Current Population Reports* and *America's Families and Living Arrangements: 2007,* July 2008: www.census.gov/population/www/socdemo/hh-fam/cps2007.html.

HEALTH PROMOTION STRATEGIES FOR WOMEN

A woman's ability to carry out her important roles can affect her entire family; therefore women should receive services that promote health and detect disease at an early stage. Early detection and improved treatments for disease allow women to return to work or remain working throughout the course of an illness. Although work is essential to the economic and social well-being of many women's families, the workplace itself creates physical and social stress. As more women enter the workforce and face many of the same risks and stressors as men, it is not surprising that their formerly favorable mortality and morbidity rates have been worsening.

Many women seek information that will allow them to be in control of their own health. Since the early 1970s, women have met in self-help groups to develop a better understanding of their own health needs. Some of the health behaviors that women learn in self-help groups are the importance of nutrition and exercise, breast self-examination (BSE), pregnancy testing and contraceptive awareness; recognition of the early signs of vaginal infections and STDs; and awareness of the variations in female anatomy and physiology.

For women who desire to become more knowledgeable about their own health, there are books available in bookstores, public libraries, and among the holdings of traditional women's groups such as sororities, federated women's clubs, and others. An excellent resource for women is the *FDA Consumer* (www.fda.gov/fdac/), the official magazine of the FDA, which reports on studies that cover a variety of women's health issues, such as mammography standards, menopause, treatment for STDs, eating disorders, infertility, cosmetic safety, silicone breast implants, and osteoporosis. Another resource is the U.S. Department of Health and Human Services (USDHHS) Office on Women's Health (www.WomensHealth.gov), which highlights positive health behaviors for women and girls. The community health nurse can use models such as Pender's Health Promotion Model in teaching health behaviors that lead to general health promotion among women. Pender notes that health-promoting behaviors are directed toward sustaining or increasing the level of well-being, self-actualization, and fulfillment of a given individual or group (Pender, Murdaugh, and Parsons, 2006). However, because many models were developed for the middle class, they may not be useful to community health nurses working with low-income families.

Knowledge deficits related to body awareness prevail among all women, regardless of socioeconomic or educational level. Regardless of whether a group comprises college-educated professional women or blue-collar working women, many of the questions they pose are the same. For example, a woman may ask if she will menstruate after a hysterectomy, whether she should perform a BSE, or what she can do to prevent recurrent episodes of vaginitis. Nurses can play an instrumental role in helping women develop a greater sense of self-awareness. Furthermore, community health nurses can remove the mystery surrounding the woman's body and encourage clients to ask previously unmentionable questions.

Acute Illness

Females report a greater incidence of acute conditions than males. This section describes several of the most common.

Urinary Tract Infection and Dysuria

By age 32 years, half of all women report a history of at least one urinary tract infection (UTI). Peak incidence in women is ages 20 to 24 years (Foxman and Brown, 2003). In every age group, adult women have a higher incidence of UTI than men, with an annual incidence of 12.6% compared with 3% among men. The higher incidence among women is attributed to differences in anatomy, which enhance the exposure to potential uropathogens and enhance the ability of these pathogens to colonize the urinary tract.

Women often experience dysuria, the sensation of pain, burning, or discomfort on urination. Dysuria accounts for 5% to 15% of visits to family physicians; approximately 25% of American women report acute dysuria every year. The symptom is most prevalent in women 25 to 54 years of age and in those who are sexually active. Although many physicians equate dysuria with UTI, it is actually a symptom that has many potential causes, infection being only one. Treatment with antibiotics may be inappropriate, except in carefully selected patients. Risk factors for both UTI and dysuria are female gender, advancing age, sexual activity, vaginitis, renal stone, and a history of sexual abuse, which can result in psychogenic dysuria (Bremnor and Sadovsky, 2002).

Diseases of the Reproductive Tract

Acute illnesses specific to the reproductive tract include conditions such as vulvovaginitis, pelvic inflammatory disease, and toxic shock syndrome.

Vaginitis and vulvovaginitis. Vaginitis involves inflammation of the vaginal mucosa; vulvovaginitis refers to inflammation of the vulva as well. Both may start in girls before puberty and are more common than in women of reproductive age. These conditions continue to be frequent and often acute painful problems for which thousands of women seek relief annually. Symptoms include increase in vaginal discharge, itching, burning, dysuria, and dyspareunia. The physical examination may reveal vaginal and/or vulvar edema and erythema and a discharge that varies in color, odor, and consistency (Mou, 1999). Causes include candidiasis, trichomoniasis, bacteria, chemical irritants, allergens, and foreign bodies (Schuiling and Likis, 2006).

Pelvic inflammatory disease. Pelvic inflammatory disease (PID) refers to acute infection of the upper genital tract structures in women, involving any or all of the uterus, fallopian tubes, and ovaries. It is estimated that more than 1 million women have an episode of acute PID each year (Epperly and Viera, 2005). PID is considered a community-acquired infection initiated by a sexually transmitted agent.

Women with PID often have atypical or no symptoms, which delay diagnosis and treatment. If symptomatic, a woman may have lower abdominal or pelvic pain, malodorous or new-onset vaginal discharge, abnormal uterine/vaginal bleeding, dyspareunia, dysuria, nausea, vomiting, and fever. The diagnosis of PID is often based on imprecise clinical findings. Definitive diagnosis is obtained best by laparoscopy, but this surgical procedure has risks and is hard to justify for mild cases. Despite this, diagnosis and treatment are critical to prevent serious reproductive sequelae, including ectopic pregnancy and infertility. Young women having lower abdominal pain and who are at risk for STDs should be treated with multiple antimicrobials that cover the potential microorganisms listed at the CDC STD website (www.cdc.gov/std/treatment/2006/updated-regimens.htm). Their partner(s) should also receive treatment, and all parties should be instructed to abstain from intercourse until treatment is complete.

Toxic shock syndrome. Toxic shock syndrome (TSS) is a rare but serious disorder caused by toxins released by some strains of *Staphylococcus aureus.* TSS came to public attention in 1980 on the basis of a series of menstrually associated cases (Davis et al., 1980). The number of cases of menstrual TSS has declined from nine out of 100,000 women in 1980 to one out of 100,000 women since 1986 (CDC, 1990). It is most often associated with tampon use during menses; nonmenstrual TSS risk is increased for women who use vaginal barrier methods for birth control (Cates, Ellertson, and Stewart, 2004). The incidence of TSS has declined over the years owing to product changes and media warnings about tampon use (Farley, 1994). Although rare, TSS is a serious disorder of women's health, and providers must make women aware of this acute illness and its potential consequences, encourage them to report symptoms early, and exercise caution when using tampons and vaginal family planning methods (Cates et al., 2004).

Chronic Illness

Included among chronic diseases that may affect a woman during her life span are coronary vascular disease and metabolic syndrome, hypertension, diabetes, arthritis, osteoporosis, and cancer.

Coronary Vascular Disease and Metabolic Syndrome

Evidence suggests that coronary vascular disease (and metabolic syndrome in most women are preventable. Coronary vascular disease is caused by arthrosclerosis, which results in buildup of plaque that narrows arteries, decreasing blood flow to the heart muscle. *Metabolic syndrome* is a group of risk factors that have been linked to an increased risk of cardiovascular events. These factors include abdominal obesity (waist circumference greater than 35 inches in women), dyslipidemia (elevated triglycerides and low high-density lipoprotein), insulin resistance, and elevated blood pressure. The underlying etiology of metabolic syndrome is related to the combination of inactivity, obesity, and genetics.

At-risk women will have nonmodifiable risk factors such as increasing age, race, gender, or family history of coronary vascular disease and diabetes. Where the greatest impact can be made is with the modifiable risk factors including

- Cigarette smoking
- Obesity
- Diet high in calories, total fats, cholesterol, refined carbohydrates, and sodium
- Glucose intolerance
- Elevated serum lipid levels
- Sedentary lifestyle
- Personality type
- Hypertension
- Stress
- Alcohol (AHA, 2009c)

Education by community nurses can assist women in identifying their risk of CVD and metabolic syndrome along with health behaviors that decrease modifiable risk factors. Also important are evidence-based recommendations for high-risk women with existing CVD, including aspirin therapy and omega-3 supplementation (Mosca, 2007).

Hypertension

The latest report of the Joint National Committee on Prevention, Detection, Evaluation, and Treatment of High Blood Pressure defines hypertension as blood pressure of 140/90 mm Hg or greater. The guidelines include the category, "prehypertensive," which refers to systolic pressure of 120 to 139 mm Hg and/or diastolic pressure of 80 to 89 mm Hg. Clients with prehypertension are at increased risk for progression to hypertension and require lifestyle modifications to prevent CVD (Chobanian et al., 2003). Essential hypertension is the most common type of chronic hypertensive disorder in women of childbearing age, accounting for 85% of such cases. It is also responsible for approximately one third of all hypertension cases during pregnancy. Hypertension is more common in women than in men and affects more blacks than whites. Additional factors associated with primary hypertension are age (older than 35 years), family history of hypertension, obesity, cigarette smoking, and diabetes mellitus (AHA, 2005). Hypertension usually starts with an asymptomatic phase; therefore, every woman should be screened on an average of every 2 years beginning in her teenage years. Diagnosis is crucial to prevent or modify possible complications of this disease.

Diabetes

According to the American Diabetes Association (2009), 23.6 million people (7.8% of the population) in the United States have diabetes, and the number is growing every year. Furthermore, although an estimated 17.9 million have been diagnosed, some 5.7 million people are not aware they have the disease. In previous years, community health nurses have worked to educate women to assume responsibility in their management of diabetes mellitus. More recently, community health nurses have been actively involved in education and screening programs for groups at high risk. Included in these groups are individuals who have a family history of diabetes, those who are obese, and older adults. Nurses who

design education programs need to be aware of the ethnic differences in the prevalence of diabetes. African-American, Hispanic, American Indian, and Asian women are two to four times more likely to have diabetes than their non-Latino white counterparts (American Diabetes Association, 2009).

According to Cunningham and colleagues (2005), pregnancy is potentially diabetogenic. Pregnancy may aggravate the condition, and clinical diabetes may appear in some women only during pregnancy. Consequently, screening for diabetes is routine in pregnancy.

Controversy surrounds the most effective method of screening for diabetes, but regardless of the selected method, the nurse is involved in explaining the purpose of the screening and how to prepare for the tests. In most public health settings, the nurse is responsible for explaining the results.

Arthritis

In 2006, 46 million people in the United States, nearly one in five adults, were afflicted with arthritis. The incidence of osteoarthritis is higher in women than in men: approximately 24.3 million women have the condition compared with 17.1 million men (Arthritis Foundation, 2010).

Osteoarthritis (OA) is the most common form of the disease. It is characterized by degeneration of the joints and is more common with increasing age and in women. OA of the knee is the leading cause of disability in the United States. Modifiable risk factors for OA include excess body mass, joint injury, occupation, and estrogen deficiency (CDC, 2008a).

Rheumatoid arthritis (RA) can affect anyone, but 70% of people with RA are women. Onset usually occurs between 30 and 50 years of age. RA often goes into remission in pregnant women, although symptoms tend to increase in intensity after the baby is born, and RA develops more often than expected the year after giving birth. Although women are two to three times more likely to get RA than men, men tend to be more severely affected when they do get it (Arthritis Foundation, 2010).

Arthritis is the leading cause of disability in the United States (CDC, 2007a). Nursing interventions focus on prevention of joint deformity and lifestyle modification if necessary.

Osteoporosis

Osteoporosis is a major disorder affecting women, occurring in 25% to 50% of postmenopausal women. Although men may have osteoporosis, it is four times more common among women. The Arthritis Foundation (2010) estimates that of the 10 million Americans who have osteoporosis, 8 million are women and 2 million are men. An additional 34 million Americans have osteopenia. Half of all non-Hispanic white women in the United States will sustain an osteoporosis-related fracture during their lifetime. The most serious complication of osteoporosis is hip fracture, which is experienced by 280,000 Americans annually. Approximately 24% die within a year of complications from hip fracture (USDHHS, 2000b).

Postmenopausal white women are at highest risk for osteoporosis. In women, loss of bone begins at an earlier age and proceeds twice as rapidly as in men. The recent guidelines issued by the National Osteoporosis Foundation recommend bone mineral density tests for selected post-menopausal women and the use of oral bisphosphonates as the first-line pharmacological treatment of osteoporosis. In light of the results of the women's health initiative study showing that nonestrogen therapies fail or cause intolerance to side effects, hormone replacement therapy is currently considered second-line therapy (Wei et al., 2003). Osteoporosis has no cure; therefore prevention is especially important early in life. Prevention involves an awareness of dietary practices such as maintaining a correct balance of calcium, vitamin D, and protein throughout life, in addition to regular weight-bearing, muscle-strengthening, and aerobic exercise.

Nurses in ambulatory health practices should encourage women to become more knowledgeable of the strategies to prevent osteoporosis. For women with a diagnosis of osteoporosis, nurses can assist in various aspects of management (e.g., education regarding prescribed medication, follow-up care, avoidance of complications, and dietary modifications as needed).

Breast Cancer

The incidence of breast cancer has been increasing since the 1950s. Presently, one of every eight women will acquire breast cancer sometime in her life. The chance of dying of breast cancer is about one in thirty-five. The ACS estimated that 192,370 women in the United States would be found to have invasive breast cancer in 2009. Risk factors include aging, personal or family history (especially mother or sister) of breast cancer, early age at menarche, late age at menopause, never having children, or having a first child after age 30 years. Female gender and aging are the most significant risk factors for breast cancer (ACS, 2009).

According to the results of a randomized trial of women employed in Shanghai textile factories from October 1989 through July 2000, the mortality rate from breast cancer in women who practiced BSE was no lower than in women who did not practice BSE. In the group that practiced BSE, there was a higher rate of breast biopsy that did not reveal breast cancer. These findings were confirmed by a Denmark-published study in 2009, although both studies had reported low compliance. Recent evidence demonstrated that detection of abnormality using BSE in women with high risk for breast cancer is as accurate as a mammogram or magnetic resonance imaging (MRI) (Mulcahy, 2009).

In 2009, the U.S. Preventative Task Force published recommendations based on review of scientific evidence that women should not get routine mammography screening between the ages of 40-49, and receive biennial screenings between the ages of 50-74 (Agency for Healthcare Research and Quality, 2009). This is a major shift from current recommendations of annual screening mammograms for women over the age of 40. The researchers cited this recommended change was due to improvements in mammography screening films which leads to more accurate diagnosing. Also cited were the high cost and harmful psychological effects on women related to unnecessary diagnostic testing resulting from the high number of false positive screens. The America Cancer Society and the National Cancer Institute did not respond with changing their guidelines, but by recommending an increased focus on the woman's informed choice based on her individual risk factors for developing breast cancer. The current position of the U.S. Preventative Health Services Task Force is that there is insufficient evidence to recommend for or against the teaching of BSE (Thomas et al., 2002).

The American Cancer Society (2008) recommendations for BSE are:

- BSE should be performed monthly beginning at age 20 years. BSE is only one part of a three-part early detection program, which should include mammography and clinical breast examination.
- Mammography and clinical breast examination have the greatest impact on reducing breast cancer mortality. BSE's role in early detection is a supporting but important one.
- BSE contributes to awareness, helping women be alert to changes in their breasts and to identify changes earlier. However, for women 40 years of age and older, the greatest potential to save lives from breast cancer is through early detection with mammography.

In addition to annual mammography, the annual clinical breast exam is key to screening. Other methods for detecting breast cancer involve digital mammograms, ultrasound, MRI, positron emission tomography (PET) scan, and testing for genetic mutations such as BRCA 1 and 2 (National Cancer Institute, 2009). Box 17-2 lists resources that provide information about breast cancer and early detection.

RESEARCH HIGHLIGHTS

Breast Cancer Study

A number of clinical trials in the 1990s and 2000s indicated that self breast examinations (SBEs) were not effective in increasing the survival rate in women in whom breast cancer was diagnosed. In fact, the prevailing thought has been that SBE increases patient anxiety and unnecessary biopsies. Two of those studies, done in Russia and China, demonstrated poor compliance with the SBE by the participants.

A study done in 147 women at Duke University who scored high on the GALE breast cancer risk assessment demonstrated that performing SBEs was as effective as MRI and mammography in detecting early cancer. Another retrospective study done at Harvard University showed that in a group of 628 women under the age of 40 years, 71% had detected their own breast cancer with SBE.

From American Society of Breast Surgeons 10th Annual Meeting: abstracts 9 and 20. Presented April 24, 2009.

Lung Cancer

Although breast cancer is the most common cancer among women (i.e., excluding skin cancer), cancer of the lung and bronchus is responsible for more cancer deaths. Lung cancer is responsible for more deaths yearly in U.S. women than breast cancer. In fact, lung cancer kills more women annually than breast, ovarian, and uterine cancers combined (ACS, 2009). Between 1990 and 2003, there was a 60% increase in the number of new cases of lung cancer in American women, whereas the number of men in whom lung cancer was diagnosed remained stable (Patel, 2005). The increase in the incidence of lung cancer in women is due primarily to an increase in their tobacco use: 85% to 90% of all clients in whom lung cancer develops have a history of cigarette smoking. Yet, lung cancer develops in only 20% of cigarette smokers, suggesting that the cause of lung cancer is multifactorial.

Widely accepted risk factors for lung cancer include exposure to environmental tobacco smoke, certain occupational exposures (especially asbestos), genetic predisposition, sex, gender, diet, chronic lung disease, and a history of tobacco-related cancer (Rivera and Stover, 2004). Studies have shown that the risks for development of lung cancer are different in women compared with men and that lung cancer appears to be a biologically different disease in women. Women smokers are more likely than men to have adenocarcinoma of the lung, and women who have never smoked are more likely to have lung cancer than men who have never smoked. These differences are due to hormonal, genetic, and metabolic differences between the sexes (Patel, 2005).

Although medical treatment may be similar for men and women, the symptom distress, quality of life, and demands of illness experienced by women may be different than they are for men because the competing household, child care, and other role-related demands take a toll on many women (Sarna and McCorkle, 1996). Further, women with advanced lung cancer report more psychological symptoms than men (Hopwood and Stephens, 1995).

Lung cancer is often a fatal illness because it is difficult to obtain early detection and effective treatment for advanced disease. Lung cancer at diagnosis is most commonly at an advanced stage. Women appear to have a slight survival advantage over men: the 5-year survival rate for women who have lung cancer is 15.6% compared with 12.4% for men (Patel, 2005).

The primary factor in preventing lung cancer is for individuals to never start smoking or to quit smoking. Nurses must work with other health care providers to reverse the morbidity and mortality rates related to this disease. The Agency for Healthcare Research and Quality has developed a useful guideline for health care professionals to assist women and their families in smoking cessation efforts plus summaries of more than 400 guidelines on a wide variety of topics, which can be found on its website (www.ahrq.gov).

Gynecological Cancers

About 20% of all malignant diseases in women occur in the genital tract. Carcinoma of the cervix is the most common and accounts for 21% of all new genital tract malignancies. The cervix is accessible to cytologic study; therefore the mortality rate related to cervical cancer has decreased. Risk factors for cervical cancer include coitus at an early age, multiple sexual partners, history of sexually transmitted infections with certain types of HPV, cigarette smoking, and low socioeconomic status (ACS, 2006).

The incidence of invasive cervical cancer has declined dramatically as a result of regular Pap tests that allow for identification of a precancerous condition (i.e., cervical carcinoma in situ). However, the ACS (2008) estimated that 3700 women would die of the disease.

Current guidelines recommend cervical cancer screening to begin approximately 3 years after a woman begins having vaginal intercourse, but no later than 21 years of age. Screening should be done every year with regular Pap tests every 2 years using liquid-based tests, with HPV DNA testing to be added if the Pap smear result is abnormal. HPV DNA is not recommended for routine screening in adolescent women, as the prevalence of HPV is 60% to 80% at this age, and more than 90% of those who are positive will clear the HPV within 1 to 2 years of sexual debut (Wright et al., 2006). At or after age 30 years, women who have had three normal test results in a row may get screened every 2 to 3 years. Women aged 70 years and older who have had three or more consecutive Pap tests in the past 10 years may choose to stop cervical cancer screening (ACS, 2009). Evidence is also emerging that HPV infection is linked to 30% of cancers of the anus and throat (National Cancer Institute, 2009).

According to the National Cancer Institute (2009), the incidence of carcinoma of the endometrium has declined 25% since 1974. This drop has been attributed to the decline in women using unopposed exogenous estrogen to control menopausal symptoms. It is commonly found in women during their sixth and seventh decades of life (i.e., 80% of women with this condition are postmenopausal). Approximately 7470 women in the United States died of endometrial cancer in 2009. The incidence of endometrial cancer is highest among white women, but mortality is higher among black women, suggesting disparity in diagnosis and/or treatment. Factors related to its occurrence are obesity, low parity, diabetes mellitus, and conditions in which high circulating estrogen levels are not countered by adequate progesterone levels. The most common sign of endometrial cancer, occurring in 90% of women, is abnormal vaginal bleeding. Postmenopausal women experiencing vaginal bleeding should seek immediate gynecological evaluation.

Cancer of the ovary causes more deaths than any other pelvic malignancy. In the United States, the lifetime risk of ovarian cancer is 1.48%. The incidence for ages 75 to 79 years is 57.3 in 100,000 women. In 2005, 19,842 new cases were diagnosed, and 14,874 women died (CDC, 2009f). Risk factors include increasing age, nulliparity, never having breastfed, a history of breast cancer, postmenopausal use of hormone replacement therapy, obesity, and a family history of breast and ovarian cancer. Protective factors against ovarian cancer include use of oral contraceptives, having and breastfeeding children, tubal sterilization, hysterectomy, and prophylactic oophorectomy (National Cancer Institute, 2009).

Ovarian cancer is a silent cancer. Early-stage detection of ovarian cancer is difficult; therefore it has usually reached an advanced stage once discovered. The health professional should be alert to ovarian enlargement on pelvic examination with suspicion that ovarian malignancy may be present, especially in postmenopausal women. The most common sign a woman experiences is abdominal enlargement. She may complain that her skirts and slacks are getting tighter in the waist. Any woman older than age 40 years who has vague digestive complaints that persist and are not explained by another cause must have a thorough evaluation for ovarian cancer. According to the CDC, (2010), transvaginal ultrasound and a blood test for tumor marker CA 125 may assist in the diagnosis of ovarian cancer. These are not recommended for routine screening of all women but are recommended for those with risk factors related to family history (strong family history of ovarian and breast cancer, positive test genetic mutations BRCA 1 and 2).

Mental Disorders and Stress

Various circumstances and conditions influence the mental health of women. Women face stressful decisions about career and family, and many express anxieties with these decisions.

A woman may feel pressured to make decisions regarding childbearing before she has fulfilled her career goals. Deciding to focus on a career may mean decreased authority and the suffering of stress in the workplace. Women combining motherhood and a career have additional decisions such as working during pregnancy and choice of child care. More women are occupying middle-management positions, which are known for creating stress-related illness associated with high demands and little or no power.

A woman's emotional state can be influenced by ovarian function from the onset of menstruation to the cessation of menstrual periods. Depression may be triggered or worsened by hormonal changes premenstrually. Women with a history of depression are also at increased risk for a recurrent episode of depression during the postpartum period, and they also are at risk for depression during the perimenopausal transition (Blehar, 2003). Depression is more prevalent among women than among men. In all age groups from adolescents through the elderly, approximately two thirds of those affected are women. According to Bhatia and Bhatia (1999), the higher prevalence of depression in women is most likely due to a combination of gender-related differences in cognitive styles, certain biological factors, and a higher incidence of psychosocial and economic stressors.

Mental disorders often go undiagnosed and untreated or undertreated despite the availability of effective treatments. Women may fail to recognize or correctly identify their symptoms, and even when they do, they may be reluctant to seek care because of stigma associated with mental illness (Blehar, 2003). Community health nurses are in a good position to assess women's moods in diverse aggregates and to assist in seeking and maintaining continuity of care (see Box 17-1).

Reproductive Health

Community health nurses provide a variety of services in the area of women's reproductive health from menarche through postmenopause. Nurses, in collaboration with other health care professionals, have identified a persistent group of preventable and correctable problems related to maternal-child health. *Healthy People 2010* (USDHHS, 2000b) provides numerous recommendations for improving maternal and infant health, including reduction of cigarette smoking, reduction of alcohol and other drug use, optimal nutrition, improved socioeconomic opportunities (including education), and decreased environmental hazards.

For the *Healthy People 2000* initiative, family planning objectives witnessed progress. For example, the number of unintended pregnancies decreased from 56% to 49% between 1988 and 1995. Adolescent pregnancy rates had also seen a decrease until the year 2005, but a 5% increase was seen between 2005 and 2007 (CDC, 2009c). With *Healthy People 2020* family planning objectives, the focus is on the positive that "all pregnancies should be intended." Examples of *Healthy People 2020* objectives related to family planning are shown in the *Healthy People 2020* table.

HEALTHY PEOPLE 2020

Selected Proposed Objectives for Family Planning

OBJECTIVE
FP HP2020–1: Increase the proportion of pregnancies that are intended. FP HP2020–8: Reduce pregnancy rates among adolescent females. FP HP2020–13: Increase the proportion of sexually active women who received reproductive health services in the last 12 months. MICH HP2020–25: Among women delivering a live birth, increase the percentage who receive preconception care services and practice key recommended preconception health behaviors. MICH HP2020–31a: Reduce the proportion of persons (women) aged 18-44 years who have impaired fecundity (i.e. physical barrier preventing pregnancy or carrying a pregnancy to term).

U.S. Department of Health and Human Services. Healthy People 2020 Draft Objectives 2009. http://www.healthypeople.gov/hp2020/Objectives/files/Draft2009Objectives.pdf

Nutrition

One of the most important factors in a woman's reproductive health is her total life nutritional experience from infancy through childhood and adolescence. Obesity has become a major public health concern. The community health nurse is in an advantageous position to provide nutritional counseling. The U.S. Department of Agriculture updates the dietary recommendations every 5 years based on current scientific information, and the 2005 Food Guide Pyramid stresses a personalized approach to healthy eating and physical activity. The new dietary pyramid includes the addition of the variable of activity, focusing on the importance of moderation, proportionality, and variety. It also depicts the five food groups and oils, and advocates personalization and gradual improvement. The updated guidelines encourage most Americans to eat fewer calories, be more active, and make wiser food choices (USDHHS, 2005b).

Pregnancy may provide a motivational factor for developing an awareness of proper nutrition. During the nutritional assessment of a prenatal client, the community health nurse can take the opportunity to determine dietary habits and initiate a referral to the Special Supplemental Food Program for Women, Infants, and Children (WIC). WIC provides food vouchers for pregnant or breastfeeding women, infants, and children who are at nutritional risk.

Good nutrition must include factors other than kinds and amounts of foods. Other elements to consider include age, lifestyle, economic status, and culture. For example, when counseling a pregnant adolescent, the nurse can include the primary person responsible for meal preparation. The nurse should include the adolescent in the planning of her diet, asking her to identify foods that she likes from those recommended. The nurse should make the adolescent aware of the influence of her nutrition on fetal growth and development. This information must be balanced with the young woman's individual needs.

Dysmenorrhea is another reproductive health problem affecting approximately 50% to 80% of the female population between ages 15 and 24 years (Nelson, 2004). At least 10% to 20% of women with dysmenorrhea are incapacitated for 1 to 3 days each month. Dysmenorrhea is the greatest single cause of absenteeism from school and work among young women and causes the loss of approximately 140 million working hours annually; therefore the economic influence of this condition is significant.

ETHICAL INSIGHTS

Working with Women's Health

Community health nurses working in the field of women's health will be exposed to ethical dilemmas during their career. Due to this, nurses must have a working knowledge of the principles of health care ethics. The commonly accepted principles include the following:

- Respect for autonomy
- Beneficence
- Nonmaleficence
- Justice

Nursing care revolves around moral values such as compassion, empathy, honesty, trust, and respect. Most encounters will be nonproblematic. Occasionally, nurses may be exposed to clinical situations that challenge their values and beliefs. Clients and family members may, at times, also disagree with the nurse's professional advice/plan. It is important for the nurse to keep his or her personal philosophy, politics, religion, and moral values out of clinical work with individuals and families.

Examples of potential ethical dilemmas related to women's health care are emergency contraception, abortion, assisted reproductive technology, and end-of-life issues.

Family Planning

The community health nurse has many opportunities to provide counseling in the area of family planning. Although the phrase "family planning" has come to imply planned limitation of pregnancies, another important aspect of family planning concerns couples attempting to increase their chances of conception. This is because infertility occurs in a surprising number of otherwise healthy adults. Indeed, approximately 10% to 15% of couples in the United States are unintentionally childless (Nelson and Marshall, 2004).

Community health nurses are in a strategic position to provide support and guidance for women in the area of fertility control. Numerous factors contribute to the decision of whether to use family planning methods and what methods to use. When counseling women on this matter, the nurse should use a holistic approach. The nurse must consider factors such as age, sexual activity, cost, health care access, and the woman's and her partner's values and beliefs. After a discussion with the nurse about benefits and risks, indications and contraindications, and advantages and disadvantages of the various contraception methods, the client selects a method that she believes is safe, effective, and comfortable.

Methods of family planning include hormones such as oral contraceptive pills, long-term injections, subcutaneous implants, vaginal rings, and intrauterine devices. Barrier methods such as condoms and diaphragms afford less-effective protection in terms of pregnancy prevention and are most effective when combined with spermicides. When counseling women on their method of choice it is imperative that safer sex practices such as condom use be employed if the woman is at risk for acquiring a sexually transmitted infection.

Natural family planning is a method of contraception that, in order to be effective, requires motivation by the couple. Proponents of natural family planning describe this method as natural reproductive technology, a term that is broader in scope and encompasses the health of a woman's reproductive system. Such self-knowledge encourages feelings of empowerment and a sense of control over fertility.

Women who decide that their families are large enough and do not wish to be concerned with temporary methods of fertility control may select voluntary surgical contraception (VSC) or contraceptive sterilization by tubal ligation. The VSC is one of the most effective, safe, and cost-effective methods of family planning, and developed and developing countries use it widely. Vasectomy as a VSC continues to be the simpler, safer, and less-expensive procedure than tubal ligation (Pollack, Carignan, and Jacobstein, 2004). The client's decision must be based on clear, complete information for sterilization more than any other phase of family planning. The reversibility of sterilization procedures is not dependable; if a woman has doubts about her future childbearing, the nurse should encourage her to use other methods of fertility control.

Nurses worldwide have a major role to play if the health of women and their families is to improve. Besides being knowledgeable about family planning methods and services, all nurses must work for universally accessible maternal and child health care and seek to protect the rights of couples and individuals to receive good information about family planning. In addition, nurses must be involved in shaping policy that affects every woman's reproductive health. Research in the area of family planning has provided multiple safe options designed to meet the individual needs of all women.

Sexually Transmitted Diseases and Human Immunodeficiency Virus

STDs are commonly found among U.S. women. Community health nurses and other health providers, including physicians, nurse practitioners (NPs), nurse-midwives, and social workers, must be prepared to provide age-appropriate STD prevention, education, and counseling.

Sexually transmitted diseases. In 2007, the CDC reported the most common STD was infection with *Chlamydia trachomatis* (1,108,374 cases), followed by *Neisseria gonorrhoeae* (355,991 cases). This was the largest number of chlamydia cases ever reported. Chlamydia is diagnosed three times more in women than men, most likely because of CDC-recommended routine screening for any sexually active woman of childbearing age to prevent infertility. Gonorrhea

is also diagnosed more often in women but is particularly high in black women, who have the disease diagnosed 15 times more often than do white women. The Gonococcal Isolate Surveillance Project (GISP) demonstrated that gonorrhea was becoming resistant to treatment with CDC-recommended fluoroquinolone drugs in 2007, prompting the CDC to revise treatment guidelines (CDC, 2007d).

When rates of syphilis, another STD, dropped nearly 90% between 1990 and 2000, the CDC initiated the "National Plan to Eliminate Syphilis." However, rates have increased yearly since 2001. Racial disparity in cases of syphilis has improved, from 1999 when the diagnosis was made in twenty-nine times more blacks than whites down to a rate that is now seven times higher. The major increase in syphilis since 2001 has been in men, especially men having sex with men, and less in women (CDC, 2007d).

Treatments of STDs are outlined in the CDC guidelines, which are updated regularly (www.cdc.gov/std/treatment/2006/rr5511.pdf). A vital role of the community health nurse is to follow up with the woman's sex partner(s) who requires evaluation and treatment. Partner notification and expedited treatment, along with avoiding sexual activity until they are treated/cured, are key to stopping the spread of STDs. In addition to medications, women and their partners need individualized counseling on reducing risky sexual behaviors.

Human immunodeficiency virus and acquired immunodeficiency syndrome. Today, the HIV/AIDS epidemic represents a growing and persistent health threat to women in the United States, especially young women and women of color. According to the CDC (2009b), HIV infection was the third leading cause of death for African-American women aged 25 to 44 years and was the fourth leading cause of death for those aged 45 to 54 years. Among women with a diagnosis of HIV/AIDS, 64% are black, yet blacks make up only 13% of the general population. The majority of infants born with HIV are black. For all ethnicities, primary transmission in men is through sexual contact with other men, whereas in women it is high-risk heterosexual contact. HIV disease among Hispanic women aged 25 to 44 years was the fifth leading cause of death. Worldwide, AIDS is a leading cause of death among young women (WHO, 2004).

According to the CDC (2009b), risk factors and barriers to prevention for women include the following:

- Young age at sexual initiation
- Lack of awareness regarding disease and condom use
- Sexual inequality in relationships
- Biological vulnerability and sexually transmitted infections
- Substance abuse
- Poverty, out of school
- Stigma surrounding testing and treatment
- Working in the sex trade
- Participants in unprotected sex

In November 2008, the USDHHS released the updated *Guidelines for the Use of Antiretroviral Agents in HIV-1 Infected Adults and Adolescents* (USDHHS, 2005b). Treatment guidelines continually evolve with new research and experience. The use of antiretroviral drugs has decreased the rate of death for HIV disease in women, which peaked in 1993-1994 at 6 per 100,000, down to 2.5 per 100,000 (CDC, 2009b). It is imperative that the community health nurse working with this population stay abreast of the current trends for both counseling and treatment options. Community health nurses also must target at-risk populations and campaign for the use of safer sex practices and routine testing for HIV for those at risk.

Other Issues in Women's Health
Unintentional Injury or Accidents

Although unintentional injury affects women less commonly than it does men, several areas of concern still exist for women. For example, older women are at increased risk for accidents such as falls. Falls account for the majority of serious unintentional injuries and lead to 40% of all deaths from injury in people older than 75 years of age. Factors that may be responsible for this major cause of injury among older adults are an unsteady gait, reduced vision, or a hazardous environment. Older women experience an increasing number of falls; therefore the nurse must identify the preventable factors. Nurses, whether working with older adults in the home or in institutional settings, must be knowledgeable of hazards that may be corrected to decrease the incidence of falls.

Domestic violence is the single largest cause of injury to women between the ages of 15 and 44 years in the United States—more than muggings, car accidents, and rapes combined. Each year 4.8 million women are battered. In 2004, 1158 of these women died of their injuries. Two thirds of women are abused by a current or former intimate partner (CDC, 2008d).

Abuse in women is often explained as accidental injury. Approximately 6% of visits made by women to emergency departments are because of injuries that result from physical battering by their husbands, former husbands, boyfriends, or lovers. Domestic violence includes physical, sexual, and psychological attacks and economic coercion (Warshaw, Ganley, and Salber, 1995). Reports of teen dating abuse indicate that one in five teens report some sort of abuse and one in four girls report being sexually coerced (CDC, 2008d).

Nurses employed in community health settings need to know how to make assessments, provide support, and make referrals to agencies dealing with domestic violence. Understanding the state laws related to reporting known or suspected domestic violence is important. The American Medical Association and American Nurses Association advocate that all women should be assessed for intimate partner violence. Questions should be posed privately, in nonjudgmental specific terms (i.e., "Do you feel safe?" "Have you ever been hit, punched, slapped, or kicked?") with follow-up questions if the woman responds "yes" (Kovach, 2004). However, according to Blair (1999), barriers can interfere with such screening, including frustration when clients fail to leave the abusive situation after intensive intervention or counseling. Also, many nurses are past or current victims of abuse; assessing abuse with clients can evoke painful emotions that the nurse may not be ready to confront. Chapter 27 contains additional information about domestic violence.

Disability

More women than men have disabilities resulting from acute conditions, but women experience fewer disabilities resulting from chronic conditions because they report their symptoms earlier and receive necessary treatment. According to the U.S. Census Bureau (2000), of the 2.7 million disabled persons, 48% are men and 52% are women. Women report proportionately more days of restricted activity than men. Women average 16.1 days of disability per year compared with 12.7 days for men (U.S. Census Bureau, 2000).

Disabling conditions limit the physical functional abilities of many women, but the health care delivery system has often overlooked the unique needs of this aggregate. In planning care for disabled women, community health nurses should focus attention on enabling women to strengthen their capabilities. In addition, nurses should be sensitive to barriers in the clinical setting that affect the access of disabled women to health care services. Chapter 21 discusses the needs of disabled people in greater detail.

MAJOR LEGISLATION AFFECTING WOMEN'S HEALTH

Several legislative acts have a direct or indirect influence on the health of women. Many changes have been made in the past two decades that have the potential for improving the health and welfare of all women.

Public Health Service Act

The Public Health Service (PHS) Act, passed in 1982, provides biomedical and health services research, information dissemination, resource development, technical assistance, and service delivery. In the area of women's health, the PHS Act supports activities related to general health issues, reproductive health, social and behavioral issues, and mental health. Aggregates of women targeted by the PHS Act include those disabled by specific diseases, victims of sexual abuse and domestic violence, recent immigrants, and occupational groups.

Title X of the PHS Act is the Family Planning Public Service Act, which helped 5 million women obtain family planning services in 2008. Since 1970, federally subsidized family planning funds have been available to clinics and health departments throughout the country. These facilities provide not only access to contraception but also routine preventive health services, education, and counseling. The program is an important part of the public effort to prevent low birth weight through addressing the relationship between lack of family planning and those at greatest risk for low-birth-weight infants (women who are adolescents, single, and/or low income) (Office of Population Affairs, 2009).

Civil Rights Act

Title VII of the Civil Rights Act of 1964 prohibits discrimination based on sex, race, color, religion, or national origin in determining employment eligibility or termination, wages, and fringe benefits. The Act was amended to prohibit discrimination against pregnant women or conditions involving childbirth or pregnancy. This landmark legislation makes it unlawful for employers to refuse to hire, employ, or promote a woman because she is pregnant. In addition, employee benefit plans that continue health insurance, income maintenance during disability or illness, or any other income support program for disabled workers must include disabilities resulting from pregnancy, childbirth, and other related conditions. If employers allow disabled employees to assume lighter or medically restricted assignments, the same considerations must extend to pregnant women.

The amendment does not require employers to pay health insurance benefits for abortions or abortion-related care unless the mother's life is endangered or she has medical complications after an abortion. Employers are prohibited from firing or refusing to hire a woman because she had an abortion.

Sexual harassment is a violation of the Civil Rights Act. Sexual harassment is "conduct of a sexual nature…unwelcome by the target…severe or pervasive enough to create an intimidating work environment" (Women Employed Institute, 1994). Female and male workers may face unwelcome sexual advances or requests for sexual favors or other verbal or physical conduct of a sexual nature. Awareness of sexual harassment in the workplace has increased dramatically over the past decade, but sexual harassment has not been eliminated.

Social Security Act

The Social Security Act provides monthly retirement and disability benefits to workers and survivor benefits to families of workers covered by Social Security. Full retirement benefits are available after 10 years of covered employment, and workers can collect partial benefits beginning at age 62 years and full benefits after age 67 years.

The Social Security Act permits a divorced person to receive benefits based on a former spouse's earning record when that spouse retires, becomes disabled, or dies if the marriage lasted at least 10 years. Since January 1985, a woman who has been divorced for at least 2 years can receive spousal benefits at age 62 years, if her former husband is eligible for benefits, regardless of whether he is actually receiving them.

Medicare and Medicaid also resulted from the Social Security Act. Medicare is the insurance plan that covers the majority of the health care expenses of older adults, including payments for hospital care, physicians, home health care, and other services and supplies after co-payments and deductibles. Medicaid covers health care for indigent and eligible children and includes family planning, obstetric care, and preventive cancer screening for women, such as mammography and Pap smears. Chapters 11 and 12 describe Medicare and Medicaid in detail.

Occupational Safety and Health Act

The Occupational Safety and Health Act, enacted in 1970, helps ensure safe and healthful working conditions for workers throughout the United States. Although there is an increasing emphasis on the study of the health of women workers, gaps in knowledge exist. For example, little is known about women who work in cottage industries, as domestic workers, as prostitutes, in agriculture, and in the garment industry. In addition, the work of some women is classified as "women's work" and includes such things as housework, child care, caregiver of the sick, and farming (Misner, Beauchamp-Hewitt, and Fox-Levin, 2004). These women experience physical demands and hazards, yet government economic reports have not recognized these individuals as workers. Investigations of factors that influence the health of these women workers are needed. Table 17-6 lists specific positions in which a large number of women are employed and the potential for health hazards within these positions.

Community health nurses, occupational health nurses, and NPs need to be cognizant of environmental hazards wherever they find women at work. In taking health histories, the nurse should collect data regarding the client's occupational environment to assess the potential risk to emotional, general, and reproductive health. In addition, nurses must work individually and as an aggregate with their legislatures to maintain strong worker health and safety programs to protect the health of all women.

Family and Medical Leave Act

Enacted in 1993, the Family and Medical Leave Act (FMLA) allows an employee a minimum provision of 12 weeks unpaid leave each year for family and medical reasons such as personal illness; an ill child, parent, or spouse; or the birth or adoption of a child. In 2008, FMLA was updated to include family

TABLE 17-6	HAZARDOUS OCCUPATIONS IN WHICH WOMEN ARE EMPLOYED
OCCUPATION	**HEALTH HAZARD**
Clerical workers	Organic solvents in stencil machines, correction fluids, rubber cement, and ozone from copying machines
Textile and apparel workers	Cotton dust, skin irritants, and chemicals
Hairdressers and beauticians	Hair, nail, and skin beauty preparations
Launderers and dry cleaners	Heat, heavy lifting, and chemicals
Electronics workers	Solvents and acids
Hospital and other health care workers	Infectious diseases, heavy lifting, radiation, skin disorders, and anesthetic gases
Laboratory workers	Biological agents; flammable explosive, toxic, or carcinogenic substances; exposure to radiation; and bites from and allergic reactions to research animals

providing care to members of the Armed Forces injured in the line of duty. This act guarantees the employee the same or equivalent job with the same pay and benefits upon the employee's return to work. In addition, health benefits must continue throughout the leave. Approximately 20% of the U.S. workforce needed some form of FMLA-covered leave after the law was enacted (Gilinson, 1999).

The FMLA is particularly important to female workers because they are more likely to use leave to care for seriously ill family members, whereas male workers more often use leave for personal illness (Gilinson, 1999). Employees who must be away from work for family and medical reasons lose income with the most significant impact on those without job-protected leave. The FMLA is an important step toward equitable leave policies, but more change is needed.

HEALTH AND SOCIAL SERVICES TO PROMOTE THE HEALTH OF WOMEN

Medicaid is a health insurance program that was instituted in 1965 for the poor. It is funded jointly by the federal and state governments but is administered by individual states. It is the largest source of funding for medical and health-related services for people with limited income, regardless of age eligibility. Medicaid is classified into five broad coverage groups: children, pregnant women, adults in families with dependent children, individuals with disabilities, and individuals 65 years or older.

Many of the pregnant women who are eligible for Medicaid are at high risk for poor pregnancy outcome, including low birth weight. Ideally, a maternity care provider should examine women with high maternal risk immediately after conception. However, too often these women seek prenatal care late in the pregnancy or arrive at the emergency department when delivery is imminent without having previously received prenatal care. This case is not unusual. Barriers limit access to prenatal care among those most in need. Medicaid allows some access to care. Greater public awareness of facilities and maternity care providers who accept Medicaid is necessary. Recent changes in payment plans that allow billing for care at higher rates have increased the number of providers who accept Medicaid clients.

Clinical Example

Anita Rogers, a 16-year-old unemployed single woman, arrived at the Family Services Health Center seeking initial prenatal care at 36 weeks' gestation. She stated that for a few days she noted some brown discharge from her vagina. She told the nurse she knew she should have begun prenatal care earlier, but, when she called several physicians' offices, the receptionist told her she should bring $1000 for her first visit. She said that neither she nor her parents had that much money. Her father was unemployed, and her mother worked at a café as a waitress. She also had difficulty with transportation. Anita was sent to the hospital immediately for an ultrasound examination. The sonogram revealed triplets, but two of them had died in utero. Anita was hospitalized and began to hemorrhage. She delivered a 3-lb infant.

Women's Health Services

Since the mid-1970s, women have sought health services beyond the conventional mode of care delivery. Many self-help groups have emerged, and new approaches to women's health services have been accepted. Women desire a participatory role in their health and have become more assertive. Health care facilities have recognized the importance of meeting women's health needs. A notable evolution has been in maternity care, where the demands of women as consumers lead to the emergence of freestanding and hospital-based birth centers and family- and sibling-attended births.

However, health care needs of women go beyond their reproductive status and include their primary health care needs. The health care needs of women must be addressed more effectively and should include services for the following (Star, Shannon, and Lommel, 2004):

1. Eating disorders
2. All forms of abuse
3. Disease prevention, including smoking cessation
4. Health promotion focusing on nutrition, exercise, and stress management

The National Women's Health Network has been a strong advocate for women's concerns and has provided testimony before congressional hearings dealing with women's issues. This organization is concerned with women's rights, environmental safety, reproductive rights, warnings regarding the effects of alcohol and drugs on the developing fetus, safety in relation to medical devices, and drug safety, especially that may have teratogenic or carcinogenic effects. Examples of its work include recall of the Dalkon Shield intrauterine device, identification of women who may have been exposed to diethylstilbestrol in utero, and promotion of well-women's health care.

Other Community Voluntary Services

Networking, a system of interconnected or cooperating individuals, has been one of the major movements during the past two decades. It is a means by which women seek to advance their careers, improve their lifestyles, and increase their income while helping other women become successful. Networks in business, professional support, politics and labor, arts, sports, and health have been established throughout the United States. These multiple networks have enabled women to develop new identities and become empowered to achieve mutual goals.

Many private voluntary organizations spend money, time, and energy in attempting to increase health awareness among their members and provide direct services to the public. Most urban areas have crisis hotline services in which women volunteer to provide counseling to battered women, battering parents, rape victims, those considering suicide, and those with multiple needs. One of the most effective, lowest-cost, voluntary efforts to assist abused women involves shelters and safe houses scattered throughout the United States. One of the goals of *Healthy People 2020* relates to this issue, as many women needing shelter are often denied emergency housing.

Women's organizations have a long history of voluntary involvement with the community. An increasing number have added activities to their agenda to improve pregnancy outcomes, prevent teen pregnancy, and support older women's rights. Organizations such as the Older Women's League, United Methodist Women, other religious denomination women's groups, Urban League, sororities, Junior League, YWCA, National Association of Colored Women's Clubs, and many others have made women's health a major item on their agenda.

LEVELS OF PREVENTION AND WOMEN'S HEALTH

Primary Prevention

The focus of primary prevention is preventing disease from occurring. Women should recognize the risk of disease and target their health care behaviors accordingly. Types of primary prevention include never smoking, following a nutritious diet, having safe sex practices, avoiding drugs, limiting alcohol consumption, and staying physically active.

Consider Jackie, a 39-year-old woman with three first-order relatives in whom breast and/or ovarian cancer was diagnosed. She is at risk for hereditary cancer and should seek genetic counseling and possibly testing. If genetic testing is positive, she should be given information on measures that could prevent cancer from occurring, which constitutes primary prevention. These measures include lifestyle choices (early childbearing/breastfeeding), prophylactic surgical procedures (oophorectomy/mastectomy), and medical treatment (contraceptive pills, tamoxifen). Vigilant screenings (pelvic ultrasound with CA 125/breast MRI) to detect cancer early would be considered secondary prevention.

Secondary Prevention

The focus of secondary prevention is detecting the disease once it has begun but before it appears clinically. Examples of this level of prevention would be routine screening for cervical cancer through Pap smears and for chlamydial infections through nucleic acid amplification tests either by urine or cervical specimen, and clinical breast examination and mammogram.

Tertiary Prevention

Tertiary prevention seeks to stop further complications after a disease has become clinically evident. For example, Sandra Smith, a 55-year-old Native American, has had diabetes mellitus for the past 3 years. She attended an urban clinic for monitoring her diabetes. After the physician examined her, he suggested that she have her annual pelvic examination. She was overdue for this and agreed to be seen by the women's health care NP. Ms. Smith described symptoms of a yeast infection (e.g., increase in vaginal discharge and itching) to the nurse. Her examination and a wet mount confirmed the diagnosis of *Candida albicans* infection, a common problem among women with diabetes. The woman learned about the nature, predisposing factors, and treatment of the infection.

CASE STUDY APPLICATION OF THE NURSING PROCESS

John Lawrence, an educator at the state women's correctional center, contacted Donna Williams, a women's health care nurse practitioner and faculty member at the College of Nursing, and expressed concern for the health of an inmate, Lela Marvin. According to Mr. Lawrence, Lela, a 19-year-old pregnant primigravida woman, was being seen at the state-supported hospital for antepartal care; however, she was not permitted to attend perinatal education classes. He stated that other pregnant women in the facility could benefit from perinatal education. In fact, approximately 6.1% of female state prison inmates are pregnant when admitted to prison and could benefit from perinatal education (Snell, 1994).

Lawrence's call was followed by a call from Herman Martin, an RN who also expressed concern for the other women's needs for information regarding their personal hygiene. Although an RN, Mr. Martin was not knowledgeable of women's health because his primary clinical focus was emergency and trauma care. He indicated that many of the women were overweight, cared little about themselves, and lacked a general knowledge of how to maintain their health.

Assessment

After gaining clearance by the prison officials, Ms. Williams made an assessment of health care information needs and started offering classes for the inmates. The immediate need was for perinatal education for women in the last weeks of pregnancy. Lela said she wanted to learn about labor because she had heard only horror stories from other women. Donna noted that three other women were close to term and they also seemed eager to learn. Donna knew that students' readiness to learn was key to the course's success. Success of this course would be crucial to future course offerings.

The traditional perinatal education course was designed to promote healthy birth outcomes and an emotionally satisfying birth experience. These goals are also important to pregnant women in a correctional facility; however, perinatal education should be modified to meet this group's special needs. For example, information on newborn care is not appropriate because the infant is usually placed with the mother's family or in foster care.

Assessment of nonpregnant women provided opportunities for other health education classes. The next spring and each spring thereafter, junior nursing students under the guidance of Ms. Williams were assigned to develop and carry out a 1-hour weekly health education and awareness session at the correctional facility. Although each student expressed some initial anxiety toward the experience, each evaluated it as being worthwhile.

Diagnosis

After assessment, the community health nurse developed community and aggregate diagnoses, which served as the basis for the care plan.

Individual
- Inadequate preparation for childbirth related to lack of resources in prison (Lela)
- Lack of family support related to separation secondary to incarceration (Lela)
- Potential for feelings of loss related to separation from infant after birth (Lela)

Family
- Lela's family visits were rare; therefore she looked for others to provide support during her pregnancy. Lela told Ms. Williams that her cellmate, Julieanna, offered to be her labor support person.
- Lack of knowledge of her role as a labor support person (Julieanna)

CASE STUDY APPLICATION OF THE NURSING PROCESS—cont'd

Community

- Deficient knowledge of adequate health-seeking behaviors of women in the correctional facility (i.e., pregnant and nonpregnant women)
- Lack of programs to promote health and prevent diseases among women prisoners

Planning

After validating the nursing diagnosis with the individual, family, or community, the plan of care is developed. Examples of long- and short-term goals follow.

Individual

Long-Term Goal
- Individual family members will have a positive birth experience (Lela).

Short-Term Goal
- Family member or friends will help Lela use relaxation techniques to cope with discomforts of labor.

Family

Long-Term Goal
- The family members will be strengthened through their newly acquired knowledge and skills.

Short-Term Goal
- The family members will demonstrate increased ability to perform role as labor support people.

Community

Long-Term Goal
- The health and well-being of incarcerated women (i.e., pregnant and nonpregnant) will improve.

Short-Term Goal
- Health education programs will be instituted to individuals, families, and aggregates in the correctional facility.

Intervention

The community health nurse works with the individual, family, or community to achieve mutually established goals. Intervention is aimed at empowering individuals and groups to take responsibility for themselves and form links with others to accomplish goals.

Individual

Providing a perinatal education program for Lela is Ms. Williams' first priority. In addition, counseling related to feelings of loss after birth may be appropriate. Referral to a counselor may be necessary, and Ms. Williams must become familiar with available resources.

Family

Teaching the family the roles and responsibilities of a labor support person is an important intervention. In the correctional facility, interventions must ensure that Lela has a labor support person to practice her relaxation techniques and be available. In this case, Lela's cellmate, Julieanna, was willing to act in this role, and the nurse must negotiate with prison officials to allow this arrangement.

Community

Specific interventions with a group of pregnant women in the correctional facility are based on the specific needs of the group. The community health nurse must identify prison officials who are supportive of health education programs and request input as to which women should be targeted for such programs. Then the nurse meets with targeted women to assess level of knowledge and skills regarding women's health. For example, the nurse should survey what the woman perceives as learning needs (e.g., well-women's care, women's anatomy and physiology, self-care in health promotion, health protection, and disease prevention). Then the nurse tailors an intervention that is compatible with the community. Ms. Williams asked each nursing student to select a topic based on the survey and develop a teaching plan for presentation to female prisoners (i.e., pregnant and nonpregnant) at least once during the spring semester.

Evaluation

The community health nurse compares the actual and predicted outcomes to determine the efficacy of the plan of care and make revisions.

Individual

For example, Lela learned necessary relaxation techniques that were useful to her in labor and assisted in making the birth experience positive. Follow-up of Lela's psychosocial concerns in postpartum was also important.

Family

Evaluation of this nontraditional family would include their level of satisfaction with their role in the birth experience. Evaluation would also include learning how this interaction between family members (i.e., Lela and Julieanna) prepared them for other situations.

Community

The aggregate evaluation focuses on the community. For example, in health education programs designed for pregnant and nonpregnant women in the correctional facility, it is important to do the following:
- Maintain attendance records.
- Seek feedback from women, the referring nurse-educator, and prison officials regarding changes in self-care behavior regarding health.
- Obtain student response to learning experience.
- Make changes in health education programs based on evaluation.

Levels of Prevention

The following are examples of the three levels of prevention as applied to the individual, family, and community.

Primary

- Assessment and teaching perinatal education course to pregnant inmates
- Assessment and teaching health education classes to nonpregnant inmates
- Teaching the family the roles and responsibilities of a labor support person

Secondary

- Screening at the community level (correctional facility) of what is perceived as learning needs
- Educating the family and community of the signs of postpartum depression

Tertiary

- Educating HIV-positive pregnant inmates on the need of antiviral treatment and delivery by cesarean section
- Educating family members and foster parents about the need of neonatal follow-up with regard to HIV status
- Assessing available community resources for counseling and treatment of postpartum depression

ROLES OF THE COMMUNITY HEALTH NURSE

Direct Care

The community health nurse provides direct care in a variety of settings. Often, this is considered the "hands-on" nursing care given to a client in the home or a clinic.

Educator

The nurse encounters many opportunities for teaching. To be successful with health education, the nurse must attempt to gain trust and be sensitive to any cultural issues present. The nurse must also be aware of the emotional and physical state of the client. If the client is anxious or in pain, teaching may be ineffective.

Counselor

The counseling role of the nurse occurs in almost every interaction in the area of women's health. Before beginning counseling in the area of reproductive health, it is essential for effective intervention that the nurse becomes aware of his or her value system, including how biases and beliefs about human sexual behavior affect the counseling role.

RESEARCH IN WOMEN'S HEALTH

Women have long been the major users of the health care system. Research involving women is beginning to provide information enabling prediction, explanation, or description of phenomena affecting health. In the past, medical treatment for women was based on research with male subjects exclusively, even in conditions that cause more deaths in women. Since the federal mandate regarding women and research was instituted, research efforts to include women in studies have grown. If women are not included in research, a rationale must be given for their exclusion.

The National Institutes of Health (NIH) established the Office of Research on Women's Health (ORWH) in 1990. Through a special task force, recommendations were made for the research agenda for women's health for the next two decades. In addition, nurse researchers are encouraged to test interventions and question rituals in nursing by conducting research. The following are some of the areas for exploration and research among women:

- Alcohol, tobacco, and other drug use
- Domestic violence
- Heart disease
- Health behaviors
- Genetic screening and breast cancer
- Bone and musculoskeletal disorders
- Cancer prevention, screening, diagnosis, and treatment
- Health education at various literacy levels
- Wellness across the life cycle
- Differences among women having menopausal symptoms
- Dysmenorrhea
- Safe and effective contraception
- Promotion of breastfeeding
- Infertility
- Coping with chronic illness, such as systemic lupus erythematosus or arthritis
- Discomforts of pregnancy, including morning sickness
- Strengths of single, female heads of households
- Adolescent sexuality
- Multiple-role adaptation
- Menstrual cycle variations
- Control of obesity
- Substance abuse and its effect on pregnancy
- HIV infection and pregnancy
- Influence of diet on osteoporosis
- Effect of socialization on role
- Gender differences in pharmacology

Currently, research on the financing and delivery of health services for women has been supported. The American Recovery and Reinvestment Act of 2009 provided funding to the NIH to support research in women's health by the ORWH. Overarching themes in women's health research identified by the ORWH include:

- Developmental, psychological, spiritual, and physiological factors' effect on life span
- Female determinants such as genetics and gender expectations' effect on health
- Health disparities and diversity
- Diseases and conditions affecting women
- Career development and advancement of women in the sciences

With the increased emphasis on community health, community health nurses can make significant contributions toward the improvement of women's health through scholarly research, either as principal investigators or through data gathering. Furthermore, they can become consumers of research and develop nursing interventions based on sound research and recommendations.

SUMMARY

Women's health care has multiple facets. Many areas for community health nursing intervention exist. Nurses are advocates and activists for women's health through their involvement in health policy making as a profession. Along with other multidisciplinary and consumer groups, professional nurses are in the forefront of making changes in the health care delivery system that will promote an overall quality and research-based health plan for women. Women are at the center of the health of the United States; therefore, if better models are developed for improving the health of women, the health of the entire nation will benefit.

LEARNING ACTIVITIES

1. Identify examples from everyday life that support or encourage violence against women (e.g., magazines, books, and television advertisements). Share findings with classmates.

2. Survey lay magazine advertisements and estimate the percentage of total pages that use a woman's image, including aging, menopause, overweight and obesity, and sexuality to sell products. Share these with classmates.

3. Discuss the need for cancer screening with female relatives; refer to the ACS guidelines.

4. Discuss with female relatives the need for a heart-healthy nutritional plan based on AHA guidelines.

5. Identify resources for mammograms and Pap smears for low-income women.

6. Visit with a women's group in the community (e.g., business, church, sorority, and Parents Without Partners, Red Hat Society) to discuss members' health care needs and concerns. From these data, develop research questions.

7. Call a family planning clinic and determine the population served (i.e., eligibility), available services, and costs.

8. Review county or state health department statistics for leading causes of death among women of varying ethnic or racial groups.

REFERENCES

Adams PF, Barnes PM, Vickerie JL: Summary health statistics for the U.S. population: National Health Interview Survey, 2007, *Vital Health Stat* 10(238):2008.

Agency for Healthcare Research and Quality, U.S. Preventative Services Task Force Recommendations: *Screening for breast cancer*, 2009. http://www.ahrq.gov/clinic/uspstf09/breastcancer/brcansum.htm. Accessed March 9, 2010.

American Academy of Pediatrics: *Family pediatrics: report of the task force on the family*, Elk Grove Village, IL, 2005, The Author.

American Cancer Society: *Cancer facts and figures 2006*, Atlanta, 2006, The Author. www.cancer.org.

American Cancer Society: *Guidelines for the early detection of cancer*, 2008, American Cancer Society Prevention and Early Detection. March 5, www.cancer.org/docroot/PED/content/PED_2_3X_ACS_Cancer_Detection_Guidelines_36.asp?sitearea=PED. Accessed April 25, 2009.

American Cancer Society: *Cancer statistics 2009*, www.cancer.org/docroot/PRO/content/PRO_1_1_Cancer_Statistics_2009_Presentation.asp. Accessed May 8, 2009.

American College of Nurse Midwives Position Statement: *Elective primary cesarean section*, Dec. 2005, www.midwife.org/siteFiles/position/Elective_Primary_CS.pdf. Accessed May 14, 2009.

American Diabetes Association: *Total prevalence of diabetes & pre-diabetes, All about diabetes*, 2009, www.diabetes.org/diabetes-statistics/prevalence.jsp. Accessed May 22, 2009.

American Heart Association: *Heart disease and stroke statistics, 2005 update*, Dallas, Texas, 2005, The Author. www.americanheart.org.

American Heart Association: *Heart disease and stroke statistics 2009 update: A report from the American Heart Association Statistics Committee and Stroke Statistics Subcommittee: Circulation* 119:e50, 2009a.

American Heart Association: *Cardiovascular disease statistics, Learn and live*, February 16, 2009b, www.americanheart.org/presenter.jhtml?identifier=4478. Accessed May 20, 2009.

American Heart Association: *Risk factors and coronary heart disease*, 2009c. www.americanheart.org/presenter.jhtml?identifier=4726. Accessed May 21, 2009.

American Psychological Association: *Women and depression*, 2005, www.apa.org/about/gr/issues/women/depression.aspx.

Arthritis Foundation: Disease center, *Women and arthritis*, 2010, www.arthritis.org/women.php. Accessed March 9, 2010.

Bhatia SC, Bhatia SK: Depression in women: diagnostic and treatment considerations, *Am Fam Physician* 60:225, 1999.

Blair T: Domestic abuse: What is the ob/gyn nurse's role? *Ob Gyn Nurse Forum* 7(2):1, 1999.

Blehar M: Public health context of women's mental health research, *Psychiatr Clin North Am* 26:781–799, 2003.

Bremnor JD, Sadovsky R: Evaluation of dysuria in adults, *Am Fam Physician* 65:1589–1596, 2002.

Cates W, Ellertson C, Stewart F: Abortion. In Hatcher RA, et al: *Contraceptive technology*, ed 18, New York, 2004, Ardent Media.

Centers for Disease Control and Prevention: *Arthritis, Newest estimates for specific forms of arthritis*, January 8, 2007a. www.cdc.gov/arthritis/misc/new_estimates.htm. Accessed May 22, 2009.

Centers for Disease Control and Prevention: *HPV: Gardasil and GBS, CDC Immunization Safety Office*, August 15, 2007b. www.cdc.gov/vaccines/vpd-vac/hpv/downloads/hpv-gardasil-gbs.pdf. Accessed May 3, 2009.

Centers for Disease Control and Prevention: *Leading cause of death in females, Women's Health*, September 10, 2007c. www.cdc.gov/Women/lcod/04all.pdf. Accessed April 30, 2009.

Centers for Disease Control and Prevention: *MMWR: Update to CDC's Sexually Transmitted Diseases Treatment Guidelines, 2006: fluoroquinolones no longer recommended for treatment of gonococcal infections*, Atlanta, GA, 2007d, The Author.

Centers for Disease Control and Prevention: *Arthritis types—overview, Arthritis*, June 8, 2008a. www.cdc.gov/arthritis/arthritis/osteoarthritis.htm. Accessed May 22, 2009.

Centers for Disease Control and Prevention: *Number of people with diabetes increases to 24 million, Online Newsroom*, June 24, 2008b. www.cdc.gov/media/pressrel/2008/r080624.htm. Accessed May 4, 2009.

Centers for Disease Control and Prevention: *Age-adjusted hospital discharge rates for diabetes as any-listed diagnosis per 1,000 diabetic population, by sex, United States, 1980–2005, Diabetes Data and Trends*, September 29, 2008c. www.cdc.gov/diabetes/statistics/dmany/fig5.htm. Accessed May 4, 2009.

Centers for Disease Control and Prevention: *Pregnancy related mortality surveillance: United States—1991–1999, MMWR Morb Mortality Wkly Rep* 52(SS2):2003.

Centers for Disease Control and Prevention: *Understanding intimate partner violence, Violence prevention*, October 21, 2008d. www.cdc.gov/ViolencePrevention/pdf/IPV-FactSheet.pdf. Accessed April 20, 2009.

Centers for Disease Control and Prevention: *National diabetes fact sheet: general information and national estimates on diabetes in the United States, 2007, Diabetes data and trends*, 2008e. www.cdc.gov/diabetes/pubs/pdf/ndfs_2007.pdf.

Centers for Disease Control and Prevention: *Age-adjusted incidence of diagnosed diabetes per 1,000 population aged 18–79 years, by sex, United States, 1980–2007*, February 27, 2009a, www.cdc.gov/diabetes/statistics/incidence/fig4.htm. Accessed May 4, 2009.

Centers for Disease Control and Prevention: *Death rates* for human immunodeficiency virus (HIV) disease among women, by race and age group United States, 1987–2005, MMWR*, March 27, 2009b. www.cdc.gov/mmwr/preview/mmwrhtml/mm5811a4.htm. Accessed April 22, 2009.

Centers for Disease Control and Prevention: *Birth rates for teens aged 15–19 years, by age group—United States, 1985–2007, MMWR*, April 3, 2009c. www.cdc.gov/mmwr/preview/mmwrhtml/mm5812a5.htm?s_cid=mm5812a5_e. Accessed April 23, 2009.

Centers for Disease Control and Prevention, Early Release of Selected Estimates Based on Data from the 2008 National Health Interview Survey: *Lack of health insurance and type of coverage*, June, 2009e. www.cdc.gov/nchs/data/nhis/earlyrelease/200906_01.pdf. Accessed March 9, 2010.

Centers for Disease Control and Prevention: *Prevalence and most common causes of disability among adults—United States, 2005, MMWR Weekly*, May 1, 2009d. www.cdc.gov/mmwr/preview/mmwrhtml/mm5816a2.htm#tab1. Accessed May 21, 2009.

Centers for Disease Control and Prevention: Reduced incidence of menstrual toxic-shock syndrome, United States 1980–1990, *MMWR Morb Mortality Wkly Rep* 39:421–424, 1990.

Centers for Disease Control and Prevention, Women's Reproductive Health: *Hysterectomy Fact Sheet, Hysterectomy in the United States 2000–2004*, Sept. 22, 2008g. www.cdc.gov/reproductivehealth/WomensRH/00–04–FS_Hysterectomy.htm. Accessed May 20, 2009.

Centers for Disease Control and Prevention Gynecologic cancers: *Ovarian cancer*, 2009f. www.cdc.gov/cancer/ovarian/statistics/index.htm. Accessed May 18, 2009.

Centers for Disease Control and Prevention Gynecologic cancers: *Ovarian cancer information for health care providers*, 2010. www.cdc.gov/cancer/ovarian/healthcare/index.htm. Accessed March 9, 2010.

Chadwick BA, Heaton TB, editors: *Statistical handbook on the American family*, Phoenix, 1992, Oryx Press.

Chang WC, et al: Impact of sex on long-term mortality from acute myocardial infarction vs. unstable angina, *Arch Intern Med* 163:2476–2484, 2003.

Cheung BM, Ong KL, Cherny SS: Diabetes prevalence and therapeutic target achievement in the United States, 1999 to 2006, *Am J Med* 122:443, 2009.

Choi M: Preamble to a new paradigm for women's health, *Image (IN)* 17:14, 1985.

Chobanian AV, et al: The seventh report of the joint national committee on prevention, detection, evaluation, and treatment of high blood pressure, *JAMA* 289(19):2003.

Cunningham FG, et al: *Williams' obstetrics*, ed 21, Norwalk, CT, 2005, Appleton & Lange.

Davis JP, et al: Toxic-shock syndrome: epidemiologic features, recurrence, risk factors, and prevention, *N Engl J Med* 303:1429–1435, 1980.

DeFrances C, Lees K, Kazk J, Hall M, Pokras B: *National Hospital Discharge Survey (NHDS) and National Survey of Ambulatory Surgery (NSAS), 2006 Data Users Conference*, Hyattsville, MD, 2006, Centers for Disease Control and Prevention.

Department of Reproductive Health and Research: *Maternal mortality in 2005: estimates developed by WHO, UNICEF, UNFPA, and the World Bank*, Geneva, Switzerland, 2005, World Health Organization.

Downs J, Clearfield M, Weis S: Primary prevention of acute coronary events with lovastatin in men and women with average cholesterol levels: results of AFCAPS, *JAMA* 279:1615–1622, 1998.

Elders J: *Public Health Practice Symposium, Public health leadership to improve the health of young people*, Ann Arbor, MI, 2009, University of Michigan.

Farley D: Preventing TSS: tampon labeling allows women to compare absorbencies. In U.S. Department of Health and Human Services, *FDA consumer special report: current issues in women's health*, ed 2, Rockville, MD, 1994, The Author.

Evans DL, et al: Depression in the medical setting: biopsychological interactions and treatment considerations, *J Clin Psychiatry* 60(Suppl 4):40, 1999.

Epperly AT, Viera AJ: Pelvic inflammatory disease, *Clinics in Family Practice* 1(7):67–68, 2005.

Finkel ML, Finkel DJ: The effect of a second opinion program on hysterectomy performance, *Med Care* 28:776, 1990.

Food and Drug Administration: *FDA licenses new vaccine for prevention of cervical cancer and other diseases in females caused by human papillomavirus*, June 8, 2006. http://www.fda.gov/bbs/topics/NEWS/2006/NEW01385.html. Accessed May 3, 2009.

Foxman B, Brown P: Epidemiology of urinary tract infections transmission and risk factors, incidence, and costs, *Infect Dis Clin North Am* 17:227–241, 2003.

Gamble SB, Strauss LT, Parkere WY, Cook D, Zane SB, Hamdan S: *Abortion surveillance, United States, 2005, MMWR*, November 14, 2008. www.cdc.gov/mmwr/preview/mmwrhtml/ss5713a1.htm Accessed April 5, 2009.

Gilinson T: Know family, medical leave rights for yourself, your patients, *Am Nurse* 31(14):0098–1486, 1999.

Hamilton BE, Martin JA, Ventura M: Births: preliminary data for 2007, National Center for Health Statistics, *Natl Vital Stat Rep* 2009. March 18. www.cdc.gov/nchs/data/nvsr/nvsr57/nvsr57_12.pdf Accessed May 20, 2009.

The Henry J. Kaiser Family Foundation: *Kaiser daily women's health policy, Kaisernetwork*, August 27, 2007. www.kaisernetwork.org/daily_reports/rep_index.cfm?hint=2&DR_ID=47116. Accessed May 4, 2009.

Heron M, Hoyert DL, Murphy SL, et al: *Deaths: final data for 2006*, Hyattsville, MD, 2009, US Department of Health and Human Services, Centers for Disease Control and Prevention, National Center for Health Statistics.

Hopwood P, Stephens RJ: Medical Research Council (MRC) Lung Cancer Working Party: Symptoms at presentation for treatment in patients with lung cancer: implications for the evaluation of palliative treatment, *Br J Cancer* 71:633, 1995.

Hoyert D: Maternal mortality and related concepts, *Vital Health Stat* 3(33):8–10, 2007.

Jacobs A: Coronary revascularization in women in 2003: sex revisited, *Circulation* 107:375–377, 2003.

Kovach K: Trauma nursing: intimate partner violence, *RN* 67:38, 2004.

Kuehn J, McMahon P, Creekmore S: Stopping a silent killer, *AWHONN Lifelines* 3(2):31–35, 1999.

Kung H-C, Hoyert DL, Xu J, Murphy SL: Deaths: final data for 2005, *Natl Vital Stat Rep* 56(10):4–10, 2008.

Levine E, Ghai V, Barton J, Strom C: Mode of delivery and risk of respiratory diseases in newborns, *Obstet Gynecol* 97:1635–1638, 2001.

Martin R, et al: Gender disparities in common sense models of illness among myocardial infarction victims, *Health Psychol* 23:345–353, 2004.

Matthews S, Power C: Socio-economic gradients in psychological distress: a focus on women, social roles and work-home characteristics, *Soc Sci Med* 54:799–810, 2002.

Misner ST, Beauchamp-Hewitt JB, Fox-Levin P: Occupational issues in women's health. In *National Center for Health Statistics: Health, United States, 2004, with chartbook on trends in the health of Americans*, Hyattsville, MD, 2004, The Author.

Mosca CL: Evidence-based guidelines for cardiovascular disease prevention in women: 2007 update, *Circulation* 115:1481–1501, 2007.

Mou SM: Gynecologic infections. In Seltzer VL, Pearse WH, editors: *Women's primary health care*, ed 2, New York, 1999, McGraw-Hill.

Mulcahy N: *ASBS 2009: breast self-exam as accurate as mammography, MRI in high-risk women, Medscape Nurses*, April 24, 2009. www.medscape.com/viewarticle/701881?src=mp&spon=16&uac=72588CN. Accessed May 20, 2009.

National Cancer Institute: *Surveillance epidemiology and end results*, April 15, 2009. http://seer.cancer.gov/csr/1975_2006/index.html. Accessed May 12, 2009.

National Center for Health Statistics: *Health, United States, 2004, with chartbook on trends in the health of Americans*, Hyattsville, MD, 2004, The Author.

National Center for Health Statistics: *Health, United States, 2007 with chartbook on trends in the health of Americans*, 2007, www.cdc.gov/nchs/hus.htm. Accessed April 28, 2009.

National Center for Health Statistics: *Health, United States, 2008 with chartbook*, Hyattsville, MD, 2009, The Author.

National Institutes of Health, Office of Research on Women's Health, *American Recovery and Reinvestment Act of 2009*. http://orwh.od.nih.gov/recovery/index.html. Accessed March 5, 2010.

Nelson AL: Menstrual problems and common gynecologic concerns. In Hatcher RA, et al: *Contraceptive technology*, ed 18, New York, 2004, Ardent Media.

Nelson AL, Marshall JR: Impaired fertility. In Hatcher RA, et al: *Contraceptive technology*, ed 18, New York, 2004, Ardent Media.

Norhammar A, Stenestrand UJ, Lindbäck J, Wallentin L: Women younger than 65 years with diabetes mellitus are a high-risk group after myocardial infarction: a report from the Swedish Register of Information and Knowledge about Swedish Heart Intensive Care Admission (RIKS-HIA), *Heart* 94:1565–1570, 2008.

Office of Population Affairs: *Family planning, US Department of Health and Human Services*, 2009. www.hhs.gov/opa/familyplanning/index.html. Accessed May 2, 2009.

Patel JD: Lung cancer in women, *J Clin Oncol* 23(14):3212–3218, 2005.

Pender NJ, Murdaugh CL, Parsons MA: *Health promotion in nursing practice*, ed 4, Upper Saddle River, NJ, 2006, Prentice Hall.

Pleis JR, Lucas JW, Ward BW: Summary health statistics for U.S. adults: National Health Interview Survey, 2008. National Center for Health Statistics, *Vital Health Stat* 10(242):2009.

Pollack AE, Carignan CS, Jacobstein R: Female and male sterilization. In Hatcher RA, et al: *Contraceptive technology*, ed 18, New York, 2004, Ardent Media.

Rhodes DJ: Identifying and counseling women at increased risk for breast cancer, *Mayo Clinic Proc* 77:355–361, 2002.

Rivera MP, Stover DE: Gender and lung cancer, *Clin Chest Med* 25:391–400, 2004.

Safe Motherhood Organization: *Safe motherhood initiative*, 2005. www.safemotherhood.org/resources/pdf/e_facts.pdf.

Sarna L, McCorkle R: Burden of care and lung cancer, *Cancer Pract* 4:245, 1996.

Schuiling KD, Likis FE: *Women's gynecologic health*, Sudbury, MA, 2006, Jones and Bartlett.

Schulman KA, Berlin JA, Harless W, Kerner JF, Sistrunk S, Gersh BJ, Dubé R, Taleghani CK, Burke JE, Williams S, Eisenberg JM, Escarce JJ, Ayers W: The effect of race and sex on physicians' recommendations for cardiac catheterization, *N Engl J Med* 340:618–626, 1999.

Snell T: *Survey of state prison inmates: 1991—women in prison*, Washington, DC, 1994, US Department of Justice, Bureau of Justice Statistics, US Government Printing Office.

Star WL, Shannon MT, Lommel LL: *Women's primary care: protocols for practice*, San Fransisco, 2004, UCSF Nursing Press.

Stewart SL, King JB, Thompson TD, Friedman C, Wingo PA: *Cancer mortality surveillance United States, 1990–2000:* Morbidity and Mortality Weekly Report, *Centers for Disease Control* 53(03):1–108, 2004.

Thibos M, Lavin-Loucks D, Martin M: The feminization of poverty, *The J. McDonald Williams Institute and the YWCA*, Dallas, 2007, Dallas Indicators.

Thomas B, et al: Randomized trial of breast self-examination in Shanghai: final results, *J Natl Cancer Inst* 94(19):1445–1447, 2002.

Urbanic JC: Depressive disorders. In Urbanic JC, Groh CJ, editors: *Women's mental health: a clinical guide for primary care providers*, Philadelphia, PA, 2009, Wolters Kluwer.

U.S. Census Bureau: *Single-parent households showed little variation since 1994, Census Bureau reports (news release)*, Washington, DC,

2007, U.S. Department of Commerce, Public Information Office.

U.S. Census Bureau: *As baby boomers age, fewer families have children under 18 at home (news release)*, Washington, DC, 2009, US Department of Commerce, Public Information Office.

U.S. Census Bureau American Community Survey: Class of worker by sex and median earnings in the past 12 months for the civilian employed population 16 years and over, 2008a, http://factfinder.census.gov/servlet/STTable?_bm=y&-state=st&-qr_name=ACS_2008_3YR_G00_S2408&-ds_name=ACS_2008_3YR_G00_&-redoLog=true&-_caller=geoselect&-geo_id=01000US&-format=&-_lang=en. Accessed May 21, 2009.

U.S. Census Bureau: Disability status by sex: 2000, http://factfinder.census.gov/servlet/QTTable?_bm=y&-geo_id=D&-qr_name=DEC_2000_SF3_U_QTP21&-ds_name=D&-_lang=en.

U.S. Census Bureau American Fact Finder: *Selected social characteristics in the United States: 2006–2008*, 2008b, http://factfinder.census.gov/servlet/ADPTable?_bm=y&-geo_id=01000US&-qr_name=ACS_2008_3YR_G00_DP3YR2&-ds_name=ACS_2008_3YR_G00_&-_lang=en&-_sse=on. Accessed March 9, 2010.

U.S. Department of Health and Human Services: *Public Health Service: Healthy People 2010: national health promotion and disease prevention objectives*, Washington, DC, 2000b, US Government Printing Office.

U.S. Department of Health and Human Services: *Guidelines for the use of antiretroviral agents in HIV-1 infected adults and adolescents*, 2005b, http://www.aidsinfo.nih.gov/guidelines.

U.S. Department of Labor: *Women in the labor force: a databook*, Washington, DC, 2005, The Author.

U.S. Department of Labor, Women's Bureau: *Quick stats on women workers, 2008*. May 25, 2008: www.dol.gov/wb/stats/main.htm. Accessed May 20, 2009.

Vaccarino V, Lin ZQ, Kasl S, et al: Sex differences in health status after coronary artery bypass surgery, *Circulation* 108(143):2642–2647, 2003.

Vogel WH: The advance practice nursing role in a high-risk breast cancer clinic, *Oncol Nurs Forum* 30:115–122, 2003.

Warshaw C, Ganley AL, Salber PR: *Improving the health care response to domestic violence: a resource manual for health care providers*, San Francisco, 1995, Family Violence Prevention Fund.

Wei G, et al: Osteoporosis management in the new millennium, *Prim Care* 30:711–741, 2003.

Wenger NK: You've come a long way, baby: cardiovascular health and disease in women: problems and prospects, *Circulation* 109:558–560, 2004.

Wexler DJ, et al: Sex disparities in treatment of cardiac risk factors in patients with type 2 diabetes, *Diabetes Care* 28:514–520, 2005.

Whiteman MK, Hillis SD: Inpatient hysterectomy surveillance in the United States, 2000–2004, *Am J Obstet Gynecol* 198:1–7, 2008.

Women Employed Institute: *Sexual harassment: the problem that isn't going away*, Chicago, 1994, The Author.

World Health Organization, *Department of Reproductive Health and Research: Maternal mortality in*, 2000, Geneva, 2004a, The Author. www.WHO.int/reproductivehealth/publications/maternal_mortality2000/.

World Health Organization: *Joint United Nations programme on HIV/AIDS*, 2004, www.who.org.

World Health Organization: *International statistical classification of diseases and related health problems, 10th revision*, ICD version 2007, http://apps.who.int/classifications/apps/icd/icd10online/.

Wright TC Jr, Massad LS, Dunton CJ, et al: 2006 consensus guidelines for the management of women with abnormal cervical cancer screening tests, *Am J Obstet Gynecol* 197:346–355, 2006.

Zeidenstein L: Health issues of lesbian and bisexual women. In Varney H, editor: *Varney's midwifery*, ed 4, Sudbury, MA, 2004, Jones and Bartlett.

Men's Health

Carrie Morgan

Additional Material for Study, Review, and Further Exploration

evolve WEBSITE

http://evolve.elsevier.com/Nies

- Quiz
- Case Studies
- Glossary
- WebLinks

OBJECTIVES

Upon completion of this chapter, the reader will be able to do the following:

1. Identify the major indicators of men's health status.
2. Describe physiological and psychological factors that have an impact on men's health status.
3. Discuss barriers to improving men's health.
4. Discuss factors that promote men's health.
5. Describe men's health needs.
6. Apply knowledge of men's health needs in planning gender-appropriate nursing care for men at the individual, family, and community levels.

KEY TERMS

acute condition	illness orientation	morbidity
androgen	life expectancy	mortality
chronic condition	medical care	

OUTLINE

It is common knowledge that women live longer than men and that health care use is greater among women than men. Death rates for men are higher than for women in the major causes of death. Although the overall interest in health promotion and illness prevention has increased, men's health issues remain largely unaddressed (Baerlocher and Verma, 2008). Women's health has become a specialty practice with courses and programs available in many colleges of nursing. A specialty in men's health has not been established.

This chapter focuses on exploring the health needs of men and the implications for community health nursing. Specific areas that are discussed include the current health status of men, physiological and psychological theories that attempt to explain men's health, factors that impede men's health, factors that promote men's health, men's health needs, and planning gender-appropriate care for men at the individual, family, and community levels.

MEN'S HEALTH STATUS

Traditional indicators of health for all persons include rates of longevity, mortality, and morbidity. Reviewing these rates provides nursing students with a better understanding of the community aggregate.

Longevity and Mortality in Men

Major gender differences in longevity and mortality rates reveal that men remain disadvantaged despite advances in technology. Although women are more likely to use health services and have higher morbidity rates, mortality rates for men remain higher. Gender differences are generally associated with both physiological and behavioral factors, which place men at greater risk of death. These behavioral factors, together with men's reluctance to seek preventive and health services, have marked implications for community health nursing.

STANDARDIZED TERMINOLOGY

In the fields of demography and sociology, the following terms are standardized:

People of all ages: Males and females
Children younger than 18 years of age: Boys and girls
Adults 18 years of age or older: Men and women
Sex: The biological distinction between males and females
Gender: The attitudes and behavior of men and women that are shaped by socialization and have a potential to be changed
Role: The part one plays in society

Modified from Skelton R: Man's role in society and its effect on health, *Nursing* 26:953, 1988; Verbrugge LM, Wingard DL: Sex differentials in health and mortality, *Women Health* 12:103, 1987.

Longevity

Rates of longevity are increasing for both men and women. People can now expect to live more than 20 years longer than their forefathers and foremothers lived at the turn of the nineteenth century. Infants born in the United States in 1996 can expect to live 77 years, whereas those born in

1900 lived an average of 47.3 years when the death rate was highest. Life expectancy for both males and females has increased; however, since the 1970s this gender gap in longevity has decreased (Table 18-1). Between 2005 and 2006, men gained 0.2 year of longevity while females gained 0.3 year of longevity (National Center for Health Statistics [NCHS], 2009). This change in male longevity may be attributed to the advances in treatment of heart disease and cancer, which have been the major causes of death in U.S. males (Table 18-2).

Factors that influence the incongruencies between males and females are race or ethnic origin, social economic status, and education. Reported by race, gender mortality rates show that less-advantaged populations in the United States, especially minorities, live significantly fewer years. African-American males live 6 years less than white males (NCHS, 2009). Native American males live an average of 4 years less than white males. Hispanics have a life expectancy comparable with that of their white counterparts.

Mortality

The United States lags behind several other countries in mortality rates for males. In 2005 only four countries had mortality rates higher than the United States: Hungary, the Netherlands, Poland, and Slovakia (Organisation for Economic Co-operation and Development [OECD], 2007). In the United States, as in most industrialized countries, males lead females in mortality rates in each leading cause of death. Although males were the primary source of medical data before the 1970s, and most of the treatment advances have been developed from these data, gender-related disparity in death rates continues. Other factors also account for this mortality gender gap.

The gender disparity for disease-related deaths has narrowed. Heart disease remains the leading cause of death, but the ratio of death for heart disease decreased by 2.8 between 2005 and 2006. During this same period of time, male-to-female deaths increased by 1.4. Since the 1990s, female, cancer-related deaths have declined at a slower rate than men's. Lifetime risk for lung cancer among males is estimated to be 9.8%, and 3.8% for females (Lynch, 2008). The death rate for chronic lower respiratory tract disease among females increased 150% between 1980 and 2002, whereas death rates for males increased 7% (NCHS, 2004b). This may be associated with the increase in incidence of lower respiratory disease among the elderly (Lynch, 2008). Unintentional injury deaths due to accidents, suicide, or homicide for the whole population have increased by 1.8 from 2005-2006. Males continue to be at risk for death due to unintentional injury. Males aged 15 to 64 years are two to three times more likely to die as a result of unintentional injury than females of the same age. Men are five times more likely to commit suicide. Males over age 85 years are eleven times more likely to die as a result of suicide.

Race and ethnic background also are factors to be considered when evaluating male mortality rates. Black men between ages 45 and 64 years are more than ten times as

TABLE 18-1   LIFE EXPECTANCY AT BIRTH ACCORDING TO SEX AND RACE, UNITED STATES: 1900, 1950, 2000, 2005, 2006

YR	ALL RACES BOTH SEXES	MALE	FEMALE	WHITE BOTH SEXES	MALE	FEMALE	BLACK BOTH SEXES	MALE	FEMALE
1900	47.3	46.3	48.3	47.6	46.6	48.7	33.0	32.5	33.5
1950	68.2	65.6	71.1	69.1	69.1	72.2	62.1	59.6	64.8
2000	76.8	74.1	79.3	77.3	74.7	79.9	72.0	68.4	75.2
2005	77.4	74.9	79.9	77.9	75.4	80.4	72.8	69.3	76.1
2006	77.7	75.1	80.2	78.2	75.7	80.4	73.2	69.7	76.5

Data from National Center for Health Statistics: *Health, United States: 2004,* Hyattsville, MD, 2006, US Public Health Service.

TABLE 18-2   LEADING CAUSES OF DEATH IN MALES, UNITED STATES, 2004

	PERCENT
All Males, All Ages	
1. Heart disease	27.2
2. Cancer	24.3
3. Unintentional injuries	6.1
4. Stroke	5.0
5. Chronic lower respiratory diseases	5.0
6. Diabetes	3.0
7. Influenza and pneumonia	2.3
8. Suicide	2.2
9. Kidney disease	1.7
10. Alzheimer's disease	1.6
White Males, All Ages	
1. Heart disease	27.7
2. Cancer	24.6
3. Unintentional injuries	6.1
4. Chronic lower respiratory diseases	5.3
5. Stroke	4.9
6. Diabetes	2.8
7. Influenza and pneumonia	2.3
8. Suicide	2.3
9. Alzheimer's disease	1.7
10. Kidney disease	1.6
Black Males, All Ages	
1. Heart disease	24.8
2. Cancer	22.2
3. Unintentional injuries	5.9
4. Stroke	5.2
5. Homicide	4.7
6. Diabetes	3.8
7. HIV disease	3.3
8. Chronic lower respiratory diseases	2.8
9. Kidney disease	2.4
10. Influenza and pneumonia	1.9
Asian or Pacific Islander Males, All Ages	
1. Cancer	26.7
2. Heart disease	25.4
3. Stroke	7.6
4. Unintentional injuries	5.5
5. Chronic lower respiratory diseases	3.5
6. Diabetes	3.3
7. Influenza and pneumonia	2.8
8. Suicide	2.5
9. Kidney disease	1.7
10. Homicide	1.2

TABLE 18-2   LEADING CAUSES OF DEATH IN MALES, UNITED STATES, 2004—cont'd

	PERCENT
Hispanic Males, All Ages	
1. Heart disease	21.9
2. Cancer	19.0
3. Unintentional injuries	11.4
4. Stroke	4.7
5. Diabetes	4.2
6. Homicide	4.1
7. Chronic liver disease	3.5
8. Suicide	2.7
9. Chronic lower respiratory diseases	2.4
10. Perinatal conditions	2.2

From Centers for Disease Control and Prevention, Office of Women's Health, Department of Health and Human Services, 2008: www.cdc.gov/men/lcod/index.htm.

likely to die of human immunodeficiency virus (HIV) infection as white males. Among males aged 15 to 24 years, African-American males are twice as likely to die of vehicle accidents and seven times more likely to die of homicide (NCHS, 2004b). Hispanic males fare somewhat better but are twice as likely to die as a result of homicide as white males.

Morbidity

Despite the differences in mortality rates, men tend to perceive themselves to be in better health than women do (Brown and Bond, 2008). In the National Health Interview Survey of 2003 (NCHS, 2004b), which asked people to rate their health status, men were more likely to rate their health as excellent or very good as opposed to fair or poor. Morbidity rates, or rates of illness, are difficult to obtain and have been available usually only in Western industrialized countries. For example, in the United States, reports of analyses of morbidity rates by gender lag several years behind analyses of mortality rates by gender. Gender differences in morbidity rates reflect the latest available reports. The following are common indicators of morbidity rate:

- Incidence of acute illness
- Prevalence of chronic conditions
- Use of medical care

Although variations exist, women are more likely to be ill, whereas men are at greater risk for death.

Acute Illness

According to the National Health Interview Survey, an acute condition is a type of illness or injury that usually lasted less than 3 months and either resulted in restricted activity (e.g., causing a person to limit daily activities for at least half a day) or caused the patient to receive medical care. The incidence rate for acute infective and parasitic disease, digestive system conditions, and respiratory conditions is higher for women than for men (Benson and Marano, 2001-2002). The only exception is for injuries, which were 1.5 times greater for men in 2006 (National Vital Statistics Reports, 2009). In addition, the severity of these injuries is reported to be greater in men than in women. When conditions associated with childbearing are excluded from the list of acute illnesses, the incidence rate for women remains 18% greater than for men.

Women reported that they slowed their activities and rested more often than men. The number of restricted-activity days associated with acute conditions per 100 people is 33% greater for women than for men; similarly, the number of bed days associated with acute conditions per 100 people is 38% greater for women than for men (Benson and Marano, 2001).

Chronic Conditions

A chronic condition is a condition that persists for at least 3 months or belongs to a group of conditions classified as chronic regardless of time of onset, such as tuberculosis, neoplasm, or arthritis. In general, women have higher morbidity rates than men. Women are more likely than men to have a higher prevalence of chronic diseases that cause disability and limitation of activities but do not lead to death. However, men have higher morbidity and mortality rates for conditions that are the leading causes of death.

SOURCES OF DATA

Health, United States: Submitted by the Secretary of the Department of Health and Human Services, *Health, United States* is a report of the health status of the nation. The data are compiled by the National Center for Health Statistics and the Centers for Disease Control and Prevention. The National Committee on Health and Vital Statistics reviews the report (www.cdc.gov/nchs/data/hus/hus04.pdf).

National Center for Health Statistics (NCHS): Through the National Vital Statistics System, the NCHS collects data from each state, New York City, the District of Columbia, the U.S. Virgin Islands, Guam, and Puerto Rico on births, deaths, marriages, and divorces in the United States (www.cdc.gov/nchs/Default.htm).

National Health Interview Survey: Directed by the National Center for Health Statistics of the Centers for Disease Control and Prevention, the National Health Interview Survey is a continuing, nationwide sample survey in which data are collected by personal interviews about household members' illnesses, injuries, chronic conditions, disabilities, and use of health services (www.cdc.gov/nchs/nhis.htm).

USE OF MEDICAL CARE

Medical care, the use of ambulatory care, hospital care, preventive care, or other health services, also illustrates the different gender patterns.

Use of Ambulatory Care

Men seek ambulatory care less often than women. According to the 2003 National Health Interview Survey (NCHS, 2004b), the physician's office is the primary setting for ambulatory care for both men and women. In this report, males visited physician offices, outpatient departments, or emergency departments less often than women in all age groups, with the exception of males over age 75 years. Men were likely to visit a physician only if a specific health-related symptom was experienced (Brown and Bond, 2008). Injury-related visits to hospital emergency departments are higher for males than females. Males aged 18 to 24 years are twice as likely to visit hospital emergency departments for unintentional injuries as females in the same age range. Even though gender differences in ambulatory care utilization are lessening, males continue to delay medical treatment, resulting in men being sicker when they do seek health care. Because they are sicker, they require more intensive medical care. Physicians see men more frequently than women for the chronic diseases that are more prevalent among them. Males are twice as likely to visit specialists (Singh-Manoux, et al., 2008).

Use of Hospital Care

The literature indicates that hospitalization rates also vary by sex. In 2003, rates of discharges from short-stay hospitals were lower for males (102 per 1000) than for females (133 per 1000), even when discharges for deliveries were excluded. However, males had a longer length of stay in the hospital than females (4.3 vs. 3.8 days). Discharge rates increase for both men and women after 45 years of age; however, rates for men increase more rapidly. After 65 years of age, men's discharge rates continue to be higher than women's rates (NCHS, 2004b).

Use of Preventive Care

Preventive examinations and appropriate health protective behavior are necessary for health promotion and early diagnosis of health problems. Men do not engage in these health protective behaviors at the same frequency as females (Brown and Bond, 2008). Most men do not have routine checkups. National health surveys indicate that women are more likely than men to receive physical examinations (NCHS, 2004b). Men are twice as likely to report no usual source of care although eligibility for primary care in males exceeds that for females (Lynch, 2008).

Use of Other Health Services

Admission for serious mental disease accounts for the largest number of hospital admissions for men aged 45 to 74 years. Women of the same age are more likely to be admitted for disease of the heart. Women are also more likely to reside in nursing homes because they have a longer life expectancy.

Men are more likely than women to be admitted for psychiatric services in state and county mental hospitals (NCHS, 2004b).

THEORIES THAT EXPLAIN MEN'S HEALTH

As discussed previously, a gender gap exists in health. The data reviewed raise many questions for community health nurses to explore, regarding gender differences in health and illness. Although men have shorter life expectancy and higher rates of mortality for all leading causes of death, women have higher rates of morbidity, including rates of acute illness and chronic disease and use of medical and preventive care services. Verbrugge and Wingard (1987) asked why "females are sicker, but males die sooner" (p. 135). Several explanations exist for this paradox.

Nurses traditionally use developmental theories to explain individual behavior. Erickson's model was not gender specific (Levinson focused somewhat on male development). There remains a need for literature detailing the factors and combinations of factors that influence gender differences in the health and illness of populations.

The following explanations proposed by Waldron (1995a, 1995b, 1995c, 1995d, 1995e) and Verbrugge and Wingard (1987) attempt to account for gender differences in this important area:

- Biological factors, including genetics, effects of sex hormones, and physiological differences, which may be influenced by genetics, hormones, and environment
- Socialization
- Orientations toward illness and prevention
- Data collection of health behavior

Biological Factors

Several biological factors influence sex differences in mortality and morbidity rates, including genetics, effects of sex hormones, and physiological differences, which may be influenced by genetics, hormones, and environmental factors (Waldron, 1995a, 1995b, 1995c, 1995d, 1995e). The embryo is unisexual until the seventh week of gestation. Androgen, a hormone from the Y-chromosome coupled with the maternal androgen source, results in the development of the male sex. More male births occur than female births. In 2003, 1049 male births occurred for every 1000 female births. However, infant mortality rate for males was 9% higher than for females, thus reducing this ratio. Sex ratios at birth appear to be lower for births to older fathers, black fathers, higher-order births (i.e., second, third, or fourth births), and births after induced ovulation.

Whether sex ratios at birth are influenced by sex ratios at conception or sex differentials in mortality rates before birth is unknown. Current evidence suggests that more than two out of three prenatal deaths occur before clinical recognition of the pregnancy. Embryonic research shows excess male fetuses in early pregnancy and less male delivery at term. Males' experience of higher mortality rates for perinatal conditions is attributed to biological disadvantages

such as males' greater risk of premature birth, higher rates of respiratory distress syndrome, and infectious disease in infancy resulting from the influence of male hormones on the developing lungs, brain, and possibly the immune system of the male fetus (National Vital Statistics Reports, 2009). Sex chromosome–linked diseases, such as hemophilia and certain types of muscular dystrophy, are more common among males than females (Waldron, 1995d).

Biological advantages for females may also exist later in life because the mechanism produced by estrogen protects against heart disease. Some evidence supports the hypothesis that men's higher testosterone levels contribute to men's lower high-density lipoprotein levels. Body fat distribution, specifically the tendency for men in Western countries to accumulate abdominal body fat versus the tendency for women to accumulate fat on the buttocks and thighs, may also contribute to sex differences in development of metabolic syndrome (Kirby et al., 2006). Men's higher levels of stored iron also may contribute to risk for ischemic heart disease. Some additional physiological gender differences are the following (Tanne, 1997):

- During the process of aging, men's brain cells die faster than women's brain cells. This may explain why men are more often hospitalized for serious mental disease.
- Male immune systems are weaker than women's.

Socialization

A second theory for explaining sex differences in health is socialization, especially within the area of masculinity. Society emphasizes assertiveness, restricted emotional display, concern for power, and reckless behavior in males. Pursuit of these attributes results in increased risks in work, leisure, and lifestyle. Internalization of these norms of masculinity reduces the likelihood of engaging in health promotion behaviors for fear these behaviors might be interpreted as a sign of weakness. Gender-role socialization may influence these differences. Peer pressure plays an important role in adhering to masculine norms. Men enculturate their sons to believe that risking personal injury demonstrates masculinity (Brown and Bond, 2008).

According to the National Institute for Occupational Safety and Health *Workers Health Chartbook* (2004), 54.2% of U.S. workers are males. Male workers account for 66.1% of the reported occupational injuries and 92% of work-related fatalities. Men's higher exposure to carcinogens at the work site is associated with high rates of mesothelioma and coal worker's pneumoconiosis. In the United States, men score higher than women on measures of hostility and lack of trust of others, which may place them at higher risk of ischemic heart disease. Although occupational hazards to women's health are being identified, evidence indicates that, unlike for men, employment of U.S. women outside the home has a positive effect.

Popular male leisure, sports, and play activities place men at high risk for injury. Males between the ages of 18 and 24 years are twice as likely as women to visit a hospital emergency department because of motor vehicular accidents, stabs, or intentional injury (NCHS, 2004b). Statistics show that men drive faster than women, receive more traffic violations, and are less likely to wear seat belts, all of which contribute to a greater number of motor vehicle fatalities. Although prevalence of smoking is decreasing, 25.5% of males smoke (NCHS, 2004b); 68% of men consume alcohol, and men are five times more likely than women to drink heavily. Males have a greater use of illegal psychoactive substances and are three times more likely to be involved in criminal activity (NCHS, 2004b).

Men are more likely to be involved in violent crimes, and violence is a typical precursor to homicide. Men are victims in four out of five homicides. Black males are involved in a homicide seven times more often than European-American males (NCHS, 2004a).

Many barriers exist that prohibit positive male health behavior changes, but female family members were seen as facilitators. Cheatham and colleagues (2008) reported that several studies showed males to be more likely to change health behaviors when these changes were suggested and supported by female family members who they thought were concerned about the well-being of the man.

FOUR DIMENSIONS OF STEREOTYPED MALE GENDER-ROLE BEHAVIOR

No Sissy Stuff: The need to be different from women
The Big Wheel: The need to be superior to others
The Sturdy Oak: The need to be independent and self-reliant
Give 'em Hell: The need to be more powerful than others, through violence if necessary

Modified from David DS, Brannon R: The male sex role: our culture's blueprint of manhood, and what it's done for us lately. In David DS, Brannon R, editors: *The forty-nine percent majority: the male sex role*, Reading, MA, 1976, Addison-Wesley.

Orientation Toward Illness and Prevention

Illness orientation, or the ability to note symptoms and take appropriate action, also may differ between the sexes. Most diseases, injuries, and deaths prevalent among men are preventable. However, the stereotypical view of men as strong and invulnerable is incongruent health promotion. Boys are socialized to ignore symptoms and "toughen up." Surveys done by *Men's Health* reveal that 9 million men have not seen a health care provider in 5 years. Men may be aware of being ill, but they make a conscious decision not to seek health care to avoid being labeled as "sick." Brown and Bond (2008) suggest that men lack the somatic awareness and are less likely to interpret symptoms as indicators of illness. There may be a desire to rationalize symptoms and denial of susceptibility to disease that contributes to the delay in treatment (Brown and Bond, 2008).

Health protective behavior, or the ability to take action to prevent disease or injury, also may vary between the sexes. Perhaps as a result of the contraceptive developments of the 1970s, women have a higher likelihood to seek preventive examinations. Routine reproductive health screening (i.e., the Pap test and breast examination) has been expanded to include some general screening, such as testing blood pressure, urine,

and blood for chronic problems. Men do not have routine reproductive health checkups that include screening, which would detect other health problems at an early stage. Among respondents to the National Health Interview Survey (NHIS) of Health Promotion and Disease Prevention, more women than men reported wearing seat belts, receiving blood pressure checks, having their blood cholesterol checked, and seeking help for an emotional or personal problem in the past year (NHIS, 2002a). Men reported spending more time in leisure activities than women, including playing sports regularly. The rapid growth of gymnasiums and health spas indicates a growing interest in maintaining physical fitness. Only 4.9% of male respondents and 5.5% of female respondents reported knowing that exercise periods of 20 minutes per session three times per week are necessary to strengthen the heart and lungs.

The survey results also revealed that in other areas of preventive health behaviors, men are less likely than women to visit a dentist, and 26.1% of men over age 65 years have no natural teeth. Males tend to participate in exercise, but 68% of men over 20 years of age are overweight. Men consume more fatty foods and are less likely than women to change their eating habits.

Gender differences in preventive health behavior are a fertile ground for continued research. Meryn (2009) reported that 21% of research was devoted to men's health compared with 53% for female health. He suggests that large-scale research in this area would add to the small evidence bases of health promotion behaviors among men. Specific national health objectives have only recently addressed the health care needs of this aggregate. Uniformly recognized preventive screening programs for males have only recently been developed. With the advent of managed care, men who are eligible for coverage will have access to these routine health screenings. However, it is undetermined whether men will take advantage of these programs. Box 18-1 discusses matters related to men's reproductive health needs.

Reporting of Health Behavior

Data regarding health behaviors are collected from a variety of sources, such as interviews, surveys, questionnaires, or reports. Data from these sources may not be accurate because males are less likely than females to participate in the data collection process. Men may be less willing to talk, may not recall health problems, and may lack a health vocabulary. Men may be more hesitant to talk about their illness. Not only do women participate in the data collection process but they also are often solicited in health surveys to report the health behavior of men. In this manner, women are proxies, and proxies have a tendency to underreport behavior. The accuracy of the data does increase with male participation, but men may not want to participate in the socialization of sickness and will make light of health problems. Males with an extreme conception of masculinity are less likely to express their health problems and may conceal or suppress pain in an effort to appear strong (Naslindh-Ylispanger, Sihvonen, and Kekki, 2008). Males are far less likely than women to

BOX 18-1   MEN'S REPRODUCTIVE HEALTH NEEDS

Reproductive health needs are beginning to be recognized as important to men's health and to women's health. Usually the term reproductive health is applied to women of childbearing age. Used here, the term applies to the health of reproductive organs, which develop in utero and with which a person is born, in both males and females, regardless of whether a person has sex or reproduces. Males may have reproductive health needs whether child or adult, straight or gay, or virgin or sexually experienced.

Many sexually transmitted diseases (STDs) are at epidemic proportions in the United States and are a major health hazard for many men and women. Acquired immunodeficiency syndrome (AIDS) in the United States is twice as likely to occur in males as in females. In 2002, death due to HIV in African-American males was 49.9 per 100,000, and African-American females' deaths due to HIV were 25.9. Less well known, perhaps, is that many STDs are considered intrinsically "sexist" because clinical evidence, more overt in men, is more likely to facilitate a correct diagnosis in men than in women. These STDs are easier to detect in men because men are more likely to be symptomatic, laboratory tests are more reliable in men, efficiency of transmission is greater from male to female, and men are more likely to seek care for STDs that are symptomatic. For example, incidence rates for chlamydia in 2003 for males was 134.6 per 100,000; for females, the rate was 468.1 per 100,000. The rate of gonorrhea was slightly lower among men (113.3 per 100,000 population) than among women (119 per 100,000 population). Only syphilis was more common in men than in women (4.2 per 100,000 males; 0.8 per 100,000 females) (Centers for Disease Control and Prevention, 2003).

Testicular cancer represents only 1% of cancers in males and is the most common cancer to affect young men between ages 15 and 35 years. Cancer of the prostate is a leading cause of death from cancer in men, was estimated to account for 171 deaths per 100,000 population in 2002, and remains twice as common in African-American males as in white males. The increase in the incidence of prostate cancer has been attributed to factors such as improved methods of detection and increased exposure to environmental carcinogens.

Mortality rates for all cancers remain high, especially in males over 75 years of age. Men over age 85 years are twice as likely to die of cancer as those aged 75 to 84 years.

Many occupational and environmental agents associated with adverse sexual and reproductive outcomes in men have been identified, including pesticides, anesthetic gases in the operating room and dental office, inorganic lead from smelters, paint, printing materials, carbon disulfide from vulcanization of rubber, inorganic mercury manufacturing and dental work, and ionizing radiation from x-rays (Whorton, 1984). Nonchemical agents have also been identified as hazardous in men; for example, hyperthermia experienced by firefighters has been linked to male infertility.

Many pharmacological agents, including prescription, over-the-counter, and recreational drugs, have been found to affect the reproductive outcomes or sexual functioning of men. Examples include drugs from the following categories: antihypertensives, antipsychotics, antidepressants, hormones, sedatives, hypnotics, stimulants, chemotherapy agents used in cancer treatment, amphetamines, opiates, alcohol, marijuana, cocaine, barbiturates, and lysergic acid diethylamide (LSD). Erectile dysfunction has become a "socially acceptable" topic of discussion since many high-profile men, such as Senator Bob Dole, former National Football League coach Mike Ditka, and retired General Norman Schwarzkopf have openly discussed their problem. Pharmaceutical companies market their products for treatment of this disorder via mass media. Controversy has arisen as to the use of public funding for these products.

A focus on homosexual men's health has come about largely through the advent of AIDS. Today, homosexuality encompasses not only the male but also the entire family. The community health nurse should develop nonjudgmental assessment skills that foster honest and open expression for all members of the community. Nurses may need specialized skills to work with these individuals.

---

seek counseling. Socialization to suppress expressiveness may represent the explanation for gender differences in reporting health behaviors.

Discussion of the Theories of Men's Health
Interpreting the Data

Community health nurses should be aware of gender disparity when collecting and interpreting data. To avoid bias, the community health nurse should consider the following things:

- Gender-specific interview techniques may be necessary to obtain the most accurate health history. Men respond better to direct questioning rather than open-ended questions.
- How do data obtained by male nurses differ from those obtained by female nurses? Is there personal gender bias in data collection?
- The accuracy of secondary sources of information is skewed toward the interpretation of the source. How do the data provided by women about male health behavior compare with the data collected from males regarding these same behaviors?
- Men are not enculturated to be caregivers. Men need assistance to learn how to provide support to the caregiver or to develop a caregiver role.

In response to the question of why "females are sicker, but males die sooner," several reasons can be provided. Conditions that affect morbidity rates (e.g., arthritis and gout) do not significantly affect mortality rates. Conditions that affect mortality rates may not significantly affect day-to-day activity until the condition is advanced. Men tend to delay seeking health care until their condition is advanced. Although mortality rates are, in large part, the outcome of inherited or acquired risks, gender differences in illness and health promotion behaviors, as well as the reporting of health behaviors, suggest that social and psychological factors also affect morbidity rates. Although males have higher prevalence and death rates for "killer" chronic diseases, injuries, and accidents, females have higher prevalence rates for a greater number of nonfatal chronic conditions.

Gender-Linked Behavior

The largest gender differences in mortality rates occur for causes of death associated with gender-linked behavior and suggest that gender-linked behavior, which is more prevalent and encouraged in men, correlates with the following major categories of death:

- *Tobacco use:* Lung cancer, bronchitis, emphysema, and asthma

- *Substance abuse:* Cirrhosis, accidents, and homicide
- *Poor preventive health habits and stress:* Heart disease
- *Lack of other emotional channels:* Cirrhosis, suicide, homicide, and accidents

Physical conditions can be seriously affected by social and environmental conditions, such as occupational hazards (e.g., carcinogens and stress), unemployment, and massive advertising campaigns that use gender and gender roles to sell alcohol and tobacco. These lifestyle factors are compounded by men's lack of willingness to seek preventive care such as screening and to seek health care when a symptom arises. To counter these types of factors, research is needed to determine gender-specific methods of data collection, education, and practice that are aimed at health promotion, illness prevention, and political processes for males.

RESEARCH HIGHLIGHTS

Doctors and Patients: Gender Interaction in the Consultation

Much research on gender differences in medicine has centered on women as better communicators, more egalitarian, more patient-centered, and more involved with psychosocial problems, preventive care, and female-specific problems. Little research has examined the interaction between a health care provider and the patient's gender. Anecdotal evidence says that women prefer to see women doctors. Research indicates that men as well as women are more satisfied with the care given by a woman doctor. This leads to the question of why this is so.

Research indicates that women doctors demonstrate more "humanitarian" and "patient-care values." They conduct longer consultations and manage more problems of a psychosocial nature. Women doctors tend to use a conversational style of communication that is egalitarian and encourages participation, whereas men doctors tend to be more dominant and directive. Clearly, men and women have different styles of consultation. Does this imply that consultation outcomes are influenced by a doctor's gender? Does the patient's gender influence the doctor's management? In other words, do men and women doctors treat men and women patients equally?

A study was planned that tested a cohort of medical students to see whether their gender interacted with that of their patients, influencing the outcome of the consultation. The study examined the perceptions of medical students and the comfort levels of patients during consultation. This cross-sectional study used a self-administered questionnaire to survey 132 final-year medical students at one school in 1999. It tested students' patient-centeredness, "patient-care" values, and degree of comfort in performing certain intimate physical examinations.

The study showed that women medical students were more patient-centered than were men medical students. Both genders were more attuned to the concerns of patients of their own gender, were more comfortable with personal rather than sexual issues, and were more uncomfortable with performing more intimate examinations upon the opposite gender. Using comparable case studies, it was also shown that the female student-female patient dyad had significantly greater "patient care" values than did the male student-male patient dyad.

The study showed that medical students did not behave in a gender-neutral way in the consultation. There is a powerful interaction between a health provider's gender and a patient's gender.

From Zaharias G, Piterman L, Liddell M: Doctors and patients: gender interaction in the consultation, *Acad Med* 79(2):148-155, 2004.

FACTORS THAT IMPEDE MEN'S HEALTH

Many factors present as barriers to men's health, including their risk-taking behavior and infrequent use of the health care system. In addition, gaps in preventive health behavior and differences in illness and health orientations and reporting health behavior all contribute to a diminished health status for men. Several other barriers have been proposed, including the patterns of medical care provided in the United States, access to care, and lack of health promotion.

Medical Care Patterns

Although the data that serve as a foundation for medical treatment were collected from males, the concept of a health care provider that specializes in men's health is a relatively recent phenomenon. Many health professionals provide care for men with complex health needs in a wide variety of settings. A specialist to which a male could go to for care that "feels right" for him has not been developed. Little effort has been made to create a male-specific health care climate (Haines and Wender, 2006). Urologists, who may see men for genital abnormalities or diseases of the prostate, became the proxy "male health specialist." The medical specialty andrology, which originated in Europe to treat problems of fertility and sterility, is considered too narrow in focus to treat "the whole man." Without a primary care specialty that focuses specifically on men's needs and gender-role influences on health and lifestyle, the gender disparity will continue. Currently, male health concerns are addressed by specialists and generalists who have not received gender-specific training that would enable them to focus on men's health needs. In the current era of managed care, men will still be left without a gender-specific primary care provider with training focused specifically on men's needs.

Access to Care
Mission Orientation

Historically, society's interest in men's health has focused on efforts necessary to maintain an effective workforce. Men are socialized to view health as a commodity or resource that enables the body to work. Mission-oriented health care is a priority for large industries and organized sports. Industries provide workers with preventive health care to maintain workplace productivity. Mission-oriented health care in the sports arena has given birth to the specialty of sports medicine. Insurance programs such as health maintenance organizations (HMOs) may provide more comprehensive health care to men. Perhaps the most complete care is currently offered by the military; however, marked deficiencies exist in the lack of a focus on prevention and health promotion at the individual and aggregate levels and inattention to policy regarding environmental hazards.

Financial Considerations

Another barrier to health care for men is financial ability. A man may receive an annual physical examination if he belongs to an HMO or if he is an executive or an airline pilot, but many private insurance companies will reimburse more fully for a diagnosed condition (e.g., for pathology) and less fully for preventive care. A man is more likely insured for acute or chronic illness conditions than for health education, counseling, or other types of preventive health care. Women have annual gynecological examinations that include screening for other conditions and allow a woman to express other physical or psychological needs; however, men have lacked entrée to the health care system for a physical examination on a routine basis. With the advent of managed care and societal interest in preventive health focus, gender differences in routine physical examinations for preventive reasons have narrowed. However, socialization has a marked influence on behavior, and current trends may prevail despite attitudinal changes in health care delivery. Men must become advocates for programs that meet their own health care needs (Porche, 2009).

Time Factors

Historically, medical care could be accessed between the hours of 9:00 AM and 5:00 PM Monday through Friday. Men were reluctant to take time from work for a medical visit, especially for reasons other than illness. Fear of loss of income or the stigmatization of being "weak," "ill," or "less of a man" inhibited medical care access for males. Men in the lower socioeconomic group may be too exhausted from working to access health care, especially preventive health care (Haines and Wender, 2006). Variety in the times and locations of care delivery clinics should increase male access. More walk-in primary care clinics that provide evening and weekend appointments have appeared. These clinics may be housed in occupational settings, malls, and even grocery stores. Data need to be collected regarding male utilization of these additional health care sites.

Lack of Health Promotion

Limiting the concept of health as merely absence of disease eliminates health promotion. Using traditional mortality and morbidity rates as reflective of the state of "health" of a population represents only a biological basis of health. To provide the community health nurse with a clearer picture of male health, the presence of behavioral risk factors such as smoking, alcohol consumption, obesity, and sedentary lifestyle should be considered. When asked, men describe "healthy" people as those with proportional body weight and height who do not engage excessively in behaviors detrimental to health. Physical recovery after impairment, illness, or injury is also considered a factor in men's definition of "healthy." Disease prevention and health promotion are not often reflected in a man's perception of health. Addressing and limiting the precursors of death is a recent health care phenomenon (Box 18-2). Interventions by many disciplines are needed to prevent current health problems. Nursing can play a pivotal role in the contribution to practice and research in this area of concern.

The continued focus on disease cure in the present health care system reinforces men's perception of health. Coronary heart disease, cancer, and stroke are three conditions that account for two thirds of all deaths and require the greatest

BOX 18-2 PRECURSORS OF DEATH

The following precursors of death are frequently unaddressed by the present health care system:
- Heart disease and stroke
- Hypercholesterolemia
- Hypertension
- Diabetes mellitus
- Obesity
- Type A personality
- Family history
- Lack of exercise
- Cigarette smoking
- Cancer
- Sunlight
- Radiation
- Occupational hazards
- Water pollution
- Air pollution
- Dietary patterns
- Alcohol
- Heredity
- Certain medical conditions

use of health care resources. The increase in life expectancy exhibits the effect these medical advances have had on mortality rates from these diseases. These advances have resulted in an increase in years of disability, which may account for the increase in suicide among males over the age of 65 years (NCHS, 2004b). An increase in health care costs has also resulted.

SOCIAL DEMOGRAPHY AND SOCIAL EPIDEMIOLOGY

Epidemiology is the method of research used to determine the nature and distribution of a health problem in a community. Social demographers and social epidemiologists study social and psychological factors that affect the distribution of health problems in a community. Factors associated with the occurrence of the problems can be identified, and resources can be focused on prevention. Social epidemiologists have identified men as a population at risk for premature death. Concentrated efforts can improve men's health.

ETHICAL INSIGHTS
Social Justice Versus Market Justice Ethics

Community health nurses should be involved in political activities that develop health policies that will make a difference in the health of males and the entire population. Such activities are congruent with the philosophy of public health as "health for all" and a commitment to a social justice ethic of health care rather than a market justice ethic of health care. Examining men's health gives the community health nurse an opportunity to observe the market justice ethic of health care's influence on men's health in the United States from men's traditional roles in the family, the health of women, family, and community. The community health nurse can play a vital role in contributing to a social justice ethic of health care, particularly in relation to promoting men's health. Nurses must focus on health promotion and prevention at the aggregate and population levels rather than focus on treatment and cure.

Financial resources are invested in traditional disease curative care rather than health promotion action. An inordinate amount of funding is poured into the health care system each year, with only minimal amounts allotted to public health promotion, as discussed in earlier chapters. In 2002, total health expenditures accounted for 14.1% of the gross domestic product. Of every dollar spent on health care in 2002, more than half went to hospital care and physician services, which are, in large part, curative in focus. The current health care system is making limited advances in addressing the precursors of death. It is questionable whether medical care, or another medical specialty, is the answer to men's health needs when social, occupational, environmental, and lifestyle factors continue to place men at risk.

Healthy lifestyles are not a matter of free choice but rather a result of opportunities that are not always equally available to people. Although available, prevention and health promotion are not uniformly applied at the aggregate and population levels. Health policies shape these opportunities for a healthy lifestyle for individuals and aggregates. Policies related to environmental and occupational changes beyond an individual's control are required to significantly impact the health of the population (Meryn, 2008).

MEN'S HEALTH CARE NEEDS

DeHoff and Forrest (1984) delineated men's health care needs that draw from the biological and the psychosocial causes of men's distinctive health situation, and these health care needs continue today. According to these authors, men need the following:

- Permission to have concerns about health and talk openly to others about their concerns
- Support for the consideration of gender-role and lifestyle influences on their physical and mental health
- Attention from professionals regarding factors that may result in illness or influence a man's expression of illness, including such things as occupational factors, leisure patterns, and interpersonal relationships
- Information about how their bodies function, what is normal, what is abnormal, what action to take, and the contributions of proper nutrition and exercise
- Self-care instruction, including testicular and genital self-examination
- Physical examination and history taking that include sexual and reproductive health and illness across the life span
- Treatment for problems of couples, including interpersonal problems, infertility, family planning, sexual concerns, and sexually transmitted diseases (STDs)
- Help with fathering (i.e., being included as a parent in child care)
- Help with fathering as a single parent, in particular with a child of the opposite sex, in addressing the child's sexual development and concerns
- Recognition that feelings of confusion and uncertainty in a time of rapid social change are normal and that they may mark the onset of healthy adaptation to change

- Adjustment of the health care system to men's occupational constraints regarding time and location of health care sources
- Financial ways to obtain these goals

Additional health care needs of men are for primary prevention, and for secondary and tertiary prevention at the individual, family, and community levels, to address the precursors of death that influence males so greatly. Men are less likely to be consumers in the health care system than are women; therefore alternative approaches must be developed that address their health needs. The most significant approaches in the future will be those that reach men in the community, schools, the workplace, and public settings. These approaches call for political processes that set policy, for health marketing techniques, and for advocacy (Meryn, 2009).

COMMUNITY HEALTH NURSING SERVICES FOR MEN

A male can be seen by a community health nurse in a well-baby clinic, by a school nurse, by an occupational health nurse, and by a community health nurse or home health nurse on a home visit for follow-up of a chronic disease. However, men are less likely than women to be seen by a community health nurse. Not only is maternal and child health a major focus of many health departments, but neither a medical nor a nursing specialty within a health department routinely exists to specifically address men's health. Preventive reproductive health care (i.e., family planning, prenatal care, and cancer screening) and associated general screening are not routinely available for men. The hours of services offered by health departments usually do not provide convenient access for men. The community health nurse's commitment to health for all requires an increased awareness of men's health issues in their social and cultural context and individual and group action that will improve men's physical, psychological, and social well-being.

Meeting men's health care needs can be viewed in a traditional public fashion. By viewing the problem from a primary, secondary, and tertiary intervention method, the nurse can look at the problem in a holistic manner. Factors that promote men's health are in the community, including interest groups in men and men's health, men's increasing interest in physical fitness and lifestyle, policy related to men's health, and health services for men.

GAINING SKILLS NECESSARY TO ADDRESS MEN'S HEALTH NEEDS

Assessment skills necessary to carry out screening activities with men to detect reproductive health needs may be lacking in nursing education. One community health nurse who worked in a rural health department felt unable to respond to male partners' requests for genital examinations when couples came to seek family planning services. This community health nurse requested to work for specified periods of time with a urologist and in an STD clinic in a large urban area to gain the necessary skills. On return to the rural health department, she felt comfortable with male patients and taught the skills she had learned to nurse colleagues. Cheatham et al. (2008) suggests that providers make efforts to establish a positive patient-provider relationship using nonjudgmental verbal and nonverbal communication techniques. Engage the male and the female significant other in a manner that is easily understood.

PRIMARY PREVENTIVE MEASURES

Health Education

Health care professionals, including the community health nurse, find that health education is the cornerstone of prevention. Although criticized by some as too narrow, health education can be a means of empowerment that assists individuals to make behavioral changes. Education about male health issues should begin early. At school, boys should learn the anatomical and physiological aspects of their bodies and the social aspects of taking responsibility for their health. Coeducational discussion classes that cover a variety of social and personal topics can be a venue to encourage boys to talk about their bodies and their feelings. Adolescent males are shown to lack the use of language when compared with their female counterparts. This may lead to a less self-conscious attitude toward health seeking when boys reach adulthood.

Access to health education should follow males into the workplace. Many employers have experienced benefits such as lower health care costs when their employees receive health education programs coupled with health screening. Government and private insurance incentives given to employers who provide such programs would provide further impetus. Men who are not in the workplace can access health education in other areas, such as shopping malls, barbershops, and local senior centers. Some health care professionals are concerned about this informal dispersion of health literature, citing concern about the literacy level of the population. Government benefits programs can be a medium for health education by including such in their benefit mailing. More control over the readability and the information included can be exerted over this material. Educational material should be written in the context of male interests and should focus on making healthy living relevant to the male (Cheatham, Barksdale, and Rodgers, 2008).

Interest Groups for Men and Men's Health

Unlike the consumer movement that occurred on behalf of women's health in the 1960s and early 1970s, a consumer movement has not taken place advocating men's health. However, a viable men's consumer movement is forming. The National Organization for Men Against Sexism is interested in redefining the male role, particularly those aspects of the male role that are detrimental to health and growth. The American Assembly for Men in Nursing sponsors annual meetings that address issues such as men's health, men's work environments, research on men's health, and networking and support among male nurses. Researchers are beginning to define and study men's health beyond men's occupational role (e.g., reproductive health). Marketing has changed to include male health promotion public service announcements. Peer-reviewed journals such as *International Journal of Men's Health* and *American Journal of Men's Health* are providing scholars with avenues to disseminate men's health concerns.

Men's Increasing Interest in Physical Fitness and Lifestyle

Although cardiovascular diseases (CVDs) are a major health hazard for men, research on the validity and usefulness of preventive and treatment modalities is an issue of considerable debate (Harvard Men's Health Watch, 2009). Men's interest in altering behavior that places them at risk for cardiovascular and other major diseases is increasing, especially among older males (Shapiro and Yarborough-Hayes, 2008). For example, men's smoking behavior has changed dramatically. In 1965, more than 50% of males smoked compared with 25% in 2002. Today, 59.4% of men report exercising three times a week or more, compared with 52.1% of females (NCHS, 2004b).

However, those health behaviors that have reported the greatest change in a positive direction have been those most influenced by legislative action (e.g., seat belt use, use of smoke detectors, and drunk driving). Even with these legislative actions, males remain three times less likely to use a seat belt as females of the same age. In the Southeast, pickup truck usage of seat belts was 25% compared with greater than 75% for other vehicles. The states of Alabama, Florida, Georgia, Kentucky, Mississippi, North Carolina, South Carolina, and Tennessee have begun a campaign called "Buckle Up in Your Truck." The campaign's centerpiece is the use of targeted television and radio advertisements to encourage seat belt use. Intensive enforcement mobilizations in the form of Selective Traffic Enforcement Programs (STEPs), like "Click It or Ticket," will immediately follow the periods of pickup truck advertisements.

The Southeast's "Buckle Up in Your Truck" campaign is a 16-month campaign, whereby program processes and outcomes will be measured and documented. Progress will be measured using a number of data collection methods (Preusser Research Group, 2003).

Policy Related to Men's Health

Policies related to any group of people should include the opinions and perceptions of those directly affected. Policy related to men's health should include the male perception of health. Community health nurses can encourage and assist males to be advocates for policies regarding their health care. Male nurses can be extremely instrumental in this endeavor. Liaisons between male consumers and policy planners should be formed.

SECONDARY PREVENTIVE MEASURES

Health Services for Men

Fewer health care clinics are tailored to men's special needs than to women's special needs. The "well-man clinics" set up in the 1980s were designed to identify lifestyle risk factors, not to provide screening clinics like the women's clinics. Once identified, a method or resolution for these lifestyle risk factors is formulated. Although many well-man clinics exist in the United Kingdom, male usage of these clinics is far below female usage of women's clinics (Roberts and

Gerber, 2003). Although not based on the medical model, Australia's Men's Shed provided men with the socialization needed to make positive health behavior changes. Male screening methods typically have been limited to detecting high blood cholesterol levels and cancers such as prostate cancer, skin cancer, and testicular lumps. The era of managed care may not encourage the concept of gender-specific care, as men and women receive primary care from the same health services.

Screening Services for Men

The U.S. Preventive Services Task Force (2004) outlines the kinds of screening tests the population should receive. According to the Task Force, healthy men under age 50 years should have the following:

- Dental examination: Yearly
- Eye examination: Every 3 to 5 years
- Blood pressure check: Every 2 years
- Blood cholesterol check for men aged 53 years and older: Yearly
- Prostate examination: Every year after age 50 years; blacks every year after age 40 years
- Colorectal screening: Every 3 to 5 years
- Tobacco use and cessation information every year
- One-time screening for abdominal aortic aneurysm for men 65 years old if the male has smoked

Community health nurses should be familiar with these recommended screening test frequencies and should take every opportunity to encourage men to have these screenings. Through the institution of male health care fairs and other organized screenings, nurses are able to work with other health care providers to ensure these routine screenings are performed.

TERTIARY PREVENTIVE MEASURES

Sex-Role and Lifestyle Rehabilitation

Traditional health services for males are available in both private and governmental arenas. The emphasis of these services is on diagnosis and treatment. The traditional male role may change dramatically from treatment modalities. Rehabilitation services for males must include counseling on lifestyle, role changes, and job retraining. Men must be given permission to express their emotions, such as fear and anxiety, over the resultant change (Cheatham et al., 2008).

Goal setting and possible methods for achievement must be acceptable to the man. For example, after a heart attack, a man may be told to stop smoking and begin an exercise program. To be successful, the male must be an active partner in the formation of the plan. (He may be able to exercise, for example, by walking to the nearest automotive shop to talk with friends rather than spending time on a stationary bicycle at a local gym.)

Time away from work due to occupational injuries should be kept to a minimum. Males should be encouraged to return to work in an altered capacity rather than remaining away from work until the injury is completely healed. Occupational

accommodation for the treatment regimen will help ensure compliance. Provision of medical care, supportive physical and occupational therapies, and "light-duty" jobs at the worksite help preserve the masculine persona.

DOOR OPENERS: WAYS TO ADDRESS MEN ABOUT HEALTH CONCERNS

Strategies to address men about health concerns include the following:

- Ask a man to talk about the last time he had a physical examination, what was done, why it was done, where it was done, and what the recommendations were.
- Ask a man how he feels about his health insurance coverage. If he lacks health insurance, ask about the resources he used to obtain medical care for himself and for his family.
- Ask a man about how he spends his leisure time, what he is doing to take care of himself, and what his usual physical activities are.
- Observe a man for signs of stress such as moist palms, nail biting, posture, and nervous movements. If signs of stress are present, ask about how he is coping with an identified health problem, family problem, or being unemployed.
- Observe a man for difficulty clearing airway (e.g., from smoking) and flushing of the face (e.g., from alcohol). Inquire as to habits of smoking and drinking and whether these habits have increased since the occurrence of the particular health or social problem.
- Involve men in decision making about health care to instill a sense of control over events.

New Concepts of Community Care

Specific services for men within health departments continue to be lacking in the United States. With the exception of STD clinics and selected family planning service models, male health concerns remain unaddressed. Two male health visitors (the British term for public health nurses) from the National Health Service (NHS) started an innovative public health nursing program directed at men in Glasgow, Scotland. Health visitors Bill Deans and Bob Hoskins established a nurse-run well-man clinic with the help of the NHS and the Scottish Council for Health Education. During home visits with mothers and infants, Deans and Hoskins observed that fathers excused themselves and went to the local pub when they arrived.

Any intervention regarding men's health needs must include men as willing participants (Lynch, 2008). Noting characteristics of the male population in their community (e.g., overweight, heavy smoking, drinking, and high unemployment), Deans and Hoskins decided to modify their practice to serve their clients' needs. One afternoon per week, the clinic, which is based on a nursing model rather than a medical model, offers health screening, health education, and primary prevention to men. Marketing is important, and men are referred from general practitioners' and specialists' practices and recruited through newspaper advertisements. Clients with clinical signs and symptoms are referred back to their physicians. Lifestyle counseling and education are offered in areas such as fat and fiber content in diet, smoking, alcohol use, and exercise.

Deans and Hoskins consider the clinic a way to extend the health visitor's role in the NHS's efforts in health education with an aim to "nip potential diseases in the bud." Deans and Hoskins are concerned that the NHS does not provide male services and are clear that "the unemployed chain-smoking husband needs as much care and health education from the health visitor as do his wife and baby" (Sadler, 1979, p. 18). The well-man clinic and the well-woman clinic models can now be found in several communities throughout Great Britain and have been expanded to serve inmates in prison (Ballinger, Talbot, and Verringer, 2009; Woodland and Hunt, 1994). After 10 years in existence, the well-man clinics in Great Britain are only sporadically used by males. Even when the services were expanded to the home, nurses found that men were purposely absent at the appointment time. Usage was highest with informal evening clinics directed by male nurses (Roberts and Gerber, 2003). An attempt to evaluate these nationally funded clinics was undertaken in 2003. It was suggested from the data that a collaborative approach to these interventions is a slow process and adequate time should be provided prior to evaluation (Reid et al., 2009).

In Australia, Men's Shed is a community-based health promotion initiative in men's health. Based on the social rather than medical model, these sheds promote well-being among older males by providing them with accepted and respected activities, as well as providing a male-friendly space for socialization. Ballinger and colleagues (2009) found that participants in these activities reported an increase in recognition of the importance of health determinants and a sense of well-being.

Public health nurses working in the Benton County Health Department in Corvallis, Oregon, responded to the challenge of teen pregnancy in the 1970s by launching a community-wide effort that included developing a men's health clinic and marketing reproductive health services directly to teenage boys and men. An early effort established an advisory committee that included people from churches, schools, and health care facilities. A public health nurse health educator launched an extensive education program in the high school, which focused on decision-making processes and services available in the community. Later efforts involved the establishment of a clinic for men. Teenage boys were members of a consumer advisory committee established by the nurses that recommended the wording and format for advertisements about the clinic that ran in the high school newspaper. The advisory committee also recommended a flyer format that would be attractive to males. Specifically, they requested a card with information about the clinic and how to use condoms that would discreetly fit into their wallets and be available to share with peers.

The nurses have expanded their focus to create inclusive service environments in which teenage girls and boys and adult men and women will feel accepted and comfortable. Particular attention is given to the clinic decor and advertising, reading materials, and posters to transmit a message that includes offering health care for males and females. Clinic staff will see males or females at any time; however, a room in which staff members see men has decor geared toward men (e.g., no gynecological stirrups on the examining table) and pamphlets available for men on topics such as testicular cancer and chewing tobacco. Integrated services exist in the areas of family planning, STDs, and HIV counseling and testing.

CASE STUDY APPLICATION OF THE NURSING PROCESS

Community health nurses are in an ideal position to address the health needs of men at the individual, family, and community levels. The community health nurse may promote self-care in male members of the family, facilitate men's health by addressing needed changes at the family level, buttress women's roles as caregivers of the family's health, and bring about change that influences policies that affect men at the community level.

Planning gender-appropriate care for males is outlined in the following case study, which is an application of the nursing process at the individual, family, and aggregate levels initiated in a home visit, and applies the previous discussions about the levels of prevention, roles of the community health nurse, research, and men's health.

Application of the nursing process to aggregates is facilitated by the use of systems theory, in which the nurse identifies the system and subsystems involved. The nurse may use a deductive or an inductive approach. A deductive approach would involve carrying out a community assessment and identifying an area or areas, such as a program needed by the community. Planning, implementation, and evaluation of the program would be carried out at the family or group level. An inductive approach would involve entering the community system through a person or client via a referral about a problem or concern. Assessment of the individual would be followed by identification of those groups to which the client belongs, such as family and community, and assessment of those groups.

Beth Lockwood, a community health nursing student at a health department, received a referral from the high school nurse to visit the Connors family to assess Richard Connors' mental health status. Richard was a 16-year-old sophomore whose academic work in school had declined rapidly after the premature death of his 46-year-old father. He died of a myocardial infarction, which he had while cleaning the garage with Richard one evening after school. Richard and the neighbors failed to revive Mr. Connors, and Richard carries feelings of guilt. Household members include Mrs. Connors, age 44 years, and Richard's sister Yvonne, age 12 years.

Assessment
The referral to assess the Connors family called for an inductive approach to assessment. Beth used a deductive approach later, when her experience with the Connors family piqued her concern about the status of men's health in her community. Beth assessed Richard, his mother, and his sister as household members of the family. However, she could not stop with the immediate family; she had to continue to identify the other groups within the community to which each individual family member belonged. Viewing the community as a system and focusing on systems and subsystems helped Beth organize the data she collected during assessment. Knowing that "the whole is greater than the sum of its parts," Beth prepared for her visit by reviewing adolescent theories of development and family theory. Beyond individual assessment, she noted factors related to the development of sex-role–related behavior that may influence health. Examples of assessment areas include the following:
- Family configuration, traditional or nontraditional
- Sex-role-related behavior of parents, including work patterns in and out of the home, division of household labor, and decision-making patterns

- Patterns of parenting: mothering, fathering, and substitute father figure(s)
- Ability of male children to disclose feelings to family members and others
- Degree of assertiveness in female children
- Ability of family members to give emotional and physical support during crises and noncrises
- Ability of family members to trade off role-related behavior during crises and noncrises
- Risk-taking health behaviors
- Processing stress and grief
- Communal lifestyle patterns that place the individual or family at risk (e.g., lack of exercise, poor diet, smoking, and drinking)
- Family history of death and illness
- Health care–taking patterns of family members
- Preventive health behaviors
- Leisure activities

Assessment of other groups includes neighborhood and other peer groups, school environments, sports, and church and civic activities.

Diagnosis

Through induction, the nurse makes a diagnosis for each individual and each system component, including family and the community. The following are examples of diagnoses.

Individual

- Loss of interest or involvement in an activity, related to conflicting stages of grief process secondary to premature death of father (Richard)
- Expressed dissatisfaction with parenting role, related to feelings of helplessness and hopelessness secondary to premature death of husband (Mrs. Connors)
- Risk of interpersonal conflict, resulting from prolonged, unrelieved family stress secondary to premature death of father (Yvonne)

Family

- Decreased ability to communicate, related to family stress secondary to premature death of father
- Risk of family crisis, related to disequilibrium

Community

- Inadequate systematic programs for linking families in crisis to community resources
- Inadequate systematic programs for populations at risk of premature death, related to inadequate planning among community systems

Planning

Planning involves contracting and mutual goal setting and is an outcome of mutually derived assessment and diagnosis. A contract with the family alone is shortsighted and may provide little community benefit over time. The following are examples of other aggregates with which a contract may be established:

- The school subsystem that does not provide ongoing counseling, but will meet periodically to evaluate pupil progression with family members
- The school subsystem that provides physical education in football, basketball, and baseball (i.e., nonaerobic, nonlifetime sports), but offers extramural aerobic, lifetime sports such as swimming and track after school hours
- The American Red Cross, which does not offer cardiovascular pulmonary resuscitation (CPR) courses on evenings or weekends, but offers to consider doing so for a defined minimum-size community.

Mutual goal setting requires collaboration regarding long- and short-term goals. Again, mutually defined needs and diagnoses are important to this process. Regardless of the diagnosis, each individual in the family and the subsystem must participate in developing a care plan. The following are examples of goals.

Individual
Long-Term Goal

- Individual family members will be able to trade off role-related behavior.

Short-Term Goal

- Individual family members will express feelings related to abandonment and loss.

Family
Long-Term Goal

- The family will exhibit an increased ability to handle crisis, as evidenced by ability to discuss roles and interdependencies.

Short-Term Goal

- The family will identify specific ways to recognize and use support services.

Community
Long-Term Goal

- Systematic programs, with ongoing program evaluation, will be established for populations at risk of premature death from coronary heart disease, as evidenced by local planning bodies.

Short-Term Goals

- Dissemination is provided to individuals, families, groups, and planning bodies in the community about the incidence of coronary heart disease.
- Existing programs are identified that address coronary heart disease.
- Existing programs are coordinated to bridge gaps and avoid duplication of effort.

Intervention

The nurse, family, and other aggregates carry out interventions contracted during the planning phase to meet the mutually derived goals. Most important, the nurse empowers the family and community to develop the networks and linkages necessary to care for themselves.

Individual

Individual counseling regarding loss and grief may be beneficial to each family member, but options may need to be explored and referrals may need to be reevaluated for members of the rural family. Education regarding preventive measures that combat risk factors for heart disease include those aimed at individual family members and address areas such as diet, exercise, smoking, alcohol use, and stress management.

Family

Examples of interventions with the family include counseling, education, and referral aimed at family self-care promotion. For example, Beth's interventions with the Connors family were dependent on the family's ability to solve problems, investigate community resources, and create linkages between the family and resources. Periodic family conferences at school and more inclusive family therapy may enable the family to work through the death of Mr. Connors; this results in the development of new roles and the communication necessary to maintain family equilibrium. Education regarding preventive measures to combat risk factors for heart disease may need discussion at the family and individual levels (e.g., diet, exercise, smoking, alcohol use, and stress management).

Continued

Community

The nurse must also carry out interventions with other aggregates. These may involve activities such as educating, facilitating program expansion, or tailoring programs to meet community needs. Intervention at the aggregate level calls for group and community work. The nurse carries out interventions at this level in several ways (e.g., by communicating community statistics from a community analysis, relating anecdotes from families served, or linking family experience to program need by acting as an advocate and bringing family members to board meetings or hearings on community health issues).

Education regarding preventive measures to combat risk factors for heart disease also includes those interventions aimed at the community. A rationale for the development of lifetime aerobic sports is needed not only by Richard, but also by school districts. Exploration of options with the school nurse and review of the school district health education curriculum would be beneficial. A community assessment of heart disease awareness, including determination of the availability of resources such as emergency response and CPR courses, is an aggregate intervention. Taking the outcome of the assessment in the form of statistics and the anonymous anecdotal story of the Connors family to planning bodies in the community is also intervention at the aggregate level. Creative programs other communities used (e.g., teaching CPR within the school system) should be investigated and proposed.

Evaluation

Evaluation is multidimensional and ongoing. Using a systems approach to evaluation, the nurse evaluates each component of the system, from individual family member to family and community, in terms of goal achievement. Evaluation includes noting degrees of equilibrium established, degree of change, how the system handles change, whether the system is open or closed, and patterns of networking. Ongoing evaluation includes noting referrals and follow-up of the individual, the family, and other aggregates in resource use.

Individual

Use of resources such as support groups by the individual family member may be noted. These resources may include a teen support group, a women's support group, support groups for those experiencing the loss of a spouse or other family member, reentry programs for women at a local junior college or university, and Parents Without Partners.

Family

Evaluation of the Connors family would include follow-up of their use of support services specifically for the family, such as counseling options for the family as a unit. Evaluation would also focus on the family's ability to handle crises in the future.

Community

Aggregate evaluation would focus on the community. For example, to what extent do school programs encourage sports options that promote lifetime aerobic activities and prevent premature death from heart disease? Are programs systematically planned in the community for populations that are at risk of premature death from heart disease?

Levels of Prevention

Society's expectations of men and women are in transition. Application of levels of prevention by the community health nurse must take into account men's health status, men's socialization, men's use of health care services, men's primary needs for prevention and health promotion, and the role of women as caregivers in family health.

Primary

Men are more likely to engage in risk-taking behavior than women and are less likely to engage in preventive behaviors; therefore, primary prevention must be marketed specifically to men. Examples of primary prevention for the Connors family are applied at the following individual, family, and community levels:

Individual

- Assessment, teaching, and referral related to diet and exercise behaviors

Family

- Assessment and teaching related to food selection and preparation at home and fast-food restaurant food selection
- Teaching and role-modeling gender roles that allow male members of the family to use alternative expressions of emotion

Community

- Provision of CPR courses for members of the community; consultation with schools regarding need for aerobic activities in physical education and sports programs

The nurse must pull men from the family, workplace, or other aggregates into involvement with family planning, education, antepartum and postpartum care, parenting, dental prophylaxis, and accident prevention. In addition, assessment of need for immunizations and classes (e.g., retirement preparation) is considered action aimed at primary prevention.

Secondary

Men have higher mortality, morbidity, and health care use rates for many of the leading causes of death, but they are second to women in overall use of health care services, including preventive physical examinations and screening; therefore, early diagnosis and prompt intervention must also meet men's needs. Examples of secondary prevention regarding the Connors family include the following:

Individual

- Screen for risk factors related to CVD in the individual, such as how the individual handles stress.

Family

- Screen for risk factors related to CVD in the family, such as how the family processes stress.

Community

- Organize screening programs for the community, such as health fairs.

The nurse must screen individuals and aggregates of men according to lifestyle risk factors, mortality rates at different age levels, morbidity rates, and occupational health risks.

Tertiary

Activities that rehabilitate individuals and aggregates and restore them to their highest level of functioning are aimed at tertiary prevention. The nurse in the community is ideally situated to locate people in need of rehabilitation services. The nurse may provide evaluation and physical, mental, and social restoration services. Men in need of rehabilitation may have special needs because their disability influences them, their families, and ultimately their communities. Financial assistance and vocational counseling, training, and placement may be priorities for the well-being of the family. Socialization causes men to have difficulty admitting they need help. Community health nurses who teach men with chronic disease to rest at specified periods during the day or continue with medical regimens or speech or occupational therapy are providing tertiary prevention. Working with couples as a unit is also important because caregiving patterns may shift as a result of chronic disease and disability. Encouraging men to express their concerns about their health, families, and jobs and frustration with themselves is important. The following are examples of tertiary prevention with the Connors family.

Individual
- Assist individual family members in dealing with grief from the loss of the father and husband.

Family
- Assist family in dealing with grief and assuming alternative roles.

Community
- Assist the community in dealing with loss of a fully functioning family by providing grief support services that include males or target males and females.

SUMMARY

As the information within this chapter shows, women do get sick and men die. There is gender disparity when comparing all areas of disease and health entities. Things are changing as there is more and more attention provided to the health of men.

LEARNING ACTIVITIES

1. Examine the vital statistics in the community and compare the gender-specific differences in mortality rates.
2. During a 1-week period, determine the frequency of newspaper articles in the local major newspaper that identify the top twelve causes of death for men.
3. Survey the billboards in the community and determine the frequency of those that depict gender-linked behavior of men associated with risk-taking behavior.
4. Survey local businesses and industries in the community to determine what health promotion and pre-

vention programs are available and used by men and women.
5. Select a family that has a man in the household who is accessible. Select two "door openers" appropriate to initiate discussion of health concerns with this man. Devise a gender-appropriate nursing care plan that includes primary, secondary, and tertiary prevention for this man as an individual, for his family, and for his community.
6. Select a family that has a man in the household who is not readily accessible. Interview the female caregiver in the household and obtain information by proxy about the man's health. If possible, arrange to meet the man for lunch, at work, or after work and obtain information about his health. Compare the information obtained by proxy with that obtained from the client.
7. Review major nursing texts (e.g., medical-surgical); examine the tables of contents and the indexes for content on men's health versus women's health.

REFERENCES

Baerolcher MO, Verma S: Men's health research: under researched and under appreciated, *Meidal Schience Monitor* 14:Part 3, 2008.

Ballinger M, Talbot L, Verrinder G: More than a place to do woodwork: a case study of a community-based Men's Shed, *J Men's Health* 6(1):20–27, 2009.

Benson V, Marano MA: *Current estimates from the National Health Interview Survey, 2001–2002,* www.cdc.gov/nchs/data/10_190_1.pdf.

Brown L, Bond M: An examination of influences on health protective behaviors among Australian men, *Int J Men's Health* 3(7):274–287, 2008.

Cheatham C, Barksdale D, Rodgers S: Barriers to health care and health seeking behaviors faced by black men, *J Am Acad Nurse Pract* 20:555–562, 2008.

Dehoff JB, Forrest K: Men's health. In Swanson J, Forrest K, editors: *Men's reproductive health*, New York, 1984, Springer.

Haines C, Wender R: Men's health, *Prim care: Clinics in office practice* 33(1):xiii–xv, 2006.

Harvard Men's Health Watch, Volume 13: Number 8, March 2009, (no author)

Kirby R, Kirby M, Aoroso P, Dean J, Gould D: Steps by which better overall health for men could be achieved, *BJU Int* 98(2):285–288, 2006. www.bjui.org/ContentFullItem. aspx?id=81&SectionType=5.

Lynch L: Men's Health, *Ir Med J* 101(1):5–6, 2008.

Meryn S: Global man and health, *J Men's Health* 6(1):2–3, 2009.

Naslindh-Ylispangar A, Sihvonen M, Kekki P: Health, utilization of health services, "core" information and reasons for non-participation: a triangulation study among non-respondents, *J Clin Nurs* 17:2972–2978, 2008.

National Center for Health Statistics [NCHS], 2009: National Vital Statistic Report Volume 57, Number 14, April 2009. www.cdc. gov/nchs/data.

National Center for Health Statistics: 2004a. www. cdc.gov/nchs/fastats/mens_health.htm.

National Center for Health Statistics: *Health, United States, 2004*, Hyattsville, MD, 2004b, US Public Health Service.

National Health Interview Survey: 2002a. www.cdc.gov/nchs/nhis.htm.

National Health Interview Survey: 2002b. www. cdc.gov/nchs/data/series/sr_10_222.pdf.

National Institute for Occupational Safety and Health: *NIOSH workers health chartbook*, NIOSH publ 2004–146, 2004, www.chc.gov/ niosh/doc./chartbook.

National Vital Statistic Report: *Natl Vital Stat Rep* 57(14):April 2009 http://cdc.gov/nchs/data/ hus/hus08.pdf.

Organisation for Economic Co-operation and Development: *Health at a glance*, 2007.

www.oecd.org/document/16/0,3343,en_2649_ 34631_2085200_1_1_1,00.html.

Porche D: Men's health: building the science, *Am J Men's Health* 3(2):92, 2009.

Preusser Research Group: 2003, www.pickup safetybelt.com/index.php.

Reid G, van Teijlingen E, Douglas F, Robertson L, Ludbrook A: The reality of partnership working when undertaking an evaluation of national well men's service, *J Men's Health* 1(6):36–49, 2009.

Roberts A, Gerber L: *Nursing perspective on public health programming in Nunavut*, Iqaluit, Nunavut, 2003, Department of Health and Social Services. www.gov.nu.ca/ health/Report%20on%20Nursing% 20Perspectives%20on%20Public%20Heatlh% 20Programming%20in%20Nunavut.pdf.

Shapiro A, Yarborough-Hayes R: Retirement and older men's health, *Generations: Journal of the American Society on Aging* 32(1):49–53, 2008.

Singh-Manoux A, Gueguen A, Ferrie J, et al: Gender differences in the association between morbidity and mortality among middle-aged men and women, *Am J Public Health* 98(12):2251–2257, 2008.

Tanne JH: Medicine's new motto: one sex does not fit all, *American Health for Women* 16(5): 54–58, 1997.

U.S. Preventive Services Task Force: Men: Stay Healthy at 50+. Checklists for Your Health.

Agency for healthcare research and quality, 2004. /www.ahrq.gov/ppip/men50.htm.

Verbrugge LM, Wingard DL: Sex differentials in health and mortality, *Women's health* 12:103, 1987.

Waldron I: Changing gender roles and gender differences in health behavior. In Gochman DS, editor: *Handbook of health behavior research*, New York, 1995a, Plenum.

Waldron I: Contributions of changing gender differences in behavior and social roles to changing gender differences in mortality. In Sabo D, Gordon DF, *Men's health and illness: gender, power and the body*, Thousand Oaks, CA, 1995b, Sage.

Waldron I: Contributions of biological and behavioral factors in changing sex differences in ischaemic heart disease mortality. In Lopez A, Caselli G, Valkonen T, editors: *Adult mortality in developed countries: from description to explanation*, New York, 1995c, Oxford University Press.

Waldron I: Contributions of changing gender differences in behavior and social roles to changing gender differences in mortality. In Sabo D, Gordon D, editors: *Men's health and illness: gender, power, and the body*, Thousand Oaks, CA, 1995d, Sage.

Waldron I: Factors determining the sex ratio at birth. In United Nations, editors: *Sex differentials in infant and child mortality*, New York, 1995e, United Nations.

Whorton MD: Environmental and occupational reproductive hazards. In Swanson J, Forrest K, editors: *Men's reproductive health*, New York, 1984, Springer.

Woodland A, Hunt C: Healthy convictions… well-man clinic for the inmates of Lindholme prison, *Nurs Times* 90:32, 1994.

Senior Health

Mary Ellen Trail Ross, Edith B. Summerlin

Additional Material for Study, Review, and Further Exploration

evolve WEBSITE

http://evolve.elsevier.com/Nies
- Quiz
- Case Studies
- Glossary
- WebLinks

OBJECTIVES

Upon completion of this chapter, the reader will be able to do the following:

1. Discuss the aging process.
2. Discuss the demographic characteristics of the elderly population.
3. Describe psychosocial issues related to aging.
4. Describe physiological changes due to aging.
5. Recognize *Healthy People 2020* wellness goals and objectives for older adults.
6. Describe health/illness concerns common to the elderly population.
7. Identify nursing actions that address the needs of older adults.
8. Identify resources available to older adults.

KEY TERMS

advance directives
aging
alternative housing options
Alzheimer's disease
anxiety disorder
crime

depression
elder abuse
falls
glaucoma
guardianship
macular degeneration

Medicaid
Medicare
Social Security
suicide

OUTLINE

Concept of Aging
Theories of Aging
Demographic Characteristics
  Population
  Racial and Ethnic Composition
  Geographic Location
  Gender
  Marital Status
  Education
  Living Arrangements
  Sources of Income
  Poverty and Health Education
Psychosocial Issues
Physiological Changes
Wellness and Health Promotion
  Healthy People 2020

Recommended Health Care Screenings and
  Examinations
Physical Activity and Fitness
Nutrition
Common Health Concerns
  Chronic Illness
  Medication Use by Elders
Additional Health Concerns
  Sensory Impairment
  Hearing Loss
  Dental Concerns
  Incontinence
Elder Safety and Security Needs
  Falls
  Driver Safety
  Residential Fire–Related Injuries

In America, individuals aged 65 years or older are an important and growing segment of the population. Life expectancy is increasing; thus, larger numbers of people are reaching 65 years of age and older. In view of the increasing number of seniors who potentially will remain living in the community, the role of the community health nurse becomes very important in helping these seniors to continue to live independently and to increase their years of healthy life. For community health nurses to assist older adults, they must be familiar with the characteristics of seniors, their socioeconomic situations, their health behaviors, health status, health risks, and available community resources. This chapter discusses these issues and gives suggestions as to how community health nurses might address them.

CONCEPT OF AGING

Aging is a natural process that affects all living organisms. The concept of aging is most often defined chronologically. Chronological age refers to the number of years a person has lived. In the United States, an older adult is generally defined as one who is 65 years of age or older. However, it is important to remember that older adults cannot be grouped collectively as just one segment of the population. The older adult population is a heterogeneous group. The young-old (aged 65 to 74 years), the middle-old (aged 75 to 84 years), the old-old (aged 85 to 99 years), and the elite-old (more than 100 years old) are four distinct cohort groups (Ebersole et al., 2008).

Functional age, on the other hand, refers to functioning and the ability to perform activities of daily living (ADLs), such as bathing and grooming, and instrumental activities of daily living (IADLs), such as cooking and shopping. This definition of aging is a better measure of age than chronological age. After all, most older adults are more concerned with their functional ability than their chronological age. Assisting older adults to remain independent and functional is a major focus of nursing care.

THEORIES OF AGING

Since early times, scientists have attempted to explain why humans age. There are many biological and psychosocial theories of aging. Biological theories of aging answer questions such as "How do cells age?" and "What triggers the actual aging process?" (Miller, 2009). The biological theories can be subdivided into two main divisions: stochastic and nonstochastic. Stochastic theories explain aging as events that occur randomly and accumulate over time, whereas nonstochastic

BOX 19-1 BIOLOGICAL THEORIES OF AGING

Stochastic Theories
Error Theory
The error theory proposes that an accumulation of errors in protein synthesis occurs over time, resulting in impaired cellular function. Defective cells are produced, which eventually interfere with biological function (Orgel, 1963).

Somatic Mutation Theory
This theory is similar to the error theory but also suggests that when cells are exposed to x-ray radiation or chemicals, alteration of DNA occurs, increasing the incidence of chromosomal abnormalities and decreasing cellular and organ function. The deleterious effects appear in later life (Morley, 1995).

Free Radical Theory
Free radicals are highly reactive molecules that possess an extra electric charge (free electron) that can damage protein membranes, enzymes, and DNA. The body produces antioxidants that scavenge the free radicals (Hayflick, 1996).

Cross-Link Theory
This theory posits that aging causes body chemicals (proteins, lipids, nucleic acid, and carbohydrates) to become cross-linked. This causes abnormal metabolic activity and waste products to accumulate in the cells. The result is poor functioning of body tissues and structures (Hayflick, 1996).

Wear-and-Tear Theory
This theory describes a human as similar to a machine in that the human body eventually wears out because of decline in cellular function, death of cells, and mechanical injury and use (Hayflick, 1996).

Nonstochastic Theories
Programmed Theory
This theory postulates that normal cells divide a specific number of times. The number of cell divisions is proportional to the life span of the species. Human cells double 40 to 60 times before the ability to replicate is lost and cellular death occurs (Hayflick, 1996).

Immunologic Theory
There is alteration of the B and T cells, which causes a loss of a self-regulatory pattern between the body and the cell. Autoaggression occurs when cells normal to the body are misidentified as alien and are attacked by the body's immune system (Miller, 1996).

theories view aging as predetermined. Some of the popular biological theories are included in Box 19-1.

The three classic psychosocial theories of aging are behavioristic and examine how humans experience late life. The disengagement theory, proposed by Cumming and Henry

(1961), states that aging is inevitable, with mutual withdrawal or disengagement common; this results in decreased interaction between the aging person and others. The activity theory posits that activity is necessary to maintain life satisfaction and a positive self-concept (Lemon, Bengston, and Peterson, 1972; Maddox, 1963). The continuity theory suggests that a person continues through life in a similar fashion as in previous years (Havighurst, Neugarten, and Tobin, 1968).

Concepts gleaned from the various theories are useful to nurses as they care for older adults. For example, knowledge that the immune system is affected by aging implies the need for nurses to be vigilant about preventing infections (Miller, 2009). Psychosocial theories of aging point out the uniqueness of older individuals as they age and make life adjustments. Knowledge of these theories may help nurses to dispel common myths of aging.

DEMOGRAPHIC CHARACTERISTICS

Population

Americans are living longer than ever before, and it is expected that the older population will continue to grow. Presently, people who survive to age 65 years can expect to live an average of nearly 18 more years. The life expectancy of people who survive to age 85 years today is about 7 more years for women and 6 more years for men. Life expectancy varies by race, but the difference decreases with age. In 1900, people aged 65 years and older made up 4% of the population. In 2006, nearly 37 million people aged 65 years and over lived in the United States, accounting for just over 12% of the total population. The oldest-old population (those 85 years and older) grew from just over 100,000 in 1900 to 5.3 million in 2006 (Federal Interagency Forum on Aging-Related Statistics, 2008). There are about 40,000 centenarians in the United States (Ebersole et al., 2008).

The baby boomers (individuals born between 1946 and 1964) will start turning 65 years old in 2011, and the number of older adults will increase dramatically. By 2030, the number of Americans aged 65 years and older is expected to be twice as large as their counterparts in 2000, growing from 35 million to 71.5 million, and will represent nearly 20% of the total U.S. population. The greatest growth will occur in the population aged 85 years and older, whose numbers are projected to grow from 5.3 million in 2006 to nearly 21 million by 2050 (Federal Interagency Forum on Aging-Related Statistics, 2008).

Racial and Ethnic Composition

In addition to growing larger, the older population is becoming more diverse, as is the rest of the population. In 2006, non-Hispanic whites accounted for nearly 81% of the U.S. older population. Blacks made up 9%, Asians made up 3%, and Hispanics (of any race) accounted for 6% of the older population. The older population will grow among all racial and ethnic groups; however, the older Hispanic population is projected to grow the fastest (Federal Interagency Forum on Aging-Related Statistics, 2008).

Geographic Location

The proportion of the population aged 65 years and over varies by state. In 2006, Florida had the highest proportion of people aged 65 years and over (17%). Pennsylvania and West Virginia also had high proportions, each slightly over 15% (Federal Interagency Forum on Aging-Related Statistics, 2008). The nine states with the largest number of elderly individuals (1 million or more) are California, Florida, New York, Texas, Pennsylvania, Ohio, Illinois, Michigan, and New Jersey (Administration on Aging, 2001).

Gender

Older women outnumber older men in the United States. In 2006, women accounted for 58% of the population aged 65 years and over and 68% of the population aged 85 years and over (Federal Interagency Forum on Aging-Related Statistics, 2008).

Marital Status

Older men are more likely than older women to be married. In 2007, more than three quarters (78%) of men aged 65 to 74 years were married, compared with more than half (57%) of women in the same age-group. The proportion married is lower at older ages: 38% of women aged 75 to 84 and 15% of women aged 85 years and over were married. Widowhood is more common among older women than older men. Women aged 65 years and over were three times as likely as men of the same age to be widowed: 42% compared with 13%. In 2007, 76% of women aged 85 years and over were widowed, compared with 34% of men. Relatively small proportions of older men (8%) and women (10%) were divorced in 2007, and a small proportion of the older population has never married (Federal Interagency Forum on Aging-Related Statistics, 2008).

Education

Educational attainment has increased among older adults. In 2007, 76% of older adults were high school graduates (compared with 24% in 1965). Older blacks and Hispanics aged 65 years and older completed high school at lower rates than their white and Asian counterparts (58% and 42%, compared with 81% and 72%). In 2007, 19% of older adults had a bachelor's degree or higher (compared with 5% in 1965). Older Asians had the highest proportion with a bachelor's degree or higher (32%), compared with 21% for non-Hispanic whites, 10% for blacks, and 9% for Hispanics. Older men attained a bachelor's degree more often than older women (25% compared with 15%); however, the gender gap in completion of a college education is narrowing (Federal Interagency Forum on Aging-Related Statistics, 2008).

Living Arrangements

As age increases and widowhood rates rise, the percentage of the population living alone increases accordingly. In 2007,

73% of older men lived with their spouse, whereas fewer than one half (42%) of older women did. In contrast, older women were more than twice as likely as older men to live alone (39% and 19%, respectively). Older Hispanic (33%), black (32%), and Asian (30%) women were more likely than white women (14%) to live with relatives other than a spouse. Older white and black women were more likely than women of other races to live alone (approximately 40% each, compared with about 20% for Asian and 26% for Hispanic women). Older black men (29%) lived alone more than three times as often as older Asian men (8%). Older Hispanic men were more likely (17%) than men of other races and ethnicities to live with relatives other than a spouse (Federal Interagency Forum on Aging-Related Statistics, 2008).

Housing and Residential Services

Older adults typically prefer to "age in place" or live in their own home for as long as possible. In 2005, 93% of Medicare enrollees aged 65 years and over resided in traditional community settings. Two percent of the Medicare population aged 65 years and over resided in community housing with at least one service available, such as meal preparation, housekeeping, laundry, and assistance with medication. Approximately 5% resided in long-term-care facilities. The percentage of people residing in community housing with services and in long-term-care facilities was higher for the older age-groups. For example, among older adults aged 85 years and older, 76% resided in traditional housing, whereas 7% resided in community housing with services and 17% resided in long-term-care facilities (Federal Interagency Forum on Aging-Related Statistics, 2008).

Alternative Housing Options for Older Adults

The significant majority (93%) of older adults aged 65 years and older reside in the traditional, single-family home; however, some choose to downsize to smaller housing, such as townhouses or condominiums, where maintenance needs are eliminated or minimized. As mentioned, in 2005, only about 2% of elders aged 65 years and over resided in community housing with at least one service available. The types of alternative housing options included retirement communities or apartments, continuing-care retirement facilities, assisted-living facilities, and board and care facilities/homes. Services at these facilities include meal preparation, housekeeping, laundry, and medication administration. Approximately 5% of older adults reside in long-term-care facilities that provide 24-hour personal and/or skilled care, 7 days a week. The percentage of people residing in community housing with services and in long-term-care facilities is higher for individuals aged 85 years and older. These older adults generally have more functional limitations (Federal Interagency Forum on Aging-Related Statistics, 2008). It is important to note that many older adults who would like to change current living arrangements find that organized senior housing is too expensive for middle-class and lower-middle-class citizens. On the other hand, these individuals often have too many assets to qualify for subsidized housing.

Although not considered a housing option, adult day care provides a safe and supportive environment during the day for adults who cannot or choose not to stay alone. This service is often needed for caregivers who work during regular hours or need respite. Socialization, recreational activities, medication supervision, and meals are provided on-site. Often transportation to and from the facility is provided.

Sources of Income

In 2006, the median household income of older adults was $27,798. Aggregate income for the population aged 65 years and over came largely from four sources: Social Security provided 37%, earnings accounted for 28%, pensions provided 18%, and asset income accounted for 15%. Among older Americans in the lowest fifth of the income distribution, Social Security accounts for 83% of aggregate income, and public assistance accounts for another 8%. For those whose income is in the highest income category, Social Security, pensions, and asset income each account for about one fifth of aggregate income, and earnings account for the remaining two fifths (Federal Interagency Forum on Aging-Related Statistics, 2008).

With aging, a good percentage of income is spent on health care. Most older adults have Medicare, which provides health insurance for those who are 65 years of age or older, disabled, or have end-stage renal disease. Medicare is funded, in part, by Social Security contributions from employers, employees, and the self-employed. Medicare Part A is a hospital insurance plan that covers acute care, short-term rehabilitative care, and some costs associated with hospice and home health care. For 2009, the Part A deductible for acute care was $1068 for the first 60 days of a hospital stay per benefit period. This amount increases for longer hospital stays. Rehabilitative care generally provided in skilled nursing facilities is only covered if it occurs after a 3-day hospital stay and requires "skilled care" provided by a licensed nurse or by a physical or occupational therapist. Medicare Part A will pay 100% of the first 20 days of a nursing home stay, with a daily co-pay for days 21 to 100 and no coverage after that (U.S. Department of Health and Human Services [USDHHS]/Centers for Medicare and Medicaid Services [CMS], 2006).

Medicare Part B covers the costs for physician and nurse practitioner services; outpatient services, such as diagnostic procedures (e.g., laboratory and x-ray); qualified physical, speech, and occupational therapy; ambulance services; durable medical equipment; and some home health care services. Charges are paid by Medicare at a rate of 80% of what Medicare considers an "allowable charge." The client is responsible for the remaining 20% of the charge. In addition, the client is responsible for an annual Part B deductible ($135.00 in 2009) and a monthly premium of $96.40. This amount is generally deducted directly from the monthly Social Security check. Most individuals purchase Medigap policies, which cover the deductibles and co-pays. Another option is to join a Medicare Advantage Plan, which often provides more choices and benefits such as extra days in the hospital. To join a Medicare Advantage Plan, an older adult must have Medicare Part A and Part B. In addition to the Part B premium, there may be an additional monthly premium for the extra benefits provided (USDHHS/CMS, 2006).

The newest component of Medicare is the prescription drug coverage that became available in January 2006. The prescription drug plan is designed to help lower prescription drug costs. The individual chooses the drug plan and pays a monthly premium (about $37/month) and an annual deductible ($250 in 2006—this may increase in subsequent years). After the plan participant meets the deductible, he or she is responsible for 25% co-pay up to $2250. The individual is responsible for 100% of the next $2850, or a total out-of-pocket cost of $3600. At that point, the plan will pay 95% of prescription drug costs (USDHHS/CMS, 2006).

For older adults with low incomes, Medicaid may be available to offset the Medicare deductibles and co-pays and to provide additional health benefits. Each state establishes its own eligibility criteria within the broad guidelines established by the federal government. Medicaid generally covers more services than Medicare, including custodial care in nursing homes, without deductibles or co-pays.

Poverty and Health Education

To determine who is considered poor, the U.S. Census Bureau compares family income (or an unrelated individual's income) with a set of poverty thresholds that vary by family size and composition and are updated annually for inflation. By 2006, the proportion of the older population living in poverty had decreased dramatically to 9%. Older women (12%) were more likely than older men (7%) to live in poverty. Older people who live alone have higher rates of poverty than those who are married. Race and ethnicity are also related to poverty among the older population. In 2006, older whites were far less likely than older blacks and Hispanics to be living in poverty (about 7% compared with 23% and 19%, respectively) (Federal Interagency Forum on Aging-Related Statistics, 2008).

Community nurses will be increasingly called upon to care for older adults of diverse backgrounds who reside in various living arrangements. Although educational attainment has increased among the elderly population, many older adults have less than a high school education; therefore nurses must be sensitive and creative when providing instruction and teaching. Nurses cannot assume that an older adult has had a formal education. In addition, instructions may need to be given at a slower pace. It may also be imperative to include family or significant others when providing instruction. Also, written information may be sent home for further reference.

On the other hand, increased educational levels of current and future elders also provide a challenge for the community health nurse. These elders are, and will be, more informed and will make greater demands for current and scientifically based information, thus requiring the community health nurse to be knowledgeable about the latest developments in health care. Last, nurses must be aware of community programs and services that address the needs of a diverse older population. Many of these resources are discussed in this chapter.

PSYCHOSOCIAL ISSUES

In addition to adjusting to physiological changes related to aging and health concerns (discussed later in this chapter), older adults must cope with psychosocial and role changes such as retirement, relocation, widowhood, loss of family and friends, and possibly raising their grandchildren. Retirement may be a happy occasion when voluntary; however, the opposite may be true if it is involuntary. When older adults retire, they inevitably must cope with a change in social status and possibly income level; this may be especially difficult for people whose self-concept is related to job status. For retirees who are married, the spouse must also adjust to the changes related to retirement. Indeed, the adjustment may be more difficult for the spouse than the retiree as the retiree's leisure time will be increased. For elders who have no hobbies or interests, this extra leisure time may be a source of boredom. Nurses should encourage older retirees to pursue old hobbies and interests or establish new ones.

Relocation is another psychosocial issue that many older adults must manage. Often, relocation occurs as a result of health and functional impairment, lack of ability to maintain one's home, unsafe neighborhoods, and lack of assistance with ADLs or IADLs. The relocation may be prompted by the older adult's desire to be closer to family or medical care, or interest in moving to a new location or more supportive housing (as discussed in the section Alternative Housing Options for Seniors).

RESEARCH HIGHLIGHTS

Recognizing the Needs of the Elderly

Tsai (2005) examined factors that predicted distress and depression among elders with arthritis. Performing secondary analysis of data from 234 people aged 65 years and older (mean age 74.1 years), she determined that elders with higher levels of disability, more financial hardship, less social support, and younger age were more likely to have higher levels of distress than those who did not share these characteristics. Furthermore, distress, along with pain and disability, significantly predicted depression. She concluded that nurses should recognize the needs of elders with arthritis, considering a number of both physical (e.g., pain, level of disability) and psychosocial (e.g., social support, financial hardship) factors that might lead to depression, and intervene where appropriate and feasible.

From Tsai P: Predictors of distress and depression in elders with arthritic pain, *J Adv Nurs* 51:158-165, 2005.

Widowhood is an event experienced by most older adults, especially elderly women. According to Miller (2009), common consequences of widowhood are loss of one's sexual partner; loss of companionship and intimacy; feelings of grief, loneliness, and emptiness; increased responsibilities and dependency on others; loss of income and less efficient financial management; and changes in relationships with children, married friends, and other family members. Widowhood may be especially traumatic for elders who have been married for many decades. In addition to the loss of a spouse, older adults must also cope with loss of family members (sometimes their own children) and friends.

On the other hand, many older adults are faced with the responsibility of raising their grandchildren. Substantial increases have occurred in the number of children under age 18 years living in households maintained by their grandparents, often without the presence of the grandchildren's parents. Antecedents to children being raised by grandparents include neglect related to parental substance abuse, abandonment, emotional and physical abuse, parental death, mental and physical illness, incarceration, teen pregnancy, and grandparents assisting adult children who work or attend school. This arrangement may contribute to both physical and psychological problems. For example, Ross and Aday (2006) investigated the degree of stress in 50 African-American grandparents and found that 94% of the grandparents reported a "clinically significant" level of stress. Use of professional counseling, special school programs, and length of care giving greater than 5 years were associated with less stress. From

this study it was noted that coping strategies that were significantly correlated with less stress included accepting responsibility, confrontive coping, self-control, positive reappraisal, planful problem solving, and distancing.

The role of the community health nurse is to identify, support, and assist older adults experiencing various psychosocial changes and role adjustments. In addition, the nurse should provide information about various community resources and make referrals to agencies that might be helpful.

PHYSIOLOGICAL CHANGES

Normal physiological aging changes occur in all body systems. However, it is important to note that the rate and degree of these changes are highly individualized. These changes are influenced by genetic factors, diet, exercise, the environment, health status, stress, lifestyle choices, and many other elements. Table 19-1 depicts common physiological changes that occur with aging.

TABLE 19-1   NORMAL PHYSIOLOGICAL CHANGES ASSOCIATED WITH AGING

PHYSIOLOGICAL CHANGES	NURSING INTERVENTIONS
Sensory Changes	
Vision	
Decreased visual acuity	Use large print for teaching
Decreased visual accommodation	Encourage adequate lighting (e.g., nightlights)
Increased opacities	Encourage use of corrective lenses as prescribed
Increased sensitivity to glare	Decrease glare
Decreased ability to discriminate within blue-green color range caused by yellowing of the lens	Advise to use caution with blue-green color range (e.g., when taking medications and selecting clothing)
	Advise use of contrasting colors, reds, and yellows
Hearing	
Decreased ability to hear—presbycusis	Decrease extraneous sounds
Decreased ability to hear consonants with high-frequency sounds	Use concise sentences and speak slowly and distinctly in low-pitched voice
	Face person when talking; use gestures
	Encourage hearing examination (see Hearing Loss section)
	Encourage use of hearing aid if needed
Taste	
Diminished taste sensation	Encourage well-balanced meals
Decreased saliva production	Advise to drink plenty of fluids
Increased sensitivity to bitterness	Observe for overconsumption of sweets and salt
Decreased sensitivity to sweetness and salt	Give options for seasoning other than salt
	Teach about good oral hygiene
Smell	
Decreased smell acuity	Advise to use other senses and other people to assist with monitoring the environment for safety (e.g., spoiled food and gas fumes)
Touch	
Decreased sensitivity to touch	Provide a safe environment
	Monitor for extreme temperature changes in the environment (e.g., water temperature)
	Maintain adequate room temperature
	Ensure adequate clothing is worn for body warmth
Nervous System	
Decrease in brain weight	Assess neurological status
Reduction in neurons and cerebral blood flow	Ensure frequent position changes

TABLE 19-1 NORMAL PHYSIOLOGICAL CHANGES ASSOCIATED WITH AGING—cont'd

PHYSIOLOGICAL CHANGES	NURSING INTERVENTIONS
Slower autonomic and voluntary reflexes	Assess for pain and unique responses to pain
Reduced capacity to sense pain and pressure	
Increase in amount of senile plaque and neurofibrillary tangles	
Cognitive Changes and Changes in Balance	
Slower reaction time	Allow adequate time for response; teach fall precautions (see Falls section)
Slower learning time	Break instructions into small units
Memory: long-term memory better than short-term memory	Use shorter teaching sessions; Use cues and gestures
Intelligence: little change	Relate education to prior experience
Personality consistent with earlier years	Allow adequate time for completing tasks
Sleep	
Decrease in Stages 3 and 4 sleep pattern	Avoid interruptions at night
Increase in arousals during the night	Allow naps as needed
Total sleep time is slightly reduced	Avoid sleep medication use if possible
	Provide quiet environment for sleep
	Avoid stimulants and caffeine
	Assess quantity and quality of sleep
Cardiovascular System	
Decrease in tone and elasticity of aorta and great vessels	Pace activities
Thicker and stiffer heart valves	Allow rest periods
Slowing down of heart's conduction system	Encourage use of ambulation aids when appropriate
Myocardium slower to recover its contractility and irritability	Monitor for activity intolerance
Decreased cardiac reserve	Prevent or eliminate stressors
Decreased cardiac output	Monitor heart rate and blood pressure
Decreased ability to increase heart rate when stress occurs	Encourage regular exercise program
Increased peripheral resistance and pulse pressure	
Increased systolic blood pressure	
Respiratory System	
Reduced size of lungs, lung expansion, activity, and recoil	Encourage influenza and Pneumovax vaccinations
Increased rigidity of lungs and thoracic cage	Encourage regular exercise
Decreased cough response	Auscultate lung sounds
Decreased vital capacity	Encourage adequate fluid intake
Decreased number of alveoli and gas exchange	Monitor oxygen administration
Increased anterior:posterior chest diameter	
Musculoskeletal System	
Atrophy and decrease in muscle fibers	Prevent immobility
Decreased muscle mass and strength	Encourage regular exercise program
Reduced bone minerals and mass, causing porous and brittle bones	Teach safety precautions to prevent falls (see Falls section)
Shortening vertebra, causing shrinkage in height	Encourage adequate calcium intake
Kyphosis more common	
Gastrointestinal System	
Teeth become more brittle	Encourage good dental health (see Dental Concerns section)
Decreased esophageal/colonic peristalsis	Encourage diet that is well balanced and has adequate protein and vitamins
Decreased stomach motility	Encourage adequate fluids
Decreased production of saliva, HCl, and digestive enzymes	Encourage fiber in the diet
Decreased absorption of fat and vitamins B_1 and B_{12}	Advise to eat slowly and assess for indigestion
Decrease in thirst response	Monitor diet for deficiencies
	Encourage toileting schedule and monitor frequency of bowel movements
Renal	
Decreased size of kidneys	Monitor drugs—smaller doses may be needed
Decrease in number of nephrons	Observe for adverse responses to drugs
Reduced renal blood flow and tubular function	Monitor electrolytes and lab values
Decrease in glomerular filtration rate	Prevent dehydration
Decreased ability to concentrate urine	

Continued

TABLE 19-1   NORMAL PHYSIOLOGICAL CHANGES ASSOCIATED WITH AGING—cont'd

PHYSIOLOGICAL CHANGES	NURSING INTERVENTIONS
Genitourinary System	
Weakening of bladder muscle, causing increased urinary frequency, urgency, and nocturia	Assess bladder function and assist with frequent toileting
Decreased bladder capacity	Encourage bladder training program, exercises, and medication when needed
Increased retention	Observe for signs of urinary tract infection
Increased nocturia	
Women	
Atrophy of vulva and flattening of labia	Differentiate between changes due to normal aging, disease, and medications
Vaginal drying	Advise about use of lubricants for comfort during intercourse
Atrophy of cervix and ovaries	Provide education in normal reproductive changes
Shrinkage of uterus	Recommend breast examinations and mammograms
Ovulation ceases	
Decreased amount and elasticity of breast tissue	
Men	
Decreased elasticity of scrotal skin	Differentiate between changes due to normal aging, disease, and medications
Decrease in size and firmness of testes	Recommend prostate examination
Takes 2-3 times longer to achieve an erection, but able to maintain a long erection without ejaculation	
Venous and arterial sclerosis of the corpus spongiosum	
Prostatic enlargement	
Endocrine System	
Increased fibrosis and nodularity of thyroid gland	Recommend pneumococcal, influenza, and tetanus vaccinations
Shrinkage of thymus and pituitary glands	Monitor electrolytes and glucose
Decline in natural antibodies	Prevent infection
Decrease in adrenal gland secretion of glucocorticoid	Encourage good nutrition
Decreased levels of aldosterone	Observe for hypoglycemia or hyperglycemia
Delayed insulin release	
Reduced peripheral sensitivity to insulin	
Reduced ability to metabolize glucose	
Decrease in testosterone, estrogen, and progesterone	
Integumentary System	
Decreased skin elasticity	Encourage frequent position changes and inspect skin
Generalized thinning and dryness	Be careful of skin tears, bruising, and pressure ulcers
Atrophy of sweat glands	Recognize need for less frequent bathing; avoid harsh soaps; use lotion
Decline in natural insulation	Advise to eat a good diet, exercise, and limit exposure to harmful radiation
Variation in pigmentation (age spots)	Ensure adequate clothing and comfortable room temperature
Hair thins and grays on head and becomes thicker in nose, ears, and eyebrows (men)	
Increased facial hair on women	
Fingernails are fragile and brittle and grow more slowly	

From Eliopoulos C: *Gerontological nursing,* ed 7, Philadelphia, 2010, Lippincott Williams & Wilkins.

WELLNESS AND HEALTH PROMOTION

Health promotion and illness prevention interventions for older adults may be beneficial in reducing death and disability and improving quality of life. These are goals of *Healthy People 2020*. To address these goals, health care professionals must inform and educate elders about the benefits of health care screenings and examinations, physical activity and fitness, and good nutrition.

Healthy People 2020

A primary goal of *Healthy People 2020* is to increase the quality and years of healthy life. Although people are living longer, many older adults have chronic illnesses that interfere with the quality of their lives. To address this issue, *Healthy People 2020* includes specific objectives related to increasing health promotion programs and decreasing morbidity and mortality in older adults.

HEALTHY PEOPLE 2020

Selected Proposed Objectives for Older Adults

OBJECTIVE
AOCBC HP2020–8: Reduce the proportion of adults with osteoporosis.
AOCBC HP2020–10: Reduce hip fractures among older adults.
C HP2020–15: Increase the proportion of adults who receive a colorectal cancer screening based on the most recent guidelines.
ECBP HP2020–9: Increase the proportion of older adults who have participated during the preceding year in at least one organized health promotion activity.
ENT-VSL HP2020–3b: Increase the proportion of persons who have had a hearing examination on schedule; adults aged 70 years and older who have had a hearing examination in the past 5 years.
HDS HP2020–11: Reduce hospitalization of older adults with heart failure as the principal diagnosis.
IID Hp2020–24: Increase the proportion of adults who are vaccinated annually against influenza and ever vaccinated against pneumococcal disease.
IVP HP2020–26b: Reduce fall-related deaths; Adults age 65 and older.
OA HP2020–3: Increase the proportion of older adults with one or more chronic health conditions who report confidence in managing their conditions.
OA HP2020–7: Increase the number of States and Tribes that publically report elder maltreatment and neglect.
RD HP2020–2c: Reduce hospital emergency department visits for asthma; adults aged 65 years and older.

From US Department of Health and Human Services: *Healthy People 2020*: 2009 draft objectives. Accessed from www.healthypeople.gov/HP2020/Objectives/TopicAreas.aspx.

Recommended Health Care Screenings and Examinations

Many organizations such as the American Cancer Society, the American Heart Association, and the USDHHS Preventive Services Task Force have established recommendations for health promotion screenings and examinations. Box 19-2 depicts some of the more widely agreed-on screenings and examinations for older adults. These established recommendations might be very useful to community nurses when educating older adults about the benefits of screening and early detection of disease. Frequently, earlier detection of disease allows better treatment, lower health care costs, and the possibility of cure.

Physical Activity and Fitness

Physical activity is beneficial for the health of people of all ages, including older adults. Although there are various types of exercises, walking is one of the best forms of exercise, and it is free. Many older adults engage in walking, swimming, dancing, yoga, and tai chi for exercise. Regular exercise improves functional status, reduces blood pressure and cholesterol, decreases insulin resistance, prevents obesity, strengthens bones, and reduces falls. Despite known benefits of exercise, two thirds of adults between 65 and 75 years of age are inactive. Barriers to exercising that have been identified in older adults include lack of access to safe areas to exercise, pain, fatigue, and impairment in sensory function and mobility (Mauk, 2010).

Proposed objective PAF-6 of *Healthy People 2020* recommends that health care providers work to "increase the proportion of adults who meet current federal physical activity guidelines for aerobic physical activity and for muscle

strength training" (USDHHS, 2009). Nurses may help older adults accomplish this goal by assessing their understanding of the beneficial effects of exercise. Nurses should also educate, encourage, and assist older adults with exercise. When applicable, anti-inflammatory medications may be administered before physical activity to address accompanying pain.

Nutrition

In *Healthy People 2020*, nutrition was identified as a priority area of health promotion for people of all ages. Similar to patterns among other age groups, poor nutrition in the elderly population is common. An inappropriate diet is related to constipation, dental disease, physical inactivity, and depression. Normal physiological changes related to aging affect nutritional status. Fewer calories taken in may result in a decreased intake of essential nutrients. A diminished sense of smell may reduce the enjoyment of eating. Gastrointestinal changes can interfere with absorption of vitamin B_{12} and folic acid, leading to anemia. A diminished thirst sensation may lead to dehydration. Other factors that can affect the nutritional status of the elderly are income, functional status, taking multiple medications, social isolation, lack of transportation, and dependence on others for grocery shopping and cooking. The nutrition checklist presented in Table 19-2 lists warning signs and risk factors of poor nutritional health described by the mnemonic DETERMINE.

The new U.S. Department of Agriculture's (USDA's) food pyramid, known as MyPyramid, is a personalized approach to healthy eating and physical activity (Figure 19-1). Each person can find the amounts of food he or she should eat daily by going to http://www.MyPyramid.gov. Figure 19-2 depicts a sample food plan for a 70-year-old female who engages in 30 to 60 minutes of physical activity per day. Tips are provided

BOX 19-2 RECOMMENDED EXAMINATIONS FOR HEALTH PROMOTION AND DISEASE PREVENTION IN OLDER ADULTS

Examinations/Tests for All Older Adults

Complete physical: Annually

Blood pressure: Annually, more frequently if hypertensive or at risk

Serum cholesterol: Every 5 years; more frequently if high risk

Fecal occult blood test: Annually

Sigmoidoscopy: Every 5 years; or

Colonoscopy: Every 10 years

Visual acuity and glaucoma screening: Annually

Dental examination: Annually for those with teeth; cleaning every 6 months, every 2 years for denture wearers

Hearing test: Every 2 to 5 years

Women

Breast self-examination: Monthly

Clinical breast examination: Annually

Pelvic examination and Pap smear: Not needed if aged 65 years or older and not otherwise at risk

Digital rectal examination: Annually with pelvic examination

Mammogram: Every 1 to 2 years if aged 40 years or older

Men

Digital rectal examination and prostate examination: Annually

Prostate specific antigen (PSA) blood test: Annually

Immunizations for All Older Adults

Tetanus-diphtheria: Every 10 years

Influenza/flu vaccine: Annually

Pneumonia vaccine: Once after age 65 years; ask physician about booster every 5 years

Hepatitis A and B: For those at risk

Herpes zoster (shingles): One-time dose

From American Cancer Society: *Cancer facts & figures*, Atlanta, GA, 2008, The Author; and Centers for Disease Control and Prevention: Recommended adult immunization schedule, U.S., 2009, *MMWR Morb Mortal Wkly Rep* 59(1), 1-4, 2010.

on how to incorporate foods from each food group. The 2005 Dietary Guidelines remain the current guidance until the 2010 guidelines are published.

The community health nurse should use the nutrition checklist (see Table 19-2) to evaluate the nutritional status and needs of the elderly. A copy of a personalized food pyramid can be obtained and then used to assess the current eating patterns of the elderly. This may also be useful in making recommendations for dietary changes. The physical and mental status of the individual must be taken into account when making recommendations. For example: Can he or she shop for groceries? Can he or she prepare meals? Can he or she make logical choices related to food? Also, the social and cultural factors influencing nutritional choices need to be considered. The benefits of good nutrition are an important factor in helping to maintain independence and quality of life.

COMMON HEALTH CONCERNS

Chronic Illness

Chronic diseases are the leading causes of death among persons 65 years and older (Table 19-3). The prevalence of chronic diseases increases with aging, and most older adults have more than one chronic illness. The ten leading chronic conditions affecting the population aged 65 years and older are arthritis, hypertension, heart conditions, diabetes, hearing impairment, vision impairment, orthopedic impairments, chronic sinusitis, hay fever/allergic rhinitis (without asthma), and varicose veins (National Center for Health Statistics, 2003). Chronic illnesses are a major cause of disability and may cause limitations with ADLs and IADLs.

Medication Use by Elders

The high prevalence of chronic diseases in the elderly population causes this group to use a large number of medications. According to the Center for Medicare Education (2002), older adults consume slightly more than one third of all prescription drugs and spend billions annually on medications. Older adults also consume many over-the-counter medications, as well as "folk" or herbal remedies.

The elderly population is vulnerable to the effects of drugs because of normal aging changes (see Table 19-1) and age-related differences in pharmacokinetics and pharmacodynamics. Polypharmacy may also make older adults vulnerable to drug interactions and dangerous adverse reactions. During a 12-month period (1999 to 2000), Gurwitz and colleagues (2003) studied Medicare enrollees (30,397 person-years of observation) cared for by a multispecialty group practice. The researchers found 1523 identified adverse drug events, of which 27.6% (421) were considered preventable. Of the adverse drug events, 578 (38%) were categorized as serious, life-threatening, or fatal; 244 (42.2%) of these more severe events were deemed preventable, compared with 177 (18.7%) of the 945 significant adverse drug events. Errors associated with preventable adverse drug events occurred most often at the stages of prescribing and monitoring (i.e., the same medication[s], or different medications for the same condition, being prescribed by different health providers). Errors involving client adherence also were common. The most common medication categories associated with preventable adverse drug events were cardiovascular medications (24.5%), followed by diuretics (22.1%), nonopioid analgesics (15.4%), hypoglycemics (10.9%), and anticoagulants (10.2%). The most common types of preventable adverse drug events were electrolyte/renal (26.6%), gastrointestinal tract (21.1%), hemorrhagic (15.9%), metabolic/endocrine (13.8%), and neuropsychiatric (8.6%). The researchers concluded that prevention strategies should target the prescribing and monitoring stages of pharmaceutical care and that interventions should focus on improving client adherence to prescribed regimens.

TABLE 19-2	NUTRITION CHECKLIST FOR OLDER ADULTS: WARNING SIGNS OF POOR NUTRITIONAL HEALTH	

POSSIBLE PROBLEM	QUESTION TO ANSWER	SCORE FOR "YES" ANSWER (CIRCLE IF "YES")
Disease	Do you have an illness or condition that makes you change the kind and/or amount of food you eat?	2
Eating poorly	Do you eat fewer than two meals per day?	3
	Do you eat few fruits, vegetables, or milk products?	2
	Do you have three or more drinks of beer, liquor or wine almost every day?	2
Tooth loss/mouth pain	Do you have tooth or mouth problems that make it hard for you to eat?	2
Economic hardship	Do you sometimes have trouble affording the food you need?	4
Reduced social contact	Do you eat alone most of the time?	1
Multiple medications	Do you take three or more prescribed or over-the-counter drugs a day?	1
Involuntary weight loss/gain	Have you lost or gained 10 lb in the last 6 months without trying?	2
Needs assistance in self-care	Are you sometimes physically not able to shop, cook, or feed yourself?	1
Elder years >80 yr	Are you over 80 years old?	1
	TOTAL:	

Scoring:
- *0-2:* Good!
  Recheck your nutritional score in 6 months.
- *3-5:* You are at moderate nutritional risk.
  See what can be done to improve your eating habits and lifestyle. Your office on aging, senior nutrition program (e.g., Meals on Wheels), senior center, or health department can help. Recheck your nutritional score in 3 months.
- *6 or more:* You are at high nutritional risk.
  Bring this checklist the next time you see your physician/nurse practitioner, dietitian, or other qualified health or social service professional. Talk with them about any problems you may have. Ask for help to improve your nutritional health.

From Virginia Department for the Aging, *The Nutrition Screening Initiative,* Washington, DC, 2007, The Author: http://www.vda.virginia.gov/pdfdocs/Nutritional_chklst.pdf.

One of the roles of community health nurses is to closely monitor medication use in the home to ensure safety. An easy-to-use pill organizer may be helpful to older adults. In addition, older adults should be educated about potential adverse reactions, as well as drug-drug and drug-food interactions.

ADDITIONAL HEALTH CONCERNS

Sensory Impairment

Visual and hearing impairment are among the most common age-related conditions affecting the elderly population. Vision and hearing impairments were reported by 35% and 42% of respondents in the Longitudinal Study of Aging (LSOA). Further, dual sensory impairment affects more than one fifth (21%) of adults 70 years and older in the United States (Lighthouse International, 2005).

Visual acuity and visual accommodation normally decrease with age. Presbyopia, loss of elasticity of the lens of the eye causing difficulty with near vision, generally occurs in the 40s. Among older adults, the three most common pathologic eye conditions are cataracts, macular degeneration, and glaucoma. Among people aged 65 years and older who reported trouble seeing, 44% reported having had cataracts in the past 12 months, 16% reported having macular degeneration, and 16% reported having glaucoma (Federal Interagency Forum on Aging-Related Statistics, 2008).

Cataracts

Cataracts are the leading cause, as well as the most reversible cause, of visual impairment in older adults. A cataract is a clouding of the normally clear lens of the eye. Age is the single greatest risk factor for cataracts. By age 65 years, some degree of lens clouding has developed in half of all Americans, although it may not impair vision. Other risk factors that increase a person's risk of cataracts include diabetes, family history of cataracts, previous eye injury or inflammation, prolonged use of corticosteroids, excessive exposure to sunlight, and smoking. Older adults should have annual eye examinations. This examination will allow early detection and tracking of cataract development. The only effective treatment for a cataract is surgical removal of the clouded lens and replacement with a clear lens implant (Mayo Clinic Staff, 2004a).

Macular Degeneration

Macular degeneration causes severe loss of vision in older adults in the United States and other developed countries. Macular degeneration is a chronic eye disease that occurs when tissue in the macula, the part of the retina responsible for central vision, deteriorates. The retina is the layer of tissue on the inside back wall of the eyeball. Degeneration of the macula causes blurred central vision or a blind spot in the center of the visual field. Annual eye examinations can detect early signs of macular degeneration before the disease leads to vision loss. Any change to central vision or in the ability

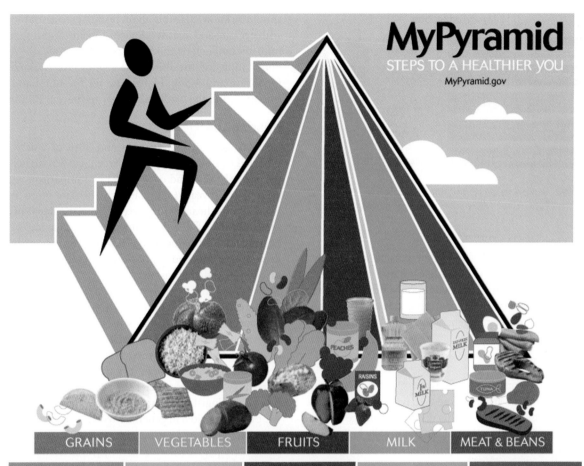

MyPyramid
STEPS TO A HEALTHIER YOU
MyPyramid.gov

GRAINS	VEGETABLES	FRUITS	MILK	MEAT & BEANS

GRAINS Make half your grains whole	VEGETABLES Vary your veggies	FRUITS Focus on fruits	MILK Get your calcium-rich foods	MEAT & BEANS Go lean with protein
Eat at least 3 oz. of whole-grain cereals, breads, crackers, rice, or pasta every day 1 oz. is about 1 slice of bread, about 1 cup of breakfast cereal, or ½ cup of cooked rice, cereal, or pasta	Eat more dark-green veggies like broccoli, spinach, and other dark leafy greens Eat more orange vegetables like carrots and sweetpotatoes Eat more dry beans and peas like pinto beans, kidney beans, and lentils	Eat a variety of fruit Choose fresh, frozen, canned, or dried fruit Go easy on fruit juices	Go low-fat or fat-free when you choose milk, yogurt, and other milk products If you don't or can't consume milk, choose lactose-free products or other calcium sources such as fortified foods and beverages	Choose low-fat or lean meats and poultry Bake it, broil it, or grill it Vary your protein routine — choose more fish, beans, peas, nuts, and seeds

For a 2,000-calorie diet, you need the amounts below from each food group. To find the amounts that are right for you, go to MyPyramid.gov.

Eat 6 oz. every day	Eat 2½ cups every day	Eat 2 cups every day	Get 3 cups every day; for kids aged 2 to 8, it's 2	Eat 5½ oz. every day

Find your balance between food and physical activity
- Be sure to stay within your daily calorie needs.
- Be physically active for at least 30 minutes most days of the week.
- About 60 minutes a day of physical activity may be needed to prevent weight gain.
- For sustaining weight loss, at least 60 to 90 minutes a day of physical activity may be required.
- Children and teenagers should be physically active for 60 minutes every day, or most days.

Know the limits on fats, sugars, and salt (sodium)
- Make most of your fat sources from fish, nuts, and vegetable oils.
- Limit solid fats like butter, stick margarine, shortening, and lard, as well as foods that contain these.
- Check the Nutrition Facts label to keep saturated fats, *trans* fats, and sodium low.
- Choose food and beverages low in added sugars. Added sugars contribute calories with few, if any, nutrients.

MyPyramid.gov
STEPS TO A HEALTHIER YOU

U.S. Department of Agriculture
Center for Nutrition Policy and Promotion
April 2005
CNPP-15

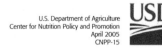

USDA is an equal opportunity provider and employer.

FIGURE 19-1 USDA Food Pyramid. (US Department of Agriculture: MyPyramid, 2005: www.mypyramid.gov.)

My Pyramid Plan

▶ Grains	6 ounces	tips
▶ Vegetables	2.5 cups	tips
▶ Fruits	1.5 cups	tips
▶ Milk	3 cups	tips
▶ Meat & Beans	5 ounces	tips

FIGURE 19-2 Sample food plan for 70-year-old woman. (From US Department of Agriculture: MyPyramid, 2005: http://www.mypyramid.gov.)

to see colors and fine detail should be reported to one's eye care specialist. An Amsler grid is a simple test that may be used to detect changes in vision. Treatment options depend on the location and the extent of the abnormal blood vessels. Damage already caused by macular degeneration cannot be reversed (Mayo Clinic Staff, 2004c).

Glaucoma

Glaucoma is sometimes referred to as the silent thief because it can slowly diminish vision before one realizes anything is wrong. The common feature of this disease is damage to the optic nerve, usually accompanied by an abnormally high pressure inside the eyeball. The most common form of glaucoma, primary or chronic open-angle glaucoma, develops gradually without warning and progresses with few or no symptoms until the condition reaches an advanced stage. The drainage angle formed by the cornea and the iris remains open; however, the aqueous humor drains too slowly. This leads to fluid backup and a gradual buildup of pressure within the eye. Increased eye pressure continues to damage the optic nerve, and more and more peripheral vision is lost. If left untreated, tunnel vision develops, followed by total vision loss (Mayo Clinic Staff, 2004b).

Nurses should educate clients about recommended vision screening. To determine the influence of visual impairment, the nurse should inquire about activity limitations associated with poor vision. Determining whether the client is using visual assistive devices such as glasses, contact lenses, magnifying lenses, or large-print books can be beneficial in recognizing the degree of adaptation. The community health nurse should be knowledgeable about resources to assist older adults with eye care and assistive devices. Organizations that provide information include the National Eye Institute, the American Foundation for the Blind, the Lighthouse National Center for Vision and Aging, Lighthouse for the Blind and Visually Impaired, and the National Society to Prevent Blindness.

Hearing Loss

In 2006, 48% of elderly men and 35% of elderly women reported trouble hearing. The percentage was higher for people aged 85 years and over (62%) in comparison with elders aged 65 to 74 years (32%). Elderly men are more likely than women to be hearing impaired. Eighteen percent of all older men and 10% of all older women reported having ever worn a hearing aid. Consequences of hearing loss may include withdrawal, isolation, and depression (Federal Interagency Forum on Aging-Related Statistics, 2008).

Nurses should assess older adults for hearing loss by using a tuning fork to detect hearing impairments and to differentiate between conductive and sensorineural loss. An otoscopic examination also should be done to examine the external ear canal and the tympanic membrane. If there is an abnormal accumulation of cerumen, it may need to be removed. The nurse may also need to refer the client for further assessment by an audiologist or otolaryngologist, who might recommend use of hearing aids. In general, Medicare and Medicaid do not cover the costs of hearing aids. Box 19-3 contains tips for health care providers who work with older adults with hearing difficulties.

Dental Concerns

The dental health of elderly individuals is often neglected with advanced age because of inadequate dental care, limited mobility and transportation, poor nutrition, the myth that it is natural for older adults to become edentulous, and lack of finances and reimbursement (Medicare and some states' Medicaid programs do not provide adequate reimbursement for dental needs). These risk factors predispose older adults to periodontal disease and tooth loss.

Serious dental problems are related to both age and income. The prevalence of edentulism (having no natural teeth) was higher for people aged 85 years and over (32%) than for people aged 65 to 74 years (23%). Thirty-nine percent of older people with family income below the poverty line reported no

TABLE 19-3	**LEADING CAUSES OF DEATH FOR PERSONS 65 YEARS OF AGE AND OLDER**				
WHITE	**BLACK**	**AMERICAN INDIAN**	**ASIAN OR PACIFIC ISLANDER**	**HISPANIC**
1. Heart disease	1. Heart disease	1. Heart disease	1. Heart disease	1. Heart disease
2. Cancer	2. Cancer	2. Cancer	2. Cancer	2. Cancer
3. Stroke	3. Stroke	3. Diabetes	3. Stroke	3. Stroke
4. COPD	4. Diabetes	4. Stroke	4. Diabetes	4. Diabetes
5. Alzheimer's disease	5. COPD	5. COPD	5. Pneu/influenza	5. COPD

From Gorian Y, Hoyert D, Lentzner H, Goulding M: *Trends in causes of death among older persons in the United States. Aging Trends,* No 6, Hyattsville, MD, 2006, National Center for Health Statistics: www.cdc.gov/nchs/data/ahcd/agingtrends/06olderpersons.pdf.
COPD, Chronic obstructive pulmonary disease; *Pneu,* pneumonia.

BOX 19-3 WORKING WITH OLDER ADULTS WITH HEARING DIFFICULTIES

- Include people with hearing loss in the conversation.
- Find a quiet place to talk to help reduce background noise, especially in restaurants and social gatherings.
- Stand in good lighting and use facial expressions or gestures to give clues.
- Face the person and talk clearly.
- Speak a little more loudly than normal, but don't shout.
- Speak at a reasonable speed; do not hide your mouth, eat, or chew gum.
- Repeat yourself if necessary, using different words.
- Try to make sure only one person talks at a time.
- Be patient. Stay positive and relaxed.
- Ask how you can help.

From National Institute on Aging: *Age page: hearing loss,* July 2009: www.nia.nih.gov/HealthInformation/Publications/hearing.htm.

natural teeth, compared with 26% of people above the poverty threshold (Federal Interagency Forum on Aging-Related Statistics, 2008).

Nurses should routinely assess their clients' oral and dental health. Gums should be inspected for color and palpated for lesions and swelling. If the client wears dentures, proper fit should be assessed, as well as excessive wear and rough spots. The teeth should be inspected for looseness, caries, and lost fillings. The tongue and mucous membranes should also be inspected for color, swelling, lesions, and moistness (Ebersole et al., 2008). The nurse should teach the client or their caregiver proper dental care, including brushing at least twice a day and flossing once a day. The nurse may also be helpful in providing referrals to dentists and periodontists.

Incontinence

Aging does not cause incontinence; however, at least one in ten people aged 65 years or older has this problem (National Institute on Aging, 2008). Incontinency is a symptom of underlying problems. Urinary incontinence can occur for many reasons. Urinary tract infections, vaginal infection or irritation, constipation, and certain medicines can cause short-term bladder control problems. Weak bladder muscles, overactive bladder muscles, blockage from an enlarged prostate, or damage to nerves that control the bladder may cause longer-lasting incontinence. However, in most cases, urinary incontinence can be treated or controlled, if not cured.

The choice of treatment depends on the type of bladder control problem. Types of urinary incontinence are stress incontinence, urge incontinence, and overflow incontinence or functional incontinence. One of the treatments that health care providers may suggest is Kegel exercises. These exercises strengthen the muscles that are used to stop urination.

An individual may also experience fecal incontinence. Loss of control of the bowels leads to stool leakage from the large intestine. Medical evaluation to determine the cause should

be recommended. Treatment varies, depending on the cause. Self-treatment is rarely successful (American Academy of Family Physicians, 2005).

ELDER SAFETY AND SECURITY NEEDS

Injuries and violence are serious threats to seniors, and older adults are at higher risk for injuries that can lead to death or disability. According to the National Center for Injury Prevention and Control (2005), the injuries and violence that pose the greatest threat to seniors are elder abuse and maltreatment, falls, driving, residential fire–related injuries, suicide, and traumatic brain injury. The leading cause of death due to unintentional injuries for seniors is fall-related injuries. Indeed, hip fracture is a major contributor to death, disability, and diminished quality of life. Seniors who experience a hip fracture are likely to die in the first year following that injury.

Falls

Many of the physiological changes that normally occur with aging, as well as a variety of chronic illnesses, can affect balance and make falls more likely. Medications such as blood pressure pills, heart medicines, diuretics, and tranquilizers may increase the risk of falling. Osteoporosis, a disease that causes a gradual loss of bone tissue or bone density, makes bones more susceptible to breaking. There is a link between osteoporosis and broken bones from falls. A person who falls and sustains a fracture may become afraid of falling again and thus will limit his or her activities. Seniors living independently before a fall may be institutionalized for as long as a year after their fracture. Loss of footing and loss of traction are factors that can lead to a fall. Uneven surfaces such as sidewalks, curbs, or floor elevations, wet or slippery ground, and climbing up on household items not intended for climbing can result in loss of footing or loss of traction. In addition, drinking alcoholic beverages increases the risk of falling because alcohol slows reflexes and response time; causes dizziness, sleepiness, or lightheadedness; and alters balance.

Steps can be taken to reduce the chance of falls. The Falls Free National Action Plan developed by leading fall prevention experts in March 2005 serves as a guide for reducing fall-related injuries and fatal falls among older adults (Centers for Disease Control and Prevention [CDC] and Merck, 2007). The community health nurse can educate seniors regarding measures they can take to lessen the risk of falls. Adequate amounts of calcium and vitamin D, exercising several times a week, obtaining a bone density test, and taking medications that are available for slowing bone loss are activities that can help. Simple exercises that strengthen leg muscles and exercises that can improve balance are recommended (Box 19-4). Seniors can also improve their environment in order to reduce their risk of falling by checking floor surfaces and curb heights; identifying weather-related problems before venturing outside; wearing supportive, low-heeled shoes; making sure that rooms are well lit; and ensuring that safety equipment is installed in bathrooms and stairwells. In the event of a fall, if the senior remembers to fall forward or backward or

Focus on the Following Areas

Muscle strengthening exercises.

Obtain maximum vision correction.

When using bi-trifocal glasses, practice looking straight ahead and lowering the head.

Practice balance exercises daily.

Balance Exercises

While holding on to a stable item like a chair or counter, practice standing on one leg at a time for a minute.

Gradually increase time, try balancing with eyes closed, and try balancing without holding on to anything.

Practice standing on toes, then rock back to balance on heels.

Hold for count of 10.

Hold on to stable item with both hands, then make a big circle to the left with hips.

Repeat to the right.

Do not move shoulders or feet.

Repeat five times.

From National Institutes of Health Osteoporosis and Related Bone Diseases, National Resource Center: *Preventing falls and related fractures,* Bethesda, MD, 2005, The Author: www.niams.nih.gov/Health_Info/Bone/Osteoporosis/Fracture/preventing_falls.asp.

to land on his or her hands to break a fall, it will lessen the risk of hip fracture. Another factor older adults should consider is having a cellular phone with them at all times to call for help directly. Telephone systems providing personal emergency response services may be available on a subscription basis thus allowing seniors to be monitored. If no answer is received, then help can be sent.

Traumatic Brain Injury

Traumatic brain injury (TBI), also called acquired brain injury or simply head injury, occurs when a sudden trauma causes damage to the brain. TBI can result when the head is suddenly and violently hit, or when an object pierces the skull and enters brain tissue (National Institute of Neurological Disorders and Stroke, 2005). TBI results in a number of deaths and cases of permanent disability. Men have consistently composed about three quarters of the number of TBI cases. Motor vehicle crashes account for 48.3%, and falls, the next most common cause of TBI, account for 18.5% (Millis and Wood, 2006). People 75 years of age and older have the highest rates of TBI-related hospitalizations and death (CDC, 2008). Prevention of TBI is directly related to measures taken to prevent falls and driving accidents.

TBI symptoms may be mild, moderate, or severe. Symptoms of mild TBI include headache, confusion, lightheadedness, dizziness, blurred vision or tired eyes, ringing in the ears, bad taste in the mouth, fatigue or lethargy, and a change in sleep patterns or thinking. Moderate or severe TBI may demonstrate the same symptoms as mild TBI plus a headache that gets worse or does not go away, repeated vomiting or nausea, convulsions or seizures, an inability to awaken from sleep, dilation of one or both pupils of the eyes, slurred speech, weakness or numbness in the extremities, loss of coordination, and increased confusion, restlessness, or agitation (National Institute of Neurological Disorders and

Stroke, 2005). Medical attention should be sought for monitoring and treatment of symptoms. Referral for rehabilitation may be required for persons with disabilities resulting from TBI.

Driver Safety

One of the quality-of-life factors that is important to the senior is the ability to drive. Many older adults depend on driving in order to maintain independence and personal mobility. Seniors overwhelmingly prefer to drive as their means of transportation, with being a passenger their second preferred option. Over the next 30 years, the number of drivers over the age of 85 years is expected to be four to five times greater than it is today. Seniors are generally safe drivers. Unfortunately, they are more likely than other age groups to be injured or killed in an accident (Tucker, 2004).

Age alone should not be the determining factor of whether or not a senior can drive safely. Driving skills vary from one elderly person to another, and aging-related physiological and psychological changes and medical, physical, and mental illnesses may interfere with an individual's ability to drive safely. There are certain functional capabilities that are essential for safe driving. These functional capabilities include body strength, range of motion, and coordination (Russo-Meek, 2004). In addition, hearing and vision are essential for responding safely to the driving environment. Most older drivers monitor their own driving ability and gradually limit or stop driving; others risk personal injury rather than give up their driver's license.

The community health nurse should be alert to signs of driving impairment in older clients and offer practical advice so that the driver may either continue to drive safely or be encouraged to find alternative transportation. The nurse can discuss issues with the senior driver, family, or friends and refer them to multiple resources available for identifying the warning signs of when someone should begin to limit driving or to stop altogether.

The American Association of Retired Persons (AARP) (2004) provides a list of fifteen warning signs to help identify unsafe older drivers (Box 19-5). These drivers can be encouraged to take a driver safety program or be educated to make changes in their behavior that might help them to continue driving safely.

Some interventions older adults could implement are limiting their driving to daylight hours, planning their trips to avoid rush hour, not listening to the radio, or avoiding talking with passengers. The driver should also be encouraged to find other methods of transportation such as family and friends or public transportation, taxis, or other private transportation options available in the community. A helpful booklet that offers many suggestions as to what the individual can do to prolong the ability to drive safely is "Driving Safely While Aging Gracefully" (National Highway Traffic Safety Administration, 2005).

When the question of driving safely becomes personal, elderly drivers might get very defensive. Therefore it is important

BOX 19-5 WARNING SIGNS FOR DRIVING CESSATION

- Feeling less comfortable and more nervous or fearful while driving
- Difficulty staying in the lane of travel
- More frequent close calls (i.e., almost crashing)
- More frequent dents, scrapes on the car or on fences, mailboxes, garage, doors, curbs, etc.
- Trouble judging gaps in traffic at intersections and on highway entrance and exit ramps
- Other drivers honking at you more often; more instances when you are angry at other drivers
- Friends or relatives not wanting to ride with you
- Getting lost more often
- Difficulty seeing the sides of the road when looking straight ahead (i.e., cars or people seem to come "out of nowhere" more frequently)
- Trouble paying attention to or violating signals, road signs, and pavement markings
- Slower response to unexpected situations; trouble moving foot from gas to brake pedal or confusing the two pedals
- Easily distracted or hard to concentrate while driving
- Hard to turn around to check over shoulder while backing up or changing lanes
- Medical conditions or medications that may be increasingly affecting your ability to handle the car safely
- More traffic tickets or "warnings" by traffic or law enforcement officers in the last year or two

that elderly persons, if at all possible, be involved in the decision-making process of identifying their ability and deciding what should be done. However, if the individual is greatly impaired and, therefore, is dangerous to himself or herself and others, it may be necessary to involve the family, family physician, or department of motor vehicles in determining whether to suspend or revoke an older person's license. In addition, it may be necessary to take the keys, disable the car, or move it to a location beyond the individual's control to protect the senior and others from injury or accidents.

Residential Fire–Related Injuries

In the United States, more than 1000 older adults aged 65 years and older die each year in home fires, and more than 2000 are injured. In addition, older adults are two times more likely to die in a residential fire than the rest of the population. This risk may be attributed to reduced sensory abilities such as smell, touch, vision, and hearing, diminished mental faculties, slower reaction time, increased disabilities, and economic and social concerns that may prevent necessary home improvements that could reduce fire risk. The predominant causes of fires that result in injuries to older adults are cooking, open flames, smoking, and heating (National Fire Data Center, 2006). Community health nurses making home visits can assess their elderly client's home for fire risk and teach fire safety, including the importance of home smoke detectors and fire extinguishers. In many communities, the fire department will install free smoke detectors for older adults. In addition to

the U.S. Fire Administration's public information campaign, A Fire Safety Campaign for People 50-Plus, organizations such as the National Fire Protection Association and the American Burn Association have active fire prevention and education programs for older adults.

Cold and Heat Stress
Cold Stress Disorders

Hypothermia is the most serious of the cold stress–related disorders and is the one elderly individuals might experience in the home because of failure of their heating system or lack of financial resources to pay for sufficient heat. Factors that contribute to the development of hypothermia are age, health, nutrition, exhaustion, exposure and duration of exposure, wind, temperature, wetness, and medications that may decrease heat production or increase heat loss or interfere with thermostability.

Initial management is to prevent further loss of heat. Rewarming of the core temperature at a safe, slow rate is important in order to avoid lethal side effects. The reason for rewarming the core first is to prevent vasodilatation that would place the individual in ventricular fibrillation. Measures that can be taken are: (1) remove the individual from the cold area as soon as possible; (2) add more clothing, especially to the head (e.g., use a hat or scarf); (3) provide a warm sweetened drink (no coffee or tea); and (4) apply mild heat to the head, neck, chest, and groin areas using hot water bottles or warm moist towels. Medical help is imperative, and hospitalization may be needed depending on the stage of hypothermia. Other cold stress disorders are frostbite and trench foot, which occur from long exposure to extremely cold temperatures.

Heat Stress Disorders

The heat stress disorders are heatstroke, heat syncope, heat exhaustion, and heat cramps. As the environment becomes warmer, all methods of heat elimination become less effective. These conditions should be taken seriously and require immediate medical attention; heatstroke is life threatening. Heat cramps are painful spasms of muscles of the arms, legs, or abdomen that occur during or after work. Heat exhaustion signs and symptoms are fatigue, nausea, headache, and giddiness. The skin is clammy and moist, and the complexion may be pale, or flushed. The individual may faint on standing with a rapid, thready pulse and low blood pressure. Heatstroke signs and symptoms are hot dry skin, which is usually red, mottled, or cyanotic. Confusion, loss of consciousness, or convulsions might occur. All of these may occur in the home without fans or air conditioning, or from being in the sun for prolonged periods of time, either in recreation or working in extremely hot temperatures and humidity. In all instances, the individual should be moved to a cooler environment and made to lie down and rest. With heatstroke, immediate and rapid cooling with chilled water or by wrapping in a wet sheet, as well as removing to a cooler area, should be done while seeking immediate medical attention.

Elder Abuse

Elder abuse is a serious problem throughout the United States. It is important to remember that abuse is not only a health concern but also a legal problem. States have laws defining abuse and identifying who is required to report abuse to Adult Protective Services. Abuse is generally defined as the willful infliction of pain, injury, or debilitating mental anguish; unreasonable confinement; or deprivation by a caretaker of services that are necessary to maintain mental and physical health. The categories of abuse are domestic, institutional, or self-neglect. Domestic abuse is that which occurs in the home. Institutional abuse is that which occurs in a nursing home or other residential care facility. Self-neglect is that which occurs when a person living alone threatens his or her own health or safety.

There are four common types of elder abuse. One is physical abuse, which includes slapping, pushing, pinching, and beating; physical restraint that results in broken bones, sprains, dislocations, bruises, black eyes, cuts, and rope marks; or sexual assault. Second is psychological or emotional abuse, which includes humiliation, intimidation, threats, and destruction of belongings (e.g., broken glasses). The third type of abuse is financial or material exploitation, which refers to the improper or illegal use of the resources of an older person without consent (e.g., use of ATM card). The final type is neglect. Signs of neglect might include dehydration, malnutrition, untreated health problems, bedsores, unclean or inappropriate clothing, and weight loss.

Elder abuse affects approximately 2 million elderly each year; an accurate number is unknown because it is estimated that for every case reported, five go unreported. This problem will steadily increase as more and more elderly are living longer and remaining in their homes. Abuse of the elderly is underreported for a number of reasons, including denial, fear of further abuse, no other place to go, love of the abuser and not wanting the abuser locked up, dependence on an abuser, and shame and embarrassment that someone they love could act in an abusive manner. Another reason is that elder abuse is often not recognized by health care providers (Meeks-Sjostrom, 2004).

Diagnosis is very difficult because many of the signs and symptoms may truly be the result of normal physiological aging. Ways to tell the difference include conflicting stories about how physical injuries were obtained, "physician shopping," clusters of signs and symptoms, increasing depression of the elder, new poverty, poor personal care, malnutrition, unresponsiveness, hostility, anxiety, confusion, new health problems, improper medication, dehydration, and longing for death.

The abuser is frequently the spouse, sibling, child, friend, or caregiver. The family member profile of an abuser is an individual who is middle-aged or older, a daughter or son of the elder, someone with low self-esteem and impaired impulse control. Caregiver behavior to look for is aggression, defensive or increasingly resentful attitude toward the elder, blames the victim for an injury, and treats the elder like a child; or, if the caregiver shows new affluence while withholding food or medication from the elder. Factors that lead to abuse are a lack of knowledge about normal aging, caregiver exhaustion, anger and frustration with the elder, financial problems, and drug and alcohol use of the caregiver. Elders who are most vulnerable are older females who are widows, single, and over 75 years of age; those dependent on a caregiver for their shelter and food; those with incontinence; and individuals who are frail or who have illness or mental disability.

Prevention activities include professional training of health care personnel, public education about elder abuse and its seriousness, and development of reliable assessment tools for the detection of abuse appropriate for the categories of abuse. Nurses should report suspected abuse to Adult Protective Services through their state's hotline. Suggestions the community health nurse can give to the elder are to stay sociable, maintain friendships, and participate in senior citizen activities; have pension and Social Security checks deposited directly into bank accounts and obtain a durable power of attorney when no longer able to manage property and assets; consider co-guardians so more than one person knows and can act on the elder's behalf; ask for help if needed; keep records, property, and a will in order; and plan ahead for possible disability. Community health nurses also should advise elders to avoid leaving cash, jewelry, and other valuables lying around visible; refuse to sign a document unless someone the elder trusts reviews it first; and resist letting anyone isolate them from others. Additional resources that can be used for further information are the Administration on Aging (www.aoa.gov) and the National Center on Elder Abuse (www.ncea.aoa.gov).

Crime

According to the National Center for Injury Prevention and Control (2006), serious violent crimes of the elderly include rape and sexual assault, robbery, and aggravated assault. Older adults are less likely to be victims of crime than are teenagers and young adults; however, if an older person becomes a victim of a crime, the result is that the individual is more likely to be seriously hurt than someone who is younger. Crime against the elderly occurs in the form of robbery, purse snatching, pocket picking, car theft, and home repair scams (National Institute on Aging, 2003).

The key for crime prevention for the senior is to be careful and alert to what is going on in the environment and to the types of crimes to which elders are vulnerable. Measures can be taken to lessen the risk of crime happening to the elderly person. In the home, safety measures include making sure that door and window locks are strong. Bars on doors and windows need to be installed with caution because they may increase the risk of harm in the event public officials need to access the home because of fire or to assist the elderly person who may be ill or injured from a fall. The use of a safe deposit box should be recommended to store a list and pictures of expensive belongings and other important documents, such as a copy of the individual's will. Installation of a monitored alarm system with its accompanying outdoor security sign would also help deter criminals. Caution should always be used before answering the door. The elder should note who is at the door before opening the door and, if it is a stranger, have the person show identification. Nurses should remind elders that if they are uneasy about the visitor, they should not answer the door.

When out in the community, measures that should be observed are to stay away from unsafe places, keep car doors locked and windows up at all times, and park in well-lit areas. Do not open the car door or roll down the window for strangers. Use inside pockets of clothing for valuables such as a wallet, money, or credit cards. A purse should be carried close to the body and kept closed. Credit cards and money should be kept separately so that, if a thief steals a purse, the credit card signature cannot be used to forge a signature for illicit use of checks. Only carry what is needed at the time. In addition, the elderly person should be advised not to resist the thief, but to hand over immediately what the person is requesting.

Fraud is the crime that frequently is mentioned in the media as happening to elders. Older people are subject to con games, insurance scams, home repair scams, and telephone scams. Types of Internet fraud include auction fraud, non-delivery of products ordered, securities fraud, credit card fraud, identity theft, bogus business opportunities, and unnecessary professional services. One strategy to recommend to seniors to prevent fraud from happening to them is to hang up the phone on telephone salespeople. Today, the elder can get caller identification service for the telephone; if no number or individual is identified, the elder may choose not to answer the call. No personal or financial information should be given over the phone unless the elder made the phone call. When in doubt about an inquiry or opportunity, the elder should be encouraged to say no and in this way protect himself or herself. The elder should check the references of anyone seeking to do home repairs and be sure to get, in writing, the details of the work to be completed, as well as the cost. A job should never be paid for in advance.

Identity theft is on the increase, and elderly individuals are particularly vulnerable. To avoid this problem, Social Security and monthly pension checks should be deposited directly into a bank account. Any information that is sent to the home with credit card offers, personal information, and so forth should be shredded so that the information cannot be used illegally. All cancelled and new checks should be kept in a safe place. The elder should check carefully the bank statement and credit card account statements for any discrepancies and report them immediately to the respective business. Caution should be used in using the Internet for buying products or paying bills, because of websites without security.

PSYCHOSOCIAL DISORDERS

Psychosocial disorders account for a significant number of suicides, especially among older men. Depression is likely to lead to suicides. Alzheimer's disease becomes more common with age. Alcohol and drug abuse are less common in older individuals; however, this is still a concern. Depression and abuse of drugs and alcohol can coexist with one or more anxiety disorders. These conditions are discussed in the following section.

Anxiety Disorders

Anxiety is a normal human emotion that everyone experiences at one time or another. For elderly individuals, normal age-related worries experienced are financial concerns, health problems, and reduced social interactions due to loss of friends because of death and relocation, but these do not mean that the individual has an anxiety disorder. An anxiety disorder is diagnosed only if symptoms are excessive, uncontrollable, create significant distress, or interfere with normal activities (Grayson, 2005).

However, anxiety disorders are a very real and relatively common problem among older adults. Some older adults with anxiety disorders may have had the problem for a long time, whereas others may experience anxiety problems only later in life. Studies have shown that among older adults, anxiety disorders occur anywhere from two to seven times more often than depression problems. It is possible that depression and abuse of drugs or alcohol can coexist with one or more anxiety disorders. Generalized anxiety disorder, social phobia, and agoraphobia seem to be the most common types of anxiety in the elderly; obsessive-compulsive disorder, panic disorder, and posttraumatic stress disorder also occur in the elderly but at a lower rate.

Generalized anxiety disorder is characterized by excessive, exaggerated anxiety and worry about everyday events and is accompanied by physiological problems, including headaches, muscle tension, nausea, trembling, and frequent trips to the bathroom (Grayson, 2005). The worry is often unrealistic or out of proportion to the real situation because anxiety dominates the individual's thinking to such a point that it interferes with daily activities. Social phobia involves overwhelming worry and self-consciousness about everyday social activities. Worry centers on fear of being judged by others or fear of behaving in a way that might cause embarrassment. Agoraphobia is a fear of leaving the familiar setting of home that is so invasive that the individual avoids social situations or enters into life situations reluctantly. Symptoms vary depending on the type of anxiety; as noted earlier, an anxiety disorder is diagnosed only if the symptoms are excessive, uncontrollable, create significant distress, or interfere with daily living.

Anxiety disorders cannot be prevented. Some things that can be suggested to control or lessen symptoms are to stop or reduce consumption of caffeine, check over-the-counter medicines or herbal remedies for any chemicals that can increase anxiety symptoms, exercise daily and eat an adequate nutrient-based diet, and seek counseling and support after experiencing a traumatic or disturbing event (Haines, 2005). All anxiety disorders are serious medical conditions, and elderly clients should be referred to their physician for evaluation and treatment. The nurse can help elders realize that what they are experiencing does not need to interfere with their lives if they seek medical help.

Depression

Everyone has times when they are unhappy with their lives. Feelings of sadness are not a weakness or a character flaw. These feelings can happen at any time and to anyone, and they are not necessarily related to an unhappy event. Depression can affect people of all ages, backgrounds, and ethnic groups.

Many myths exist concerning depression. Depression may last for days, weeks, months, or even years without treatment. Treatment is not just for those who are threatening suicide but also for anyone with symptoms that last more than 2 weeks. Depression is a serious condition that lasts longer and increases the risk of death in the elderly population. For example, depression is likely to lead to suicide. Elderly white men are at greatest risk. Suicide rates in people aged 80 to 84 years are more than twice that of the general population. Also, depression is associated with increased risk of death following a heart attack, and depression may coexist with other medical illnesses and disabilities such as diabetes, stroke, cancer, chronic lung disease, Alzheimer's disease, Parkinson's disease, and arthritis. Health care providers may miss the diagnosis of depression associated with one of these diagnoses, as well as depression in general (Healthy Place. com, 2000-2004).

Depression refers to a lasting (2 weeks or longer) sad mood or loss of interest or pleasure in most activities. People may experience several or all of the following symptoms: changes in appetite or weight, changes in sleep patterns, restlessness, loss of energy, feelings of worthlessness or guilt, and repeated thoughts of death or suicide. If any of these symptoms exist, the client should be referred to his or her physician for diagnosis. Only a physician can make a diagnosis of clinical depression, which calls for the presence of five or more of the symptoms mentioned above. Clinical depression usually interferes with a person's work, social life, or daily life. Seniors with depression usually do not complain of depressed mood or a loss of interest in previous areas of activity; family or friends usually observe these symptoms. Elders who are no longer able to live independently are at great risk for suicide (Scanlon, 2006). Treatment is available and is helpful. The physician and the individual determine which treatment would be used. There is medication alone or medication with psychotherapy. How long depression lasts depends a great deal on identifying the condition early and seeking treatment early. Depression is often undiagnosed or underdiagnosed. Delay in treatment in the elderly can be very dangerous, as noted before.

Thus, the community health nurse can play an important part in recognizing individuals who may be experiencing depression and who need to be referred for medical diagnosis and supervision. There are a number of checklists, including the Geriatric Depression Scale short form (Healthy Place. com, 2000-2004), which can be used to help the nurse recognize those at risk.

Substance Abuse

Data from the Substance Abuse and Mental Health Services Administration's (SAMHSA) National Survey on Drug Use and Health conducted from 2002 to 2003 revealed that 13.7 million (17.1%) persons aged 50 years or older smoked cigarettes and 36 million (45.5%) drank alcohol during the month prior to responding to the survey. Approximately 12.2% of older adults reported binge alcohol use, and 3.2% reported heavy alcohol use. A binge drinker is defined as a person who drinks five or more drinks on the same occasion on at least 1 day in the past 30 days. Among older adults, 1.4 million (1.8%) used an illicit drug during the past month. Marijuana was the most commonly used illicit drug, followed by prescription-type drugs used nonmedically and cocaine (SAMHSA, 2005).

Many older adults with substance abuse problems are continuing a pattern of behavior or addiction that began earlier in life. Substance abuse that begins in later life may be due to losses associated with aging. The warning signs of abuse are less obvious in older adults. For example, many older adults are retired and drink alone at home, so they are less likely to be noticed or get into trouble. Also, many of the diseases caused by substance misuse (e.g., hypertension, stroke, dementia, or ulcers) are common disorders in later life, so health care providers and family members may not recognize substance abuse as an underlying cause (American Geriatrics Society, 2009).

As a result of normal physiological changes (discussed earlier in this chapter), older adults generally experience increased sensitivity and decreased tolerance to alcohol and drugs. Because of loss of body mass, decreased absorption rate in the gastrointestinal system, slower kidney function, and slower metabolism, drugs and alcohol remain in the body longer and at higher rates of concentration, thus prolonging and increasing their effects. The problem is compounded when alcohol and illicit drugs interact with prescribed or over-the-counter medications. This may be dangerous and results in the medications having a stronger or weaker effect on the body.

Careful screening must include a thorough review of factors that may be directly affecting substance use and abuse. Several instruments have been utilized with the population of elderly individuals including the CAGE, the Michigan Alcohol Screening Test—Generic Version (MAST-G), and the Alcohol Use Disorders Identification Test (AUDIT). The CAGE is an easy-to-use, four-question interview. The MAST-G (twenty-three questions) and AUDIT (ten items) are screening instruments that provide a more detailed description of alcohol use. All three of these instruments rely on client self-report.

Alcoholics Anonymous (AA) is a community peer self-help group that may be very beneficial; however, elderly individuals may believe that they do not fit into the group or have differing concerns from those of younger members. In addition, they may have age-related mobility or hearing problems that prevent participation in peer self-help groups.

It is important that nurses recognize, assess, and screen for substance abuse in older adults so that they can refer these individuals to appropriate community resources. Nurses are in a prime position to educate clients about the dangers of substance abuse.

Suicide

Suicide, the act of intentionally taking one's own life, is a serious health concern related to the elderly, who account for

19% of all suicides. Elder suicide may be underreported (40% or more). Omitted are "silent suicides," for example, deaths from medical noncompliance or overdoses, self-starvation or dehydration, and "accidents." As mentioned, elders at highest risk are white males over the age of 85 years; the second highest are American Indian and Native Alaskan men (CDC, 2004). Elderly individuals have a high success rate for suicide because they use firearms, hanging, and drowning. "Double suicides" involving spouses or partners occur frequently among the aged.

Elder suicide is associated with depression, chronic illness, physical impairment, unrelieved pain, financial stress, loss and grief, social isolation, and alcoholism. Depression is tied to low serotonin levels. Serotonin is a neurotransmitter that limits self-destructive behavior. Serotonin levels decrease with age, predisposing elders to depression.

Warning signs to watch for in the elderly are loss of interest in things or activities that are usually found enjoyable; cutting back from social interactions, self-care, and grooming activities; not following medical regimens (e.g., going off diets, not taking prescriptions); experiencing or expecting a significant personal loss (e.g., spouse or friend); feeling hopeless or worthless; putting affairs in order; giving things away; making changes in will; and stockpiling medications or obtaining other lethal means for committing suicide. The most significant warning sign is any expression of intent. Risk factors that should also be considered in determining whether an elder might be at risk are previous suicide attempts, history of mental disorders, alcohol and substance abuse, family history of suicide, and local epidemics of suicide.

Prevention activities include dispelling any myths that exist relating to suicide. Many think that winter holidays are linked to suicide, but, in fact, suicide rates in the United States are lowest in the winter and highest in the spring (CDC, 2004). Other myths that need to be discussed and banished are that those who kill themselves must be crazy, asking someone about suicide can lead to suicide, pain goes along with aging so nothing can be done, those who talk about suicide rarely actually do it, and, if someone is determined to kill himself or herself, no one can stop that person. Other prevention concepts are to promote awareness, develop broad-based support, reduce stigma associated with aging and being a consumer of mental health, urge use of substance abuse and suicide prevention services, develop community-based suicide prevention programs if none exist, reduce access to lethal means of self-harm, promote participation in education programs related to recognition of at-risk behaviors, and, last, promote and support research.

Alzheimer's Disease

Alzheimer's disease is a slowly progressive brain disorder that begins with mild memory loss and progresses through stages to total incapacitation and eventually death. Diagnosing whether an individual has Alzheimer's disease is very difficult because it mimics other conditions such as depression and other types of dementia. Usually, a tentative diagnosis is reached after all other conditions have been ruled out. The only sure way to diagnose Alzheimer's disease is by autopsy. There is no cure, and limited treatment options are available.

The estimate of Americans who have the disorder is 3 to 4 million; however, the exact number is unknown because of difficulty in diagnosing dementia of the Alzheimer's type. The numbers are expected to increase to 7 million as people are living longer. As age increases, so does the risk of Alzheimer's disease. The percentage of individuals with the disease doubles every 5-year period beyond 65 years of age (Alzheimer's Disease Education and Referral Center, 2005). Many of these individuals live in their homes and are taken care of by family members or friends.

Wolf-Klein and colleagues (1989) studied 312 active outpatient geriatric clients to measure the validity of the clock drawing test in screening individuals with probable Alzheimer's disease. They found that clients with Alzheimer's disease were unable to draw a normal clock and demonstrated five characteristically abnormal patterns. As a test for Alzheimer's disease, clock drawing had a sensitivity of 86.7% and a specificity of 92.7%. There was correct identification in 97.2% of healthy individuals. The researchers reported that the findings indicate that the clock drawing test, an easily administered, low-cost screening tool, can be useful to health care professionals in characterizing cognitive loss in a general geriatric clinic population. Research is ongoing for developing a diagnostic test that could improve recognition of the disease in early stages, encouraging better management using available drugs and therapies. The Food and Drug Administration has approved four drugs for people in the mild to moderate stages of the disease. They are Pazadyne (formerly Reminyl), Exelon, and Aricept. Cognex (tacrine) is rarely prescribed today because of safety concerns. Drugs used for moderate to severe cases are Namenda and Aricept (Alzheimer's Disease Education and Referral Center, 2010). These drugs appear to slow down some of the symptoms, but they do not stop the progression of the disease. Research continues related to diagnosis, causes and risk factors, and treatment and care issues.

The behavioral and physical changes from Alzheimer's disease create many challenges for caregivers, family, and friends. If the individual is living alone and develops short-term memory loss, problems such as fires from leaving the stove on, having the electricity turned off because bills have not been paid, or leaving to go to the store and forgetting how to get home are just some of the problems that might occur. Some of the behavioral symptoms are agitation, aggression, wandering, and sleep disturbances.

Management strategies for caring for the individual with Alzheimer's disease should be elicited from the Alzheimer's Association's many publications, experts, and local chapter programs. Medical supervision of the physical condition and medications (if clinically indicated) is essential. In addition,

Alzheimer's disease centers throughout the country offer diagnosis and treatment; provide information about the disease, services, and resources; and provide volunteers an opportunity to participate in drug trials and other research projects. Any number of resources is available for respite for the caregiver, support groups for both client and family, and day care facilities for the client. These resources can be found by contacting the local chapter of the Alzheimer's Association. If wandering is a problem, the local police should be informed of the potential problem, current pictures of the individual should be available, and safety measures such as locks, bells on the doors, or other means to ensure safety should be installed.

END-OF-LIFE ISSUES

Advance Directives

Decision making at the end of life is complex. It is recommended that all adults have advance directives. Older adults often experience multiple chronic illnesses, some life threatening; therefore it is especially imperative that this population have advance directives. An older person who is approaching death may not be able to make end-of-life decisions. In this case, confusion as to how to provide appropriate care may develop.

The Patient Self-Determination Act is a federal law that requires health care facilities that receive Medicare and Medicaid funds to inform patients in writing of their rights to execute advance directives concerning end-of-life care. In the absence of written advance directives, oral advance directives may be challenged legally if family members are not in agreement about the person's wishes (Hooyman and Kiyak, 2007).

The most common type of advance directive is a living will. Living wills are legal documents whose purpose is to allow individuals to specify what type of medical treatment they would or would not want if they became incapacitated or had an irreversible terminal illness. Living wills can direct physicians to withhold life-sustaining procedures and can assist family members in making decisions when they are unable to consult a comatose or medically incompetent relative. An individual must be competent to initiate a living will, and he or she can revoke or change it at any time (Miller, 2009).

A durable power of attorney is another type of advance directive that authorizes someone to act on an individual's behalf with regard to property and financial matters. A durable power of attorney for health care is an advance directive that allows an individual to designate a health care proxy or surrogate to make decisions about medical care if the person is unable to make them for himself or herself. When an individual has no advance directive, is incompetent, or unable to handle his or her affairs adequately, a guardian may be appointed by the court to direct the individual's medical treatment, housing, personal needs, finances, and property. Because the guardian manages all the individual's affairs and assumes legal rights, a guardianship is generally considered a last resort (Hooyman and Kiyak, 2007).

Last, a do-not-resuscitate (DNR) order is another kind of advance directive. A DNR order is a request not to have cardiopulmonary resuscitation (CPR) if an individual's heart stops or if the person stops breathing. Persons should place their request on an advance directive form or tell their physician. Afterward, a DNR order is placed in the medical chart by the physician.

Advance directives not only make a person's wishes known, but they may also decrease the stress of decision making experienced by family members at the end of a loved one's life. State-specific advance directives can be ordered from the national organization, Caring Connections, or downloaded from its website (www.partnershipforcaring.org).

The Nurse's Role and End-of-Life Issues

The nurse is encouraged to discuss and educate clients about end-of-life issues. These include advance directives and pre-funeral considerations when death is imminent. When a client enters a health care facility with an advance directive, nurses should ensure that it is current and reflects the client's wishes. The nurse should inform other members of the health care team and make sure that the document is visible and accessible in the client's chart. Nurses should also encourage clients to discuss with their family their wishes regarding decisions in these documents. Clients should provide copies of advance directives such as living wills to their family members in case of emergency. Furthermore, clients should discuss the living will with their physician so that this document is made a part of their medical record. A copy of advance directives should also be kept in the individual's automobile.

⚖ ETHICAL INSIGHTS

Making End-of-Life Decisions When the Client Cannot

The Terri Schiavo case, which riveted the nation for weeks in 2005, demonstrated a worst-case scenario in an end-of-life situation. The case involved a brain-damaged client without a written advance directive and a family bitterly divided on what to do. In the end, the court ruled in favor of Schiavo's husband, who won the right to have her feeding tube removed over her parents' objections.

Similar situations occur with regularity in caring for elders who are near the end of their lives. According to Erlen (2005), family members sometimes do not agree with specific wishes of their family member regarding continuation of treatment and/or providing comfort through palliative care. Even though health care providers want to respect their clients' wishes, this is not always easy. Factors to consider are whether the client has provided written advance directives, the vulnerability of the client, whose interests and wishes should prevail, and quality of life.

CASE STUDY   APPLICATION OF THE NURSING PROCESS

Mrs. Darren, a 75-year-old widow, was referred to the community health nurse by her physician, who did not believe she could care for herself sufficiently. Her diagnoses were hypertension, mild congestive heart failure, arthritis, and occasional confusion after transient ischemic attacks.

During the initial home visit, the nurse observed that Mrs. Darren lived in a run-down house in an inner-city neighborhood. The roof leaked, and the house had no functioning heat unit. A rat was scrambling in the garbage. Mrs. Darren told the nurse that she did not have children and her only relative was a sister who lived with her family in another state. She was used to the neighborhood and knew her neighbors, but she was frightened of the teenagers who lingered when she took the bus to the supermarket to cash her Social Security check.

Mrs. Darren received Supplemental Security Income, Medicare, Medicaid, and food stamps. She ate mostly bread and butter and drank coffee, but she enjoyed fried chicken and oranges after going to the supermarket. Constipation was sometimes a problem, and she took a laxative every night. She said she did not always remember whether she took her medication and held out a small bottle containing an assortment of pills of different colors, shapes, and sizes.

Assessment

With Mrs. Darren as the system, or central planning focus, the nurse identified her biopsychosocial subsystem strengths and weaknesses and looked for actual or potential connections to her family and community suprasystems. Considering aging theories, the nurse believed Mrs. Darren was undergoing disengagement from her physical and social circumstances and decided that this might reverse if her health could be maintained and her links to the community strengthened. On a practical level, the nurse also checked with Mrs. Darren's physician regarding the prescriptions and identified the assortment of pills by taking them to the pharmacist who filled the prescriptions.

The nurse used a problem-solving approach to data gathering and identified Mrs. Darren's assets as the following:
- Being basically able to care for herself
- Receiving medical treatment
- Receiving income from various sources
- Being accustomed to the neighborhood and knowing her neighbors

Her liabilities were more extensive, as follows:
- Inadequate nutrition
- Confusion with medications and improper use of laxatives
- Condition of the house, which was not supportive of health
- Threat of violence in neighborhood and possibility of attack for her Social Security money
- Physical impairment resulting from age and illness
- No children or other family living nearby
- Probable progression of confusion
- Possibility of a major stroke at home while unattended

Diagnoses

Diagnoses and related short- and long-term goals address Mrs. Darren's situation. The nurse wrote plans at the three levels of prevention for the diagnoses and included suggestions for intervention with families.

Individual
- Imbalanced nutrition: less than body requirements, which was related to difficulty or inability to procure food
- Risk for injury related to inadequate housing, possibility of robbery for Social Security money, aging, and progression of disease

Family
- Risk for injury to family unit related to unanticipated loss of interaction with Mrs. Darren because her health is declining and her residence is distant

Community
- Deficient knowledge of nutritional services, related to lack of publicity of available nutritional programs for older adults
- Lack of support programs for medication consistency related to unrecognized need
- Lack of programs and resources for older adult residents of limited income related to cost of services and competition for limited funds

Planning
Individual
Long-Term Goals
- Mrs. Darren will maintain a nutritionally adequate diet through self-care and use of community programs as evidenced by a steady weight and normal tests for nutritional status during physical examinations.
- Mrs. Darren will avoid inconsistency in her medication regimen related to forgetfulness and mild confusion.
- Mrs. Darren will continue to take medications as ordered, as evidenced by stabilization of disease processes and intermittent demonstration to a nurse.
- Mrs. Darren will explore sheltered housing for older adults and continue contact with a community health nurse and neighborhood friends.

Short-Term Goals
- Mrs. Darren will improve her diet to include a recommended daily allowance of nutrients, including fiber and fluids, as evidenced by diet recall, and she will report regular bowel habits without use of laxatives.
- Mrs. Darren will utilize memory aids for consistent medication regimen.
- Mrs. Darren will identify medications and know when to take them, as evidenced by demonstration to a nurse.
- Mrs. Darren will improve her home to allow healthy habitation, avoid robbery by varying her routine and using banking services, expand her social network, and maintain health care appointments.

Family
Long-Term Goal
- Mrs. Darren will maintain family contact by mail, telephone, or possible visits.

Short-Term Goal
- Family members' addresses are included in Mrs. Darren's record to facilitate emergency contact.

Community
Long-Term Goals
- Promote publicity campaign to advertise nutritional services for older adults in the community.
- Support community pharmacists in the campaign to increase public awareness of the need to take medications as prescribed.
- Identify and support programs that will assist with provision of prescribed medications for people who have difficulty obtaining prescriptions because of a lack of insurance, money, transportation, or other problems.
- Community groups work together to maximize use of resources.

CASE STUDY   APPLICATION OF THE NURSING PROCESS—cont'd

Short-Term Goal
- Identify existing programs for older adults in the community.

Intervention
Individual

When the nurse discussed the nursing diagnoses and plans with Mrs. Darren, Mrs. Darren agreed with the short-term goals, but she was not sure that she wanted to leave her home for other housing or meet other people through community activities. She agreed, however, to try. During the course of the next few visits, the nurse explained basic nutritional principles and helped make a shopping list and menus for 1 week. Together, they developed a plan to assist with medication scheduling.

The nurse encouraged Mrs. Darren to talk about her earlier life during the nurse's visits. She had been widowed soon after her marriage when her husband was killed serving in the army overseas, and she had never remarried. She lived in the neighborhood where she grew up, although it had deteriorated over the years. She had worked as a secretary until her retirement and had no pension plan.

Family

Because Mrs. Darren's family did not live close by, the nurse designed a plan to increase Mrs. Darren's social contacts by introducing her to a group that met frequently and offered several activities she might enjoy. If she were unexpectedly absent, the group would check on her. A neighbor invited her to a senior center, where she became involved in a domino-playing group. Mrs. Darren allowed her name to be put on the waiting list for an apartment for older adults. With the other changes, the apartment was no longer a priority, and Mrs. Darren could make a decision when an apartment became available.

Community

Referrals initiated by the nurse resulted in a greatly improved living situation. A financial advisor from the city's Supportive Services to the Elderly program encouraged Mrs. Darren to open a bank account for the direct deposit of her checks and showed her how to use it. A home health aide from the same program came for half a day each week to assist with shopping and cleaning. The sanitation department of the health district exterminated the rats, the local Area Agency on Aging fixed the roof, and a church-sponsored group painted the house and cleaned the yard. A small heater was purchased from the Salvation Army store, and application was made to the utility company for help with bills during the winter months.

Evaluation
Individual

With the nurse as intermediary and coordinator of community services, Mrs. Darren easily accepted help with the problems related to security and survival. When her home improvements were completed, Mrs. Darren was able to maintain herself more comfortably with the help of the weekly visit from the home health aide.

Family

In the absence of family support, the establishment of an orderly routine, the companionship at the nutrition site, and safer financial arrangements increased Mrs. Darren's feelings of belonging and self-esteem. The nurse reduced her home visits but maintained contact with Mrs. Darren during her visits to the health clinic for blood pressure checks and preventive health care to supplement her medical care.

Community

Discussion with the home health aide informed the nurse of proposed funding cuts to the city's Supportive Services to the Elderly program, which would result in reduced services. The nurse spoke to the president of the district branch of the professional nurses'

association, who notified the state level of the association to monitor funding on the state level. The association also assisted the nurse in working with other local agencies for older adults to establish a publicity campaign against proposed funding cuts through writing letters to the editors of local newspapers, speaking at public hearings on the city budget, and speaking at city council meetings. Although funds were reduced, the cuts were much less severe than they would have been without the campaign, and most services were able to continue, although with increased waiting time for admission of new clients.

Levels of Prevention
Primary

Goal: Promote good nutrition.

Individual
- Instruct about nutritional needs.
- Plan a shopping list and menus incorporating a prescribed diet for health problems.

Family
- Instruct about nutritional needs of family members by age, sex, or special needs.

Community
- Increase nutrition information where food is sold.

Goal: Promote safety and prevention of injury.

Individual
- Provide immunizations as appropriate.
- Provide community services for assistance to maintain property and prevent deterioration.
- Encourage a network of friends and family members.

Family
- Provide services of community health nurse or case manager.
- Provide counseling.
- Provide respite care.

Community
- Provide community education programs for older adults.
- Be aware of potential hazards for older adult residents and provide intervention as needed.

Secondary
Goal: Assess and treat nutrition-related disorders.

Individual
- Provide referral for assessment of possible nutrition-related disorders.
- Provide hospitalization or prescribed nutritional supplements for illness resulting from inadequate nutrition.

Family
- Provide referral for nutritional assessment and counseling.

Community
- Encourage emergency food supplies.

Goal: Diagnose and treat medication-related injuries.

Individual
- Provide referral for apparent overmedication or undermedication symptoms.
- Diagnose and treat drug or food reactions.

Continued

CASE STUDY   APPLICATION OF THE NURSING PROCESS—cont'd

Family
- Reassess the client's understanding of medications.

Community
- Provide a 24-hour poison hotline.
- Provide an emergency department with 24-hour response.
- Provide medical services.

Tertiary
Goal: Maintain improved nutrition.

Individual
- Encourage use of community services.

Family
- Encourage exchange of family recipes.
- Encourage attendance of home economics classes.

Community
- Provide campaigns for nutritional awareness and healthy eating.
- Encourage the eating of healthy snacks in food machines.

- Encourage use of funding of community food services for aggregates or emergencies.
- Encourage use of services providing access to food (e.g., food banks, Meals on Wheels, and food stamps).
- Encourage use of transportation to grocery stores or nutrition services.

Goal: Be consistent with prescribed medications and prevent medication error.

Individual
- When medications are dispensed, provide written and oral instructions at the level of understanding and in the language of the client.
- Have the client repeat instructions to the health care provider.

Family
- Have the client repeat instructions to family members.

Community
- Provide a community education program about understanding medications.

SUMMARY

Increasing life expectancy, coupled with aging baby boomers, will cause a dramatic and continual rise in the number of older adults. In addition to longevity, older adults desire to function independently for as long as possible. This chapter has described aging, demographic characteristics, normal aging changes, health promotion and illness prevention interventions, common health and psychosocial concerns, end-of-life issues, and various resources that may assist older adults. Community health nurses should be aware of and address these issues and concerns so that they may help elders have a better quality of life.

LEARNING ACTIVITIES

1. Interview an elderly person you know to assess his or her physical activity level and nutritional status using the nutrition checklist and food pyramid. Review the results with the person and help the person plan a nutritious menu for 1 day. What factors hindered or enhanced interaction with this person?
2. Find the names, addresses, and phone numbers of local resources for someone interested in, for example, exercise programs for the elderly, smoking cessation programs, and so forth.
3. Devise a nursing care plan for an elder with a visual disturbance (i.e., cataracts, glaucoma, or macular degeneration).

4. You are asked to lead a 1-hour discussion (see topics below) for a group of ten seniors at a senior citizens center. What would be your goal? What physiological aspects would you include? What psychosocial aspects would you consider?
   - Issues related to urine control
   - Fall prevention
   - Prevention of influenza and pneumonia
   - Medications and aging
   - Normal aging changes
5. Speak with police officers in a local community about elder abuse and crimes against elders. Identify community strengths and weaknesses. Discuss needs and solutions.
6. The family of your elderly client is considering taking the keys from him. They asked you how to decide whether their loved one should stop driving. How would you respond?
7. Your 80-year-old client has become very frail and needs assistance with several activities of daily living. There are no family members who are able or willing to take care of him full-time. The family has asked you for advice. What information would you share with them about alternative housing options?
8. Your elderly client has a terminal illness. You note that she does not have an advance directive. What issues surrounding this topic would you discuss with her?

REFERENCES

Administration on Aging: *Geographic distribution: a profile of older Americans*, Washington, DC, 2001, The Author: www.aoa.gov/aoa/stats/profile/2001/6.html.

Alzheimer's Disease Education and Referral Center: *Alzheimer's disease fact sheet*, Silver Spring, MD, 2010, The Author: Accessed March 24, 2010 at www.nia.nih.gov/Alzheimers/Publications/medicationsfs.htm.

American Academy of Family Physicians: *Fecal incontinence*, 2005, http://familydoctor.org/067.xml?printxml.

American Association of Retired Persons: *Keeping safe: when to stop driving*, Washington, DC, 2004, The Author: www.aarp.org/life/drive/safetyissues/Articles/a2004-06-21-whentostop.html.

American Geriatrics Society Foundation for Health in Aging: *Substance abuse*, 2009, www.healthinaging.org/agingintheknow/chapters_print_ch_trial.asp?ch=36.

Center for Medicare Education: Prescription drug coverage for people with Medicare: issue brief, *Center Medicare Educ* 3(9):1, 2002.

Centers for Disease Control and Prevention (CDC): *Suicide fact sheet*, 2004, Accessed March 24, 2010 at www.cdc.gov/ncipc/factsheets/suifacts.htm.

Centers for Disease Control and Prevention: *CDC features: Help older adults live better, longer: Prevent falls and brain injury*, Atlanta, GA, 2008, The Author: www.cdc.gov/Features/FallsandBrainInjury.

Centers for Disease Control and Prevention and The Merck Company Foundation: *The state of aging and health in America*, Whitehouse Station, NJ, 2007, The Author: www.cdc.gov/aging and www.merck.com/cr.

Cumming E, Henry W: *Growing old*, New York, 1961, Basic Books.

Ebersole P, Hess P, Touhy T, et al: *Toward healthy aging: human needs and nursing response*, ed 7, St. Louis, 2008, Mosby

Erlen JA: When patients and families disagree, *Orthop Nurs* 24(45):279–282, 2005.

Federal Interagency Forum on Aging-Related Statistics: *Older Americans 2008: key indicators of well-being*, Washington, DC, 2008, US Government Printing Office. www.agingstats.gov.

Grayson CE: *Mental health: anxiety disorders*, WebMD, April 2005, http://my.webmd.com/content/article/60/67142.htm.

Gurwitz J, et al: Incidence and preventability of adverse drug events among older persons in the ambulatory setting, *JAMA* 289(9):1107–1116, 2003.

Haines C: *Mental health: generalized anxiety disorder*, WebMD, July 2005, http://my.webmd.com/content/article/60/67148.htm.

Havighurst RL, Neugarten BL, Tobin SS: Disengagement and patterns of aging. In Neugarten BL, editor: *Middle age and aging*, Chicago, 1968, University of Chicago Press.

Hayflick L: *How and why we age*, New York, 1996, Ballantine Books.

Healthy Place.com, Depression Community: *Geriatric depression scale (GDS) short form*, 2000–2004, The Author: www.healthyplace.com/communities/depression/elderly_2a.asp.

Hooyman NR, Kiyak HA: *Social gerontology: a multidisciplinary perspective*, ed 8, Boston, 2007, Allyn and Bacon.

Lemon BW, Bengston VL, Peterson JA: An exploration of the activity theory of aging: activity types and life satisfaction among in movers to a retirement community, *J Gerontol* 27:511, 1972.

Lighthouse International: *Dual sensory impairment among the elderly*, 2005, www.lighthouse.org/research/archive/dual.

Maddox G: Activity and morale: A longitudinal study of selected elderly subjects, *Soc Forces* 42:195, 1963.

Mauk K: *Gerontological nursing competencies for care*, ed 2, Boston, 2010, Jones and Bartlett.

Mayo Clinic Staff: *Cataracts*, 2004a, www.mayoclinic.com/health/cataracts/DS00050.

Mayo Clinic Staff: *Glaucoma*, 2004b, www.mayoclinic.com/health/glaucoma/DS00283.

Mayo Clinic Staff: *Macular degeneration*, 2004c, www.mayoclinic.com/health/macular-degeneration/DS00284.

Meeks-Sjostrom D: A comparison of three measures of elder abuse, *J Nurs Scholarsh* 36:247–250, 2004.

Miller CA: *Nursing for wellness in older adults: theory and practice*, ed 5, Philadelphia, 2009, Lippincott Williams & Wilkins.

Miller RA: The aging immune system: primer and prospectus, *Science* 273:70, 1996.

Millis S, Wood K: 2005, *Database update*, TBI National Data Center. Accessed from www.tbindc.org.

Morley A: The somatic mutation theory of aging, *Mutat Res* 338(1–6):19–23, 1995.

National Center for Health Statistics: *Vital and health statistics*, 2003, www.cdc.gov/nchs/data/hus/tables/2002.

National Center for Injury Prevention and Control: *Injuries among older adults*, 2006, www.cdc.gov/ncipc/olderadults.htm.

National Fire Data Center: *Fire and the older adult*, 2006, www.usfa.fema.gov/downloads/pdf/publications/fa-300.pdf.

National Highway Traffic Safety Administration: *Driving safely while aging gracefully*, 2005, www.nhtsa.dot.gov/people/injury/olddrive/Driving%20%Safely%20Aging%20Web/.

National Institute on Aging: *Age page: hearing loss*, September 2002, www.nia.nih.gov/HealthInformation/Publications/hearing.htm.

National Institute on Aging: *Age page: crime and older people*, May 2003, www.nia.nih.gov/HealthInformation/Publications/crime.htm.

National Institute on Aging: *Age page: urinary incontinence*, June 2008, www.nia.nih.gov/HealthInformation/Publications/urinary.htm.

National Institute of Neurological Disorders and Stroke: *NINDS Traumatic brain injury information page*, 2005. www.ninds.nih.gov/disorders/tbi/tbi.htm.

Orgel LE: The maintenance of the accuracy of protein synthesis and its relevance to aging, *Proc Natl Acad Sci* 49:517–521, 1963.

Ross MET, Aday L: Stress and coping in African-American grandparents who are raising their grandchildren, *J Fam Issues* 27:912–932, 2006.

Russo-Meek PA: Nurses can help older drivers steer clear of trouble, NurseWeek November 15, 2004: www.nurseweek.com.

Scanlon B: *Recognizing depression in later years*, 2006, http://healthyplace.healthology.com/printer_friendlyAR.asp?b=healthyplace&f=healthyaging&c=aging_depression.

Substance Abuse and Mental Health Services Administration: Substance use among older adults: 2002 and 2003 update, *National Survey on Drug Use and Health Report* April 22, 2005: www.oas.samhsa.gov/2k5/olderadults/olderadults.htm.

Tsai P: Predictors of distress and depression in elders with arthritic pain, *J Adv Nurs* 51:158–165, 2005.

Tucker LE: *Community based approach to promoting older driver safety*, 2004, National Association of Area Agencies on Aging: www.n4a.org.

U.S. Department of Agriculture: *My pyramid*, 2005, www.mypyramid.gov.

USDHHS: Healthy People 2020: Draft Objectives. 2009. http://www.healthypeople.gov/hp2020/Objectives/Files/Draft2009Objectives.pdf.

U.S. Department of Health and Human Services: *Healthy People 2010:* National health promotion and disease prevention objectives, Washington, DC, 2000, US Government Printing Office: www.health.gov/healthypeople.

U.S. Department of Health and Human Services/Centers for Medicare and Medicaid Services (USDHHS/CMS): *Medicare and you*, Baltimore, MD, 2006, The Author: www.medicare.gov/publications/pubs/pdf/10050.pdf.

Wolf-Klein G, Silverstone FA, Levy AP, Brod MS: Screening for Alzheimer's disease by clock drawing, *J Am Geriatr Soc* 37:730–734, 1989.

Family Health

Beverly Cook Siegrist

Additional Material for Study, Review, and Further Exploration

evolve WEBSITE

http://evolve.elsevier.com/Nies

- Quiz
- Case Studies
- Glossary

- WebLinks
- Resource Tools
  - 20A: Family Health Assessment Form

OBJECTIVES

Upon completion of this chapter, the reader will be able to do the following:

1. State a definition of family.
2. Identify characteristics of the family that have implications for community health nursing practice.
3. Describe strategies for moving from intervention at the individual level to intervention at the family level.
4. Describe strategies for moving from intervention at the family level to intervention at the aggregate level.
5. Discuss a model of care for families.
6. Apply the steps of the nursing process to individuals within the family, the family as a whole, and the family's aggregate.

KEY TERMS

cohabitation
contracting
ecological framework
ecomap
expressive functioning
external structure

family
Family Health Assessment
family health tree
family interviewing
gay or lesbian family
general systems theory

genogram
instrumental functioning
internal structure
network therapy
nuclear family
transactional model

OUTLINE

The four families described below depict broad contemporary definitions of family and are examples of families carried in caseloads by undergraduate community health nursing students. Assessments made by students during home, office, and hospital visits with these families triggered interventions that linked the families to resources provided by the community and, in turn, triggered questions about health needs of groups of families or larger aggregates living in the same communities.

Clinical Example

Rebecca Martin is a 72-year-old widow of 10 years who lives in a rural town in Tennessee. She resides in the home that she and her husband purchased before his death. Her primary source of income is her deceased husband's Social Security benefits, and she also receives a small income from providing child care for infants at her church. Medicare benefits are her only source of payment for health care. Her only child, a daughter from whom she has been estranged for many years, recently died. The daughter was a never-married, single mother of an 8-year-old, medically fragile child with asthma. As the only surviving relative, Rebecca has become the custodial parent for her granddaughter.

Clinical Example

Joe Hudson is a 74-year-old alcoholic who is being treated at an outpatient department in a large medical center. He lives in a hotel room in downtown Salt Lake City, Utah. He has one living relative, a 76-year-old brother. Mr. Hudson states, "I had a falling out with my brother 20 years ago. I never hear from him. I reckon he's still in Boston, if he's alive at all." Mr. Hudson frequently falls out of bed, dislodging the telephone that the desk clerk has placed precariously close to the bed, which signals the desk clerk that something is amiss. The clerk then goes to Mr. Hudson's room and puts him back in bed. Mr. Hudson's source of income is a check sent to him the first day of each month by a minister who lives in a town 75 miles away. The desk clerk cashes Mr. Hudson's check and assists him in paying his bill from the hotel, which provides congregate dining facilities.

Clinical Example

Lai Chan is a refugee from Vietnam who moved with her family to San Francisco 3 months ago. Mrs. Chan is a single parent; Mr. Chan died in an automobile accident shortly after arriving in the United States. Mrs. Chan has two children, an 11-year-old son and a 5-year-old daughter. The family resides in a one-room efficiency apartment in the Tenderloin district in downtown San Francisco.

Clinical Example

Jaime Gutierrez, a 72-year-old Mexican-American man, lives with his 36-year-old son, Roberto; his 34-year-old daughter-in-law, Patricia; and his three grandchildren who are 14, 13, and 12 years of age. Mr. Gutierrez was in good health until he fell from a tree while helping his son make roof repairs on the house in 1995. He suffered a concussion, right hemothorax, and fracture of vertebrae T-11 and T-12. Confined to bed, he is receiving home health care. He requires intermittent catheterization but feels uncomfortable when the nurse suggests that his daughter-in-law is willing to carry out this procedure for him. Therefore Roberto quit work to provide this personal care to his father. Consequently, the family of six lives on Mr. Gutierrez's retirement income, which consists of $239 from Social Security and $244 from a pension plan per month. Roberto would like to increase his job skills while at home. He has finished the fourth grade and has failed the Graduate Equivalency Degree (GED) examination twice. Patricia also would like to return to school and pursue job training. Although agreeable to Patricia's interests, Roberto is hesitant to support active steps taken by Patricia to initiate her plan.

Working with families has never been more complex or rewarding than now. Nurses understand the actual and potential impact that families have in changing the health status of Americans. Additionally, families have challenging health care needs that are not usually addressed by the health care system. Instead, the health care system most frequently addresses the individual. This holds true for nursing interventions within the health care system. This chapter will assist the nurse in understanding and addressing complex issues that impact family health and suggest methods to improve family health.

UNDERSTANDING FAMILY NURSING

Family nursing is not a new concept and has been taught in schools of nursing since Nightingale's "district nursing" concept (Cook, 1913) and Lillian Wald's (1904) principles on how to nurse families in the home. The National League for Nursing (NLN) has emphasized the importance of family nursing in standard curriculum guides for schools of nursing since 1917 (Beard, 1999; NLN, 1937). Early NLN publications directed nurses in "household science" and later required that 10 to 15 hours of study should be directed toward understanding the "modern family," in which the nurse must consider the family as a unit (NLN, 1937). Modern nurse theorists such as Newman, King, Orem, Roy, and others extensively discuss the family and its importance to individuals and society. Previously, nurses defined the family conceptually in the following ways: as the environment affecting individual clients; as small to large groups of interacting people; as a single unit of care with definable boundaries; or as a unit of care within a specific environment of a community or society. Current family theorists recognize the diversity of American families. Hanson and Kaakimen (2005) defines family as "two or more individuals who depend on one another for emotional, physical, and economical support. The members of the family are self-defined" (p. 6). Wright and Leahey (2000) state, "the family is who they say they are" (p. 70). Current advocacy groups find these definitions even too narrow. The Human Rights Campaign (2009) urges that health professions acknowledge all types of families including gay, lesbian, and even grandparents as heads of family by using this definition:

"Family" means any person(s) who plays a significant role in an individual's life. This may include a person(s) not legally related to the individual. Members of "family" include spouses, domestic partners, and both different-sex and same-sex significant others. "Family" includes a minor patient's parents, regardless of the gender of either

parent...without limitation as encompassing legal parents, foster parents, same-sex parent, step-parents, those serving in loco parentis, and other persons operating in caretaker roles (Human Rights Campaign, 2009, Inclusive Definitions of Family).

These later definitions are perhaps more useful to the nurse and allow the focus on the needs of the family. Family nursing care may be focused on the individual family member, within the context of the family, or the family unit. Regardless of the identified client, the nurse establishes a relationship with each family member within the unit and understands the influence of the unit on the individual and society.

The family is composed of many subsystems and, in turn, is tied to many formal and informal systems outside the family. The family is embedded in social systems that have an influence on health (e.g., education, employment, and housing). Many disciplines are interested in the study of families; interdisciplinary perspectives and strategies are necessary to understand the influence of the family on health and the influence of the broader social system on the family. Traditionally, nursing, and even community health nursing, has relied heavily, if not solely, on theoretical frameworks for intervention with families from the disciplines of psychology or social psychology, which target individuals (Cody, 2000; Duvall, 1977; Erikson, 1963; Maslow, 1970). This chapter addresses how community health nurses work with families within communities to bring about healthy conditions for families at the family, social, and policy levels. This chapter focuses on the following five areas:

1. The changing family
2. Approaches to meeting the health needs of families
3. Family theory approach to meeting the health needs of families
4. Extending family health intervention to larger aggregates and social action
5. An example of the nursing process applied to a family

THE CHANGING FAMILY
Definition of Family
Many definitions of family exist, from the traditional U.S. Census—"a family consists of two or more people, one whom is the householder, related by birth, marriage, or adoption and residing in the same housing unit" (2005) to the more inclusive. The nurse's definition of *family* is influenced by personal involvement with his or her own family and clinical experiences. Definitions of *family* vary by professional discipline and type of family described. For example, psychologists may define *family* in terms of personal development and intrapersonal dynamics; the sociologist has used a classic definition of *family* in terms of a "social unit interacting with the larger society" (Johnson, 2000). Other professionals have classically defined *family* in terms of kinship, marriage, and choice: "a family is characterized by people together because of birth, marriage, adoption, or choice" (Allen, Fine, and Demo, 2000, p. 7). Friedman, Bowden, and Jones (2003) incorporate the

idea of many nontraditional definitions: "a family is two or more persons who are joined together by bonds of sharing and emotional closeness and who identify themselves as being part of the family" (p. 10). Again, this definition supports the idea of letting the family define their composition and relationships (Wright and Leahey, 2005). The National Institute of Mental Health (2005) defines family simply as a "network of mutual commitment" (p. 2).

In the past, the dominant American definition focused on the intact nuclear family. African-American families focus on a wide network of kin and community. The "nuclear" family does not exist for Italians. To them, *family* means a strong, tightly knit three- or four-generational family, which includes godparents and old friends. The Chinese go beyond this and include in their definition of *family* multigenerational family members and ancestors (Li, Lin, and Cao, et al., 2009).

The community health nurse interacts with communities made up of many types of families. When faced with great diversity in the community, the community health nurse must formulate a personal definition of *family* and be aware of the changing definition of *family* held by other disciplines, professionals, and family groups. The community health nurse who interacts with Mr. Hudson, the alcoholic who lives in a hotel, must have a broad conceptualization of the family. Both the surveillance activity of the hotel manager and the financial support of the minister could be accounted for in the definition of McDaniel and colleagues: "we define family as any group of people related either biologically, emotionally, or legally. That is, the group of people that the patient defines as significant for his or her well-being" (2005, p. 2).

Regardless of the definition of *family* accepted, what is evident is the importance of the family unit to society. The family fulfills two important purposes. The first is to meet the needs of society, and the second is to meet the needs of individual family members (Friedman et al., 2003). The family meets the needs of society through procreation and socialization of family members. "The basic unit (family) so strongly influences the development of an individual that it may determine the success or failure of that person's life" (Freidman et al, p. 4). The family is the "buffer" between individuals and society. The family meets individual needs through provision of basic needs (food, shelter, clothing, affection). The family supports spouses or partners by meeting affective, sexual, and socioeconomic needs. For children, the family is the "first teacher," instructing the children in societal rules and providing values needed for growth and development.

Characteristics of the Changing Family
The characteristics of the U.S. family continue to change. Historically the typical family, the nuclear family, has been defined as "the family of marriage, parenthood, or procreation; it is composed of a husband, wife, and their immediate children—natural, adopted or both" (Friedman et al., 2003, p. 10). The stereotypical view of this family as father, mother, and nonadult children while present currently represents only a portion of U.S. families (Annie E. Casey Foundation, 2009). In 1970, 85% of children younger than 18 years of age

were living with two parents, defined as "mother and father."
In 2007, 74% of children younger than 18 years of age were
living with two parents, defined as two adults including
grandparents, same-sex partners, and other adults as parents
(Annie E. Casey Foundation, 2009). In the last decade, recognition of various types of kinship families has resulted in
available data that describe common types of families found
in the United States. Table 20-1 presents significant family
information.

Cohabitation, which is defined as "a living arrangement
in which an unmarried couple live together in a long-term
relationship that resembles a marriage," has also increased
over time (McLanahan and Percheski, 2008, p. 259). The
number of cohabiting unmarried people increased from
523,000 in 1970 to 4.85 million in 2005 (U.S. Census Bureau,
2008). In 2007, 4,849,000 of the cohabiting-couple households included children (Annie E. Casey Foundation, 2009).
Wydick (2007) found that 52% of American women currently in their 30s reported that their first relationship was
cohabitation. Although these women generally reported that
cohabitation was a prescreening situation before marriage,
they reported lower relationship satisfaction when compared with the general population of married women and
a higher divorce rate when marriage followed cohabitation.
Hohmann-Marriott and Amato (2008) analyzed data
from the Fragile Families and Child Well-being Study and
reported that cohabiting partners were more likely to be
what they termed "interethnic." Interethnic couples were of
either different ethnic or different racial backgrounds and
were more likely to have relationship difficulties because of

complications caused by different values and cultures. This
did not mean the couples were less likely to be successful as
partners, just that they were considered at risk or fragile. The
nurse should be aware of the potential need for family support and intervention.

Single parenting has also increased over time. The
increase in the teenage birth rate among this group raises
concern. During the years 1980 to 2006, the birth rate for
unmarried women 15 to 17 years of age increased from 21
to 41.9 per 1000 in the United States, representing a rise in
26 states (Centers for Disease Control and Prevention,
2009). The majority of teen parents raise their children
alone. The proportion of children younger than 18 years
of age who are living with their grandparents remains
constant. In 2007, grandparent-headed families comprised 5% of all families. The American Academy of Child
& Adolescent Psychiatry (2009) suggests that this is "due
to serious societal issues and problems including increasing numbers of single parent families, the high rate of
divorce, teenage pregnancies, AIDS, incarcerations of parents, substance abuse by parents, death or disability of parents, parental abuse and neglect" (p. 3). The gay or lesbian
family is made up of a cohabiting couple of the same sex
who have a sexual relationship. The homosexual family
may or may not have children. Estimates of the number
of children who live in lesbian- or gay-parented families,
including children conceived in heterosexual marriages,
range from 6% to 11% of children (Women's Educational
Media, 2005). These numbers are estimates because the
U.S. Census Bureau does not count the number of lesbians
and gay men. The University of California at Los Angeles
(2009) reports that "more than one in every three lesbians
have given birth and one in six gay men have fathered or
adopted a child. An estimated 14,100 foster children are
living with same-sex couples" (p. 8).

Single parenting is associated with greater risk associated
with lesser social, emotional, and financial resources, which
affect the general well-being of children and families. In 2007,
32% of all U.S. children lived in single-parent homes. Single
parenting is a key indicator of well-being in children (Annie
E. Casey Foundation, 2009). Table 20-2 shows statistics for
single-parent families by ethnic group, and Table 20-3 shows
teen birth rates by ethnic group.

TABLE 20-1	A COMPARISON OF FAMILIES BY TYPE IN THE UNITED STATES, 2003-2007	
FAMILY TYPE	2003	2007
Married couple households	50,130,111 (68%)	49,932,000 (69%)
Father only households	4,425,000 (6%)	5,076,000 (7%)
Mother only households	21,138,000 (31%)	22,282,000 (32%)
Children in care of grandparents	3,194,000 (4%)	3,457,000 (5%)
Children living with co-habiting domestic partners	4,186,000 (6%)	4,343,000 (6%)
Children living with neither parent	4,126,000 (6%)	4,343,000 (6%)
Children living in married-couple immigrant families	10,935,000	12,774,000
Children living in single-parent immigrant families	2,944,000	3,680,000
Children living in single-parent immigrant families (U.S. born children)	17,967,000	18,602,000

From Annie E. Casey Foundation: *National Kids Count key indicators,* 2009: www.kidscount.org.

TABLE 20-2	PERCENTAGE OF U.S. FAMILIES THAT ARE SINGLE-PARENT FAMILIES BY ETHNIC GROUP, 2007
Non-Hispanic white	23%
Black or African American	65%
American Indian	49%
Asian and Pacific Islander	17%
Hispanic or Latino	37%
Total	32%

From Annie E. Casey Foundation: *Kids Count data center,* 2009: www.kidscount.org.

TABLE 20-3	TEEN BIRTH RATE (PER 1000) AGES 15-17 YEARS BY ETHNIC GROUP
Non-Hispanic white	26
Black or African American	62
American Indian	53
Asian or Pacific Islander	17
Hispanic or Latino	82
Total	40

From Annie E. Casey Foundation: *Kids Count data center*, 2009: www.kidscount.org.

APPROACHES TO MEETING THE HEALTH NEEDS OF FAMILIES

Community health nursing has long viewed the family as an important unit of health care, with awareness that the individual can be best understood within the social context of the family. Observing and inquiring about family interaction enables the nurse in the community to assess the influence of family members on each other. However, direct intervention at the family rather than the individual client level is a new frontier for many nursing students, most of whom have experience in acute care settings before the community setting. A family model, largely a community health nursing or psychiatric–mental health intervention model, also includes the areas of birthing and parent-child interventions, adult day care, chronic illness, and home care. Nursing assessment and intervention must not stop with the immediate social context of the family, but it must also consider the broader social context of the community and society. Friedman et al. (2003, pp. 5-6) suggest reasons why it is important for nurses to work with families:

- "The family is a critical resource." The importance of the family in providing care for its members has already been established. In this caregiver role, the family can also improve individual members' health through health promotion and wellness activities.
- "In a family unit any dysfunction (illness, injury, separation) that affects one or more family members will affect the members and unit as a whole." Also referred to as the "ripple effect," changes in one member cause changes in the entire family unit. The nurse must assess each individual and the family unit.
- "Case finding" is another reason to work with families. As the nurse assesses an individual and family, he or she may identify a health problem that necessitates identifying risks for the entire family.
- "Improving nursing care." The nurse can provide better and more holistic care by understanding the family and its members.

Moving from Individual to Family

Community health and home care nurses have traditionally focused on the family as the unit of service. With the move to managed care throughout the United States, most of these nurses continue to focus their practice on individuals residing in the home. As a result of the current era of cost containment, constraints on the community health nurse and on nurses working within hospitals and in other settings will increase. For example, reimbursement, which is almost entirely calculated for services rendered to the individual, is a major constraint toward moving toward planning care for the family as a unit. Various creative approaches to meeting the health needs of families are needed, reflecting interventions appropriate to the needs of the population as a whole.

Family Interviewing

Approaches to the care of families are needed and must be creative, flexible, and transferable from one setting to another. Community health nurses are generalists who bring previous preparation in communication concepts and interviewing to the family arena. Wright and Leahey (2005) proposed the realm of family interviewing rather than family therapy as an appropriate model. In this model, the community health nurse uses general systems and communication concepts to conceptualize the health needs of families and a family assessment model to assess families' responses to "normative" events such as birth or retirement or to "paranormative" events such as chronic illness or divorce. Intervention is straightforward, as in helping parents educate prepubescent teenage family members about sex by providing appropriate educational materials or making a referral to another health professional, if the level of intervention is beyond the preparation of the nurse. For the purposes of this text, the model is extended to include intervention at the level of the larger aggregate. For example, the index of suspicion based on the health needs of a particular family would prompt the community health nurse to assess the need for similar information and the resources for intervention with other families in the community, schools, churches, or other institutions. Family interviewing requires thinking "interactionally," not only in terms of the family system but also in terms of larger social systems.

Wright and Leahey (2005) identify the following critical components of the family interview: manners, therapeutic conservation and questions, family genogram (and ecomap when indicated), and commendations. With experience, they believe that the family interview can be accomplished in 15 minutes.

Manners

Manners are common social behaviors that set the tone for the interview and begin the development of a therapeutic relationship. Wright and Leahey (2005) believe that erosion of these social skills prevents the family nurse from collecting essential data. Many nurses argue that too much formality establishes artificial barriers to communication; however, studies identify that the essentials of a therapeutic relationship begin with manners. The nurse introduces himself or herself by name and title, always addresses the client (and family members) by name and title (i.e., Mr., Mrs., or Ms., unless otherwise directed by client), keeps appointments, explains the reason for the interview or visit, and brings a positive attitude. Other behaviors (manners) that invite rapport include being honest with the client and checking attitude (the nurse's) before each client encounter.

Therapeutic conversations. The second key element in the interview is the therapeutic conversation. This type of conversation is focused and planned and engages the family. The nurse must listen and remember that even one sentence has the potential to heal or help a family member. The nurse encourages questions, engages the family in the interview and assessment process, and commends the family when strengths are identified. Every encounter, whether brief or extended, has "healing potential." Therapeutic conversation may initiate further discussion that brings the family together on issues (Wright and Leahey, 2005).

Genogram and ecomap. The genogram and ecomap constitute the third element and are described in detail later in this chapter. These tools provide essential information on family structure and are an efficient way to gather information, such as family composition, background, and basic health status, in a way that engages the family in the interview process.

Therapeutic questions. Therapeutic questions are key questions that the nurse uses to facilitate the interview. The questions are specific for the context or family situation but have the following basic themes (Wright and Leahey, 2005): family expectations of the interview or home visit; challenges, concerns, and problems encountered by the family at the time of the interview; and sharing information (e.g., who will relate the family history or information).

Commending family or individual strengths. The fifth element of the family interview is commending the family or individual strengths. Wright and Leahy (2005) suggest identifying at least two strength areas and, during each family interview, sharing them with the family or individual. Sharing strengths reinforces immediate and long-term positive relationships between the nurse and family. Interviews that identify and build upon family strengths tend to progress toward more open and trusting relationships and often allow the family to reframe problems, thereby increasing problem solving and healing (Wright and Leahey, 2005).

Issues in family interviewing. Creative family interviewing requires interviewing families in many types of settings. The prediction of decreased hospitalization, supplemented by a wide variety of health care settings ranging from acute to ambulatory to community centers, calls for flexible, transferable approaches. Clinical settings for family interviewing are reviewed by Wright and Leahey (2005) and include inpatient and outpatient ambulatory care and clinical settings in maternity, pediatrics, medicine, surgery, critical care, and mental health. According to Wright and Leahey, community health nurses have many opportunities besides the traditional home visit to engage the family in a family interview. Community health nurses are employed in ambulatory care centers, occupational health and school sites, housing complexes, day care programs, residential treatment and substance abuse programs, and other official and nonofficial agencies. At each of these sites, community health nurses meet families and can assess and intervene at the family and community levels.

The community health nurse can implement preventive programs for family units. The family is particularly appropriate because it experiences similar risk factors (i.e., physiological, behavioral, and environmental). Studies have documented the familial predisposition to the three major diseases resulting in morbidity and mortality in the United States: cardiac disease, cancer, and diabetes. Family health practices also influence lifestyle habits among family members. Recognizing the importance of a family health history related to individual and public health, the U.S. Surgeon General initiated the National Family History Initiative in 2003 with a goal to educate individuals about inherited predispositions to disease (McNeill et al., 2008). A study by Ehrensaft (2009) documented how the family of origin influenced antisocial or aggressive behaviors among family members. Such programs can occur in community health settings and demonstrate the need to go beyond intervention with the individual family to groups of families, serving the population as a whole.

Another example would be a Hispanic-American family in which a family member has diabetes; the nurse could implement a family health promotion plan based on the needs of the individual within an at-risk family. The family plan for diabetes prevention is based on the nurse's understanding that the National Institutes of Health (NIH) reports that this group has the highest rate of diabetes among a nonwhite ethnic group in the United States (NIH, 2009).

Involving family members in newborn assessments can aid the community health nurse in determining the family's adjustment to the newborn and parenthood. The nurse can do this in the home, clinic, or other health care center. Family members should be involved during the first contact or visit, and, if they do not attend, a telephone call explaining the nurse's interest in them should take place (Wright and Leahey, 2005).

The community health nurse working with single-parent families may face particular challenges. Single-parent families report a higher incidence of children's academic and behavioral problems and health problems than do two-parent families (Spencer, 2005). Children and parents in these families need a chance to express their concerns; the family interview is important and may provide the nurse with necessary information needed to care for these families.

School Nurse

The school nurse has a unique opportunity to compare the child in the school system with the child in the family system. The school nurse is becoming increasingly involved in planning special programs in the schools. Astute assessment of children's needs within the context of their families in interviews at school or in the home can lead to innovative interventions such as support groups for children with chronic illness. Other areas of assessment and intervention that benefit from a family approach include learning or behavioral problems and absenteeism (Wright and Leahey, 2005).

Occupational Health Nurse

The nurse in the occupational health setting also can use a family approach to improve the health of the worker and contribute to overall productivity. For example, alcohol and chemical abuse account for much absenteeism in the workplace. Effective intervention with these families has been demonstrated. Assessment of occupational hazards may involve conducting reproductive histories in an effort to determine the effects of a chemical or agent on the reproductive capacity of the couple. Toxic agents can also transfer to family members from the workplace via clothes and equipment.

An awareness and a high degree of suspicion about the risks of occupational hazards in community industry are necessary. Obtaining an occupational history from all family members who have entered the workplace and obtaining referrals for family members' screening and health education will contribute to unraveling occupational hazards and effects in the future. In addition, the community health nurse should be aware of the many family-related work issues that may trigger stress-related illness, such as job promotion, job loss, or shift work.

Intervention in Cases of Chronic Illness

Perhaps as many as 80% of families are dealing with chronic illness in a family member (Hopia, Paavilainen, and Astedt-Kurki, 2004). Also significant is the fact that resources such as third-party reimbursement cause most of these families to learn to manage the chronic problems with limited or infrequent intervention by health professionals. The community health nurse working with families coping with chronic illness in a child, adult, or older adult is aided by the family interview. As Glaser and Strauss (1975) stated, chronic illness interjects change into various areas of family life:

Sex and intimacy can be affected. Everyday mood and interpersonal relations can be affected. Visiting friends and engaging in other leisure time activities can be affected. Conflicts can be engendered by increased expenses stemming from unemployment and the medical treatment… different illnesses may have different kinds of impact on such areas of family life, just as they probably will call for different kinds of helpful agents. (p. 67)

Changes in family patterns, fears, emotional responses, and expectations of individual family members can be assessed in the family interview. Special needs of the primary caretaker (i.e., often the spouse, daughter, or daughter-in-law) can be assessed. The community health nurse making family visits to older adults and the terminally ill is able to assess intergenerational conflict and stress and influence family interaction positively (Wright and Leahey, 2005).

Moving from Family to Community

The health of families can affect the health of society as a whole, in both positive and negative ways. The health of a community is measured by the well-being of its people and families. Circumstances such as low-birth-weight infants, lack of health insurance, homelessness, violence, poverty, and low employment rates provide a description of families and nations. Community health nurses provide family nursing to improve individual and family health; however, the potential

result is that of improving the health of society. The care of entire populations is the major focus, as stated by Freeman in her classic work (1963).

The selection of those to be served…must rest on the comparative impact on community health rather than solely on the needs of the individual or family being served…. The public health nurse cannot elect to care for a small number of people intensely while ignoring the needs of many others. She must be concerned with the population as a whole, with those in her caseload, with the need of a particular family as compared to the needs of others in the community. (p. 35)

The challenge to the community health nurse is to provide care to communities and populations and not to focus only on the levels of the individual and family. The community health nurse, who traditionally carries a caseload of families, extends his or her practice to the community. To do so, an aggregate, community, and population focus must serve as a backdrop to the entire practice.

For example, families must be viewed as components of communities. The community health nurse must know the community. As stated in previous chapters, a thorough community assessment is necessary to practice in the community. By way of review, the nurse must remember that communities must be compared not only in terms of different health needs but also in terms of different resources to effect interventions that influence policies and redistribute resources to ensure that community and family health needs are met.

Community health nurses must then compare city data with county data and then county data, state data, and national data. In addition, they may need to compare local census tract data and areas of a city or county with other areas of the city or county.

For example, community health nursing students in San Antonio, Texas, who were planning home visits to families of pregnant adolescents attending a special high school, compared local, state, and national statistics on infant mortality rates as a part of a community assessment. They found higher rates of infant mortality in San Antonio in census tracts on the south side of the city in which the population was predominantly Mexican American. They also found the population to be younger, to have a higher rate of functional illiteracy among adults, to be less educated, to be more likely to drop out of high school, to have higher fertility rates, to have higher birth rates among adolescents, and to be more likely to be unemployed. They found that specific health needs varied among census tracts. Common major health needs of this subpopulation were identified from the community assessment, which assisted the students in planning care for these families. For example, their goals were broadened from carrying out interventions at the individual level to interventions at the family and community levels. In addition to targeting good perinatal outcomes for the individual teenage parent, nursing students planned to include assessments of functional literacy at the individual and family levels and arranged for group sessions in clinic waiting rooms that informed and referred individuals and family members to alternative resources to enable teenage parents to complete school, take classes in English as a second language, and use resources for family planning and employment at the community level.

In addition to the cross-comparison of communities, the community health nurse also cross-compares the needs of the families within the communities and sets priorities. The nurse in the community finds that specific health needs vary among families. The nurse must account for time spent with families and choose those families on the basis of their needs compared with the needs of others in the community.

♥ HEALTHY PEOPLE 2020

Access to Health Care

In relation to improving family health, all of the leading health indicators listed as priority in *Healthy People 2020* can serve as a guide for family nursing interventions. Access to quality health care affects every aspect of family nursing. The objectives for measurement of this goal are:
- Increase the proportion of persons with health insurance.
- Increase the proportion of insured persons with coverage for clinical preventative services.
- Increase the proportion of persons with a usual primary care provider.
- Increase the proportion of persons who have a specific ongoing care.

In this chapter, we have discussed the disparities that exist among families and populations with regard to health care access. The community nurse should use political skills, advocacy, and education to influence policy that will result in increased access to health care. The nurse can educate families about available resources and help communities develop resources to improve health care access.

From US Department of Health and Human Services: *Healthy People 2020,* Draft Objectives, 2009 http://www.healthypeople.gov/hp2020/Objectives/files/Draft2009Objectives.pdf

Delegation of Scarce Resources

Although the community health nurse serves the community or population as a whole, fiscal constraints hold the nurse accountable for the best delegation of scarce resources. Time spent on home visits has traditionally allowed the community health nurse to assess the environmental, social, and biological determinants of health status among the population and the resources available to them. Fiscal accountability, nevertheless, means setting priorities. In 1985, Anderson, O'Grady, and Anderson listed the factors that influence public health nursing practice, especially home visits, as "the need to justify personnel costs in a time of fiscal constraint, the increasing number of medically indigent who turn to local public health services for primary care, and the change in reimbursement mechanisms by the federal government and some states" (p. 146). Anderson's observations still hold true. In 2009, more than 46 million Americans, including 9 million children, lacked health insurance (Robert Wood Johnson Foundation, 2009). Many of these individuals are Americans working in low-paying jobs and their families. The Children's Health Insurance Program (CHIP) of 1997 has greatly increased access to health care for many low-income children. When the

CHIP program was initiated, there were 10 million children in the United States and 14% were uninsured; in 2008, 7.4 million children were enrolled in state CHIP plans (Centers for Medicare and Medicaid Services, 2009). The majority of these children lived in families with working, low-income parents. On February 4, 2009, President Obama signed the Children's Health Insurance Program Reauthorization Act (CHIPRA), which renews and expands coverage of the CHIP from 7 million children to 11 million children (2009).

Double standard in public health. A double standard is tolerated in public health. Although the government is responsible for the maintenance of health, a minimal amount of health care is guaranteed to each person because public resources are limited.

A minimum is established for all; however, as demonstrated with Medicare and Medicaid, unequal care exists as a result of differences in income (i.e., Medicare) and geographic location (i.e., Medicaid). In a market system, the wealthy can purchase all the health care services they desire and the poor cannot afford these services. The few supplemental resources provided by the government to ensure a minimum for all vary among communities, states, administrations, and counties.

In a period of cost containment, the focus of community health nurses on prevention and health maintenance, which are difficult areas to justify, must carefully legitimate home visiting services by identifying aggregates in need of care.

Prioritizing groups at highest risk and using home visits in conjunction with planning for larger aggregates' needs are necessary. Working for social and policy changes to alter the conditions that place these families at high risk goes hand-in-hand with this activity. More research needs to be done that documents the importance of family nursing through home visits or community-based programs.

Many populations at high risk benefit from family nursing through home visits. Cornell University's Family Life Development Center houses the Prenatal/Early Infancy Project. This project began in 1977 and involves a home visiting program for high-risk families having their first child. Registered nurses provide supportive and educational services. Nurse researchers reviewing the program noted that, among the participants, the program outcomes included 46% fewer verified reports of child abuse or neglect, 31% fewer subsequent births, 30 months less use of federal aid, 44% fewer behavioral problems from alcohol and substance abuse, and 69% fewer maternal arrests (Cornell University, 2009).

APPROACHES TO FAMILY HEALTH

Many schools of thought regarding the approaches to meeting family health needs exist among community health, community mental health, and public health nursing professionals. Dreher (1982) stated that the traditional basis for community health nursing intervention has a focus that has long endorsed psychological and social-psychological theories to explain variations in health and patterns of health care, such as those set forth by Erikson (1963), Maslow (1970), and Duvall (1977). Dreher (1982) stated that what is needed are "more encompassing theories which explain the relationship between society and health [and]the policies which will be most effective in assuring health and health care" (p. 508). To help bridge this gap, four frameworks are presented (i.e., meeting family health needs through the application of family theory, systems framework, structural-functional conceptual framework, and developmental theory).

Clinical Example

Ten-year-old Jean Wilkie was referred by her teacher to the school nurse. She was withdrawn, had no school friends, and was dropping behind in her schoolwork. The school nurse talked to Jean in her office. Jean said that she had no friends because the other girls stayed overnight with one another "all the time" and that she did not want to bring her friends home because her father "drank all the time." The school nurse decided that Jean's problems needed assessment within the context of the family and arranged to visit the family at home. The father refused to participate in the family interview, but Jean's mother, her 13-year-old brother Peter, and Jean expressed concerns that the father had changed jobs several times in the past year, was frequently absent from work, and had been in two recent car accidents while "drinking." The school nurse was able to verify the family context as the basis of Jean's "problems," continue her family assessment, and plan for intervention at the family level. In addition, she was prompted to assess the community's preventive efforts directed toward drinking and the ability to provide ongoing care for families of alcoholics.

Family Theory

Many reasons exist for why the community health nurse should work with families. Friedman (1998) listed the following six reasons:

1. Any "dysfunction" (e.g., separation, disease, or injury) that affects one or more family members probably affects other family members and the family as a whole.
2. The wellness of the family is highly dependent on the role of the family in every aspect of health care, from prevention to rehabilitation.
3. The level of wellness of the whole family can be raised through care that reduces lifestyle and environmental risks by emphasizing "health promotion, 'self-care,' health education, and family counseling" (p. 5).
4. Commonalities in risk factors and diseases shared by family members can lead to case finding within the family.
5. A clear understanding of the functioning of the individual can be gained only when the individual is assessed within the larger context of the family.
6. The family as a vital support system to the individual member needs to be incorporated into treatment plans.

Nurses have relied heavily on the social and behavioral sciences for approaches to working with families. These approaches include psychoanalytical, anthropological, systems or cybernetic, structural-functional, developmental, and interactional frameworks (for reviews, see Friedman, 1998;

Wright and Leahey, 2005). The use of a framework for assessing families is useful to help the nurse understand the health potential for the family. Three conceptual frameworks (systems, structural-functional, and developmental), often used by nurses in providing health care to families, are described. These models help the nurse empower the family in the process of family health promotion.

Systems Theory

The systems approach has been used in such diverse areas as education, computer science, engineering, and communication. General systems theory (Minuchin, 2002; von Bertalanffy, 1968, 1972, 1974) has been applied to the study of families. General systems theory is a way to explain how the family as a unit interacts with larger units outside the family and with smaller units inside the family (Friedman, 1998). The family may be affected by any disrupting force acting on a system outside the family (i.e., suprasystem) or on a system within the family (i.e., subsystem). Parke (2002) stated that there are three subsystems of the family that are most important: parent-child subsystem, marital subsystem, and sibling-sibling subsystem. Allmond, Buckman, and Gofman (1979) compared the family as a system to a piece of a mobile suspended from the air that is in constant movement with the other pieces of the mobile. At any time, the family, like any piece of the mobile, may be caught by a gust of air and become unbalanced, moving "chaotically" for a time; however, eventually, the stabilizing force of the other parts of the mobile will reestablish balance. An understanding of systems theory is still important for the nurse working with families today. Dunst and Trivette (2009) review 20 years of systems theory and the importance to early childhood interventions, adding that systems theory provides direction in understanding how health care providers can expand family capacity by changing parenting, and therefore changing child behaviors. Table 20-4 presents the major definitions from the systems approach.

Characteristics of Healthy Families

Otto (1973) and Pratt (1976) characterized healthy families as "energized families" and provided descriptions of healthy families to guide in assessing strengths and coping. DeFrain (1999) and Montalvo (2004) helped to identify healthy families. These authors suggest the following traits of a healthy family:

- Members interact with each other; they communicate and listen repeatedly in many contexts.
- Healthy families can establish priorities. Members understand that family needs are priority.
- Healthy families affirm, support, and respect each other.
- The members engage in flexible role relationships, share power, respond to change, support the growth and autonomy of others, and engage in decision making that affects them.
- The family teaches family and societal values and beliefs and shares a religious core.

TABLE 20-4   MAJOR DEFINITIONS FROM SYSTEMS THEORY

TERM	DEFINITION
System	"A goal-directed unit made up of interdependent, interacting parts which endure over a period of time" (Friedman, 1992, p. 115). A family system is not concrete. It is made up of suprasystems and subsystems and must be viewed in a hierarchy of systems. The system under study at any given time is called the focal, or target, system. In this chapter, the family system is the focal system.
Suprasystem	The larger system of which the family is a part, such as the larger environment or the community (e.g., churches, schools, clubs, businesses, neighborhood organizations, and gangs).
Subsystem	Smaller unit within the family, such as the relationship between spouses, parent and child, sibling and sibling, or extended family.
Hierarchy of systems	The levels of units within the system and its environment, which, in their totality, make up the universe. Higher-level units are composed of lower-level units (e.g., the biosphere is made up of communities, which are made up of families). Families are made up of family subsystems, and, in turn, family subsystems are made up of individuals, who are made up of organs, which are made of cells, which are made of atoms.
Boundary	An imaginary definitive line that forms a circle around each system and delineates the system from its environment. Auger (1976) conceptualized the boundary of a system as a "filter" that permits the constant exchange of elements, information, or energy between the system and its environments. "...The more porous the filter, the greater the degree of interaction possible between the system and its environment" (p. 24). Families with rigid boundaries may lack necessary information and resources pertinent to maintaining family health or wellness.
Open system	A system that interacts with its surrounding environment and gives outputs and gets inputs necessary to survival. An exchange of energy occurs. All living systems are open systems. However, if a boundary is too permeable, the system may be too open to input new ideas from the outside and may be unable to make decisions on its own (Wright and Leahey, 1994).
Closed system	A system that theoretically does not interact with the environment. This is a self-sufficient system; no energy exchange occurs. Although no system has been found that exists in a totally closed state, if a family's boundaries are impermeable (i.e., less open as a system), needed input or interaction cannot occur. An example is a refugee family from Vietnam living in San Francisco; they may remain a closed family for some time because they have differences in culture and language.
Input	Information, matter, or energy that the open system receives from its environment that is necessary for survival.
Output	Information, matter, or energy dispensed into the environment as a result of receiving and processing the input.
Flow and transformation	The system's use of input may occur in two forms. Some input may be used in its original state, and some input may have to be transformed before it is used. Both original and transformed input must be processed and flow through the system before being released as output (Friedman, 1992).
Feedback	"The process by which a system monitors the internal and environmental responses to its behavior (i.e., output) and accommodates or adjusts itself" (Friedman, 1992, p. 117). The system controls and modifies inputs and outputs by "receiving and responding to the return of its own output" (Friedman, 1992, p. 117). Internally, the system adjusts by making changes in its subsystems. Externally, the system adjusts by making boundary changes.
Equilibrium	A state of balance or steady state that results from self-regulation or adaptation. As with the concept of a system as a mobile in the wind, balance is dynamic and, with change, is always reestablishing itself.
Differentiation	The tendency for a system to actively grow and "advance to a higher order of complexity and organization" (Friedman, 1992, p. 117). Energy inputs into the system make this growth possible.
Energy	Energy is needed to meet a system's demands. Open systems will require more input through porous boundaries to meet high energy levels needed to maintain high levels of activity.

- Healthy families foster responsibility and value service to others.
- Healthy families have a sense of play and humor and share leisure time.
- Healthy families have the ability to cope with stress and crisis and grow from problems. They know when to seek help from professionals.

Structural-Functional Conceptual Framework

With the structural-functional conceptual framework approach to the family, the family is viewed according to its structure, or the parts of the system, and according to its functions, or how the family fulfills its roles.

Structural

Wright and Leahey (2000, 2005) stated that three aspects of family structure can be examined (internal structure, external structure, and context). Internal structure of the family refers to the following five categories:

1. Family composition, the family members, and changes in family constellation
2. Gender
3. Rank order, or positions of family members by age and sex
4. Subsystem or labeling of the subgroups or dyads (e.g., spouse, parental, and interest) through which the family carries out its functions

5. Boundary, or who participates in the family system and how they participate (e.g., a single-parent mother who does not allow her 17-year-old son to have his girlfriend spend the night in their home)

External structure refers to the extended family and larger systems (Wright and Leahey, 2005). It includes the following two categories:

1. Extended family, including family of origin and family of procreation
2. Larger systems, including work, health, and welfare

Context refers to the background or situation relevant to an event or personality in which the family system is nested (Wright and Leahey, 2005). It includes the following five categories:

1. Ethnicity
2. Race
3. Social class
4. Religion
5. Environment

Clinical Example
Role Relationships

When Edna Smith, a 64-year-old client with severe arthritis, received a diagnosis of diabetes, her longtime friend, Frank Gardens, a widower of several years, moved in with her and assumed a caregiver role. The community health nurse assessed the dietary habits of Mr. Gardens and Mrs. Smith and found that Mr. Gardens did the shopping and the cooking because Mrs. Smith's mobility was severely restricted from her arthritis. Mr. Gardens did the cooking; therefore he purchased canned fruits and vegetables rather than fresh or frozen. Mr. Gardens perceived cooking, which was a new role for him, as demanding. After several visits, he disclosed to the nurse that his resistance to preparing fresh or frozen fruits and vegetables came from "the time it takes to clean the darn things, cook 'em, store 'em, and clean up the fridge when they go bad on ya." He stated unequivocally that it was stressful caring for Mrs. Smith and that he wanted to do it, but it was "much easier" to just "open a can" and "heat it in a pan" than to take the time and energy that preparation of fresh or frozen foods would require. The shift in roles that is often required of couples when a chronic illness is diagnosed in one can have an influence on the health of the family. Miller (2000) provides additional reading about how couples manage with chronic illness.

Functional

Wright and Leahey (2005) also dichotomized family functional assessment, or how family members behave toward one another, into two categories (instrumental functioning and expressive functioning). Instrumental functioning refers to routine activities of daily living (e.g., elimination, sleeping, eating, or giving insulin injections) (Box 20-1). This area takes on important meaning for the family when one member of the family becomes ill or disabled and is unable to carry out daily functions and must rely on other members of the family for assistance. For example, an older adult may need

---

BOX 20-1	SUMMARY OF FAMILY FUNCTIONAL ASSESSMENT

I. Instrumental functioning (i.e., activities of daily living)
II. Expressive functioning
   a. Emotional communication
   b. Verbal communication
   c. Nonverbal communication
   d. Circular communication
   e. Problem solving
   f. Roles
   g. Influence
   h. Beliefs
   i. Alliances and coalitions

Data from Wright LM, Leahey M: *Nurses and families: a guide to family assessment and intervention,* ed 2, Philadelphia, 1994, FA Davis.

---

assistance getting into the bathtub, or a child may need to have medications measured and administered.

The second type of family functional assessment is expressive functioning, or affective or emotional aspects. This aspect has nine categories, which follow:

1. Emotional communication: Is the family able to express a range of emotions, including happiness, sadness, and anger?
2. Verbal communication focuses on the meaning of words. Do messages have clear meanings rather than distorted meanings? Wright and Leahey (2000, 2005) gave the example of masked criticism when a father states to his child, "Children who cry when they get needles are babies."
3. Nonverbal communication, which includes sounds, gestures, eye contact, touch, or inaction. An example is when a husband remains silent and stares out the window when his wife is talking to him.
4. Circular communication is commonly observed between dyads in families. A common example is the blaming, nagging wife and the guilty, withdrawn husband.
5. Problem solving refers to how the family solves problems. Who identifies problems? Someone inside or outside the family? What kinds of problems are solved? What patterns are used to solve and evaluate tried solutions?
6. Roles refer to established patterns of behavior for family members (Wright and Leahey, 2000). Roles may be developed, delegated, negotiated, and renegotiated within the family. It takes other family members to keep a person in a particular role. Traditional roles are being challenged and are evolving with economic and feminist changes; many women are entering the workforce outside the home. Formal roles, with which the larger community agrees, may come into conflict with roles set by family members and influenced by religious, cultural, and other belief systems.
7. Influence refers to methods used to affect the behavior of another. Instrumental influence refers to the use of reinforcement via objects or privileges (e.g., money or watching television). Psychological influence refers to the influence of behavior through the use of communication

or feelings. Corporal control refers to use of body contact (e.g., hugging and spanking).

8. Beliefs refer to assumptions, ideas, and opinions that are held by family members and families as a whole. Beliefs shape the way families react to chronic or life-threatening illness. For example, if a family of a person with colon cancer believes in alternative treatments, then acupuncture may be a viable option.

9. Alliances and coalitions are important within the family. What dyads or triads appear to occur repeatedly in the family? Who starts arguments between dyads? Who stops arguments or fighting between dyads? Is there evidence of mother and father against child? When does this change to parent and child against the other parent? The balance and intensity of relationships between subsystems within the family are important. Questions may be asked regarding the permeability of the boundary. Does it cross generations?

Developmental Theory

Nurses are familiar with developmental states of individuals from prenatal through adult. Duvall (Duvall and Miller, 1985), a noted sociologist, is the forerunner of a focus on family development. In her classic work, she identified stages that normal families traverse from marriage to death (Box 20-2).

To assess the family, the community health nurse must comprehend these phases and the struggles that families experience while going through them. Wright and Leahey (2000, 2005) called attention to the need to distinguish between "family development" and "family life cycle." They stated that the former is the individual, unique path that a family goes

---

BOX 20-2	FAMILY LIFE CYCLE

1. Leaving home
2. Beginning family through marriage or commitment as a couple relationship
3. Parenting the first child
4. Living with adolescent
5. Launching family (youngest child leaves home)
6. Middle-aged family (remaining marital dyad to retirement)
7. Aging family (from retirement to death of both spouses)

Data adapted from Duvall EM, Miller BC: *Marriage and family development,* ed 6, New York, 1985, Harper and Row; Carter B, McGoldrick M: *The expanded family life cycle: individual, family, and social perspectives,* 2005, Pearson Allyn & Bacon.

---

through, whereas the latter is the typical path many families go through.

The developmental categories listed in Box 20-3 outline the six stages of the middle-class North American family life cycle (Carter and McGoldrick, 1988; Wright and Leahey, 2005) and the tasks necessary for the family's resolution of each stage. Nurses may use the stages to delineate family strengths and weaknesses.

The profiles of families living in North America and in many other parts of the world are changing dramatically from what they have been in the recent past, in both structure and form (Wright and Leahey, 2005). Language used in reference to the family should be inclusive of many kinds of "families," including those headed by dual-career parents, single parents, unmarried couples, gay or lesbian couples, or remarried couples. The nurse should no longer use terms such as *working mother, children of divorce,* or *fatherless home* when speaking of the family.

RESEARCH HIGHLIGHTS

Adolescent Mothers: Resilience, Family Health Work, and Health-Promoting Practices

The dominant perspective of adolescent mothering is that it is an immense social problem. The complexities of adolescent development combined with parenting challenges are thought to place adolescent mothers and their children at high risk for poor health and developmental outcomes. However, findings of some qualitative studies suggest that, although some adolescent mothers struggle as parents, others embrace their parenting responsibilities with optimism and determination. Given that relatively little is known about the successes of these young women in caring for themselves and their children, the purpose of this study was to examine how an adolescent mother's strengths affect her health promotion efforts.

The study was conducted with a convenience sample of 41 adolescent mothers recruited through a variety of strategies. Mothers were asked to provide verbal responses to items on three study instruments: the Resilience Scale, the Health Options Scale, and the Health Promoting Lifestyle Profile. This study examined the relationships among the mother's resilience, family health promotion, and the mother's health-promoting lifestyle practices in single-parent families led by adolescent mothers by testing hypotheses derived from the Developmental Model of Health and Nursing. The Developmental Model of Health and Nursing (DMHN) gives a perspective from which to understand health promotion in

families led by adolescent mothers. The DMHN focuses on process and emphasizes family strengths. Health is seen as a characteristic of the family—a way of living that develops over time within the context of everyday family life. In the DMHN, family health is a composite of four distinct but interrelated concepts: health work, health potential, competence in health behavior, and health status. Health work, the central concept of the theory, is a process of active involvement through which families learn ways of coping with health challenges and of using strengths and resources to achieve goals for individual and family development.

Study findings support the premise that resilience is a critical source for single adolescent mothers. Both mother's resilience and health work predicted health-promoting lifestyle practices, suggesting that both of these variables play an important role in creating a family context in which health is nurtured. Adolescent mothers have been found to be at increased risk for a variety of social, psychological, and physiological problems, including poverty, domestic violence, abuse, and low educational attainment. Giving that resilience is an internal strength that develops in the context of adversity, it is not surprising that levels of resilience were relatively high since half of the participants reported some type of past abuse. The results raise issues for nurses working with adolescent mothers and provide a basis for developing their nursing practice.

From Black C, Ford-Gilboe M: Adolescent mothers: resilience, family health work and health-promoting practices, *J Adv Nurs* 48(4):351-360, 2004.

BOX 20-3 STAGES AND TASKS OF MIDDLE-CLASS NORTH AMERICAN FAMILY LIFE CYCLE

I. Launching: single young adult leaves home
   a. Coming to terms with the family of origin
   b. Development of intimate relationships with peers
   c. Establishment of self: career and finances
II. Marriage: joining of families
   a. Formation of identity as a couple
   b. Inclusion of spouse in realignment of relationships with extended families
   c. Parenthood: making decisions
III. Families with young children
   a. Integration of children into family unit
   b. Adjustment of tasks: child rearing, financial, and household
   c. Accommodation of new parenting and grandparenting roles
IV. Families with adolescents
   a. Development of increasing autonomy for adolescents
   b. Midlife reexamination of marital and career issues
   c. Initial shift toward concern for the older generation
V. Families as launching centers
   a. Establishment of independent identities for parents and grown children
   b. Renegotiation of marital relationship
   c. Readjustment of relationships to include in-laws and grandchildren
   d. Dealing with disabilities and death of older generation
VI. Aging families
   a. Maintenance of couple and individual functioning while adapting to the aging process
   b. Support role of middle generation
   c. Support and autonomy of older generation
   d. Preparation for own death and dealing with the loss of spouse and/or siblings and other peers

Data from Wright LM, Leahey M: *Nurses and families: a guide to family assessment and intervention*, ed 2, Philadelphia, 1994, FA Davis.

Alterations in Family Development: Divorce and Remarriage

Alterations to the life cycle occur, as seen in previously reviewed statistics of separation, divorce, single-parent families, and remarriage. The family must engage in emotional work as a result of divorce, a process that may occur suddenly or may be long and drawn out. In her classic study, Stern (1982) interviewed stepfather families in their homes and conceptualized the integration of the blended family, once remarriage occurs, as the integration of two distinct family cultures. In addition, Stern identified a set of affiliating strategies that families can learn to establish stepfather-child friendship.

ASSESSMENT TOOLS

Many tools exist for the community health nurse to use in assessing the family (Friedman et al., 2003; Wright and Leahey, 2005; Butler, 2008). Reviewed here are the genogram, family health tree, and ecomap.

Genogram

The genogram is a tool that helps the nurse outline the family's structure. It is a way to diagram the family (Figure 20-1). Generally, three generations of family members are included in a family tree, with symbols (Figure 20-2) denoting genealogy. Children are pictured from left to right, beginning with the oldest child.

The community health nurse may use the genogram during an early family interview, starting with a blank sheet of paper and drawing a circle or a square for the person initially interviewed. The nurse tells the family that he or she will ask several background questions to gain a general picture of the

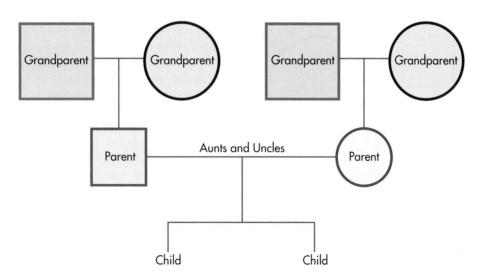

FIGURE 20-1 Simple genogram. (Redrawn from Wright LM, Leahey M: *Nurses and families: a guide to family assessment and intervention*, Philadelphia, 2005, FA Davis.)

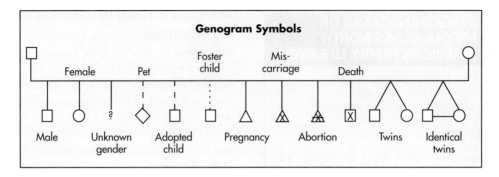

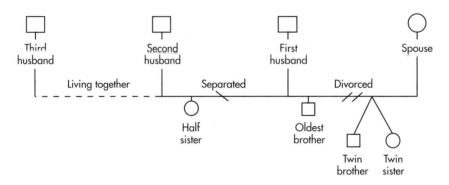

FIGURE 20-2 Commonly used genogram symbols. (Redrawn from Genopro Software: Symbols used in genograms, 2009: www.genopro.com.)

family. The nurse may draw circles around family members living in separate households.

For example, as depicted in the case study (Figure 20-3), family order across generations can be illustrated and specific personal characteristics can be noted in the drawing. Mr. and Mrs. Garcia are non–English speaking, a factor that will be of importance to the nurse as he or she plans nursing interventions. At times, the usefulness of the genogram is limited by how freely the family member relates significant information

such as divorces and remarriages, or family health concerns. Other families may be sensitive to the sharing of such information, particularly when it is shown to recur with each generation. For example a family history of alcohol or substance abuse or depression may be a sensitive issue. For other families, the development of the genogram is an excellent opening to the discussion of family history or hereditary health problems, or highlights the need for health education and promotion.

Family Health Tree

The **family health tree** is another tool that is helpful to the community health nurse. Based on the genogram, the family health tree provides a mechanism for recording the family's medical and health histories (Diekelmann, 1977; Friedman, 1992; U.S. Department of Health and Human Services, 2005, 2010). The nurse should note the following on the family health tree:

- Causes of death of deceased family members
- Genetically linked diseases, including heart disease, cancer, diabetes, hypertension, sickle cell anemia, allergies, asthma, and mental retardation
- Environmental and occupational diseases
- Psychosocial problems, such as mental illness and obesity
- Infectious diseases
- Familial risk factors from health problems
- Risk factors associated with the family's methods of illness prevention, such as having periodic physical examinations, Pap smears, and immunizations
- Lifestyle-related risk factors (i.e., by asking what family members do to "handle stress" and "keep in shape")

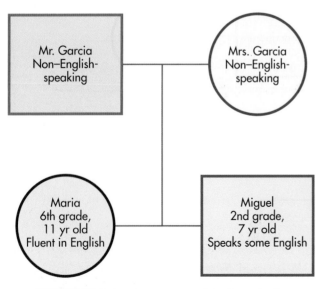

FIGURE 20-3 Sample genogram of the Garcia family.

The family health tree can be used in planning positive familial influences on risk factors such as diet, exercise, coping with stress, or pressure to have a physical examination. The U.S. Department of Health and Human Services (2005), under the direction of U.S. Surgeon General Richard Carmona, launched the "Family History Initiative." Included in this initiative is an online interactive tool "My Family Health Portrait" to help families learn about their risk for disease (www.hhs.gov/familyhistory). Included are questions to ask family members about common diseases, questions that suggest health promotion activities and goals as established in *Healthy People 2020*. When completed, the "family tree" can be printed. This tool could be incorporated into the family assessment and utilized by the nurse to plan family interventions to improve health.

Ecomap

The ecomap (Figure 20-4) is another classic tool that is used to depict a family's linkages to their suprasystems (Hartman, 1979; Wright and Leahey, 2000, 2005). As originally stated by Hartman:

> The eco-map portrays an overview of the family in their situation; it depicts the important nurturant or conflict-laden connections between the family and the world. It demonstrates the flow of resources, or the lacks and deprivations. This mapping procedure highlights the nature of the interfaces and points to conflicts to be mediated, bridges to be built, and resources to be sought and mobilized. (p. 467)

As with the genogram, the nurse can fill out the ecomap during an early family interview, noting people, institutions, and agencies significant to the family. The nurse can use symbols used in attachment diagrams (see Figure 20-2) to denote

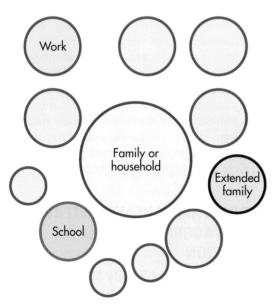

FIGURE 20-4 Ecomap. (Redrawn from Hartman A: Diagrammatic assessment of family relationships, *Soc Casework* 59:496, 1978.)

the nature of the ties that exist. For example, in Figure 20-5, which presents a sample ecomap of the Garcia family, the ecomap suggests that few contacts occur between the family and the suprasystems. The community health nursing student was able to use the ecomap to discuss with the Garcia family the types of resources in the community and the types of relationships they wanted to establish with them.

The nurse can use these tools for family assessment with families in every health care setting. They help increase the nurse's awareness of the family within the community and help guide the nurse and the family in the assessment and planning phases of care.

FAMILY HEALTH ASSESSMENT

Many agencies in the community have developed guidelines for assessment of the family that help practitioners identify the health status of individual members of the family and aspects of family composition, function, and process. Often included in family health assessment guidelines is information about the environment, or community context, and information about the family. A Family Health Assessment form can be used as a guide to assist the nurse in data collection and organization of the data collected from families over time. (See **Resource Tool 20A**, Family Health Assessment Form on the book's Evolve site.)

The nurse can obtain information for the Family Health Assessment through interviews with one or more family members individually, interviews of subsystems within the family (e.g., dyads of mother-child, parent-parent, and sibling-sibling), or group interviews with more than two members of the family. The nurse can also obtain information through observation of individual family members, dyads, and the entire family and observation of the environment in which the family lives, including housing, the neighborhood, and the larger community.

Family assessment tools have been developed by nurses and other professionals, such as sociologists, social workers, and psychologists working with families, to assess a range of dimensions of the family, such as marital satisfaction, parental coping abilities, and family dysfunction.

The Family Health Assessment addresses family characteristics, including structure and process and family environment (i.e., residence, neighborhood, and community). Not all dimensions on the Family Health Assessment will be appropriate for every family; therefore the nurse should modify content of the assessment guideline and adapt it as necessary to fit the individual family. The guidelines should serve as a guide only, as a means to record pertinent information about the family that will assist the nurse in working with the family. The nurse should gather information in the assessment spontaneously over several contacts with the family and various members and dyads within the family. It should also include multiple forays into the community, neighborhood, and home in which the family resides. Several contacts with the family will be required to complete the Family Health Assessment.

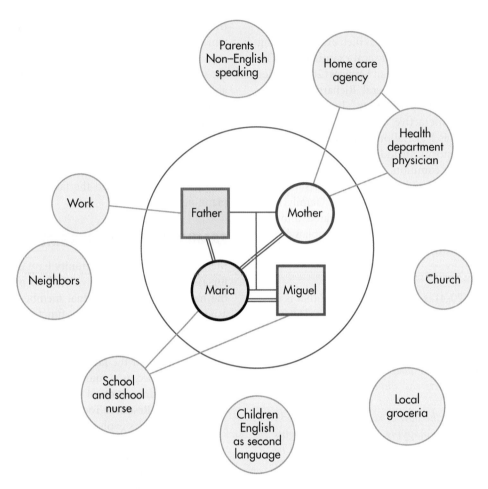

FIGURE 20-5 Sample ecomap of the Garcia family.

Social and Structural Constraints

In addition to the tools just reviewed, an important aspect of family assessment and planning for intervention is the need to make note of the social and structural constraints that prevent families from receiving needed health care or achieving a state of health. These constraints explain why some families differ in mortality rates, ability to achieve "integrity" rather than "despair," or ability to "self-actualize." Social and structural constraints are usually based in social and economic causes, which affect a wide range of conditions (e.g., literacy, education, and employment) associated with major health indicators (i.e., mortality and morbidity rates). Families most frequently served by the community health nurse are disadvantaged in that they are unable to buy health care from the private sector. However, constraints to obtaining needed health and social services are well documented and may come from characteristics of health and social services rather than individual family limitations. The nurse can note these constraints on the ecomap because they influence each family's ability to interact with a specific agency. For example, in addition to noting the strength of the relationship between family and agency or institution, the nurse should note those constraints that prevent use or full use of the resource. Constraints include hours of service, distance and transportation, availability of

interpreters, and criteria for receiving services (e.g., age, sex, and income barriers). Specific examples include the different guidelines posed by each state for Medicaid and by each community for home-delivered meals to the homebound.

Helping families understand constraints and linking them to accessible resources is necessary, but intervention at the family level is not sufficient. The common basic human needs of families in a community add up, and the community health nurse must tally structural constraints faced repeatedly by families and compare them with families in other communities. The nurse can then plan and implement interventions at the aggregate level. The following section is an overview of how community health nurses can extend intervention at the family level to larger aggregates and social action.

EXTENDING FAMILY HEALTH INTERVENTION TO LARGER AGGREGATES AND SOCIAL ACTION

Institutional Context of Family Therapists

Many theories exist to help bridge the gap between the application of nursing and family theory to the family and broader social action on behalf of communities of families.

Most family theorists view the family as a system that interfaces with outside suprasystems or institutions only when a problem is to be addressed, such as in the school or a courtroom. The following three approaches go beyond the family as a system to address the interaction between the family and the larger social system:

- Ecological framework
- Network therapy
- Transactional model

Ecological Framework

The ecological framework is a blend of systems and developmental theory with an individual's understanding of his or her environment. This approach indicts the specialization and fragmentation seen in the social and health service structure based on Western concepts of time and space. It focuses on providing a more complex and flexible structure. For example, Kogan and others (2004) investigated parent–health care provider discussions of family and community health risks during well-child examinations. Additionally, they studied the gaps in issues discussed by the practitioner and the information the parent desired. Based on the results of the National Survey of Early Childhood Health, health topics for discussion were identified: family financial difficulties, the presence of a support partner, parent's emotional support, alcohol and/or drug use in the home, cigarette smoking in the home, the parent's physical health, and community violence. Cigarette smoking was discussed nearly 80% of the time, and alcohol and drug use was discussed 45% of the time; however, community violence was discussed less than 10% of the time and financial needs 12%. The results indicate the need for better communication and education between health care providers and clients.

Network Therapy

Network therapy involves changing the network of families, be it extended family or friends, who tend to maintain a dysfunctional status quo in the nuclear family. This is done by replacing the network with others from the wider system that would be able to provide more support and enhance the functioning of the family. The concept of social network is related to social support. "Social network refers to a web like structure comprising one's relationships and social support focuses on the nature of the interactions taking place within social relationships" (Friedman et al., 2003, p. 462). A family's social network includes friends, community groups, church, and agencies. Social network also can be explained as the structure of relationships and social support as the function of relationships. Examples of network therapy are drawn from community mental health.

In a 2005 study, Voorhees, Murray, Welk, and others studied the relationship between peer social network and physical exercise in adolescent girls. The study found that younger adolescent girls were more active than older girls and that physical activity was significantly increased in both groups when it was supported by peer networks. The study supports the idea of building support systems for at-risk populations, as proposed by social network theory.

Transactional Model

In the transactional model, the term *transaction* refers to a system that focuses on process as opposed to a linear approach. This may lead to blaming or labeling. The family as an institution, along with other institutions (e.g., religious, educational, recreational, or governmental), is culturally anchored (i.e., each holds a distinct set of beliefs and values about the nature of the world and human existence). An awareness of culture (e.g., beliefs and values) as it is expressed in each system is important (i.e., as it is expressed in mainstream U.S. values vs. the value patterns of the family).

VanderValk and colleagues (2007) used a transactional model to explore the relationship of parental marital distress and adolescent emotional adjustment. In a 6-year prospective study of 531 parent-adolescent dyads, they found a relationship especially for late adolescent and young adult girls and less so for males. The findings suggest that "girls' greater sensitivity to interpersonal problems may be reciprocal and that the parental marriage is still associated with adjustment for girls in late adolescence and early adulthood" (p. 130).

Models of Social Class and Health Services

Social class places major limitations on access to medical care. In 1997, 15% of children had no health coverage of any kind. This accounts for 10.7 million children in the United States. In 2008, the uninsured rate for children was 13.8% (Children's Defense Fund, 2008). Approximately 60% of Americans were covered by employment-based health insurance plans in 2003. In 2006 this number had dropped to 57.9% (Gould, 2007). During this time, there was also an increase in the number of people covered by Medicare and Medicaid. Medicaid coverage increased to 13% and Medicare to 14.3% (U.S. Census Bureau, 2008).

Most children in poverty are white and non-Hispanic; however, the percentages of black or Hispanic children living in poverty are higher than that of white families. Figure 20-6 illustrates the percentages of American children living in poverty.

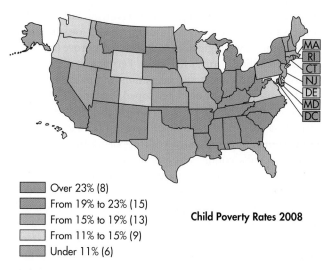

Child Poverty Rates 2008

Over 23% (8)
From 19% to 23% (15)
From 15% to 19% (13)
From 11% to 15% (9)
Under 11% (6)

FIGURE 20-6 Percentage of American children living in poverty: 2008. (From National Conference of State Legislators: [2009] www.ncsl.org/default.aspx?tabid=18557.)

Brownstein (1999) stated that the 1980s and 1990s were a time when the "rich got rich and the poor got poorer." The result has been a shift in the distribution of money and resources. Since the 1990s, there has been a decrease in the number of social programs designed to target the poor, especially the working poor. The nature of poverty continues to change, with increased numbers of the working poor in the lower class (Seccombe, 2001). With the current economic crisis, all socioeconomic levels have been affected. The U.S. Department of Labor Statistics reports that unemployment rates have increased in all 50 states (U.S. Department of Labor Statistics, 2009). With unemployment, additional Americans enter the medically uninsured category. Families need more support and resources than ever before but have greater financial and systems barriers, which prevent them from using the current health care system. Evidence supports the findings that unequal use of health care is likely the result of the system of care rather than of individual characteristics of people seeking care. Unexpected unemployment affects everyone in the family. The effects of job loss can be economic, emotional (anger and grief are common reactions), and social (more disagreements among family members coping with the stressors) (Kalil, 2005).

Models of Care for Communities of Families

Models exist to guide the community health nurse in providing care to communities of families in special need of services that improve access, equality between consumer and provider, and sensitivity to human need. There is generally an increase in the number and type of models that emerge, as traditional public and private models of health care decline due to funding and shrinking resources. Many of the programs develop as the result of community efforts or partnerships with existing health care providers. The following are examples of models.

The Kentucky Partnership for Farm Family Health and Safety

The Kentucky Partnership is a community coalition, originally funded by WK Kellogg Funds, involving farm families, universities, and various community-based organizations. The coalition was originally established to improve the health of farm families in rural Kentucky. Farming is identified as one of the most dangerous occupations in the United States, and few resources have been developed to support the unique needs of farm families. The Partnership identified farm women as the primary "health officers" for farm families. The farm women were provided with opportunities to develop leadership skills, conflict resolution, and team-building skills. Nurse educators and nursing students provided health education and assisted the farm women in developing a self-sustaining structure to support their efforts to improve family health. Cardiopulmonary resuscitation and first aid classes, the development of unique emergency medical subsystems, and other activities helped improve the health of the farm families. The local members reported an increase in personal knowledge, self-esteem, and personal satisfaction through the Partnership efforts. The Kentucky Partnership for Farm

Family Health and Safety continues to affect the health of farm families in south central Kentucky. The efforts are supported through the help of the South Central Kentucky Area Health Education Center at Western Kentucky University. The coalition has been replicated in three states (Texas, Louisiana, and Florida) and continues to connect universities and farm families in research efforts. Outcome assessment research was conducted to evaluate the impact of the coalition efforts on farm family health (Palermo and Ehlers, 2001; Siegrist and Jones, 2005). This organization continued in 2009 as a positive force improving the health of farm families.

The Health Access Nurturing Development Services Program

The Health Access Nurturing Development Services (HANDS) program is a voluntary home visitation program for new and expectant parents. Implemented through interdisciplinary teams consisting of social workers, nurses, and parent resource persons, the program serves first-time pregnant mothers and their families. HANDS was originally funded through tobacco settlement monies allocated through the state legislature to the Kentucky Cabinet for Health and Family Services. The program services are provided through district health departments and currently are available throughout the Commonwealth of Kentucky. Counseling, education, and support services are provided until the child reaches school age (4-5 years of age). Referrals to the program can be made through any primary care provider such as obstetricians-gynecologists, family physicians, and/or family nurse practitioners. The HANDS team completes an assessment to identify at-risk, first-time mothers, for example, teen mothers, older first-time mothers, pregnant women lacking social support or networks, mothers with substance abuse in the home, or mothers in abusive relationships. Such women qualify as candidates for HANDS services. Regardless of the risk level, all first-time mothers may receive the services. The goal is to support families in developing successful parenting. The program is based on evidence-based interventions that result in healthy families and children. Specific outcomes of this program have not been identified; however, the growth of the program supports the need for home visitation programs such as HANDS (Kentucky Cabinet for Health and Family Services, 2009).

These alternative health programs are strategies to change the structural barriers that prevent low-income families' access to care. Professional role functions changed as nurses, rather than physicians, provided health care. Active self-care was promoted, and health and medical knowledge was shared. Assistance by family and social networks was encouraged. Both of these programs address aspects of the health needs of populations at risk, but they do not "address the social determinants of disease." Neither program addresses the health-damaging conditions that poor people face, such as poor housing, malnutrition, and environmental hazards at the workplace and in the community. Although these programs represent steps in the right direction, changes in access to medical and health services are not enough. Social changes also are necessary.

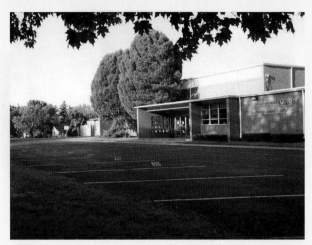

The school nurse, Jana, works with multiple city schools including this inner-city school. The school has a low-income, ethnically diverse population.

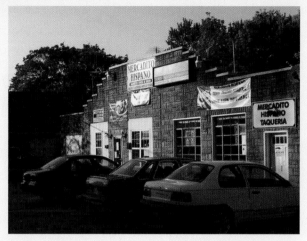

Jana assesses the community as she drives to the Garcias' home, noting the availability of resources such as the local groceria.

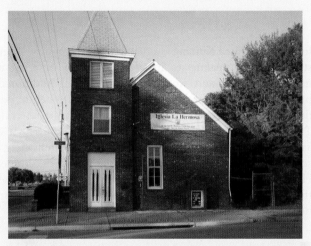

Local churches are a community resource, offering socialization and spiritual support for immigrant families such as the Garcia family in the United States.

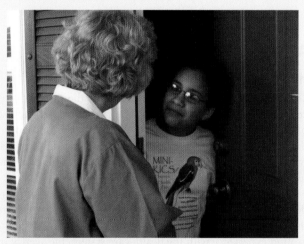

Jana arrives at the Garcias' home. Maria answers the door and invites Jana in.

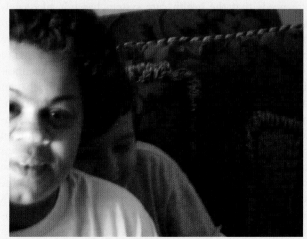

Miguel hides behind Mrs. Garcia shyly during the completion of the family assessment. Jana tries to include all family members present in the completion of the family assessment in order to develop a comprehensive family assessment.

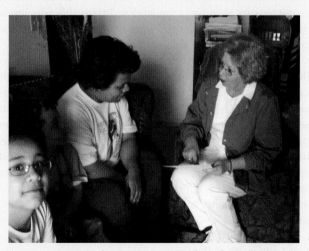

Jana completes the family assessment of the Garcia family with the help of Maria as interpreter for Mrs. Garcia. Mrs. Garcia listens intently as Jana asks questions about the family's health needs.

Jana reviews the plan of care and confirms the family's commitment to the plan of care developed with Jana.

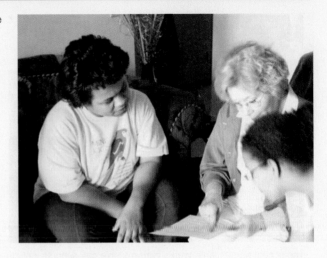

APPLYING THE NURSING PROCESS

Home Visit

The case study presents the application of the nursing process to a family on a home visit. The example notes the use of the home visit to identify health needs of the family within the community and programs planned to meet those needs, which ultimately will benefit a population of families in the future.

The home visit is a crucial experience for the nursing student and family (Friedman et al., 2003). Important factors that may influence the home visit include the family's background experience with the health care system, the agency in which the nursing student is working, the family's experience with previous nursing students who have visited the family, and the student's background. For example, nursing student characteristics may vary; the student brings differing levels of knowledge of medical and nursing practice, self, and the community.

The nursing student brings previous learning about families, family-related theory, the growth and development of members of different ages within a family, disease processes, and access to the health care system. Curricula within schools of nursing vary; therefore some students will also bring preparation in all specialties—medical-surgical nursing, childbearing, parent-child nursing, and psychiatric and mental health nursing—to the experience. Others may be taking basic clinical courses, such as pediatrics and psychiatric–mental health nursing, concurrently with community health. Thus the need for review of appropriate theory, health education, and standard assessment tools for individuals and families will vary.

The nursing student's knowledge of self, previous life experiences, and values also are important in planning for home visits. Nursing students must recognize their strengths and weaknesses in preparation for entering a new community and working with families. Additional preparation by all nursing students is necessary before the first home visit, depending on the content of the referral. The student should gather referral information, review assessment forms, and gather intervention tools (e.g., screening materials, supplies) before going to the home. Flexibility is important in working with families because the nursing student will not know the family's priority needs until the home visit.

SUMMARY

This chapter highlighted the community health nurse's work with families and identified the major family-related health care needs that the health care system has not adequately addressed. The nature of the family is changing and challenging traditional definitions and configurations. Approaches to meeting the health needs of families must go beyond that of the traditional health care system, which addresses the individual as the unit of care. Strategies were given in this chapter for expanding notions of care from the individual to the family and from the family to the community. To guide intervention with families, nurses have traditionally relied on common theoretical frameworks from the disciplines of psychology or social psychology. These frameworks often target individuals; frameworks are needed that go beyond the individual to the family and community and address social and policy changes needed to alter the social, economic, and environmental conditions under which families must function. This chapter provided tools for assessing the family and the family within the community and gave examples of the extension of family health intervention to larger aggregates, which involves social action to overcome constraints to accessing health services. Nonnursing and community health nursing models of care provided for communities of families were presented and critiqued. The nursing process was applied at the individual, family, and community levels on a home visit. Examples of interventions by the community health nurse at individual, family, and community levels were presented.

Families remain the core of society, with diversity as the constant for families in the United States. Family nursing must be understood and practiced by community health nurses. An understanding of family theory provides a mechanism for assessing and intervening with families to improve their level of wellness and increase the health of the community as a whole.

CASE STUDY   APPLICATION OF THE NURSING PROCESS

Jana Parks is a community health nurse employed by the District Health Department. She is a school health nurse, providing services for six schools in a moderately sized community. After receiving a referral from school officials related to a student's absenteeism, Jana plans to assess the student and family. (See the Photo Novella on pp. 398-399 for photos that depict this case study.)

Assessment

Jana knows that the school is located in the inner city, with approximately 360 students in the first through sixth grades; nearly 75% have a median family income at or below the federal poverty level. The school population is significantly more ethnically diverse than the overall community; the surrounding neighborhood frequently houses newly immigrated families. English is the second language for approximately 25% of the students, and 5% are not fluent in spoken or written English. Each year, more than 20% of the student body moves into or out of the school district.

She reviews the school records for the student, Maria Garcia, and learns that this is the first year of enrollment for the sixth grader and her second-grade brother, Miguel. Maria's family moved to the area 6 months ago from the Dominican Republic. School records note that the girl is adequately fluent in spoken English but that the parents do not speak English. The student's father works part-time at a local furniture manufacturer. There has been a noticeable decline in grades over the previous quarter, there have been no disciplinary actions, and teacher comments are positive regarding the student's classroom performance. The health record indicates that she is up-to-date with required immunizations; no chronic illnesses are noted on the school physical examination record. Jana notes that Maria's brother does not have the same school absence pattern.

Jana contacts the family and identifies her role as school health nurse. She explains the need for a meeting with the student and family to discuss concerns about Maria's school attendance. A time is scheduled when both parents and the student are available. She confirms the home address and directions.

As she drives through the neighborhood, Jana notes both single-family and multifamily dwellings; the streets are lined with parked vehicles, trash bins, and household items. As she approaches the student's home, she observes that an older model sedan is parked in the drive. The house is in need of paint and some windows have been replaced with cardboard; however, the yard is free of clutter and there are containers of blooming plants on the small porch.

Jana knocks on the door and, after a moment, states, "It's Jana Parks, the school nurse." Maria Garcia opens the door, and Jana enters a small, dimly lit room. As the student makes introductions, Mr. Garcia stands and greets Jana with a nod and handshake while Mrs. Garcia remains recumbent on the sofa but raises her hand in greeting. Mrs. Garcia's appearance surprises Jana, as she appears much older than Mr. Garcia. Her skin color is pale, eyes are sunken, and she appears frail, with a distended abdomen and generalized muscle wasting.

Jana is aware that the exchange of social conversation is important in establishing a relationship with Hispanic clients. She mentions the beautiful picture in the room and learns that a family member painted it as a wedding gift for the Garcias. Jana learns that the family has no other relatives in the community and moved to the city through the work of a refugee assistance organization. She asks where they would like her to sit and, after a few minutes, begins to transition to a focused question interview. In this interview, Jana plans to collect information related to individual, family, and/or community functioning.

Throughout the conversation, Jana has noted that both Maria and Mr. Garcia appear tense; Mrs. Garcia is quiet and rarely speaks or smiles. Maria has translated throughout the conversation, although Jana senses that the parents may have limited understanding of spoken English. To lessen anxiety, Jana begins the interview by saying, "I am here because the school and I are concerned about Maria's absences. I want to learn why Maria misses school and to see if there are ways that the school can help."

Through the interview process, Jana learns that Maria likes school and has made friends there. She observes that Miguel stays close to Maria and frequently hides his face into her shoulder when Jana speaks to him. She also notes that Mr. and Mrs. Garcia rarely look at each other, and Mr. Garcia chooses a seat on the opposite side of the room. The family rents the home, and the father has been able to supplement his part-time income by working as a day laborer for a lawn service. The family was beginning to establish connections at a local church and with neighbors when Mrs. Garcia had an abdominal tumor diagnosed that has required numerous surgeries over the past 3 months. She is still receiving home care visits for a surgical wound that has not healed. Although Medicaid has covered most physician and hospital expenses, the family has experienced out-of-pocket expenses for noncovered medications. These problems have contributed to family financial stress. Mr. Garcia has to drive his wife to medical appointments; as a result, he is in danger of losing his job. Maria also attends these appointments to serve as the interpreter, resulting in her frequent school absences.

In addition, Jana learns that Maria has assumed responsibility for the household cooking, cleaning, and laundry since her mother's illness. Mr. Garcia shops at a small neighborhood groceria. Jana determines that with food stamps the family has adequate resources to purchase food, although Maria admits that she is still learning to cook. The family eats the evening meal together, frequently rice and beans. Maria and Miguel are eligible for subsidized breakfast and lunch at school. Maria believes that it is her responsibility to help Miguel complete his homework, get to bed on time, and attend school regularly. Mr. Garcia disciplines both children. Jana asks questions regarding family health practices and learns that they see a provider at the health department only when ill or for school requirements and do not seek dental care. She observes a number of medication bottles on a table near the sofa.

Diagnosis
Individual

- Caregiver role strain related to time-consuming activities, insufficient finances, and insufficient recreation (Mr. Garcia and Maria)
- Risk for injury related to improperly stored medications (Miguel)

- Deficient knowledge related to language and cultural differences (Mr. and Mrs. Garcia)
- Ineffective health maintenance related to lack of routine dental hygiene (Mr. and Mrs. Garcia, Maria, and Miguel)

Family

- Risk for interrupted family processes related to change in Mrs. Garcia's ability to function, financial burden of treatments for ill family member, and disruption of family routines
- Impaired parenting related to mother's illness
- Risk of family crisis secondary to mother's prolonged illness

Community

- Inadequate systematic programs for linking Hispanic families to community resources

Planning

A plan of care is developed to meet the needs of the individuals, family, and community. Planning involves mutual goal setting between the nurse and family; mutual setting of objectives to meet goals; prioritizing, or setting short- and long-term goals with the family; contracting, or establishing the division of labor between nurse and family that will meet the objectives; and evaluation of the process and outcome.

Individual
Long-Term Goals

- Mr. Garcia will recognize appropriate roles and responsibilities for Maria. He will identify and use resources to allow her to resume suitable educational, social, and family duties.
- Mr. Garcia will identify and use community resources to assist with transportation needs and medication costs.
- Jana noted a long-term need to discuss dental care.
- Mr. and Mrs. Garcia will improve their English comprehension and speaking skills.

Short-Term Goals

- Relieve Maria of interpreting at medical appointments by identifying alternate interpretive resources.
- Store medications in a secure location.

Family
Long-Term Goal
The family will be able to find and use appropriate services for physical and social support.

Short-Term Goal
The family will learn to appropriately express their feelings related to the mother's illness, social isolation, role strain, and/or fear.

Community
Long-Term Goal
The community will establish programs to support immigrant family needs for transportation, interpretation, and enculturation to the American medical system.

Short-Term Goal
Mr. Garcia will identify existing programs available to support Hispanic immigrants.

Intervention
Jana recognizes that many interventions must be carried out at the individual, family, and community levels.

Individual

- Education regarding safe medication storage
- Referral to the Refugee Assistance Society or local churches for interpretive assistance

Family
Direct nursing interventions directed at family functioning include the following levels:

- Cognitive: New information is provided to the family that promotes problem solving by the family. An example is referring the Garcias to the community free clinic for medical and dental care.
- Affective: Families are encouraged to express their feelings that may be blocking their efforts at problem solving. An example of this would be Jana's planned validation of Mr. Garcia's concerns regarding finances and the threat of losing employment.
- Behavioral: Tasks are negotiated to be carried out either during the family interview or as homework between visits. An example is Mr. Garcia's planned call to the Refugee Assistance Society.

Community
Jana recognizes that her referral of Mr. Garcia to the Refugee Assistance Society to obtain support through existing programs is also an intervention at the community level. She engages in ongoing parafamily work to identify how the community can be mobilized to provide physical, mental, and social support to immigrant families. Does anyone at the community free clinic speak Spanish? Are interpreters available at health care facilities? Where do most immigrant families receive health care and social support? Are classes on English as a second language free of charge for Hispanic families? Are job skill training or courses available for Mr. Garcia? Questions such as these bring up many areas of assessment that Jana will need to make with the Garcia family and the community in the future.

Evaluation
Individual/Family
Jana assists the Garcias to obtain a small lockable box in which to store medication. Mr. Garcia establishes contact with a local church that provides a volunteer interpreter and driver for medical visits and twice-weekly delivery of meals. Mr. Garcia takes Maria and Miguel to the free clinic where dental sealants are applied to molars. The social worker at the community's free clinic meets with Mr. Garcia to offer him assistance in obtaining low-cost medications. Through this conversation, Jana identifies his reluctance to ask for financial assistance. He states that he should provide for his family and that Maria should not have to assume the role of mother for Miguel. However, he does not see any other options at this time. She identifies that Mr. Garcia may be in need of ongoing support and suggests that he talk with a counselor about his concerns. Mr. Garcia refuses to see a counselor but agrees that he will talk to the pastor of his church. Maria and Miguel meet with the school counselor as needed to discuss feelings related to the mother's illness and resulting family strain.

Community
Jana identified that many community resources are available to immigrant families; however, information is limited and not readily accessible. She contacts the director of the Refugee Assistance Society, and together they initiate a community coalition to address this issue.

Continued

CASE STUDY APPLICATION OF THE NURSING PROCESS—cont'd

Levels of Prevention

Society's expectations of the family are in transition. Application of the levels of prevention to families by the community nurse must take into account the changing family configuration; the financial, emotional, and physical burdens often compounded in the single-parent family; and the lack of resources such as nonexisting health insurance or inadequate health insurance.

Primary Prevention

This chapter has established the importance of the family to individuals and society. Primary prevention with families becomes an essential element of any comprehensive family health plan. From the family perspective, health education must address actual and potential challenges to health such as immunizations of all family members, educating about resources to support the family financially and emotionally, encouraging exercise and activity, and empowering the family to build upon strengths. An example is using the family genogram to teach the family about predisposition to diseases and helping the family develop a health prevention plan.

Secondary Prevention

The focus of secondary prevention for the family includes assuring that the family has continued access to health care and resources for individual and family health problems. The changing economy in the United States has "closed the door" to regular health providers for some families. The challenge to the nurse is helping the family locate and access continued care and teaching the family to move through the system of government assistance, which may be new and unacceptable for the family. The nurse must be politically active in lobbying legislators for continued resources to support families.

Tertiary Prevention

Tertiary prevention for family includes assuring that the needed resources are available to support long-term care of each family member. An example of a community-based organization established and funded solely by volunteers is the Kelly Autism Program (KAP). KAP is "designed to provide services to adolescents and young adults diagnosed along the Autism Spectrum Continuum, as well as their families, while serving as a training opportunity for future professionals in a variety of disciplines. KAP has programs for middle school, high school and post-secondary participants including higher education, vocational training, and job support" (Western Kentucky University, 2009, p. 1, Vision). It includes a comprehensive screening program and one-on-one support for young adults with autism capable of living and studying on a university campus.

Developed by Mary Kovar, RN, MSN, and Barbara Minix, RN, MSN.

■ LEARNING ACTIVITIES

1. Define the term *family* with a group of three colleagues. Compare definitions and list similarities and differences. Develop a list of criteria for being a member of a family.
2. Complete a personal genogram. What are the high-risk factors in the family history? Current risk factors? Categorize current risk factors into physical, interpersonal, and environmental. Identify needed health education and determine who needs the education. Identify sources of appropriate screening in the community for the identified risk factors.
3. Complete a personal ecomap. Is the family an "open" or "closed" family system? What resources do families currently use for mental, physical, emotional, social, and community health? What referrals are needed?
4. Identify family types or situations (e.g., families of different cultures, gay or lesbian families, or never-married-mother families) that elicit "discomfort" in working situations. Identify ways to overcome barriers in working with these types of families.

REFERENCES

Allen DR, Fine MA, Demo HD: An overview of family diversity: controversies, questions, and values. In Demo DH, Allen KR, Fine MA, editors: *Handbook of family diversity*, New York, 2000, Oxford Press.

Allmond BW, Buckman W, Gofman HF: *The family is the patient*, St. Louis, 1979, Mosby.

American Academy of Child & Adolescent Psychiatry: *Grandparents raising grandchildren*, 2009. www.aacap.org/cs/root/facts_for_families/grandparents_raising_grandchildren.

Anderson MP, O'Grady RS, Anderson IL: Public health nursing in primary care: impact on home visits, *Public Health Nurs* 2:145, 1985.

Annie E. Casey Foundation: Kids Count Faststats data book online, 2009, www.aecf.org/kidscount/databook/indicators.htm.

Auger JR: Behavioral systems and nursing, *AJN* 77(11):1856–1857, 1977.

Beard M: Home nursing, *Public Health Nurs Q* 7:44–51, 1999.

Brownstein R: Government should work harder to help those left behind by booming economy, *Los Angeles Times* A5, Oct 11, 1999.

Butler JF: The family diagram and genogram: comparisons and contrast, *Am J Family Therapy* 36:169–180, 2008.

Carter E, McGoldrick M, editors: *The changing family life cycle: a framework for family therapy*, ed 2, New York, 1988, Gardner Press.

Centers for Disease Control and Prevention: *Faststats: Teen births*, 2009, www.cdc.gov/nchs/fastats/teenbrth.htm.

Centers for Medicare and Medicaid Services: *The children's health insurance program*, 2009, www.cms.hhs.gov/LowCost HealthInsFamChild/.

Children's Defense Fund: *Why children's health insurance matters*, 2009. www.childrensdefense.org/helping-americas-children/childrens-health/health-coverage-for-all-children-campaign/uninsured-children.html.

Cody WK: Nursing frameworks to guide practice and research with families, *Nurs Sci Q* 13(4):277–284, 2000.

Cook E: *The life of Florence Nightingale*, vol 2, London, 1913, Macmillan.

Cornell University: *Family life center: Elmira nurse family partnership*, 2009. www.human.cornell.edu/che/fldc/programs/Elmira-Nurse-Family-Partnership.cfm.

DeFrain J: Strong families, *Family Matters* 53:6–13, 1999.

Diekelmann N: *Primary health care of the well adult*, New York, 1977, McGraw-Hill.

Dreher MC: The conflict of conservatism in public health nursing education, *Nurs Outlook* 30:504, 1982.

Dunst CJ, Trivette CM: Capacity-building family-systems intervention practices, *Journal of Family Social Work* 12(2):119–143, 2009.

Duvall EM: *Marriage and family relationships*, ed 5, Philadelphia, 1977, JB Lippincott.

Duvall EM, Miller BC: *Marriage and family development*, ed 6, New York, 1985, Harper and Row.

Erikson E: *Childhood and society*, ed 2, New York, 1963, WW Norton.

Freeman R: *Public health nursing practice*, ed 3, Philadelphia, 1963, WB Saunders.

Friedman MM, Bowden VB, Jones EG: *Family nursing: research, theory and practice*, ed 2, Upper Saddle River, NJ, 1992, Prentice Hall.

Friedman MM: *Family nursing: theory and assessment*, ed 3, East Norwalk, CT, 1998, Appleton-Lange.

Friedman MM, Bowden VB, Jones EG: *Family nursing: research, theory and practice*, ed 3, Upper Saddle River, NJ, 2003, Prentice Hall.

Glaser B, Strauss AL: *Chronic illness and the quality of life*, St. Louis, 1975, Mosby.

Gould E: The erosion of employment-based insurance: more working families left uninsured, EPI Briefing Paper No. 203, 2007, www.epi.org.

Hanson S, Kaakimen J: *Family health care nursing: Theory & practice*, ed 3, Philadelphia PA, 2005, FA Davis.

Hartman A: *Finding families: an ecological approach to family assessment in adoption*, Beverly Hills, CA, 1979, Sage.

Hohmann-Marriott AP: Relationship quality in interethnic marriages & cohabitation, *Soc Forces* 87(2):825–855, 2006.

Hopia H, Paavilainen E, Astedt-Kurki P: Promoting the health for families of children with chronic conditions, *J Adv Nurs* 48(6):575–583, 2004.

Hohmann-Marriott BE: Relationship quality in interethnic marriages and cohabitations, *Soc Forces* 87(2):276–286, 2008.

Human Rights Campaign: *Marriage and relationship recognition*, 2009, www.hrc.org/issues/marriage.asp.

Kalil A: Unemployment and job displacement: the impact on families and children, *Ivey Business Journal*, July/August: 1–5, 2005.

Kentucky Cabinet for Health and Family Services: *HANDS program*, Frankfort, KY, 2009, The Author: http://chfs.ky.gov/dph/ach/hands/htm.

Kogan MD, et al: Routine assessment of family and community health risks: parent views and what they receive, *Pediatrics* 113:1934–1943, 2004.

Li L, Lin C, Cao H, Lieber E: Intergenerational and urban-rural health habits in Chinese families, *Am J Health Behav* 33(2):172–180, 2009.

Maslow A: *Motivation and personality*, ed 2, New York, 1970, Harper and Row.

McDaniel SH, Campbell TL, Hepworth J, et al: *Family-oriented primary care*, ed 2, New York, 2005, Springer.

McLanahan S, Percheski C: Family structure and the reproduction of inequalities, *Annu Rev Sociol* 34:257–276, 2008.

McNeill JA, et al: Family history: value-added information in assessing cardiac health, *AAOHN* 56(7):297–305, 2008.

Miller FM: *Coping with chronic illness: overcoming powerlessness*, Philadelphia, 2000, FA Davis.

Minuchin P: Looking toward horizon: present and future in study of family systems. In McHale JP, Grolnick WS, editors: *Psychological study of families*, Mahwah, NJ, 2002, Lawrence Erlbaum.

Montalvo B: Useful coincidences and family strengths, *Contemp Fam Ther* 26(2):117–119, 2004.

National Institute of Mental Health: NIMH International scientific conference on the role of families in preventing and adapting to HIV/AIDS, 2005, www.nimh.nih.gov/scientific meetings/hivaids2005.cfm.

National League for Nursing: *A curriculum guide for schools of nursing*, New York, 1937, The Author.

National Institute of Health: *Better diabetes care for systems change: Cultural competency tips 2009*, http://betterdiabetescare.nih.gov/ISSUESculturalcompetencytips.htm.

Otto H: A framework for assessing family strengths. In Reinhard A, Quinn M, editors: *Family-centered community health nursing*, St. Louis, 1973, Mosby.

Palermo T, Ehlers J: *Coalitions: building partnerships to promote agricultural health and safety*, Washington DC, 2001, National Institutes for Occupational Health and Safety, www.cdc.gov/nasd/doc/d001701-d001774.html.

Parke RP: Family & peer systems, *Psychol Bull* 128(4):596–601, 2002.

Pratt L: *Family structure and effective health behavior*, Boston, 1976, Houghton Mifflin.

Robert Wood Johnson Foundation: *Let's cover the uninsured*, 2009, http://covertheuninsured.org/.

Saksvig B, Jobe JB: The role of peer social network factors and physical activity in adolescent girls, *Am J Health Behav* 29(2):183–190, 2005.

Seccombe K: Families in poverty in the 1990s: trends, causes, consequences, and lessons learned. In Milardo RM, editor: *Understanding families into the new millennium*, Minneapolis, Minn, 2001, National Council on Family Relations.

Siegrist B, Jones S: *Nursing education beyond classroom walls: Service learning through collaboration with community partners*, WKU Center for Excellence in Teaching, 2005, www.wku.edu/Dept/Support/AcadAffairs/CTL/booklets/serviclrn.htm.

Spencer N: Does material disadvantage explain the increased risk of adverse health, educational, and behavioural outcomes among children in lone parent households in Britain? A cross sectional study, *J Epidemiol Community Health* 59(2):152–157, 2005.

Stern PN: Conflicting family culture: an impediment to integration in stepfather families, *J Psychosoc Nurs Ment Health Serv* 20:27, 1982.

University of California at Los Angeles, The Williams Institute: *Adoption and foster care by gay and lesbian parents in the United States*, March 2009, www.law.ucla.edu/williamsinstitute/publications/FinalAdoptionReport.pdf.

U.S. Census Bureau: *Population profile of the nation: dynamic version 2005*, Washington, DC, April 2005, The Author, www.census.gov/population/www/pop-profile/profiledynamic.html.

U.S. Census Bureau: *Income, poverty and health insurance: coverage in the US in 2007*, 2008, www.census/prod/2008/pub/p60.

U.S. Department of Health and Human Services: New family history tool promotes prevention, *Nations Health* 34(10):33, 2005.

U.S. Department of Health and Human Services: *My family health portrait: A tool from the US Surgeon General 2010*, https://familyhistory.hhs.gov/fhh-web/home.action.

U.S. Department of Labor Statistics: *Labor Force Statistics from the Current Population Survey 2009*, www.bls.gov/cps/.

VanderValk I, de Goede M, Spruijt E, et al: A longitudinal study on transactional relations between parental marital distress and adolescent emotional adjustment, *Adolescence* 42: 165:116–136, 2007.

Vorhees CC, Murray D, Welk G, et al: The role of peer social network factors and physical activity in adolescent girls, *Am J Health Behav* 29(2):183–190, 2005.

von Bertalanffy L: *General systems theory: foundations, development, applications*, New York, 1968, George Braziller.

von Bertalanffy L: The history and status of general systems theory. In Klir G, editor: *Trends in general systems theory*, New York, 1972, Wiley.

von Bertalanffy L: General systems theory and psychiatry. In Arieti S, editor: *American handbook of psychiatry*, New York, 1974, Basic Books.

Wald L: The family as a unit of care: a historical review, *Public Health Nurs* 3:427–428, 515–519, 1904.

Western Kentucky University: *Kelly Autism Program*, 2009, http://kap.wku.edu/vision_mission.html.

Women's Educational Media: *It's elementary: why address gay issues with children*, 2005, www.womedia.org/ie_whyaddress.htm.

Wright LM, Leahey M: *Nurses and families: a guide to family assessment and intervention*, Philadelphia, 1994, FA Davis.

Wright LM, Leahey M: *Nurses and families: a guide to family assessment and intervention*, Philadelphia, 2000, FA Davis.

Wright LM, Leahey M: *Nurses and family: a guide to family assessment and intervention*, ed 4, Philadelphia, 2005, FA Davis.

Wydick B: Grandma was right: why cohabitation undermines relationship satisfaction but is increasing anyway, *KYKLOS* 60:617–645, 2007.

Populations Affected by Disabilities

Linda L. Treloar

Additional Material for Study, Review, and Further Exploration

evolve WEBSITE

http://evolve.elsevier.com/Nies
- Quiz
- Case Studies
- Glossary
- WebLinks

OBJECTIVES

Upon completion of this chapter, the reader will be able to do the following:

1. Differentiate between medical model and social construct definitions for disability.
2. Describe historical attitudes and perspectives surrounding disability that have contributed to devaluation and disempowerment of people with disabilities.
3. Compare and contrast short- and long-term, health-related, disabling conditions.
4. Discuss key federal legislation applicable to people with disabilities.
5. Identify selected health care and social issues that influence the ability of people with disabilities to live and thrive in the community.
6. Apply narrative experience to disability that integrates a holistic focus and promotes the health and well-being of people with disabilities and their families.

KEY TERMS

activities of daily living (ADLs)
ADA Amendments Act of 2008
Americans with Disabilities Act (ADA)
children with a disability (CWD)
disability
functional activities
handicap

impairment
Individuals with Disabilities Education Act (IDEA)
individualized education plan (IEP)
instrumental activities of daily living (IADLs)
intellectual disability (ID)

people with disabilities (PWD)
reasonable accommodations
Social Security Disability Insurance (SSDI)
Supplemental Security Income (SSI)

OUTLINE

Self-Assessment: Responses to Disability
Definitions and Models for Disability
    National Agenda for Prevention of Disabilities Model
    Four Models for Disability
    Differentiating Illness from Disability
Characteristics of Disability
    Measurement of Disability
    Prevalence of Disability
    Health Status and Causes of Disability
    Aging and Personal Assistance

Disability and Public Policy
    Legislation Affecting People with Disabilities
    Public Assistance Programs
Costs Associated with Disability
    Economic Well-Being and Employment
***Healthy People 2020* and the Health Needs of People with Disabilities**
    Health Disparities in Quality and Access
    People with Intellectual Disabilities: Undervalued and Disadvantaged

After having an incomplete spinal cord injury following an automobile accident, a 29-year-old man named Jim progressed from visible physical disability and paralysis to continued disability without the use of a wheelchair. Jim explained his progression, which follows:

You know it's really weird. In some ways it's hard to enter into that wheelchair life, to go into that life and then come back out of it again. I entered into a whole other realm [life with paralysis] that I'd only observed. I stepped into the unknown and pulled back out of it again. Yet, one foot is still in that world. (Treloar, 1999a, p. 189)

According to Jim, disability may create a "whole other realm," or an "unknown" world. Like Jim, most people lack awareness of the divergence of perceptual worlds that disability creates and the historical, sociopolitical context and culture that surround disability. Nurses may think they understand disability, but this may not be true. Attitudes toward disability influence people's responses to and care for others. Before reading further, consider the following self-assessment.

SELF-ASSESSMENT: RESPONSES TO DISABILITY

What comes to mind when you think of *someone with a disability*? Focus on those sights, sounds, and smells. List characteristics using adjectives or short phrases. What values, customs, and traditions may be promoted or blocked for individuals with disabilities?

Picture yourself as a *person with a disability*. How do others respond to you? Who or what kinds of supports are available to help? Consider your health care concerns and needs. How might health care professionals devalue or disempower you? How can nurses and other caregivers convey respect and concern for you: to acknowledge insights gained through living with a disability, while helping to fill in the gaps where you lack wisdom?

Imagine yourself as a *nurse with a visible disability*, or the client receiving care from a nurse with a disability. What thoughts and feelings flood your mind? Would anything change if the nurse were invisibly disabled? Consider a scenario in which you apply as a preprofessional student with a disability to a college of nursing. Your disability requires additional time to achieve performance-based tasks. What might concern nursing program staff and faculty about this situation?

Think about living in a *family affected by disability*. Consider the impact of a child with a disability on sibling and parental activities and family roles. What if you were an active, growing child in a family where mom or dad is disabled? Although it may seem easier to focus on difficulties, consider possible benefits, to include positive learning and growth in family members. What kinds of social and personal supports do you have, or find are inadequate or lacking altogether? What do you wish others understood about living in a family affected by disability?

Finally, what is the experience of *living with disability within your community*? What social or environmental barriers related to disability exist? How can nurses and an interdisciplinary team form alliances with the client and family to reduce or eliminate these barriers? Health care professionals are taught to assess and provide interventions that promote health, and they usually believe they know what people with disabilities need. However, the actions of providers may convey different messages to people with disabilities and their families. Regardless of their professional experience or familiarity with disability, clients may question providers' ability to understand their experience.

Disability affects people irrespective of class, culture, race, or economic level. Depending on the term's definition, disability affects nearly one out of every five Americans. Disability increases with age, often influencing a person's ability to maintain self-care, which is essential to living in his or her preferred living environment.

People who grow up with a disability describe their lived experience with disability somewhat differently from those who become disabled as the result of a health condition. For example, people having a sensory disability (blind/deaf), or a physical disability from birth, adapt to the world as they know it. Compare this situation with that of a 20-year-old who becomes blind, deaf, or paralyzed because of an accident. The loss may never be fully grieved. Adaptation may be delayed by the psychological impact of what is gone and its meaning. If an 80-year-old becomes blind because of diabetes-induced retinopathy, the loss of sight was chronic, progressive, and predictable. There will be loss and grief, but it occurs as part of the aging process. Rather than seeing people with disabilities (PWD) as "all the same," nurses must be able to see each person with a disability as unique, having different goals, knowledge, and experiences.

This chapter provides content that nurses can use in a variety of settings to provide knowledgeable, appropriate care for people with disabilities and their families. Throughout your reading, consider: What implications exist for health care policy and research related to disability?

DEFINITIONS AND MODELS FOR DISABILITY

The International Classification of Functioning, Disability and Health (ICF) (World Health Organization [WHO], 2001) defines the following key terms. A disability, resulting from an impairment, involves a restriction or an inability to perform an activity in a normal manner or within the normal range. An anatomical, mental, or psychological loss or abnormality is an impairment. A handicap is a disadvantage resulting from an impairment or a disability that prevents fulfillment of an expected role. In comparing these concepts, an impairment affects a human organ on a micro level, disability affects a person on an individual level, and a handicap involves society on a macro level of analysis (Batavia, 1993). Table 21-1 compares and contrasts these definitions related to disability.

The "old" paradigm for viewing disability was based on the Nagi model, which used functional limitations to determine whether an individual was disabled (Pope and Tarlov, 1991). Although the WHO and Nagi frameworks recognize that a person's ability to perform a socially expected activity reflects characteristics of the individual and the larger social and physical environment, they are commonly criticized for their medical emphasis and definitional inconsistencies. Impairments do not necessarily result in disabilities, and disabilities do not necessarily produce handicaps. Whether a person is viewed as disabled varies according to the environmental barriers and the perspectives of the onlooker.

National Agenda for Prevention of Disabilities Model

The Committee on a National Agenda for the Prevention of Disabilities (NAPD) conceptualized a model for disability (Figure 21-1) that extends the ICF and Nagi frameworks. In the NAPD model, disability occurs when a person's physical or mental limitations, in interaction with physical and social barriers in the environment, prevent the person from taking equal part in the normal life of the community (Pope and Tarlov, 1991). Furthermore, disability develops through a complex, interactive process involving biological, behavioral, and environmental (i.e., social and physical) risk factors and quality of life (QOL). In this social model for disability, bodily impairments and functional limitations are not necessarily

accompanied by disability. Disability may be preventable, and preventive measures can promote an improved QOL and reduce costs related to dependence, lost productivity or unemployment, and medical care.

The Disabling Process

The NAPD model provides an alternative framework for viewing four related and distinct stages in the disabling process. Pathology at the cellular and tissue level may produce an impairment in structure or function at the organ level. An individual with an impairment may experience a functional limitation, which restricts his or her ability to perform an action within the normal range. The functional limitation may result in a disability when certain socially defined activities and roles cannot be performed.

Although the model appears to indicate unidirectional progression from pathology, to impairment, to functional limitation, to disability, stepwise or linear progression may not occur. Disability prevention efforts can address any of the risk factors or stages in the disabling process. Health promotion efforts include primary prevention of disability, secondary reversal of disability and restoration of function, and tertiary prevention of complications.

Quality of Life Issues

Accessing environmental and social barriers to needed services can frustrate and exhaust many PWD and their families. Barriers to access may include transportation to a needed service, the cost of care, appointment challenges, language barriers, financial issues (e.g., family has no phone to make or confirm appointments), and migrant/noninsured issues. Denied or delayed access to needed health services can negatively affect the health and well-being of any person. A PWD with an accompanying health concern may change a chronic concern into an acute problem. The Clinical Example (as follows) illustrates an attitudinal barrier and how it influences living with disability.

Community nurses can partner with clients and families affected by disabilities to remedy barriers that negatively affect QOL for this population. Most important, nurses must look beyond health-related concerns, a significant challenge in the current managed-care environment. Nurses cannot

TABLE 21-1	TERMINOLOGY FOR IMPAIRMENT, DISABILITY, AND HANDICAP		
CHARACTERISTIC	IMPAIRMENT	DISABILITY	HANDICAP
Definition	Physical deviation from normal structure, function, physical organization, or development	May be objective and measurable	Not objective or measurable; is an experience related to the responses of others
Measurability	Objective and measurable	May be objective and measurable	Not objective or measurable; is an experience related to the responses of others
Illustrations	Spina bifida, spinal cord injury, amputation, and detached retina	Cannot walk unassisted; uses crutches and/or a manual or power wheelchair; blindness	Reflects physical and psychological characteristics of the person, culture, and specific ircumstances
Level of analysis	Micro level (e.g., body organ)	Individual level (e.g., person)	Macro level (e.g., societal)

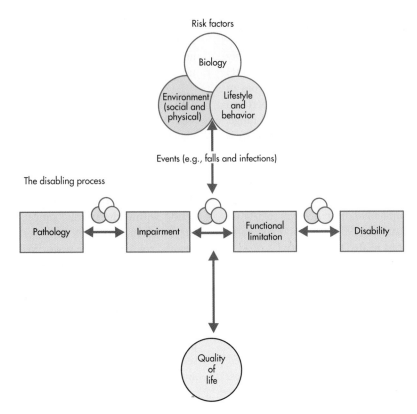

FIGURE 21-1 Model of disability. (Reprinted with permission from Pope AM, Tarlov AR, editors: *Disability in America: toward a national agenda for prevention*, Washington, DC, 1991, Institute of Medicine, National Academy Press. Copyright 1991 by the National Academy of Sciences. Courtesy National Academy Press, Washington, DC.)

remedy health concerns without attending to interacting systems such as knowledge and educational background, personal and family belief systems, religious/spiritual beliefs and supports, finances, social networks, physical resources, and cultural influences.

Clinical Example

Cathy sought an eye examination at an optical center in a local department store where she did much of her shopping. Although the receptionist advised her that no one could see her for several months, she noted that the woman in line behind her received an appointment for the following day. Cathy left the store feeling puzzled and angry. She called several optical offices and advised them that, unless their equipment could accommodate her motorized wheelchair, someone would need to lift her into the examining chair and hold her upright throughout the eye examination. The limitations of the optical equipment required someone to assist Cathy during the examination. After she contacted several potential providers, Cathy finally obtained an appointment.

One optometrist chose to see Cathy when the others failed. Physically disabled himself, the optometrist had a mobility impairment as evidenced by a limp. Although his functional limitations and the extent of his disability were much less severe than Cathy's, he also experienced societal bias and discrimination related to disability. Unfortunately, when people saw Cathy's wheelchair or heard about her potential need for accommodation, their attitudes may have transformed her disability into a handicap.

Four Models for Disability

Disability is a socially constructed issue, and how it is perceived and understood often relates to perspective. Four models for viewing disability are described here:

1. *Medical model*—Disability is a defect in need of cure through medical intervention.
2. *Rehabilitation model*—A defect to be treated by a rehabilitation professional.
3. *Moral model*—Connected with sin and shame.
4. *Disability model*—Socially constructed.

The medical and rehabilitation models would attempt to correct Cathy's disability, whether that was indicated or desirable. The moral model would blame her for having a disability. Cathy had a college "friend" who repeatedly asked what "sin" in her life was unconfessed to God to remain unhealed. The socially constructed disability model recognizes that whether Cathy is perceived as able-bodied or disabled depends on the lenses through which she is viewed and the barriers that promote or prevent her participation to an equal extent with any other person.

Disability: A Socially Constructed Issue

Disability is a complex, multifaceted culturally rich concept that cannot be readily defined, explained, or measured (Mont, 2007). Whether the inability to perform a certain function is seen as disabling depends on socioenvironmental barriers, for example, attitudinal, architectural, sensory, cognitive, and economic, and inadequate support services and other factors (Kaplan, 2009).

Much of the complexity in defining disability stems from its socially constructed nature.... Because disability is more usefully conceptualized as the inability to perform important life functions, it becomes a product of interaction between health status and the demands of one's physical and social environment. Thus, using a wheelchair is disabling in a workplace with steps and narrow doorways, but much less so in one with ramps and wide passageways. Similarly, cultural beliefs and attitudes shape the extent to which an impairment is disabling, and the extent to which people with physical or mental impairments are able to function in jobs and more broadly in public life. (Scotch, 1994, p. 172)

Differentiating Illness from Disability

The nurse must be able to differentiate between the person who has an illness and becomes disabled secondary to the illness, and the person who has a disability but may not need treatment. A disability is not necessarily accompanied by, nor related to, an illness; neither is an illness necessarily accompanied by, nor related to, a disability. Rather than assuming a need for treatment, the nurse should ask whether the client wants assistance, ask the client/family to describe the goal(s), and ask how and in what way(s) the nurse can help.

Hayes and Hannold (2007) wrote:

Although some persons with disabilities have recurrent health complications secondary to disability, the sole assignment of a disability label or diagnosis does not necessarily warrant the need for ongoing medical surveillance. Historically however, disabilities have been equated with sickness, and people with disabilities have been viewed as patients. The medicalization of disability has often relegated people with disabilities into a "sick-role" in which they are exempt from social role obligations and expectations of productivity, and instead, are viewed only as passive recipients of health care resources.

Persons with disabilities often confront "medicalization" issues when others view them in the "sick role" rather than as people first. Nurses who demonstrate understanding of these issues should approach PWD and their families on an eye-to-eye level; listening to understand, collaborating with the person/family, and making plans and goals that meet the other's needs and that draw on strengths and improve weaknesses. This collaboration empowers and affirms the worth and knowledge of the person/family with a disability. This promotes self-determination and allows choices that foster personal values and preferences.

RESEARCH HIGHLIGHTS

Hayes and Hannold (2007) provide a historical perspective on the medicalization of disability. They claim that medicine and health care professionals (HCP) have oppressed persons with disabilities (PWD) through a medical/knowledge power differential, reinforcement of the "sick role," and objectification of PWD. Clients who refused to follow HCP recommendations have been viewed as noncompliant, uncooperative, resistant, and/or deviant. Because PWD seek medical treatment when sickest and most in need of care, HCP form skewed opinions about their capabilities and potential, lacking data for baseline comparison. Appropriately "aggressive" therapies may not be offered, particularly if no one can advocate for the client. The authors state that health care management, wellness, and prevention of further disability should be emphasized, as opposed to treatment that intends to cure or normalize.

From Hayes J, Hannold EM: The road to empowerment: a historical perspective on the medicalization of disability, *J Health Hum Services Admin* Winter 2007: http://findarticles.com/p/articles/mi_m1ylz/is_3_30/ai_n25014454/. Accessed July 3, 2009.

CHARACTERISTICS OF DISABILITY

Whether someone has a disability depends on the criteria used. The Americans with Disabilities Act of 1990 (ADA) and the Rehabilitation Act of 1973 define a disability by the limitations in carrying out a major life activity. Physical disabilities, sensory disabilities (e.g., being deaf or blind), intellectual disabilities (i.e., preferred terminology for mental retardation), serious emotional disturbances, learning disabilities, significant chemical and environmental sensitivities, and health problems such as acquired immunodeficiency syndrome (AIDS) and asthma are examples of disabilities that may substantially limit at least one major life activity. Major life activities include the ability to breathe, walk, see, hear, speak, work, care for oneself, perform manual tasks, and learn. The U.S. Census Bureau (2006) defines *disability* as a long-lasting physical, mental, or emotional condition that creates a limitation or inability to function according to certain criteria.

Measurement of Disability

To monitor changes in socioeconomic conditions for the general population, as well as for special populations, the government administers four household surveys. As definitions for disability change, so must measurement criteria. For example, the Survey of Income and Program Participation (SIPP) includes an extensive set of disability questions that include limitations in functional activities (e.g., seeing, hearing, speaking, walking, using stairs, and lifting and carrying items), activities of daily living (ADLs) (e.g., getting around inside the home, getting in and out of a bed or chair, bathing, dressing, eating, or toileting), and instrumental activities of daily living (IADLs) (e.g., going outside the home, shopping, tracking money or bills, light housecleaning, and preparing meals). It gathers data on whether an individual uses an adaptive mobility device (e.g., wheelchair, cane, crutches, or walker) for 6 or more months; has a mental or emotional disability; has an impairment that produces on-the-job limitations or the inability to perform housework, or that involves the disability status of children (Brault, 2008).

The American Community Survey (ACS), having undergone extensive recent improvement, asks respondents whether they have a disability limitation that affects a certain function or activity, such as sensory perception, physical activities, mental and emotional state, self-care, ability to leave home, and employment options (U.S. Census Bureau, 2009). The Current Population Survey (CPS), while not specifically designed to measure disability, asks questions to determine whether people are less able or unable to work because of a health condition or disability. Limited data relative to disability are collected from the Decennial Census of Population and Housing.

Prevalence of Disability

In 2005, approximately 54.4 million (18.7%) of the 291.1 million civilian noninstitutionalized population aged 5 years and older had a long-lasting condition or disability (Brault, 2008). Of those with a disability, 35 million (12%) had a "severe" disability. Further, it is important for health care policymakers and health care providers to recognize that the prevalence of disability is increasing.

Disability Prevalence by Race and Sex: 2005

U.S. Census Bureau SIPP data, June-September 2005 (Brault, 2008), indicate prevalence differences by race and sex. Blacks (20.5%) had a higher rate of disability when compared with Asians (12.4%) and Hispanics (13.1%), although it was not statistically different from that of non-Hispanic whites (19.7%). Females had a higher disability rate (20.1%) than males (17.3%) across all racial groups. However, higher disability rates in females can be explained by proportionally larger groups of older women as compared with older men.

Selected Measures of Disability

The U.S. Census Bureau collects data related to disability in communications, mental, and physical domains. Wheelchair users (15 years and older) comprised 1% of the population with a disability (Brault, 2008). An additional 3% of the population used a cane, crutches, and/or walker. In comparison, about 8 million people reported hearing and visual disabilities, a rate approximately twice that of wheelchair users. Collectively, more than 16 million people experienced a mental disability as defined by one or more of the following: a learning disability, intellectual disability, cognitive disability (dementia), other mental/emotional condition, and/or difficulty managing money/bills. An emotional disability, experienced by nearly 8.4 million people, included one or more of the following: depression and/or anxiety, interpersonal challenges, concentration difficulties, and/or difficulty coping with stress (Brault, 2008).

Prevalence of Disability in Children

According to the National Center for Health Statistics (U.S. Department of Health and Human Services [USDHHS], 2008) about 21.8% of households with children have at least one child with a special health care need (disabling condition). Children with special health care needs received a broad range of comprehensive health services, including prescription medications (86%), specialty medical care (52%), vision care (33%), mental health care (25%), specialized therapies (23%), and medical equipment (11%). Preventive dental care was an unmet need reported by 16% of parents of these children.

Among school-aged children, almost 13% had a disability as defined by a communication-related difficulty, mental or emotional condition, difficulty with regular schoolwork, difficulty getting along with other children, difficulty walking or running, use of some assistive device, and/or difficulty with ADLs. Further, in this population, 4.4% had what would be termed a severe disability. Not being capable of doing regular schoolwork was the most prevalent disability affecting children (7.0%), and almost 6% had one or more selected developmental conditions. These included a learning disability, 2.8%; mental retardation (intellectual disability), 0.5%; other developmental disability, such as autism or cerebral palsy, 1.0%; and other developmental conditions that required therapy or diagnostic services, 2.9% (Brault, 2008).

Recommendations for the nurse. Community nurses who listen to parental concerns about their children establish what may be the most important bond they will have with a health care provider. Nurses should pay attention, particularly when parents intuitively whisper, "Something is not right." A well-meaning health care provider may attempt to reassure a concerned mother. However, this kind of response may create silence and delay further questions by the parent. Rather than decrease parental concern, it may increase anxiety. The nurse can serve as an intermediary, working among the family and the health care team, to address parental concerns and client goals.

Whether working in a school or an office setting, the nurse should regularly assess for key developmental milestones and compare current status with predicted values. The school-aged child with developmental delays or disabilities should work with a team of resource providers, following an individualized education plan (IEP). If a child is not making progress, a parent has the right to ask for a change in the plan. Parents of children with disabilities frequently complain of fatigue associated with fighting "bureaucracies" tangled in rules that fragment, delay, or make services difficult to obtain. Similarly, parents may feel they are at "war" with schools when parental and organizational goals or plans for the child are in conflict.

Student learning activity. Parents taught their autistic son Tim to use sign language to communicate at home. However, public school staff rejected this communication mode. At age 8 years, Tim was mainstreamed, and, predictably, he was unable to use verbal communication. The child regressed, and his behavior deteriorated. The parents withdrew Tim when the school refused to modify the IEP. They planned to homeschool Tim, even though he required 24-hour-a-day supervision because he lacked safety awareness. Consider the family's need for support. Other members include his father, who works 50 hours a week, and 6-year-old brother Roger who helps mom with Tim (Treloar, 1999b).

Break into small groups, and select one person to play the role of the mom. The highest priority goals should consider what key element? Establish three priority nursing diagnoses based on mom's verbalized concerns and your assessment. Family and community resources should be assessed from a holistic perspective.

Mom's assessment includes the following concerns:

- The family cannot locate a church that will provide supervision for Tim while they attend the worship service. Initially this was not a concern until Tim became too large to be accepted in the church's nursery. This is a significant disappointment to them.
- Mom mentions that she and her husband have not had any time alone in years. She wonders if Roger will be "normal" because he always shares her time with Tim. Although they qualify for State Developmental Disability Respite Services, services are offered only in an institutional setting. The family believes this would upset Tim.
- How can the family provide 24-hour-a-day care for Tim, who is severely disabled with autism, and support the health and well-being of each family member and the family system?

RESEARCH HIGHLIGHTS

Spiritual beliefs and religious practices bring meaning and purpose, emotional and practical support, and friendships with other believers, among other benefits. Families affected by disabilities who find places of worship are inaccessible or unfriendly lose on many levels. A person affected by a disability or another difficult situation can understand the value of believing in God who can provide strength and wisdom to make it through another day, another night. Faith communities must explore the multiple barriers against inclusion, increase disability access, and include PWD as integral to the mission of faith communities as a national public health imperative.

From Cunningham JL, Mulvihill BA, Speck PM: Disability and the church: how wide is your door, *J Christ Nurs* 26:3, 140-147, 2009.

Health Status and Causes of Disability

Chronic health problems are associated with aging and functional disability. Commonly, chronic respiratory conditions, hearing and vision disabilities, stroke, and fractures (both pathological, caused by osteoporosis, and accidental, from falls) increase with aging. Cognitive impairments, such as dementia, are recognized for their disabling potential. Americans in all age groups and cultures who are sedentary and overweight or obese are more likely to have type 2 diabetes develop. The nurse's involvement in health promotion and disease prevention is critical. Regardless of the cause of disability, the nurse must see beyond the disabling impairment, carefully assessing affected persons' perceptions of the disability experience. Ultimately, the personal belief system of the individual and the family and the traditions of the community influence the individual's lived experience with disability and his or her participation in health care.

Aging and Personal Assistance

Disability prevalence and disability severity levels increase with aging. Thus, disability accompanies the "graying" of our elderly population, which is proportionately increasing as the "baby boomer" generation turns 65 years and older. In 2005, half (51.8%) of people aged 65 years and older had a disability, and 36.9% of people 65 years and older had a severe disability (Brault, 2008). The highest incidence of disability (71%) occurred in people 80 years and older; of these, 56% had a severe disability and 29.2% needed personal assistance. Not surprisingly, people in nursing facilities have a disability prevalence of 97.3% and a median age of 83.2 years.

Notably, the need for assistance with one or more ADLs or IADLs increases as severity of disability increases. In 2005, 11 million people needed personal care services (ADLs) and/or light housework assistance (IADLs). Community nurses are ideally qualified to provide care to individuals, families, and community neighborhoods through the use of strategies including evidence-based practice research application, case management, and team leadership.

DISABILITY AND PUBLIC POLICY

Early American public policy viewed people with disabilities as "deserving poor" who required governmental protection and provision, with little capacity for self-support or independence (Rubin and Millard, 1991). Contemporary disability policy minimizes disadvantages and maximizes opportunities for people with disabilities to live productively in their communities. Public policy on disability includes civil rights protections (e.g., Title 504 of the Rehabilitation Act and the ADA), skill enhancement programs (e.g., special education, vocational rehabilitation, Ticket to Work and Work Incentives), and income and in-kind assistance programs (e.g., Social Security Disability Insurance [SSDI], Medicare, and Medicaid). Box 21-1 contains foundational values and ideologies that underlie public policy related to people with disabilities.

Legislation Affecting People with Disabilities

Consistent with historical and social changes and the recognition of barriers and discrimination, key federal legislation supports the rights of people with disabilities. The following section describes a few of the most significant acts.

The Individuals With Disabilities Education Act (IDEA)

The Individuals with Disabilities Education Act (IDEA) (PL 94-142) ensures a free appropriate public education to children with disabilities, based on their needs in the *least restrictive setting* from preschool through secondary education. Addressing special education needs requires appropriate evaluation and transition services. Parents, students, and

BOX 21-1 PUBLIC POLICY VALUES RELATED TO DISABILITY

Equal protection: All deserve equal protection under the law.
Egalitarianism: Regardless of differences in abilities, all people should receive equal treatment through equal opportunities.
Normalization: People with disabilities should be treated like nondisabled people, minimizing differences wherever possible.

professionals join together to develop an IEP that includes measurable special educational goals and related services for the child. See the IDEA website (http://idea.ed.gov/) for additional information.

The Americans with Disabilities Act of 1990 and ADA Amendments Act of 2008

The Americans with Disabilities Act (ADA) (PL 101-336) became law in July 1990. This landmark civil rights legislation prohibits discrimination toward people with disabilities in everyday activities (U.S. Department of Justice, 2009). The ADA guarantees equal opportunities for people with disabilities related to employment, transportation, public accommodations, public services, and telecommunications. It provides protection to people with disabilities similar to those provided to any person on the basis of race, color, sex, national origin, age, and religion. The U.S. Equal Employment Opportunity Commission (EEOC) is charged with enforcement for the employment provisions found in Title I of the ADA.

The ADA refers to a "qualified individual" with a disability as a person with a physical or mental impairment that substantially limits one or more major life activities or bodily functions, a person with a record of such an impairment, or a person who is regarded as having such an impairment. The ADA prohibits discrimination against people who have a known association or relationship with an individual with a disability. A qualified individual with a disability must meet legitimate skill, experience, education, or other requirements of an employment position. The person must be able to perform the essential functions of the job, such as those contained within a job description, with or without reasonable accommodation(s). Qualifying organizations must provide reasonable accommodations unless they can demonstrate that the accommodation will cause significant difficulty or expense, producing an undue hardship.

Over time, judicial decisions eroded the ADA rights of people whose disabilities were intermittent, nonvisible, or manageable with medications, prosthetics, and/or medical equipment. On January 1, 2009, the ADA Amendments Act of 2008 (PL 110-325), a bipartisan bill supported by disability advocates and employers, became effective, making it easier for a person "seeking protection under the ADA to establish that he or she has a disability within the meaning of the ADA" (U.S. Department of Justice, 2009). For additional information, see the ADA website (www.ada.gov/).

The community health nurse should develop a resource network that includes disability resource center specialists, public interest law firms, and legal advocacy groups. High-priority interventions include helping people with disabilities learn about their rights and empowering them to act on their own behalf.

Ticket to Work and Work Incentives Improvement Act

Historically, national public policy has defined disability as the inability to work. Typically, people with disabilities could only qualify for such benefits as health care, income assistance programs, and personal care attendant services if they chose not to work. To address employment and benefit issues for persons with disabilities, in December 1999, the Ticket to Work and Work Incentives Improvement Act (TWWIIA) was signed into law. The TWWIIA reduced PWD's disincentives to work by increasing access to vocational services and provided new methods for retaining health insurance after returning to work. Congressional efforts through the TWWIIA demonstrated evolution of attitudes and interest in PWD's ability to work, potential economic contributions, and decreased reliance on public funds (Ticket to Work and Work Incentives Advisory Panel, 2007).

TICKET TO WORK, SOCIAL SECURITY DISABILITY INSURANCE, AND SUPPLEMENTAL SECURITY INCOME ELIGIBILITY

What is a Ticket?

A Ticket to Work increases a person with a disability's available choices when obtaining employment services, vocational rehabilitation services, and other support services needed to get or keep a job. It is a free and voluntary service. A ticket may be used for its purpose, held for future use, or not used.

Where can a Ticket be used?

The program is available in all fifty states and ten U.S. territories. Many SSDI and Supplemental Security Income (SSI) disability beneficiaries may obtain services from a state vocational rehabilitation (VR) agency or contracted employment network.

Where can I find more information?

Contact the SSA Ticket Program Operations Support Manager, MAXIMUS, at its toll-free numbers: 1-866-YOURTICKET (1-866-968-7842) or for TTY/TDD call 1-866-833-2967 between 8 AM and 10 PM Eastern time (Monday through Friday). Online information can be found at www.ssa.gov/work/aboutticket.html, www.yourtickettowork.com, or www.socialsecurity.gov/work/receiving-benefits.html (Social Security Administration, 2009c).

Clinical Example
The Dilemma of Choosing Employment Versus Health Care and Community Support Assistance

John uses a power wheelchair because he experiences "spastic quadriplegia" from cerebral palsy. John is college educated and chooses not to work. John weighed his options and acknowledged that, if he worked, he would lose the state-supported social service benefits that provide his health care services and attendant caregiver services (Treloar, 1999a).

John, similar to many PWD, remains locked in poverty. John's situation remains the "norm" despite the potential held by the TWWIIA. Complexity of rules, lack of awareness of work incentive provisions, fear of loss of health care and other support systems needed for work, and distrust associated with governmental operational issues are primary reasons the TWWIIA is poorly utilized (Ticket to Work and Work Incentives Advisory Panel, 2007). Change seems certain because Social Security Trust Fund resources will be inadequate to meet the needs of a rapidly aging baby boomer generation.

Public Assistance Programs

Public assistance programs include cash assistance (e.g., SSI, Social Security, and other cash assistance), food stamps, and public/subsidized housing. For people 25 to 64 years of age, participation in public assistance programs increased with severity of disability, consistent with the highest poverty levels. In 2005, 57% of people with a severe disability received public assistance, compared with 16.3% of people with a non-severe disability, whereas only 7.3% of people with no disability received public assistance (Brault, 2008).

TABLE 21-2	INFLUENCE OF DISABILITY ON EMPLOYMENT	
LEVEL OF DISABILITY	PERCENTAGE OF PERSONS AGES 21-64 YEARS WHO ARE EMPLOYED
Any disability	46.6%
Non-severe disability	75.2%
Severe disability	30.7%
No disability	83.5%

From Brault MW: Americans with disabilities: 2005, *Curr Popul Rep* 70-117, 2008, US Census Bureau: www.census.gov/2008pubs/p70-117.pdf. Accessed June 20, 2009.

SUPPLEMENTAL SECURITY INCOME AND SOCIAL SECURITY DISABILITY INSURANCE

The Social Security Administration (2009a) defines *disability* as the "inability to engage in any substantial gainful activity (SGA) because of a medically determinable physical or mental impairment(s) that is expected to result in death, or that has lasted or is expected to last for a continuous period of not less than 12 months." Most people who receive disability benefits qualify based on their personal inability to work because of a disability; however, exceptions include people who are blind or have low vision, benefits for widows or widowers who are disabled, and benefits for children who are disabled.

Differentiating SSI from SSDI The *SSI* program is funded through general tax revenues, whereas the *SSDI* program receives disability trust fund monies (Social Security taxes paid by workers, employers, and self-employed workers). To qualify for *SSI*, the PWD must have limited income and resources; for *SSDI*, the PWD must be "insured" through FICA earnings of self, parents, and/or spouse. *SSI* disability benefits are payable to adults and children who are disabled or blind and are eligible, whereas *SSDI* disability benefits are payable to workers or widow(er)s who are disabled or adults who have been disabled since childhood and are eligible. *SSI* program recipients receive Medicaid health benefits, whereas *SSDI* recipients receive Medicare health benefits. Income varies according to a specific formula depending on whether the PWD receives SSI or SSDI. Some states may elect to pay a state supplement to some PWD in SSI programs, whereas PWD in SSDI programs are never provided with state supplements (Social Security Administration, 2009b).

Information about **Supplemental Security Income (SSI)** and **Social Security Disability Insurance (SSDI)** can be accessed online (www.ssa.gov/disability/) or obtained at a Social Security office.

COSTS ASSOCIATED WITH DISABILITY

People with disabilities continue to lag behind nondisabled Americans in most basic areas of life. These include gaps in employment, income, education, access to transportation, attendance at religious services, and so forth. People with no disability earn the most, are more likely to be employed, and are least likely to live in poverty, whereas people with a severe disability earn the least, are less likely to be employed, and are most likely to live in poverty.

Economic Well-Being and Employment

For people 25 to 64 years of age in 2005, 12% with a non-severe disability and 27.1% with severe disabilities lived in poverty (Brault, 2008). People with no disability were most likely to be employed, and those having a severe disability

were least likely to be employed. Among individuals from 21 to 64 years, only 45.6% of people with a disability and 30.7% with a severe disability were employed (Table 21-2).

Determining the actual number of PWD who are employed or unemployed at any time is challenging at best. Research outcomes vary depending on survey design, population size and characteristics, aims of the study, interpretation of the variables, and so forth. Rates of employment for PWD, compared with nondisabled counterparts, remain at significantly lower levels. What can be done to promote employment opportunities for PWD? Employers willing to hire PWD may receive monies provided through the American Recovery and Reinvestment Act (2009). Although this is a noteworthy effort, consider the impact of the TWWIIA on employment levels described in the section on Public Policy. Little improvement in employment levels has been realized, keeping many PWD in poverty, fearing loss of health care benefits and social supports.

HEALTHY PEOPLE 2020 AND THE HEALTH NEEDS OF PEOPLE WITH DISABILITIES

Persons with disabilities are one of several populations that receive poorer quality health care. The next section describes health disparities and provides application to *Healthy People 2020*.

Health Disparities in Quality and Access

The National Healthcare Disparities Report of 2008 (NHDR) explains that, within the scope of health care delivery, disparities are due to differences in access to care, provider biases, poor provider-patient communication, poor health literacy, and other factors (Agency on Healthcare Research and Quality, 2009). Congress mandated the NHDR to identify differences or gaps where some populations receive poor or worse care than others and to track how the gaps change over time. Because PWD experience a higher rate of chronic illness, pneumococcal vaccination of adults aged 65 years and older is a *Healthy People 2020* objective used as a quality of care monitor. In 2006, only 54.4% of all adults 65 years and older had a pneumococcal vaccination compared with 63.1% of PWD with basic activity limitations. Although PWD were immunized at a significantly higher rate than nondisabled elders, both populations must make significant gains to approach 90% immunization levels desired.

Without appropriate support, PWD and their families are at increased risk for medical, physical, social, emotional, and/or spiritual secondary issues. Goals for relief aim to improve quality and access to care that promotes health and well-being, prevents secondary conditions, and provides support for long-term health conditions. *Healthy People 2010* established goals to eliminate health disparities between people with disabilities and the U.S. population. This work continues in *Healthy People 2020*.

Student Learning Activity

Break into small groups and select one or more of the following learning activities:

A. Can a client who uses a wheelchair obtain mammography for breast cancer screening, or is the lack of adaptive equipment a barrier to her or his participation? What is the availability and cost of accessible transportation to the screening site? Can a woman get onto an exam table for a Pap smear? Although office staff and equipment *should* accommodate people's limitations, how many actually do? Think about the office where you receive health care. Consider the imaging laboratories in the area where you live. Can any of them accommodate someone in a wheelchair? How can you find out?

B. In a physical medicine specialty office where pain management is practiced, several clients who are morbidly obese are unable to sit down on the toilet and hold a cup required to collect a urine drug screen (UDS). Rather than send the patient to an outpatient lab, how can the nurse assist the client to collect the UDS sample on-site?

C. Your client needs an eye exam. Are there any providers with equipment that will allow a client to remain in a wheelchair for an eye exam? If not, how will the eye center handle the accommodation issue? Divide students into small groups, each group representing a different geographic area. Each student will role-play being a client who uses a wheelchair. Go to the appointment desk of an eye center in a retail setting and make an appointment for a future eye exam. Describe your experience. What happened? What did you observe? How did you feel? How did staff respond to your request for accommodation?

People with Intellectual Disabilities: Undervalued and Disadvantaged

Worldwide, unrecognized health care problems frequently are untreated in people with intellectual disabilities (ID) who cannot easily communicate their symptoms and demonstrate varied participation in shared decision-making. Indeed, Walsh (2008) explored health literature to determine how people with ID compared on health measures with the general population and concluded that adults with ID were consistently undervalued and disadvantaged. Socioeconomic disadvantage accounted for a "significant proportion" of variation in health status apart from personal characteristics or other circumstance.

For example, women with ID often experience disparities in primary care services, particularly in women's health issues. Because osteoporosis develops at higher rates in women with ID, recommendations include screening at earlier and more frequent intervals, special gynecological exam techniques, and "thoughtful well-coordinated" care from primary care physicians (Wilkinson and Cerreto, 2008). Further, because the likelihood of accessing special health services increases with both higher family income and insurance coverage, those with special health care needs such as ID often have less access to health services (Porterfield and McBride, 2007). Clients with ID may exhibit behavioral problems that discourage health care providers from caring for them, or they may resist others' attempts to care for them because of their discomfort or unfamiliarity with the health care setting or equipment. Other problems include difficulties in obtaining a client history and in determining the nature and cause of a problem, along with inexperience and inadequate training by health care providers in specific health care problems that accompany ID (Jansen, Krol, and Post, 2004). Health care providers, whether nurse's aide, nurse, therapist, or physician, would benefit from increased education that addresses issues on caring for people with ID.

Health care for people with disabilities must incorporate remedies that address issues surrounding access to health care and the removal of environmental and social barriers that prevent full participation in society. The community health nurse will use a range of support systems that promotes the health of the person with a disability and the health of his or her family. Figure 21-2 illustrates these support systems. The importance of governmental public policies, including disability legislation and financial support, cannot be overemphasized. It is only when the nurse considers a broad approach to disability that he or she can realize the objectives of *Healthy People 2020*, including caring for those who may be undervalued and disadvantaged.

A HISTORICAL CONTEXT FOR DISABILITY

Current models and definitions for disability cannot be understood apart from their historical-sociopolitical context. As cultures changed, and with them images of beauty and value, "exceptional" people have experienced a wide range of treatment. They have been loved as mascots and fascinating freaks. In other cases, people with disabilities have been isolated, ridiculed, and discriminated against, or worse, marked for extermination. The following section explores some of the images and attitudes that surround people with disabilities.

Early Attitudes Toward People with Disabilities

Societal bias toward people with disabilities has ancient roots. Since the beginning of recorded history, people with disabilities were set apart from others and viewed as different or unusual. Carvings on the walls of Egyptian tombs contain pictures of dwarfs and blind or disabled musicians and singers. Early Greek and Roman cultures emphasized bodily and intellectual perfection. Babies who were sick, weak, or born with obvious disabilities were commonly killed or left to die (Barnes, 1996). In Biblical times, people with disabilities were

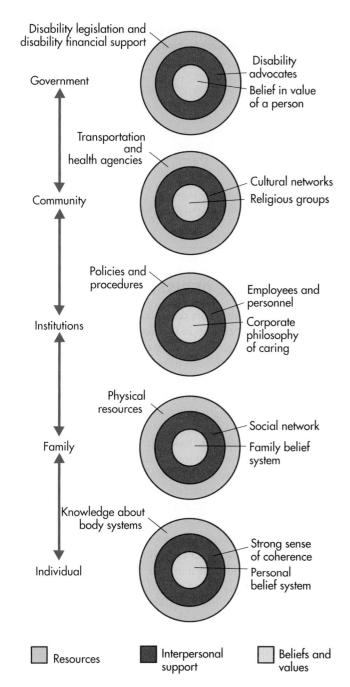

Government — Disability legislation and disability financial support — Disability advocates — Belief in value of a person

Community — Transportation and health agencies — Cultural networks — Religious groups

Institutions — Policies and procedures — Employees and personnel — Corporate philosophy of caring

Family — Physical resources — Social network — Family belief system

Individual — Knowledge about body systems — Strong sense of coherence — Personal belief system

□ Resources ■ Interpersonal support □ Beliefs and values

FIGURE 21-2 Systems of support for people with disabilities.

often viewed as unclean and/or sinful. However, the Jewish culture prohibited infanticide based on sanctity of life beliefs. In European history, people with disabilities sometimes served as entertainers, circus performers, and sideshow exhibitions.

Attitudes Toward People with Disabilities in the Eighteenth and Nineteenth Centuries

In the absence of a scientific model for understanding and treating disability, people saw disability as an irreparable condition caused by supernatural agency (Longmore, 1987). People with disabilities were viewed as sick and helpless, following a "medical model." They were expected to participate in whatever treatment was deemed necessary to cure

or produce a reasonable level of social or vocational performance. Although contemporary perspectives for disability in Western civilizations do not support these ancient views, they persist to varying degrees, depending on culture and world location.

During the nineteenth century, the Industrial Revolution stimulated a societal need for increased education. People who were unable to achieve the equivalent of a contemporary third-grade education (e.g., those with ID) were labeled as "feebleminded" (Pfeiffer, 1993). Soon, the label was applied to people with vision, hearing, speech, and mobility impairments. Schools for people who were deaf and blind were established in the early 1800s. Although these early efforts demonstrated that people with disabilities could be educated and integrated into society, institutionalization and segregation of people with disabilities was the norm.

Disability in the Twentieth Century

Special interest groups for PWD began to develop in the twentieth century. The first federal vocational rehabilitation legislation was passed in the early 1920s and focused on limitations in the amount or type of work that people with disabilities could perform (Longmore, 1987). In the early 1900s, social Darwinism and the Eugenics Movement conducted involuntary sterilization of many people with intellectual disabilities (Pfeiffer, 1993). A few years later, the Association for Retarded Children (Arc) began to advocate for children with intellectual disabilities. Today, the Arc of the United States reportedly is the "world's largest community-based organization of and for people with intellectual and developmental disabilities" (Arc, 2009).

One of the most horrendous tragedies of World War II occurred during Adolf Hitler's euthanasia or "good death" program in which at least 5000 mentally and physically disabled children, birth to age 17 years, were killed by starvation or lethal overdoses. Soon the killing, through use of six gassing installations, extended to adults with mental or physical disabilities who lived in institutional settings. Following widespread public and private protest, especially by the German clergy, Hitler cancelled the adult euthanasia program in late 1941. By that time, he had killed 70,273 adults with disabilities between January 1940 and August 1941. This was in addition to the minimum 5000 children killed over the war years. Killing resumed in August 1942 and continued until the last days of World War II, although in a more concealed manner than previously. An estimated 200,000 people were exterminated through Hitler's euthanasia program since they were "life unworthy of life" (U.S. Holocaust Memorial Museum, 2009).

Stimulated by the deinstitutionalization movement in the 1960s and 1970s, parents' groups and professionals improved institutional care and established community-based Independent Living Centers for PWD. Although some PWD moved into a limited number of community settings, most people with ID and others with severe disabilities remained in institutional settings.

Contemporary Conceptualizations of People with Disabilities

Stereotypical images of people with disabilities and their families remain common in contemporary literature and the media. People with disabilities are seldom presented with a full range of personalities and abilities. However, when the media portrays people with disabilities as fully functioning, integral members of society, the public views this as unusual or unexpected. Although some progress is evident, the population is primarily portrayed as a burden to society, or from pity/pathos or heroic/"supercrip" perspectives (Martiniello, 2009).

Stigmatizing influences shape our perceptions of disability. Murphy (1990), a tenured university anthropologist who became a wheelchair user after he had a spinal tumor, reports the following in *The Body Silent*:

> One cannot…shelve a disability or hide it from the world. A serious disability inundates all other claims to social standing, relegating to secondary status all the attainments of life…it is an identity, a dominant characteristic…just as the paralytic cannot clear his mind of his impairment, society will not let him forget it. (Murphy, 1990, p. 106)

Many parents teach their children not to look at a person who is obviously disabled, which reinforces "deviance disavowal" of disability. A community health nurse describes societal stigma experienced by the families of children with disabilities, which follows:

> It's a huge amount. The teasing in schools. Kids are brutal to normal kids. We try to run some groups on teasing and how to cope with that….Families talk about going to the grocery store and being sick of answering questions or having people stare at the child. I don't know that any of the families really always know how to deal with that. (Treloar, 1999b)

The words and actions of others reveal their regard for people with disabilities. Table 21-3 describes more and less desirable language related to disability. Box 21-2 lists common misconceptions surrounding disability. Finally, Table 21-4 makes recommendations that promote effective interactions between people with and without disabilities.

TABLE 21-3 LANGUAGE USAGE SURROUNDING DISABILITY

LESS DESIRABLE LANGUAGE	MORE DESIRABLE LANGUAGE
Confined to a wheelchair; wheelchair-bound	Uses a wheelchair
Afflicted with or suffers from cerebral palsy	Has cerebral palsy
The blind, the deaf, and the disabled	People who are blind, deaf, or disabled
Mentally handicapped or mentally retarded	People with intellectual disabilities
Handicapped students and normal classmates	Students who are disabled and nondisabled or students with and without disabilities
The spinal-cord injury in room 232	John, in room 232, has a spinal cord injury

BOX 21-2 MISCONCEPTIONS SURROUNDING DISABILITY

- Disability = cannot have fun
- Disability = want to be pitied
- Disability = cannot live in the community
- Disability = menace to society
- Clear voice = clear mind
- You can always tell if someone has a disability by looking at the person.
- All parents want to care for a child with a disability.
- Wheelchair = hard of hearing
- Wheelchair = mentally retarded
- Mentally retarded = cannot learn
- People with disabilities do not know when someone makes fun of them.
- Most disabilities and disabling diseases are contagious.

THE EXPERIENCE OF DISABILITY

Persons with disabilities are commonly thought to constitute the largest minority group in the United States. In fact, most people whose lives do not end abruptly will experience disability. Regardless of the condition associated with disability, many experiences are common to lived experience with disability. However, the personal meaning of disability differs significantly, based on the timeframe and the event or disease process. Table 21-5 compares differences among short-term and long-term conditions characterized by disability.

Those who have a temporary disability, such as a sprained or broken ankle, have a very different experience than those who are permanently disabled. Although they may experience the frustrations of mobility associated with the use of a wheelchair or crutches, they do not enter the world of people with disabilities, because they know they will soon reenter society as able-bodied. They often do not develop the skills of living with a disability, such as walking on crutches expertly, obtaining a disabled parking placard, and learning to perform daily activities with a disability. They view it as a temporary problem and a temporary setback.

In contrast, those who have a permanent disability from an accident or disease process, such as a stroke, must learn to incorporate the modifications required for living into their daily routine and identity. "Their difference from other people is inescapable and can be concealed—if at all—only at formidable cost to their energy and self esteem" (Silvers, Wasserman, and Mahowald, 1998, p. 2). Franklin D. Roosevelt, the nation's thirty-second president, hid his disability from most Americans with the cooperation of the press. He began using a wheelchair at age 21 years after contracting polio, yet only two photographs show him profiled in a wheelchair, rather than from the waist up (Health Media Lab, 2004).

People who become disabled from the progressive decline of a chronic illness may be reluctant to use assistive devices that would make life easier for them. They believe that accepting the device would mean accepting the label of being disabled. Unfortunately, many falls could be prevented by use of a walker or cane that is declined because the person did not want to appear disabled.

TABLE 21-4   DOs AND DON'Ts FOR INTERACTIONS WITH PEOPLE WITH DISABILITIES

DON'T	DO
Assume anything or offer expert advice or assistance based on what you think the person needs or can do	Ask if the person needs help and how to assist; listen and follow his or her instructions; allow him or her to do what he or she can
Ignore or exclude the person	Treat him or her like any other person or friend; approach and include him or her
Be afraid of joking with or offending the person	
Be afraid to ask questions	Recognize that educating others helps remove attitudinal barriers; children who ask are less likely to be afraid of people with disabilities
Focus on differences	See the person as able; accept differences and be patient; seek out similarities and shared interests
Lean on or move the person's wheelchair	Respect a wheelchair as part of the person's personal space; sit or kneel at eye level when communicating with the person
Assume that a person who is blind knows who is speaking or who is present	Inform the person who is present; say good-bye when leaving
Grab the arm of a person who is blind	Let the person take your arm so he or she does not lose balance
Become impatient and complete the speech or the action of the person	Acknowledge that the person has something important to say or do; take time to listen and understand
Repeat loudly what you want to say	Face the person; speak distinctly and slightly more slowly (this is particularly important for the person who lip-reads)
Pet a working dog; there are service dogs for people with physical, hearing, or visual disabilities	Ask for permission to pet the dog; better yet, do not interrupt the dog's work
Assume that the person can participate	Consider possible environmental obstacles (e.g., sensory, architectural, colognes or fragrances for people with chemical sensitivities)
Assume that "bad" parenting explains children's behavior	Recognize that autism and other invisible disabilities influence behavior
Assume that disability and failure to be healed reflects unresolved sin and lack of faith in God	Recognize that humans as holistic beings benefit from interventions that address spiritual meaning for disability

TABLE 21-5   CONCEPTUALIZATION OF CHRONIC HEALTH CONDITIONS

DIMENSION	SHORT-TERM CONDITIONS ACUTE ILLNESS	LONG-TERM CONDITIONS		
		MODEL CASE CHRONIC ILLNESS	RELATED CASE DISABLING CONDITION	CONTRARY CASE LIFE-THREATENING ILLNESS
Cellular	Inflammation	Inflammation; degeneration	Destruction or atrophy	Proliferation
Time	Short	Long	Long	Short or long
Purpose of Rx	Rx to remove problem (i.e., cure)	Rx to alleviate symptoms	Rx to improve functioning	Rx to kill cancer cells (i.e., cure)
Examples of immediate effect of treatment	Severe pain of surgery; immobility	Weight gain of prednisone therapy; dietary restrictions	Discomfort of splinting; pain of retraining muscles	Loss of hair, nausea, and weight loss
Anticipated outcome	Cure expected	Cure not expected	Cure not expected	Cure hoped for or death feared
Trajectory	Short	Exacerbations and remissions; slow progressive decline; shortened life span	Steady	Remission or cure or death
Effect on ADLs	Severe during Rx or none after	Regimen required	Modifications required	Severe during Rx or none during remission or cure
Mental outlook	Temporary problem	Depression or challenge	Stigma or challenge	Fear or hope
Metaphorical interpretation	A temporary setback	Chain binding; a prisoner of uncertainty because body is unreliable	Obstacle to overcome	Sword hanging over head; a sentence

In many progressive diseases, a benchmark event forces the person to accept the label of disabled, for example, a driving accident caused by failing eyesight or mental capacity, a leg amputation from diabetic complications, or a fall when a degenerative disease such as multiple sclerosis impairs mobility and the person's body becomes unreliable. The person can no longer plan daily activities and expect to accomplish them independently. Because chronic illness and disability increase with longevity, many elderly persons experience benchmark disabling changes.

When people with disabling symptoms are unable to return to work, they may lose their jobs and their benefits and exhaust personal resources. They apply for state and federal disability benefits, feeling fully qualified, but are warned to expect to be rejected. They may lose their homes; some will become homeless. Some will adapt to their experience, choosing to live with pain, whereas others will fight their discomfort, expecting relief. Community nurses may find their best tool is use of self and assisting the client through the life-altering experience. Nurses may show they care through listening, presence, and use of holistic and spiritual resources. Finally, nurses may assist clients to connect with personnel at neighborhood centers that provide comprehensive social services.

Family and Caregiver Responses to a Child with a Disability

Those who have limited experience caring for children with disabilities (CWD) may wonder how parents cope with the responsibility. All members of the family are affected. Parents will redefine their image and expectations for the child, and also themselves as individuals, parents, marital partners, and members of a culture and society. Sibling responses to a brother/sister who is disabled may be influenced by such factors as age of sibling, reservoir of coping strategies, strength of peer relationships, perception of parent's burden in caring for the CWD, desire of sibling to protect parents from their concerns about the CWD, and the impact of the CWD on family plans and social activities. The comments of a mother with two children, the youngest one with serious disabilities, illustrate these points (Dwight, 2001):

> My first son, Timmy...had taught my husband, Phil, and me many things....But I don't think I came face to face with the true meaning of motherhood until Aidan entered our lives [p. 18]....As I poured over the books and talked with these other parents, I found the factual side of Down Syndrome fairly easy to piece together....Of course, there was nothing in those reference books that could fully explain the other side of the story—the ups and downs of raising a child with Down Syndrome in our society [pp. 34–35]....In many ways, our lives have been transformed. We have found loving support from people who used to be strangers. We look at the world differently....We have an appreciation for a slower pace....And we have a newfound understanding of the preciousness of all people. (p. 37)

Family Research Outcomes

In the past, research of children with disabilities has emphasized pathology, personal deficits, and impaired family functioning (Cuskelly, 2009). Contemporary research, on the other hand, clearly establishes various benefits, amid challenges in families who care for disabled children. These families' lives resemble those of other families, exhibiting variability comparable with that of the general population with respect to outcomes, including parenting stress, family

function, and marital satisfaction (Ferguson et al., 2000; Ferguson, 2002). Related research describes lived experience marked by joy amid chronic sorrow (Kearney and Griffin, 2001). Families quickly learn that neither governmental social support nor private health plans offer adequate community-based or in-home assistance for disabled family members. Parents with satisfying emotional support by families, friends, and professionals, however, tend to experience fewer potentially negative effects of unplanned or distressing events (Treloar, 2002).

Parents of a child with a disability grieve the loss of the idealized or expected child over time. Whether or not parent(s) anticipated the child's disability, the birth of any child with a disability is a shock, and denial may result. Parents are likely to be sad and may eventually embrace the child, although in some cases, the child will be rejected (more commonly by one parent).

Nurses can help parents and families adjust to disability in a child by establishing a supportive relationship, educating them about the child's condition based on their readiness to learn, and referring them to a case manager for a support group, and for pastoral/spiritual care. Empowering and enabling parent(s) for decision making on behalf of the CWD and establishing a partnership between the parent and health care team are other important strategies.

"Knowledgeable Client" and the "Knowledgeable Nurse"

A person who lives with a disability commonly becomes an expert at knowing what works best for his or her body. This case differs significantly from the person with a new disabling injury or the parent of a CWD who needs information and time to adapt to disability. The Intersystem Model (Artinian, 1997) refers to the first person as the "Knowledgeable Client." In this case, a client has been living with disability for an extended time and has become sensitive to the needs of his or her body. The nurse must ask the client what works best for him or her and what goals the client is pursuing. The client wants the nurse to listen to his or her concerns and may benefit from a referral to health-related resources. However, if the nurse attempts to tell the Knowledgeable Client what to do, the client may become angry and seek help from other sources.

The clients in the second situation need the services of the "Knowledgeable Nurse" (Artinian, 1997). The client with a newly diagnosed condition can benefit from the nurse's information about the disability and the available community and governmental resources. If the nurse is unable to help a client with a new diagnosis learn how to manage the disability and accept himself or herself as disabled, the nurse may compromise the client's adaptation and future client/nurse interactions. Table 21-6 applies this information to the Disability Paradigm.

Active collaboration by client and nurse are required to develop a plan of care that both will find acceptable. Sometimes the nurse must be flexible in his or her expectations. In the

TABLE 21-6 DISABILITY PARADIGM INFLUENCES POLICY AND ACTIONS

DEFINING CHARACTERISTIC	MEDICAL MODEL	SOCIAL CONSTRUCT
Framework or paradigm	Disability as pathology; emphasizes functional limitations; physical limitations are primary source of problems	Disability as expected (i.e., normal); emphasizes minority-group model (i.e., discrimination and oppression) related to social attitudes and other barriers
Focus of concern	Person	Environment
Problem	Personal deficits (e.g., an impairment, lack of a vocational skill, poor adjustment, or lack of motivation)	Environmental barriers (e.g., attitudinal, architectural, sensory, economic, and inadequate social supports)
Person with a disability	Patient in need of professional help	Person is expert, knowledgeable about self, may or may not seek professional assistance
Role of the health professional	Expert and expects advice to be followed	Collaborating partner; mutually negotiated role reflects needs and desires of person and resources of professional
Perspective of discipline	Medicine, nursing, rehabilitation, medical sociology and psychology, special education, and allied health	Disability studies and disability policy
Model for decision making	Hierarchical (i.e., professional on top)	Collaboration for empowerment of person
Plan of care	Professional-centered	Person-centered
Desired outcomes	Reflect professional's goals	Reflect person's goals

final analysis, the client will only accomplish what he or she agrees to accomplish. As one nurse observed,

> *Sensitivity is being able to listen, being able to hear families, being able to respond to where they're at. Not your own agenda, and that's real hard for nurses…what you think you need to do for health care and you really lose track of where the family is.…They may not do it the way we want, but they're experts in their own child's care. (Treloar, 1999b)*

⚖ ETHICAL INSIGHTS

Advances in neonatology are responsible for increasing numbers of very-low-birth-weight babies, at high risk for cognitive disorders and other serious health problems (Reichman, Corman, and Noonan, 2008). Consider the health care implications for caring for the infant and growing child in the home. High-quality primary and specialized, highly technological comprehensive care on a long-term basis will be required. What kinds of community resources will be needed? What anticipated challenges/obstacles may arise in obtaining necessary services? (See National Dissemination Center for Children with Disabilities [NICHCY], www.nichcy.org/Pages/Home.aspx).

As the child grows, early intervention services will be utilized prior to mainstreaming into public education. Consider economic issues, because families having children with disabilities across all income levels are significantly more challenged by food, housing, and health issues.

STRATEGIES FOR THE COMMUNITY HEALTH NURSE IN CARING FOR PEOPLE WITH DISABILITIES

Nurses who partner with people with disabilities and their families provide nursing care using a number of strategies in a variety of community sites. The individual, his or her family, and the community may be the primary client. People affected by disabilities have health care needs and resources common to people without disabilities; others are

unique. Lawthers et al. (2003) identified five major quality of care issues for PWD: underutilization of age-appropriate preventive health care; undertreatment of comorbid health care conditions; inadequate health care provider knowledge of appropriate and effective treatments; barriers to effective communication between client, family, and providers; and risk factors for accidental injury.

The nurse's role should reflect the needs and resources of the client and his or her family. Data from interviews conducted with nurses who provide care to this population and people with physical disabilities illustrate the following guiding principles (Treloar, 1999b):

- *Do not assume anything.* The nurse should collect data from the perspective of the person and family with a disability. A nurse case manager for families with disabled children explains:
  Look at each person, client, family, each situation as a totally new and different one.…There are cultural things that you would want to respect. But, do not assume anything.…listen to what is not said. I watch people.…You go into a home and you can learn a tremendous amount by not even asking any questions.
- *Adopt the client's perspective.* If the nurse operates from his or her agenda or personal cultural norms rather than from those of the client, less productive and satisfactory outcomes will result. More important, the nurse will fail to establish a relationship that respects the client as expert in his or her own health status. Further, what appears to be a barrier or a limitation may not reflect the true situation, or the client's perspective (priorities).
- *Listen and learn from the client. Gather data from the perspective of the client and family.* If the client has severe mental disabilities and cannot offer reliable information, ask the family or caregiver. Nurses must establish relationships that are responsive to the person's methods

and the family's methods for dealing with disability. An experienced nurse, who explained that she does not consider herself the expert, stated:

That parent or caretaker is the one that is there for that child all the time. They know that child far better. I may know something medical that they do not know....That is where you get down to sharing those kinds of things. Teach me. I am always there to learn.

- *Care for the client and the family, not the disability.* The style and intent of client and provider communication influences the acceptability of the interaction. A "conversational" style that establishes an equal partnership with the client is preferable to an "open up the textbook" approach that tells the client "here is what you need to do." The nurse should ask what the client needs help with, what the client is capable of doing, what the client would like to do, and how he or she can help. A community health nurse illustrates these ideas in working with families of children with disabilities:

Are they able to develop a health care plan of their own for their child? This, again, may not be ours [plan]. Are they able to follow through on the important pieces of health care for their child, or at least identify that they don't have the resources to do that?...At times we make families feel that if they don't follow our plan, then they're bad parents.

- *Be well informed about community resources.* Learning about resources by reading a community manual is less helpful than meeting with the staff and agencies in person. People often respond differently to requests by someone they know and respect; therefore, it may be beneficial for the community health nurse to contact agency personnel about a client and family need. Lawthers and colleagues (2003) describe care coordination as the "lubricant" that facilitates links for all areas of quality for a person with a disability and provides the most significant opportunity for improvement in care delivery by multidisciplinary health care providers.

- *Become a powerful advocate.* The community health nurse's advocacy for the person affected by a disability extends beyond a resource and referral coordinator role or speaking on the other's behalf. People with disabilities want to speak for themselves. They want to be in control of their lives and their health care. One person with a disability stated:

They [health care providers who act in an advocacy role] provide the information, but they leave the choice up to the person. And then even if the person chooses against what has been suggested, they still provide the same support.

The community health nurse's perspective on disability will influence the nursing role and the level of care he or she provides to people with disabilities and their families. A variety of systems, ranging from government, community, institutions, family, to the individual (see Figure 21-2), influence the experience of living with a disability. Whether the nurse chooses to work in a setting that specializes in health care services for people affected by disabilities, disability is a common experience that all practicing nurses will encounter.

ETHICAL ISSUES FOR PEOPLE AFFECTED BY DISABILITIES

People with disabilities and their families are concerned about the same contemporary ethical and legal issues that concern nondisabled people. However, some of the associated issues carry particular interest for people with disabilities and their families, including questions and problems surrounding definitions of personhood, respect for human beings, and the rights of people with disabilities.

Associated issues include choosing between abortion and continuing the pregnancy when prenatal screening suggests the presence of impairments and health problems and determining appropriate medical care for infants, children, and adults with disabilities. In 2009, parents filed a $14 million malpractice suit when prenatal testing failed to correctly diagnose Down syndrome. They stated that an accurate test would have led them to end the pregnancy, and, although the child is a "dear," they fear public perception of them as "heartless" for their actions (Green, 2009). The Prenatally and Postnatally Diagnosed Awareness Act of 2008 (PL 110-374) uses federal resources to produce and distribute information about prenatally and postnatally diagnosed conditions (Dresser, 2009). Because health care professionals may convey negative attitudes about life with a disability, accurate and balanced information must be provided. The bill received wide support for its emphasis on information disclosure.

People's spiritual perspectives play an important role in decision making when there is a change in health status or life-threatening illness. People who establish hope and meaning in their lives may choose to positively reframe the difficulties associated with functional limitations that others may find intolerable. Holistic caregiving requires the nurse to assess and promote spiritual health, along with physical and psychological well-being as illustrated in Box 21-3.

Differences in quality of life and justice perspectives intersect with concerns about the control of health care costs. For example, people with disabilities and their families may be concerned with how many and what kind of health care services they should be entitled to receive; whether or not these expenditures should be capped; and, if so, under what criteria. Many people with lifelong disabilities establish a "disability identity" in their adaptation to their limitations and may desire (costly) life-sustaining treatment. In contrast, people who are either newly disabled or nondisabled may see future life as a disabled person as so burdensome that they may refuse extraordinary medical treatments and/or actively seek to end their lives (Hahn and Belt, 2004).

Newer genetic technologies offer hope for the prevention and cure of disease. However, people with disabilities caution that these scientific advances could be used to eliminate people with disabilities. Advocacy groups, such as Not Dead Yet, have taken a strong stance against physician-assisted suicide,

BOX 21-3   SPIRITUAL ISSUES AND DISABILITY

Assessment: Theresa is a 29-year-old, single, separated mother of two children, an 8-year-old daughter and a 5-year-old son. Her husband left her shortly after the premature birth of Joseph. He has cerebral palsy with serious intellectual and physical disabilities. In the months and early years following Joseph's birth, Theresa experienced an intense and prolonged questioning of God. Theresa remarks:

> In the beginning, I used to ask Him, "Why me?" I was upset. I had little hope, little faith, but I stuck to it. I knew it was going to get better, I just didn't know when....It's been tough for me as a single parent. What I've been through has made me stronger. Now I thank God for my boy. But when he was born, I thought God was punishing me....I didn't understand how God could give me a problem like this, when I had so many problems to begin with. (Treloar, 1999a, p. 111)

Nursing Diagnosis: Spiritual distress related to establishing meaning for disability as manifested by repeated questioning and blaming of God

Commentary: Disability is an unexpected event, often with what feel like tragic consequences. While disability may not be easy to adapt to, declining capabilities more commonly occur with aging and chronic illness. However, we do not expect disability to strike in the prime of our lives, or with the birth of a new child.

Regardless of our religious perspectives, we are all spiritual beings who seek meaning for the events that occur in our lives. Even people with established spiritual beliefs may question their relationship with God. Community health nurses who are comfortable with their own spirituality should assess for spiritual needs and provide appropriate spiritual care for people affected by disabilities. In talking directly with the person or family about these needs, the nurse does not push his or her version of spiritual beliefs. The nurse creates a climate that invites people to incorporate religious rituals, connect with clergy, and address spiritual needs according to their preferences. However, when people's spiritual needs are unrecognized and unmet, spiritual distress may linger, causing disruption in other parts of their lives.

---

fearing it will lead to the early or forced death of people with disabilities. Parents who seek cochlear implants for their deaf children often encounter opposition by deaf advocacy groups. These groups argue that people should accept deafness because deafness benefits the client through deaf culture and additional skills, such as sign language. Similarly, the use of methylphenidate (Ritalin) and other stimulant medications for children or adults with attention deficit hyperactivity disorder carries pro and con arguments that include ethical considerations.

People with disabilities who need assistance with ADLs and IADLs commonly find that social welfare programs have limited funding for community-based living, finding it less expensive to place PWDs in long-term care settings. According to Hahn and Belt (2004), the disability rights movement was started by the students who refused to live in nursing homes.

Like any ethical problem, issues related to disability do not have easy solutions. However, societal attitudes and bias toward people with disabilities may negatively influence policies and decisions related to the interests and fair treatment of PWD. Disability rights proponents recognize that the devaluation of PWD may promote their unnecessary and untimely deaths. In 2009, plans for health care reform heightened their concerns, knowing they may be viewed as "life unworthy of life" or "burdens upon society" (Ne'eman, 2009). Ethical decision making cannot be separated from discussions that include the meaning associated with life and life's accompanying challenges. The case of Terri Schaivo described in the Ethical Insights box illustrates some of these issues.

⚖ ETHICAL INSIGHTS

When Is Life Worth Continuing?

The world watched while Terri Schaivo's situation unfolded amid numerous legal and legislative challenges surrounding whether her feeding tube should be discontinued, and conflict developed between her parents and her husband and guardian, Michael. Disability rights groups and right-to-life advocates kept vigil for weeks outside the nursing home where Terri resided. Terri, a 41-year-old brain-damaged woman, died on March 31, 2005, 7 years after experiencing an anoxic event that led to her condition. Although previous court decisions have clearly established a person's right to discontinuation of treatment, including the provision of food and fluids, there was no documentation or advanced directive indicating Terri's wishes. Terri's parents offered to assume guardianship of their daughter, believing her to be both responsive to her environment and desiring life in her current condition. Michael fought to have her feeding tube removed, stating that in previous discussions Terri said that, in a similar situation, she would not want to continue living. Medical discussions focused on the extent of her "vegetative state" and capacity to respond to her environment. Seven years later, amid numerous court challenges and Michael's obtaining a reported million-dollar-plus malpractice settlement designated for his wife's care, the court ordered that Terri's feeding tube and all hydration be stopped as requested by her husband. She died several days later.

What do you think? When is life meaningless? What are the relevant issues when families are in conflict about what medical treatment the person with a severe disability would want in the absence of written advanced directives? What values and ethical principles should be considered? Williams (2005), a physician, suggests that a key question to be considered is "How should we have looked at Terri? Was she a person (or nonperson) in a persistent vegetative state, perhaps with diminished rights, or was she a severely handicapped person with rights that were not considered fairly?" When medical care is futile (i.e., useless or burdensome), it *should* be stopped; however, what guides our practice when treatment, such as artificial nutrition through a feeding tube, is withdrawn because a life is seen to have no value or care of that person is excessively burdensome?

Many hoped that the Patient Self-Determination Act of 1990 would motivate people to prepare advance directives for decision making in life-threatening illness. However, many people do not consider these issues, leaving families as surrogates to decide what the individual would want. Hopefully Terri's case, which polarized the nation on what should be done in her situation, may stimulate people to think through, discuss with loved ones, and complete advance directives that are communicated to a health care provider.

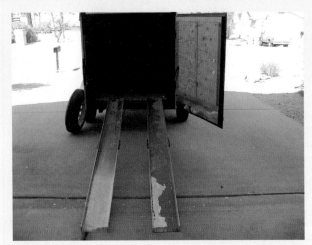

Creative wheelchair transport. People with disabilities and their families become experts at adapting to their environment. The author's husband, Bob, built these folding ramps for use with daughter Joy's wheelchair. Unfortunately, many families lack easy access to a vehicle equipped with a wheelchair lift, or accessible public transportation. This affects their ability to obtain health care, to accomplish instrumental activities of daily living, and to compete with others on an equal level.

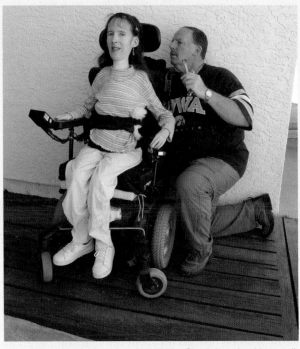

Father Bob adjusting Joy's wheelchair. Obtaining durable medical equipment that fits properly and meets a disabled person's specific needs often challenges therapist and client alike. Commonly, families with disabled members learn to modify and repair wheelchairs and other adaptive equipment. This illustrates another aspect in which family and client become experts in the care of the person with a disability.

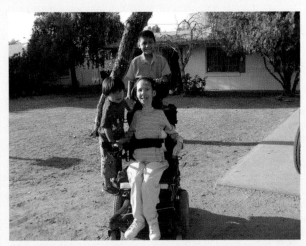

I want a ride, too! Joy rents a home that she shares with her caregiver family. The Hispanic couple's children began riding on Joy's lap in a carrier harness when they were babies. As young children, they delight in climbing onto Joy's wheelchair and helping her shop for groceries at the corner fruit and vegetable market. Joy comments: "When children see me they ask questions out of curiosity, while adults practice avoidance." Joy comments further: "Being in a wheelchair is one part of me—it doesn't define who I am. After a while, people don't see my wheelchair."

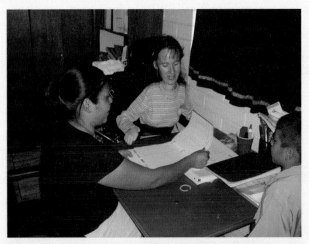

Preparing teacher lesson plans. Joy teaches underprivileged students in an inner-city grade school. As a college student, she faced bias by education faculty who questioned the appropriateness of her dream to be a teacher. Admittedly, they lacked experience in working with a teacher or student with a disability. A few advocated for her, and she persevered and fulfilled her career goal. Despite the ADA, discrimination and misunderstanding continue to influence the lives of people with disabilities, stimulating some to fight, while others give up.

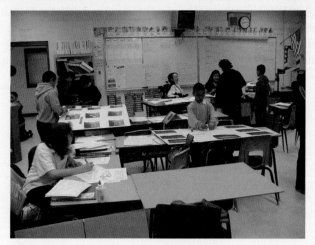

Science fair preparations.

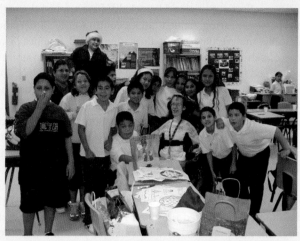

Teacher Joy and her class. Joy's students like the fact that they are at her eye level (although some tower over her). Students quickly learn to actively help their teacher and one another. Joy uses a variety of resources to teach concepts that may be challenging because of her physical limitations. This includes the use of volunteers like Joy's dad (Bob) who assist students with science experiments.

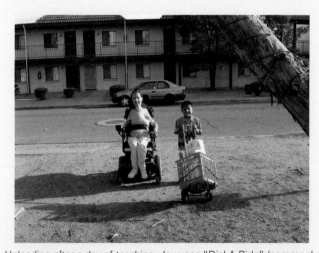

Unloading after a day of teaching. Joy uses "Dial-A-Ride" (commonly described as "Dial-A-Wait") to travel to and from her job and to run errands. Local bus service is another option, but can be problematic due to bus route scheduling, broken-down lifts, and sometimes surly bus drivers.

Photos taken by Dr. Linda Treloar, of her family.

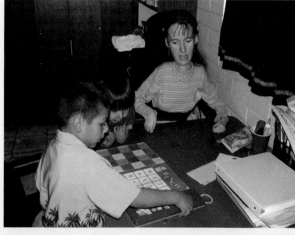

Wieners go with everything, even bingo! Joy lives in a multicultural world where Spanish is the dominant language spoken by people in her home and at school. Joy contributes to and benefits from being part of two families—that of her parents (the author) and her Hispanic caregiver family. Nurses with a community focus recognize and support human networks that encourage and move one another toward well-being.

When the Nurse Has a Disability

Under the ADA, nursing education programs and employers must provide reasonable accommodations for qualified students and nurses, unless this would present an undue burden or hardship on the institution or employer as established by law. A qualified student or nurse must be able to meet the requirements of the clinical experience or job with reasonable accommodations, removal of barriers, and provision of appropriate aids (e.g., amplified stethoscope for someone with a hearing impairment) and services (e.g., scribe or translator). Institutions are not expected to lower their standards for an unqualified student or nurse.

Because "technical" aspects of nursing practice (e.g., bed making) tend to discriminate against nurses with physical or sensory disabilities, nursing should emphasize its "humanistic" capacities (Carroll, 2004). The art and science of nursing practice reflect a specialized knowledge base applied through interpersonal caring. Skilled nurses continuously gather and critically analyze data about their clients and families. The type of setting influences whether a nurse with a disability is qualified to perform the essential functions of the job. For example, a nurse with serious physical disabilities may be qualified to practice nursing when providing telephone triage. However, the same nurse may be unqualified to practice nursing in a medical-surgical setting or emergency department, where physical lifting and similar movements are essential functions of the job.

Although concerns about client safety and competing rights (individual vs. societal) must be considered, people with disabilities are excluded too often from nursing educational programs and practice, based on what the person cannot do, rather than how or where access could be created to practice

nursing. Nurses must consider how personal attitudes toward people with disabilities influence not only their client care but also their responses to nursing students and colleagues with disabilities. Sowers and Smith (2004) surveyed eighty-eight nursing faculty members in eight programs on their perceptions, knowledge, and concerns regarding nursing students with disabilities. They write:

> Perhaps the most positive and hopeful finding of this study was that respondents recognized that they needed to learn more about disability issues and how to teach and accommodate students with disabilities....There is still a desperate need for faculty training, not only about the law, but also about the ability of people with disabilities to successfully complete nursing school and to be practicing nurses, as well as about the strategies that are effective in making this a reality for them. (p. 218)

CASE STUDY   APPLICATION OF THE NURSING PROCESS

Assessment

The narrative report on lived experience in an acute care setting provides community-based nurses with rich material for application as a case study.

Situation: Joy from the Photo Novella on pp. 421-422 is 33 years old. Joy went to her primary care physician (PCP) on June 30, 2008, who sent her for a swallowing test when she experienced progressive swallowing difficulties. She shares her story:

> I already knew the diagnosis. I'd had the beginning of symptoms since October of 2007. The swallowing test on July 2 confirmed the epiglottis no longer functioned and advised me to be NPO. There was no surgeon appointment for a week, so the PCP recommended I go to the ER the evening of July 4 and faxed the records for a feeding tube to be placed that evening.
>
> Upon reaching the ER, the doctor chose to give me IV sedation for the PEG tube placement, but I stopped breathing. After that my heart stopped as well. They resuscitated me. They tried to put a tube down my mouth for the ventilator, but couldn't, so they did a tracheotomy. I went into a coma. They told Cristofer (my caregiver) to go home; that I wouldn't wake up. The doctors did not give any hope, but Cristofer came back to the house and spent the night praying for me. He called my mom the next morning. When I came out of the coma the following day, I was swollen all over with fluid. Cristofer provided me with the details of what was happening and communicated my wishes with the staff. His priority was to honor my wishes and support me completely in all ways. I was in the ICU for 1 week, and then transferred to a smaller hospital where I began the process of weaning off the ventilator.
>
> A week later they attempted with twilight anesthesia to put the tube down my throat in order to place the PEG tube, but they were unsuccessful. A week later, they placed a J tube through radiology without anesthesia. I didn't want to be put asleep which was against their recommendations, but I didn't want the risk of my lungs or heart stopping even though I was on a ventilator. So I signed a consent

with a stipulation that I was not to be under anesthesia. [Q: How bad was the pain?] Horrible, like nothing you can imagine, but better than the risk. They tried to give me pain medication or things to relax me but I refused. I choose to live without medication, with the constant support of my caregivers and their creativity in making me comfortable and content.

> Now a balance had to be found for the continuous feed formula used in the feeding tube. I am allergic to milk and milk products, so special food had to be ordered. Despite signs and reports to avoid milk in my formula, a mistake was made causing continual abdominal pain and nausea. We looked at the formula can in the trash and discovered the cause. It contained milk products. On another occasion, a change was made in the formula, increasing the fat content from 3% to 35% so that my body could more effectively store and use proteins and amino acids due to my lack of muscle tissue. However, my body could not digest this level of fat, and this again resulted in abdominal pain and nausea. Hospital staff did not realize this was the cause of my reaction. I refused the new formula and asked for the old formula, suspecting this was the cause. It was. However, I could not stay on 3% fat without long-term damage to my liver and pancreas. So, my dad and I made a simple plan to mix the formulas. The dietary staff wanted the plan to use only the 35% fat formula in the future, but I have chosen to stay on the 50%/50% of each formula for a 17% daily fat intake. My weight remains stable on that formula.

> My only means of communication was by someone reading my lips or speaking with an alphabet board. Cristofer made an alphabet board on paper when I was in ICU so that I could communicate my wants and needs. Within a matter of days, he learned to read my lips, allowing us to communicate for a couple of hours at a time. This allowed me to express myself beyond just my basic physical needs. Each evening I moved from the hospital bed to a recliner chair brought from my home, which allowed me to change positions and be more comfortable for a time. This was possible due to my caregiver being with me every night

Continued

and moving me. With support and encouragement, God provided people in my life to give me the strength for each step in my recovery.

I weaned off the ventilator in about 6 weeks, despite medical beliefs that it was not possible due to poor lung function. I liked my pulmonologist. He was willing to look outside the box and consider how my body reacted and trust my instincts and my knowledge about my own body.

When in the hospital, even after weaning off the ventilator, I was unable to speak audibly. I was given a Passy-Muir Valve, but was unable to tolerate it without choking in order to speak. About 6 weeks after coming home, I was able to use the valve for a few hours at a time. Gradually, I increased the time of usage.

After 2 months in the hospital, I went home using a feeding tube, 2 L oxygen, and a custom Jackson trach, which had to be cut and shaped to fit in my trachea. When I left the hospital, the recommendation was a nursing home but I did not consider that as an option. I was going home and had live-in caregivers responsible for my care. Equipment and supplies were delivered and my room was set up with all the things I would use. My caregiver family took responsibility for my 24-hour care, always having someone with me.

Two months after arriving home, I stopped using oxygen and the humidified air. I have always struggled with breathing when it is humid. Despite warning [from medical personnel] that humidity is necessary for the trach, I discontinued its use because it stimulated the overproduction of secretions and required continual suctioning due to choking. Shortly after, my need for suctioning decreased to a few times a week. I made this decision, as all others, with the support of my caregivers, without doctor consent.

Although I am unable to return to teaching classes in person, I am still able to provide knowledge and experience to others through the computer and Internet. This provides distraction for me and a sense of normalcy. People in my community assist me with these activities, while others share the responsibility of my 24-hour care.

Author's note: The author assumed the role of community-based nurse in assisting Joy to write her plan of care.

Diagnosis
Individual
- Lifestyle adaptation required related to inability to resume role responsibilities
- Impaired verbal communication related to weakened respiratory muscles (speaking requires expiring adequate air through Passy-Muir Valve over trach)
- Readiness for enhanced comfort related to thin body habitus, immobility, and bed rest
- Risk for ineffective airway clearance related to collection of secretions in trach
- Risk for imbalanced nutrition: less than body requirements related to formula mixture and/or feeding tube

Caregiver Family
- Risk for caregiver role strain related to 24-hour care of Joy

Community
- Effective community therapeutic regimen related to history of support

Planning
Joy considers the recommendations of health care providers; alters care based on knowledge of what works best for her with the support of caregivers.

Individual
Long-Term Goals
- Joy will verbalize acceptable adaptation to limitations related to immobility, trach, and feeding tube as indicated by, "I am still able to provide knowledge and experience to others."
- Joy will report ability to verbally communicate 3 hours at a time related to trach as indicated by increasing ease and time of use for Passy-Muir [speaking] Valve over trach.
- Joy will verbalize an acceptable level of comfort related to thin body habitus, immobility, and bed rest.
- Improved airway clearance related to trach as indicated by reduced collection of secretions and frequency of suctioning.
- Nutritional status, balanced related to feeding tube as indicated by maintenance of weight and absence of GI upset.

Short-Term Goals
- Joy will resume limited activities (e.g., educational) of 1–2 hours as tolerated within 6 weeks after hospital discharge.
- Joy will report an additional 15 minutes of verbal communication per week using the trach speaking valve until able to tolerate periods of 3 hours.

Caregiver Family
Long-Term Goal
- Effective family therapeutic regimen related to caring for Joy and family unit as indicated by harmonious, collaborative relationship with clear roles, intact boundaries, etc.

Short-Term Goals
- Caregivers and Joy make collaborative decisions based on needs of Joy, caregivers on ongoing basis.
- Caregivers and Joy verbalize mutual benefits of their relationship within 1 month.

Community
Long-Term Goal
- Joy's neighborhood community will provide caregivers and assistance as needed.

Short-Term Goal
- Caregivers, in collaboration with Joy, will educate other caregivers, as needed.

Intervention and Evaluation
Individual
- *Intervention:* Within 6 weeks following hospital discharge, Joy reduced the feeding tube rate from 55 mL/hr to 40 mL/hr due to abdominal discomfort.
- *Evaluation:* She reports feeling "less overfull," but not hungry.
- *Intervention:* Within 6 weeks following hospital discharge, Joy discontinued use of Prevacid (for reflux) after it repeatedly plugged the feeding tube.
- *Evaluation:* Joy no longer experiences acid reflux with the lower feeding tube rate.
- *Evaluation:* One year after being home, Joy's trach typically requires weekly suctioning unless there is increased humidity.
- *Intervention:* Joy comments, "On most weekends, one of my caregivers carries me from my bed to a recliner in the living room so that I can be in a different position and setting. The equipment is moved as well."

CASE STUDY   APPLICATION OF THE NURSING PROCESS—cont'd

- *Evaluation:* This promotes Joy's personal well-being and provides additional comfort and normalcy. "My care is based on my needs and my schedule, rather than on a predetermined generic plan. One size does *not* fit all."

Caregiver Family
- *Intervention:* Cristofer learned suctioning and trach care in the hospital and taught other caregivers.
- *Evaluation:* Joy and caregivers adapted her care to meet her needs.

Community
- Joy budgets and directs the use of her disability benefits to provide for self (e.g., includes household rent and expenses) and pay caregivers.

Levels of Prevention
Primary

Prevention of choking and potential aspiration through 24 hr/day caregivers and oral suctioning as needed (primary level modified based on situation).

Secondary

Inspect skin and change position no less than every 2 hours to prevent skin breakdown secondary to immobility.

Tertiary

Caregivers' priority is to maintain Joy as head of household, providing information required for fully informed decisions.

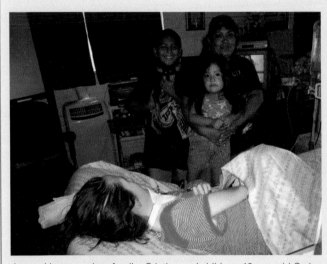

Joy and her caregiver family: Cristina and children, 10-year-old Carlos holding Paco, and 2½-year-old Alejandra.

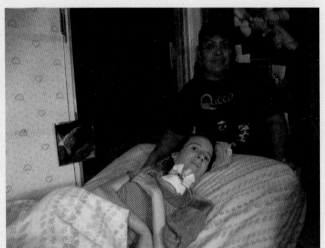

Joy and caregiver Cristina.

Photos taken by Dr. Linda Treloar.

SUMMARY

Community health nurses must recognize that there are a variety of personal and societal perspectives on disability with accompanying moral or ethical issues. They should practice holistic nursing care that incorporates mind, body, and spiritual care considerations into health care practice. To this end, nurses can do the following:

- Become familiar with a variety of ethical frameworks for decision making, and learn a strategy to analyze ethical problems related to health care for people with disabilities.
- Help the client and family access needed information from the health care team to make informed decisions that reflect their interests and priorities.
- Help educate the public on health care issues within the nurse's scope of practice and knowledge and skill level.
- Participate in the development of institutional policies and procedures for ethical and legal issues related to disability.
- Take a position on an ethical issue with political implications.
- Work to influence governmental policies and laws related to disability.

LEARNING ACTIVITIES

1. Interview a person with a disability or his or her family member about their experiences with health care providers and the health care system.
2. Shadow a nurse in a community health clinic that serves children with disabilities. Observe the roles and the interactions of the multidisciplinary team members. Follow a family through clinic. If possible, meet the family at their home before clinic and observe their preparations before coming to clinic. Accompany them from clinic check-in to departure. After returning to their home, ask them for their thoughts on the clinic experience.
3. Interview a community resident with a serious disability. How does the resident view himself or herself? What challenges or concerns does the resident mention? Interview a caregiver about the caregiving experience.
4. Ask an experienced nurse about his or her encounters with people with disabilities. Listen to his or her language and perceptions of disability. Compare these with the perspectives reflected in the social construct model for disability.

5. Visit with the residents and staff in a community-based living environment for people with disabilities. Assist with caregiving for the residents.
6. Visit one or two community agencies that provide services to people with disabilities. How do families gain access to services and what services are offered? How do available services and resources address the needs of a person with a disability and his or her family?
7. Spend time in the home of a family who has a child with intellectual disabilities. Note the family relationships. Interview the parents and siblings about their experiences with the child. Spend time with the child.

REFERENCES

Agency on Healthcare Research and Quality: National healthcare disparities report 2008: http://www.ahrq.gov. Accessed June 29, 2009.

American Recovery and Reinvestment Act of 2009: *Enable America, economic stimulus bill benefits PWD,* www.disabled-world.com/disability/employment/usa/stimulus-bill.php. Accessed July 3, 2009.

Arc of the United States: *The first 50 years,* 2009. www.thearc.org/NetCommunity/Page.aspx?pid=269. Accessed August 5, 2009.

Artinian BM: Overview of the Intersystem Model. In Artinian BM, Conger M, editors: *The Intersystem Model: integrating theory and practice,* Thousand Oaks, CA, 1997, Sage.

Barnes C: Theories of disability and the origins of the oppression of disabled people in Western society. In Barton L, editor: *Disability and society: emerging issues and insights,* New York, 1996, Longman.

Batavia AI: Relating disability policy to broader public policy: understanding the concept of "handicap," *Policy Stud J* 21(4):735–739, 1993.

Brault MW: Americans with disabilities: 2005, *Curr Popul Rep* 70–117, December 2008, US Census Bureau www.census.gov/2008pubs/p70-117.pdf. Accessed June 20, 2009.

Carroll SM: Inclusion of people with physical disabilities in nursing education, *J Nurs Educ* 43(5):207–212, 2004.

Cuskelly M: Challenging the myths and redressing the missteps in family research, *Journal of Policy Practice in International Disabilities* 6(2):86–88, 2009.

Dresser R: Prenatal testing and disability: a truce in the culture wars? *Hastings Cent Rep* 39(3):7–8, 2009.

Dwight V: Aidan's gift. In Klein SD, Schive K, editors: *You will dream new dreams: inspiring personal stories by parents of children with disabilities,* New York, 2001, Kensington, pp 31–37.

Ferguson PM: Mapping the family: disability studies and the exploration of parental response to disability. In Albrecht GL, Seelman KD, Bury M, editors: *Handbook of disability studies,* Thousand Oaks, CA, 2002, Sage, pp 373–395.

Ferguson PM, Gartner A, Lipsky DK: The experience of disability in families: a synthesis of research and parent narratives. In Parens E, Asch A, editors: *Prenatal testing and disability rights,* Washington, DC, 2000, Georgetown University Press, pp 72–94.

Green A: Prenatal testing goes to court, OregonLive.Com June 14, 2009: www.oregonlive.com/news/oregonian/index.ssf?/base/news/1244872511325030.xml&coll=7&thispage=3. Accessed June 18, 2009.

Hahn H, Belt TL: Disability identity and attitudes toward cure in a sample of disabled activists, *J Health Soc Behav* 45:453–464, 2004.

Hayes J, Hannold EM: The road to empowerment: a historical perspective on the medicalization of disability, *J Health Hum Serv Adm.* http://findarticles.com/p/articles/mi_m1YLZ/is_3_30/ai_n25014454/. Accessed July 3, 2009.

Health Media Lab: Franklin Delano Roosevelt (1933–1945), the dying president, 2004. www.healthmedialab.com/html/president/roosevelt.html. Accessed August 16, 2009.

Jansen DE, Krol B, Post D: People with intellectual disability and their health problems: a review of comparative studies, *J Intellect Disabil Res* 48(Pt 2):93–102, 2004.

Kaplan D: The definition of disability, The Center for an Accessible Society, www.accessiblesociety.org/topics/demographics-identity/dkaplanpaper.htm. Accessed June 19, 2009

Kearney PM, Griffin T: Between joy and sorrow: being a parent of a child with developmental disability, *J Adv Nurs* 34:582–592, 2001.

Lawthers AG, Pransky GS, Peterson LE, et al: Rethinking quality in the context of persons with disability, *Int J Qual Health Care* 15(4):287–299, 2003.

Longmore PK: Uncovering the hidden history of people with disabilities, *Rev Am Hist* 15(3):355–364, 1987.

Martiniello N: Disability in the media [see chapters 6–8], 2009, www.trinimex.ca/disabilityinmedia/lesson8.htm. Accessed August 22, 2009.

Mont D: Measuring health and disability, *Lancet* 369:1658–1663, 2007.

Murphy RF: *The body silent,* New York, 1990, Henry Holt.

National Dissemination Center for Children with Disabilities: Home page: www.nichcy.org/Pages/Home.aspx. Accessed August 12, 2009.

Ne'eman A: Health care reform and the disability community, The Huffington Post May 21, 2009. www.huffingtonpost.com/ari-neeman/health-care-reform-and-th_b_206492.html. Accessed August 26, 2009.

Pfeiffer D: Overview of the disability movement: history, legislative record, and political implications, *Policy Stud J* 21(4):724–734, 1993.

Pope AM, Tarlov AR, editors: *Disability in America: toward a national agenda for prevention,* Washington, DC, 1991, Institute of Medicine, National Academy Press.

Porterfield SL, McBride T: Effect of poverty and caregiver education on perceived need and access to health services among children with special healthcare needs, *Am J Public Health* 97(2):323–329, 2007.

Reichman NE, Corman H, Noonan K: Impact of child disability on the family, *Matern Child Health J,* www.medscape.com/viewarticle/581577. Accessed August 16, 2009. October 15, 2008.

Rubin SE, Millard RP: Ethical principles and American public policy on disability, *J Rehabil* http://findarticles.com/p/articles/mi_m0825/is_n1_v57/ai_10684712/?tag=content;col1. Accessed July 19, 2009. January-March 1991.

Scotch RK: Understanding disability policy: varieties of analysis, *Policy Stud J* 22(1):170–175, 1994.

Silvers A, Wasserman D, Mahowald MB: *Disability, difference, discrimination: perspectives on justice in bioethics and public policy,* Lanham, MA, 1998, Rowman & Littlefield.

Social Security Administration: *Definition of disability, 2009 Social Security Administration Redbook,* 2009a, www.ssa.gov/redbook/eng/overview-disability.htm#5. Accessed June 29, 2009.

Social Security Administration: *Differentiating SSI from SSDI, 2009 Social Security Administration Redbook,* 2009b, www.ssa.gov/redbook/eng/overview-disability.htm#4. Accessed June 29, 2009.

Social Security Administration: *Ticket to Work, SSDI and SSI Eligible, 2009 Social Security Administration Redbook,* 2009c, www.socialsecurity.gov/redbook/eng/ssdi-and-ssi-employments-supports.htm#5. Accessed June 29, 2009.

Sowers J, Smith MR: Nursing faculty members' perceptions, knowledge, and concerns about students with disabilities, *J Nurs Educ* 43(5):213–218, 2004.

Ticket to Work and Work Incentives Advisory Panel: Annual report to the President, Congress, and the Commissioner of SSA, Year Eight, December 2007, www.ssa.gov/work/panel/panel_documents/FORMAT%20-%20Final%20Report--121707.pdf. Accessed August 15, 2009.

Treloar LL: *Perceptions of spiritual beliefs, response to disability, and the church,* Unpublished doctoral dissertation, Cincinnati, Ohio, 1999a, Union Institute and University.

Treloar LL: Unpublished interviews, 1999b.

Treloar LL: Disability, spiritual beliefs and the church: the experiences of adults with disabilities and family members, *J Adv Nurs* 40(5):594–603, 2002.

U.S. Census Bureau: *Definition of disability varies by survey, Housing and Household Economic Statistics Division*, May 2006, http://www.census.gov/hhes/www/disability/disab_defn.html#CPS. Accessed June 20, 2009.

U.S. Census Bureau: *American community survey*, April 2009, http://www.census.gov/acs/www. Accessed June 20, 2009.

U.S. Department of Health and Human Services: The National Survey of Children with Special Health Care Needs Chartbook 2005–2006,

Health Resources and Services Administration, Maternal and Child Health Bureau, 2008, http://mchb.hrsa.gov/cshcn05/index.htm. Accessed August 26, 2009.

U.S. Department of Justice: ADA home page, July 2009, www.ada.gov/. Accessed July 20, 2009.

U.S. Holocaust Memorial Museum: *Euthanasia program, Holocaust Encyclopedia*, 2009, www.ushmm.org/wlc/article.php?lang=en&ModuleId=10005200. Accessed August 22, 2009.

Walsh PN: Health indicators and intellectual disability, *Curr Opin Psychiatry* 21(5):474–478,

2008: www.medscape.com/viewarticle/581738?src=emailthis. Accessed July 4, 2009.

Wilkinson JE, Cerreto MC: Primary care for women with intellectual disabilities, *J Am Board Fam Med* 21:215–222, 2008.

Williams H: Afterthoughts on Terri Schaivo, *Center for Bioethics and Culture Electronic Newsletter* May 5, 2005, www.thecbc.org/enewsletter/index.html.

World Health Organization: *The international classification of functioning, disability and health*, Geneva, 2001, The Author, www.who.int/classifications/icf/en/. Accessed August 28, 2009.

Homeless Populations

Nellie S. Droes, Diane C. Hatton

Additional Material for Study, Review, and Further Exploration

evolve WEBSITE

http://evolve.elsevier.com/Nies

- Quiz
- Case Studies
- Glossary
- WebLinks

OBJECTIVES

Upon completion of this chapter, the reader will be able to do the following:

1. Discuss two meanings of the term *homeless*.
2. Describe the scope of homelessness in the United States.
3. Analyze factors that contribute to homelessness.
4. Identify major health problems among various homeless aggregates.
5. Discuss access to health care for the homeless.
6. Analyze the health problems of the homeless using upstream thinking and a social justice perspective.
7. Apply knowledge about the homeless when planning community health services for this aggregate.

KEY TERMS

acceptability
accessibility
accommodation
acquired social consciousness

affordability
availability
awakened social consciousness
expanded social consciousness

market justice
social consciousness
social justice

OUTLINE

The presence of homeless people continues a trend that began in the early 1980s. The number of homeless individuals has increased, and the demographic profile of this population has changed. Late in the twentieth and early twenty-first century, the "traditional" homeless, predominantly composed of single males, were joined by new groups of homeless, including families (Wright, Rubin, and Devine, 1998). At the time of this writing, the global recession including the mortgage foreclosure crisis has added to an increase in family homelessness (National Alliance to End Homelessness, 2009; Sermons and Henry, 2009).

The purpose of this chapter is to describe the scope of this problem. The chapter presents definitions, prevalence, and demographic characteristics of homelessness; analyzes factors that contribute to homelessness; and describes the health status of various aggregates of the homeless population. The chapter also addresses issues of health care access, explores conceptual approaches to understanding health among the homeless, and proposes community health nursing strategies for the primary, secondary, and tertiary prevention of homelessness and its associated problems.

DEFINITIONS, PREVALENCE, AND DEMOGRAPHIC CHARACTERISTICS OF HOMELESSNESS

Definitions of Homelessness

Many meanings exist for the term *homeless*. Official governmental agencies, the professional literature, and lay people use the term in various ways. Some view the term *home* as a synonym for the place where an individual's family resides. People without family ties, such as those living in single-room–occupancy hotels without family contacts, are, from this perspective, "homeless" (Jencks, 1995; Smith and Smith, 2001). However, government agencies' definitions of *homeless* focus on living quarters, or more specifically sleeping places of individuals, and not family ties. Official governmental reports continue to use the statutory definition put forth by the federal McKinney-Vento Homeless Assistance Act, which was originally authorized in 1987 and defines *homeless* in two different sections.

One section defines homeless as the following (U.S. Department of Housing and Urban Development, 2007):

1. *an individual who lacks a fixed, regular, and adequate nighttime residence; and*
2. *an individual who has a primary nighttime residency that is the following:*
   A. *a supervised publicly or privately operated shelter designed to provide temporary living accommodations (e.g., welfare hotels, congregate shelters, and transitional housing for the mentally ill);*
   B. *an institution that provides a temporary residence for individuals intended to be institutionalized; or*
   C. *a public or private place not designed for or ordinarily used as a regular sleeping accommodation for human beings.*

The education subtitle of the McKinney-Vento Homeless Education Assistance Improvements Act of 2001 as amended by the No Child Left Behind Act of 2001 (U.S. Department of Education, 2004) contains definitions that relate to children and youth.

2. *The term homeless children and youths*
   A. *means individuals who lack a fixed, regular, and adequate nighttime residence (within the meaning of section 103(a)(1)); and*
   B. *includes*
      i. *children and youths who are sharing the housing of other persons due to loss of housing, economic hardship, or a similar reason; are living in motels, hotels, trailer parks, or camping grounds due to the lack of alternative adequate accommodations; are living in emergency or transitional shelters; are abandoned in hospitals; or are awaiting foster care placement;*
      ii. *children and youths who have a primary nighttime residence that is a public or private place not designed for or ordinarily used as a regular sleeping accommodation for human beings (within the meaning of section 103(a)(2)(C));*
      iii. *children and youths who are living in cars, parks, public spaces, abandoned buildings, substandard housing, bus or train stations, or similar settings; and*
      iv. *migratory children (as such term is defined in section 1309 of the Elementary and Secondary Education Act of 1965) who qualify as homeless for the purposes of this subtitle because the children are living in circumstances described in clauses (i) through (iii).*

In addition to these statutory definitions of homelessness, federal agencies administratively define another category of homeless persons—the chronically homeless individual. According to the federal government, a chronically homeless person is "an unaccompanied homeless individual with a disabling condition who has either been continuously homeless for a year or has had at least four (4) episodes of homelessness in the past three (3) years" (U.S. Department of Health and Human Services, 2003b).

Other meanings of homeless are found in the professional literature, where individuals or families are frequently categorized according to the duration and number of episodes of homelessness. Those experiencing a relatively infrequent and short duration may be designated as *crisis, first time, transitionally,* or *temporarily* homeless; those who experience longer and more frequent periods are referred to as *episodically* or *intermittently* homeless individuals; and families who are homeless for a year or with more episodes over several years are classified as *chronically* homeless (Burt, Aron, and Lee, 2001; Kuhn and Culhane, 1998; Lambert and Caces, 1995; U.S. Department of Health and Human Services, 2003a, 2003b).

However, many Americans use another definition of *homelessness*. This colloquial usage reflects the more traditional view of the homeless as the shabbily dressed people they notice in public places during the day (O'Flaherty, 1996). Homeless advocates argue that it is also important to consider those who are poor and tenuously housed. This includes those who are without their own shelter but have "doubled up" with a family member or friend. An estimate of this population is difficult at best. Definitions of *homelessness* vary and consequently give rise to many interpretations and considerable confusion regarding research findings and policy implications (Shinn and Baumohl, 1999).

Prevalence of Homelessness

The homeless are intrinsically difficult to count. Past efforts to enumerate the homeless included the U.S. Census Bureau's collections of national data on the homeless population in Census 1990 and Census 2000 and an Urban Institute study, conducted in 1996. More recent efforts are those based on responses to requirements of the U.S. Department of Housing and Urban Development (HUD). Both the earlier Census Bureau and the more recent HUD efforts are outlined next.

Early Efforts to Count the Homeless

A brief description of the Census Bureau's efforts, including the limitations, in enumerating the homeless population is presented first. The description of the Census Bureau's efforts is followed by a brief account of an Urban Institute study including an estimate of homeless prevalence in 1996.

The earliest effort by the U.S. Census Bureau (Smith and Smith, 2001) to collect data related to the homeless population occurred during Census 1990. On "Shelter and Street Night (S-Night)" in March 1990, the U.S. Census Bureau enumerators counted people in shelters, which served adults, youth, and abused women, and were visible in preidentified street locations. Although the Bureau had indicated the results of this 1990 effort were limited and not to be used as a count, "census stakeholders and data users" (p. 1) expressed concern as to the meaning and use of the data.

Attempting to indicate clearly that Census 2000 would not produce a count of the homeless population, the Bureau used the term "people without conventional housing." On March 27, 2000, enumerators gathered information from individuals located in emergency and transitional shelters, including hotels and motels used to provide shelter for people without conventional housing. The next day, March 28, enumerators counted people at soup kitchens and mobile food vans. On March 29, 2000, the Bureau enumerated people at targeted, nonsheltered outdoor locations. The Bureau's report of the Census 2000 efforts is limited to the data obtained on the first night, March 27, with one very important exception. The "report does not include data for the population counted in shelters for abused women or shelters against domestic violence" (Smith and Smith, 2001). Consequently, these reports, due to severe limitations, are not an appropriate source of valid information regarding the homeless population.

The Urban Institute's 1996 study (Burt et al., 2001), although more than 10 years old, remains as an important source of national data on the homeless population. This

federally funded study was a *point prevalence study*. In other words, it obtained data during a limited point in time, in contrast to collecting data over an extended period. On the basis of data collected during the study, the researchers estimated the number of homeless for a 1-week period to be between 444,000 and 842,000. On the basis of the 444,000, they projected that 2.3 million people experienced a spell of homeless and used homeless assistance programs over the course of a year. Care should be used in interpreting this last number. It does not mean that there were 2.3 million people homeless at one time in 1996 (Burt et al., 2001).

Recent Efforts to Count Homeless

Reports from three different agencies provide recent information related to homeless prevalence. These reports are (1) *The Third Annual Homeless Assessment Report (AHAR)* (HUD, Office of Community Planning and Development, 2008); (2) National Alliance to End Homelessness' *Homeless Counts* (Sermons and Henry, 2009); and (3) the U.S. Conference of Mayors' *Hunger and Homelessness Survey 2008* (U.S. Conference of Mayors, 2008a). The first two reports use HUD's generated data; the third uses data from the annual survey of member cities. A brief sketch of the federal data is outlined next.

The federal government, in 2004, implemented two strategies designed to coordinate efforts to reduce homelessness—implementation of (1) the Continuum of Care (CoC) concept, and (2) the Homeless Information Management System (HMIS). CoCs are local systems responsible for providing a range of housing and related services that meet HUD guidelines for persons experiencing homelessness, including emergency and preventive responses, and implementing and managing the HMIS (HUD, 2009). In response to HUD requirements, CoCs conduct point in time (PIT) counts of homeless persons on one night in January of every other year. In addition to the PIT counts that occur during January, CoCs are required to report the number of homeless persons who use emergency shelters or transitional housing throughout each federal fiscal year: October-September. Data submitted by the CoCs for the October 1, 2006–September 30, 2007 reporting period form the basis for HUD's third AHAR.

As structured, the AHAR provides national estimates of the number of homeless according to two different time intervals: (1) a 1-night PIT count conducted by CoCs in January 2007 and (2) an annual estimate based on CoCs reports of service use occurring between October 1, 2006, and September 30, 2007. It is important to note that the PIT count included both sheltered and unsheltered persons—those who were sleeping in shelters or transitional housing and those who were on the streets or in other places not meant for human habitation. In contrast, the annual estimated counts of the homeless population include only those who were in shelters or transitional housing.

Estimates based on the PIT count indicate that nationally there were 672,000 (sheltered and unsheltered) homeless persons on any one night in January 2007. Of this total, 423,400 (63%) were individuals and 248,500 (37%) were persons in families (one adult with at least one child). Of the total (sheltered and unsheltered) homeless population, there were 123,833 individuals classified as chronically homeless (HUD, Office of Community Planning and Development, 2008). These PIT-based estimates provide a "snapshot" picture of the homeless population. When one uses a different lens—the annual estimate—another picture appears.

According to the reports that CoCs submitted to HUD, there were an estimated 1,589,000 persons who used emergency shelters or transitional housing at some time between October 1, 2006, and September 30, 2007. Included in this total were 1,115,000 (70%) individuals and 474,000 (30%) persons who were in families (HUD, Office of Community Planning and Development, 2008).

In order to interpret the information related to counts of homeless persons, it is essential to note that the two different methods, the PIT and annual survey, generate different results. The National Alliance to End Homelessness (NAEH), using HUD-generated data, provided another report on the number of homeless (Sermons and Henry, 2009). A brief summary of NAEH's reported changes in counts over a 2-year period follows.

According to Sermons and Henry (2009) estimates, between 2005 and 2007 there was, at the national level, a 10% decline across all groups of homeless. They also note that there was a larger decline in family and chronically homeless adult subpopulations. However, this decline, occurring between 2005 and 2007, was not uniform across all reporting levels. Local and state levels, 44% and 36% respectively, reported increased rates of homelessness. Importantly, the authors note that (1) these changes occurred between 2005 and 2007, a period of relative economic stability, and (2) recent economic conditions in the United States and globally (the increasing mortgage foreclosure and unemployment rates) are predicted to increase the number of households who are homeless or at risk for homelessness (Sermons and Henry, 2009).

HUD's and NAEH's reports are based on PIT and annual counts of homeless persons from data generated through the HUD-directed HMIS. In addition to these reports, the survey conducted by the U.S. Mayors' Conference provides a perspective on homelessness prevalence from a local level.

The U.S. Conference of Mayors provided information on homeless in the cities that are members of the U.S. Conference of Mayors Taskforce on Hunger and Homelessness. According this report, during 2007-2008, homelessness increased by an average of 12% (unweighted) in the twenty-five reporting cities. Los Angeles and Cleveland were the only two cities to report a decrease in family homelessness; three cities reported no change. The majority of the cities (sixteen of twenty-one) that responded to the survey in family homeless reported an increase. As with other efforts to enumerate homelessness, the authors of the Mayors' report indicate caution in interpreting the information. They note that the cities reporting are not a representative sample of cities and hence are not a national report (U.S. Conference of Mayors, 2008a).

Attempting to grasp the various nuances involved in counting the homeless, Wright and colleagues (1998) offer the following helpful metaphor:

Given the episodic nature of much homelessness, trying to count the homeless is a little like trying to count the number of flies in a house whose windows and doors are wide open. At any one moment, there is a definite number of flies in the house and that number is theoretically countable. Practically speaking, however, the rapid movement of flies in and out means that no count can be definitive or even very useful. Likewise, while there is some finite and theoretically countable number of literally homeless people in the United States at any one time, they are but a fraction of a much larger number of persons who are at risk of homelessness and who are destined to be homeless at some other time. In this sense, the number of flies or of homeless people is a less pertinent question than the transition probabilities that govern movement in and out of the condition being counted. (p. 63)

In summary, Kozol (1988) argued more than 20 years ago:

We would be wise to avoid the numbers game. Any search for the "right number" carries the assumption that we may at last arrive at an acceptable number. There is no acceptable number. Whether the number is "1 million or 4 million," there are too many homeless people in America. (p. 10)

Demographic Characteristics

Based on data collected during the January 2007 1-night counts, the third AHAR report identifies the following sheltered homeless subpopulations: domestic violence victims, persons with serious mental illness, unaccompanied youth, veterans, persons with substance abuse problems and persons living with human immunodeficiency virus/acquired immunodeficiency syndrome (HIV/AIDS). Among all sheltered homeless persons, 13% were victims of domestic violence and 28% were persons with serious mental illness. Unaccompanied youth comprised 2% of the total sheltered homeless population. Veterans and persons with substance abuse problems comprised 15% and 39% respectively of all sheltered homeless adults. Persons living with HIV/AIDS represented 4% of sheltered adults and unaccompanied youth (HUD, Office of Community Planning and Development, 2008).

In addition to the information based on the PIT January 2007 count, the third AHAR includes descriptions of homeless people who were sheltered at some time during October 2006 to September 2007. The report uses two categories of homeless persons: individual and family. Individuals accounted for 70% of the sheltered homeless population. Among this group, 69% were men, 25% were women, and 5% were unaccompanied youth. Individuals whose ages ranged from 31 to 50 years comprised 55% of the sheltered homeless individual population as compared with 24% of nonhomeless persons living alone in poverty. African Americans represented 33%

of the sheltered individuals, a larger number compared with 18% of nonhomeless poverty population (HUD, Office of Community Planning and Development, 2008).

Presented next are the characteristics of sheltered family members (composed of at least one adult and one child). Of the total number of people in sheltered homeless families, children are 62%; adults are 38%. Women account for 82% of adult members, which is a larger percentage than the 67% of women in poor families. Adults in homeless families are younger than the adults in poor families, as 55% of homeless adult family members are between 18 and 30 years of age in contrast to 42% of adults in nonhomeless poor families. Sheltered homeless children are young, as 87% are under 12 years of age; more than half (51%) are under 6 years of age. African Americans make up 55% of the sheltered homeless population compared with 26% of nonhomeless poor (HUD, Office of Community Planning and Development, 2008).

This section has presented the federal definition of homelessness, a discussion of the challenges in obtaining a count of homeless populations, and a brief outline of selected demographic characteristics. A discussion of factors contributing to homelessness follows.

FACTORS THAT CONTRIBUTE TO HOMELESSNESS

In the larger society, there are three broad factors that contribute to homelessness: (1) shortage of affordable housing, (2) incomes insufficient to meet basic needs, and (3) inadequate and scarce support services. The interaction among these factors has been largely responsible for the continuation of homelessness.

Shortage of Affordable Housing

Housing is considered affordable if it costs a renter or an owner no more than 30% of his or her income. HUD operates, in cooperation with state and local governments and nonprofit housing organizations, programs that provide financial housing assistance to low-income families. This assistance may be provided as (1) direct payment to apartment owners, who in turn lower rents for low-income tenants; (2) access to an apartment located in a public housing facility; or (3) housing choice vouchers, which may be used by low-income persons to "pay" all or part of the rent. The third option continues to be more commonly known as "Section 8 housing." Although these programs are intended to alleviate housing problems for low-income renters, the demand for these assisted housing programs has far exceeded the supply.

Factors contributing to the shortages include market forces that inhibit the private housing sector's production of affordable rental housing, decreases in the federal government's spending on assisted housing for low-income families, and the increasing inequality of incomes among groups within the larger population. The foreclosure crisis that began in 2007 has exacerbated the obstacles that people with low incomes face in obtaining affordable housing (Khadduri, 2008; Rice and Sard, 2009; HUD, Office of Policy Development and Research, 2007; Wardrip, Pelletiere, and Crowley, 2009).

Income Insufficiency

Burt and colleagues, more than 10 years ago, documented that insufficient incomes and lack of employment prevented people from leaving homelessness (Burt et al., 2001). The U.S. Census Bureau's report (DeNavas-Walt, Proctor, and Smith, 2008) reveals that, in 2000, the real median household income was $50,557 (adjusted to reflect 2007 dollars); in 2007 it was $50,223. Although the 2007 level reflects an increase compared with 2005 and 2006 levels, it is still less than the 2000 level. During the same period, 2000-2007, both the number of people in poverty and the poverty rate increased. Overall, the percentage of people living below the poverty line increased from 11.3% in 2000 to 12.7% in 2007, and during this same period, the number increased from 31.5 million to 37.0 million. The poverty rate among children younger than 18 years increased from 16.2% to 18.0% between 2000 and 2007. Moreover, in 2007, among the poor, 41.8% were in extreme poverty—classified as those having an income below half of the poverty line (DeNavas-Walt et al., 2008).

As a consequence of the shortage of affordable housing and insufficient income, an increasing number of low-income people end up paying much more than they can afford for rent. In many areas of the country, wages needed to afford housing are three to five times higher than the federal minimum wage of $7.25 (as of July 2009) per hour. This increase was the last increase of a three-step process. The wage first increased in July 2007 from the previous $5.15 per hour, which had been in effect since 1997; the second increase, to $6.55, occurred in July 2008 (U.S. Department of Labor, Employment Standards Administration, Wage and Hour Division, 2007). Paying too much of their income for rent leaves low income people without adequate resources for other necessities, such as food, clothing, and health care, and increases the risk of homelessness (Children's Defense Fund, 2008).

Inadequacy and Scarcity of Supportive Services

Accompanying the previously described factors, shortage of affordable housing and insufficient income, is the scarcity of supportive services for low-income people who need them. Some low-income people need services to maintain their housing status, whereas others need services in order to work and earn money. Those that need services to maintain their housing status include those with serious chronic mental health and/or substance abuse problems. In addition to needing income assistance, this group requires comprehensive and accessible health care, both physical and behavioral.

There are other homeless people who, without the serious physical and mental disabilities of the former group, are able to function in the workforce. These people need assistance in the forms of child care, transportation, and vocational training.

What the two groups have in common is the need for affordable health care, that is, health care in its broadest sense as outlined by the World Health Organization (WHO) (1948).

Unfortunately, the proportion and number of people in the general population without health insurance increased during the period 2000-2007. In 2000, 13.7% (38.4 million) were not covered by health insurance; in 2007, 15.3% (45.7 million) were not covered. Among those whose incomes are below federal poverty levels, 24.5% were without health insurance in 2007. Among homeless clients receiving health care services, the rates of uninsured are even higher than among the nonhomeless poor (Kidder, Wolitski, Campsmith et al., 2007; Pearson, Bruggman, and Haukoos, 2007). Consequently, lack of health insurance is a significant factor in preventing people from leaving homelessness and may, indeed, be a major risk factor for homelessness. A serious illness or disability can lead to a downward spiral into homelessness as a result of job loss, use of savings to pay for care, and inability to pay rent (Burt et al., 2001; DeNavas-Walt et al., 2008).

The three broad factors contributing to homelessness—shortage of affordable housing, insufficient income, and scarcity of supportive services—are conditions in society. Singularly and more important, the interaction among these factors has serious consequences for low-income people. These conditions potentiate the vulnerability factors found among certain individuals and families and increase the probability of homelessness.

HEALTH STATUS OF THE HOMELESS

As discussed in Chapter 1, the WHO has defined health from a broad perspective. This classic definition, which purports that health is "a state of complete physical, mental, and social well-being and not merely the absence of disease or infirmity" (WHO, 1948), is particularly useful when considering the health status of the homeless. For these individuals, a continual interaction exists among these three dimensions (physical, mental, and social) that has enormous consequences for health. The boundaries of these dimensions overlap; therefore, it is difficult, if not impossible, to address health among the homeless without a concomitant analysis of physical, mental, and social dimensions. Therefore, this section addresses the health status of various homeless aggregates from this broad WHO interpretation. Specifically, the subgroups discussed include men, women, children, and adolescents. Special groups considered are homeless families and homeless individuals with mental health and substance abuse problems, including the chronically homeless.

Homeless Men

From a historical perspective, much of the earliest information on the health status of men was provided by data from the National Health Care for the Homeless Program, an initiative funded by the Robert Wood Johnson Foundation and the Pew Charitable Trust Fund in the late 1980s. Although dated, these data nevertheless stand as major sources of information on the health status of the homeless population (Institute of Medicine, 1988; Wright, 1990). The more recent reports cited in the following sections substantiate this earlier report.

Homeless men experience physical health problems, both acute and chronic, at higher rates than men in the general population. Acute physical health problems occurring at higher rates in homeless men include respiratory infections, trauma, and skin disorders (Bargh, Hoch, Hwang et al., 2007; Bucher, Brickner, and Vincent, 2006; Hwang, Colantonio, Chiu et al., 2008). Chronic disorders including hypertension, musculoskeletal disorders, diabetes, respiratory problems (asthma, chronic bronchitis, emphysema), neurological disorders including seizures, and poor dentition are also more prevalent among homeless populations (Schanzer, Dominguez, Shrout et al., 2007; Zlotnick and Zerger, 2009). In addition, HIV and AIDS, tuberculosis, hepatitis C, and sexually transmitted diseases (STDs) occur at higher rates in homeless men than in the general population. (Kidder et al., 2007; U.S. Department of Health and Human Services, Centers for Disease Control and Prevention, 2008).

Many of these acute and chronic conditions are exacerbated by alcoholism, which occurs more frequently among homeless than nonhomeless men; alcoholism may be the single most prevalent health problem among the homeless. Likewise, serious mental illnesses occur more frequently among the homeless than in the general population. In addition, minor emotional problems (e.g., personality disorders) are also more frequent among homeless than nonhomeless men. Drug abuse, like alcohol abuse, occurs more frequently among the homeless, and considerable overlap of alcohol and drug abuse exists. Men are more likely than women to report alcohol abuse (Eyrich-Garg, Cacciola, Carise et al., 2008; Fazel, Khosla, Doll et al., 2008; Goldstein, Luther, Jacoby et al., 2008; Greenberg and Rosenheck, 2008a, 2008b; Padgett, Henwood, Abrams, et al., 2008).

Studies comparing homeless and housed poor people indicate that homeless adults are more likely to be male and have veteran status than the housed poor. Homeless adults are more likely to be unemployed, or if employed, the job is temporary or at a low wage and without benefits. Consequently, their income is insufficient to maintain housing costs. Although a lack of monetary resources is a variable related directly to becoming and remaining homeless, additional deficits in social resources contribute to the condition. Many of the homeless have relied on social support from families and friends to provide housing. Homelessness results when both monetary resources and social support are exhausted (National Coalition for the Homeless, 2008).

Homeless Women

The National Survey of Homeless Assistance Providers and Clients (NSHAPC) has identified the following three subgroups among women experiencing homelessness: 38% have a minor child, 47% are by themselves, and 15% are with another person/not a minor child ("other clients"). Women from all three groups report health and nutrition needs that far exceed those of women in the general population. Women with minor children and single women are more likely to use shelters and less likely to sleep on the streets; women designated as "other clients" are the least likely to receive services. The latter are the most reclusive of the three subgroups—generally avoiding shelters and soup kitchens (Burt et al., 2001).

An accumulation of research evidence indicates that when compared with men, single women report more stressful life events, foster care as children, intimate partner violence as adults, and hospitalizations for psychiatric problems (Caton, Wilkins, and Anderson, 2007). Homeless women have higher rates of pregnancy, including unintended pregnancy, than their housed counterparts, and researchers have demonstrated that the severity of homelessness increases the likelihood of preterm births and low-birth-weight infants. Although increased access to prenatal care may improve the health of pregnant women, preventing homelessness in the first place is even more critical for birth outcomes, as women bring to pregnancy stressors that have a cumulative effect over the life course for reproductive health (Gelberg, Lu, Leake et al., 2008; Stein, Lu, and Gelberg, 2000).

In the 1990s, research clearly documented the extraordinary histories of violence, from childhood through adulthood, among women experiencing homelessness (Anderson, 1996; Bassuk, Buckner, Weinreb et al., 1997; Bassuk, Melnick, and Browne, 1998). Bassuk, Weinreb, Buckner, and colleagues (1996) reported that an estimated 92% of homeless women have experienced physical or sexual assault sometime in their lives. Researchers continue to document rape and other assaults among homeless women. Clearly, sexual assaults are associated with worse physical and mental health outcomes including use/abuse of alcohol and other drugs (Austin, Andersen, and Gelberg, 2008; Wenzel, Leake, and Gelberg, 2000). As may be expected, women living in unsheltered locations on the street have increased risk for victimization over women living in shelters. Unsheltered women also have greater odds of having multiple sexual partners and are less likely to utilize health services. Other factors that increase risk of physical and sexual victimization include history of mental illness, substance use/abuse, and engaging in survival strategies including selling sex and drugs (Nyamathi, Leake, and Gelberg, 2000; Wenzel et al., 2000). The Welfare Reform Act has impacted women's homelessness in a variety of ways. Some stay in abusive relationships because of anticipated difficulty in accessing Temporary Aid to Needy Families (TANF) under this legislation. Others who do access TANF find it difficult to manage small children and fulfill work obligations: "exempting battered homeless women from participating in welfare-to-work activities exists in principle but for many women…does not exist in reality" (Roschelle, 2008). In addition, researchers report workplace violence in the lives of women who are homeless. Many of the women are reluctant either to report the violence or to leave the job because of financial needs (Anderson, 2008).

Social support influences women's physical and mental well-being and their ability to access health services. Women who are homeless report a disconnectedness beginning in childhood that continues in adult life (Anderson, 1996). As adults, they score lower than their housed counterparts on measures of social support, as well as intimacy and reciprocity (Anderson and Rayens, 2004). They have fewer persons in their social networks, and these persons often experience similar emotional distress and have high-risk behaviors (Bassuk et al., 1996; Nyamathi, Flaskerud, and Leake, 1997). Women who have substance nonusers in their social support networks report better psychosocial status and increased health services utilization than those who have only substance users (Nyamathi, Leake, and Keenan et al., 2000).

It is impossible to separate women who are homeless from the context in which they live. Promoting lasting change in their lives requires not only addressing specific physical and mental health needs, but imbedding programs into their particular communities and assuming that women may need programs for a long term (Smyth, Goodman, and Glenn, 2006). Others suggest that because of the high numbers of women reporting histories of foster placement as children, as well as exposure to violence as both children and adults, assistance requires gender-specific interventions; pointing to the large numbers of women who have lost custody of their children in this aggregate, they also advocate programs that support and preserve families (Caton et al., 2007).

Finally, women who are homeless have an increased risk for incarceration. Incarceration risk is related to the public nature of homelessness and the likelihood of arrest for misdemeanors and other minor crimes. Shelters, jails, and prisons have become part of an "institutional circuit" that houses people, replacing more stable, community-based living situations (Caton et al., 2007; Hatton and Fisher, 2008; Metraux, Caternia, and Cho, 2007). Moreover, access to housing upon release to the community is a key predictor for decreasing recidivism among formerly incarcerated women (Freudenberg, Daniels, Crum et al., 2005).

Over a decade ago, Dr. Ellen Bassuk, president of the National Center on Family Homelessness, summarized the health-related problems from which homeless women suffer. They do not differ from the problems that impede many women in the United States, she argued, although their problems are likely to be more intense, frequent, and apt to occur in concert. Often, homeless women have limited education, limited earning power, and fragmented support networks. Trapped by a lack of economic and social opportunities, homeless women profoundly experience society's inequities (Bassuk, 1993).

Homeless Children

At the national level, the National Alliance to End Homelessness reported that the number of homeless families with children decreased between 2005 and 2007 (Sermons and Henry, 2009). In contrast, the National Center on Family Homelessness (2009), reported that the extent of child homelessness was worsening. Differences in the two accounts are mainly due to the use of two different definitions of homelessness. As indicated in a previous section of this chapter, the statutes and regulations governing HUD define homelessness more narrowly than those that govern the Department of Education (Vissing and Hudson, 2008). Whether the decreasing trends noted by the report using the HUD definition will continue is questionable, given the economic and housing crisis that began in 2007 (Duffield and Lovell, 2008). An overview of studies that provide information about homeless children's health status follows. Included is information about broad aspects of the health of homeless children—physical and mental health and educational attainment.

In an extensive review of studies of homeless children, Buckner (2008) divided the research according to two periods: those published before and since 1991. He also noted whether the studies included comparisons of homeless children with housed poor children and/or the general population of children. The earlier studies conducted in the 1980s when family homelessness was emerging as a national problem were mainly descriptive, indicating the homeless children's characteristics and needs. Later studies used more sophisticated research and statistical methods and provided answers to more complex questions.

Studies comparing homeless children with children located in the general population report that homeless children are more apt to experience physical health problems including asthma, iron deficiency, anemia, and obesity. Homeless children experience higher rates of mental health problems, including behavior problems and developmental delays, than rates reported for children in the general population (Grant, Shapiro, Joseph et al., 2007; Rog and Buckner, 2007; Shinn, Schteingart, Williams et al., 2008; Yu, North, LaVesser et al., 2008).

The previously outlined physical, mental, and developmental problems interact and adversely affect homeless children's educational achievement on standardized tests covering reading, language usage, and/or mathematics. Missing days of school because of family mobility, homeless children are more likely than other children to repeat grades. Homeless children may lack resources for clothing and school supplies and access to facilities for personal hygiene maintenance. As a consequence, they may be at risk of nonacceptance or teasing by other students, thereby compounding the effects of their physical and mental problems (Duffield and Lovell, 2008; Dworsky, 2008; Obradovic, Long, Cutulia et al., 2009).

Although homeless children had higher rates of physical, mental health and behavior, and educational problems than children in the general population, when compared with poor but housed children, the rates were similar. In other words, the difference in housing status was not a contributing factor. Other authors report that there are significant differences within the population of homeless children. There is a subpopulation of homeless children that is doing well, while another subpopulation is experiencing multiple problems (Huntington, Buckner, and Bassuk, 2008; Obradovic et al., 2009).

Homeless Adolescents and Youth

This next section describes the population of homeless adolescents and youth. The wide range of ages and categories designating adolescents and youth is outlined, and the health problems in both the general and homeless adolescents and youth are presented. The health problems of several homeless adolescent subpopulations are also included.

Studies, policies, and programs related to homeless adolescents and youth use varying ages and overlapping categorical descriptors. Ages may range from 13 to 25 years. Categories used in studies and reports include *runaway, throwaway, street,* and *system* adolescent and/or youth. *Runaways* have left home without permission; *throwaways* have been forced out of the home; *street* adolescents and youth live primarily on the street; *system* adolescents and youth have been wards of the state (foster care, juvenile justice system) (Burt, 2007; Fernandes, 2007; Slesnick, Dashora, Letcher et al., 2009).

As indicated by several substantial reports and reviews of studies, adolescents and youth from all sectors of society engage in health-risk behaviors that result in serious health problems (Centers for Disease Control and Prevention, 2008). These problems include unintended pregnancy, STDs (including HIV/AIDS), alcohol and drug abuse, depression, and suicide. For the most part, these problems are related to risk-taking behaviors. However, homeless adolescents experience these problems at higher rates than the general adolescent population (Burt, 2007; National Research Council and Institute of Medicine, 2009; Toro, Dworsky, and Fowler, 2007; Zerger, Strehlow, and Gundlapalli, 2008).

Homeless adolescents experience STDs, physical and sexual abuse, skin disorders, anemia, drug and alcohol abuse, and unintentional injuries at higher rates than adolescents in the general population. Depression, suicidal ideation, and disorders of behavior, personality, or thought also occur at higher rates among homeless adolescents. Family disruption, school failures, prostitution or "survival sex," and involvement with the legal system indicate that homeless adolescents' social health is severely compromised (Burt, 2007; Busen and Engebretson, 2008; National Research Council and Institute of Medicine, 2009; Rew, Grady, Whittaker et al., 2008; Rew, Rochlen, and Murphey, 2008; Tevendale, Lightfoot, and Slocum, 2009; Toro et al., 2007).

Homeless adolescents and youth who are pregnant, engage in prostitution, or identify themselves as gay, lesbian, bisexual, or transgender experience more health problems than other homeless adolescents. Pregnant homeless adolescents and youth have more severe mental health problems and use alcohol and drugs more than nonpregnant homeless peers. Not surprisingly, they have higher rates of negative pregnancy outcomes than nonhomeless adolescents and youth (National Research Council and Institute of Medicine, 2009; Rew et al., 2008).

Runaway or homeless adolescents and youth, both female and male, make up a large percentage of all youth involved in prostitution. Many become involved because they need money to meet subsistence needs, which is the source of the term "survival sex." They are more likely to have serious mental health problems and to be actively suicidal. Alcohol and drug use occurs at higher rates among this group than among homeless adolescents and youth not engaged in prostitution. Those involved in prostitution are more likely to report histories of physical and sexual abuse (Fernandes, 2007; Molino, 2007; National Research Council and Institute of Medicine, 2009).

Rates of attempted suicide are higher among gay homeless adolescents and youth. A large majority of males involved in survival sex identify themselves as gay or bisexual. Many of these young people are on the streets because of effects of homophobia and prejudice. Facing problems similar to those of other homeless adolescents and youth, the gay-identified face an additional set of problems as a result of others rejecting them because of their sexual orientation (National Research Council and Institute of Medicine, 2009).

Adolescents and youth in the general population are at risk, those who are homeless are at even higher risk, and the special subpopulations of adolescents and youth—including those who are gay-identified, those who are pregnant, and those who are practicing survival sex—are particularly vulnerable. Health for many of these groups is severely jeopardized.

Homeless Families

In the 1980s, much discussion ensued about the "old homeless" and the "new homeless"—a situation whereby young families with children joined the "homeless population" previously composed of mostly single men with substance use disorders living on the streets (Rossi, 1990). Many thought the improved economic conditions of the 1990s would eventually eradicate this problem. Yet, family homelessness persists and has actually worsened in recent years. Research has shown that women heading homeless families in 2003 reported more physical health problems, major depressive illness, and posttraumatic stress disorder than women in 1993 (Weinreb, Buckner, Williams et al., 2006).

In 2008, when the U.S. Conference of Mayors released its annual report on hunger and homelessness, the Task Force emphasized the increased risk for hunger and homelessness among the nation's working families because of the weak economy and the high cost of food and fuel (U.S. Conference of Mayors, 2008b). More specific causes of family homelessness identified in the report were lack of affordable housing (72%), poverty (52%), unemployment (44%), low-paying jobs (36%), domestic violence (28%), family disputes (20%), mental illness (12%), and substance abuse (12%). Of the twenty-two major U.S. cities responding to the Mayors' annual survey, sixteen cities reported an increase in family homelessness, two reported a decrease, and four cities had no change (U.S. Conference of Mayors, 2008a).

The Mayors' report indicates that families experiencing homelessness are less likely to be living on the street than other homeless populations, with twenty-three cities reporting that, on an average night, 543 of the persons homeless in families were on the streets, 9930 were in emergency shelters, 12,862 in transitional housing, and 10,710 in permanent housing. The average stays in these settings were 69 days (emergency shelter), 175 (transitional housing), and 556 (permanent supportive housing). The report warns that because families without housing usually double up with others before using shelters, the data probably do not reflect the actual level of housing need for families.

A systematic review of the research on homelessness concludes that families comprise approximately 34% of the homeless population; are frequently headed by single women with young, preschool children; and disproportionately represent ethnic minority groups. Families are commonly separated when they become homeless; shelters may not allow male children; and children may go to live with other family members or friends. Mothers report poorer mental and physical health than their domiciled counterparts, and they have incomes significantly below the federal poverty level. Without subsidies, their incomes are too low to obtain housing. Social networks have shown some protection from homelessness for poor families, but networks characterized by interpersonal conflict increase a family's risk for homelessness. This systematic research review concludes with recommendations that include targeting families at imminent risk of homelessness, as well as mobilizing other prevention efforts, such as affordable housing policies and other measures that lift families out of poverty (Rog and Buckner, 2007).

Homeless Individuals with Mental Health and Substance Use Problems

This section describes problems experienced by homeless individuals with mental and substance use disorders and examines inherent risks for health status. A brief description of the characteristics of the available information is included.

Several authors (e.g., Fazel et al., 2008; Folsom and Jeste, 2002; Wright et al., 1998), in substantial reviews of multiple studies on homelessness and the mentally ill, note that the rate of mental disorders is higher among the homeless compared with the domiciled population. Estimates of mental disorders have varied from 20% to 90%.

In a 1996 national survey of clients of homeless service providers, 45% of respondents self-reported experiences with mental health problems in the previous year (Burt et al., 2001). Fazel and colleagues (2008) systematically reviewed surveys of the prevalence of mental and substance disorders among the homeless in Western countries (United States, United Kingdom, Germany, Australia, Netherlands, France, and Greece) that were conducted between 1979 and 2005. The pooled prevalence of psychotic disorders among homeless persons was 12.7%, with a range of 3% to 42%, which is a higher rate than found in housed populations.

Recent reports from the U.S. Conference of Mayors (2008a) and HUD (2008) indicate that 26% to 28% of the homeless population had a serious mental illness. Other studies conducted at local or regional levels also report that the prevalence of mental disorders is higher in homeless populations than comparative groups within the general population (Forney, Lombardo, and Toro, 2007; Goldstein et al., 2008; North, Eyrich, Pollio et al., 2004).

Estimates of the rates of the use of legal and illegal substances among homeless populations are higher than rates found in comparative groups. Wright et al. (1998) allege that the estimated rate of alcohol abuse exceeds 40% among the nations' homeless and is near 50% among homeless men. Fazel et al. (2008) estimated that alcohol dependence ranged from 8.5% to 58.5% with a pooled estimate of 38%, and other types of substance dependence ranged from 4.7% to 54.2%

with a pooled estimate of 24%. In the previously mentioned 1996 national survey (Burt, Aron, Douglas et al., 1999; Burt et al., 2001), 46% of the adult respondents reported problems with alcohol, and 38% reported problems with other substances within the previous year. HUD's report indicated that 39% of sheltered adults were persons with chronic substance abuse problems (HUD, Office of Community Planning and Development, 2008).

Substance use carries considerable health risks. Alcohol abuse and dependence are associated with a wide range of health problems involving the liver, nervous system, and heart. The loss of economic productivity, vulnerability to accidents, and victimization are common outcomes. Substance use involving intravenous administration carries risks of infections (e.g., hepatitis); STDs (e.g., HIV); and significant social, legal, and economic problems (Forney et al., 2007; Kim, Daskalakis, Plumb et al., 2008; Wolitski, Kidder, and Fenton, 2007).

Moreover, for a sizable proportion of the homeless, severe mental illness exists concomitantly with the problems of alcohol or other types of substance use. Terms used to denote this phenomenon include co-occurrence disorders, comorbidity, and dual diagnosis (Forney et al., 2007; Mares, Greenberg, and Rosenheck, 2008; U.S. Department of Health and Human Services, Substance Abuse and Mental Health Services Administration, Center for Substance Abuse Treatment, 2007).

As noted by the reporting authors, there is considerable variation in prevalence rates for mental and substance use disorders. This variation is attributed to differences that include diagnostic criteria, sampling methods, participation rates, definitions of homelessness, and geographic locations. Much of the available information is based on data collected in the previous two decades. Current information regarding the prevalence of mental and substance use disorders among homeless people is only recently available. The *Third Annual Homeless Assessment Report* (AHAR) (HUD, Office of Community Planning and Development, 2008) was the first based on a full year of the HMIS data. HUD expects this report to provide a baseline for subsequent annual reports.

Chronically Homeless

As noted in the previous section, many homeless individuals experience both mental and substance disorders. These are the individuals included in the federal definition of the chronically homeless. More specifically, these are unaccompanied adults who are homeless for extended or numerous periods and have one or more disabling conditions. The disabling conditions that chronically homeless people experience are very often severe mental and substance use disorders (Caton, Dominguez, Schanzer et al., 2005; Caton et al., 2007; Larimer, Malone, Garner et al., 2009; Sadowski, Kee, VanderWeele et al., 2009). This subpopulation is also at increased risk for the health problems outlined in previous sections on the health status of men and women.

As of January 2007, the chronically homeless represented 18% of the total sheltered and unsheltered homeless population. Two thirds of the chronically homeless were

unsheltered, sleeping on the street or in places not meant for human habitation. Advocates that support focusing on this subpopulation of the homeless cite studies that indicate the chronically homeless, although comprising a relative smaller proportion of all homeless persons, use a disproportionate amount of homeless services. Others, although not discounting the problems of this group, indicate that the federal definition is too narrow. The policy excludes children, parents, youth, with or without disabilities, and adults whose housing status does not meet the required duration or frequency (Kertesz and Weiner, 2009; Larimer et al., 2009; Rosen, 2009; Sadowski et al., 2009).

ACCESS TO HEALTH CARE FOR THE HOMELESS

The work of Penchansky and Thomas (1981) in clarifying "access" as it relates to health care services provides a framework for exploring access to health care by people who are poor but housed, homeless people in general, and special aggregates of the homeless. Noting that *access* is a general concept that represents the "degree of 'fit' between the clients and the system" (p. 128), Penchansky and Thomas identified the following five specific areas of "fit between the patient and the health care system" (p. 128):

1. Availability refers to the relationship between the amount (i.e., number of providers and facilities) and type of health care services and the amount and type of client needs.
2. Accessibility connotes the relationship between the location of the services and the client's location.
3. Accommodation indicates the relationship between how services are organized (e.g., hours of operation and appointment systems) and the client's ability to accommodate to these factors. The client's perception of the appropriateness of these factors is a component of accommodation.
4. Affordability refers to the price of provider services or payment requirements and the client's ability to pay.
5. Acceptability represents the relationship between the client's attitudes about providers and providers' attitudes about acceptable client characteristics.

Poor but housed people experience considerable problems related to each of the five access dimensions; however, the primary problem is affordability. Many poor people lack any form of health insurance, including Medicaid or State Children's Health Insurance Program (SCHIP). For those who do meet the eligibility requirements, the low reimbursement rates and cumbersome requirements tend to discourage or prohibit health care providers from participating. As a consequence of the inability to afford the services of a market-driven system, those who are excluded from the private fee-for-service arrangement must rely on health care safety net providers—community health centers or hospital systems' outpatient clinics, emergency departments, and inpatient services. Heavy demands on these less-than-adequately funded facilities frequently result in less-than-desirable or appropriate accommodations. Long waits for services in overcrowded, uncomfortable settings may discourage people from seeking care at an earlier and more easily treated stage (Blanchard, Ogle, Thomas et al., 2008; DeVoe, Graham, Angier et al., 2008; Grossman, Legedza, and Wee, 2008; Hoffman and Paradise, 2008; Shields, McGinn-Shapiro, and Fronstin, 2008).

Notwithstanding such difficulties, these facilities are frequently situated relatively remote from the person's location. Frequently, individuals are without the financial, familial, or social resources to get to the provider. For example, inner-city residents may access such facilities through a public transportation system; those individuals who reside in rural areas lack such services and must find other resources (e.g., relatives, neighbors, and friends) or do without health care. Many providers in the safety net systems are under considerable stress working in less than optimal conditions with heavy workloads, and they find it difficult to provide care to poor clients who frequently have complex problems and different cultural and language expectations. Consequently, these clients may find such services unacceptable and may fail to seek care until illnesses are intolerable (Aday, 2001; Institute of Medicine, 1988; Silverstein, Lamberto, DePeau et al., 2008; Wright, 1990).

Like people who are poor but housed, homeless people experience considerable difficulty accessing the health care system. However, the homeless face more severe problems than the housed poor. Eligibility for many services frequently requires forms of documentation that homeless people find difficult to provide because they are homeless. Lacking secure storage space makes it difficult to protect personal papers from loss, theft, or weather. Frequently, homeless people must walk to service sites because public transportation is unavailable or too costly. Consequently, accessibility is even more problematic for the homeless than for those who are housed and have a more intact system of transportation (e.g., vouchers, relatives, neighbors, and friends). Without a permanent mailing address or message center, accommodating a health care system that relies on mailed notification of appointments or the results of health care procedures is unlikely. Furthermore, the hours of service may force the homeless to choose between obtaining health care and obtaining food and shelter (Blanchard et al., 2008; Reid, Vittinghoff, and Kushel, 2008).

Special aggregates within the homeless population experience additional problems in obtaining health care services. The following section describes the problems of homeless people who are chronically mentally ill and homeless pregnant women.

Although physical health services available to the poor are inadequate, mental health services are even less available. Several researchers have investigated access to mental health and substance abuse services by homeless adults. As a group, homeless people with chronic mental illness or substance abuse continue to have trouble in obtaining access to needed services. These researchers stress that attention to systems-level features is necessary to provide access for this especially vulnerable group of homeless people. The historic conditions of deinstitutionalization, whereby community-based mental health services failed to materialize, and the current policy, whereby insurance plans reimburse less for mental health services than for physical health services, result in the need for mental health services for homeless mentally ill clients to far exceed the supply (Aron, Honberg, Duckworth et al., 2009; Martens, 2001; Street Health, 2009).

The homeless mentally ill also require physical health services. Obtaining such care from these two disconnected and complex systems requires considerable skill in negotiation. The nature of the illness frequently compromises this skill. Notwithstanding the lack of services, the chronically mentally ill, from the intrinsic nature of their health problems, frequently experience significant problems related to dimensions of accommodation and acceptability. Frequently distrustful of established institutions, the chronically mentally ill find the traditional services provided by mental health agencies inappropriate. Many providers find their bizarre manner of dress, lack of personal hygiene, and inappropriate physical appearance difficult to accept (Martins, 2008).

Given the conditions of homelessness and the necessity of obtaining food and shelter, pregnant homeless women frequently find seeking early prenatal care a lesser priority. Compounding the lower priority are the problems of obtaining prenatal and obstetric care. Some obstetric providers refuse to see or limit the number of women on Medicaid they will see because low reimbursement rates, complex billing requirements, and increased risk associated with malpractice suits exist. Consequently, the availability of prenatal and obstetric services is severely compromised. Long waits for initial appointments and long waits at each visit impose considerable stress on homeless women obtaining prenatal care. Many providers find the unhealthy lifestyles, lack of compliance with provider advice, and failure to keep appointments unacceptable (Aday, 2001; Bloom, Bednarzyk, Devitt et al., 2004; Gelberg et al., 2008; Institute of Medicine, 1988).

CONCEPTUAL APPROACHES TO HEALTH OF THE HOMELESS

The following discussion provides a conceptual and theoretical framework for exploring health care of the homeless and outlines the market justice and social justice approaches to the distribution of benefits and burdens. It provides an explanation of social justice as the absence of structural violence, discusses upstream versus downstream approaches to homeless health care, and outlines a model of nursing positions related to social justice.

Models of justice provide a blueprint for considering the health problems of the homeless. Beauchamp (1979) distinguished between the two types of justice (i.e., market justice and social justice) that influence public health policy in the United States. Market justice has been the dominant model and purports that people are entitled to valued ends (i.e., status, income, and happiness) according to their own individual efforts. Moreover, this model stresses individual responsibility, minimal collective action, and freedom from collective obligations other than respect for another person's fundamental rights. In contrast, under a social justice model, all people are equally entitled to key ends (i.e., access to health care and minimum standards of income). Consequently, all members of society must accept collective burdens to provide a fair distribution of these ends. Moreover, social justice is a foundational aspect of public health (Krieger and Birn, 1998). More recently, others have noted the limits of the market approach. Citing the many problems inherent in the current health care system, they call for the need of a social justice approach to health care (Budetti, 2008; Pauly, MacKinnon, and Varcoe, 2009).

Additional explication of social justice is found in Galtung's analysis of violence. Distinguishing between physical and structural violence, Galtung (1969) defined violence as "present when human beings are being influenced so that their actual somatic and mental realizations are below their potential realization" (p. 168). The difference is between the actual and the possible. He further distinguished between physical and structural violence according to whether a person who acts is present. Galtung noted that when an actor is present who commits the violence, this is personal or direct violence. In contrast, structural violence is indirect because it lacks an actor. More specifically, the violence is built into the social structure and is displayed as unequal power and unequal life chances. Stated differently, resources are unevenly distributed (e.g., access to medical services from ability to pay or from location). Presence of structural violence is also known as social injustice. Conversely, its absence is social justice.

McKinlay's (1979) use of the metaphor depicted illness as a river; health workers focus exclusively on pulling people out of the river rather than going upstream to find out why people are in the river. Hence, the predominant mode of approaching societal problems is a downstream mode of intervention.

As McKinlay and Marceau (2000) note, a social philosophy that is focused on an individualistic approach is the dominant approach to public health problems in the United States. In this approach, individual people are the center of concern. Collectivism is a contrasting approach that focuses on "categories (age, sex, social class, race/ethnicity) or places and social positions in society" (p. 26), which is the more dominant theme in Europe.

McKinlay and Marceau (2000) argue that the market justice model, accompanied by an individualistic social model, results in a downstream approach to problems and contributes to structural violence. This model holds individuals responsible for their own conditions and negates the responsibility of all individuals and groups to share in the burdens of prevention. In contrast, the social justice model, which seeks to reduce the structural conditions contributing to the problem through collective action, supports upstream thinking.

Building on McKinlay's "river" metaphor, McKinlay and Marceau (2000) suggest conceptualizing homelessness as the river and the people in the river as the homeless. They purport that government and private efforts to address homeless health care problems largely focus on "pulling the bodies out of the river of homelessness." Such downstream interventions aimed at treating or alleviating health care problems such as physical disease and mental illnesses are worthy and needed. However, these interventions are far less adequate in alleviating homeless people's social health problems. To improve the social health of the homeless, it is necessary to go upstream and focus on the primary contributors to homelessness itself (i.e., lack of affordable housing, inadequate income, and insufficient services).

In contrast to the three macro-level approaches, market justice versus social justice, structural violence, and the downstream versus upstream approach to illness, Giddings' (2005) dialectical model of social consciousness provides a micro-level perspective useful in conceptualizing approaches to health care of the homeless. Based on her study of both marginalized and privileged nurses, she proposes three positions that describe relationships with social injustices—acquired, awakened, and expanded relationship. A nurse who reflects the acquired social consciousness position tends to be unaware of or does not acknowledge how people are treated differently, that is, privileged or oppressed, according to gender, class, ethnicity, sexual identity, or a differing worldview. The nurse in the awakened social consciousness position is aware of processes of unjust actions, may question dominant assumptions, and may join with others in resisting mainstream actions. When functioning in the expanded social consciousness position, the third position in Giddings' model, the nurse acknowledges that the processes of oppression place him or her in a privileged position while placing others in a subordinate marginalized role. The three positions are not mutually exclusive; one can function in more than one position simultaneously depending on the particular context.

Perspectives on the three macro-level approaches to the health of the homeless are related to the relationship of social injustice the individual nurse uses when viewing the three macro-level approaches. The nurse who operates within the socially expanded relationship to social injustice is better equipped to function in the upstream mode and identify why people are in the homeless river.

This section has presented conceptual approaches to homelessness. These include views of market and social justice influences on health care services, overviews of structural violence and its relationship with social injustice, and downstream thinking in public health. In addition, the section outlined is a model of social consciousness describing ways nurses approach social injustices.

CASE STUDY APPLICATION OF THE NURSING PROCESS

Katie Brown, a public health nurse (PHN), has just received a new referral from a transitional shelter for mothers and children located near the County Health Center where she is a member of the nursing staff. The shelter staff requests an assessment of a new client, Annie Jones, who is "having difficulty adapting to communal living." The referral indicates that Annie is a 33-year-old white mother of four children, although she currently has custody of only one child, a newborn girl. Her three other children reside in foster care.

Assessment

When Katie visits the shelter, she finds Annie sobbing in her room. Annie tells her she has a history of severe depression and has been hospitalized "many times." Annie reports that after the birth of her daughter, her physician recommended she not take her medications because she intended to breast feed the infant. Annie also informs the PHN that she has a long history of alcohol and methamphetamine use and that she left the father of the baby because he repeatedly assaulted her.

The shelter's case manager impatiently says that Annie's behavior disrupts the other shelter residents. She adds that the shelter cannot manage clients with psychiatric problems. Annie has a newborn, however, so they decided to give her special consideration. Tensions among Annie, the staff, and other clients clearly have begun to escalate, and Katie's past clinical experience reminds her that the community has few agencies that provide shelter and services to mothers with mental illness.

Diagnosis
Individual
- Client: Risk for ineffective health maintenance
- Infant: Risk for delayed development

Family
- Impaired home maintenance
- Risk for impaired parenting

Community
- Inadequate mental health services for women with children
- Inadequate affordable housing

Planning
Individual
Long-Term Goal
- Client will, in the next 6 months, engage in actions designed to maintain health of infant and self.

Short-Term Goal
- Client will, in the next week, follow through with scheduled appointments for identified health and social services.

Family
Long-Term Goal
- Client will adhere to plan she, shelter staff, and PHN formulated to assist her in adapting to shelter living and parenting.

Short-Term Goal
- Client will, in the next week, meet with shelter staff and PHN to develop a 6-month plan designed to assist her in adapting to shelter living and parenting.

Community
Long-Term Goal
- Increased capacity of mental health agencies to provide services for women with comorbidities and their children.

Short-Term Goal
- Enhanced ability of shelter staff to assist women who have comorbidities and are accompanied by children.

Interventions
Individual and Family
Katie consults with colleagues in the community who have experience working with persons who have co-occurring disorders (substance use disorder and other mental illness) and identifies resources for treatment. She discusses the importance of managing mental health problems with Annie and the case manager. Based on Annie's desires for care for herself and baby, Katie contacts the family nurse practitioner (FNP) at the County Health Center and arranges for an appointment the next day for health maintenance care for both Annie and her baby.

For psychiatric evaluation and treatment, Katie refers Annie to a community mental health agency that provides services to low-income and homeless persons. This agency has services especially designed for individuals with co-occurring disorders. Annie's case manager facilitates her care by assisting her to reestablish her Medicaid eligibility and begins to explore her eligibility for disability benefits under Supplemental Security Income (SSI).

Katie develops specific guidelines with Annie's case manager to monitor her progress in the shelter.

Community
Katie continues to work with the shelter staff to develop strategies for caring for Annie and her newborn. One strategy that Katie and staff used to provide care was to identify clear expectations for Annie in the shelter, including household tasks, management of her illness, and care of her newborn. As Annie gradually adapts to shelter living, Katie and staff assist her in keeping appointments for health and social services.

As a member of the local Interagency Council on Homelessness, Katie volunteered to serve on an ad hoc committee formed to identify housing needs of women with mental illness and substance use problems with special emphasis on women who had young children.

Evaluation
Individual and Family
Over the 6-month period, the case manager, Annie, and Katie met on a biweekly basis to review the overall situation and address any concerns that emerged.

Annie attended parenting classes with other shelter residents and weekly Narcotics Anonymous meetings. She also enrolled in the shelter's program that addresses intimate partner violence. Annie left her infant for short periods in the shelter's day care facility and attended a day treatment program at the community mental health agency. She resumed a prescribed antidepressant and initiated formula-feeding her baby. Gradually she adapted to shelter living. Having successfully met her goals, Annie was, at the end of 6 months, beginning to plan for moving to a more independent living facility.

Community
At the shelter's manager's request, Katie, in collaboration with colleagues at the Community Health Center, developed an in-service educational program for shelter staff. The program was designed to enhance the staff's skills in assisting women residents who had mental illness and substance use problems and who had young children. Staff indicated, in their self-reported evaluations, that the program provided helpful information. Katie also noted that the shelter was now providing services to several more women with problems similar to Annie's.

CASE STUDY   **APPLICATION OF THE NURSING PROCESS—cont'd**

The Interagency Council on Homelessness ad hoc committee completed the needs survey related to housing needs of women with mental illness and substance use problems. The committee has recommended to the Council that advocating for an increase in the supply of available housing for this at-risk population deserves a high priority, as it has the potential of preventing homelessness at all levels—primary, secondary, and tertiary.

Levels of Prevention
Primary
- Immunizations for Annie and her infant
- Promotion of policies designed to increase supply of affordable and accessible housing, health, and social services

Secondary
- Provision of services that enhance Annie's ability to maintain a residency for herself and her infant at the transitional shelter
- Periodic health screening services for Annie and her infant
- Advocating for policies and programs to assist homeless persons

Tertiary
- Treatment for Annie's mental illness and substance use disorder in order to prevent further deterioration

RESEARCH AND THE HOMELESS

Numerous circumstances complicate research on homelessness. Many of the data on individuals who are homeless are collected at only one point in time, and longitudinal studies are more limited because of factors such as the cost of research and the transient nature of homelessness. The presence of substance use disorders, other mental illnesses, and additional physical comorbidities compounds the difficulty of conducting research with this vulnerable population. To improve studies with difficult-to-reach and hidden populations, researchers have described specific strategies for locating participants over time, using incentives for participation, developing rapport with participants and community agency staff, and training peer-to-peer data collectors (Anderson and Hatton, 2000; Hatton and Kaiser, 2004; McKenzie, Tulsky, Long et al., 1999).

In spite of obstacles, a considerable body of research related to homelessness has developed over the past two decades from a variety of disciplines, including nursing. Offering both clinical and research perspectives, nurse scientists have considerable expertise to conduct research with this aggregate. Dr. Adeline Nyamathi and her colleagues at the Center for Vulnerable Populations Research, University of California Los Angeles, have examined drug and alcohol use, social support, HIV prevention education, perception of health status, victimization, and acculturation among individuals who are homeless (Nyamathi, Leake, and Gelberg, 2000; Nyamathi, Leake, Keenan et al., 2000; Nyamathi, Wenzel, Lesser et al., 2001; Nyamathi, Longshore, Galaif et al., 2004).

More recently, they have evaluated the effectiveness of nurse–case-managed interventions related to hepatitis A and B vaccines among adult shelter residents (Nyamathi, Liu, Marfisee et al., 2009) and adherence to latent tuberculosis infection treatment (Nyamathi, Nahid, Berg et al., 2008). Researchers from nursing and medicine also have advocated innovative research approaches and developed theoretical perspectives to guide studies of homelessness (Flaskerud and Winslow, 1998; Flaskerud, Lesser, Dixon et al., 2002; Gelberg, Andersen, and Leake, 2000).

In the last decade, homelessness research has become increasingly sophisticated and advocates have promoted a shift from research about individual characteristics to system change. Additionally, experts have argued for an increased emphasis on the evaluation of program effectiveness and service outcomes, especially programs geared toward individuals most at risk for homelessness, such as those with mental illness and other disabilities (Caton et al., 2007). Particularly important is the evaluation of services required by individuals who are chronically homeless and use a disproportionately larger share of public services. These types of investigations are difficult because of the complexity of designing community-based studies that include randomized control trials. In spite of these concerns, evidence from the evaluation of existing programs is critical for increased understanding of how to provide "evidence-based care" with persons experiencing homelessness.

Another development in the homelessness research literature is the increased documentation of the link between homelessness and incarceration. Recently, the Pew Center on the States (2008) reported that one in 100 persons in the United States is in jail or prison. For several decades, advocates have noted the disproportionate number of persons with mental illness in jails and prisons (Abram, Teplin, and McClelland, 2003; Blitz, Wolff, and Shi, 2008; Peternelj-Taylor, 2003; Peternelj-Taylor and Johnson, 1995; Steadman and Veysey, 1997; Teplin, Abram, and McClelland, 1996).

Recently, scientists have published several reports indicating that a history of homelessness before and after incarceration is far more common among prisoners than among the general population (Copeland, Miller, Welsh et al., 2009; Greenberg and Rosenheck, 2008a, 2008b; Metraux et al., 2007). Evidence also suggests that women prisoners are more likely to have a history of homelessness than men (Freudenberg, Moseley, Labriola et al., 2007). Advocates recommend that future research in this area focus on a clearer understanding of the association between homelessness and incarceration; the effectiveness of interventions aimed at preventing incarceration and homelessness; and consideration of incarceration and homelessness as they impact not only individuals, but also families (Metraux et al., 2007).

Farmer (1999, 2003) reminds us that research must not have an undue emphasis on the psychological or cultural peculiarities of vulnerable persons; he argues that an individualistic focus can limit our research to the effects of larger societal problems rather than on their causes. Although past homelessness research has focused on the study of individual characteristics and risk factors for homelessness, experts now point to the urgent need to evaluate best practices and consider how we change systems of care. The former U.S. Surgeon General, David Satcher (2006), in challenging the status quo, noted that:

We must keep in mind that America leads the world in science and that Americans have been awarded almost 50% of the Nobel Prizes in Medicine. We invest more in research, publicly and privately than any other country in the world. In spite of this, there are tremendous gaps here between what we know and what we do. (p. xii)

Many programs to prevent or reduce homelessness among individuals and families have demonstrated their effectiveness, but, most often, it is a lack of political will that impedes their implementation.

SUMMARY

Homelessness evolves from the interaction of complex factors at the societal level and among vulnerable individuals. Consequently, these individuals and families find themselves living in the streets, abandoned buildings, other public places, and shelters. Homeless people are heterogeneous, difficult to count, and suffer from a variety of complex health problems.

Their access to health care is problematic at best, and interventions to deal with this enormous problem represent largely downstream endeavors. Future research with members of this aggregate, which explores the complexity of their lives from a variety of methodological perspectives, will generate the knowledge necessary for more upstream community health nursing interventions.

LEARNING ACTIVITIES

1. Compare the information contained in the most recent U.S. Conference of Mayors Annual Report on Hunger and Homelessness with the information contained in the previous 3 years. What has changed?
2. Analyze at least three or four factors that contribute to homelessness in the United States.
3. Discuss common health problems found among homeless men, women, children, and adolescents.
4. Identify two special subgroups of the homeless and describe their health problems.
5. Describe the five specific areas of access identified by Penchansky and Thomas (1981). What is the significance of these areas for community health nursing practice with homeless individuals and families?
6. Use a market justice model and a social justice model to analyze how the United States has approached the health problems of the homeless.

REFERENCES

Abram KM, Teplin LA, McClelland GM: Comorbidity of severe psychiatric disorders and substance use disorders among women in jail, *Am J Psychiatry* 160(5):1007–1010, 2003.

Aday LA: *At risk in America : The health and health care needs of vulnerable populations in the United States*, ed 3, San Francisco, 2001, Jossey-Bass Publishers.

Anderson DG: Homeless women's perceptions about their families of origin, *West J Nurs Res* 18(1):29–42, 1996.

Anderson DG: Women, poverty, and workplace violence [Abstract], *Southern Online Journal of Nursing Research* 8(2):2, 2008.

Anderson DG, Hatton DC: Accessing vulnerable populations for research, *West J Nurs Res* 22(2):244–251, 2000.

Anderson DG, Rayens MK: Factors influencing homelessness in women, *Public Health Nurs* 21(1):12–23, 2004.

Aron L, Honberg R, Duckworth L, et al: *Grading the states 2009: A report on America's health care system for adults with serious mental illness*, Arlington, VA, 2009, National Alliance on Mental Illness. www.nami.org/gtsTemplate09. cfm?Section=Grading_the_States_ 2009&Template=/ ContentManagement/ContentDisplay. cfm&ContentID=75459.

Austin EL, Andersen R, Gelberg L: Ethnic differences in the correlates of mental

distress among homeless women, *Womens Health Issues* 18(1):26–34, 2008.

Bargh GJ, Hoch JS, Hwang SW, et al: Group A streptococcal carriage among residents of an urban homeless shelter, *The Canadian Journal of Infectious Diseases & Medical Microbiology* 18(5):316–317, 2007.

Bassuk EL: Social and economic hardships of homeless and other poor women, *Am J Orthopsychiatry* 63(3):340–347, 1993.

Bassuk EL, Buckner JC, Weinreb, et al: Homelessness in female-headed families: childhood and adult risk and protective factors, *Am J Public Health* 87(2):241–248, 1997.

Bassuk EL, Melnick S, Browne A: Responding to the needs of low-income and homeless women who are survivors of family violence, *J Am Med Wom Assoc* 53(2):57–64, 1998.

Bassuk EL, Weinreb LF, Buckner JC, et al: The characteristics and needs of sheltered homeless and low-income housed mothers, *JAMA* 276(8):640–646, 1996.

Beauchamp DE: Public health as social justice. In Jaco EG, editor: *Patients, physicians, and illness*, ed 3 New York, 1979, Free Press.

Blanchard J, Ogle K, Thomas O, et al: Access to appointments based on insurance status in Washington, DC, *J Health Care Poor Underserved* 19(3):687–696, 2008.

Blitz CL, Wolff N, Shi J: Physical victimization in prison: the role of mental illness, *Int J Law Psychiatry* 31(5):385–393, 2008.

Bloom KC, Bednarzyk MS, Devitt DL, et al: Barriers to prenatal care for homeless pregnant women, *J Obstet Gynecol Neonatal Nurs* 33(4):428–435, 2004.

Bucher SJ, Brickner PW, Vincent RL: Influenza like illness among homeless persons, *Emerg Infect Dis* 12(7):1162–1163, 2006.

Buckner JC: Understanding the impact of homelessness on children, *Am Behav Sci* 51(6):721–736, 2008.

Budetti PP: Market justice and US health care, *JAMA* 299(1):92–94, 2008.

Burt MR: Understanding homeless youth: numbers, characteristics, multisystem involvement and intervention options, June 19, 2007. Testimony: Subcommittee on Income Security and Family Support, U.S. House Ways and Means, www.urban.org/ UploadedPDF/901087_Burt_Homeless.pdf.

Burt MR, Aron LY, Douglas T, et al: Homelessness: Programs and the people they serve: A summary report of the findings of the national survey of homeless assistance providers and clients, Washington, DC, 1999, Urban Institute. www.urban.org/url.cfm?ID=310291.

Burt MR, Aron LY, Lee E: Helping America's homeless: emergency shelter or affordable housing? Washington, DC, 2001, Urban Institute Press.

Busen NH, Engebretson JC: Facilitating risk reduction among homeless and street-involved youth, *J Am Acad Nurse Pract* 20(11):567–575, 2008.

Caton CL, Dominguez B, Schanzer B, et al: Risk factors for long-term homelessness: findings from a longitudinal study of first-time homeless single adults, *Am J Public Health* 95(10):1753–1759, 2005.

Caton CL, Wilkins C, Anderson JA: People who experience long-term homelessness: Characteristics and interventions. Paper presented at Toward Understanding Homelessness: The 2007 National Symposium on Homelessness Research, Washington DC, 2007, http://aspe.hhs.gov/hsp/homelessness/symposium07/caton/report.pdf.

Centers for Disease Control and Prevention: Surveillance summaries: Youth risk behavior survey U.S. 2007, *MMWR Morb Mortal Wkly Rep* 57(SS–4), 2008.

Children's Defense Fund: *The state of America's children 2008: Annual report*, Washington, DC, 2008, Children's Defense Fund. www.childrensdefense.org/child-research-data-publications/data/state-of-americas-children-2008-report.pdf.

Copeland LA, Miller AL, Welsh DE, et al: Clinical and demographic factors associated with homelessness and incarceration among VA patients with bipolar disorder, *Am J Public Health* 99(5):871–877, 2009.

DeNavas-Walt C, Proctor BD, Smith JC: Income, poverty, and health insurance coverage in the United States: 2007, Curr Popul Rep No. P60-235. Washington, DC, 2008, U.S. Census Bureau. www.census.gov/prod/2008pubs/p60-235.pdf.

DeVoe JE, Graham AS, Angier H, et al: Obtaining health care services for low-income children: A hierarchy of needs, *J Health Care Poor Underserved* 19(4):1192–1211, 2008.

Duffield B, Lovell P: *The economic crisis hits home*, Minneapolis, MN, 2008, National Association for the Education of Homeless Children. First Focus: www.naehcy.org/dl/TheEconomicCrisisHitsHome.pdf.

Dworsky A: Educating homeless children in Chicago: A case study of children in the family regeneration program, 2008, www.chapinhall.org/sites/default/files/ChapinHallDocument(2).pdf. Accessed May 15, 2009.

Eyrich-Garg K, Cacciola JS, Carise D, et al: Individual characteristics of the literally homeless, marginally housed, and impoverished in a US substance abuse treatment–seeking sample, *Soc Psychiatry Psychiatr Epidemiol* 43(10):831–842, 2008.

Farmer P: *Infection and inequalities: The modern plagues*, Berkeley, CA, 1999, University of California Press.

Farmer P: *Pathologies of power: Health, human rights, and the new war on the poor*, Berkeley, CA, 2003, University of California Press.

Fazel S, Khosla V, Doll H, et al: The prevalence of mental disorders among the homeless in western countries: systematic review and meta-regression analysis, *PLoS Medicine/Public Library of Science* 5(12):e225, 2008.

Fernandes AL: *Runaway and homeless youth: demographics, programs and emerging issues*, (No. RL33785). Washington, DC, 2007, Congressional Research Services.

Flaskerud JH, Lesser J, Dixon E, et al: Health disparities among vulnerable populations: evolution of knowledge over five decades in nursing research publications, *Nurs Res* 51(2):74–85, 2002.

Flaskerud JH, Winslow BJ: Conceptualizing vulnerable populations health-related research, *Nurs Res* 47(2):69–78, 1998.

Folsom D, Jeste DV: Schizophrenia in homeless persons: a systematic review of the literature, *Acta Psychiatr Scand* 105(6):404–413, 2002.

Forney JC, Lombardo S, Toro PA: Diagnostic and other correlates of HIV risk behaviors in a probability sample of homeless adults, *Psychiatric Serv* 58(1):92–99, 2007.

Freudenberg N, Daniels J, Crum M, et al: Coming home from jail: the social and health consequences of community reentry for women, male adolescents, and their families and communities, *Am J Public Health* 95(10):1725–1736, 2005.

Freudenberg N, Moseley J, Labriola M, et al: Comparison of health and social characteristics of people leaving New York city jails by age, gender, and race/ethnicity: implications for public health interventions, *Public Health Rep* 122(6):733–743, 2007.

Galtung J: Violence, peace, and peace research, *Peace Res* 16:167–191, 1969.

Gelberg L, Andersen RM, Leake BD: The behavioral model for vulnerable populations: application to medical care use and outcomes for homeless people, *Health Serv Res* 34(6):1273–1302, 2000.

Gelberg L, Lu MC, Leake BD, et al: Homeless women: who is really at risk for unintended pregnancy? *Matern Child Health J* 12(1):52–60, 2008.

Giddings LS: A theoretical model of social consciousness, *ANS Adv Nurs Sci* 28(3):224–239, 2005.

Goldstein G, Luther JF, Jacoby AM, et al: A preliminary classification system for homeless veterans with mental illness, *Psychological Serv* 5(1):36–48, 2008.

Grant R, Shapiro A, Joseph S, et al: The health of homeless children revisited, *Adv Pediatr* 54:173–187, 2007.

Greenberg GA, Rosenheck RA: Homelessness in the state and federal prison population, *Crim Behav Ment Health* 18(2):88–103, 2008a.

Greenberg GA, Rosenheck RA: Jail incarceration, homelessness, and mental health: a national study, *Psychiatric Serv* 59(2):170–177, 2008b.

Grossman E, Legedza AT, Wee CC: Primary care for low-income populations: comparing health care delivery systems, *J Health Care Poor Underserved* 19(3):743–757, 2008.

Hatton DC, Fisher AA: Incarceration and the new asylums: consequences for the mental health of women prisoners, *Issues Ment Health Nurs* 29(12):1304–1307, 2008.

Hatton DC, Kaiser L: Methodological and ethical issues emerging from pilot testing an intervention with women in a transitional shelter, *West J Nurs Res* 26(1):129–136, 2004.

Hoffman C, Paradise J: Health insurance and access to health care in the United States, *Ann N Y Acad Sci* 1136:149–160, 2008.

Huntington N, Buckner JC, Bassuk EL: Adaptation in homeless children: An empirical examination using cluster analysis, *Am Behav Sci* 51(6):737–755, 2008.

Hwang SW, Colantonio A, Chiu S, et al: The effect of traumatic brain injury on the health of homeless people, *CMAJ* 179(8):779–784, 2008.

Institute of Medicine: *Homelessness, health, and human needs*, Washington DC, 1988, National Academy Press.

Jencks C. *The homeless*, Cambridge, MA, 1995, Harvard University Press.

Kertesz SG, Weiner SJ: Housing the chronically homeless: high hopes, complex realities, *JAMA* 301(17):1822–1824, 2009.

Khadduri J: Housing vouchers are critical for ending family homelessness, Washington DC, January 2008, The Homelessness Research Institute, www.endhomelessness.org/files/1875_file_10976_HousingVouchers.pdf.

Kidder DP, Wolitski RJ, Campsmith ML, et al: Health status, health care use, medication use, and medication adherence among homeless and housed people living with HIV/AIDS, *Am J Public Health* 97(12):2238–2245, 2007.

Kim DH, Daskalakis C, Plumb JD, et al: Modifiable cardiovascular risk factors among individuals in low socioeconomic communities and homeless shelters, *Fam Community Health* 31(4):269–280, 2008.

Kozol J: *Rachel and her children: Homeless families in America*, New York, 1988, Crown.

Krieger N, Birn AE: A vision of social justice as the foundation of public health: commemorating 150 years of the spirit of 1848, *Am J Public Health* 88(11):1603–1606, 1998.

Kuhn R, Culhane DP: Applying cluster analysis to test a typology of homelessness by pattern of shelter utilization: results from the analysis of administrative data, *Am J Community Psychol* 26(2):207–232, 1998.

Lambert EY, Caces MF: Correlates of drug abuse among homeless and transient people in the Washington, DC, metropolitan area in 1991, *Public Health Rep* 110(4):455–461, 1995.

Larimer ME, Malone DK, Garner MD, et al: Health care and public service use and costs before and after provision of housing for chronically homeless persons with severe alcohol problems, *JAMA* 301(13):1349–1357, 2009.

Mares AS, Greenberg GA, Rosenheck RA: Client-level measures of services integration among chronically homeless adults, *Community Ment Health J* 44(5):367–376, 2008.

Martens WH: A review of physical and mental health in homeless persons, *Public Health Rev* 29(1):13–33, 2001.

Martins DC: Experiences of homeless people in the health care delivery system: a descriptive phenomenological study, *Public Health Nurs* 25(5):420–430, 2008.

McKenzie M, Tulsky JP, Long HL, et al: Tracking and follow-up of marginalized populations: a review, *J Health Care Poor Underserved* 10(4):409–429, 1999.

McKinlay JB: A case for refocusing upstream; the political economy of illness. In Jaco EG, editor: *Patients, physicians, and illness*, ed 3, New York, 1979, Free Press.

McKinlay JB, Marceau LD: To boldly go...., *Am J Public Health* 90(1):25–33, 2000.

Metraux S, Caternia R, Cho R: *Incarceration and homelessness*. Paper presented at Toward Understanding Homelessness: The 2007 National Symposium on Homelessness Research, 2007, Washington, DC, http://aspe.hhs.gov/hsp/homelessness/symposium07/metraux/report.pdf.

Molino A: *Characteristics of help-seeking street youth and non-street youth*, Washington, DC, 2007, U.S. Department of Health and Human Services, Office of the Assistant Secretary for Planning and Evaluation, http://aspe.hhs.gov/hsp/homelessness/symposium07/molino/index.htm.

National Alliance to End Homelessness: *Homelessness looms as potential outcome of recession*, Washington, DC, January 23, 2009, The Author, www.endhomelessness.org/content/article/detail/2161/.

National Center on Family Homelessness: *America's youngest outcasts: state report card on child homelessness*, Newton MA, 2009, The Author, http://www.homelesschildrenamerica.org/pdf/rc_full_report.pdf.

National Coalition for the Homeless: *Why are people homeless?*, NCH Fact Sheet No. 1. Washington DC, 2008, National Coalition for the Homeless, http://www.nationalhomeless.org/publications/facts/why.html.

National Research Council and Institute of Medicine: *Adolescent health services: missing opportunities*, Washington, DC, 2009, National Academies Press.

North CS, Eyrich KM, Pollio DE, et al: Are rates of psychiatric disorders in the homeless population changing? *Am J Public Health* 94(1):103–108, 2004.

Nyamathi A, Flaskerud J, Leake B: HIV-risk behaviors and mental health characteristics among homeless or drug-recovering women and their closest sources of social support, *Nurs Res* 46(3):133–137, 1997.

Nyamathi A, Leake B, Gelberg L: Sheltered versus nonsheltered homeless women differences in health, behavior, victimization, and utilization of care, *J Gen Intern Med* 15(8):565–572, 2000.

Nyamathi A, Leake B, Keenan C, Gelberg L: Type of social support among homeless women: its impact on psychosocial resources, health and health behaviors, and use of health services, *Nurs Res* 49(6):318–326, 2000.

Nyamathi A, Liu Y, Marfisee M, et al: Effects of a nurse-managed program on hepatitis A and B vaccine completion among homeless adults, *Nurs Res* 58(1):13–22, 2009.

Nyamathi A, Longshore D, Galaif ER, et al: Motivation to stop substance use and psychological and environmental characteristics of homeless women, *Addict Behav* 29(9):1839–1843, 2004.

Nyamathi A, Nahid P, Berg J, et al: Efficacy of nurse case-managed intervention for latent tuberculosis among homeless subsamples, *Nurs Res* 57(1):33–39, 2008.

Nyamathi A, Wenzel SL, Lesser J, et al: Comparison of psychosocial and behavioral profiles of victimized and nonvictimized homeless women and their intimate partners, *Res Nurs Health* 24(4):324–335, 2001.

Obradovic J, Long JD, Cutulia A, et al: Academic achievement of homeless and highly mobile children in an urban school district: longitudinal evidence on risk, growth, and resilience, *Dev Psychopathol* 21:493–518, 2009.

O'Flaherty B: *Making room: The economics of homelessness*, Cambridge, MA, 1996, Harvard University Press.

Padgett DK, Henwood B, Abrams C, et al: Social relationships among persons who have experienced serious mental illness, substance abuse, and homelessness: implications for recovery, *Am J Orthopsychiatry* 78(3):333–339, 2008.

Pauly BM, MacKinnon K, Varcoe C: Revisiting "who gets care?", Health equity as an arena for nursing action, *ANS Adv Nurs Sci* 32(2):118–127, 2009.

Pearson DA, Bruggman AR, Haukoos JS: Out-of-hospital and emergency department utilization by adult homeless patients, *Ann Emerg Med* 50(6):646–652, 2007.

Penchansky R, Thomas JW: The concept of access: definition and relationship to consumer satisfaction, *Med Care* 19(2):127–140, 1981.

Peternelj-Taylor C: Incarceration of vulnerable populations, *J Psychosoc Nurs Ment Health Serv* 41(9):4–5, 2003.

Peternelj-Taylor CA, Johnson RL: Serving time: psychiatric mental health nursing in corrections, *J Psychosoc Nurs Ment Health Serv* 33(8):12–19, 1995.

Pew Center on the States: *One in 100: Behind bars in America 2008*, 2008, Pew Charitable Trusts, www.pewcenteronthestates.org/uploadedFiles/8015PCTS_Prison08_FINAL_2-1-1_FORWEB.pdf.

Reid KW, Vittinghoff E, Kushel MB: Association between the level of housing instability, economic standing and health care access: a meta-regression, *J Health Care Poor Underserved* 19(4):1212–1228, 2008.

Rew L, Grady M, Whittaker TA, Bowman K: Interaction of duration of homelessness and gender on adolescent sexual health indicators, *J Nurs Scholarsh* 40(2):109–115, 2008.

Rew L, Rochlen AB, Murphey C: Health educators' perceptions of a sexual health intervention for homeless adolescents, *Patient Educ Couns* 72(1):71–77, 2008.

Rice D, Sard B: *Decade of neglect has weakened federal low-income housing programs*, Washington, DC, 2009, Center on Budget and Policy Priorities, www.cbpp.org/files/2-24-09hous.pdf.

Rog D, Buckner J: *Homeless families and children*. Paper presented at Toward Understanding Homelessness: The 2007 National Symposium on Homelessness Research, Washington, DC, 2007, http://aspe.hhs.gov/hsp/homelessness/symposium07/rog/report.pdf.

Roschelle AR: Welfare indignities: homeless women, domestic violence, and welfare reform in San Francisco, *Gender Issues* 25(3):193–209, 2008.

Rosen J: *NPACH statement on the HEARTH Act*, 2009, http://npach.org/2009/05/npach_statement_on_hearth_act_1.html. Accessed May 21, 2009.

Rossi PH: The old homeless and the new homelessness in historical perspective, *Am Psychol* 45:954–959, 1990.

Sadowski LS, Kee RA, VanderWeele TJ, et al: Effect of a housing and case management program on emergency department visits and hospitalizations among chronically ill homeless adults: a randomized trial, *JAMA* 301(17):1771–1778, 2009.

Satcher D: Challenging the status quo, *J Health Care Poor Underserved* 17(1):xii–xiv, 2006.

Schanzer B, Dominguez B, Shrout PE, et al: Homelessness, health status, and health care use, *Am J Public Health* 97(3):464–469, 2007.

Sermons W, Henry M: *Homelessness counts: Changes in homelessness from 2005 to 2007*, Washington, DC, 2009, National Alliance to End Homelessness, Homelessness Research Institute.

Shields AE, McGinn-Shapiro M, Fronstin P: Trends in private insurance, Medicaid/State children's health insurance program, and the healthcare safety net: implications for vulnerable populations and health disparities, *Ann N Y Acad Sci* 1136:137–148, 2008.

Shinn M, Baumohl J: *Rethinking the prevention of homelessness*. Paper presented at Practical Lessons: The 1998 National Symposium on Homelessness Research, Arlington, VA, 1999, http://aspe.hhs.gov/homeless/symposium/13-Preven.HTM.

Shinn M, Schteingart JS, Williams NC, et al: Long-term associations of homelessness with children's well-being, *Am Behav Sci* 51(6):789–809, 2008.

Silverstein M, Lamberto J, DePeau K, et al: "You get what you get": Unexpected findings about low-income parents' negative experiences with community resources, *Pediatrics* 122(6):e1141–e1148, 2008.

Slesnick N, Dashora P, Letcher A, et al: A review of services and interventions for runaway and homeless youth: moving forward, *Children & Youth Services Review* 31(7): 732–742, 2009.

Smith AD, Smith DI: *Emergency and transitional shelter population 2000, special reports* (No. CENSR/01-2), Washington, DC, 2001, U.S. Census Bureau, www.census.gov/prod/2001pubs/censr01-2.pdf.

Smyth KF, Goodman L, Glenn C: The full-frame approach: a new response to marginalized women left behind by specialized services, *Am J Orthopsychiatry* 76(4):489–502, 2006.

Steadman HJ, Veysey BM: *Providing services for jail inmates with mental disorders* (Research in Brief No. NCJ 162207). Washington DC, 1997, U.S. Department of Justice, www.ncjrs.gov/pdffiles/162207.pdf.

Stein JA, Lu MC, Gelberg L. Severity of homelessness and adverse birth outcomes, *Health Psychol* 19(6):524–534, 2000.

Street Health: *The street health report 2007: Homelessness, mental health, & substance use,* Research Bulletin No. 4. Toronto, 2009, The Author, www.streethealth.ca/Downloads/SHResearchBulletin-4.pdf.

Teplin LA, Abram KM, McClelland GM: Prevalence of psychiatric disorders among incarcerated women. I. Pretrial jail detainees, *Arch Gen Psychiatry* 53(6):505–512, 1996.

Tevendale HD, Lightfoot M, Slocum SL: Individual and environmental protective factors for risky sexual behavior among homeless youth: an exploration of gender differences, *AIDS Behav* 13(1):154–164, 2009.

Toro P, Dworsky A, Fowler P: *Homeless youth in the United States: Recent research findings and intervention approaches.* Paper presented at the 2007 National Symposium on Homelessness Research, Washington, DC, 2007, http://aspe.hhs.gov/hsp/homelessness/symposium07/Toro/report.pdf.

U.S. Conference of Mayors: *Hunger and homelessness survey 2008: A status report on hunger and homelessness in America's cities,* 2008a. Retrieved from www.usmayors.org/pressreleases/documents/hungerhomelessnessreport_121208.pdf.

U.S. Conference of Mayors: *Mayors examine causes of hunger, homelessness,* 2008b. http://usmayors.org/pressreleases/documents/hungerhomelessness_121208.pdf.

U.S. Department of Education: *Education for homeless children and youth,* 2004, http://www.ed.gov/policy/elsec/leg/esea02/pg116.html#sec725. Accessed March 30, 2009.

U.S. Department of Health and Human Services: *Ending chronic homelessness,* Washington, DC, 2003a, http://aspe.hhs.gov/hsp/homelessness/strategies03/index.htm.

U.S. Department of Health and Human Services: *Secretary's work group on ending chronic homelessness: Strategies for action, Chapter 2,* Washington, DC, 2003b, http://aspe.hhs.gov/hsp/homelessness/strategies03/ch.htm#ch2.

U.S. Department of Health and Human Services, Centers for Disease Control and Prevention: *Reported tuberculosis in the United States, 2007,* Atlanta, GA, 2008, The Author, www.cdc.gov.jproxy.lib.ecu.edu/tb/.

U.S. Department of Health and Human Services, Substance Abuse and Mental Health Services Administration, Center for Substance Abuse Treatment: *Addressing co-occurring disorders in non-traditional service settings,* 2007, COCE overview paper No. 4. DHHS Publication No. (SMA) 07-4277, www.coce.samhsa.gov/cod_resources/PDF/OP4-SpecialSettings-8-13-07.pdf.

U.S. Department of Housing and Urban Development: *Federal definition of homeless,* 2007, www.hud.gov/homeless/definition.cfm. Accessed March 30, 2009.

U.S. Department of Housing and Urban Development: *Homeless information management systems (HMIS),* 2009, www.hud.gov/offices/cpd/homeless/hmis/. Accessed May 15, 2009.

U.S. Department of Housing and Urban Development, Office of Community Planning and Development: *The third annual homeless assessment report,* Washington, DC, 2008, www.hudhre.info/documents/3rdHomelessAssessmentReport.pdf.

U.S. Department of Housing and Urban Development, Office of Policy Development and Research: *Affordable housing needs 2005: Report to Congress,* Washington, DC, 2007, The Author, www.huduser.org/Publications/pdf/AffHsgNeeds.pdf.

U.S. Department of Labor, Employment Standards Administration, Wage and Hour Division: *Handy reference guide to the Fair Labor Standards Act,* WH Publication No. 1282. Washington, DC, 2007, The Author, www.dol.gov/esa/whd/regs/compliance/wh1282.pdf.

Vissing YM, Hudson C: *Issues in enumerating homeless children and youth.* Paper presented at the NAEHCY 2008 Annual Conference, Crystal City, VA, 2008, www.naehcy.org/conf/2008_conf_sess_mat.html.

Wardrip KE, Pelletiere D, Crowley S: *Out of reach 2009,* Washington, DC, 2009, National Low Income Housing Coalition, www.nlihc.org/oor/oor2009/oor2009pub.pdf.

Weinreb LF, Buckner JC, Williams V, et al: A comparison of the health and mental health status of homeless mothers in Worcester, MA, 1993 and 2003, *Am J Public Health* 96(8):1444–1448, 2006.

Wenzel SL, Leake BD, Gelberg L: Health of homeless women with recent experience of rape, *J Gen Intern Med* 15(4):265–268, 2000.

Wolitski RJ, Kidder DP, Fenton KA: HIV, homelessness, and public health: critical issues and a call for increased action, *AIDS Behav* 11:S167–S171, 2007.

World Health Organization: *WHO definition of health, preamble to the constitution of the World Health Organization as adopted by the International Health Conference, New York, 19–22 June, 1946; signed on 22 July 1946 by the representatives of 61 states (Official records of the World Health Organization, no. 2, p. 100) and entered into force on 7 April 1948,* 1948, World Health Organization, www.who.int/entity/governance/eb/who_constitution_en.pdf.

Wright JD: Poor people poor health: the health status of the homeless, *J of Soc Issues* 46:49–64, 1990.

Wright JD, Rubin BA, Devine JA: *Beside the golden door: policy politics and the homeless,* New York, 1998, Aldine de Gruyter.

Yu M, North CS, LaVesser PD, et al: A comparison study of psychiatric and behavior disorders and cognitive ability among homeless and housed children, *Community Ment Health J* 44(1):1–10, 2008.

Zerger S, Strehlow AJ, Gundlapalli AV: Homeless young adults and behavioral health, *Am Behav Sci* 51(6):824–841, 2008.

Zlotnick C, Zerger S: Survey findings on characteristics and health status of clients treated by the federally funded (US) health care for the homeless programs, *Health Soc Care Community* 17(1):18–26, 2009.

Rural and Migrant Health

*Patricia L. Thomas, Patti J. Shoe**

Additional Material for Study, Review, and Further Exploration

evolve WEBSITE

http://evolve.elsevier.com/Nies
- Quiz
- Case Studies
- Glossary
- WebLinks

OBJECTIVES

Upon completion of this chapter, the reader will be able to do the following:
1. Compare and contrast characteristics of rural and urban communities.
2. Describe features of the health care system and population characteristics common to rural aggregates.
3. Discuss the impact of structural and personal barriers on the health of rural aggregates.
4. Identify factors that place farmers and migrant workers at risk for illness and accidents.
5. Discuss the importance of the informal care network to rural health and social services.
6. Describe the characteristics of rural community health nursing practice.
7. Apply an upstream perspective to health promotion and illness prevention for rural and migrant populations.

KEY TERMS

disparities
frontier
metropolitan

migrant farmworkers
pesticide
rural

seasonal farmworkers
urban

OUTLINE

*The authors would like to acknowledge the contribution of Kathleen Chafey, Wade G. Hill, and Glenna R. Burg, who wrote this chapter for the previous edition.

RURAL UNITED STATES

There are many different versions of rural America, in that each rural area is unique in some respects but shares certain features with other rural regions. Geographic, demographic, environmental, economic, and social factors all influence health, access to health care, and quality of health care. When aggregated, these characteristics may be contrasted with those of urban populations. In this section, we present a "snapshot" of rural population and health characteristics that contribute to challenging health disparities for many of the people living in the most rural areas of America.

Although the urban growth rate has been steadily climbing since 1890, with numbers of urban dwellers surpassing those in rural areas around 1920, the number of rural residents is the highest in the country's history (U.S. Department of Agriculture [USDA], 2008). The number and size of rural counties are highest in the South (35%), followed by the Midwest and West (23%), and Northeast (19%) (USDA, 2007). Current census estimates are that 18% of the nation's children under age 18 years live in rural areas (USDA, 2005), as do 15% of the nation's elderly, and more than 50% of the nation's poor (USDA, 2007).

The economic base of rural America is changing rapidly. Whereas rural residents have long been thought to be family farmers and ranchers, today rural America is a diverse and important marketplace to marketers of consumer products, and demographers and economists consider trends in farm and farm-related employment much more broadly. They characterize agriculture as a "food and fiber system" that encompasses all aspects of agriculture, from core materials sectors (farm, food processing, textiles, and other manufacturing) to wholesale and retail trade and the food service sector (Edmondson, 2004). Despite the shrinking number of family farms and full-time farmers, agriculture continues to be an important part of the rural and U.S. economy.

Poverty, a key health determinant, continues to be greater in rural America than in urban areas. Whereas the metropolitan population had a poverty rate of 11% in 2002, the rural population had a poverty rate of 14%. This overall gap may not seem large, but when the degree of rurality or the poverty rate for particular subpopulations (e.g., minorities, children under 18 years of age, or the elderly) is examined, the gap increases greatly. For example, the poverty rate for non-Hispanic blacks in nonmetropolitan areas in 2002 was 33%, compared with a rate of 23% for the same group in metropolitan areas. The poverty rate for people in the rural South was 18%, versus 13% for Southerners living in and around metropolitan areas (USDA, 2005).

Not only is the economic base shifting, the age composition is as well. Many rural areas are growing, especially in the West and South, and many rural counties, especially in the Great Plains states, are losing population because of a decline in agricultural and manufacturing jobs. Younger people are leaving rural areas for jobs in urban centers, so that those who remain behind are increasingly older and isolated and have diminished access to health care (Whitener and McGranahan, 2003). Recent demographic changes in rural areas have also included an influx of retirees and others from urban areas, who are able to live in rural areas and conduct business through telecommunication and travel (Malecki, 2003). Recent demographic data indicate that rural persons aged 60 years and older comprise 20% of the population of nonmetropolitan areas, in contrast to 15% of the population of urban areas (Rogers, 2002). Of the nation's rural elderly, the largest clusters live in the South (45%) and the Midwest (31%) (Rogers, 2002). The trends of "aging-in-place, out-migration of young adults, and immigration of older persons from metro areas" (Rogers, 2002, p. 2) present challenges to already stressed communities that must provide adequate health care, housing, transportation, and other human services.

The rural population is also becoming more ethnically diverse. Generations ago, many families began farming when they came to the United States as European immigrants. In the 1990s, new immigrants began buying and operating their own small family farms, and others found employment in rural agriculture and manufacturing. Today, nearly one half of rural Hispanics live outside the Southwest, and "high-growth Hispanic counties" are mostly in the South and Midwest (Kandel and Newman, 2004). Hispanics are now the most rapidly growing demographic group in rural and small-town America.

Policies and programs developed to close the health disparities gap must take a population health view of the special circumstances of rural life. Although 75% of U.S. counties are classified as rural, they contain only 20% of the U.S. population. Members of rural populations also are more likely to be older, to be less educated, to live in poverty, to lack health insurance, and to experience a lack of available health care providers and access to health care. Only 10% of U.S. physicians practice in rural counties (Crouse, 2007), and the ratio of medical specialists to rural population size is forty per 100,000 people (compared with 134 per 100,000 in urban settings) (Berkowitz, 2004).

Rural residents more often assess their health as fair or poor and have more disability days associated with acute conditions than their urban counterparts. Rural people also tend to have more problems related to negative health behaviors (e.g., obesity and alcohol, tobacco, and drug use) that contribute to excess deaths and chronic disease and disability rates. The literature suggests, for example, that the highest death rates for children and young adults were in the most rural counties. Residents of rural areas are nearly twice as likely to die of unintentional injuries, including motor vehicle accidents, when compared with their urban counterparts (National Rural Health Association [NRHA], 2008).

Noting a prominent and persistent pattern of risky health behaviors in rural dwellers, Hartley (2004) has suggested that "rural culture" may itself be a key determinant of health in rural communities and these behaviors vary along the rural-urban continuum and within rural populations by geographic areas. These behaviors, including unintentional injury, smoking, and suicide will be discussed in more detail in the section titled Composition: Health Disparities Related to Persons.

Defining Rural Populations

Multiple definitions of rural populations have been formulated to describe the characteristics of low-population-density areas. Previous definitions have simply included either those towns with a population of less than 2500 or towns located in open country as rural. This definition has often been further differentiated into subcategories of farm and rural nonfarm. A second classification of interest used the term *rural* for populations with fewer than forty-five persons per square mile, and the term frontier for geographic areas with fewer than six people per square mile (Rural Health Assistance Center, 2010). Many counties of the Great Plains, Intermountain West, and Alaska are designated frontier.

The rural-urban continuum distinguishes counties by population and adjacency to metropolitan areas. Residences can range from small towns to large metropolitan areas. Statistical reporting has been in use since 1990. Census maps and statistical reports in use since the 1990s used the term *Metropolitan Statistical Areas (MSAs)* to differentiate nonmetropolitan and metropolitan areas. In June 2003, however, the Office of Management and Budget (OMB) released a new classification scheme, developed in 2000, to better reflect trends in population distribution across the nation (OMB, 2008). The MSA designation has been replaced by county-level *Core Based Statistical Areas (CBSAs)*, which make up a new classification scheme to simplify the multilevel designations in use since 1990. The new CBSA system includes two categories of counties: *metropolitan* areas and *micropolitan* areas. Counties that are neither metropolitan nor micropolitan are called "outside CBSAs," also known as noncare areas. Within CBSAs, metropolitan areas are those counties that contain at least one urbanized area of 50,000 or more people. A micropolitan area contains a cluster of 10,000 to 50,000 persons. Because the MSA classification is used extensively for congressional policymaking and funding

decisions, the change could have serious ramifications for health care financing within rural market areas.

Describing Rural Health and Populations

Rural populations differ in complex geographic, social, and economic areas. Although older, poorer, and less-educated people are usually overrepresented in rural areas, this may not apply to all rural areas or to everyone in a particular rural area.

The health profiles discussed below are shared by rural areas in general and may be contrasted with overall patterns of health, health habits, and health care in urban settings. However, the reader should note that it is difficult to interpret differences between urban and rural health. First, statistically significant differences between urban and rural health indicators may seem small when data are aggregated to "rural areas" in general. The differences tend to become larger when data are available for particular rural areas (e.g., certain counties), particular rural subgroups (e.g., minorities), or specific characteristics (e.g., percentage of uninsured children). Second, heterogeneity of race, age, economic status, regional distribution, and cultural groupings makes health data for rural populations useful only as estimates of individual health. For example, there were 37.3 million people in poverty in 2007, up from 36.5 million in 2006. The family poverty rate was 9.8%, unchanged from 2006. Furthermore, the poverty rate and the number in poverty showed no statistical change between 2006 and 2007 for the different types of families (U.S. Census Bureau, 2008b).

Infant mortality, a major health status indicator, varies greatly by geographic area, even within rural areas, and dramatizes the importance of both contextual and compositional data. For non-Hispanic whites, the rates of infant deaths per 1000 live births continued a downward trend. For black Americans, the rate of infant deaths is 2.5 times that of whites and Hispanics. In both the South and West, rural counties experienced the highest rates (24% and 30% higher than fringe areas of large metro areas) (Hoyert, Kung, and Smith, 2005). Infant mortality rates ranged from 10.32 per 1000 live births for Mississippi to 4.68 per 1000 live births for Vermont. The highest rate noted (11.42) was for the District of Columbia. Overall, the infant mortality rate declined 10% from 1995 until 2004 (7.57); however, the rate has not declined much since 2000. From 2000 until 2005, small declines were observed for all races and ethnic groups. Significant decreases were noted for infants of Central and South American (4.68), Asian or Pacific Islander (8.06), and Mexican (5.53) (Centers for Disease Control and Prevention [CDC], 2008).

Mortality for white infants in rural areas adjacent to a population center with fewer than 2500 people varied from a high of 9.85 per 1000 in the South, to 6.46 per 1000 in the West. Although the infant mortality rates have changed since 1993, infant mortality data provide insight into the heterogeneity of rural populations and show why national or even regional data may or may not reflect the status quo for a particular county or local population.

One might also consider the health disparities that exist among rural racial and ethnic minorities. Although limited because the phenomenon has only recently been studied, research findings support the conclusion that rural racial and ethnic minorities—Native Americans, Alaska Natives, Hispanics/Latinos, and African Americans—concentrated in the South and West are more disadvantaged, not only relative to rural majority members, but also relative to urban racial and ethnic minorities. The disparities include employment, income, education, health insurance, mortality, morbidity, and access to care (Probst, Moore, Glover et al., 2004).

Because population numbers are small, national rural data, limited as the data are, can only suggest the health needs of a particular area, racial or ethnic mix, or age distribution, for example. Program planners will still need to determine whether certain health or health care delivery problems apply to their specific service area. Useful data sources include state, county, and census tract level data on health and demographics available from state and federal government agencies, such as those cited in the reference section of this chapter. In planning for health-related programs, nurses can also gather community-level data from health care providers, local records, focus groups, and older residents who know the area's history.

RURAL *HEALTHY PEOPLE 2020*

Minority Health and *Healthy People 2020*

Healthy People 2020 represents the health promotion and disease prevention agenda for the nation (Office of Disease Prevention and Health Promotion, U.S. Department of Health and Human Services [USDHHS], nd). Additionally, *Healthy People 2020* is the United States' contribution to the World Health Organization's Health for All program. The framework for *Healthy People 2020*, developed through public consensus, builds upon the national health program established since the 1980s. It includes the broad goals of increasing quality of life and years of life, eliminating disparities in health among different population groups, and increasing access to preventive health services.

Healthy People 2020 is based on the premise that the health of the individual is almost "inseparable from the health of the larger community and that the health of every community in every State and territory determines the overall health status of the Nation" (USDHHS, 2000, p. 2). The new 10-year plan takes a bold step forward by presenting only one set of standards for the health of all racial, ethnic, income, gender, and age-groups. The new goal is to eliminate health disparities, achieve access to preventive health services, and add years of life for all groups. The challenges are great, but public health professionals and planners in every state have, or soon will have, a plan patterned on *Healthy People 2020* goals to direct their efforts. A three-volume companion document to *Healthy People 2010*, entitled *Rural Public Health 2010*, has been published. These reports are designed to "better inform readers on current rural health conditions, provide insights into possible points of attack, and offer examples of models that might be employed in practice to improve health conditions" (Gamm and Hutchison, 2004, p. vi).

Rural Health Disparities: Context and Composition

To better understand the health of populations and health disparities, there is also a growing emphasis on the distinction between context, which is defined by the characteristics of places of residence, and composition, which are the collective health effects that result from a concentration of persons with certain characteristics (Probst et al., 2004). Most public health problems include elements of both context and composition, though they may be predominately one or the other (Phillips, 2004; Probst et al., 2004).

Health issues in rural areas are contextual when they derive from characteristics of place. Characteristics of place include not only natural features of geography and environment, but also the political, social, and economic institutions that build and support communities within given geographic areas. For example, limited economic opportunities, low wages, or agricultural accidents might be considered to have contextual effects on the health of populations. Problems in rural areas are compositional when they derive from individual characteristics of groups of people residing in rural settings. Examples of compositional sources of health disparities include such characteristics as age, education, income, ethnicity, and health behaviors.

Consideration of both context and composition enables us to take a more deliberate and refined approach to study, plan programs, and deliver health care services to rural populations. Although the overall health of rural Americans is worse when compared with that of urban Americans, the relationship between rurality and health is not necessarily linear. Many differences exist between rural areas in both the nature and extent of health problems. Furthermore, some rural populations share more in common with people in urban core areas than with other rural areas. Effective planning depends on understanding and documenting needs that take into account context, composition, and their interaction (Eberhardt and Pamuk, 2004). The next section presents data for problems of both contextual and compositional sources of health disparities in rural America.

Context: Health Disparities Related to Place

Regardless of their diverse demographic and geographic attributes, rural groups share certain health patterns, difficulties, and delays in obtaining health care (Ethical Insights box). Many of the contextual issues that contribute to rural health disparities are described in the introduction to the chapter (Rural United States). Many rural regions that are already sparsely populated are losing residents, which often triggers a downward spiral. People leave and services are lost; the local drugstore closes; the tax base will not support an ambulance service; most seriously ill persons must be transported long distances to get health care; jobs become scarce and younger people leave the area. Retirees may be attracted to the lower costs, but they need public health and other services provided by counties without the tax base to support them. Racial and ethnic minorities are migrating to rural areas to find employment opportunities. Structural, financial, and personal barriers to accessing health care services exist in all environments, but rural residents are unique in how they experience structural barriers.

⚖ ETHICAL INSIGHTS

Racial and Ethnic Disparities in Health Care

Because public health is a societal approach to protecting and promoting health that usually acts through social rather than individual means (Kass, 2001), many of the most pressing ethical dilemmas are considered in public domains. Perhaps no more important ethical challenge faces our public today than that which revolves around the just distribution of health care resources.

For example, among 34.6 million rural minority adults in 2000, 32% of black, 35% of "other" race persons, and 45% of Hispanics were uninsured, compared with only 18% of whites (Glover et al., 2004). These data may help explain why minorities are more likely to be denied authorization for care (Lowe, 2001), use less prenatal care (Barfield, Wise PH, and Rust FP: 1996), and have fewer visits to physicians (Tai-Seale, Freund, and LoSasso, 2001).

Differences in care resulting from patient or care process–level variables (e.g., patient attitudes, preferences, or expectations; provider bias, stereotyping, or uncertainty) are problems of professional ethics. *Disparities in care* resulting from system-level variables, such as financing, accessibility, and geographic location, are problems of justice (Institute of Medicine, 1988). Subsequently, solutions for justice issues in *disparities in care* require public discourse aimed at solving system-level problems.

From an ethical perspective, the theory of justice as fairness was formulated to specify terms of social cooperation that are "fair" and ensures that people of equal basic liberties have equal opportunity (Daniels, Kennedy, and Kawachi, 1999). The Civil Rights Act of 1964 specifically bars discrimination in health care for all entities that receive federal funds, and both the American Nurses Association and American Medical Association codes of ethics endorse the principle of justice. However, despite overall agreement that justice is an important practice concept, difficulty arises in implementing changes in the health system to address *disparities in care*.

Solutions to disparities in care have been suggested by the Institute of Medicine (2003) and include the following policy, health system, and patient education and empowerment interventions:

- Policy interventions
  1. Medical care financing should discourage fragmentation of health care into separate tiers of providers that adhere to different standards of care and serve separate racial and ethnic minority segments of society. Government programs that require enrollment in managed care should be prepared to pay plans at rates comparable with those for privately insured patients.
  2. Strengthen the stability of patient-provider relationships in publicly funded health plans and create policy to create consistency, limit patient loads for providers, and provide reasonable time allowances for initial and follow-up visits.
  3. Increase the proportion of underrepresented U.S. racial and ethnic minorities among health professionals.
  4. Apply the same managed-care protections to publicly funded HMO enrollees that apply to private HMO enrollees.
  5. Provide greater resources to the USDHHS Office for Civil Rights to enforce civil rights laws.
- Health systems interventions
  1. Promote the consistency and equity of care through evidence-based guidelines. These guidelines should be published to allow public and professional scrutiny.
  2. Construct payment systems to enhance available services to minority patients, and limit provider incentives that may promote disparities.
  3. Enhance patient-provider communication and trust by providing financial incentives for practices that reduce barriers.
  4. Support the use of interpretation services where community need exists.
  5. Institute programs that use community health workers among medically underserved and racial and ethnic minority populations.
  6. Support greater use of multidisciplinary treatment and preventive care teams to improve and streamline care for racial and ethnic minority patients.
- Patient education and empowerment interventions
  1. Implement patient education programs to increase patients' knowledge of how to access care and participate in treatment decisions.

Barfield WD, Wise PH, and Rust FP: Racial disparities in outcomes of military and civilian births in California, *Arch Pediatr Adolesc Med* 150(10):1062-1067, 1996; Daniels N, Kennedy BP, Kawachi I: Why justice is good for our health: the social determinants of health inequalities, *Daedalus* 128:215-251, 1999; Glover S et al: Disparities in access to care among rural working-age adults, *J Rural Health* 20(3):193-205, 2004; Institute of Medicine: *Unequal treatment: confronting racial and ethnic disparities in healthcare*, Washington, DC, 1988, National Academy Press; Kass NE: An ethics framework for public health, *Public Health Matters* 91(11): 1776-1782, 2001; Lowe RA et al: Effect of ethnicity on denial of authorization for emergency department care by managed care gatekeepers, *Acad Emerg Med* 8(3):259- 266, 2001; Tai-Seale M, Freund D, LoSasso A: Racial disparities in service use among Medicaid beneficiaries after mandatory enrollment in managed care: a difference-in-differences approach, *Inquiry* 38(1):49-59, 2001.

Access to Care

In a survey of 90 national and state rural health experts, Gamm and Hutchison (2004) reported that access to health care was the number one priority identified by the majority (73%) of rural health care leaders. Access was the leading priority regardless of rural region (Northeast, Midwest, South, West) and regardless of type of organization represented in the survey (state organization, public health units, centers and clinics, or rural hospitals).

Primary care. Rural areas have fewer primary care physicians than urban areas, fueling concerns about inadequate access and gaps in U.S. health care equity in many rural areas. It is estimated that rural residents have fifty-three primary care physicians (PCPs)—internists, family/general practitioners, and pediatricians—per 100,000 people compared with seventy-eight PCPs per 100,000 urban residents (Reschovsky and Staiti, 2004; Ferrer, 2007). Only 10% of physicians, 22% of nurse practitioners (NPs), 13% of psychiatric NPs, and 23% of physician assistants practice in rural areas (Hanrahan and Hartley, 2008). The pattern distribution of these practitioners has begun to resemble the distribution of physicians and other clinicians with heavy concentrations in urban areas and a growing shortage in rural and underserved areas (Ricketts, 2008). In a joint statement, the National Rural Health Association and the American Academy of Family Physicians (AAFP) said medicine has become specialized, centralized, and urban, and challenged educators to be responsive to the needs of rural underserved communities (National Rural Health Association and AAFP, 2008).

99999999999

55555555555555

Availability of providers and health care facilities in rural areas is an important determinant of the quality of the health care delivery system and the likelihood of positive health outcomes for rural residents (Agency for Healthcare Research and Quality, 2004). A good example of the lack of specialists is the lack of mental health services available for rural dwellers of any age. The incidence of mental illness in rural areas is the same as that of urban areas, but there is far less access to mental health services in rural areas. Additionally, primary care doctors, nurses, and physician assistants, rather than mental health specialists, provide most of the mental health care in rural regions (Hanrahan and Hartley, 2008).

General health services. Population decline in rural areas, in the Great Plains and lower South for example, has resulted from an out-migration of younger people, leaving a greater concentration of older people in a dwindling population. A recent Institute of Medicine (IOM) study reported rural medical access problems in these areas, with some hospital and pharmacy closures, greater distances to travel for physician services, and limited if any choice of providers (IOM, 2005). Lack of local access to primary care and health care facilities forces rural residents to either go without or travel long distances—often over rural roads in dangerous weather conditions—to access needed care. Access to health care may become a particularly challenging and expensive proposition for the elderly who do not drive and are dependent on limited public transportation. Geography, health care costs, and lack of available services also are contextual problems that keep many rural adults and children from obtaining needed primary, secondary, and tertiary preventive services.

Health insurance. With economic decline and rising costs of health care, health insurance, or more importantly the lack of health insurance, for Americans has become a major issue for the health of the nation. An estimated 45.7 million people were without health insurance in 2007 (U.S. Census Bureau, 2008a).

As with poverty and unemployment data, insurance coverage varied with race and ethnicity coverage in 2007, as did age and residence (rural or urban). For example, 10.4% of non-Hispanic whites, 19.5% of blacks, and 16.8% of Asians were uninsured for all or part of 2007; young adults were more likely to lack health insurance than older persons; and 18% of poor or near-poor children lacked coverage (U.S. Census Bureau, 2008a). Lack of insurance coverage was greatest in the South (14.2%) and West regions (12%) in 2007, and, in general, rural residents were more likely than urban residents to lack insurance (20% vs. 17%) (IOM, 2005). Two thirds of the persons living in the most rural counties are low-income families, and 30% are children (USDA, 2004b).

Health insurance coverage influences health patterns. For example, in a study by Becker, Gates, and Newsome (2004), those who had some form of health insurance much more frequently reported the influence of physicians and health education programs in self-care regimens than did those who were uninsured. In addition, obtaining health insurance can pose a financial barrier to adequate health care for rural dwellers. Research points to a "strong nexus between health insurance status, chronic illnesses and poverty" (Bolin and Gamm, 2003, p. 19). Rural people are often employed in industries characterized by seasonal work, economic uncertainty and decline, high unemployment risk, and occupational accidents and death (e.g., agriculture, mining, forestry, and fisheries). Rural industries are often small and offer low wages, thereby contributing to the increasing number of uninsured rural families. For example, self-employed farm families need to purchase private health insurance; however, in periods of hardship they often cannot afford the increasingly high premium costs (Center on Budget and Policy Priorities, 2001). Farm families also tend to be two-parent households, so they are less likely to qualify for Medicaid, even with incomes below the federal poverty level.

Health insurance has been identified as one of the ten leading health indicators because it is generally a reliable predictor of overall health status (Cohen and Bloom, 2005). Public health professionals and health planners are most concerned with the impact of increasing numbers of uninsured children. In 1998 the overall percentage of children who were uninsured was 13.2% (Cohen and Bloom, 2005). Of the uninsured, 21% were rural children (Dunbar and Mueller, 1998). In the absence of health insurance, poverty becomes an even more powerful predictor of poor health for all age groups, and particularly for children.

In 1997, the State Children's Health Insurance Program (SCHIP) was enacted to improve health insurance coverage of children under 19 years of age in poor and near-poor families (see the Legislation and Programs Affecting Public Health in Rural Areas section in this chapter). In the years following passage of this program, 1997–2005, the overall percentage of children who were uninsured fell from 20% to 9%, and the number of uninsured children declined from 8.7 million (11.7%) in 2006 to 8.1 million (11.0%) in 2007 (U.S. Census Bureau, 2009). Gains in rural coverage were so great that rural children were actually at lower risk for being uninsured than children in urban areas. With the passage of SCHIP, some states included provisions to insure adults; however, this has not had a significant influence on rates of insured adults (Maine Rural Health Research Center, 2009). Health insurance coverage of children as well as adults varies from state to state and is influenced by employment patterns, the percentage of children in the population, state Medicaid policies, poverty levels, and racial and ethnic composition.

Composition: Health Disparities Related to Persons

To review, health problems in rural areas are compositional when they result from a concentration of persons with certain characteristics (Probst et al., 2004). Examples of compositional sources of health disparities include such characteristics as income, health behaviors, education, occupation, gender, and ethnicity. In the Rural *Healthy People 2010* survey cited previously, 73% of respondents listed access to health care as the top rural health priority (Bolin and Gamm, 2003). An additional thirteen priorities listed by respondents as leading health problems are largely compositional but may also have a contextual dimension. For example, such problems as obesity, chronic pulmonary disease, and higher levels of infant mortality have a strong compositional component because their variation is related to the health behaviors and educational, socioeconomic, racial, and ethnic characteristics of the rural groups. The variation may also be contextual, because the groups have fewer educational opportunities, have low-wage jobs, lack insurance, or have genetic propensities for certain health problems.

Income and Poverty

Income, education, and type of employment help determine socioeconomic status, and in the aggregate, rural dwellers have lower educational levels, higher unemployment rates, higher poverty rates, and lower income levels than urban aggregates (Probst et al., 2004). The poverty rate is one of the most important indicators of the health and well-being of all Americans, regardless of where they live (see Ethical Insights box p. 450). The USDA's Economic Research Service (ERS) tracks economic trends and demographic characteristics of rural dwellers to help develop policies and services. In the most recent report, the ERS contrasted the economic growth and downward trend in poverty rates during the 1990s with those of the current decade. In the previous 10 years, rural poverty declined on average from a decade high of 17% (1993) to a low of 11% (2000). Since 2000, the rate of rural poverty has been climbing. In 2003, 14% of the general rural population lived in poverty (compared with 12% of urban dwellers) (USDHHS, 2005). Poverty rates for rural people have always been higher than those of urban dwellers (Figure 23-1). As noted earlier in this section, however, data averaged across all rural counties in the United States do not give planners and providers much information about their own counties, or even regions. On the following pages are examples of data that are available to make an analysis of local and regional conditions and characteristics.

Rural poverty: regional differences. Consistent with the idea that there are many rural Americas in rural America, rural poverty varies by rural region (Box 23-1). For example, rural counties make up 340 of 386 (88%) counties with persistent poverty rates in the United States (persistent poverty is defined as counties in which 20% of the population has been in poverty over the last 30 years). Of the 340 rural counties with persistent poverty, 280 (82%) are in the South and 60 (18%) in the West and Midwest (USDA, 2004b). Poverty is also highest in the most rural areas. In completely rural counties (i.e., not adjacent to any metropolitan counties) the poverty rate is 16.8%.

Rural poverty: racial and ethnic minorities. When poverty rates among rural dwellers are analyzed by race, ethnicity, age, and family structure, the statistics on poverty are even more dramatic than for residence or region. Racial and ethnic minorities (mainly nonwhite Hispanics, blacks, and Native Americans) constituted 17% of the rural population, according to the 2000 Census (USDA, 2004b). This segment of the rural population has grown 30% in the last decade, largely due to the dramatic increase in nonwhite Hispanics (up 70.4% from 1990 to 2000) (IOM, 2005). In 2002, according to the ERS, poverty rates among rural and racial minorities were two to three times higher than poverty rates for rural whites (11%) (USDA, ERS, 2004).

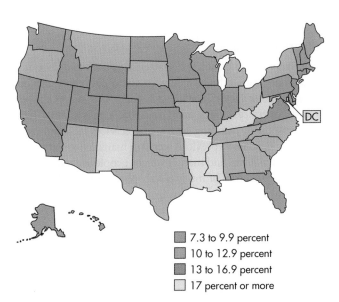

FIGURE 23-1 Percentage of total population in poverty, 2007. (Prepared by the ERS using U.S. Census Bureau data. The U.S. poverty rate in 2007 was 13%. Accessed from www.ers.usda.gov/data/povertyrates/.)

Legend:
- 7.3 to 9.9 percent
- 10 to 12.9 percent
- 13 to 16.9 percent
- 17 percent or more

BOX 23-1	**THE 2009 HEALTH AND HUMAN SERVICES POVERTY GUIDELINES**

In concept, the poverty guidelines are determined by estimating the minimum income level needed by a family or individual to just meet the basic needs of food, shelter, clothing, and other essential goods and services. Official poverty guidelines adjusted for family size and composition are set by the Department of Health and Human Services (DHHS) for use by all federal agencies to determine financial eligibility for certain federal programs (e.g., Medicaid). Some programs (e.g., State Children's Health Insurance Program) also use multiples of the guidelines to determine eligibility of participants. For example, participants may be eligible for programs if they are classified as being at or near poverty, where poverty is defined as 100%, and near poverty as 125% or 150% of the poverty level. Poverty guidelines are adjusted periodically by DHHS to reflect price changes, and are published in the *Federal Register*. The 2009 guidelines reflect just the size of the "family unit" rather than the family composition. The poverty level for a family unit of one, for example, was $2,460; it was $5,360 for a family unit of four, and $2,560 for a family of eight. Each household's cash income (including pretax income and cash welfare assistance, but excluding in-kind welfare assistance, such as food stamps and Medicare) is compared to the poverty line for the household.

From U.S. Department of Health and Human Services: *The 2009 HHS poverty guidelines: one version of the [U.S.] federal poverty measure,* 2009: http://aspe.hhs.gov/poverty/09poverty.shtml.

Rural poverty: family composition. Families with two or more adults are less likely to be poor, whether in rural or urban areas, because they are more likely to have multiple sources of income. Families with more than one adult have lower out-of-pocket child care costs and are less likely to have to limit their working hours. More than 75% of rural families are headed by a married couple, and these constitute only 7% of families living in poverty. On the other hand, people living in female-headed families (15%) have the highest poverty rates (37%), which is 10 percentage points greater than in female-headed families in metropolitan areas. The ERS attributes the high rate of poverty for female-headed families to "lower labor force participation rates, shorter average work weeks, and lower earnings" (USDA, 2004b).

Rural poverty: children. Children are particularly vulnerable to outcomes of poverty and are among the poorest citizens in rural America, constituting 36% of the overall population of rural poor in 2003. The heaviest concentrations of child poverty are in the South and West. Understanding how poverty is distributed in rural populations is important for planning and delivering programs that ameliorate the impact of poverty, such as food stamps, school lunch programs, school health nursing interventions, and health insurance coverage (USDA, 2005).

When race and ethnicity are taken into account, the poverty profile of children worsens dramatically. Racial and ethnic minorities fare far worse than the general rural population of children from birth to 18 years of age. When family composition is taken into account, we find that almost half of non-Hispanic black children, 34% of Native American children, and 18% of rural children who live in a female-headed household are poor (USDA, 2005).

Health Risk, Injury, and Death

Health behaviors vary along the rural-urban continuum and within rural populations by geographic area. For example, researchers have noted that adults in nonmetropolitan areas use seat belts less often and are less likely to use preventive screening (although the latter trend is confounded by access problems). Elliot, Ginsburg, and Winston (2008) studied the prevalence of unlicensed teenaged drivers when compared with licensed drivers and found that they were more likely black or Hispanic and live in rural areas. Rural teens are equally likely as or more likely than both suburban and urban teens to report being victims of violent behavior, to have suicide behaviors, and to use drugs (Johnson et al., 2008). Rural residents in the Southern states are more likely to be obese, smoke more heavily if they do smoke, use smokeless tobacco, and engage in sedentary lifestyles. In the rural West, rates of smoking, seat belt use, and obesity are lower, and alcohol and smokeless tobacco use are higher (Eberhardt et al., 2001). For example, 19% of adolescents living in the most rural counties are smokers, compared with 11% in large metropolitan counties. Among adults living in the most rural counties, 27% of women and 31% of men smoke, compared with 20% of women and 25% of men in large metro areas. Tobacco use is increasing for men and women in the South.

Unintentional injuries are the leading cause of death in the United States for both sexes, for all races and ethnicities, and for all age groups from ages 1 to 44 years. Overall, unintentional injuries occur most often as the result of driving a vehicle (automobile, ATV, bicycle). In the latest available reports, unintentional injuries continue to be higher in rural areas of the United States. The mortality rate for unintentional injuries reported in the *Urban and Rural Health Chartbook* was 54.1 per 100,000 rural residents, which is twice the rate for large metropolitan counties (CDC Chartbook, 2007). Unintentional injuries are highest among males and in rural counties with the lowest population densities (Peek-Asa, Zwerling, and Stallones, 2004).

According to the CDC's National Center for Health Statistics (NCHS), unintentional injuries were ranked fifth in the leading causes of death in 2004. This category of death includes "transport accidents," including motor vehicle accidents, and "non-transport accidents," including falls, firearm accidents, drowning, fire-related deaths, accidental poisoning, and other accidental deaths (Hoyert et al., 2005). Males aged 15 to 24 years are the most likely victims of unintentional injuries.

In four of the least-populated states, the percentage of deaths from unintentional injuries was much higher than the national average, with 7.7% in Idaho, 8.0% in Montana, 9.1% in Wyoming, and 14.3% in Alaska. Overall, deaths from unintentional injuries were approximately 80% to 85% higher for females and males in the most rural counties than for suburban areas of metropolitan counties in 1996 to 1998, and highest of all in the West (Eberhardt et al., 2001). Driving at high speeds, driving long distances, driving in winter conditions, not using seat belts, and consuming alcohol have been cited as contributing to greater levels of injury deaths and disability by rural residents in the West. Lack of ready access to counseling, emergency medical services, and rehabilitation is also thought to be a contributing factor to these high levels.

Vulnerable Groups

Demographic and personal characteristics, such as age, education, gender, race, ethnicity, language, and culture, round out the examples of factors that affect health and may block access to existing services (Wang and Luo, 2005). Age is an important consideration in planning health care services for rural communities. As noted in previous sections, many retirees are moving into rural areas, and many younger people are moving out. Because the incomes of many elderly people may be lower, the tax base of counties and municipalities may be inadequate to cover the disproportionate share of the health care services used by the elderly (aged 65 years and over) (Eberhardt et al., 2001).

The population of elderly people is expected to double by 2050. Elderly women tend to live at or near the poverty level and achieve poverty status twice as often as men (USDA, 2005). Along with educational attainment, this is a critical indicator of well-being for the elderly and the young. The elderly poor tend to be isolated and lack access to support services, health care, prescription drugs, adequate nutrition, and transportation.

The number of children in rural areas increased by 3% in the decade from 1990 to 2000 (USDA, 2005). In addition to population growth, racial and ethnic diversity increased in the 1990s. Today, the proportion of Hispanic children is the fastest-growing component of the rural population, regardless of region. The population of black children has remained steady, and the majority of rural black children are still concentrated in the South. Native American children constitute only 3% of the total nonmetropolitan population, although in areas of the country (mainly West and Central) with high concentrations of Native Americans, this percentage is, of course, much higher. Evidence suggests that fetal, infant, and maternal mortality are slightly higher in nonmetropolitan than metropolitan areas and that care in the later prenatal stages is problematic. Nonmetropolitan children, like adults, are more likely to live in poverty, and proportionately fewer rural children were covered by health insurance in 2001 (Kandel and Cromartie, 2003; USDA, 2005).

Education and Employment

Research on the socioeconomic determinants of health has revealed a strong positive correlation between health and length of schooling (CDC, 2009). As Swanson (1999, p. 2) discussed, "Demographic characteristics of a minority group both affect and result from their economic and social status. Age structure and education combine as an indication of the level of employment a group might be able to enjoy." For the aged and for ethnic and racial minorities, a pattern of lower educational attainment and unfavorable economic circumstances emerges with increasing rurality. Although the education picture is changing, many elderly women in their 70s and 80s grew up before public education was mandatory. Families could not afford to send them to school, or they were simply expected to learn to read and write, seek employment, and marry. Education, with its links to economic and health variables, is still a serious problem for rural America. Low education and employment levels characterize all rural minority groups except Asians. "Children of all racial and ethnic groups who live in precarious economic conditions have additional challenges to doing well in school and remaining in school through high school graduation" (Swanson, 1999, p. 4). In 2000, 77% of rural dwellers held high school diplomas or General Educational Development diplomas (GEDs) (compared with 70% in 1990) (USDA, 2005). The major difference between these two groups was in the percentage of rural students who held college degrees. The college completion rate of rural students was almost half that of urban students. There are also large gaps in educational completion by region, race, and ethnicity, with the West and Midwest students exceeding the high school completion rates of students in the rural South (USDA, 2005). Rural and central city students, especially minorities other than Asians, lag behind suburban children on most indicators of adequate progress in schools (IOM, 2005). Low educational attainment is a challenge in rural America. Skill requirements for rural employment continue to rise, lack of education is correlated with persistent poverty, and poverty is a predictor of poor health.

Furthermore, counties that have a low-wage economy have difficulty providing the infrastructure needed to provide education, public health, and health care services for low-wage families. They also have difficulty attracting new employers who might contribute to the economic development of a rural area, but need a more highly educated workforce.

Occupational Health Risks

In the United States, approximately 65,000 workers die each year of work-related illnesses and injuries (Herbert and Landrigan, 2000). Fatal occupational injuries declined 23.1% from 1992 to 2002. The rate (number of fatal injuries per 100,000 workers) decreased from 5.2 in 1992 to 4.0 in 2002 (National Institute for Occupational Safety and Health [NIOSH], 2004).

Occupational injuries, fatalities, and illnesses play a significant role in rural health, because rates of disabling injuries and injury-related mortality are dramatically higher in the rural population, particularly in the West and South (NIOSH, 2004). Industries with the highest death rates were mining, agriculture, forestry, and fishing, followed by construction, transportation, and public utilities (Eberhardt et al., 2001). The majority of job-related deaths due to workplace injuries in 2003 were in the following categories: transportation-related motor vehicle accidents, machinery-related events, homicides, falls, electrocution, and chemical and thermal injuries. Two industries accounted for more than 40% of fatal occupational injuries in 2002: construction (22.6%) and transportation and public utilities (18.3%). Three Western states, Alaska, Wyoming, and Montana, had the highest fatality rates (more than ten per 100,000 persons) for 2002 (Eberhardt et al., 2001).

Occupational death and disability can also be attributed to nonfatal injuries, and occupational diseases, such as cancer, asbestosis, silicosis, and anthracosis associated with both organic and inorganic exposures (NIOSH, 2004). Work-related injuries, deaths, and illness data must be interpreted with caution. Although surveillance of occupational injuries, illnesses, and fatalities has improved through the collaboration of the states and NIOSH, data still come from many sources, and underreporting continues to be problematic.

Perceptions of Health
Gender, Race, and Ethnicity

Both rural men and women are less likely than metropolitan residents to report their health as good or excellent. Rural areas, particularly in the rural South, have higher incidents of heart disease and cancer. Higher prevalence of chronic disease is consistent with the composition of rural populations, which tend to be older, poorer, and less educated (Gosschalk and Carozza, 2003). Rural men and women also smoke or use smokeless tobacco more. In the aggregate, they exercise fewer preventive behaviors, have less contact with physicians, and often have less access to care than people with similar problems in urban areas (Gamm, Castillo, and Pittman, 2003). Rural men and youths are also more likely to die or become disabled from unintentional injuries due to risky behavior or work-related causes and are more likely to commit suicide than women or urban men and youths.

Although rural populations overall are at lower risk for most cancers, certain rural subpopulations are at greater risk. For example, Appalachia has a much higher rate than the national figure. Residents in low-income areas and the uninsured, particularly African Americans, tend to have more late-stage cancer diagnoses; and rural residents in general may have less access to quality health care, including both medical care and screening and prevention programs (Gamm et al., 2003). A particularly serious problem for minorities and the elderly is the lack of cancer screening, including breast and cervical cancer for women and prostate cancer for men. Preventive care is especially important for African-American men, for whom prostate cancer is higher than for any other racial or ethnic group.

From 1987 to 2005, the age-adjusted percentage of women over 40 years of age who had a mammogram improved from 29% to 70.3% according to the CDC's NCHS (CDC/NCHS, 2008). The percentage was lower for all racial and ethnic minorities, with 67.8% for African-American women and 47.3% for American Indian and Alaska Native women. Use of mammography was the lowest among the poor, most particularly in the 40- to 49-year-old age bracket (47.4%), and among the least educated (CDC/NCHS, 2008). Health objectives for the year 2010 called for at least 80% of American women aged 40 years and older to have received a mammogram and clinical breast examination in the previous 2 years (USDHHS, 2000). Similarly, women who are poor, elderly, and less educated are less likely to receive Pap tests. In racial and ethnic groups, the percentages of women who get Pap tests are lower for Hispanics, American Indians, and Alaska Natives. The lowest percentage is found in Asian women.

Rural-dwelling men suffer the long-term effects of having poor health habits, lacking consistent primary health care, and participating in hazardous occupations, as mentioned previously. Rural men in the South have higher rates of ischemic heart disease and cancer. Adult males on the whole were twice as likely as females to lack a usual source of health care in 2000 to 2001. In the West, the percentage of adults without a usual source of care was 19.4% in 2001 to 2002 and has changed little over the past 10 years (NCHS, 2008). In fact, among rural working-age adults, 45% of Hispanics, 32% of blacks, and 18% of whites were uninsured, and similar percentages had not visited a health care provider in the previous year (Glover et al., 2004).

Interacting with poverty and lack of access to care, rural minorities are among the nation's least healthy citizens. African-American and Native American children and children of migrant workers are among the poorest of rural residents. By almost any measure or index (e.g., acquired immunodeficiency syndrome [AIDS] incidence, birth weight, blood pressure, cholesterol level, cancer incidence, and substance abuse), rural poor African Americans, Hispanics, American Indians, and Alaska Natives are less healthy than whites. They also have food insecurity and hunger more frequently and have less access to quality health care (Probst et al., 2004).

The Indian Health Service, whose per capita expenditure for American Indian and Alaska Native health services is about half that of the U.S. civilian population, is the only source of health care funding for many rural American Indians. Marked disparities persist between American Indians and whites. American Indians have a death rate that is 1.5 times that of whites, and they are more likely to have a chronic health condition. These higher rates of morbid conditions use significant medical resources from both primary and specialty care physicians. In addition, rural American Indians are less likely to have private health insurance coverage, less likely to use health services, and more likely to have transportation difficulties. Among perceived barriers to rural American Indians' access to important specialty services, financial constraints top the list (Baldwin et al., 2008).

The percentage of Hispanics and Latinos in the U.S. population was about equal to that of African Americans (12.5% vs. 12.3% during the year 2000), and Hispanics will soon become the largest minority group in the United States. They are already the predominant minority in the West. Hispanics have a diverse culture, history, and socioeconomic health status. The largest Hispanic subgroups are of Mexican, Cuban, and Puerto Rican descent, although Mexican is the largest by far (58% of the Hispanic population living in the United States). In nonmetropolitan areas, the population of Hispanics has doubled, and almost half of all Hispanics who live in rural areas are living outside the traditional areas of settlement in the Southwestern states. As emphasized previously, this growing segment of the population continues to be overrepresented among the rural poor. In 1999, the U.S. Census Bureau reported that just over 25% of Hispanics live below the federal poverty level, compared with 8.2% of the white, non-Hispanic population. Of those under age 18 years, the percentage living below the poverty level was 34% for Hispanics, compared with 10.6% of white non-Hispanics. The elderly were also 2.5 times more likely to live below the poverty line than white non-Hispanics. Hispanics are most likely to report barriers in obtaining needed health care and are least likely to have a usual source of care; for those blacks and Hispanics reporting a usual source of care, the source is most likely to be hospital based (Kass, Weinick, and Monheit, 1999).

SPECIFIC RURAL AGGREGATES

Agricultural Workers

Health Disparities

An example of health disparities among agricultural workers is the group of farm workers that support fruit and vegetable production. In general, migrant and seasonal farmworkers (MSFW) may have the poorest health of any aggregate in the United States and the least access to affordable health care. Eighty-five percent of the MSFW are Hispanic, Latino, or African American. The rest are largely white seasonal workers who follow the harvests to drive combines or haul crops from the fields to storage, market, or seaports. These populations, estimated between 3 and 5 million people each year, are vulnerable to a host of health problems and diseases that center on occupational and environmental hazards and other health correlates, as described in the section about agricultural workers (USDA, 2008).

Accidents and Injuries

Working in highly variable environmental conditions (e.g., temperature extremes, a wide variety of work tasks, and unpredictable circumstances) is associated with an increased frequency of accidents and fatalities. Farm-related activities are extremely heterogeneous and vary significantly with the season, types of crops produced, and types of machinery used. Farmers are located in geographically isolated areas and often work alone. This constellation of factors places farmers and their families at increased risk for accidental injury and delayed access to emergency or trauma care.

The 2001 to 2002 rate of fatal injury for those employed in the agricultural sector was 21.3 per 100,000 workers, compared with a rate of 4.2 per 100,000 for all types of U.S. workers. According to NIOSH, agricultural machinery is the most common cause of fatalities and nonfatal injuries of U.S. agricultural workers, including on-farm fatalities among youth under 20 years (NIOSH, 2004). Tractor-related accidents, especially rollovers, are the most frequent causes of farm accidents and account for more than one fourth of farm fatalities. The actual causes of death and serious injury are associated with rollovers of equipment that lack rollover protective structures and seat belts (Struttmann et al., 2001). It is easy to see why accident prevention programs for farm children and families have focused heavily on tractor safety awareness.

Acute and Chronic Illnesses

Several types of farming activities are associated with higher than expected occurrences of acute and chronic respiratory conditions. Individuals with long-term exposure to grain dusts, such as grain elevator workers and dairy workers, have diminished respiratory function and increased frequency of respiratory symptoms (Pahwa et al., 2006; Cotton et al., 1989). Occupational asthma and more exotic fungal or toxic gas–related conditions also occur in higher frequency in agricultural than nonagricultural populations (Warren, 1989). Community health nurses, who are familiar with local farming practices in rural areas, often make links between farm work and respiratory symptoms. In such situations, the role of the nurse is to refer patients to appropriate health care providers and provide support and education for affected people and their families.

Exposure to pesticides, herbicides, and other chemicals is also a major concern for farmers and their families. From an occupational perspective, farming is unusual because the home and the work site are the same. Exposure risks to children and spouses may be heightened when farmers wear contaminated clothing and boots into the home. Homes are often located in close proximity to fields and animal containment facilities, which are treated with a variety of chemicals.

Nurses in rural emergency departments or other ambulatory care settings may be the first providers to encounter farmers and others with acute pesticide poisoning. During discussions with farmers, ranchers, or other high-risk groups (e.g., nursery workers and tree planters), community health nurses may note a pattern of headaches and nausea that occur during planting or spraying seasons. In such an instance, the nurse can serve as an important resource by obtaining a careful history of signs and symptoms, the temporal nature of symptom occurrence, and the types of pesticides and personal protection used (e.g., respirators and protective clothing). When evidence suggests pesticide-related illness, appropriate referral and follow-up are imperative to ensure the safety of the affected person and the family.

Signs and symptoms of acute pesticide poisoning are fairly clear, and most health providers in rural communities would recognize them. Common symptoms include headache, dizziness, diaphoresis, nausea, and vomiting. If left untreated, those affected may experience a progression of symptoms including dyspnea, bronchospasm, and muscle twitching. Deaths are relatively uncommon, but they do occur.

Altermanan et al. (2008) studied ethnic, racial, and gender variations among U.S. farmers and found a prevalence of musculoskeletal discomfort, followed by respiratory problems, hearing loss, and hypertension. Latino and Asian-American operators had lower prevalences of health problems than white non-Latino and white farmers. Hypertension and osteoarthritis were other risk factors include alcohol use (higher in rural areas and highest among persons living in the most rural areas, and more common among men than women), obesity (higher in rural areas, most particularly rural areas of the South), and physical inactivity during leisure time, which varies by level of urbanization and also by region for both men and women (highest level of inactivity in the South and in central counties of large metro areas of the Northeast) (Eberhardt et al., 2001).

Intentional injuries are most often the result of firearms usage. This can be against oneself or another. In rural counties, nonfatal firearm injuries occur most often at home compared with urban counties where injuries occur most often in the streets. Furthermore, numerous studies have noted that firearm suicide in rural counties is an important public health problem (Branas et al., 2005), and, according to the CDC, firearms are the most commonly used method of suicide among males.

Suicide is also a major public health problem in rural areas. In rural areas adjacent to a small city, suicide rates were 31% higher than suburban rates and 43% higher in rural areas that were not adjacent to small cities (Eberhardt et al., 2001). Nationally, suicide was the eleventh leading cause of death overall, eighth for males, and seventeenth for females. Little regional variation was found, except in the most rural parts of the West (especially in the least-populated states of Wyoming, Alaska, Montana, and Idaho), where rates were 80% higher than those in metropolitan areas. There was also variation by race and ethnicity. Decreased access to mental health services for treatment of depression may contribute to these higher rates (Eberhardt et al., 2001). Among suicide victims, racial and ethnic disparities exist. Suicide rates among American Indians and Alaska Natives aged

15 to 34 years are 2.2 times higher than the national average for that age group, and Hispanic female high school students in grades 9 through 12 reported more suicide attempts (14.0%) than white, non-Hispanic (7.7%) or black, non-Hispanic (9.9%) students (CDC, 2008). The suicide rate for non-Hispanic white men 65 years of age and over is higher than in other groups. In 2004, the suicide rate for older non-Hispanic white men was about two to three times the rate for older men in other race or ethnicity groups and nearly eight times the rate for older non-Hispanic white women (CDC Chartbook, 2007).

Hypertension and osteoarthritis were more prevalent in black farmers, but they had a lower prevalence of hearing loss, skin problems, or heart problems. Cancer was less prevalent in black farmers than in white. In American Indian or Alaska Native farmers, musculoskeletal problems, skin problems, and hypertension were the most common.

Migrant and Seasonal Farm Workers

Although the discussion of agricultural issues has focused primarily on farmers and farm families, it is important to understand the role of migrant (i.e., migrate to find work) and seasonal (i.e., reside permanently in one place and work locally when farm labor is needed) farmworkers in U.S. agricultural production and the health risks to this population. Older references to farmworkers often referred to three "migrant streams," in which workers entered the country through Mexico and migrated north. The present reality is that migrant workers enter the country through a variety of access points and follow any route necessary to obtain work. Seasonal workers permanently reside in agricultural areas and take various farm jobs during harvesting times. For example, a seasonal worker may be employed in restaurant work during the winter and may spend the summer months picking apples or working in a local apple shed or cannery (Branas et al., 2005).

MSFWs comprise a vulnerable population in regard to health risks because they have low income and migratory status. In many rural areas, community health nurses form the central link between farmworkers and health services. Through standing or mobile clinic sites, nurses have established a leadership role in the provision of episodic and preventive services for workers and their families. Lacking access to many types of preventive services, farmworkers often visit a migrant clinic with any number of health problems including severe dental problems, unresolved communicable diseases, and untreated injuries. In addition to the direct provision of care, nurses in many communities have served as important advocates on behalf of farmworkers and have worked to ensure health care access to those traveling through their areas.

Cultural, linguistic, economic, and mobility barriers all contribute to the nature and magnitude of health problems observed in farmworkers. Cultural and linguistic barriers are the most overt because many of the communities where farmworkers work consider them outsiders. In many settings, migrant workers live isolated from the agricultural communities they serve. Although some workers travel in extended family groups and have the support that comes with being together, other workers leave their families at home. Often these are male workers who work and live together. A common misconception among U.S. health care providers is that these farmworkers are from Mexico and Spanish is their primary language. Farmworkers originate from many communities in Mexico, the Caribbean, and Central and South America, and they may speak English, the language of their home country, or several languages.

Enumeration of Migrant and Seasonal Farmworkers

To increase access to primary and preventive care for MSFW populations, information is needed on the numbers and distribution of farmworkers at the national, state, and local levels. Because MSFWs move frequently for work, census estimates generally provide a poor assessment of needs for health care services for this population. Additionally, the legislation that created the Migrant Health Program (MHP) (Section 330g of the Public Health Service Act), under the direction of the Bureau of Primary Health Care (BPHC) (2000) and the Health Resources and Services Administration (HRSA), requires that priorities be established based on where the greatest need exists. Hence the MHP has supported the ongoing and comprehensive assessment of the numbers of MSFWs and published the most recent estimates in the Migrant and Seasonal Farmworker Enumeration Profile Study (MSFWEPS) (Bureau of Primary Health Care, 2000).

Enumeration data from the MSFWEPS is available for Arkansas, California, Florida, Louisiana, Maryland, North Carolina, Mississippi, Oklahoma, Texas, and Washington. Although population sizes of MSFWs range from relatively small numbers in such states as Maryland and Oklahoma, to very large numbers in California and Washington, it is important to recognize that primary and preventive care services must be appropriately planned for those not engaged in farm and seasonal work, including other household members and children. For example, the state of California has an estimated population of 732,109 MSFWs, but an additional 570,688 nonfarmworkers must be considered in planning and evaluating services.

Health Needs and Opportunities for Preventive Care

Similarities in exposure and work practices make some of the farmworkers' health needs similar to those of farmers and their families. Generally, these health needs reflect the increased rates of accidents and injuries, dermatological conditions, and pulmonary problems observed in both populations. However, there are additional challenges in both the identification and treatment of farmworkers with health problems. One of the biggest problems that nurses face in designing health programs is understanding the full magnitude of their problems. Many farmworkers who become ill eventually return to their countries of origin to obtain treatment and to be with family. This phenomenon makes it difficult to get complete, reliable numbers about disease rates. A variety of public health indicators are likely to undercount farmworkers as a group, ranging from tumor registries to Workers' Compensation injuries (Schenker, 1995). In addition, farmworkers may be less likely to seek treatment for health problems that do not require emergency treatment or surgery.

Studies of farmworkers' health status have provided data indicating that farmworkers are less likely to receive preventive care from any health source (Schenker, 1995). Preventive needs include dental care, vision screening and treatment, and gynecological and breast examinations. In addition, children of farmworkers are likely to receive incomplete sets of immunizations by the age of 5 years (Schenker, 1995). Many farmworkers, because they move from community to community, are often unaware of clinical and social services they could receive at reduced or no cost to low-income families.

Hearing Farmworkers' Voices

Several studies and pilot projects have used focus groups, community meetings, or other qualitative research methods to listen to farmworkers' concerns and give these concerns a voice through publication and advocacy. Several years ago, the Farmworker Justice Fund brought female farmworkers together in a national effort to give them a forum for their concerns and their impressions of health needs. The women identified priority concerns in the areas of child and family issues, health care services, workplace issues, and empowerment. The group's recommendations in the area of health care included keeping clinics open during evening hours, providing transportation to clinics, increasing access through mobile health units, providing social and health services in one building, increasing home visits by students, encouraging careers in farmworker health, enhancing nutrition education to families, teaching first aid, enforcing farm labor health laws, and giving farmworkers a copy of the record after each clinic visit (Farm Worker Fund, 2006).

Involving MSFWs as active participants in the planning and provision of care may become more challenging since the terrorist attacks of September 11, 2001. Following this unprecedented event, policymakers began discussing broad changes to current immigration laws to protect the United States by securing the borders. In short, discussions have focused on limiting access of foreign workers to jobs in the United States and providing those already here with limited provisions for continuing in their current role. Concerns raised by public health advocates center around the idea that an increasingly punitive system of immigration will discourage seasonal workers and farmworkers from accessing health care or encourage them to lie to health care providers about critical issues (Mautino, 2004).

APPLICATION OF RELEVANT THEORIES AND "THINKING UPSTREAM" CONCEPTS TO RURAL HEALTH

Upstream and prevention-oriented approaches have several implications for nurses in rural practice. Three strategies for upstream interventions follow: attack community-based problems at their roots, emphasize the "doing" aspects of health, and maximize the use of informal networks.

Attack Community-Based Problems at Their Roots

Upstream approaches to community health problems direct the nurse toward an understanding of the precursors of poor health within populations of interest. Individual nurses can be effective forces in uncovering and enhancing community awareness of health-endangering situations. Environmental health issues in rural communities, such as pesticide exposure or health hazards from point-source factory emissions, are more effectively assessed and remedied on a community level than on a case-by-case basis. Nurses' involvement in helping people understand health problems in a larger context can be the genesis of change. Nurses and other community members can take social action on behalf of those affected. For example, by heightening awareness of sulfur dioxide levels from a local refinery and the relationship of those emission levels to respiratory problems in vulnerable populations, nurses can help citizens gain an understanding of the collective rather than individual burden of the refinery on their community's health.

Emphasize the "Doing" Aspects of Health

There are consistent differences between the ways rural and nonrural residents perceive health. The primary one may be the relative importance of "work" and "being able to work" in self-reported definitions of health (Weinert and Long, 1987). Rural attitudes generally emphasize the "doing" aspects of health by functioning and performing the daily activities fundamentally important in their daily lives. The high value placed on "being able to do" can provide astute nurses with intervention opportunities for both families and communities. Examples of nursing intervention strategies that capitalize on this include accident prevention programs for children, exercise and nutrition programs for seniors, and local industry participation in risk reduction programs for workers. Active involvement of the target population in all phases of program planning and implementation is key to the success of these programs.

Maximize the Use of Informal Networks

Recognizing and using informal networks in the community is essential to the "doing" concept of prevention programs. The name used, such as empowerment models or community action models, is less important than soliciting the involvement of informal networks and local leaders in planning health interventions. As most people who have been involved in community empowerment programs will attest, involvement of these important entities is not easy or straightforward. Turf issues and collateral agendas can obstruct rather than facilitate change. However, failure to elicit community involvement in population-based health interventions will result in unfavorable consequences. Frequently, superimposed change tends to fit poorly with the community it is intended to serve. Rural change strategies will be short-lived unless community members understand them and invest in their own well-being.

RURAL HEALTH CARE DELIVERY SYSTEM

Health Care Provider Shortages

The Bureau of Health Professions (2003) states that the size and characteristics of the future health workforce are determined by the interaction of various forces acting on the health environment, including economic factors, technology, regulatory and legislative actions, epidemiological factors, the health care education system, and demographics. Current shortages of health care professionals in rural areas are likely to become worse with increased demand caused by population aging and increasing racial and ethnic diversity. In actual numbers, the shortage has been growing since 1990. Although approximately 25% of the U.S. population lives in nonmetropolitan counties, only 18% of registered nurses (RNs) practice there. In addition, the supply of physicians has not equaled service need in rural areas (Ferrer, 2007). For nonphysician primary care professionals, such as nurse practitioners (NP), physician assistants (PAs), and certified nurse-midwives (CNMs), trends are similar to those for physicians except for PAs. Hanrahan and Hartley (2008) report that 22% of NPs and 23% of PAs practice in urban areas. This pattern distribution has begun to resemble the distribution of physicians and other clinicians with heavy concentrations in urban areas and a growing shortage in rural and underserved areas.

Clearly, the growing nursing shortage will affect all of America. This is both a supply and a demand shortage. Declining school enrollments, retirement of current nurses, and the increased need for care of an aging population make the situation especially critical (Sigma Theta Tau International, 2006). A survey by the American Organization of Nurse Executives found that in small hospitals, usually located in rural areas, it takes significantly longer to fill vacancies than in larger urban facilities (Thrall, 2007). Rural nurses earn less than their urban counterparts, which compounds recruitment difficulties. Nurses with baccalaureate and master's degrees, other than master's-prepared NPs, are compensated less for this additional education (Thrall, 2007).

A solution proposed for the shortage of health care providers is for rural communities to "grow their own." A rural community, a group of small communities, or a county could support local students attending college and recruit students currently attending professional schools. The students make a commitment to work in the community in return for monetary support for their educations (Thrall, 2007). Tuition reimbursement and access to distance learning programs can assist practicing nurses. Continuing education and baccalaureate and master's degrees are available through e-mail, Internet-based courses, interactive video classes, and by-mail videos. Some programs are provided exclusively via the Internet. Nebraska rural communities are enthusiastic about the University of Nebraska College of Nursing Internet courses. The program is helping them grow their own nurses. Research shows that nurses educated in rural communities are more apt to stay and work there than those who move away to attend school (Pullen, 1998; Thrall, 2007).

Managed Care in the Rural Environment

Managed care has recently changed health care delivery in the United States. In rural areas, health care delivery networks with managed-care elements are being developed. Potential benefits and risks of managed care to rural areas have been identified, recognizing the difficulty for rural providers to deliver the cost-effective, complex health care needed from solo or small group practices. Possible benefits to managed care include lowering primary care costs, improving the quality of care, and stabilizing the local rural health care system. Risks are also apparent, including probable high start-up and administrative costs, and the volatile effect of large, urban-based for-profit managed-care companies (Allender, Rector, and Warner, 2010; Ricketts and Heaphy, 1999).

Outside of Medicaid, managed care has yet to become a major presence in much of rural America because of small dispersed populations, few visits per individual, and large numbers of elderly on Medicare with low-level reimbursements that do not make the aggregate financially attractive to a managed-care organization (MCO). In fact, despite the existence of federally qualified health centers that provide care to underserved populations through Medicare, Medicaid, or sliding fee scales, the reality is that there were few rural people enrolled in sponsored health plans (Allender et al., 2010). Providers in rural markets face severe financial constraints as HMOs increasingly cope with smaller numbers of enrollees and continue to decrease provider reimbursement (IOM, 2005). Communities that make the most progress toward partnerships or integration are those whose local leaders and providers have strong incentives to work together and are motivated to bring about change to the health care system. Authorities in rural health and managed care report that it is too soon to know whether managed care will become a significant way of delivering health care in rural areas, as it has become in urban America (Allender et al., 2010; IOM, 2005).

COMMUNITY-BASED CARE

In the mid-1990s, the phrase *community-based care* became a popular term for the myriad of services provided outside the walls of an institution. Health care services are no longer provided exclusively in the hospital setting. Community-based care includes services that are provided where individuals live, work, or go to school. Examples of community-based services are home health and hospice care, occupational health programs, community mental health programs, ambulatory care services, school health programs, faith-based care, and elder services, such as adult day care. The concept also includes community participation in decisions about health care services, a focus on all three levels of prevention, and an understanding that the hospital is no longer the exclusive health care provider.

Home Care and Hospice

Home health and hospice programs vary in structure. In a national study on Medicare hospice use, only one third of rural counties have a hospice based within the county, but nearly two thirds of urban counties do (Virnig et al., 2004). Urban hospices are more likely to be freestanding, whereas rural hospices tend to be hospital based. Larger communities may support a hospital-based home care agency with hospice service, a freestanding, full-service agency, or both. In sparsely populated rural locations, home health and hospice services may be contracted from a larger regional agency, with a local nurse hired to provide services.

Virnig et al. (2004) found that the more remote the rural environment, the less likely hospice services were used. Nurse case management and development of local resources, using the county extension services as a bridge for outreach services, can improve home care for these patients and provide support for their families. A partnership between the public health nurse and county extension service could provide support and information groups and caregiving classes for the important informal provider network. Chapter 33 discusses home health and hospice in greater detail.

Faith Communities and Parish Nursing

Rural residents are perceived as having strong traditional values. At the heart of these values is a strong sense of community, family life, and religious faith (W. K. Kellogg Foundation, 2001).

Since the conceptualization of parish nursing in the early 1980s, RNs have developed and expanded the role. Parish nurses integrate nursing expertise and faith-based knowledge to provide holistic care to members of congregations. More than 7000 nurses have completed formal training programs in parish nursing. The exact number of parish nurses working as paid and unpaid staff in both urban and rural faith communities is not known, because many nurses have not been formally prepared for the role (International Parish Nurse Resource Center, nd). Both professional nursing and parish nursing are based on health and healing (American Nurses Association, 2005).

In a comparison of experiences of rural and urban parish nurses, Chase-Ziolek and Striepe (1999) found rural nurses more likely to be involved in case management and coordination of services than their urban counterparts. In urban settings, contact with parishioners was primarily at the church, whereas contacts in rural settings were most often in the home, on the phone, or in other community-based settings. Collaboration between faith communities and other organizations can help extend limited rural community health resources. Such partnerships have been promoted by federal and state governments to enhance the public health efforts (Zahner and Corrado, 2004). Chapter 32 provides an in-depth discussion of faith community nursing.

Informal Care Systems

Limited availability and accessibility of formal health care resources in rural areas combined with self-reliance and self-help traits of rural residents have resulted in the development of strong rural community informal care and social support networks. Rural residents are more apt to entrust care to established informal networks than to new formal care systems (Weinert and Long, 1987, 1990). One study reported that rural residents sustain a higher level of social health than urban residents. They attributed this social health to their higher level of family and community involvement (Eggebeen and Lichter, 1993), which may contribute to the formation and use of informal systems.

Informal care systems or networks include people who have assumed the role of caregiver based on their individual qualities, life situations, or social roles. People who participate in these networks may provide direct help, advice, or information. Rural residents identify spouses, adult children, other family members, friends, and neighbors as informal providers of care (Buckwalter et al., 2002).

Informal caregivers often find themselves in stressful circumstances. Rural residents who are in need of assistance are usually elderly, have chronic illness, have few resources, and must travel long distances for health care. Rasheed and Rasheed (2004) suggest that by 2050, 21% of all Americans will be members of a minority group. Existing disparities in the physical and mental health status, service availability, service access, and socioeconomics impact Americans in rural communities. Coupled with the "helping tradition" in the black community, there has been a great reliance on community-based informal care systems for the elderly black population.

Van Exel, de Graaf, and Brouwer (2008) studied caregiver attitudes toward respite care and found those who could potentially benefit were reluctant to seek it for various reasons. This has enormous implications for nursing practice. Because informal health care is an important, cost-effective component of the health care systems, different forms of respite care have been implemented to support caregivers. Not only do many patients have a preference for receiving care from someone familiar in their home environment, but in many cases it will help them to avoid long-term-care placement. Nurses have a role in discussing the potential benefits of support for both the family and the care recipient.

Rural Public Health Departments

There are more than 2800 local health departments in the United States. Many of these serve populations of fewer than 50,000 people (Rosenblatt, Casey, and Richardson, 2002). The purpose of *Healthy People 2010* objective 23-11 was to increase the proportion of state and local public health departments that meet national performance standards for public health services (USDHHS, 2000). The standards are based on the core public functions of assessment, policy development, and assurance. Data from 2004 indicate that only 11% of 2315 local public health agencies used the national standards, with only 3% fully or substantially meeting the model national standards (USDHHS, 2004).

In 2002, approximately 3.3% of all money spent on health care in the United States was spent on public health services. Public health expenditures have steadily decreased since 1960. This trend is unlikely to improve given limited public resources, the aging of the population with the subsequent need for acute illness care, and changing Medicaid from public to private providers (NIOSH, 2004).

In a study of 99 local health departments in three rural states, Rosenblatt et al. (2002) found that public health nurses were the core provider of public health services. Many smaller local health departments do not have the economic base to employ other professional public health providers, such as physicians, epidemiologists, sanitarians, and nutritionists at the local level. Frequently, these services are provided at the state level or collaboratively between groups of local health departments. A local physician may serve as a part-time, unpaid health officer. The lack of additional on-site public health providers poses two problems. First, the ability to collaborate with others about potential or actual public health problems is decreased or nonexistent. Second, the ranges of services provided are less comprehensive. Often, these small facilities can only offer federally funded programs with few locally funded services. Environmental health, maternal and child health, and communicable disease control are the three highest priority programs of rural local health departments (Berkowitz, 2004).

Rural Mental Health Care

The economic crisis that affected much of the rural population in the 1980s contributed to mental health problems (American Psychological Association, 1995). Natural disasters, such as drought and flood, and economic downturns in the late 1990s have contributed to continuing chronic stress. Those affected are most apt to work in the traditional ranching, farming, mining, forestry, and fishing industries. They have not enjoyed the good economic times generated by the information and technology age (NRHA, 2007, IOM, 2005). Although mental health disorders widely affect rural and urban residents across the life span, factors such as poverty, race, age, and rural dwelling lower the prospect of accessing mental health services (Gamm, Stone, and Pittman, 2003). Clearly, large sections of at-risk rural populations are without mental health care (NRHA, 2007).

There are three key factors that have been identified as contributing to mental illness in rural areas (Gamm et al., 2003). First, there is a lack of specialized mental health providers in rural areas. The most recent figures show that 75% of rural counties with populations between 2500 and 20,000 do not have a psychiatrist, and 95% do not have a child psychiatrist. Next, because of the lack of qualified mental health care providers, rural residents often receive services from primary care providers. McCabe and Macnee (2002) found that many rural primary care providers are ill equipped to provide mental health services. Both specialized mental health care and primary health care providers are confronted with barriers related to rural practice. These include a more diverse practice, fewer opportunities for ongoing education, and fewer professionals to consult than their colleagues in urban practice.

Last, rural residents often do not seek mental health services because of perceived stigma. They do not always recognize a need for mental health services (Gamm et al., 2003).

Emergency Services

Access to emergency medical services (EMS) has been identified as one of the most significant health care issues for rural residents (Rawlinson and Crews, 2003). EMS include prehospital care, hospital or health center–based emergency care, and trauma systems.

Rural residents depend on EMS because of their high risk for unintentional injury. Low population density has been shown to be a strong predictor of increased injury-related morbidity and mortality rates in rural areas (Peek-Asa et al., 2004). In medically underserved areas, EMS systems play an increasingly important role in decreasing the morbidity and mortality of individuals needing emergency care. Getting patients from the place of injury to the trauma center within the "golden hour" is frequently not possible in rural areas because distance, terrain, climatic conditions, and communication methods produce barriers. Some rural facilities are more than 1 hour away by air from the nearest trauma center or tertiary care hospital, and, according to Branas et al. (2005), of the 46.7 million Americans who have no access within an hour, most live in rural areas. For those rural residents the death rate remains twice that of urban residents.

Challenges faced by rural EMS systems include a shortage of volunteers, a lower level of training than among urban providers, training curricula that often do not reflect rural hazards (e.g., farm equipment trauma), lack of guidance from physicians, and lack of physician training and orientation to the EMS system (Rawlinson and Crews, 2003). Low population density; large, isolated, or inaccessible areas; severe weather; poor roads; and lower density of telephones or other communication methods also contribute to difficult public access for emergency care. These problems make the challenges of developing EMS in rural areas substantial (Branas et al., 2005).

LEGISLATION AND PROGRAMS AFFECTING RURAL PUBLIC HEALTH

Programs That Augment Health Care Facilities and Services

Several programs are particularly important for meeting the public health needs of rural people. One is the Community Health Centers (CHC) program, administered by the U.S. Public Health Service (USPHS). The CHC program benefits underserved areas and populations by providing primary health care and, in some cases, supplemental secondary and tertiary health care, such as hospital care, long-term home health care, and rehabilitation. Rural health clinics (RHCs) are designed to improve access to primary care. As an incentive to rural communities to apply for RHCs, Medicare and Medicaid are reimbursed at a higher rate than usual.

The Migrant Health Clinic (MHC) program and the Migrant Health Program (MHP) also come under the Division of Community and Migrant Health and HRSA. The MHC program provides comprehensive nursing and medical care and support services to migrant and seasonal farmworkers and their families. The centers provide culturally sensitive care to a racially and culturally diverse farm labor force from many countries in Latin America and the Caribbean.

Bilingual, bicultural health personnel, including lay outreach workers, use culturally appropriate protocols for providing primary care, preventive health care, transportation, dental care, pharmaceuticals, and environmental health. The MHCs must provide the same services as the CHC and may also offer supplemental services, such as environmental health services, infectious disease and parasite control, and accident prevention programs.

Medicare's Rural Hospital Flexibility (RHF) grant program replaces earlier demonstration programs during the 1990s. According to information provided by the Office of Rural Health Policy (ORHP), the RHF program "allows small hospitals the flexibility to reconfigure operations and be licensed as Critical Access Hospitals (CAHs)" (Office of Rural Health Policy, nd). The program also provides cost-based reimbursement for inpatient Medicare and outpatient service. Grants are also awarded for planning, implementing, and establishing networks of care and improving EMS.

Primary care cooperative agreements facilitate the development of primary care services and attract primary care providers to rural HPSAs. Special legislation for HPSAs has also created programs to provide acute care facilities and services. The Rural Transition Grants Program, administered by HCFA, helps small rural communities with nonprofit hospitals adjust to changes in clinical practice patterns and in-hospital use, shifts from hospital- to community-based care, and changes in emergency care delivery patterns.

RURAL COMMUNITY HEALTH NURSING

Perhaps a more accurate title than rural community health nursing would be "community health nursing along the rural continuum." Nonmetropolitan areas are at one end of the continuum, whereas metropolitan areas are at the other end.

Practice in a rural area may require working as the only nurse at a health department in a remote Western Great Plains frontier county with a population of 6000, at a full-service health department in a town of 50,000 people, or at a large health department in a rural area next to an urban population. A practice in a rural area adjacent to a large metropolitan area often appears to have more in common with the urban end of the continuum in terms of agency size, distances, and resources. For the purposes of this discussion, the practice setting is at the more "rural" end of the continuum.

The following definition illustrates the broad-based, generalist focus of the modern rural community health nurse. It includes the important geographic and cultural environment where community health practice is implemented and helps define appropriate nursing interventions.

Rural nursing is the practice of professional nursing within the physical and sociocultural context of sparsely populated communities. It involves the continual interaction of the rural environment, the nurse, and his or her practice. Rural nursing is the diagnosis and treatment of a diversified population of people of all ages and a variety of human responses to actual (or potential) occupational

hazards or actual or potential health problems existent in maternity, pediatric, medical/surgical and emergency nursing in a given rural area. (Bigbee, 1993, p. 132)

Characteristics of Rural Nursing

The uniqueness of rural nursing practice has been in question. Some believe that nursing care for rural clients is the same as for other individuals, and health problems and patient care needs are similar regardless of the setting. Others argue that rural practice should be designated as a specialty or subspecialty area because of factors such as isolation, scarce resources, and the need for a wide range of practice skills that must be adapted to social and economic structures. Whether generalist or specialist, nurses prepared for rural practice must be equipped with other community health assessment skills (Thrall, 2007, IOM, 2005).

Bowlby (2002) states increased interest in public health has brought community nurses greater respect. Nurses cite feeling valued as a resource and the ability to change behavior in a community as positive aspects of the profession. Autonomy, professional status, and being valued by the agency and community have been reported components of positive job satisfaction (Davis and Droes, 1993; Dunkin et al., 1992).

Of those components identified as negative, agencies and professional organizations are most actively addressing professional isolation. The use of distance education technologies is one way to address the isolation many rural nurses experience. University degree programs and continuing education courses are readily available online or by full-motion interactive television. Using these technologies, rural nurses are able to update their skills and network with other nurses without having to leave their home communities.

Scharff (1998) discussed the distinctive nature of the rural nurse's practice. She found that the rural nurse is a generalist, and generalist is not synonymous with boring. Interviews with rural nurses show that they feel an "intensity of purpose" that makes rural nursing distinctive. Nurses living and practicing in the same place have a strong sense of integration and continuity between practice and community.

The newcomer practices nursing in a rural setting, unlike the more experienced nurse, who practices rural nursing. Somewhere between these extremes lies the transitional period of events and conditions through which each nurse passes at her or his own pace. It is within this time zone that nurses experience rural reality and move toward becoming professionals who understand that having gone rural, they are not less than they were, but rather, they are more than they expected to be. Some may be conscious of the transition, and others may not, but in the end, a few will say, "I am a rural nurse." (Scharff, 1998, p. 38)

Rural community health nursing is rewarding and challenging. Services can include maternal and child health, elder health, school health, mental health, and occupational health. The nurse practicing with the autonomy common in rural practice brings knowledge and competence in other clinical

Rural Health Priorities from Rural Healthy People 2010

RURAL PRIORITIES (IDENTIFIED BY 25% OR MORE)	PERCENTAGE OF RESPONDENTS (N = 44)
Access to health care (includes one of the following):	73
Access to emergency medical services	32
Access to health workforce	29
Access to health services (general)	29
Access to health insurance	26
Access to primary care	24
Mental health	49
Oral health	41
Educational and community-based programs	29
Diabetes	26
Injury and violence prevention	26
Nutrition and overweight	21
Public health infrastructure	21
Tobacco	21
Maternal, infant, and child health	18
Occupational safety and health	18
Cancer	15
Environmental health	15
Heart disease and stroke	15

Data from Gamm LD, Hutchison L, Dabney RJ, Dorsey AM, editors: Rural *Healthy People 2010: a companion document to Healthy People 2010*, vols 1-3, College Station, TX, 2003, The Texas A&M University System Health Science Center, School of Rural Public Health, Southwest Rural Health Research Center.

specialties. The work requires a discriminating, solid practitioner who can perform general nursing at a skill level beyond that of the outdated "mile wide and inch deep" general nursing. The rural nurse must be an "expert generalist."

RURAL HEALTH RESEARCH

Contemporary developments in the health care delivery system and advances in science suggest the need for an active agenda in rural health research. Berkowitz, Ivory, and Morris (2002) comment that rural health policy and research agendas must at the very least address the following issues:

1. The capacity of rural public health to manage improvements in health
2. Information technology capacity in rural communities
3. Developing and monitoring performance standards in rural public health
4. Developing leadership and public health workforce capacity within rural public health
5. Interaction and integration of community health systems, managed care, and public health in rural America

Capacity of Rural Public Health to Manage Improvements in Health

Healthy People 2020 (USDHHS, 2009) outlines health-related objectives for Americans and forms the rationale for efforts to intervene with trends in disease to improve health. The status of health indicators, such as rates of morbidity, mortality from common diseases or injury, and perhaps more important, access to health care services, allows for priorities to be determined for which improvements in health are needed. Importantly, *Healthy People 2020* objectives have been analyzed for rural-urban disparities that may exist along geographic, demographic, and cultural dimensions to provide

a more specific picture of potential research priorities concerning improvements in health for rural areas alone (Gamm et al., 2003, vol. 1). The *Healthy People* table presents data from a survey of forty-four national and state rural health experts that identify percentages of respondents indicating priority status for various health issues.

Research questions directed toward improving health may be suggested along any of the *Healthy People 2020* objectives but may have the greatest potential to address salient rural trends if they relate to issues of access to care, mental health, oral health, educational and community-based programs, diabetes, or injury and violence prevention. Additionally, investigators may want to consider how these established rural priorities may be consistent or different within specific populations of concern. Because availability of surveillance data is often limited as researchers concern themselves with increasingly smaller populations (e.g., from state to county), efforts to gather additional primary data may be needed to set research priorities for improvements to health.

Information Technology in Rural Communities

As the distribution of technology expands across rural populations, more research is needed to examine the impacts of readily accessible information to both rural citizens and the health care delivery system. Rural patients are able to access specialty services such as radiological or dermatological exams through telemedicine, and rural people are increasingly taking advantage of the World Wide Web to access information to make health decisions. Recent federal efforts directed toward disaster and terrorism preparedness have strengthened rural technological infrastructure so that communication pathways remain open during times of need. Just as patients access health care services from isolation, rural citizens are accessing health education through

RESEARCH HIGHLIGHTS

Defining Rural Areas: Old and New Classifications

Old system (before Census 2000)
Metropolitan (metro) areas:
- Cities of 50,000 or more residents, or
- Urbanized areas of 50,000 or more residents and total area population of 100,000 or more

Nonmetropolitan (nonmetro) areas:
- All counties not classified as metro

New core-based system (starting with Census 2000)
Metropolitan (metro) areas:
- Central counties with 50,000 or more residents, regardless of total area population. Includes outlying counties with 25% or more of the employed population commuting daily.

Micropolitan (micro) areas:
- Central counties with one or more urban clusters of 10,000-50,000 persons. Includes outlying counties with 25% or more of the employed population commuting daily.

Noncore areas:
- All counties not meeting the new "metro" or "micro" classification are classified as "outside core based statistical areas."

From Slifkin RT, Randolph R, Ricketts TC: The changing metropolitan designation process and rural America, *J Rural Health* 20(1):1-6, 2004.

distance programs for both continuing education and entry-level and advanced degree programs in various health sciences. The need to address new research questions has grown alongside rapid expansion of information technology (IT), and questions abound relating to the application and evaluation of technology for improving both systems of care and care outcomes (Research Highlights box). Berkowitz et al. (2002) suggest that the following questions be answered with respect to IT for public health in rural areas:
- What is the role of telehealth in public health?
- What impact is distance learning having on the skills of rural public health professionals?
- What are the costs and infrastructure implications of ensuring access to IT in rural areas?
- How can IT be used to fill the gaps in epidemiology and surveillance capacity in rural health departments?

Performance Standards in Rural Public Health

The National Public Health Performance Standards Program (NPHPSP) is a collaborative effort, organized through the CDC, the mission of which is to improve the quality of public health practice and the performance of local public health systems by providing and evaluating standards of performance.

The NPHPSP utilizes the Ten Essential Public Health Services to establish three assessment instruments that can be used by local and state public health systems for evaluation and improvement. Standards describe an optimal level of performance by public health systems, which include all public, private, and voluntary entities that contribute to activities directed toward public health in an assessment area. The assessment can be used to improve collaborations among key public health partners, educate participants about public health, strengthen the network of public health partners, identify strengths and weaknesses, and provide benchmarks for public health practice improvements (CDC, 2004a). Research questions that need to be addressed in rural areas may focus on the extent to which state and local performance assessments outlined by NPHPSP have been carried out, as well as the ability of rural public health systems to respond to needed changes to comprehensively address essential services. Additionally, rural areas may benefit from research examining resource constraints and the need to expand partnerships to address essential services that may be challenging to provide within isolated populations.

CASE STUDY   APPLICATION OF THE NURSING PROCESS

All three levels of prevention (i.e., primary, secondary, and tertiary) are reflected in rural practice. These are applied to individuals, families, and aggregates. The generalist nature of the rural community health practice gives the nurse an excellent opportunity to assess health needs and help improve health status at all levels of prevention. The following case study includes short-term individual and family approaches. It also focuses on upstream interventions developed to handle the identified problems. Upstream interventions focus on population and prevention. They deal with political, economic, and environmental factors that are precursors to health problems.

At 4:30 PM on a hot fall day, community health nurse Mary Fieldson, RN, drove up a narrow gravel township road 40 miles from her office in the county courthouse. She had just completed her sixth home health visit. By the time Mary returned home, she had traveled more than 150 miles, but she enjoyed the drive. She worked in a rural county of 6000 where she grew up. She made a skilled visit to Joe Lingh, the father of a high school friend. On her way home, she traversed the valley where she once lived. She recently returned "home" after a 15-year absence to live, work, and raise her 12-year-old daughter.

When she approached the Connelly farm, Mary saw Eliza Connelly standing by the road waving her down. Mary stopped to say hello. Eliza said, "I called Ruth Lingh and she said you had just left. How is Joe's leg?" Mary was aware that this was a friendly inquiry about a neighbor of 40 years, but she was mindful of the need for confidentiality. Mary told Eliza that Joe was glad to be home from the hospital. Eliza asked if Mary had heard about her husband's accident Monday evening. "He cut his hand up in the silage chopper and is in the hospital in Spring City," she told Mary tearfully. "I just knew something was going to happen someday. I worry so much about them working with all that machinery and the men work in the fields alone so much. I feel about ready to fall apart. Thank God Jim [their son] was working with him when it happened!"

Mary had a cup of coffee with Eliza, who regained her composure. Eliza continued to talk about long-standing fears for the safety of her family in doing the farm work. She asked Mary to stop by and check on her husband, Austin, when he returned home the following week. Mary told Eliza to request a referral from the primary care physician so insurance would pay for the visits. At 5:30 PM Mary began the drive back to her office in Wolsey, the county seat.

Monday afternoon, Mary received a telephone call from Dr. Lobban, the local primary care physician. He requested weekly skilled nursing visits for Austin for the next 3 weeks to assess the wound for infection and to teach Eliza how to change the dressings and recognize signs and symptoms of infection. Austin was discharged from the Spring City hospital the following day, 6 days after the injury. Dr. Lobban sent Mary the emergency department records and the hand specialist's discharge summary.

Assessment

The medical records provided the following information. The first finger was severed at the metacarpophalangeal joint (i.e., the third joint) and reattached. The second, third, and fourth fingers were severed distal to the proximal interphalangeal joints (i.e., between the first and second joints). The severed portions of the second, third, and fourth fingers could not be reattached because they were too badly mangled. At discharge, infection was not evident. The injuries were healing well.

The Connelly family provided additional information about the circumstances of the accident. At approximately 6:30 PM, Austin and his son, Jim, were chopping oats for silage. Seeing rain clouds on the horizon, Jim and Austin hurried to finish before rain fell on the unchopped grain. The silage chopper was not working well. Austin shut it off and hurriedly reached into the inspection hole. The still-turning blades caught his right hand, severing the fingers. Jim wrapped his father's hand tightly in his shirt, retrieved the fingers, and drove his father to their house 2 miles away. Jim went back to the field to finish chopping the oats. Eliza drove her husband 23 miles to the primary care hospital emergency department. The family physician cleaned and dressed Austin's hand, gave him medication for pain, and packed the severed fingers for transport to the hand specialist in Spring City. A family friend and his son drove Mr. and Mrs. Connelly 150 miles to the Spring City hospital where Austin was admitted and underwent surgery. Eliza went home with their friend and his son after the surgery. She spoke to Austin by telephone daily and drove to Spring City on Tuesday to bring him home.

On her first home visit Mary assessed the following:
- Individual client, Austin, for signs and symptoms of infection, pain control, and functional positioning
- Eliza's comfort level and knowledge of dressing changes and signs and symptoms of infection (i.e., she is the primary caregiver)
- Stress and grief processing of all family members
- Ability of family members to provide physical and emotional support during crisis resolution
- Risk-taking behaviors, especially those related to work, of all family members
- Assessment of neighborhood groups and neighbors who can provide support and help the family with the fall harvest work

Diagnosis
Individual
- Risk for infection, pain, and loss of hand function (Austin)
- Risk for grief related to loss of fingers, some use of hand, and decreased ability to do farm work (Austin)
- Anxiety related to ongoing fear of injury of family members (Eliza)
- Stress related to new responsibilities for farm management (Jim)

Family
- Risk for family crisis related to instability caused by the injury

Community
- Inadequate programs for farm injury prevention
- Nonexistent EMS or first-response service

Planning
A plan of care is developed at the individual, family, and community levels. Mutual goal setting and contracting are essential if the outcomes are to be optimal.

Individual
Long-Term Goal
- Client will experience successful rehabilitation.

Short-Term Goals
- Client will remain free of infection.
- Individual family members will be able to express grief.

Family
Long-Term Goals
- Family will demonstrate coping skills appropriate to the crisis.
- Family will identify risky behavior related to farm work.

Short-Term Goals
- Identify support to help with farm work.
- Identify ways to keep in contact with each other when family members are working alone in the fields.

Community
Long-Term Goal
- Program will be established for farm injury prevention education for populations at risk.

Short-Term Goals
- Begin the health planning process to put into place a farm injury primary prevention program.
- Explore the potential for a volunteer EMS response team.

Intervention
Mutual goal setting between Mary Fieldson and the Connelly family made it possible for them to carry out interventions collaboratively.

Individual
Mary taught Eliza how to change dressings and monitor Austin's hand for infection and function. Austin was involved in his care during healing and was able to monitor and manage the pain. He was most concerned about rehabilitation. He especially wanted to know when he could return to work and how disabled he would be. The local physician monitored Austin's progress. With Austin and Eliza present, the local physician consulted with the hand specialist by two-way interactive video conferencing. This enabled them to confer, thereby eliminating a 150-mile trip to Spring City. The home care physical therapist (PT) visited the farm once to set up a program of hand exercises. Austin, who plays the piano, wanted to know if piano playing would be a good exercise. "Playing 'Moonlight Serenade' would sure stretch that right hand," he told the therapist. The therapist told him that he should play three times a day as part of the rehabilitation care plan.

Family
Mary worked with the family to find ways to finish the fall work. They decided to hire part-time help, and two workers helped full-time until the crop was harvested. While in the hospital, Austin was able to assist his son by supporting his ability to make the necessary decisions about farm management. After discharge, he also

(Continued)

was able to participate in the process. The family identified the need for more awareness about the dangers of farm work. They immediately purchased a cellular phone to take to the field. Eliza felt this would relieve her anxiety about being out of touch with Austin and Jim and not knowing why they were later than expected for meals. There was much discussion about the cost of the telephone and service. Eliza convinced the men that her peace of mind was worth the cost.

The stress and grief reactions were minimal. Most of the stress centered on getting the fall farm work done and seeing that Austin recovered enough to work "the way he is used to doing." Support from neighbors and the rehabilitation program helped them deal with stress and grief.

Community

When an accident happens in a small rural community, it brings home the dangerous nature of farm work. People begin recalling their own "close calls" and remembering friends and family members who have been injured. This period of high awareness is an excellent time to bring people together to discuss accident prevention. During the annual fall 4-H Achievement Days, Mary Fieldson set up an information booth in the exhibit hall and asked for volunteers to plan and implement a farm safety program in the county.

Austin's accident was handled appropriately by the family without EMS intervention. However, other accidents had recently required trained personnel at the site to stabilize the injured person and minimize damage during transport to the primary care hospital. For Mary, her home care visits to farm families reinforced the need for EMS in these remote areas. She met with the county health department, local physicians, and county commissioners to investigate the feasibility of establishing an EMS.

Evaluation
Individual

Individual members of the Connelly family used the home care nurse, PT, and local physician appropriately as evidenced by Austin's successful healing and rehabilitation. Austin returned to work with minimum disability. During a drop-in visit by Mary 3 months after the accident, Austin treated her to a rousing piano rendition of "Stars and Stripes Forever."

Family

With Mary's guidance, the family wrote down a list of hazards and strategies to improve safety on the farm. Interestingly, one of the items was to wear seat belts in the car and truck. The family installed seat belts in a 40-year-old farm truck still in regular

use. They purchased the cellular phone and used it to keep Eliza in touch with Austin and Jim while they were in the field. This has proved so successful that several neighbors have also bought cellular phones.

The family continued to demonstrate good coping skills as Austin progressed in his rehabilitation. Communication between father and son was excellent after the initial concern that Austin would feel like his position as farm manager was being usurped. He became involved with daily decision making as soon as he returned home from the hospital. The family effectively solved the problem of getting the fall work done by requesting the help of friends and neighbors. They borrowed money from the bank to hire a part-time farm hand until Austin could work again.

Community

Mary's information booth at the 4-H Achievement Days attracted the attention of several women from the County Extension Club. As a result of their interest, the club made farm safety education their service project for the following year. Lack of community support halted development of a volunteer emergency medical first-response team.

Levels of Prevention

The following are examples of the three levels of prevention as applied to the individual, family, and community.

Primary
- Assessment and teaching about farm accident prevention to family
- Initiation of a program of farm safety information at the community level
- Use of a cellular telephone to decrease anxiety about family members' locations and well-being

Secondary
- Infection prevention and pain management of injured hand
- Screening at family and community level for farm hazards (i.e., a component of the overall primary prevention education program)

Tertiary
- Rehabilitation of Austin to limit disability
- Assessment and counseling to help family and injured individual cope with stress and grief reactions
- Attempted development of an EMS system to facilitate stabilization and safe transport

Leadership and Workforce Capacity for Rural Public Health

In 2003, the IOM published results of a project intended to improve our understanding of what is needed to prepare the public health workforce for the twenty-first century (Gebbie, Rosenstock, and Hernandez, 2003). Workforce capacity challenges cited by the IOM report include globalization, which increases travel and allows for distribution of emerging and reemerging diseases (e.g., human immunodeficiency virus and AIDS, tuberculosis, hepatitis B, malaria, cholera, diphtheria, and Ebola); advances in scientific and medical technologies that challenge the public health workforce in areas of

ethics, data security, and communication; and demographic transformations that require new skills and services as our population ages and becomes more diverse.

The Public Health Workforce Development initiative (CDC, 2004b), created jointly by the CDC and the Agency for Toxic Substances and Disease Registry to address future challenges to public health workforce development, outlines six strategies to prepare a competent workforce that will be able to perform the essential public health services in light of new challenges. This initiative suggests that an initial strategy is to monitor workforce composition and conduct research to validate methodology for public health worker enumeration. Since that time, strides have been made, and, despite increased attention and resources, major concerns remain regarding the public health workforce. The most commonly cited concerns are (1) inadequate numbers of workers, especially for specific skilled public health occupational categories such as public health nurses; (2) impending shortages of experienced workers who are approaching retirement age, without adequate replacements; and (3) workers insufficiently trained (Gebbie and Turnock, 2006).

Interaction and Integration of Community Health Systems, Managed Care, and Public Health

The evolution of managed care into rural environments has limited the safety-net role of some local health departments to provide primary care by preventing fee-for-service reimbursement and contracting care to networks of providers or organizations. This is especially true for Medicaid-managed care, which serves that same population of people that are traditionally served with primary care services through local public health departments. As Hurley, Crawford, and Praeger (2002) note, Medicaid's importance for rural areas is likely to grow as broader health care developments, such as declining inpatient use of rural hospitals and reductions in Medicare reimbursement, provoke more interest in using the Medicaid system to support threatened rural infrastructure.

Consequently, the administration of the Medicaid program will increasingly seek the cost savings promised by managed care, and the role of rural public health departments may increasingly narrow into areas that are currently without any type of reimbursement. Because of this, Berkowitz et al. (2002) argue that finding ways to integrate public health in the rural primary care at the community level will become increasingly important. There will be many questions to be answered by additional research. What are the factors associated with successful integration of public health and managed care in rural environments? What capacity do rural health departments have for contracting arrangements with managed care organizations? What are the effects of local public health and managed-care contracts on direct provision of services?

SUMMARY

This chapter provides an overview of rural and migrant health. People who live in rural areas make up 61 million, or approximately 25%, of the U.S. population. The reader must not assume that all rural people are similar; diversity exists in age, ethnicity, income, education, and geography.

Not all rural residents are disadvantaged. The data show that in some ways they are penalized as a whole, no matter how diverse the rural population. Health care access and income levels are areas where disadvantages generally exist. Provider shortages, an ineffective health care system, hospital-based and community-based care, and few health promotion and disease prevention services represent a marginal health care network. One half of the poor in the United States live in rural areas. The combination of poor health care access and low income level results in higher morbidity and mortality rates in rural populations. The high-risk nature of such occupations as farmworkers, miners, and loggers also contributes to disability and death rates. This chapter describes the structural, financial, and personal barriers contributing to poor health care access.

Nurses who work with rural people must assess each aggregate's characteristics. A ranching community in Wyoming will have different needs than a migrant community in Arizona. Demographic information, aggregate morbidity and mortality data, emerging rural nursing theory, knowledge of barriers, and rural health care research are all necessary to plan appropriate upstream community health nursing interventions. Integrating these concepts gives nurses the tools to improve the health of rural people.

LEARNING ACTIVITIES

1. University libraries commonly subscribe to newspapers published within the state. Visit the library and select three or four small-town or rural county newspapers. Read them for information about health care activities and concerns related to the health of the individuals, families, and community.
   - Report findings to the class about rural health concerns and activities.
   - Identify one priority problem that could be researched in the community and has relevance to rural community health nursing practice.
2. Select a rural community health nurse (i.e., public health or home care), and conduct an interview in person or by telephone if distance prohibits a face-to-face meeting.
   - Identify what the nurse sees as the pros and cons of rural nursing.
   - If negative aspects of rural nursing are identified, discuss how the nurse deals with them.
   - Ask the nurse to discuss the three highest priority efforts related to his or her rural practice.
3. Choose one of the major causes of morbidity and mortality in migrant populations.
   - On the basis of risk factor and natural history, specify interventions for primary, secondary, and tertiary prevention of this problem.
   - Identify which of these interventions are examples of upstream thinking.
4. Locate a telephone book or community resource directory from a rural community.
   - List and evaluate the resources that are available for prevention, assessment, intervention, and follow-up care for the major cause of mortality and morbidity identified in Learning Activity No. 3. Would it be necessary to go outside the rural town or county for any of the needed resources? Which ones? Where might they be located?

REFERENCES

Agency for Healthcare Research and Quality: *Health care disparities in rural areas*, Washington, DC, 2004, The Author.

Allender JA, Rector C, Warner KD: *Community health nursing: promoting and protecting the public's health*, ed 7, Philadelphia, 2010, Wolters Kluwer, Lippincott Williams & Wilkins.

Altermanan T, et al: Ethnic, racial, and gender variations in health among farm operators in the United States, *Ann Epidemiol* 18(3): 179–186, 2008.

American Nurses Association: *Scope and standards of parish nursing practice*, Washington, DC, 2005, The Author.

American Psychological Association: *Office of Rural Health: caring for the rural community*, Washington, DC, 1995, The Author.

Baldwin LM, et al: Access to specialty health care for rural American Indians in two states, *Rural Health* 24(3):269–278, 2008.

Becker G, Gates RJ, Newsome E: Self-care among chronically ill African Americans: culture, health disparities, and health insurance status, *Am J Public Health* 94(12):2066–2073, 2004.

Berkowitz B: Rural public health service delivery: promising new directions, *Am J Public Health* 94(10):1678–1681, 2004.

Berkowitz B, Ivory J, Morris T: Rural public health: policy and research opportunities, *J Rural Health* 18(Suppl):186–196, 2002.

Bigbee J: The uniqueness of rural nursing, *Nurs Clin North Am* 28:131–144, 1993.

Bolin J, Gamm LG: Access to quality health services in rural areas: insurance. In *Rural Healthy People 2010: A companion document to Healthy People 2010*, vol 1. College Station, TX, 2003, The Texas A&M University System Health Science Center, School of Rural Public Health, Southwest Rural Health Research Center.

Bowlby J: *Renewed Respect, No longer on the sidelines since Sept. 11, Public health nurses take center stage in their communities*, 2002, 03/publichealth.asp. Accessed March 23, 2010.

Branas CC, MacKenzie E, Williams JC, et al: Access to trauma centers in the United States, *JAMA* 293(21):2626–2633, 2005.

Branas CC, Nance MD, Elliott MR, et al: Urban-rural shifts in intentional firearm death: different causes, same results, *Am J Public Health* 94(10):1750–1755, 2004.

Buckwalter KC, et al: Telehealth for elders and their caregivers in rural communities, *Fam Community Health* 25(3):31–40, 2002.

Bureau of Health Professions: *Changing demographics: implications for physicians, nurses, and other health workers*, 2003. ftp://ftp.hrsa.gov/bhpr/nationalcenter/changedemo.pdf.

Bureau of Primary Healthcare: *Migrant and seasonal farmworker enumeration profiles study*, 2000. http://bphc.hrsa.gov/migrant/Enumeration/EnumerationStudy.htm.

Center on Budget and Policy Priorities: *Improving rural parents health insurance coverage: a fact sheet*, 2001, www.cbpp.org/cms/?fa=view&id=539. Accessed April 14, 2009.

Centers for Disease Control and Prevention, National Center for Health Statistics: *Health*, United States, 2007, The Author, pp. 33, www.cdc.gov/nchs/data/misc/injury2007.pdf.

Centers for Disease Control and Prevention: *National Public Health Performance Standards Program*, 2004a, www.cdc.gov/od/ocphp/nphpsp/.

Centers for Disease Control and Prevention: *The public health workforce development initiative*, 2004b, http://www.phppo.cdc.gov/owpp/workforcedev.asp#Workforce%20Development%20Library.

Centers for Disease Control and Prevention: *Health*, United States, 2007, With Chartbook on Trends in the Health of Americans, www.cdc.gov/nchs/data/hus/hus07.pdf. Accessed March 21, 2010.

Centers for Disease Control and Prevention: *Recent trends in infant mortality*, 2008, Retrieved March 14, 2010 from www.cdc.gov/nchs/data/databriefs/db09.htm.

Centers for Disease Control and Prevention: *Healthy Youth*, 2009, Retrieved March 14, 2010 from www.cdc.gov/HealthyYouth/healthtopics/disparities.htm.

Chase-Ziolek M, Striepe J: A comparison of urban versus rural experiences of nurses volunteering to promote health in churches, *Public Health Nurs* 16(4):270–279, 1999.

Cohen RA, Bloom B: *Trends in health insurance and access to medical care for children under age 19 years: United States, 1998–2003*. Advance data from vital and health statistics; no 355, Hyattsville, MD, 2005, National Center for Health Statistics.

Cohen RA, Martinez ME, Hao CKK: *Health insurance coverage: estimates from the National Health Interview Survey*, January–September, 2004, Centers for Disease Control and Prevention, Division of Health Interview Statistics, National Center for Health Statistics, www.cdc.gov/nchs/nhis.htm.

Cotton DJ, et al: Grain dust and alveolar macrophages: an experimental study of the effects of grain dust on the mouse lung. In Dosman JA, Cockcroft DW, editors: *Principles of health and safety in agriculture*, Boca Raton, FL, 1989, CRC Press.

Crouse BJ: Preparing physicians for rural practice: the role of medical student education, *J Agromedicine* 12(4):2007.

Davis D, Droes N: Community health nursing in rural and frontier counties, *Nurs Clin North Am* 28:159–169, 1993.

Dunbar J, Mueller C: *Anticipating the 1997 state children's health insurance program: what's current in five rural states?* Bethesda, MD, January 1998, The Project HOPE Walsh Center for Rural Health Analysis.

Dunkin J, et al: Job satisfaction and retention of rural community health nurses in North Dakota, *J Rural Health* 8:268–275, 1992.

Eberhardt MS, et al: *Urban and rural health chartbook*, Hyattsville, MD, 2001, Department of Health and Human Services, Centers for Disease Control and Prevention, National Center for Health Statistics. National Center for Health Statistics, www.cdc.gov/nchs/pressroom/01news/hus01.htm.

Eberhardt MS, Pamuk ER: The importance of place of residence: examining health in rural and nonrural areas, *Am J Public Health* 94(10):1682–1686, 2004.

Edmondson W: *Economics of the food and fiber system*, 2004, Amber Waves, US Department of Agriculture, Economic Research Service, www.ers.usda.gov/AmberWaves/February04/DataFeature/.

Eggebeen D, Lichter D: Health and well-being among rural Americans: variations across the life course, *J Rural Health* 9:86–98, 1993.

Elliott MR, Ginsburg KR, Winston FK: Unlicensed teenaged drivers: who are they, and how do they behave when they are behind the wheel? *Pediatrics* 122(5):994–1000, 2008.

Farm Worker Fund: *Innovative outreach practices report*, 2006, www.farmworkerhealth.org/docs/IOPR2006.pdf. Accessed April 13, 2009.

Ferrer RL: Pursuing equity: contact with primary care and specialist clinicians by demographics, insurance, and health status, *Ann Fam Med* 5(6):492–502, 2007, www.aarp.org/research/health/carefinancing/reform_profiles.html.

Gamm LD, Castillo G, Pittman S: Access to quality health services in rural areas—primary care: a literature review. In Gamm LD, Hutchison L, Dabney RJ, Dorsey AM, editors: *Rural Healthy People 2010: a companion document to Healthy People 2010*, vol 2. College Station, TX, 2003, The Texas A&M University System Health Science Center, School of Rural Public Health, Southwest Rural Health Research Center.

Gamm LD, Hutchison L: Rural *Healthy People 2010*: evolving interactive practice, *Am J Public Health* 94(10):1711–1712, 2004, www.pubmedcentral.nih.gov/articlerender.fcgi?artid=1448522. Accessed April 13, 2009.

Gamm L, Stone S, Pittman S: *Mental health and mental disorders a rural challenge: a literature review. Rural Healthy People 2010: A companion document to Healthy People 2010*, vol 2, College Station, TX, 2003, The Texas A&M University System Health Science Center, School of Rural Public Health, Southwest Rural Health Research Center.

Gebbie K, Rosenstock L, Hernandez LM: *Who will keep the public healthy? Educating public health professionals for the 21st century*, Washington, DC, 2003, The National Academies Press.

Gebbie K, Turnock BJ: A two-decade trend of increasing numbers of public health workers could end if federal bioterrorism grants decrease, *Health Aff* 25(4):923–933, 2006.

Glover S, et al: Disparities in access to care among rural working-age adults, *J Rural Health* 20(3):193–205, 2004.

Gosschalk A, Carozza S: Cancer in rural areas. In Gamm LD, Hutchison L, Dabney RJ, Dorsey AM, editors: *Rural Healthy People 2010: a companion document to Healthy People 2010*, vols 1–3. College Station, TX, 2003, The Texas A&M University System Health Science Center, School of Rural Public Health, Southwest Rural Health Research Center.

Hanrahan NP, Hartley D: Employment of advanced-practice psychiatric nurses to stem rural mental health workforce shortages, Psychiatryonline.org 59(1):109–111, 2008.

Hartley D: Rural health disparities, population health, and rural culture, *Am J Public Health* 94(10):1675–1678, 2004.

Herbert R, Landrigan PJ: Work-related death: a continuing epidemic, *Am J Public Health* 90(4):541–545, 2000.

Hoyert DL, Kung HC, Smith BL: Deaths: preliminary data for 2003, *Natl Vital Stat Rep* 53(15). Hyattsville, MD, 2005, National Center for Health Statistics.

Hurley RE, Crawford H, Praeger S: Medicaid and rural health care, *J Rural Health* 18(Suppl):164–175, 2002.

Institute of Medicine: *Quality through collaboration: the future of rural health*, Washington, DC, 2005, National Academy Press.

International Parish Nurse Resource Center: *Information for clergy*. http://ipnrc.parishnurses.org/forcl.phtml. Accessed April 21, 2005.

Johnson AO, et al: Violence and drug use in rural teens: national prevalence estimates from the 2003 Youth Risk Behavior Survey, *J Sch Health* 78(10):554–561, 2008.

Kandel W, Cromartie J: *Hispanics find a home in rural America*, 2003, Amber Waves, US Department of Agriculture, Economic Research Service, www.ers.usda.gov/AmberWaves/.

Kandel W, Newman C: *Rural Hispanics: employment and residential trends*, 2004, www.ers.usda.gov/AmberWaves/June04/Features/RuralHispanic.htm. Accessed April 13, 2009.

Kass BL, Weinick RM, Monheit AC: *Racial and ethnic differences in health: 1996, MEPS Chartbook No 2, Pub No 99-0001*, Rockville, MD, 1999, Agency for Health Care Policy and Research.

Maine Rural Health Research Center: *Rural coverage gaps decline following public health insurance expansions*, 2009, http://muskie.usm.maine.edu/Publications/rural/pb/Rural-Public-Health-Insurance.pdf. Accessed April 14, 2009.

Malecki E: Digital development in rural areas: potentials and pitfalls, *Rural Studies* 9(2):201–214, 2003.

Mautino K: Law watch: the new amnesty, *Immigration Health* 6(3):101–102, 2004.

McCabe S, Macnee C: Weaving a new safety net of mental health care in rural America: a model of integrated practice, *Issues Ment Health Nurs* 23(3):263–278, 2002.

National Center for Health Statistics: *Health, United States, with chartbook on trends in the health of Americans*, 2008, Centers for Disease Control and Prevention, www.cdc.gov/nchs/data/hus/hus08.pdf. Accessed April 14, 2009.

National Institute for Occupational Safety and Health: *Worker health chartbook, 2004*. NIOSH Pub No. 2004-146, Cincinnati, Ohio, 2004, The Author.

National Rural Health Association: *Summary and action plan for implementing quality through collaboration*, 2007, www.ruralhealthweb.org/go/rural-health-topics/quality-issues/nrha-summary-and-action-plan-for-implementing-quality-through-collaboration. Accessed March 21, 2010.

National Rural Health Association: *What's different about rural health care?* 2008, www.ruralhealthweb.org/go/left/about-rural-health/what-s-different-about-rural-health-care/what-s-different-about-rural-health-care. Accessed April 13 and April 25, 2009.

National Rural Health Association and the American Academy of Family Physicians (AAFP): *A joint statement*, July 2008, www.aafp.org/online/en/home/policy/policies/r/fammedruralpractice.html. Accessed April 14, 2009.

Office of Disease Prevention and Health Promotion, U.S. Department of Health and Human Services, www.healthypeople.gov/. Accessed April 13, 2009.

Office of Management and Budget: *Metropolitan and micropolitan statistical areas*, www.census.gov/population/www/metroareas/metroarea.html. Accessed April 14, 2009.

Office of Rural Health Policy, Health Resources and Services Administration: *Rural Hospital Flexibility Grant Program*, http://ruralhealth.hrsa.gov/funding/flex.htm. Accessed April 13, 2009.

Pahwa P, McDuffie HH, et al: Longitudinal changes in prevalence of respiratory symptoms among Canadian grain elevator workers, *Chest* 129:1605–1613, 2006.

Peek-Asa C, Zwerling C, Stallones L: Acute traumatic injuries in rural populations, *Am J Public Health* 94(10):1689–1693, 2004.

Phillips CD: Health in rural America: remembering the importance of place, *Am J Public Health* 94(10):1661–1663, 2004.

Probst JC, Moore CG, Glover SH, et al: Person and place: the compounding effects of race/ethnicity and rurality on health, *Am J Public Health* 94(10):1695–1703, 2004.

Pullen C: Modern technology brings nursing education into rural students' homes, *Rural Clinician Q* 8(3):3–5, 1998.

Rasheed MN, Rasheed JM: Rural African American older adults and the black helping tradition, *J Gerontol Soc Work* April 2004, www.informaworld.com/smpp/title~content=t792304007.

Rawlinson C, Crews P: Access to quality health services in rural areas: emergency medical services. In Gamm LD, Hutchison L, Dabney RJ, et al, editors: *Rural Healthy People 2010: a companion document to Health People 2010*, vol 1, College Station, TX, 2003, The Texas A&M University System Health Science Center,

School of Rural Public Health, Southwest Rural Health Research Center.

Reschovsky JD, Staiti A: *Access and quality of medical care in urban and rural areas: does rural America lag behind?* Working paper, Washington, DC, 2004, Center for Studying Health System Change.

Ricketts TC: Education of physician assistants, nurse midwives, and nurse practitioners for rural practice, *J Rural Health* 4(6):537–543, 2008.

Ricketts TC, Heaphy P: Hospitals in rural America. In Ricketts TC, editor: *Rural health in the United States*, New York, 1999, Oxford University Press.

Rogers CC: The older population in 21st century rural America, *Rural America* 17(3):2002, www.ers.usda.gov/publications/ruralamerica/ra173/ra173b.pdf.

Rosenblatt RA, Casey S, Richardson M: Rural-urban differences in the public health workforce: local health departments in 3 Western states, *Am J Public Health* 92(7):1102–1105, 2002.

Rural Assistance Center: www.raconline.org/.

Rural Health Assistance Center: *What is rural?* 2010. Retrieved March 14, 2010 from www.raconline.org/info_guides/ruraldef/.

Scharff KE: The distinctive nature and scope of rural nursing practice: philosophical bases. In Lee HJ, editor: *Conceptual basis for rural nursing*, New York, 1998, Springer.

Schenker MA: General health status and epidemiologic considerations in studying migrant and seasonal farmworkers. In McDuffie H, et al editors: *Agricultural health and safety: workplace, environment, sustainability*, Boca Raton, FL, 1995, CRC Press.

Sigma Theta Tau International: *Facts on the nursing shortage*, 2006, www.nursingsociety.org/MEDIA/Pages/shortage.aspx. Accessed April 13, 2009.

Struttmann TW, et al: Equipment dealers' perceptions of a community-based rollover protective structures promotion campaign, *J Rural Health* 17(2):131–139, 2001.

Swanson LL: Minorities represent growing share of tomorrow's work force, *Rural Cond Trends* 9(2):9–13, 1999, www.ers.usda.gov/publications/rcat/rcat92/rcat92b.pdf. Accessed April 13, 2009.

Thrall T: Rural recruitment, *Health and Hospital News* 81(12):1–6, 2007.

U.S. Department of Agriculture, Economic Research Service: Rural poverty at a glance, 2004b, Rural Development Research Report, No 100, www.ers.usda.gov/Publications/ rdrr 100/.

U.S. Census Bureau: Historical health insurance tables, 2008a: http://www.census.gov/hhes/www/hlthins/historic/index.html.

U.S. Census Bureau: Household income rises, poverty rate unchanged, number of uninsured down, 2008b: http://www.census.gov/Press-Release/www/releases/archives/income_wealth/012528.html. Accessed April 14, 2009.

U.S. Department of Agriculture, Economic Research Service: The economics of food, farming, natural resources, and rural

America, United States farm and farm-related employment, 2002, www.ers.usda.gov/Data/FarmandRelatedEmployment/.

U.S. Department of Agriculture, Economic Research Service: Rural education at a glance, 2004a. Rural Development Research Report, No 98, www.ers.usda.gov/publications/rdrr98.

U.S. Department of Agriculture, Economic Research Service: Rural poverty at a glance, 2004b, Rural Development Research Report, No 100, www.ers.usda.gov/Publications/rdrr100/.

U.S. Department of Agriculture, Economic Research Service: Rural children at a glance, Economic Information Bulletin, No 1, March 2005, www.ers.usda.gov/Emphases/Rural.

U.S. Department of Agriculture, Economic Research Service: Measuring what is rural, 2007. http://www.ers.usda.gov/Briefing/rurality/Whatisrural. Accessed April 19, 2009.

U.S. Department of Agriculture, Economic Research Service: Rural labor and education: farm labor, 2008, www.ers.usda.gov/Briefing/LaborAndEducation/FarmLabor.htm. Accessed April 13, 2009.

U.S. Department of Agriculture, Economic Research Service, www.ers.usda.gov/Emphases/Rural/. Accessed April 14, 2009.

U.S. Department of Health and Human Services, Public Health Service: *Healthy People 2010*, vol I, Understanding and improving health 2000, 2002, US Department of Health and Human Services, Leading health indicators, www.healthypeople.gov/LHI/.

van Exel J, de Graaf G, Brouwer W: Give me a break!: Informal caregiver attitudes towards respite care, *Health Policy* 88(1):73–87, 2008.

Virnig B, Moscovice I, Durham S, Casey M, Do Rural Elders Have Limited Access to Medicare Hospice Services? *Journal of the American Geriatrics Society*, 52(5):731–735, 2004.

Wang F, Luo W: Geographies of intellectual disability, *Health Place* 11(2):131–146, 2005.

Warren CP: Overview of respiratory health risks in agriculture. In Dosman JA, Cockcroft DW, editors: *Principals of health and safety in agriculture*, Boca Raton, FL, 1989, CRC Press.

Weinert C, Long KA: Understanding the health care needs of rural families, *Fam Relat* 36:450–455, 1987.

Weinert C, Long KA: Rural families and health care: refining the knowledge base, *J Marriage Fam Rev* 15:57–75, 1990.

Whitener LA, McGranahan DA: *Rural America: opportunities and challenges*, 2003, Amber Waves, US Department of Agriculture, Economic Research Service, www.ers.usda.gov/AmberWaves/.

W.K. Kellogg Foundation: *Perceptions of rural America*, 2001, www.wkkf.org.

Zahner SJ, Corrado SM: Local health department partnerships with faith-based organizations, *J Public Health Manag Pract* 10(3):258–265, 2004.

Populations Affected by Mental Illness

Jane Mahoney, Nancy Diacon

Additional Material for Study, Review, and Further Exploration

evolve WEBSITE

http://evolve.elsevier.com/Nies
- Quiz
- Case Studies
- Glossary
- WebLinks

OBJECTIVES

Upon completion of this chapter, the reader will be able to do the following:

1. Explain the concept of mental health, and discuss the importance of mental health promotion.
2. Discuss the historical context for contemporary mental health care.
3. Describe biological, social, and political factors associated with mental illness.
4. Illustrate the impact of natural and man-made disasters on the mental health of communities.
5. Describe some of the most common types of mental illnesses encountered in community settings.
6. Discuss the problem of suicide and recognize suicide warning signs.
7. Describe different types of treatment for mental disorders, including use of psychotherapeutic medications, psychotherapy, and behavior therapy.
8. Describe the role of mental health nurses in the community.

KEY TERMS

agoraphobia
anorexia nervosa
anxiety disorders
attention deficit disorder
attention deficit hyperactivity disorder
bipolar disorder
bulimia nervosa
Community Mental Health Centers Act
deinstitutionalization

depression
generalized anxiety disorder (GAD)
major depression
mental health
mental illness
obsessive-compulsive disorder (OCD)
panic disorder

Paul Wellstone and Pete Domenici Mental Health Parity and Addiction Equity Act
phobia
posttraumatic stress disorder
Program of Assertive Community Treatment (PACT)
psychotherapeutic medications
schizophrenia

OUTLINE

Overview and History of Community Mental Health
  Age of Confinement
  Mental Health Reform
  Medicalization of Mental Illness
  Community Mental Health and Deinstitutionalization
  Decade of the Brain
Healthy People 2020 and Mental Health
Factors Influencing Mental Health
  Biological Factors
  Social Factors

Natural and Man-made Disasters and Mental Illness
  Political Factors
Mental Disorders Encountered in Community Settings
  Overview of Selected Mental Disorders
Identification and Management of Mental Disorders
  Identification of Mental Disorders
  Management of Mental Disorders
Community-Based Mental Health Care
Role of the Community Mental Health Nurse

Mental health refers to the absence of mental disorders and to the ability for social and occupational functioning. Mental health can be affected by numerous factors, such as biological and genetic vulnerabilities, acute or chronic physical dysfunction, environmental conditions, and stressors. Threats to mental health are numerous and pervasive. Indeed, the U.S. Department of Health and Human Services (USDHHS) (2007) reported that more than 25% of adults 18 years of age and older have at least one mental disorder, and approximately 5% have three or more. Additionally, visits for mental illness and substance abuse in community health centers tripled from 2004 to 2009.

Community mental health nurses face multiple challenges such as complex patient comorbidity, lack of resources, the need for a broad base of expertise, physical facility inadequacies, and the stigma of mental illness, which affects clients and clinic staff (Cristofalo, Boutain, Schraufnagel et al., 2009). The purpose of this chapter is to describe critical issues that affect the mental health of individuals, families, groups, and communities and to explore the potential influence that nurses have on these issues. It also provides basic information on mental illnesses encountered in community settings and explores the environmental, biological, social, and political factors that influence mental health. Finally, some of the most commonly encountered options for management of mental illness are discussed.

OVERVIEW AND HISTORY OF COMMUNITY MENTAL HEALTH

The 1999, the *Surgeon General's Report on Mental Health* defined mental health as a state of successful performance of mental function that results in productive activities, fulfilling relationships with others, and an ability to adapt to change and cope with adversity. Mental illness includes all diagnosable mental disorders (i.e., those health conditions characterized by alterations in thinking, mood, or behavior associated with distress and/or impaired functioning). The report emphasized the importance of the mind-body connection and the detrimental effects of the stigma of mental illness (USDHHS, 1999).

Since recorded history, communities have been caring for the mentally ill. The history of community mental health has included the Age of Confinement, mental health reform, medicalization of mental illness, deinstitutionalization, and Decade of the Brain. Historically, mental illness has been associated with behavior different from the social norm. Table 24-1 provides a snapshot of the evolutionary phases of community mental health.

Age of Confinement

The "Age of Confinement" refers to the early years of establishment of the colonies. Individuals whose behavior was inconsistent with social norms were labeled "mad," separated from their communities, and placed in the custodial care of the state. Poverty, alcoholism, seizure disorders, and mental illness created rationale for asylum placement. Conditions in the asylums were deplorable. Individuals were often restrained, whipped, ill-fed, unwashed, and treated

TABLE 24-1	EVOLUTIONARY PHASES OF COMMUNITY MENTAL HEALTH
Age of Confinement	• Affected individuals separated from their communities • Asylum conditions deplorable • Therapy included restraint, beatings, bloodletting, purgatives, forced labor
Mental health reform	• Humanistic, psychologically oriented approach • Advent of state hospitals
Medicalization of mental illness	• Association of psychiatry with neurology • Development of biomedical perspective and somatic treatment approaches • First antipsychotic medication discovered in 1950s
Deinstitutionalization	• Increased financial concerns—states could no longer afford institutional care • 1960s—mentally ill returned to families and communities with inadequate resources • 1970s—acknowledgment by federal government of relative inadequacies of the Community Mental Health Centers Act with provisions for greater support for community resources across continuum of care
Decade of the Brain	• Neuroimaging enhances understanding of structural changes related to mental illness • Increased funding resulted in expanded development of effective pharmacological agents to treat mental illness

with bloodletting, purgatives, and other "curative" therapies. Madness was attributed to idleness; therefore, treatment included forced labor (Foucault, 1965; Hunter, 1963).

Mental Health Reform

By the end of the eighteenth century, inhumane conditions in houses of confinement gained the attention of philanthropists and humanists. A belief was established that humane treatment could abate mental illness. Humanistic person-centered principles replaced indentured servitude and confinement (Grob, 1991).

In the mid-nineteenth century, Dorothea Dix took up the cause of reform in the United States. Aided by changed attitudes toward suffering and social welfare, she helped effect reform in American hospitals and prisons. She established Saint Elizabeth's Hospital in 1885 in Washington, DC, and eventually thirty-two state mental hospitals (Grob, 1983).

Medicalization of Mental Illness

After treatment reform in the mid- to late eighteenth century, collaborations were developed between the fields of psychiatry and neurology. This association proved to be pivotal for the development of psychiatry and community mental health. Scientific and political respectability for psychiatry depended on a biomedical perspective (Grob, 1983).

Numerous somatic treatments for mental illness followed biomedical theories, including lobotomy, electroconvulsive therapy, insulin shock therapy, and hydrotherapy (Deutsch, 1949). It was not until the early 1950s that the antipsychotic medication Thorazine (chlorpromazine) was discovered; this medication alleviated, in a more humane fashion, some of the most troubling symptoms experienced by individuals with psychotic disorders (Deutsch, 1949; Grob, 1991).

Community Mental Health and Deinstitutionalization

Treatment reform was based largely on the premise that mentally ill people were sick and in need of treatment. During the Great Depression of the 1930s, most states could no longer afford the expense of institutional care for the mentally ill. Caregivers, families, and communities became viable alternatives to costly institutional care.

In 1946, the National Mental Health Act established the National Institute of Mental Health (NIMH). In 1955, the Mental Health Study Act called for "an objective, thorough, nationwide analysis and reevaluation of the human and economic problems of mental health." These efforts pointed to the need for a national program to help meet the needs of the mentally ill.

The Community Mental Health Centers Act of 1964 provided federal support for mental health services. The Act supported measures to implement facilities to care for those who were mentally retarded and to construct community mental health centers. The Act also mandated deinstitutionalization, or a halt to the long-held policy of keeping the severely mentally ill hospitalized. The intention was to reduce long-term care of seriously mentally ill persons, by transferring treatment to the community (Sharfstein, Stoline, and Koran, 2002).

Individuals with serious mental illness were returned to families and communities who were ill-prepared to care for them, compounding problems. Funding did not follow the change in policy, and many individuals with mental illness found themselves homeless, in shelters, or in prisons or jails, as families and communities were ill-prepared to deal with the shift to community-based care. Shortly thereafter, the federal government recommended linking community mental health services with informal community support services to improve treatment options.

Decade of the Brain

Although legislation improved environmental conditions, treatment for mental illness remained relatively unchanged. The development of neuroimaging in the 1980s provided new data on the anatomical and neurochemical nature of the brain (Buchsbaum and Haier, 1982). These data rendered the foundation for developing new pharmacological agents to treat mental illness. In the late 1980s, Congress declared the 1990s the Decade of the Brain (USDHHS, 1999) resulting in an increase in funding for the NIMH. An increased understanding of the biomedical components of mental illnesses led to new effective psychotropic medications (Kandel, 1998).

Although great strides have been made in understanding and treating mental illness, challenges remain for those affected by mental illness and those who work with mental illness in community settings. The Centers for Disease Control and Prevention (CDC) have released data suggesting an ongoing prevalence of untreated mental illness within communities with great variability across states. It is estimated that 53.4% of individuals experiencing serious psychological distress go untreated in the United States. The percent untreated ranges from 33.3% in Alaska to 67% in Hawaii (Strine, Dhingra, Okoro et al., 2009). Factors such as social stigma or lack of transportation to facilities impact utilization of available services (Roberts, Robinson, Topp et al., 2008). Symptoms associated with mental illness may limit an individual's capacity to make use of available resources. This may contribute to a lack of treatment effectiveness when services provided do not include a residential component (Burns, Robins, Hodge et al., 2009).

HEALTHY PEOPLE 2020 AND MENTAL HEALTH

Healthy People 2020 is a broad-based collaborative effort among federal, state, and territorial governments and private, public, and nonprofit organizations to set national disease prevention and health promotion objectives to be achieved between 2010 and 2020 (USDHHS, 2009). The *Healthy People 2020* table lists several proposed objectives from *Healthy People 2020* that cover issues related to mental health.

♥ **HEALTHY PEOPLE 2020**

Proposed Objectives Related to Mental Health

OBJECTIVE
MHMD HP2020–1: Reduce the suicide rate
MHMD HP2020–3: Increase the proportion of homeless adults with mental health problems who receive mental health services
MHMD HP2020–4: Reduce the proportion of adolescents who engage in disordered eating behaviors in an attempt to control their weight
MHMD HP2020–6: Increase the proportion of children with mental health problems who receive treatment
MHMD HP2020–13: Increase the proportion of adults with mental disorders who receive treatment
MHMD HP2020–15: Increase depression screening by primary care providers

USDHHS Healthy People 2020 Draft Objectives. 2009. http://www.healthypeople.gov/hp2010/Objectives/files/Draft2009Objectives.pdf

FACTORS INFLUENCING MENTAL HEALTH

Treatment of mental disorders has dramatically improved, yet the cause of most mental illnesses is not well understood. Research has identified a number of biological and sociological factors that contribute to mental health and mental illness. Natural and man-made disasters also influence the mental health of individuals, families, and communities, and social and political factors that may be associated with development of mental illness. Some of these factors will be presented in this section.

Biological Factors

For centuries, mental illnesses were viewed as bizarre conditions that needed to be contained in institutions. Neuroscience research has provided a better understanding of the biology of mental illnesses; however, many questions remain unanswered. Biological factors associated with mental illness include genetic factors, neurotransmission, and brain structural and functioning abnormalities.

Genetic Factors

There is little information linking a specific gene to a specific disorder. Rather, the major psychiatric disorders appear to be genetically complex (Smoller, Sheidley, and Tsuang, 2008). Genetic expressions, combined with neurochemical and metabolic changes and environmental insults, may result in the display of mental disorder characteristics. A new field known as *genetic imaging* offers promise for understanding the complexities associated with gene variation, brain structure, and the physiological response to information processing (de Geus, Goldberg, Boomsma et al., 2008).

Neurotransmitters

In recent years, dysregulation in one or more neurotransmitter systems has been described in mental illness. No single neurotransmitter is implicated in any mental illness. Rather, the regulation/dysregulation of neurotransmission is complex and involves multiple intertwined neurotransmitters. For example, serotonin, dopamine, gamma-aminobutyric acid, and norepinephrine are involved in neurotransmission dysregulation associated with posttraumatic stress disorder (Olszewski and Varrasse, 2005).

Brain Structural and Functioning Abnormalities

Evidence indicates that structural brain abnormalities can be related to some mental illnesses such as schizophrenia, depression, and Alzheimer's disease. As the science of neuroimaging evolves, a more refined view of the role of brain structure and functioning is unfolding. For example, neuroimaging studies are beginning to explain the role of different central nervous system structures in regulating the hypothalamic-pituitary-adrenal axis that controls responses to stress (Pruessner, Dedovic, Pruessner et al., 2010). Scientists are also recognizing how other systems of the body can impact brain functioning. For example, in one study researchers found a greater than 60% activation of the amygdala in sleep-deprived subjects as compared with controls. This suggests that sleep plays an important role in regulation in the emotional center of the brain (Yoo, Gujar, Hu et al., 2007).

Although a number of theories of the etiology of mental disorders have been developed, information is insufficient to establish a definitive biological cause for mental illness. Scholars have concluded that mental disorders are multifactorial, complex phenomena. The important point for community health nurses to understand is that mental illnesses have a very strong biological basis, much like other chronic conditions such as diabetes or heart disease, but other factors are highly influential.

Social Factors

Social factors can contribute to the etiology of mental illness (Institute of Medicine, 2006a; 2006b). Stress associated with social phenomena such as bullying, social rejection, domestic violence, and unemployment, for example, has been identified as causing mental illness (USDHHS, 1999). Mental illness also results in social isolation, which may compound the problem. Throughout history, the symptoms of mental illness have been perceived as permanent, dangerous, frightening, and shameful. People with a diagnosis of mental illness have been described as lazy, idle, weak, immoral, irrational, and feigning illness. On the basis of these characterizations and assumptions, many people with a diagnosis of mental illness have experienced widespread social rejection (Sadler, 2009). One of the key social implications of mental illness is the impact on the job market and employment. Individuals who have serious and persistent mental illness rarely have the luxury of private medical insurance because of the difficulties they experience in maintaining employment. In one study for example, researchers found that anxiety and depression had a major impact on employment outcomes among women (Cowell, Luo, and Masuda, 2009).

Another social concern is the trend for communities to make use of prisons rather than psychiatric hospitals as a solution to the "mental health problem." The number of persons with mental illness in prison has quadrupled in the last 10 years, and nearly 50% of all inmates report mental health concerns (Human Rights Watch, 2008).

Prisons are woefully unprepared to provide adequate care to the mentally ill. To help address this problem, in 2008, Senate Bill S.2304—Mentally Ill Offender Treatment and Crime Reduction Reauthorization and Improvement Act was signed into law. This bill provided grants aimed at improving mental health treatment provided to criminal offenders with a mental illness. Other related initiatives have focused on establishing mental health courts in communities as a cost-effective means to address the needs of the community and those who are charged with a criminal offense and also experience a mental illness (Ridgely, Engberg, Greenberg et al., 2007). Thus, some progress is being made to promote social justice for the mentally ill, but there is a need for a much more intensive effort at creating structures and processes that support the treatment needs of the mentally ill in communities.

Natural and Man-made Disasters and Mental Illness

Natural and man-made disasters such as hurricanes, floods, violence, terrorism, war, and the global economic crisis are profound stress-inducing events that can lead to mental illness. Researchers reported high levels of posttraumatic stress disorder (PTSD) among survivors of Hurricane Katrina, the natural disaster that devastated New Orleans in 2005. Of those studied, 41% stated that they thought they would die; 16% witnessed someone become injured or die; 17% observed violence; and 6% experienced violence directly (Coker, Hanks, Eggleston et al., 2006). Furthermore, the levels of hurricane-related mental illness remained high years after the event (Kessler, Galea, Gruber et al., 2008). Community mental health nurses must not only be prepared to respond to the mental health needs of a community during a disaster, but also maintain vigilance in caring for survivors many years thereafter.

PTSD is highly prevalent among combat veterans returning from war to their homes and communities. PTSD is associated with extreme anxiety that can result in suicide. Male veterans in communities are twice as likely to die by suicide as their civilian counterparts (NIMH, 2007). In a report based on compiled data from sixteen states, the CDC (2005) noted approximately 1800 suicides by former or current military personnel that took place in 2005. Of those, nearly 30% had told someone of their intention to die by suicide within enough time for someone to have intervened. The tragedy of suicide to the victims, as well as to the surviving family members, friends, and community, is devastating. Early intervention is key to prevention and treatment.

The global economic crisis that began in late 2008 has led to enormous mental health consequences. The sense of hopelessness and powerlessness that accompanied the financial losses associated with dwindling retirement accounts for some, and layoffs for others, has contributed to much emotional distress throughout the world. The World Health Organization (2009) warned that the economic crisis will have a detrimental effect on the mental health of citizens of all nations and called for enhanced monitoring for indications of mental health decline.

Political Factors

Political factors can dramatically influence how mental disorders are managed. One significant factor in the politics of mental illness is parity in health care coverage, that is, the equal access to health care for physical and mental illnesses. Historically, health insurance companies have provided less access to treatment for a mental disorder than for a physical disorder. In 2008, the Paul Wellstone and Pete Domenici Mental Health Parity and Addiction Equity Act was enacted. The law requires health insurance to cover treatment for mental illness on the same terms and conditions as physical illness (Open Congress, 2008). Although this legislation is a victory for mental health, more laws are needed to provide improved mental health services to those who do not have access to health insurance.

Health care disparities have become a key issue in public health policy discussions. Members of ethnic minority groups have less access to mental health services than do their white counterparts. Minorities are more likely to delay seeking mental health care and are more likely to receive poor care when they are treated (Miranda, McGuire, Williams et al., 2008; USDHHS, 1999). There is a critical need to address this gap in health care.

MENTAL DISORDERS ENCOUNTERED IN COMMUNITY SETTINGS

The influence of untreated mental illness on communities and their social structure has been vastly understated. The NIMH estimates that the prevalence of diagnosable mental disorders in the U.S. population is about 26.2% at any given time. Approximately 6% have serious mental illness (Kessler, Chiu, Demler et al., 2005). Mental illness accounts for more than 10% of the disease burden worldwide, ranking it second, following all forms of cardiac disease (USDHHS/Substance Abuse and Mental Health Services Administration [SAMHSA], 2005). In the United States, the estimated cost of mental illness exceeds $100 billion for costs of diagnosing and treating mental disorders and $193 billion in lost productivity (NIMH, 2008).

Recognizing that most mental illnesses are identified and managed in noninstitutional settings, it is essential that community health nurses be familiar with the most commonly occurring mental disorders. There is a need for screening, referring, and follow-up for those with mental health problems in order to meet the mental health needs of the community (Unutzer et al., 2006).

Overview of Selected Mental Disorders

The *Diagnostic and Statistical Manual of Mental Disorders* (fourth edition, text revision) (American Psychiatric Association [APA], 2000), classifies mental illnesses and outlines diagnostic criteria for more than 300 disorders. This section provides a summary of some of these disorders. More detailed information about specific disorders can be found at www.psychiatryonline.com.

Clinical Example

Michael Nye, a photographer, spent hundreds of hours photographing and taping illness narratives of individuals living with serious mental illness. Viewing his photographs and listening to the accounts of those living with these conditions are valuable experiences for nurses who care for this population (http://michaelnye.org/fineline/index.html). Fleming and colleagues (2009) analyzed the photographs and narratives from the exhibit and concluded that suffering, stigma, and loss of identity were the central experiences depicted by this project.

Schizophrenia

Schizophrenia is the most serious and profound of all mental illnesses; globally, it affects about 1% of the population (NIMH, 2005). The effect of this condition on the community is enormous in terms of social and economic burden.

To the individual and families affected by schizophrenia, the impact is incalculable. It presents with (1) positive symptoms including hallucinations, delusions, disorganized thinking and speech, and bizarre behavior and (2) negative symptoms such as flat affect, poor attention, lack of motivation, apathy, lack of pleasure, and lack of energy. Onset typically occurs during late adolescence and early adulthood in males and somewhat later in females. There is an increased risk for alcohol use, depression, suicide, and diabetes among persons with schizophrenia. These factors compound the problems associated with living with a psychotic disorder.

Treatment for schizophrenia must be intensive and generally involves hospitalization (initially), antipsychotic medications, and psychotherapy/counseling. Long-term follow-up by mental health professionals is necessary to monitor medication compliance and to watch for side effects and complications, which may be severe and life threatening, and to evaluate the patient's ability to integrate into the community.

Depression

Depression is the most frequently diagnosed and one of the most disabling mental illnesses in the United States. In 2004, more than 17 million adults experienced at least one major depressive episode (USDHHS/SAMHSA, 2005). Depression often co-occurs with serious physical disorders such as heart attack, stroke, diabetes, and cancer. About 25% of women and 12% of men will have at least one episode of depression during their lifetime. Although effective treatments exist, most people (almost two thirds) with depressive illness do not seek help (NIMH, 2000). Having a family or personal history of depression, suicide attempt, or sexual abuse, or current substance abuse or chronic medical condition increases the risk for depression (APA, 2000). Health education should include risk factor identification, as well as when and how to obtain treatment. Symptoms of depression are included in Box 24-1.

BOX 24-1   SYMPTOMS OF DEPRESSION

- Persistent sad or empty mood
- Feelings of hopelessness, pessimism
- Feelings of guilt, worthlessness, helplessness
- Loss of interest or pleasure in ordinary activities, including sex
- Decreased energy, fatigue, being slowed down
- Difficulty concentrating, remembering, making decisions
- Insomnia, early-morning waking, or oversleeping
- Appetite loss, weight loss, or overeating and weight gain
- Thoughts of death or suicide; suicide attempts
- Restlessness, irritability

From National Institute of Mental Health: *Depression*, NIH Pub No 00-3561, Rockville, MD, 2000, The Author.

Depression in children and adolescents. According to the National Mental Health Association (2006), between 2% and 4% of prepubertal children and as many as 12% of adolescents may have depression. A family history of depression is a major risk factor for childhood depression. Other associated factors that may increase the risk of depression in children and adolescents include a history of verbal, physical, or sexual abuse; frequent separation from, or loss of, a loved one; poverty; mental retardation; attention deficit hyperactivity disorder; hyperactivity; and chronic illness. Children may refuse to go to school or pretend to be ill, and adolescents may appear sulky or irritable, common behaviors in this age group making identification of depression a challenge (NIMH, 2009). It should be noted that suicide is the third leading cause of death among persons 15 to 25 years and that the rate of suicide among young males is five times that among young females. Health care providers should recognize the symptoms of depression and refer for treatment as appropriate.

Treatment. Treatment for depression includes pharmacological therapy, psychotherapy, behavior therapy, electroconvulsive therapy, or a combination of these (APA, 2005; NIMH, 2009). In general, the most effective, first-line treatment is a combination of antidepressant medication and psychotherapy.

Bipolar Disorder

Bipolar disorder refers to a group of mood disorders that present with changes in mood from depression to mania. The depressed phase is manifested by symptoms seen in major depressive disorder. The manic phase is characterized by a persistent abnormally elevated or irritable mood, impaired judgment, flight of ideas, pressured speech, grandiosity, distractibility, excessive involvement in goal-directed activities, few hours sleeping, and impulsivity. These symptoms may co-occur with psychotic features such as hallucinations and delusions. Persons with bipolar disorder are at increased risk for alcohol and substance abuse, as well as increased risk for suicide. The presence of bipolar disorder results in poor occupational and social functioning.

Management of bipolar disorder must be ongoing and involve close monitoring. Treatment generally involves use of mood-stabilizing medication, often in combination with

---

RESEARCH HIGHLIGHTS

Suicidal Thoughts Among Elderly Patients

Raue, Meyers, Rowe et al. (2007) conducted a large-scale study of suicidal ideation among elderly patients who were being cared for by home health nurses. Their analysis of interviews with more than 500 older adults showed that a high prevalence (10.6%) had passive thoughts of suicide and an additional 1.2% had actively considered taking their own life. Furthermore, follow-up interviews indicated that suicidal thoughts persisted for more than a year for one third of the patients. The researchers identified several risk factors associated with suicidal ideation. These were depression, disability, multiple medical problems, and low perceived social support. It was concluded that home health care nurses have an important potential role in identification of those at high risk for suicide and initiating appropriate interventions (e.g., communication with primary care physicians and referral to mental health specialists).

From Raue PJ, Meyers BS, Rowe JL et al: Suicidal ideation among elderly homecare patients, *Int J Geriatr Psychiatry* 22(1):32-37, 2007.

antipsychotic and antidepressant therapy (APA, 2005). When working with persons with bipolar disorder, nurses need to monitor symptoms and response to psychopharmacological treatment.

Anxiety Disorder

Anxiety disorders are a group of conditions characterized by feelings of anxiety. Anxiety disorders affect up to 16% of the general population at any time. Anxiety disorders may be attributed to genetic makeup and life experiences of the individual. Some of the more commonly encountered anxiety disorders are generalized anxiety disorder, panic disorder (sometimes accompanied by agoraphobia), phobias, obsessive-compulsive disorder, and PTSD (APA, 2000). These are discussed briefly here.

Generalized anxiety disorder. Generalized anxiety disorder (GAD) is characterized by chronic, unrealistic, and exaggerated worry and tension about one or more life circumstances lasting 6 months or longer (APA, 2000). Approximately half of cases of GAD begin in childhood or adolescence, and it is more common in women than in men. Symptoms of GAD include trembling, twitching, muscle tension, headaches, irritability, sweating or hot flashes, dyspnea, and nausea. Periods of increasing symptoms are usually associated with life stressors or impending difficulties.

Panic disorder. Approximately 6 million American adults have panic disorder (Kessler et al., 2005). Panic disorder can occur at any age, but it most often begins in young adulthood (average age, 17–30 years). Panic attacks consist of a period of intense fear that develops abruptly and unexpectedly. The initial attack may occur suddenly and unexpectedly while the client is performing everyday tasks. Typically, he or she experiences tachycardia; dyspnea; dizziness; chest pain; nausea; numbness or tingling of the hands and feet; trembling or shaking; sweating; choking; or a feeling that he or she is going to die, go crazy, or do something uncontrolled. This can be extremely frightening. A diagnosis of panic disorder is made when attacks occur with some degree of frequency or regularity.

As the disorder evolves, the anxiety attacks become increasingly frequent and severe, and the individual develops anticipatory anxiety (fear of having a panic attack). During this phase, events and circumstances associated with the attack may be selectively avoided, leading to phobic behaviors (e.g., if a woman has an attack while driving, she may become anxious the next time she needs to drive, and she may begin to avoid driving and then refuse to drive altogether). In this phase, the client's life may become progressively constricted.

As the avoidance behavior intensifies, the client begins to withdraw further to avoid being in places or situations from which escape may be difficult or embarrassing or help may be unavailable in the event of a panic attack (e.g., church, elevators, movie theaters). The fear of being in these situations or places can lead to agoraphobia (literally, fear of the marketplace or open places). Individuals with agoraphobia frequently progress to the point where they cannot leave their homes without experiencing anxiety. Agoraphobia is the most common phobia leading to the use of health services, particularly when accompanied by panic attacks. Rates for co-occurring major depression range from 10% to 65% in persons with panic disorder (APA, 2000). Alcoholism is also common among individuals with panic disorders. Cognitive behavioral treatment and short-course benzodiazepines therapy are used to treat panic disorder.

Phobias. A phobia is an irrational fear of something (an object or situation), and as many as 8% of Americans are affected by phobias at any given time. Adults with phobias realize their fears are irrational, but facing the feared object or situation might bring on severe anxiety or a panic attack. Phobias may begin in childhood, but they usually first appear in adolescence or adulthood.

Social phobia, or social anxiety disorder, is a persistent and intense fear of, and compelling desire to avoid, something that would expose the individual to a situation that might be humiliating and embarrassing (APA, 2000). Its tendency is familial and may be accompanied by depression or alcoholism. The most common social phobia is a fear of public speaking. Other examples include being unable to urinate in a public bathroom and not being able to answer questions in social situations. Most people with social phobias can be treated with cognitive-behavioral therapy and medication.

Simple phobias involve a persistent fear of, and compelling desire to avoid, certain objects or situations. Common objects of phobias are spiders, snakes, dogs, cats, and situations such as flying, heights, and closed-in spaces. The person often recognizes that the fear is unreasonable but avoids the situation or endures it with intense anxiety. Systematic desensitization and normal exposure are the most effective treatments for simple phobias.

Obsessive-compulsive disorder. Obsessive-compulsive disorder (OCD) is characterized by anxious thoughts and rituals that the individual has difficulty controlling. The person with OCD feels compelled to engage in some ritual to avoid a persistent frightening thought, idea, image, or event. Obsessions are recurrent thoughts, emotions, or impulses that cannot be dismissed. Compulsions are the rituals or behaviors that are repeatedly performed to prevent, neutralize, or dispel the dreaded obsession. When the individual tries to resist the compulsion, anxiety increases. Common compulsions include hand washing, counting, checking, or touching (APA, 2000). Most individuals recognize that what they are doing is senseless but are unable to control the compulsion. About 2% of Americans are afflicted with OCD, which often appears in the teenage years or early adulthood. Depression or other anxiety disorders often accompany OCD. Behavioral therapy and medication aimed at reducing accompanying symptoms have been found to be helpful.

Posttraumatic stress disorder. Posttraumatic stress disorder (PTSD) is a debilitating condition that follows a terrifying event. It affects about 3.5% of U.S. adults (Kessler et al., 2005). Individuals with PTSD have recurring, persistent, frightening thoughts and memories of their ordeal. Incidents may include "shell shock" or "battle fatigue" common to war veterans, violent attack, serious accidents, natural disasters, or witnessing mass destruction or injury, such as an airplane crash. Sometimes the individual is unable to recall an important aspect of the traumatic event. Highest incidence of PTSD occurs among combat-experienced military personnel (Smith, Ryan, Wingard et al., 2008). About 19% of Vietnam veterans, for example, have experienced PTSD (Dohrenwend, Turner, Turse et al., 2006).

People with PTSD repeatedly relive the trauma in the form of nightmares or disturbing recollections or flashbacks during the day, resulting in sleep disturbances, depression, and feelings of detachment or emotional numbness, or being easily startled. They may avoid places or situations that bring back memories (e.g., a woman raped in an elevator may refuse to ride in elevators), and anniversaries of the event are often very difficult. PTSD occurs at all ages and may be accompanied by depression, substance abuse, and/or anxiety. It usually begins within 3 months of the trauma, and the course of the disorder varies. Some individuals recover within 6 months; the condition becomes chronic in others. Infrequently, the illness does not manifest until years after the traumatic event. Treatment includes antidepressants and antianxiety medications and psychotherapy. Support from family and friends can be very beneficial.

Eating Disorders

Eating disorders, anorexia nervosa and bulimia nervosa, are increasingly prevalent in the United States, affecting about 3 million U.S. residents. Anorexia affects about 0.5% to 3.7% of females in their lifetime (NIMH, 2009), and as many as 4% to 15% of female high school and college women have some symptoms of bulimia (Cochrane, 2005).

Eating disorders primarily affect females; males account for 5% to 10% of cases, although this may be underreported. Most clients with a diagnosis of eating disorders are white; however, this may be because of socioeconomic factors rather than race. Anorexia and bulimia are often triggered by developmental milestones (e.g., puberty, first sexual contact) or another crisis (e.g., death of a loved one, ridicule over weight, starting college).

Bulimia nervosa. Bulimia nervosa refers to binge eating, discreetly consuming an abnormally large amount of food, accompanied by maladaptive compensatory methods to prevent weight gain (APA, 2000). For example, a person with bulimia might eat an entire pie, half a cake, or a half gallon of ice cream at one sitting. Snacking throughout the day is not considered bingeing. To lose or maintain weight, the person with bulimia practices purging, which usually involves self-induced vomiting, caused by gagging, using an emetic, or simply mentally willing the action. Laxatives, diuretics, fasting, and excessive exercise may also be employed to control weight.

Bulimia nervosa typically begins in adolescence or during the early 20s, usually in conjunction with a diet. High school and college students, as well as members of certain professions that emphasize weight and/or appearance (e.g., dancers, flight attendants, cheerleaders, athletes, actors, models), are at high risk. The condition may lead to electrolyte imbalance

resulting in fatigue, seizures, muscle cramps, arrhythmias, and decreased bone density. Vomiting can damage the esophagus, stomach, teeth, and gums.

Anorexia nervosa. The person with anorexia nervosa becomes obsessed with a fear of fat and with losing weight. Anorexia nervosa often develops with a fairly gradual decrease in caloric intake. However, the decrease in caloric intake continues until the person is consuming almost nothing. Anorexia usually begins in early adolescence (12 to 14 years is the most common age-group) and may be limited to a single episode of dramatic weight loss within a few months, followed by recovery, or the illness may last for many years.

Risk factors for eating disorders are perfectionism, low self-esteem, stress, poor coping skills, sexual/physical abuse, poor self-image, dependency on others' opinions and deference to others' wishes, and being emotionally reserved (Cochrane, 2005). In response to the severely decreased caloric intake, the body tries to compensate by slowing down body processes. Menstruation ceases; blood pressure, pulse, and respiration rates slow; and thyroid activity diminishes. Electrolyte imbalance can become very severe. Other symptoms include mild anemia, joint swelling, and reduced muscle mass. Anorexia nervosa can be life threatening and has a mortality rate of 5% to 21%.

Treatment for eating disorders includes long-term nutrition counseling, psychotherapy, and behavior modification. Hospitalization may be required for clients with serious complications. Self-help groups and support groups can be very beneficial for both the client and the family.

Nurses need to be aware of the "ProAna" websites, which promote the lifestyle associated with eating disorders. Such knowledge is important, as community health nurses assess the social influences that contribute to the condition. Also, nurses who frequently work with adolescent girls and young women in community settings such as schools and clinics should be aware of the risk factors, signs, and symptoms of anorexia and bulimia and be prepared to intervene.

Attention Deficit Hyperactivity Disorder

Two of the most common conditions encountered by nurses who work with children in community settings are attention deficit hyperactivity disorder (ADHD) and attention deficit disorder (ADD). ADHD/ADD affects 4.5 million children in the United States (CDC, 2009). Behaviors that might indicate ADHD/ADD usually appear before age 7 years and are often accompanied by related problems, such as learning disability, anxiety, and depression. The three major characteristics of ADHD/ADD are inattention, hyperactivity, and impulsivity.

The cause of ADHD/ADD is not known, but it is important to note that it is not caused by minor head injuries, birth complications, food allergies, too much sugar, poor home life, poor schools, or too much television. Maternal substance use and abuse (e.g., alcohol, cigarettes, cocaine) may affect the brain of the developing baby and produce symptoms of ADHD/ADD later in life. This, however, accounts for only a small percentage of those affected. Attention disorders run in families.

Although parents may notice symptoms and signs, it is often teachers who recognize the behaviors consistent with attention deficit disorders and suggest referral for assessment and treatment (NIMH, 2009). Experts caution that diagnosis of attention disorders should be made following a comprehensive physical, psychological, social, and behavioral evaluation and not based solely on anecdotal reports from parents or teachers. The evaluation should rule out other possible reasons for the behavior (e.g., emotional problems, poor vision or hearing, physical problems) and should include input from teachers, parents, and others who know the child well. Intelligence and achievement testing may also be performed to rule out or identify a learning disability.

Symptoms of ADHD/ADD are typically managed through a combination of behavior therapy, emotional counseling, and practical support. Use of medication is becoming increasingly commonplace in the management of ADHD/ADD. It is very important, however, that children with attention disorders and their families understand that medication does not cure the disorder; it just temporarily controls symptoms.

Stimulants have been shown to be successful in treating attention disorders. The most commonly used medications are methylphenidate (Ritalin) and amphetamines (Dexedrine, Dextrostat, or Adderall). Appetite suppression and poor sleep are common side effects. Body mass index monitoring and sleep promotion strategies are important (NIMH, 2009).

Suicide

There are approximately 1 million deaths by suicide per year throughout the world, and that number is projected to remain about the same through 2015 (Mathers and Loncar, 2005). The National Center for Injury Prevention and Control (2009) reported there were more than 30,000 deaths by suicide in the United States in 2006. Suicide is the third leading cause of death among those aged 15 to 24 years. The highest rate of suicide occurs in males over 65 years of age; white males over the age of 85 years are particularly vulnerable.

In 1999, the USDHHS and the Office of the Surgeon General identified suicide as a primary public health problem of the new millennium. Consistent with the select aims of *Healthy People 2020*, the Surgeon General's Call to Action attempts to "put into place national strategies to prevent the loss of life and the suffering suicide causes" (USDHHS, 1999, p. 7) through increased public awareness, expansion of mental health services, and continuation of support of research aimed at understanding and preventing suicide in the United States.

Historically, risk and protective factors have been used to identify those at highest risk for suicide. Recently, the American Association of Suicidology (AAS) (2008) has recommended recognition of warning signs as more relevant than risk and protective factors in preventing death by suicide. The AAS has organized the warning signs according to the easily remembered mnemonic, IS PATH WARM (Table 24-2). Recognizing the suicide-related behaviors that are occurring in the moment is more useful to health care providers than understanding risk factors that may have no bearing on the

TABLE 24-2	SUICIDE WARNING SIGNS: IS PATH WARM
Ideation	Does the person state that he or she is having thoughts of suicide?
Substance abuse	Is the person demonstrating increased use of alcohol or drugs?
Purposelessness	Does the person state that he or she feels as if there is no purpose in his or her life?
Anxiety	Is the person demonstrating anxiety-related behaviors such as: talking about being overly worried about things, ruminating, difficulty concentrating, or exhibiting increased psychomotor agitation?
Trapped	Does the person state that he or she feels trapped, that there is no way out of the current situation except to die?
Hopelessness	Does the person state that he or she feels hopeless? Is the person able to describe something to look forward to?
Withdrawal	Is the person withdrawing from others such as family and friends? Is the person isolating?
Anger	Is the person demonstrating uncontrolled anger? Is the person acting with rage or seeking revenge?
Recklessness	Is the person engaged in risk-taking behaviors? Is the person acting as if he or she "doesn't care" or isn't thinking about the consequences of the risk-taking behavior?
Mood changes	Is the person experiencing dramatic mood changes?

From American Association of Suicidology: *Know the warning signs,* 2009: www.suicidology.org.

current situation and may not be modifiable. For example, if a person has a history of a previous suicide attempt, that does not mean that person is at risk of attempting suicide at any given moment. However, if a person is talking about suicide and describing feeling very anxious and trapped, the indications are much stronger that there is an imminent threat. Warning signs that indicate acute risk for suicidality may be observed in individuals who are threatening to hurt or kill themselves, attempting to identify access to lethal weapons or other means that could result in death, or communicating about dying when these thoughts or actions are out of the ordinary for them.

Risk factors include previous suicide attempts, mental illness, substance abuse, and barriers to accessing mental health treatment. Protective factors may decrease the risk of suicide and include appropriate mental health care, easy access to treatment, community support, and continuing support from medical and mental health care providers. Box 24-2 lists risk factors all community health nurses should recognize, and Box 24-3 provides prevention strategies that will help reduce the burden of suicide.

To assess for suicidality, community health nurses should question those they determine to be at risk in terms of thoughts, plans, lethality, means, and intent. In addition to

BOX 24-2 SUICIDE RISK FACTORS

- One or more diagnosable mental or substance abuse disorder(s) (greatest risk: previous suicide attempts, major depression, drug abuse, bipolar disorder)
- Impulsivity
- Adverse life events
- Family history of mental or substance abuse disorder
- Family history of suicide
- Family violence, including emotional, physical, or sexual abuse
- Prior suicide attempt
- Firearm in the home
- Incarceration
- Exposure to the suicidal behavior of others (e.g., family members, peers, and/or the media in news or fiction stories)

Compiled from National Institute of Mental Health: *Frequently asked questions about suicide*, 1999, www.nimh.nih.gov/suicideprevention/ suicidefaq.cfm; and National Institute of Mental Health: *In harm's way: suicide in America*, NIH Pub No 03-4594, 2003, www.nimh.nih.gov/publicat/ harmsway.cfm.

BOX 24-3 SUICIDE PREVENTION STRATEGIES

- Suicide is preventable. Most people want to live but sometimes can't see any other alternative.
- Learn the warning signs of suicide.
- Be direct and talk openly about thoughts of suicide. Talking about it will not give someone the idea.
- Don't ask "why." Take a nonjudgmental stance. Listen.
- Don't act shocked, and don't agree to keep the person's thoughts of suicide a secret.
- Don't tell the person he or she has much to live for.
- Be empathic.
- Remove the means and seek immediate help.

From American Association of Suicidology: *How you can help*, 2008, www. suicidology.org/web/guest/how-can-you-help.

TABLE 24-3 SUICIDE PREVENTION AND REFERRAL RESOURCES

National Suicide Prevention Lifeline	1-800-273-TALK (8255) www.suicidepreventionlifeline.org/
American Association of Suicidology	www.suicidology.org/web/guest/ home
Suicide Prevention Resource Center	www.sprc.org/
Suicide Awareness Voices of Education	www.save.org/
Suicide Prevention: A Resource Manual for the Army	chppm-www.apgea.army. mil/dhpw/readiness/suicide.aspx
US Department of Defense: Military Health System	1-800-342-9647 www.health.mil/MediaRoom/ default.aspx?id=423&currentPg=1
American Foundation for Suicide Prevention	www.afsp.org/
Local emergency resource	Dial 911

assessing for warning signs using the mnemonic IS PATH WARM, potential questions to ask, suggested by the APA (2005), include:

- Did you ever wish you could go to sleep and just not wake up?
- Have things ever reached the point that you have thought of harming yourself?
- How often have those thoughts occurred (include frequency, obsessional quality, controllability)?
- What do you envision happening if you actually killed yourself (e.g., escape, reunion with significant other, rebirth, reactions of others)?
- Have you made a specific plan to harm yourself? If so, what does the plan include?

Thus, it is important that all community health nurses become familiar with assessing for suicide warning signs and accessing appropriate resources. Whenever individuals exhibit suicide warning signs, nurses should refer the person to a mental health clinic or provider as soon as possible. This may involve taking emergency action by calling the local emergency services number in the community and staying with the person until help arrives. Table 24-3 provides a list of suicide information resources.

IDENTIFICATION AND MANAGEMENT OF MENTAL DISORDERS

Early identification, appropriate treatment, and rehabilitation can significantly reduce the duration and level of disability associated with mental disorders and decrease the possibility of relapse. Interventions to promote mental health and decrease mental disorders include focusing on decreasing stressors and/or increasing the capacity of the individual to cope with stress. Other interventions include the use of pharmacological agents and psychosocial interventions such as strengthening interpersonal, psychological, and physical resources through counseling, support groups, and psychoeducation.

The accessibility of mental health service is pivotal in promoting and maintaining the health of aggregates. Approximately 25% of community-dwelling adults would profit from mental health services. Yet, current services are inadequate to meet the needs of this population (Messias, Eaton, Nestadt et al., 2007). Decreased funding for services, managed-care limitations on mental health coverage, and the inequality of coverage by the insurance industry have caused downsizing or forced closure in the traditional places of treatment, such as community mental health and community hospitals. In most cases, the decrease in acute care services has not been balanced by an increase in community mental health services. Consequently, the accessibility to community mental health services has become an issue of significant concern. In addition, the symptoms of mental illness often interfere with an individual's ability to access services. Alterations in thoughts and perceptions, anxiety, and decreased energy are common symptoms of mental illness, and all interfere with negotiating the complex systems that currently surround mental health service provision. This section describes actions that may be taken by community health nurses to identify mental illness. It also outlines potential treatment options.

Identification of Mental Disorders

Whether the nurse is working in a physician's office, a clinic, home health, a school, occupational health, or another setting, recognition of signs and symptoms that might indicate a mental disorder is an important component of practice. For example, a student might come to the school nurse's office concerned about a friend who induces vomiting in the bathroom after lunch each day; an occupational health nurse might observe signs consistent with alcohol abuse in an employee; or a client might visit a clinic for a routine visit but mention that for the past several weeks she has been unable to sleep, has lost several pounds, and is no longer interested in her normal activities. In each of these situations, the nurse should continue to assess for other signs and symptoms that might indicate a mental disorder and be prepared to intervene, should concerns be supported.

Often, the assessment process includes direct questioning or observation. At other times, a standardized assessment tool or questionnaire might be employed. Figures 24-1 and 24-2 contain examples of instruments that are available to elicit information about symptoms of anxiety or depression. Whenever using these or other screening tools, the nurse should be prepared in advance to intervene on the basis of assessment data. Often, this incorporates referral to other health professionals for further assessment, testing, counseling, and treatment and follow-up by all health professionals involved, including the community health nurse.

For example, the nurse who suspects that a student has an eating disorder can talk with his or her parents and teachers, the school counselor, principal, and others to determine the best course of action to follow up on assessment findings and associated concerns. If a client describes signs and symptoms consistent with depression, the nurse should chart the reported information and explain to the client's physician the comments that were voiced. When an employee is suspected of alcohol abuse, the occupational nurse should follow company policy on how, when, and under what circumstances the employee and his or her supervisor should be informed of the concerns. The employee should be given information on available treatment options and support groups.

Management of Mental Disorders

The goals of treatment for mental illness are to reduce symptoms, improve occupational and social functioning, develop and strengthen coping skills, and promote behaviors to improve the individual's life. Basic approaches to the treatment of mental disorders include pharmacotherapy, psychotherapy, and/or behavior therapy (USDHHS, 1999).

Psychotherapeutic Medications

Psychotherapeutic medications do not cure mental illness; they act by controlling symptoms. As with medications for physical health problems, the appropriateness of psychopharmacological agents and their prescribed regimen depends on the diagnosis, side effects, and client response. As information about medication profiles and treatment regimens

often changes as new information becomes available, nurses should be aware of up-to-date medication information from Internet resources such as www.nlm.nih.gov/medlineplus/druginformation.html or www.rxlist.com.

Psychotherapy

Psychotherapy refers to a process of discovery that helps alleviate troubling emotional symptoms and assists individuals in returning to a healthy life (APA, 2005). In nursing, psychotherapy is an intervention used by psychiatric/mental health advanced practice nurses only. Psychotherapy involves the use of a professional, therapeutic relationship and the application of psychotherapy theories and best practices to change a client's attitudes, feelings, beliefs, defenses, personality, and behaviors. Therapy approaches vary across schools of psychotherapy and with the nature of the client's problem. Psychotherapy is often used in conjunction with medication to treat many mental disorders. Various types of psychotherapy include the following (NIMH, 2009):

- *Individual therapy* focuses on the client's current life and relationships within the family, social, and work environments.
- *Family therapy* involves problem-solving sessions with members of a family.
- *Couple therapy* is used to develop the relationship and minimize problems through understanding how individual conflicts are expressed in the couple's interactions.
- *Group therapy* involves a small group of people with similar problems who, with the guidance of a therapist, discuss individual issues and help each other with problems.
- *Play therapy* is a technique used for establishing communication and resolving problems with young children.
- *Cognitive-behavioral therapy* may be used in individual, family, couples, or group therapy. The goal is to identify and correct distorted thought patterns that can lead to troublesome feelings and behaviors.
- *Behavioral therapy* uses learning principles to change thought patterns and behaviors systematically; it is used to encourage the individual to learn specific skills to obtain rewards and satisfaction.

Psychotherapy may be short term or long term depending on the nature of the problem and the availability of resources (APA, 2005; NIMH, 2009).

COMMUNITY-BASED MENTAL HEALTH CARE

Over the past several decades, there have been a number of initiatives directed toward improving and promoting community-based care of those with mental illness. One of those initiatives is the President's New Freedom Commission on Mental Health (NFCMH) (2003).

The New Freedom Initiative was first envisioned during George W. Bush's 2000 campaign for the presidency as a promise to tear down the barriers to equality that face millions of Americans with disabilities, including those with mental illness. Following Bush's inauguration, the NFCMH was formed to study the mental health service delivery system.

During the Past Week	Rarely or None of the Time (Less than 1 Day)	Some or a Little of the Time (1-2 Days)	Occasionally or a Moderate Amount of the Time (3-4 Days)	Most or All of the Time (5-7 Days)
1. I was bothered by things that don't usually bother me.	0	1	2	3
2. I did not feel like eating; my appetite was poor.	0	1	2	3
3. I felt that I could not shake off the blues even with the help of my family or friends.	0	1	2	3
4. I felt that I was just as good as other people.	3	2	1	0
5. I had trouble keeping my mind on what I was doing.	0	1	2	3
6. I felt depressed.	0	1	2	3
7. I felt everything I did was an effort.	0	1	2	3
8. I felt hopeful about the future.	3	2	1	0
9. I thought my life had been a failure.	0	1	2	3
10. I felt fearful.	0	1	2	3
11. My sleep was restless.	0	1	2	3
12. I was happy.	3	2	1	0
13. I talked less than usual.	0	1	2	3
14. I felt lonely.	0	1	2	3
15. People were unfriendly.	0	1	2	3
16. I enjoyed life.	3	2	1	0
17. I had crying spells.	0	1	2	3
18. I felt sad.	0	1	2	3
19. I felt that people disliked me.	0	1	2	3
20. I could not get "going."	0	1	2	3

FIGURE 24-1 Center for Epidemiologic Studies depression scale. Interpretation: a total score of 22 or higher is indicative of depression when the scale is used in primary care. (From Radloff LS: The CES-D scale: a self-report depression scale for research in the general population, *Appl Psychol Meas* 1:385-401, 1977. Copyright 1977, West Publishing Company/Applied Psychological Measurement, Inc.)

This represented the first comprehensive study of the nation's mental health delivery system in 25 years. The goal of the commission was to advise the president on strategies aimed at improving the mental health system so that persons with serious and persistent mental illnesses can enjoy full access to community life. The commission determined that in a transformed mental health system (NFCMH, 2003, p. 8):

1. Americans understand that mental health is essential to overall health.
2. Mental health care is consumer and family driven.

Rank	Life Event	Mean Value	Rank	Life Event	Mean Value
1	Death of spouse	100	23	Son or daughter leaving home	29
2	Divorce	73	24	Trouble with in-laws	29
3	Marital separation	65	25	Outstanding personal achievement	28
4	Jail term	63	26	Wife begins or stops work	26
5	Death of close family member	63	27	Begin or end school	26
6	Personal injury or illness	53	28	Change in living conditions	25
7	Marriage	50	29	Change in personal habits	24
8	Fired at work	47	30	Trouble with boss	23
9	Marital reconciliation	45	31	Change in work hours or conditions	20
10	Retirement	45	32	Change in residence	20
11	Change in health of family member	44	33	Change in schools	20
12	Pregnancy	40	34	Change in recreation	19
13	Sex difficulties	39	35	Change in church activities	19
14	Gain of new family member	39	36	Change in social activities	18
15	Business readjustment	39	37	Mortgage or loan less than $10,000	17
16	Change in financial state	38	38	Change in sleeping habits	16
17	Death of close friend	37	39	Change in number of family get-togethers	15
18	Change to different line of work	36	40	Change in eating habits	15
19	Change in number of arguments with spouse	35	41	Vacation	13
20	Mortgage over $10,000	31	42	Christmas	12
21	Foreclosure on mortgage or loan	30	43	Minor violations of the law	11
22	Change in responsibilities at work	29			

Life Crisis Categories and LCU Scores*

No life crisis	0-149
Mild life crisis	150-199
Moderate life crisis	200-299
Major life crisis	300 or more

*The LCU score includes those life event items experienced during a 1-year period.

FIGURE 24-2 Social readjustment rating scale. (From Holmes TH, Rahe RH: The social readjustment rating scale, *J Psychosom Res* 11:213-217, 1967, Elsevier Science Inc.)

3. Disparities in mental health services are eliminated.
4. Early mental health screening, assessment, and referral to services are common practice.
5. Excellent mental health care is delivered, and research is accelerated.
6. Technology is used to access mental health care and information.

The commission acknowledged that mental illness comprises the only type of illness that defies a comprehensive delivery approach. This is due to the way the state and local governments organize, manage, and carry out distinct treatment systems, making comprehensive care impossible in the larger health care system. Thus, the commission called for a shift in the fragmented system to an integrated comprehensive approach to mental health care delivery. Table 24-4 provides an overview of the recommendations of the commission. One of the areas addressed by the commission pertained to the need for school-based mental health (SBMH) programs. In an overview of key elements related to SBMH, Paternite (2005)

identified the need for (1) partnerships between and among schools, families, and communities; (2) a pledge to support a full continuum of mental health services that include education, health promotion, assessment, and early intervention; and (3) services for all children and adolescents.

Subsequently, national mental health leaders were surveyed to assess the participants' perceptions of the impact of the New Freedom Commission recommendations (von Esenwein et al., 2005). Results of this survey suggested that the commission findings and suggestions for improved care had a significant influence on the mental health care organizations represented.

In another initiative, the Center for Mental Health Services (CMHS) was formed in the early 1990s to improve prevention and mental health treatment services for all Americans. The CMHS helps states improve and increase the quality and range of treatment, rehabilitation, and support for people with mental health problems, their families, and communities (SAMHSA, 2005).

Disparities in Children's Mental Health Care

Even though there is serious need for community mental health services for children, the majority of children with a mental health disorder do not receive treatment. Researchers recently examined a large database, the National Survey of American Families, to study whether living in a state with a mental health parity law impacted the use of children's mental health outpatient services. The results of the study indicated that having children's mental health parity insurance alone was not sufficient to affect the likelihood of children using mental health services. This study suggests that receiving treatment for mental health services is complex. While mental health parity is a crucial first step in providing much needed treatment, nurses and other health care leaders must advocate for a reduction in social stigma associated with mental illness, provide screenings for childhood mental illness, and educate families and communities about the importance of early intervention for affected children in need.

From Barry CL, Busch SH: Caring for children with mental disorders: do state parity laws increase access to treatment? *J Ment Health Policy Econ* 11(2): 57-66, 2008.

One of the programs promoted by the CMHS is the Community Support System. The Community Support System uses case management strategies to comprehensively provide care for those with serious mental illness. Components of the Community Support System include client identification and outreach, mental health treatment, crisis response service, health and dental care, housing, income support and entitlement, peer support, family and community support, rehabilitation services, and protection and advocacy. The case management approach serves to link the service system to the client and to coordinate their service received (Huggins and Anderson, 2006). Other initiatives and programs sponsored by the CMHS are shown in Table 24-5.

The Program of Assertive Community Treatment (PACT) is another example of a community-based initiative to help meet the needs of those with mental illness. PACT, which has been in existence since the late 1960s, has become the exemplar of community mental health treatment models. The PACT program moves the traditional 24-hour treatment model of acute care settings into the community and serves people with mental illness in a highly individualized fashion (National Alliance on Mental Illness [NAMI], 2005). The PACT model provides around-the-clock supportive therapy, mobile crisis intervention, psychiatric medications, hospitalization, education, and skill teaching for consumers and their families. PACT brings service to the consumer and is considered the model of effective community mental health treatment of the future. A NAMI PACT initiative encourages all states to have assertive community treatment. Currently, seven states and the District of Columbia have statewide PACT programs, and many more have at least one pilot project (NAMI, 2005). Box 24-4 gives additional details about PACT programs.

TABLE 24-4	GOALS AND RECOMMENDATIONS OF THE NEW FREEDOM COMMISSION ON MENTAL HEALTH
GOAL	**RECOMMENDATIONS**
1. Americans understand that mental health is essential to overall health	Advance and implement a national campaign to reduce the stigma of seeking care and a national strategy for suicide prevention. Address mental health with the same urgency as physical health.
2. Mental health care is consumer and family driven.	Develop an individualized plan of care for every adult with a serious mental illness and child with a serious emotional disturbance. Involve consumers and families fully in orienting the mental health system toward recovery. Align relevant federal programs to improve access and accountability for mental health services. Create a comprehensive state mental health plan. Protect and enhance the rights of people with mental illnesses.
3. Disparities in mental health services are eliminated.	Improve access to quality care that is culturally competent. Improve access to quality care in rural and geographically remote areas.
4. Early mental health screening, assessment, and referral to services are common practice.	Promote the mental health of young children. Improve and expand school mental health programs. Screen for co-occurring mental and substance use disorders and link with integrated treatment strategies. Screen for mental disorders in primary health care across the life span, and connect to treatment and support.
5. Excellent mental health care is delivered and research is accelerated.	Accelerate research to promote recovery and resilience and ultimately to cure and prevent mental illnesses. Advance evidence-based practices using dissemination and demonstration projects and create a public-private partnership to guide their implementation. Improve and expand the workforce providing evidence-based mental health services and supports. Develop the knowledge base in four understudied areas: mental health disparities, long-term effects of medications, trauma, and acute care.
6. Technology is used to access mental health care and information.	Use health technology and telehealth to improve access and coordination of mental health care, especially for Americans in remote areas or in underserved populations. Develop and implement integrated electronic health record and personal health information systems.

From New Freedom Commission on Mental Health: *Achieving the promise: transforming mental health care in America, Final report*, USDHHS Pub No SMA 03-3832, Rockville, MD, 2003, The Author: www.mentalhealthcommission.gov/reports/reports.htm.

TABLE 24-5 CENTER FOR MENTAL HEALTH SERVICES: EXAMPLES OF PROGRAMS AND INITIATIVES

PROGRAM/INITIATIVE	PURPOSE AND ACTIVITIES
National Strategy for Suicide Prevention	Collaborative effort of SAMHSA, CDC, NIH, HRSA, and IHS to reduce the incidence of suicide in the United States; supports and monitors state-based suicide prevention programs and provides information and resources
Center on Women, Violence and Trauma	Sponsored by SAMHSA to highlight the role of violence and trauma in the lives of people with behavioral health disorders; provides information and helps fund related studies
Youth Violence Prevention Program	Offers the Safe Schools/Healthy Students Initiative to prevent school violence and foster the healthy development of children. This is a collaborative grant program that supports community collaborations that prevent youth violence, substance abuse, suicide, and other mental and behavioral problems
Homelessness programs	Support of programs to assist people with mental illness who are homeless in obtaining treatment and other services (e.g., primary health care, substance abuse treatment, legal assistance)
State planning and mental health block grants	Awards grants to states to provide mental health services. These grants are designed to improve access to community-based health care delivery systems for people with serious mental illnesses who quickly exhaust available resources
Caring for Every Child's Mental Health Campaign	National public information and education campaign to increase public awareness about the importance of protecting and nurturing the mental health of young people, to foster recognition that many children have mental health problems, and to encourage caregivers to seek early, appropriate treatment

CDC, Centers for Disease Control and Prevention; *HRSA,* Health Resources and Services Administration; *IHS,* Indian Health Service; *NIH,* National Institutes of Health; *SAMHSA,* Substance Abuse and Mental Health Services Administration.

BOX 24-4 KEY FEATURES OF THE PROGRAM OF ASSERTIVE COMMUNITY TREATMENT

- Psychopharmacological treatment
- Individual supportive therapy
- Mobile crisis intervention
- Hospitalization
- Substance abuse treatment
- Behaviorally oriented skill teaching
- Supported employment
- Support for resuming education
- Collaboration with families and assistance to clients with children
- Direct support to help clients obtain legal and advocacy services

ROLE OF THE COMMUNITY MENTAL HEALTH NURSE

Challenges to the effective provision of mental health services in the community abound. Stigma and poverty contribute to a mistrust of health care professionals (Cristofalo et al., 2009). Lack of understanding by affected individuals and families, lack of integrated services for mental and physical health, comorbidity of mental illness and substance abuse, and symptoms of illness precluding effective utilization of available services by clients create additional complications. Funding is inadequate to meet the needs of mentally ill individuals, and public funds such as Medicaid become available only after individuals are disabled for an extended period of time.

In spite of multiple challenges, the role of a community mental health nurse can be extremely rewarding. Perhaps the most critical impact made by the nurse in a community setting is through the establishment of interpersonal relationships with clients. Establishing supportive relationships is the first step in the role of the community mental health nurse as coach for mental and physical health promotion (Adams, 2008). The importance of relationships has also been highlighted in helping homeless individuals with mental illness to exit homelessness (Slesnick, Bartle-Haring, Dashora, et al., 2008).

Community health nurses should consider mental health and mental illness as dynamic processes. Mental illness and mental health must be assessed in the context of social environments that include family, community, peer reference groups, and physical and cultural surroundings. As factors within these areas shift, the severity of mental health symptoms and sequelae will also shift. This dynamic reinforces the importance of continual reassessment of client needs.

Finally, the community mental health nurse must provide care within the context of a client's culture and beliefs (Mahoney and Engebretson, 2000; Mahoney, Carlson, and Engebretson, 2006). This requires self-assessment and ongoing acquisition of knowledge and skills. The ability to provide care within a context of culture fosters client participation in planning and accessing care and improved outcomes.

Community mental health nursing roles are multidimensional (e.g., educator and activist or practitioner and coordinator). The educator and activist improves public awareness of effective treatments and existing community resources. Community mental health nurses as educators and activists dispel myths, provide accurate information about mental illness, and influence policy and legislation advocating for those with mental illness.

As practitioner and coordinator, the nurse works directly with individuals, groups, and families. Besides intervening to assist consumers in controlling or alleviating the symptoms of mental illness, the practitioner and coordinator also helps the consumer "navigate" within the segmented

TABLE 24-6 ORGANIZATIONS THAT ADVOCATE FOR MENTAL HEALTH

RESOURCE	SERVICES	CONTACT INFORMATION
Substance Abuse and Mental Health Services Administration, National Mental Health Information Center	Website contains information and publications related to mental health issues, current events, features related to specific mental health issues (for example, child mental health, consumer/survivor issues, youth violence prevention), link to available services by state	http://mentalhealth.samhsa.gov/
National Alliance on Mental Illness	Consumer education regarding various mental health disorders, medication and treatment, research, public policy issues; links to find support at state and local level including support groups and online discussion groups; tips for becoming politically involved in mental health public policy issues	www.nami.org/
Mental Health America	Crisis hotline (1-800-273-TALK) to assist individuals in finding treatment resources; mental health public policy information including steps to become involved; online discussion groups; current issues; online depression screening	www.nmha.org/
National Institute of Mental Health	Education on mental health topics and research	www.nimh.nih.gov/index.shtml
Depression and Bipolar Support Alliance	Education on depression and bipolar disorder; current topics/events; online discussion and support groups; assistance in finding treatment resources; advocacy information	www.ndmda.org/
National Education Alliance for Borderline Personality Disorder	Education about borderline personality disorder and treatment	www.borderlinepersonalitydisorder.com/
Obsessive-Compulsive Foundation	Education about obsessive compulsive and anxiety disorders and treatment	www.ocfoundation.org/
Postpartum Support International	Education and resource information for individuals experiencing symptoms of prenatal or postpartum mood or anxiety disorders	http://postpartum.net/

web of agencies and other service providers. A list of organizations that advocate for mental health is provided in Table 24-6. Community mental health nurses not only take action to solve an immediate problem but also plan and intervene to ensure safety, continuity, and quality of care for consumers. Therefore, the practitioner and coordinator roles require skills in anticipating and evaluating the actions of other providers and communicating with consumers, families, rehabilitation services, and government or social agencies.

Within this aspect of community mental health nursing, individual-, family-, and community-level crises are anticipated, prevented, and, failing these, contained. For example, as practitioners and coordinators, nurses might organize people taking psychotropic medications to share experiences about interacting with a psychiatrist, managing side effects of medications, and enhancing their coping strategies. Such a proactive stance may help prevent problems resulting in self-discontinuation of medication and the consequences of such action. In the practitioner and coordinator roles, community mental health nurses work toward matching consumers and families with culturally appropriate and sensitive providers to achieve the "best fit."

CASE STUDY APPLICATION OF THE NURSING PROCESS

Kay Morton is a registered nurse working in a public-sponsored primary care clinic for indigent and homeless people in a large southwestern city. The clinic is housed in a center that provides comprehensive care for the poor. The center employs family practice physicians, two registered nurses, one licensed vocational nurse, a mental health nurse practitioner, two counselors, and three social workers. Residents from an area medical school provide additional medical support. In addition to meeting the health care needs of the community, the team provides assistance with job training and employment, as well as assistance with housing and child care.

Jeannie Smith is one of the clients served by the center. Jeannie is a 25-year-old single mother of three young children (ages 8, 6, and 2 years) who has been receiving public assistance for more than 8 years. During that time, her children have been in foster care on several occasions. She admits to a history of using marijuana, methamphetamine, and alcohol, as well as having multiple sexual partners. Two years ago, Jeannie received a diagnosis of bipolar disorder and is currently taking medication to manage her symptoms.

On a recent visit to the center to work with her case manager, Jeannie was also seen at the clinic. Kay greeted Jeannie and led

CASE STUDY APPLICATION OF THE NURSING PROCESS—cont'd

her to a private room for her follow-up care. During this period, she casually asked Jeannie about her children. They discussed how Jeannie was managing three children and her new job as a clerk at a local bank.

Assessment
Kay noted that Jeannie answered questions appropriately. In her notes, Kay wrote that the client stated that her work was tedious and she did not feel like she "fit in" with the other people at work. Jeannie reported that she had been generally compliant with her medication regimen, although she stated she sometimes forgets to take her morning medications because she is in a rush to get the children to school and day care and herself to work. She had not observed any side effects from the medications, and she denied using any illicit drugs or alcohol since her last visit. However, Jeannie told Kay that she was having strong urges to drink beer when she came home from work and that she was having trouble "fighting" these feelings. She also reported that Macy, her 8-year-old daughter, was having trouble in school. The teacher had noted that Macy often did not complete homework assignments, was having trouble paying attention in class, and had few friends.

Diagnosis
Individual
- History of mental illness (bipolar disorder) and substance abuse
- Potential for noncompliance with treatment regimen
- Social isolation
- Chronic low self-esteem

Family
- Potential for family dysfunction
- Potential for social isolation

Community
- Deficient knowledge regarding community resources for diagnosis and management of mental disorders

Planning
Planning for Jeannie involved reviewing her case management protocol and determining whether she was following recommendations. Agency protocols required random drug screening for all clients. For clients on certain medications (including those taken by Jeannie), blood testing was required. Then Kay talked briefly with Jeannie's case manager to determine the time scheduled for her counseling session. Kay also obtained information about the local Alcoholics Anonymous (AA) and the National Depressive and Manic Depressive Association (NDMDA) support group meeting schedules. Kay also consulted with the case manager to determine ways to improve her daughter Macy's school performance.

Individual
Long-Term Goal
- Jeannie will progress with her employment and be able to support her family without public assistance.

Short-Term Goals
- Jeannie will remain compliant with her medication and case management regimen.
- Jeannie will remain drug free.

Family
Long-Term Goals
- Jeannie and her children will maintain a stable household.
- The children will progress well in school.

Short-Term Goal
- Daughter Macy will be evaluated for a learning or an attention disorder.

Intervention
Individual
Kay collected a urine specimen from Jeannie to be sent for drug screening. To ensure that Jeannie's lithium levels were in therapeutic range, the physician asked Kay to obtain a sample of blood. Kay drew a small sample from Jeannie's right arm using careful sterile technique and paying attention to universal precautions. She reviewed the purpose of the test with Jeannie and explained that the results would be back in a couple of days. While she was working with Jeannie, Kay listened to her concerns about how she was going to pay for new clothes and shoes for the children for the upcoming school year.

Kay suggested that Jeannie plan to attend an upcoming AA meeting and reestablish herself with the group, as this had been a successful strategy in the past for managing Jeannie's urges to drink. Kay reeducated Jeannie about the purpose and effects of lithium and discussed the importance of maintaining a therapeutic level of the drug to prevent breakthrough bipolar symptoms. Kay also referred Jeannie to the NDMDA support group as a resource for illness management.

Family
Kay suggested that Jeannie make an appointment with the school counselor to discuss Macy's progress, as well as an appointment for Macy to be seen in the clinic for a physical examination. After Kay finished charting, she reported the findings to Jeannie's counselor and was careful to mention what Jeannie had told her about financial concerns. Kay arranged for a follow-up appointment with Jeannie and Macy in 2 weeks, as she was aware that Jeannie was at risk for deteriorating symptomatically and also understood the importance of assessing Macy further in order to reduce Macy's distress and identify additional community resources for her.

Evaluation
Jeannie verbalized understanding the importance of following the recommendations and left to keep her appointment with her counselor. Jeannie's counselor reported that she would assist her client in finding sources that would help pay for school clothes and supplies. Kay would watch for the results of the tests and report back to both Jeannie and her counselor. Jeannie also reported that she would talk with Macy's teacher and school counselor.

Levels of Prevention
Primary
- Assisting Jeannie in finding and maintaining employment
- Providing information on services and providers to assist with clothing and school supplies for the children

Secondary
- Evaluation of daughter Macy to determine cause of school difficulties

Tertiary
- Monitoring of Jeannie's lithium levels
- Testing Jeannie's urine for illicit drugs
- Counseling to encourage Jeannie to attend AA meetings and NDMDA support group

SUMMARY

Like all other aspects of nursing, community mental health nursing is evolving. At the beginning of the twenty-first century, conditions are in place that may promote dramatic improvement in the identification of and care for those with mental illness. Improved information and evidence-based practice may result in greater understanding of the factors that contribute to mental disorders and lead to more effective treatment. Ultimately, there should be increased attention given to prevention of mental illness and promotion of mental health.

As discussed in this chapter, the vast majority of individuals with diagnosable mental disorders are found in the community, and many, if not most, never seek professional help. The framework for community mental health nursing presented in this chapter should prove useful in improving the lives of individuals, families, and groups of people with mental illness. Further, it is hoped that all nurses will become advocates for the mentally ill and support social and political change to improve the mental health of all.

LEARNING ACTIVITIES

1. Reflect on personal experience interacting with individuals with mental illness. What thoughts or feelings did these experiences produce?
2. Locate the NAMI chapter in your community. What services does it offer? How might those services be helpful in the community mental health nursing role?
3. List five ways to act as an educator and activist for mental health issues in the community.

REFERENCES

Adams L: Mental health nurses can play a role in physical health, *Mental Health Today* 10:27–29, 2008.

American Association of Suicidology: *Know the warning signs*, 2008, www.suicidology. org/web/guest/stats-and-tools/warning-signs.

American Psychiatric Association: *Diagnostic and statistical manual of mental disorders*, ed 4, text revision, Washington, DC, 2000, The Author.

American Psychiatric Association: *Practice guideline for the treatment of patients with major depressive disorder*, ed 2, 2005, www.psychiatryonline.com.

Buchsbaum MS, Haier RJ: Functional and anatomical brain imaging, *Schizophr Bull* 14:383, 1982.

Burns A, Robins A, Hodge M, Holes A: Long-term homelessness in men with psychosis: limitation of services, *Int J Ment Health Nurs* 18:126–132, 2009.

Centers for Disease Control and Prevention: *Surveillance for violent deaths—national violent death reporting system, 16 states*, 2005, www.cdc.gov/mmwR/preview/mmwrhtml/ss5703a1.htm.

Centers for Disease Control and Prevention: *Attention deficit/hyperactivity disorder*, 2009, www.cdc.gov/ncbddd/adhd/index.html.

Cochrane C: Eating regulation response and eating disorders. In Stuart GW, Laraia MT, editors: *Principles and practice of psychiatric nursing*, ed 8, St. Louis, 2005, Mosby.

Coker AL, Hanks JS, Eggleston KS, et al: Social and mental health needs assessment of Katrina evacuees, *Disaster Manag Response* 4(3):88–94, 2006.

Cowell AJ, Luo Z, Masuda YJ: Psychiatric disorders and the labor market: an analysis by disorder profiles, *J Ment Health Policy Econ* 12(1):3–17, 2009.

Cristofalo M, Boutain D, Schraufnagel T, et al: Unmet need for mental health and addictions care in urban community health clinics: frontline provider accounts, *Psychiatr Serv* 60(4):505–511, 2009.

de Geus E, Goldberg T, Boomsma DI, et al: Imaging the genetics of brain structure and functioning, *Biol Psychol* 79:1–8, 2008.

Deutsch A: *The mentally ill in America: a history of their care and treatment from colonial times*, New York, 1949, Columbia University Press.

Dohrenwend BP, Turner JB, Turse NA, et al: The psychological risk of Vietnam for U.S. veterans: a revisit with new data and methods, *Science* 313(5789):979–982, 2006.

Fleming JA, Mahoney JS, Carlson E, et al: An ethnographic approach to interpreting a mental illness photovoice exhibit, *Arch Psychiatr Nurs* 23(1):16–24, 2009.

Foucault M: *Madness and civilization*, New York, 1965, Random House.

Grob GN: *Mental illness and American society, 1875–1940*, Princeton, NJ, 1983, Princeton University Press.

Grob GN: *From asylum to community: mental health policy in modern America*, Princeton, NJ, 1991, Princeton University Press.

Huggins M, Anderson JA: Community mental health, support and rehabilitation. In Mohr WK, editor: *Psychiatric–mental health nursing*, ed 6, Philadelphia, 2006, Lippincott Williams & Wilkins, pp 319–337.

Human Rights Watch: *US number of mentally ill in prisons quadrupled*, 2008, www.hrw.org/en/news/2006/09/05/us-number-mentally-ill-prisons-quadrupled.

Hunter RA: *Three hundred years of psychiatry: 1535–1800*, London, 1963, Oxford University Press.

Institute of Medicine: *Genes, behavior, and the social environment: moving beyond the nature/nurture debate*, Washington, DC, 2006a, National Academies Press.

Institute of Medicine: *Improving the quality of health care for mental and substance-use conditions*, Washington, DC, 2006b, National Academies of Science.

Kandel ER: A new intellectual framework for psychiatry, *Am J Psychiatry* 155:457, 1998.

Kessler RC, Chiu WT, Demler O, et al: Prevalence, severity, and comorbidity of twelve-month DSM-IV disorders in the National Comorbidity Survey Replication (NCS-R), *Arch Gen Psychiatry* 62(6): 617–627, 2005.

Kessler RC, Galea S, Gruber MJ, et al: Trends in mental health and suicidality after Hurricane Katrina, *Mol Psychiatry* 13(4):374–384, 2008.

Mahoney JS, Carlson EC, Engebretson JC: A framework for cultural competence in advanced practice in psychiatric and mental health nursing education, *Perspect Psychiatr Care* 42(4):227–237, 2006.

Mahoney JS, Engebretson JC: The interface of anthropology and nursing guiding culturally competent care in psychiatric nursing, *Arch Psychiatr Nurs* 14(4):183–190, 2000.

Mathers CD, Loncar D: *Updated projections of global mortality and burden of disease, 2002–2030*, data sources, methods and results, 2005, www.who.int/entity/healthinfo/statistics/bodprojectionspaper.pdf.

Messias E, Eaton W, Nestadt G, et al: Psychiatrists' ascertained treatment needs for mental disorders in a population-based sample, *Psychiatr Serv* 58(3):373–377, 2007.

Miranda J, McGuire TG, Williams DR, et al: Mental health in the context of health disparities, *Am J Psychiatry* 165(9): 1102–1108, 2008.

National Alliance on Mental Illness: *PACT: program of assertive community treatment*, 2005, www.nami.org/Template.cfm?Section=ACT-TA_Center&template=/ContentManagement/ContentDisplay.cfm&ContentID=28608.

National Center for Injury Prevention and Control, Centers for Disease Control and Prevention: *WISQARS fatal injuries mortality reports*, 2009, www.cdc.gov/NCIPC/WISQARS/.

National Institute of Mental Health: *Depression*, NIH Pub No 00-3561, Rockville, MD, 2000, The Author.

National Institute of Mental Health: *Schizophrenia*, 2005, www.nimh.nih.gov/healthinformation/schizophreniamenu.cfm.

National Institute of Mental Health: *Male veterans have double the suicide rate of civilians*, 2007, www.nimh.nih.gov/science-news/2007/male-veterans-have-double-the-suicide-rate-of-civilians.shtml.

National Institute of Mental Health: *National Institute for Mental Health strategic plan*, 2000, mentaldepression.nimh.nih.gov/about/strategic-planning-reports/nimh-strategic-plan-2008.pdf.

National Institute of Mental Health: *Mental health topics*, 2009, www.nimh.nih.gov/health/topics/index.shtml.

National Mental Health Association: *Children's mental health statistics*, 2006, www.nmha.org/children/prevent/stats.cfm.

New Freedom Commission on Mental Health (NFCMH): *Achieving the promise: transforming mental health care in America*, Final report, USDHHS Pub No SMA 03-3832, Rockville, MD, 2003, www.mentalhealthcommission.gov/reports/reports.htm.

Olszewski TM, Varrasse JF: The neurobiology of PTSD: implications for nurses, *Psychosoc Nurs* 43(6):41–47, 2005.

Open Congress: *Emergency Economic Stabilization Act of 2008*, 2008, www.opencongress.org/bill/110-h1424/show.

Paternite CE: School-based mental health programs and services: overview and introduction to the special issue, *J Abnorm Child Psychol* 33(6):657–663, 2005.

Pruessner JC, Dedovic K, Pruessner M, et al: Stress regulation in the central nervous system: evidence from structural and functional neuroimaging studies in human populations, *Psychoneuroendocrinology* 35(1):179–191, 2010.

Radloff LS: The CES-D scale: a self-report depression scale for research in the general population, *Applied Psychological Measurement* 1:385–401, 1977.

Ridgely MS, Engberg J, Greenberg MD, et al: *Justice, treatment, and cost: an evaluation of the fiscal impact of Allegheny County mental health court*, Santa Monica, CA, 2007, Rand Corporation.

Roberts KT, Robinson KM, Topp R, et al: Community perceptions of mental health needs in an underserved minority neighborhood, *J Community Health Nurs* 25:203–217, 2008.

Sadler J: Stigma, conscience, and science in psychiatry: past, present, and future, *Acad Med* 84(4):413–417, 2009.

Sharfstein SS, Stoline AM, Koran LM: Mental health services. In Kovner AR, Jonas S, editors: *Jonas & Kovner's health care delivery in the United States*, ed 7, New York, 2002, Springer, pp 238–262.

Slesnick N, Bartle-Haring S, Dashora P, et al: Predictors of homelessness among street youth, *Youth Adolesc* 37:465–474, 2008.

Smith TC, Ryan MA, Wingard DL, et al: Millennium Cohort Study team: New onset and persistent symptoms of post-traumatic stress disorder self reported after deployment and combat exposure: prospective population based US military cohort study, *Br Med J* 366(7640):366–371, 2008.

Smoller JW, Sheidley BR, Tsuang MT: *Psychiatric genetics: applications in clinical perspective*, Arlington, VA, 2008, American Psychiatric Publishing.

Strine TW, Dhingra SS, Okoro CA, et al: State-based differences in the prevalence and characteristics of untreated persons with serious psychological distress, *Int J Public Health* 54(Suppl 1):9–15, 2009.

Substance Abuse and Mental Health Services Administration: *Results from the 2004 National Survey on Drug Use and Health: national findings*, NSDUH Series H-28, USDHHS Pub No SMA 05-4062, Rockville, MD, 2005, Office of Applied Studies.

Unutzer J, et al: Transforming mental health care at the interface with general medicine: report for the Presidents Commission, *Psychiatr Serv* 57:37–47, 2006.

U.S. Department of Health and Human Services: *Mental health: a report of the Surgeon General*, Washington, DC, 1999, Government Printing Office, www.surgeongeneral.gov/library/mentalhealth/chapter?/sec? 1.html

U.S. Department of Health and Human Services: *Healthy People 2010*, ed 2, Washington, DC, 2000, Government Printing Office.

U.S. Department of Health and Human Services/Substance Abuse and Mental Health Services Administration: *Results from the 2004 National survey on drug use and health: national findings*, Washington, DC, 2005, The Author.

U.S. Department of Health and Human Services: *Progress review: mental health and mental disorders*, 2007, www/healthpeople.govdata/2010prog/focus18/default.htm.

von Esenwein SA, et al: A survey of mental health leaders one year after the President's New Freedom Commission report, *Psychiatr Serv* 56(5):605–607, 2005.

World Health Organization: *The financial crisis and global health*, 2009, www.who.int/topics/financial_crisis/financialcrisis_report_200902.pdf.

Yoo SS, Gujar N, Hu P, et al: The human emotional brain without sleep—a prefrontal amygdala disconnect, *Curr Biol* 17(20):R877–R899, 2007.

Communicable Disease

Deanna E. Grimes

Additional Material for Study, Review, and Further Exploration

evolve WEBSITE

http://evolve.elsevier.com/Nies
- Quiz
- Case Studies
- Glossary
- WebLinks

OBJECTIVES

Upon completion of this chapter, the reader will be able to do the following:

1. Review principles related to the occurrence and transmission of infection and infectious diseases.
2. Describe the three focus areas in *Healthy People 2020* objectives that apply to infectious diseases.
3. Describe the chain of transmission of infectious diseases.
4. Apply the chain of transmission to describing approaches to control infectious disease.
5. Review types of immunity, including herd immunity.
6. Review principles of immunization, and specify the immunization recommended for all age groups in the United States.
7. Describe the legal responsibility for control of communicable diseases in the United States.
8. Describe the chain of transmission and control for priority infectious disease.
9. Identify nursing activities for control of infectious diseases at primary, secondary, and tertiary levels of prevention.

KEY TERMS

acquired immunity
active immunity
agent
antigenicity
carriers
case
cold chain
communicable disease
communicable period
control
direct transmission
elimination
endemic
environment
epidemic
eradication
fomites
herd immunity

host
immunity
immunization
incidence
incubation period
indirect transmission
infection
infectious disease
infectivity
isolation
latency
multicausation
natural immunity
notifiable infectious diseases
outbreak
pandemic
passive immunity
pathogenicity

portal of entry
portal of exit
primary vaccine failure
quarantine
reservoir
resistance
secondary vaccine failure
subclinical infection
susceptible
toxigenicity
universal precautions
vaccination
Vaccine Adverse Events Reporting System (VAERS)
vectors
virulence

Throughout history, epidemics have been responsible for the destruction of entire groups of people. Despite amazing advances in public health and health care, control of communicable diseases continues to be a major concern of health care providers. The emergence of new pathogens, the reemergence of old pathogens, and the appearance of drug-resistant pathogens are creating formidable challenges worldwide.

Despite global eradication campaigns, malaria and other vector-borne diseases and life-threatening gastrointestinal infections continue to cause significant morbidity and mortality in the developing world. Tuberculosis infected 13.7 million people worldwide (206 cases/100,000 population) in 2007 and has become a leading killer of young adults worldwide, particularly those infected with the human immunodeficiency virus (HIV) (World Health Organization [WHO], 2009). Measles, when coupled with vitamin A deficiency, is a leading cause of blindness in many developing countries in the Eastern Hemisphere. To add to the world's growing infectious disease burden, HIV and acquired immunodeficiency syndrome (AIDS) continue to spread unchecked throughout the world, as evidenced by estimates of 33.2 million adults and children living with HIV/AIDS globally at the end of 2007, with approximately 2.7 million new infections occurring each year (UNAIDS, 2008).

Great strides have been made in the United States with respect to vaccine-preventable diseases, yet segments of the population remain unimmunized or under-immunized. Both measles and pertussis are preventable with a vaccine, and indigenous measles has virtually been eliminated in the United States, with only forty-three cases reported in 2007. In contrast, there were 10,454 cases of pertussis reported in the same year (Centers for Disease Control and Prevention [CDC], 2009a). Hepatitis A, B, and C have been significantly reduced since the 1990s, by administering vaccines for hepatitis A and B and testing the blood supply for hepatitis C. Yet these diseases persist. Treatable sexually transmitted diseases (STDs), such as syphilis and gonorrhea, had declined until 2000 but increased in 2007 for the seventh straight year. At the same time, incidence of chlamydia, another treatable STD, has increased steadily since 1995, and the number of cases reached 1,108,374 (370.2 per 100,000 people) in 2007 (CDC, 2009a). In the United States, there have been significant accomplishments in preventing food- and waterborne infections through environmental sanitation, but there appears to be increasing incidence of vector-borne infections, such as Lyme disease, Rocky Mountain spotted fever, St. Louis encephalitis, and West Nile encephalitis. Further, although the advent of effective antiretroviral treatment for AIDS in the mid-1990s briefly slowed the incidence of AIDS diagnosis, about 37,503 new AIDS cases were reported and 455,636 persons were living with AIDS in 2007 in the United States (CDC, 2009a).

Probably one of the most profound failures in infectious disease control in the United States and elsewhere is that the successes are not equally distributed in the general population. Infectious diseases continue to be differentially distributed by income and ethnic groups, and the poor and minorities continue to experience the greater burden.

BOX 25-1 DRUG-RESISTANT PATHOGENS/DISEASES

- *Acinetobacter* spp.: Nosocomial bacteremia, septicemia
- *Bordetella pertussis:* Pertussis
- *Campylobacter* (fluoroquinolone-resistant): Enteritis
- *Enterococcus* spp. (multidrug-resistant, including vancomycin-resistant [VRE])
- *Enterobacter* spp.
- HIV/AIDS
- *Klebsiella* spp.
- *Mycobacterium tuberculosis* (multidrug-resistant [MDR-TB]): Tuberculosis
- *Neisseria gonorrhoeae* (fluoroquinolone-resistant): Gonorrhea
- *Pediculus humanus capitis:* Head lice
- *Plasmodium falciparum* and *P. vivax:* Malaria
- *Pseudomonas aeruginosa*
- *Salmonella* spp.: Typhoid fever and salmonellosis
- *Staphylococcus aureus* (methicillin-resistant [MRSA], vancomycin-resistant [VRSA])
- *Staphylococcus epidermidis* (VRSE, MRSE)
- *Streptococcus pneumoniae* (multidrug-resistant): Pneumonia, meningitis, and otitis media
- *Treponema pallidum* (azithromycin-resistant): Syphilis
- Other gram-negative bacteria developing drug resistance: *Citrobacter freundii, Escherichia coli, Morganella morganii, Providencia* spp., and *Serratia* spp.

From Centers for Disease Control and Prevention: *Diseases connected to antibiotic resistance,* 2008, www.cdc.gov/drugresistance/diseases.html; and Heymann DL, editor: *Control of communicable diseases manual,* ed 18, Washington, DC, 2008, American Public Health Association.

BOX 25-2 CENTERS FOR DISEASE CONTROL AND PREVENTION LIST OF POTENTIAL BIOTERRORISM AGENTS AND DISEASES BY CATEGORY

Category A: Highest priority; easily transmitted with high mortality and social disruption
- Anthrax *(Bacillus anthracis)*
- Botulism (botulinum toxin)
- Plague *(Yersinia pestis)*
- Smallpox (variola virus)
- Tularemia *(Francisella tularensis)*
- Viral hemorrhagic fevers (Ebola, Lassa, and Marburg viruses)

Category B: Moderately easy to disseminate; high morbidity with low mortality
- Brucellosis (*Brucella* spp.)
- Cholera *(Vibrio cholerae)*
- Epsilon toxin of *Clostridium perfringens*
- Glanders *(Burkholderia mallei)*
- Melioidosis *(Burkholderia mallei)*
- Psittacosis *(Chlamydia psittaci)*
- Q fever *(Coxiella burnetii)*
- Ricin toxin
- Salmonellosis (*Salmonella* spp.)
- Shigellosis (*Shigella* spp.)
- Typhus fever *(Rickettsia prowazekii)*
- Viral encephalitis (alphaviruses)

From Centers for Disease Control and Prevention: *Bioterrorism agents/diseases,* 2009e, http://emergency.cdc.gov/agent/agentlist-category.asp.

Although there has been marked improvement, infectious and communicable diseases persist. Recent scientific discoveries on the infectious etiology of stomach ulcers, coronary artery disease, and cervical cancer, for example, suggest that infectious agents may be responsible for more morbidity and mortality than previously recognized. New concerns include the rapid proliferation of drug-resistant organisms (Box 25-1) and the recent threat that deadly pathogens will be weaponized by terrorists (Box 25-2). Other threats are emerging infectious diseases, those diseases where the incidence in humans has increased within the past two decades or threatens to increase in the near future. (For more information, see the CDC website on Emerging Infectious Diseases at www.cdc.gov/ncidod/diseases/eid/disease_sites.htm.)

This chapter is written to provide nurses with the knowledge necessary to help control infectious diseases. The terms *communicable disease* and *infectious disease* are synonymous, and will be used interchangeably (Heymann, 2008).

COMMUNICABLE DISEASE AND *HEALTHY PEOPLE 2020*

Healthy People 2020 contains several hundred objectives to improve health; these are organized into thirty-eight topic areas. Three of the topic areas (Immunization and Infectious Diseases, Sexually Transmitted Diseases, and HIV) are specific to infectious diseases (U.S. Department of Health and Human

Services [USDHHS], 2009). These objectives have been used for evaluating national prevention and control efforts and can guide local prevention and control efforts. The *Healthy People 2020* table shows examples of objectives for immunizations and infectious diseases, objectives related to sexually transmitted diseases, and a few of the objectives covering HIV/AIDS. These lists suggest strategies for prevention and control of infectious diseases. Additional information, including baseline and target data for all objectives, can be found on the *Healthy People 2020* website.

PRINCIPLES OF INFECTION AND INFECTIOUS DISEASE OCCURRENCE

Nurses in all settings must be aware of potential threats related to communicable diseases and be prepared to intervene (Ethical Insights box). To help prepare nurses for this responsibility, biological and epidemiological principles inherent in infection and infectious disease occurrence have been reviewed and major terms defined in this section.

Multicausation

During the early years of medical and nursing history, science promulgated cause-and-effect theories of disease that relied on specifying one cause for each disease. Today, it is understood that disease etiology is complex and multicausal. Infectious diseases are the result of interaction among the human host, an infectious agent, and the environment

HEALTHY PEOPLE 2020

Communicable Disease

Topic Area – Immunization and Infectious Diseases

IID HP2020 – 1: Reduce, chronic hepatitis B virus infections in infants and young children (perinatal infections).
IID HP2020 – 5: Reduce tuberculosis.
IID HP2020 – 6: Increase the proportion of all tuberculosis patients who complete curative therapy within 12 months.
IID HP2020 – 10: Reduce hospitalization caused by peptic ulcer disease in the United States.
IID HP2020 – 11: Reduce the number of courses of antibiotics for ear infections for young children.
IID HP2020 – 14: Reduce or eliminate cases of vaccine-preventable diseases.
IID HP2020 – 16: Reduce new hepatitis C infections.
IID HP2020 – 17: Increase the proportion of international travelers who receive health care advice regarding recommended preventative services before traveling to areas of risk for select infectious diseases.
IID HP2020 – 20: Maintain vaccination coverage levels for children in kindergarten.
IID HP2020 – 22: Increase routine vaccination coverage levels for adolescents.
IID HP2020 – 25: Increase the scientific knowledge on vaccine safety and adverse events.

Topic Area – Sexually Transmitted Diseases

STD HP2020 – 1: Reduce the proportion of females aged 15-44 years who have ever required treatment for pelvic inflammatory disease (PID).
STD HP2020 – 2: Reduce congenital syphilis.
STD HP2020 – 3: Reduce the proportion of adolescents and young adults with *Chlamydia trachomatis* infections.
STD HP2020 – 4: Reduce gonorrhea rates.
STD HP2020 – 5: Reduce sustained domestic transmission of primary and secondary syphilis.
STD HP2020 – 6: Reduce the proportion of adults with genital herpes infection due to herpes simplex type 2.
STD HP2020 – 7: Reduce the proportion of females with human papillomavirus (HPV) infection.

Topic Area – HIV

HIV PH2020 – 1: Reduce acquired immunodeficiency syndrome (AIDS) among adults and adolescents.
HIV HP2020 – 2: Reduce the number of new AIDS cases among adolescent and adult men who have sex with men.
HIV HP2020 – 3: Reduce the number of new AIDS cases among adolescents and adults who inject drugs.
HIV HP2020 – 4: Reduce the number of new cases of human immunodeficiency virus/acquired immunodeficiency syndrome (HIV/AIDS) diagnosed among adults and adolescents.
HIV HP2020 – 6: Increase the proportion of adults with tuberculosis (TB) who have been tested for HIV.
HIV HP2020 – 7: Reduce deaths from HIV infection.
HIV HP2020 – 9: Increase the proportion of persons surviving more than 3 years after a diagnosis with AIDS.
HIV HP2020 –10: Reduce the number of new cases of perinatally acquired HIV/AIDS diagnosed each year and perinatally acquired AIDS.
HIV HP2020 –11: Increase the proportion of sexually active persons who use condoms.
HIV HP2020 –12: Increase the proportion of HIV-infected persons who know they are infected.

USDHHS Healthy People 2020 Draft Objectives. 2009. http://www.healthypeople.gov/hp2020/Objectives/files/Draft2009Objectives.pdf

 ETHICAL INSIGHTS

Nurse's Responsibility Regarding Communicable Diseases

Rapid proliferation of drug-resistant organisms, bioterrorism, and emerging infectious diseases are all concerns that have great implications for nursing practice. Every nurse should be knowledgeable about recognizing, preventing, and controlling infectious diseases. Infectious disease control can no longer be limited to the jurisdiction of the public health department or the hospital infection control nurse; it is every nurse's responsibility.

that surrounds the human host and where transmission is occurring. This interaction is pictured in the epidemiological triad of agent, host, and environment described in Chapter 5 (Epidemiology). The principle of multicausation emphasizes that an infectious agent alone is not sufficient to cause disease; the agent must be transmitted within a conducive environment to a susceptible host.

Spectrum of Infection

Not all contact with an infectious agent leads to infection, and not all infection leads to an infectious disease. The processes, however, begin in the same way. An infectious agent may contaminate the skin or mucous membranes of a host, but not invade the host. Or it may invade, multiply, and produce a subclinical infection (inapparent or asymptomatic) without producing overt symptomatic disease. Or the host may respond with overt symptomatic infectious disease. Infection, then, is the entry and multiplication of an infectious agent in a host. Infectious disease and communicable disease refer to the pathophysiological responses of the host to the infectious agent, manifesting as an illness. Such a person, when the disease is diagnosed in him or her, would be considered a case. Once infectious agents replicate in a host, they can be transmitted from the host irrespective of the presence of disease symptoms. Some persons become carriers and continue to shed the infectious agent without any symptoms of the disease.

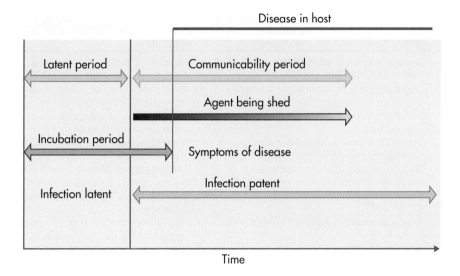

FIGURE 25-1 Stages of infection. (From Grimes DE: *Infectious diseases*, St Louis, 1991, Mosby.)

Stages of Infection

An infectious agent that has invaded a host and found conditions hospitable will replicate until it can be shed from the host. This period of replication before shedding is called the latent period or latency. The communicable period, or communicability, follows latency and begins with shedding of the agent. Incubation period is the time from invasion to the time when disease symptoms first appear. Frequently the communicable period begins before symptoms are present. Understanding the distinctions between these terms is important in controlling transmission. These stages of infection are depicted in Figure 25-1.

Spectrum of Disease Occurrence

The principles covered to this point apply to individuals and their acquisition of infections and infectious diseases. Control of infectious diseases in a population requires identifying and monitoring the occurrence of new cases (incidence) in a population. Some infectious diseases are endemic and occur at a consistent, expected level in a geographic area. Such is the case with some STDs and with tuberculosis (TB). An outbreak is an unexpected occurrence of an infectious disease in a limited geographic area during a limited period of time. Outbreaks of pertussis and salmonellosis are not uncommon. An epidemic is an unexpected increase of an infectious disease in a geographic area over an extended period of time. Epidemics are defined relative to the infectious agent and the history of the disease in the area. One case of smallpox anywhere will constitute an epidemic, whereas 1000 new cases of gonorrhea will not be considered an epidemic in an area where gonorrhea is common. A pandemic is a steady occurrence of a disease, or an epidemic, that covers a large geographic area or is evident worldwide. In July, 2009, for example, the World Health Organization designated H1N1 Influenza as a pandemic (CDC, 2009b).

CHAIN OF TRANSMISSION

Transmission is frequently conceptualized as a chain with six links, all connected, as in Figure 25-2. Each of the links (infectious agent, reservoir, portal of exit, mode of transmission, portal of entry, and host susceptibility) represents a different component that contributes to transmission. The chain of transmission and its elements are summarized in Table 25-1.

Infectious Agents

Because the process of transmission is different for every infectious agent, one might envision a different configuration of the chain and its links for each infectious agent and infectious disease that exists. Infectious agents act differently, depending on their intrinsic properties and interaction with their human host. For example, an agent's size, shape, chemical composition, growth requirements, and viability (ability

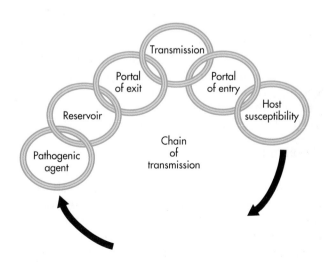

FIGURE 25-2 Chain of transmission. (From Grimes DE: *Infectious diseases*, St Louis, 1991, Mosby.)

TABLE 25-1   CHAIN OF TRANSMISSION

LINKS OF THE CHAIN	DEFINITION	FACTORS
Infectious agent	An organism (virus, rickettsia, bacteria, fungus, protozoan, helminth, or prion) capable of producing infection or infectious disease	Properties of the agent: morphology, chemical composition, growth requirements, and viability; interaction with the host: mode of action, infectivity, pathogenicity, virulence, toxigenicity, antigenicity, and ability to adapt to the host
Reservoirs	The environment in which a pathogen lives and multiplies	Humans, animals, arthropods (bugs), plants, soil, or any other organic substance
Portal of exit	Means by which an infectious agent is transported from the host	Respiratory secretions, vaginal secretions, semen, saliva, lesion exudates, blood, and feces
Mode of transmission	Method whereby the infectious agent is transmitted from one host (or reservoir) to another host	*Direct:* Person to person *Indirect:* Implies a vehicle of transmission (biological or mechanical vector, common vehicles or fomites, airborne droplets)
Portal of entry	Means by which an infectious agent enters a new host	Respiratory passages, mucous membranes, skin, percutaneous new host space, mouth, and through the placenta
Host susceptibility	The presence or lack of sufficient resistance to an infectious agent to avoid contracting an infectious disease	Biological and personal characteristics (e.g., gender, age, genetics), general health status, personal behaviors, anatomical and physiological lines of defense, immunity

to survive for extended periods of time) have an impact on transmission and the type of parasitic relationship it establishes with its host. These characteristics determine the classifications of different agents (e.g., prions, viruses, bacteria, fungi, and protozoa), and knowing the classification is helpful in understanding how specific agents are transmitted and produce disease. Also important are how the agent interacts with its host and its mode of action in the body. For example, *Mycobacterium tuberculosis* kills cells, but the spirochete that causes syphilis interferes with circulation. Or maybe it produces a toxin (toxigenicity) as does *Clostridium botulinum*, or stimulates an immune response in the host (antigenicity), as does rubella virus. Other considerations for understanding the action of agents include their power to invade and infect large numbers of people (infectivity), their ability to produce disease in those infected with the agent (pathogenicity), and their ability to produce serious disease in their hosts (virulence). Applying the above concepts, the chickenpox virus has high infectivity, high pathogenicity, and very low virulence. On the other hand, *M. tuberculosis* has low infectivity, low pathogenicity, but high virulence if untreated. Smallpox virus is high on all three concepts. Last, one must consider how adaptable an agent is to its human host and whether the agent changes, or mutates, over time, as HIV does.

Reservoirs

The environment in which a pathogen lives and multiplies is the reservoir. Reservoirs can be humans, animals, arthropods, plants, soil, water or any other organic substance. Some agents have more than one reservoir. Knowing the reservoirs for infectious agents is important because, in some cases, transmission can be controlled by eliminating the reservoir, such as eliminating the standing water where mosquitos breed.

Portals of Exit and Entry

Agents leave the human host through a portal of exit and invade through a portal of entry. Portals of exit include respiratory secretions, vaginal secretions, semen, saliva, lesion exudates, blood, and feces. Portals of entry are associated with the portal of exit and include the respiratory passages, mucous membranes, skin and blood vessels, oral cavity, and the placenta.

Modes of Transmission

Direct transmission is the immediate transfer of an infectious agent from an infected host or reservoir to an appropriate portal of entry in the human host through physical contact, such as a touch, bite, kiss, or sexual contact. Direct projections of mucous secretions by droplet spray to the conjunctiva, or mucous membranes of the eye, nose, or mouth during coughing, sneezing, and laughing is also considered direct transmission. Direct person-to-person contact is responsible for the transmission of many communicable diseases (e.g., STDs, influenza).

Indirect transmission is the spread of infection through a vehicle of transmission outside the host. These may be contaminated fomites or vectors. Fomites can be any inanimate objects, materials, or substances that act as transport agents for a microbe (e.g., water, a telephone, or a contaminated tissue). The infectious agent may or may not reproduce on or in the fomite. Substances such as food, water, and blood products can provide indirect transmission through ingestion and intravenous transfusions. Botulism is an example of an indirectly transmitted food-borne enterotoxin disease.

Vectors can be animals or arthropods, and they can transmit through biological and mechanical routes. The mechanical route involves no multiplication or growth of the parasite or microbe within the animal or vector itself. Such is the case when a housefly carries gastrointestinal agents from raw sewage to uncovered food. Biological transmission occurs when the parasite grows or multiplies inside the animal, vector, or arthropod. Examples of diseases spread by this method of transmission include arthropod-borne diseases such as malaria, hemorrhagic fevers, and viral encephalitis. Transmission from a vector to the human host is usually through a bite or sting. Such is the case with the mosquito vector that transmits St. Louis encephalitis and West Nile virus.

Fecal-oral transmission can be direct and indirect. It can occur indirectly through the ingestion of water that has been fecally polluted or by consumption of contaminated food. Direct transmission occurs through engagement in oral sexual activity. Poliovirus and hepatitis A are spread through fecal-oral routes.

Airborne transmission occurs mainly through aerosols and droplet nuclei. The timeframe in which an airborne particle can remain suspended greatly influences the virility and infectivity of the organism. The size of the particle can also determine how long it remains airborne and how successful it will be at penetrating the human lung. Aerosols are extremely small solid or liquid particles that may include fungal spores, viruses, and bacteria. Droplet nuclei, such as the spray from sneezing or coughing, may make direct contact with an open wound or with a mucous membrane, or they may be inhaled into the lung. TB is spread through inhalation of contaminated droplets.

Host Susceptibility

Not all humans are equally susceptible or at risk for contracting an infection or developing an infectious disease. Biological and personal characteristics play an important role. Just as the young are at greater risk for diphtheria, older adults are at greater risk for bacterial pneumonia. General health status is important, as evidenced by the increased risk for gastrointestinal parasites in children living in poverty. Personal behaviors certainly influence susceptibility, as does the presence of healthy lines of defense. The immune system and immunization status play important roles in the increased number of infections in unimmunized and immunocompromised persons.

BREAKING THE CHAIN OF TRANSMISSION

Picture a situation in which one of the links in the chain of transmission is broken (see Figure 25-2). Breaking just one link of the chain at its most vulnerable point is, in fact, what is done to control transmission of an infectious agent. Of course, where the chain is broken depends on all of the factors that have just been discussed—characteristics of the agent, its reservoir, portals of exit and entry, how the agent is transmitted, and susceptibility of the host.

Controlling the Agent

Controlling the agent is an area where technology and medical science have been extremely effective. Inactivating an agent

is the principle behind disinfection, sterilization, and radiation of fomites that may harbor pathogens. Anti-infective drugs, such as antibiotics, antivirals, antiretrovirals, and antimalarials, play important roles in controlling infectious diseases. Not only do they permit recovery of the infected person, but they also play a major role in preventing transmission of the pathogens to another. The first step in preventing transmission of tuberculosis and syphilis is to treat the infected person with antibiotics.

Eradicating the Nonhuman Reservoir

Common nonhuman reservoirs for pathogens in the environment include water, food, milk, animals, insects, and sewage. Treating or eliminating them is an effective method of preventing replication of pathogens, and thus preventing transmission.

Controlling the Human Reservoir

Treating infected persons, whether they are symptomatic or not, is effective in preventing transmission of pathogens directly to others. A quarantine is an enforced isolation or restriction of movement of those who have been exposed to an infectious agent during the incubation period; this is another method of controlling the reservoir. Quarantine was used effectively during the outbreak of severe acute respiratory syndrome (SARS) in 2003, when some hospitals required that their staff exposed to SARS patients remain at the hospital until proved to be symptom free at the end of the incubation period. Quarantine was selectively implemented during the H1N1 outbreak in 2009-2010.

Controlling the Portals of Exit and Entry

The transmission chain may be broken at the portal of exit by properly disposing of secretions, excretions, and exudates from infected persons. Additionally, isolation of sick persons from others and requiring that persons with tuberculosis wear a mask in public can be effective.

The portal of entry of pathogens also can be controlled by using barrier precautions (masks, gloves, condoms); avoiding unnecessary invasive procedures, such as indwelling catheters; and protecting oneself from vectors, such as mosquitoes. In response to the risk of exposure to blood-borne pathogens (e.g., HIV, hepatitis B, and hepatitis C) in the late 1980s, the CDC developed a set of guidelines, called universal precautions, to prevent transmission of diseases found in blood and other body fluids. These guidelines were developed because infected people may be asymptomatic and have no knowledge of their conditions; therefore health care workers must assume that all patients are infectious and protect themselves.

Improving Host Resistance and Immunity

Many factors, such as age, general health status, nutrition, and health behaviors, contribute to a host's resistance, or ability to ward off infections. Immunity, however, is an incredible defense against infection. There are several kinds of immunity, each providing resistance in different ways to different pathogens.

TABLE 25-2 TYPES OF ACQUIRED IMMUNITY

TYPE OF IMMUNITY	HOW ACQUIRED	LENGTH OF RESISTANCE
Natural		
Active	Natural contact and infection with the antigen	May be temporary or permanent
Passive	Natural contact with antibody transplacentally	Temporary or through colostrum and breast milk
Artificial		
Active	Inoculation of antigen	May be temporary or permanent
Passive	Inoculation of antibody or antitoxin	Temporary

From Grimes DE: Infectious diseases. In Thompson JM et al, editors: *Mosby's clinical nursing*, St Louis, 1991, Mosby.

Natural immunity is an innate resistance to a specific antigen or toxin. Acquired immunity is derived from actual exposure to the specific infectious agent, toxin, or appropriate vaccine. There are two types of acquired immunity: active and passive. Active immunity is when the body produces its own antibodies against an antigen, either from infection with the pathogen or introduction of the pathogen in a vaccine. Passive immunity is the temporary resistance that has been donated to the host through transfusions of plasma proteins, immunoglobulins, or antitoxins, or transplacentally, from mother to neonate. Passive immunity lasts only as long as these substances remain in the bloodstream. Types of acquired immunity with examples are summarized in Table 25-2.

When administered according to established guidelines and protocols, vaccines provide acquired immunity in most cases. However, there are exceptions. Primary vaccine failure is the failure of a vaccine to stimulate any immune response. It can be caused by improper storage that may render the vaccines ineffective, improper administration route, or exposure of light-sensitive vaccines to light. Additionally, some immunized persons never seroconvert, either because of failure of their own immune system or for some other unknown reason. Secondary vaccine failure is the waning of immunity following an initial immune response. This often occurs in immunosuppressed patients and organ transplant patients in whom the immune memory is essentially destroyed.

Herd immunity is a state in which those not immune to an infectious agent will be protected if a certain proportion (generally considered to be 80%) of the population has been vaccinated or is otherwise immune (Figure 25-3). This effect applies only if those who are immune are distributed evenly in the population. This is especially true for the transmission of diseases, such as diphtheria, that are found only in the human host and that have no invertebrate host or other mode of transmission. Without the presence of a susceptible population to infect, the organism will be unable to live because the vast majority of the population is immune.

PUBLIC HEALTH CONTROL OF INFECTIOUS DISEASES

Most human diseases (e.g., cancer or diabetes) can be classified as personal health problems. Individuals with a personal health problem can be treated by the health care system one person at a time. By contrast, infectious diseases are categorized as public or community health problems. Because of their potential to spread and cause community-wide or worldwide emergencies, infectious diseases require organized, public efforts for their prevention and control.

Such organized public efforts are under the jurisdiction of official public health agencies at local, state, national, and international levels. Each government unit obtains its powers through a complex array of laws. It is important to remember that in areas of health within a state, state laws usually prevail over federal law. The reason for this hierarchy is that the U.S. Constitution did not address health, and the Tenth Amendment reserved power to the states over all issues not addressed in the Constitution (Schneider, 2006). Historically, states have accepted this responsibility. For example, all states

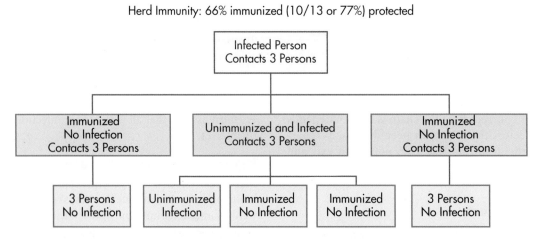

FIGURE 25-3 Example of herd immunity.

have laws addressing infectious disease control, such as what diseases must be reported and who has authority to implement quarantines. All states have a board of health and a department of health to implement state laws.

The CDC is the national public health entity responsible for infectious disease control across the states. The CDC has responsibility for monitoring infectious diseases and supporting local and state governments in control of outbreaks and epidemics, if such assistance is needed. Although there are many aspects of public health control of infectious diseases, only three are presented here—common control terminology, reporting diseases, and preventing diseases by vaccination.

Terminology: Control, Elimination, and Eradication

Control of a communicable disease, by definition, is the reduction of incidence or prevalence of a given disease to a locally acceptable level as a result of deliberate efforts (CDC, 1999a). The WHO's Expanded Programme on Immunizations (EPI) is a global attempt to control morbidity and mortality for many vaccine-preventable diseases, with each country adapting these guidelines as necessary. An example of control of pertussis would be to achieve 80% immunization coverage of children for pertussis.

Elimination of a communicable disease occurs when it is controlled within a specified geographic area such as a single country, an island, or a continent, and the prevalence and incidence of the disease is reduced to near zero. Elimination is the result of deliberate efforts, but continued intervention measures are required (CDC, 1999a). Such would be the case if no new cases of polio were reported in the United States during the year following an aggressive immunization campaign.

The International Task Force for Disease Eradication (ITFDE) defines eradication as reducing the worldwide incidence of a disease to zero as a function of deliberate efforts, without a need for further control measures (CDC, 1999a). Eradication is possible under certain conditions, which are listed in Box 25-3.

BOX 25-3   CRITERIA FOR DISEASE ERADICATION

Criteria for disease eradication include the following:
- Human host only; no host in nature
- Easy diagnosis; obvious clinical manifestations
- Limited duration and intensity of infection
- Natural lifelong immunity after infection
- Highly seasonal transmission
- Availability of vaccine, curative treatment, or both
- Substantial global morbidity and mortality rates
- Cost-effectiveness of campaign and eradication
- Integration of eradication with additional public health variables
- Eradication imperative over control measures

From Centers for Disease Control and Prevention: Recommendations of the international task force for disease eradication, *MMWR Morb Mortal Wkly Rep* 42:1-38, 1993.

Smallpox was eradicated in 1977, and the virus now exists only in storage in laboratories. Many factors contributed to the successful eradication of smallpox, including the mode of transmission of the disease, the isolated geographic distribution of the infection, the ease of administration of the freeze-dried vaccine, the establishment of an effective surveillance system, the increase of national and international political will, and tremendous community participation.

Defining and Reporting Communicable Diseases

Standardized definitions of diseases are necessary for public health monitoring and surveillance across all levels of government. Diseases are defined and classified according to confirmed cases, probable cases, laboratory-confirmed cases, clinically compatible cases, epidemiologically linked cases, genetic typing, and clinical case definition. Once defined, disease occurrence can be compared across time, populations, and geographic areas and appropriate control efforts can be implemented.

The CDC is responsible for monitoring communicable disease in the United States. Along with the Council of State and Territorial Epidemiologists, the CDC has designated notifiable infectious diseases, which health care providers who encounter these diseases must report to the local or regional health department. These notifiable diseases are listed in Box 25-4.

Because state health departments have the responsibility for monitoring and controlling communicable diseases within their respective states, they determine which diseases will be reported within their jurisdiction. Although not all nationally notifiable diseases are reportable in every state or territory, some states have notifiable disease lists that are longer than the CDC's list. So, all health professionals are advised to check the websites of their state health departments for specifics about reporting laws in their state. The processes for reporting also vary by state, and this information generally is available on the state health department's website. Generally, providers are encouraged to report cases of infectious diseases to their local or regional health departments, who will then report to the state and to the CDC.

The CDC publishes a weekly listing of notifiable diseases reported by region, state, and nation in *Morbidity and Mortality Weekly Report* (MMWR). MMWR can be found in medical libraries, local health departments, infection control departments in hospitals and medical centers, and on the Internet at http://www.cdc.gov.

VACCINES AND INFECTIOUS DISEASE PREVENTION

This section contains comprehensive information on vaccines and vaccine-preventable diseases. Diseases for which there is a vaccine are listed in Box 25-5. Recommended vaccination schedules for selected groups are available on the CDC website (Box 25-6).

BOX 25-4 NATIONALLY NOTIFIABLE INFECTIOUS DISEASES IN THE UNITED STATES: 2009

- Acquired immunodeficiency syndrome (AIDS)
- Anthrax
- Arboviral neuroinvasive and nonneuroinvasive diseases: California serogroup virus disease, eastern equine encephalitis, Powassan virus disease, St. Louis encephalitis, West Nile virus disease, and western equine encephalitis
- Botulism (food-borne, infant, and other)
- Brucellosis
- Chancroid
- *Chlamydia trachomatis*, genital infections
- Cholera
- Coccidioidomycosis
- Cryptosporidiosis
- Cyclosporiasis
- Diphtheria
- Ehrlichiosis/anaplasmosis
- Giardiasis
- Gonorrhea
- *Haemophilus influenzae* type B (Hib)
- Hansen's disease (leprosy)
- Hantavirus pulmonary syndrome
- Hemolytic uremic syndrome, postdiarrheal
- Hepatitis, acute (hepatitis A, hepatitis B, perinatal, hepatitis C)
- Hepatitis, chronic (hepatitis B and hepatitis C)
- HIV infection (adult and pediatric)
- Influenza-associated pediatric mortality
- Legionellosis
- Listeriosis
- Lyme disease
- Malaria
- Measles
- Meningococcal disease
- Mumps
- Novel influenza A virus infections
- Pertussis

- Plague
- Poliomyelitis, paralytic
- Poliovirus infection, nonparalytic
- Psittacosis
- Q fever (acute and chronic)
- Rabies (animal and human)
- Rocky Mountain spotted fever
- Rubella
- Rubella, congenital syndrome
- Salmonellosis
- Severe acute respiratory syndrome–associated coronavirus (SARS-CoV) disease
- Shiga toxin–producing *Escherichia coli* (STEC)
- Shigellosis
- Smallpox
- Streptococcal disease, invasive, group A
- Streptococcal toxic-shock syndrome
- *Streptococcus pneumoniae*, drug resistant, invasive
- *Streptococcus pneumoniae*, invasive, non–drug resistant, in children <5 years of age
- Syphilis (primary, secondary, latent, early latent, late latent, unknown duration, neurosyphilis, syphilis, late, nonneurological)
- Syphilis, congenital (syphilitic stillbirth)
- Tetanus
- Toxic shock syndrome (other than streptococcal)
- Trichinellosis (trichinosis)
- Tuberculosis
- Tularemia
- Typhoid fever
- Vancomycin-intermediate *Staphylococcus aureus* (VISA)
- Vancomycin-resistant *Staphylococcus aureus* (VRSA)
- Varicella (morbidity and death)
- Vibriosis
- Yellow fever

From Centers for Disease Control and Prevention: *Nationally notifiable infectious diseases*, 2009, www.cdc.gov/ncphi/disss/nndss/phs/infdis2009.htm.

Vaccines: Word of Caution

As with other areas of health care, information and recommendations on immunizations and vaccine usage change regularly. Therefore health care providers should seek the most current information on the CDC website. Recommendations, policies, and procedures concerning international immunization practices are determined by the WHO. In the United States, national governance is provided by the American Academy of Pediatrics Committee on Infectious Diseases and the U.S. Public Health Service Advisory Committee on Immunization Practices (ACIP). Occasionally these agencies differ in their recommendations.

Precautions must be taken when giving any immunization. The most recent recommendations regarding which immunizations to give; to whom they should be given; how they should be given; and how they are to be transported, stored, and administered can be obtained from the CDC.

The CDC produces Vaccine Information Statements (VISs) that explain the benefits and risks of a vaccine to vaccine recipients, their parents, or their legal representatives.

Federal law requires that VISs be handed out whenever (before each dose) certain vaccinations are given. VISs can be downloaded from the Internet at www.cdc.gov/vaccines/pubs/VIS/default.htm.

Types of Immunizations

Immunization is a broad term used to describe a process by which active or passive immunity to an infectious disease is induced or amplified. Immunizing agents can include vaccines, immune globulins, or antitoxins. Vaccination is a narrower term referring to the administration of a vaccine or toxoid to confer active immunity by stimulating the body to produce its own antibodies.

Vaccines can be prepared in several ways. They may be suspensions in a variety of solutions; protected with preservatives, stabilizers, or antibiotics; or mixed with adjuvants, which are used to increase immunogenicity. Vaccines can be live and attenuated, or they may be killed, or inactivated, with the virulence removed, leaving only the antigenic property necessary to stimulate the human immune system to produce antibodies. Types of inactivated vaccines include

BOX 25-5   VACCINE-PREVENTABLE DISEASES

- Anthrax
- Cervical cancer
- Human papillomavirus (HPV)
- Diphtheria
- *Haemophilus influenzae* type b (Hib)
- Hepatitis A
- Hepatitis B
- Influenza
- Japanese encephalitis (JE)
- Lyme disease
- Measles
- Meningococcus
- Monkeypox
- Mumps
- Pertussis
- Pneumococcus
- Poliomyelitis
- Rabies
- Rotavirus
- Rubella
- Shingles (herpes zoster)
- Smallpox
- Tetanus
- Tuberculosis
- Varicella (chickenpox)
- Yellow fever

From Centers for Disease Control and Prevention: *Vaccine-preventable diseases and specific vaccines*, 2009: www.cdc.gov/vaccines/vpd-vac/default.htm.

BOX 25-6   RESOURCES FOR RECOMMENDED VACCINE SCHEDULES FOR SELECTED POPULATION GROUPS

Children/adolescents	www.cdc.gov/vaccines/recs/schedules/child-schedule.htm
Adults	www.cdc.gov/vaccines/recs/schedules/adult-schedule.htm
Travelers	www.cdc.gov/travel/content/vaccinations.aspx
Pregnant women	www.cdc.gov/vaccines/pubs/preg-guide.htm
Health care workers	www.cdc.gov/vaccines/spec-grps/hcw.htm
Specific health conditions	www.cdc.gov/vaccines/spec-grps/conditions.htm
Other special groups	www.cdc.gov/vaccines/spec-grps/default.htm

TABLE 25-3   AVAILABLE VACCINES BY TYPE

VACCINES	DESCRIPTION
Live Attenuated	
Viral	Measles, mumps, rubella, oral polio, vaccinia, yellow fever, and varicella
Bacterial	BCG
Recombinant	Oral typhoid
Inactivated	
Viral	Influenza, polio, rabies, and hepatitis A
Bacterial	Typhoid, cholera, and plague
Subunit (fractional)	Influenza, acellular pertussis, typhoid Vi, and Lyme disease
Toxoid	Diphtheria and tetanus
Recombinant	Hepatitis B
Conjugate polysaccharide	*Haemophilus influenzae* type b, and pneumococcal 7-valent
Pure polysaccharide	Pneumococcal 23-valent, meningococcal, and *Haemophilus influenzae* type b

From Centers for Disease Control and Prevention: *Epidemiology and prevention of vaccine-preventable diseases (pink book)*, ed 6, Atlanta, 2000, Public Health Foundation.
BCG, Bacille Calmette-Guérin.

initiating the immune system to produce an immunogenic response. Table 25-3 presents information on types of available vaccines.

Vaccine Storage, Transport, and Handling

Vaccines should be safely stored, transported, and handled at all times to ensure the efficacy of the vaccine. A cold chain is a system used to ensure that vaccines are kept at a designated temperature from the time they are manufactured until they are used for vaccination. Failing to maintain the cold chain and exposing the vaccine to higher or lower temperatures than recommended may result in loss of potency and vaccine failure. Several methods are available for ensuring that the appropriate temperature has been maintained throughout vaccine transport and storage. These include liquid crystal thermometers, dial thermometers, recording thermometers, digital thermometers, ice pack indicators, shipping indicators that change color if the temperature exceeds or falls below the recommended level, freeze-watch indicators, and cold chain monitors. A *Vaccine Storage and Handling Toolkit* can be obtained at www2a.cdc.gov/vaccines/ed/shtoolkit/default.htm.

Vaccine Administration

The efficacy of the vaccine can be adversely affected if the vaccine is not administered appropriately. Therefore, it is important to follow the same safety procedures one would use to administer any intramuscular or subcutaneous injection (i.e., use sterile technique, use the correct size needle, avoid injecting in a blood vessel, and dispose of the needle and syringe properly). Information on the correct dosage can be found on the package insert. If more than one vaccine is being administered simultaneously, different anatomical sites should be used.

toxoids and polysaccharide vaccines. Inactivated conjugate vaccines, containing a chemically linked polysaccharide and protein and genetically engineered "recombinant" vaccines are also now being administered. Inactivated vaccines can be fractions or subunits or whole "killed" bacteria or viruses. Immune globulins and antitoxins are solutions that contain antibodies from human or animal blood and are introduced into a patient to provide passive protection without

Vaccine Spacing

Wherever possible, all children should be age-appropriately immunized and kept up-to-date according to current recommendations. The same applies to adolescents, adults, persons with chronic illness, pregnant women, health care workers, and international travelers.

The number of injections for any one immunobiological substance should be administered according to ACIP recommendations. An interruption in the schedule does not require that the entire series begin again. However, if vaccines are administered at less than the recommended intervals, they should not be counted as part of the primary series of immunization. Completion of the primary vaccine series and receiving periodic booster doses as recommended are necessary to ensure protective levels of immunity. Additional information is available at 1-800-CDC-Info (1-800-232-4636) or at www.CDC.gov/vaccines.

Vaccine Hypersensitivity and Contraindications

Although adverse reactions are not common following immunization, they can occur in some individuals. These reactions can be from vaccine components such as eggs, egg proteins, antibiotics, preservatives, and adjuvants. Patient allergies should be considered before administration of specific vaccines. For additional precautions and contraindications, the vaccine package insert and the latest instructions from the CDC should be consulted at www.cdc.gov/vaccines/recs/vac-admin/contraindications-vacc.htm.

Mild illness with or without low-grade fever is not a contraindication for vaccination. However, vaccination should be postponed in cases of moderate or severe febrile illness to avoid any confusion between a vaccine side effect and an unknown underlying cause.

Pregnancy is not a contraindication for immunization using inactivated vaccines, antitoxins, or immune globulins. However, pregnant women should avoid live vaccines, including measles-mumps-rubella (MMR), varicella, and yellow fever, unless the risk of infection is very high (see link to Guidelines for Vaccinating Pregnant Women, Box 25-6).

Immunocompromised patients should not receive live vaccines; however, MMR can be administered to asymptomatic HIV-infected people, and varicella can be given to people with humoral immunodeficiency and some HIV-asymptomatic people as determined by their physician. Killed or inactivated vaccines can be given, but they may not produce an optimal antibody response (see link to Guidelines for Vaccinating Specific Groups of People, Box 25-6).

Vaccine Documentation

Legal documentation of vaccinations is important for both the individual and the provider for future administration and follow-up of hypersensitivity reactions. Both individual and provider immunization records should be maintained. The health care provider is responsible for maintaining accurate records, including patient name, dates immunized, vaccine type, vaccine manufacturer, vaccine lot number, date of the Vaccine Information Statement (VIS), and the name,

title, and address of the person administering the vaccine. VISs can be downloaded from www.cdc.gov/vaccines/pubs/vis/default.htm.

Vaccine Safety and Reporting Adverse Events and Vaccine-Related Injuries

No drug is perfectly safe or effective, and vaccines are no exception. They are biological rather than chemical, and, when introduced into the human biological system, they can and do produce a variety of responses, both positive and negative. Furthermore, vaccines are administered to healthy people; they are given to prevent illness and not treat it; and they are given to far greater numbers of people than other pharmaceuticals.

Public concern regarding the health risk associated with vaccines has increased in recent years as the risk of contracting the diseases has declined. For example, wild virus polio has been eliminated in the United States, yet each year eight to ten cases of vaccine-induced paralysis were reported associated with use of the oral, live virus vaccine. The health risk of the oral vaccine exceeded that of the risk of the disease. This led to a change in vaccine policy from the use of the live oral vaccine to the inactivated polio vaccine (IPV) (CDC, 1999b). Likewise, whole cell pertussis vaccine has been changed to an acellular pertussis vaccine because there are adverse side effects, most notably convulsions, associated with the whole cell vaccine.

To monitor actual and potential vaccine-related problems, health care providers must report specific postvaccination "adverse events" to the Vaccine Adverse Event Reporting System (VAERS). Information and reporting forms are available at www.cdc.gov/vaccinesafety/vaers and through a 24-hour recorded telephone message at 1-800-822-7967. The National Vaccine Injury Compensation

---

RESEARCH HIGHLIGHTS

Immunization Compliance: Beliefs and Actions Among RNs

McEwen and Farren (2005) conducted a survey of 1000 RNs in Texas to analyze the nurses' beliefs and actions related to hepatitis B and influenza immunization recommendations. They learned that only 8% of the responding RNs chose to not be vaccinated against hepatitis B. The primary reasons the nurses chose to not be vaccinated were because they were not working in nursing, did not believe they were at risk of exposure, and were concerned about side effects or complications. Similarly, 86% of the RNs reported that they had ever received a flu shot and 69% noted that they had been immunized during 2 of the previous 4 years. Rationales for receiving the immunization were belief in effectiveness, belief that they were at risk of exposures, and that the vaccine was free of charge. Reasons for declining influenza immunization included concerns about side effects, lack of concern about getting the illness, and doubts about the vaccine's effectiveness.

From McEwen M, Farren E: Actions and beliefs related to hepatitis B and influenza immunization among registered nurses in Texas, *Public Health Nurs* 22(3):230-239, 2005.

Program reviews all VAERS reports and provides assistance for individuals and families who experience a vaccine-related injury, including disability and death.

VACCINE NEEDS FOR SPECIAL GROUPS

Recommendation on immunizations and schedules for vaccination are routinely updated and published by the CDC on its website. Practitioners are encouraged to check regularly for updates. Travelers can obtain the most current recommendations from the CDC through its telephone hotline 1-800-CDC-info (1-800-232-4636) or at its website at wwwnc.cdc.gov/travel/default.aspx.

HEALTHY PEOPLE 2020 FOCUS ON IMMUNIZATION AND INFECTIOUS DISEASES

Healthy People 2020 objectives, discussed earlier in this chapter, detailed three topic areas for infectious diseases. Immunization and Infectious Diseases (IID), seen previously in the *Healthy People 2020* table, highlights vaccine-preventable and other priority infectious diseases, excluding STDs and HIV. This section provides tables summarizing the chain of transmission and control of IID conditions. Table 25-4 covers childhood vaccine-preventable diseases, excluding hepatitis, which is summarized in Table 25-5. Table 25-6 summarizes tuberculosis.

HEALTHY PEOPLE 2020 FOCUS ON SEXUALLY TRANSMITTED DISEASES

Sexually transmitted diseases (STDs) include the more than twenty-five infectious organisms that are primarily transmitted through sexual activity. STDs, even those for which treatment exists, continue to be a major public health problem. The rates of STDs in the United States are among the highest in the industrialized world, approaching those in some developing countries. Indeed, an estimated 19 million cases of STDs occur each year in the United States, almost half of them in persons aged 15 to 24 years (CDC, 2009c).

Men and women of all ages, racial and ethnic backgrounds, and income levels contract STDs. However, the following populations are disproportionately affected: adolescents, young adults, women, minorities, and the poor (CDC, 2009c). Teenage girls in particular may be more susceptible to STDs because they have fewer protective antibodies to STDs and a cervix that is biologically immature. Women are at higher risk for contracting STDs than men because they have anatomical differences that enhance transmission of disease and make diagnosis difficult. In addition, they are also less likely to experience symptoms.

Further, complications from undiagnosed STDs occur more frequently and are more severe in women. For example, pelvic inflammatory disease (PID), largely resulting from an undetected STD, is diagnosed in more than 1 million women annually. Scarring from PID may lead to infertility, ectopic pregnancy, or chronic pelvic pain. An infected woman who transmits an STD to her fetus during pregnancy or childbirth may experience spontaneous abortion, premature delivery, stillbirth, neonatal death, and, in the infant, low birth weight, chronic respiratory problems, blindness, and mental retardation.

Concern over the persistence and increases in STDs led those formulating the *Healthy People 2020* objectives to create a Topic Area specific to STDs (see the *Healthy People 2020* table). For easy reference, the chain of transmission and control of STDs addressed in the *Healthy People 2020* objectives is presented in Table 25-7. The CDC regularly updates STD treatment guidelines, which are available on the CDC website.

HEALTHY PEOPLE 2020 FOCUS ON HIV/AIDS

No other infection or infectious disease in recent history has inflicted as much destruction and pain to individuals, families, and communities, and created as many challenges for health care professionals as has HIV/AIDS. Indeed, HIV stands out as the one condition that touches nurses everywhere. HIV affects persons of every age, ethnicity, socioeconomic status, gender, and occupation. Eventually, HIV/AIDS has an impact on every organ and function of the human body. Every nurse, regardless of area of practice, will eventually care for someone with HIV infection. Currently, there is no cure or vaccine, and minimal hope of stemming the continuing spread throughout the world (Figure 25-4, p. 512). It is not surprising, then, that *Healthy People 2020* objectives have an entire Topic Area specific to HIV/AIDS (see the *Healthy People 2020* Box).

HIV, a retrovirus, is the organism that causes the syndrome known as AIDS. Following initial infection, the disease is typically asymptomatic for months to years. Usually the infected person does not know that he or she is infected and continues to transmit the virus to others. The timeline for the usual course of HIV infection can be seen in Figure 25-5 on p. 512. HIV usually manifests gradually with conditions that result from inadequate immune system function, as the virus slowly attacks the body's immune system. Over time, the body loses its ability to fight illnesses, and opportunistic infections occur and become recurrent. A standardized case definition for AIDS was specified by CDC in 1993. This case definition can be found at www.cdc.gov/hiv/topics/surveillance/resources/guidelines, and the critical elements for both HIV and AIDS are summarized for easy reference in Table 25-8 on p. 513.

HIV infection is usually determined by the HIV antibody test, and the most commonly used form is the enzyme-linked immunosorbent assay (ELISA). There may be false-positive findings, so the Western blot is frequently used to verify the results. False-negative findings may also occur, especially before the body produces antibodies after exposure; therefore an exposed person should repeat the HIV antibody test at 1 month and 3 months after the original test. Additional tests are now available to detect the virus in the blood before antibodies are present.

Text continued on p.508.

TABLE 25-4 CHAIN OF TRANSMISSION AND CONTROL: CHILDHOOD VACCINE-PREVENTABLE DISEASES

	CHICKENPOX	DIPHTHERIA	PERTUSSIS	TETANUS	POLIO
Occurrence	Worldwide and universal in all populations, primarily in children	Rare where immunization rates are high; affects unimmunized children under 15 yr and adults whose immunity has waned	Worldwide and common in children; declined with immunization; some outbreaks in recent years in adults in the United States in those whose immunity has waned	Worldwide; occurs sporadically and affects all ages; more common in agricultural areas and among parenteral drug users; rare in areas with high immunization rates	Worldwide before immunization; it is now rare in countries with adequate immunization rates
Etiological agent	Human (alpha) herpesvirus 3 (varicella zoster virus)	*Corynebacterium diphtheriae,* of gravis, mitis, or intermedius biotypes	*Bordetella pertussis*	*Clostridium tetani* (an anaerobic pathogen)	Poliovirus, types 1, 2, and 3; all are paralytogenic
Reservoir	Humans	Humans	Humans	Intestines of humans and animals	Humans, particularly children with subclinical infections
Transmission	Direct and indirect contact with droplets from respiratory passage or vesicle fluid; extremely contagious	Direct or indirect contact with exudates from mucous membrane lesions of infected person or carrier; raw milk has served as a vehicle	Direct contact with droplets from respiratory passages	Tetanus spores enter body through a wound (usually puncture wound) contaminated with soil and feces; necrotic tissue favors the growth of the anaerobic bacillus	Direct and indirect contact with respiratory discharges and feces; fecal-oral route more common than respiratory transmission
Incubation period	14-16 days; range 2-3 wk; prolonged in immunocompromised persons	2-5 days; occasionally longer	9-10 days; range 6-20 days	10 days; range 3-21 days; rarely, several months	7-14 days; range 3-35 days
Communicability period	1-2 days before onset of rash to 5 days after lesions have crusted	Until bacilli have disappeared from discharges and lesions (usually 2 wk); effective antibiotic therapy interferes with shedding; a carrier may transmit for 6 mo	Highly communicable during early catarrhal and coughing stages; gradually decreasing until week 3; communicability is negligible after 5 days with effective antibiotic therapy	Not transmitted directly	Highly communicable during first days after onset of symptoms; virus is in throat secretions within 36 hr and in feces 72 hr after infection; remains 1 wk in throat and 6 wk in feces
Susceptibility and resistance	General population not previously infected or vaccinated are at risk; can be severe and fatal in adults and immunocompromised persons	General unimmunized population are at risk; infants born of immune mothers have passive immunity for 6 mo; recovery from disease or asymptomatic infection usually confers lifetime immunity; immunization confers prolonged, but not lifetime, immunity	General unimmunized population are at risk; unimmunized children under 5 yr are most susceptible; no passive immunity from mother; disease confers prolonged, but not lifetime, immunity	General unimmunized population are at risk; active immunity from tetanus toxoid persists for 10 yr; tetanus immune globulin confers temporary immunity; infants born to immune mothers are protected at birth; active disease does not confer lifetime immunity	General unimmunized population is at risk; active immunization confers lifetime immunity; disease or sublinical infection confers type-specific lifetime immunity

Prevention and control	Single dose vaccination of children 12-18 mo, and for those up to 12 yr who have not had the disease	Immunization with diphtheria toxoid boosters every 10 yr	Immunization with whole cell vaccine prophylaxis with a 7-day course of erythromycin should be given to all exposed persons, including health care workers, regardless of vaccination status	Active immunization with tetanus toxoid boosters every 10 yr, and as prophylaxis following penetrating injuries for those whose last booster was more than 10 yr ago	Active immunization with inactivated polio virus (IPV)
Disease manifestations	Sudden mild fever, and malaise, rash, or both; rash is progressive changing from maculopapular to vesicular, and then forming a crust or scab; lesions tend to be more numerous on covered parts of the body; can be on all mucous membranes and are highly pruritic; complications are more common in persons over 15 yr old, infants less than 1 yr old, and immunocompromised persons; virus can persist in a dormant state in sensory nerve endings and can reactivate causing herpes zoster, or shingles	Acute onset; usually affecting the upper respiratory tract lesions are caused by the release of a cytotoxin and manifest as a patch or patches of inflammation surrounding a grayish membrane; complications may result in severe swelling of the neck, thrombocytopenia, neuritis, and myocarditis	Pertussis (whooping cough) begins with an upper respiratory cough and proceeds into a paroxysmal stage of coughing, often ending in vomiting; paroxysmal stage may last 1-2 mo or longer; complications include seizures, pneumonia, encephalopathy, and death	Tetanus (lockjaw) is an acute neurological illness caused by an anaerobic bacterium that produces an exotoxin in the portal of entry in the human host; tetanus causes gradually worsening neurological symptoms, including painful muscle contractions and spasms; frequently resulting in death	Symptoms may range from inapparent illness to severe paralysis or death
Diagnosis	By symptoms	Bacteriological culture of nasal and throat secretions and from lesions	Bacteriological culture of nasal or throat secretions	History of injury plus clinical symptoms; bacterium is rarely found in wound cultures	Isolation of the virus from fecal or oropharyngeal specimens
Treatment	Antiviral drugs within 1 wk of exposure may modify severity; varicella-zoster immune globulin administered within 96 hr of exposure can modify or prevent the disease	Single dose of equine antitoxin followed by a full course of antibiotic therapy	Treatment with antibiotics reduces the period of infectivity and may lessen the severity of the disease if given before the paroxysmal stage	Tetanus antitoxin or tetanus immune globulin (TIG), preferably human; supportive care	Supportive care
Report to local health authority	Yes	Yes	Yes	Yes	Yes

Modified from Grimes DE, Grimes KA, Zack CM: Infectious diseases. In Thompson JM et al. editors: *Mosby's clinical nursing*, ed 5, St. Louis, 2002, Mosby. Data from Heymann DL, editor: *Control of communicable diseases manual*, ed 19, Washington, DC, 2008, APHA.

Continued

TABLE 25-4   CHAIN OF TRANSMISSION AND CONTROL: CHILDHOOD VACCINE-PREVENTABLE DISEASES—cont'd

	MEASLES (RUBEOLA)	MUMPS	RUBELLA	HAEMOPHILUS INFLUENZAE TYPE B MENINGITIS	PNEUMOCOCCAL DISEASE	INFLUENZA
Occurrence	Worldwide; endemic and epidemic occurrences where immunization rates are low; still a major killer of children worldwide	Worldwide; incidence decreasing where immunization rates are high; one third of infected persons have subclinical infections	Worldwide and endemic where immunization rates are low; epidemics occur every 5-9 yr; primarily a disease of children	Worldwide; most common in children 2 mo to 5 yr of age; rare with widespread immunization	Worldwide; most common in children 2 mo to 3 yr of age, the elderly, and immunocompromised adults	Worldwide; in pandemics, epidemics, localized outbreaks, and sporadic cases
Etiological agent	Measles virus, a paramyxovirus	Mumps virus, a paramyxovirus	Rubella virus	H. influenzae serotype B (Hib)	Streptococcus pneumoniae	Three types of influenza virus (A, B, and C), each with many subtypes
Reservoir	Humans	Humans	Humans	Humans	Humans (often found in respiratory passages of healthy persons)	Humans; some mammals and birds suspected as sources of new subtypes
Transmission	Direct or indirect contact with nasal or throat secretions; highly communicable	Direct contact with saliva (airborne or droplets) from an infected person	Direct or indirect contact with nasopharyngeal secretions of infected persons; transplacental transmission leads to congenital rubella syndrome (CRS)	Direct or indirect contact with droplets of nasopharyngeal secretions	Direct or indirect contact with droplets of nasopharyngeal secretions	Airborne spread
Incubation period	10 days until fever; 14 days until rash; range 7-18 days	16-18 days; range 14-25 days	14-17 days; range 14-21 days	Unknown; probably 2-4 days	Unknown: probably 1-4 days	1-3 days
Communicability period	1 day before the prodromal period to 4 days after appearance of the rash	2 days before to 4 days after onset of parotitis; but the range can be 7 days before to 15 days after onset; can be transmitted by persons with subclinical infections	7 days before to 4 days after onset of rash; highly communicable; infants with CRS may shed virus for months after birth	Variable as long as organisms are in nasopharynx; noncommunicable within 24-48 hr after onset of effective antibiotic therapy	As long as organism is found in nasopharynx; may be prolonged in immunocompromised persons	3-5 days from clinical onset in adults; up to 7 days in children
Susceptibility and resistance	General population who have not had disease or immunization is at risk; lifetime immunity after illness; infants of mothers who have had the disease are protected for 6-9 mo; infants of immunized mothers have variable level of passive antibody; length of immunity following immunization is unknown	Lifetime immunity develops after subclinical and clinical illness	General unimmunized or previously uninfected population is at risk; lifetime immunity after illness; infants born to immune mothers are protected for 6-9 mo; longterm immunity following immunization	General unimmunized or previously uninfected population is at risk; lifetime immunity after illness; infants born to immune mothers are protected for 6-9 mo; immunity acquired transplacentally, by infection, and by immunization	General population is probably at risk; immunity is acquired transplacentally, from prior infection or from immunization	General population is at risk; infection and immunization produces immunity to only one subtype of the virus

	Measles	Mumps	Rubella	Haemophilus influenzae type b	Pneumococcal disease	Influenza
Prevention and control	Active immunization with live, attenuated measles vaccine (Tables 23-5 to 23-7)	Active immunization with live attenuated mumps virus vaccine (Tables 23-5 to 23-7)	Active immunization with live, attenuated rubella virus vaccine in childhood (Tables 23-5 to 23-7); ensure immunity in adolescent girls	Active immunization with Hib conjugate vaccine (Tables 23-7)	Pneumococcal conjugate vaccine (PCV) for infants and children; pneumococcal polysaccharide vaccine (PPV) for high-risk groups (Tables 23-5 to 23-7)	Active immunization yearly prior to influenza season
Disease manifestations	Acute-onset fever of 101°F or higher, cough, coryza, conjunctivitis, Koplik's spots on the buccal mucosa, and a red rash lasting longer than 3 days that begins on the face and becomes generalized; measles can progress into severe complications, including pneumonia, encephalitis, and death	Acute-onset fever and painful swelling of the salivary and parotid glands; may be asymptomatic; complications range from meningoencephalitis to permanent hearing impairment and orchitis in postpubescent males, but rarely sterility	Maculopapular rash and postauricular, occipital, and posterior cervical lymphadenopathy; children are usually relatively asymptomatic, but adults may experience fever, headache, and malaise; rare complications include encephalitis and thrombocytopenia; congenital defects in fetuses of pregnant women who are infected	Hib can affect multiple organ systems, resulting in meningitis, epiglottitis, otitis media, pneumonia, arthritis, and cellulitis, with symptoms associated with those conditions; complications are serious and include septic arthritis, life-threatening airway obstruction, fulminating infection, and death	Acute-onset symptoms of meningitis or pneumonia	Acute-onset dry cough, fever, headache, myalgia, sore throat, and other generalized symptoms; symptom severity depends on the subtype of the virus; complications include pneumonia, otitis media, meningitis, Reye's syndrome, and death.
Diagnosis	Tissue culture of nasopharyngeal secretions and serological testing	Isolation of virus from oral and throat spray, urine, and spinal fluid	Serological testing	Identifying organisms in blood or spinal fluid	Isolation of the organism from the blood or other sterile body site	Isolation of virus from nasal or pharyngeal secretions, serological testing, antigen detection, gene amplification, and rapid diagnostic test
Treatment	Supportive care	Supportive care	Supportive care	10-14 days antibiotics	Antibiotics	Antiviral drugs started within 48 hr of onset of symptoms
Report to local health authority	Yes	Yes	Yes	Yes	Epidemics only	Epidemics only

Continued

Modified from Grimes DE, Grimes KA, Zack CM: Infectious diseases. In Thompson JM et al, editors: *Mosby's clinical nursing*, ed 5, St. Louis, 2002, Mosby. Data from Heymann DL, editor: *Control of communicable diseases manual*, ed 19, Washington, DC, 2008, APHA.

TABLE 25-5   CHAIN OF TRANSMISSION AND CONTROL: HEPATITIS

	HEPATITIS A	HEPATITIS B	HEPATITIS C	HEPATITIS D	HEPATITIS E
Occurrence	Worldwide; sporadic and epidemic with cyclic recurrence; outbreaks in institutions where sanitation is poor	Worldwide; endemic; highest in young adults, homosexually active men, persons engaging in unprotected sex, injection drug users, health care and public safety workers	Worldwide; directly related to prevalence of injection drug use in the population, HCV in the donated blood supply, and lack of use of parenteral precautions in health care	Worldwide; occurs epidemically and endemically in population at risk for HBV infection; declining in areas where chronic carriers of HBsAG	Epidemic and sporadic cases, particularly in developing countries; highest in young adults; rare in children or the elderly
Etiological agent	HAV	HBV; made up of a core antigen, HBcAG, and a surface antigen, HBsAG; HBV has at least 8 different genotypes	HCV with 6 genotypes and 100 subtypes	HDV, consists of a coat of HBsAG and an internal antigen, the delta antigen	HEV
Reservoir	Humans and captive primates	Humans and possibly captive primates	Humans; virus has been transmitted experimentally to chimpanzees	Humans; virus can be transmitted experimentally to chimpanzees and to woodchucks	Humans and nonhuman primates, pigs, chickens, and cattle
Transmission	Person to person by fecal-oral route; contaminated food, water, shellfish, etc.	Direct and indirect contact with blood and serum-derived fluids; sexual contact; perinatal	Parenterally; sexual and mother-to-child transmission are less likely to occur	Similar to HBV; must co-infect with HBV	Person-to-person by fecal-oral route; contaminated food or water
Incubation period Communicability period	28-30 days; range 15-50 days Latter half of incubation period to 1 wk after onset of jaundice	60-90 days; range 45-180 days During incubation period and throughout clinical course of disease; carrier state may persist for years	6-9 wk; range 2 wk to 6 mo Virus persists indefinitely	2-8 wk Throughout acute and chronic disease	26-42 days; range 15-64 days Unknown; virus has been detected in stools 14 days after onset of symptoms and 4 wk after ingestion of contaminated food or water
Susceptibility and resistance	General population is at risk; usually affects children and young adults; probable lifetime immunity following infection	General population is at risk; disease is mild in children; lifetime immunity follows infection if antibody to HBV develops and HBV is negative	General population is at risk; degree of immunity following infection is not known	All persons susceptible to HBV or who have an HBV infection and coinfected with HDV	Unknown
Prevention and control	Eliminate common sources of infection by sanitation; improve hygienic practices and handwashing; cook shellfish; immunize high-risk groups or persons in high-risk situations; for post exposure: administer vaccine and IG within 2 wk; use universal precautions	Routinely immunize infants, children, and high-risk groups; at birth give HBIG and Hep B vaccine to infants born to HBsAg-positive mothers followed by additional vaccine doses at 1 and 6 months of age; immunize persons exposed to HBV; test all donated blood for HBV antigen; practice safe sex; use universal precautions	Apply HBV control measures except immunization; no vaccine exists at this time and IG does not prevent HCV infection	Apply HBV prevention and control measures; however, HBIG, IG and hepatitis B vaccine do not prevent HDV infection for those already infected with HBV	No vaccine; IG not effective; sanitation appears to be the only effective measure of prevention

	Hepatitis A	Hepatitis B	Hepatitis C	Hepatitis D	Hepatitis E
Disease manifestations	Acute-onset fever, anorexia, malaise, dark urine, and jaundice, usually lasting 2 mo; it has a very low fatality rate and, although rare, it can last up to 6 mo	Insidious onset that ranges from asymptomatic illness to generalized nonspecific symptoms, such as anorexia, nausea, and vomiting followed by jaundice and occasionally resulting in fulminant fatal hepatitis	Like HBV, HCV has an insidious onset; symptoms vary from completely asymptomatic (80%) to the rare fulminating, fatal disease; mild symptoms are same as those for HBV; of those who are acutely ill, 75% to 85% develop chronic hepatitis	Abrupt onset with range of symptoms similar to HBV; always associated with HBV infection, either co-infection or as a suprainfection in persons with chronic hepatitis B	Clinical course similar to hepatitis A; no chronic form
Diagnosis	Serum antibodies (anti-HAV) detectable 5-10 days postexposure	Presence in sera of HBsAG, anti-HBsAG (antibodies), HBc AG and anti-HBcAG, HBeAG and anti-HBeAG	Presence of serum antibodies to HCV (anti-HCV)	Presence of serum antibodies to HDV (anti-HDV)	Eclusion of other causes of hepatitis, particularly hepatitis A; presence of serum antibodies, anti-HEV; presence of HEV RNA in feces and serum
Treatment	Supportive care	Supportive care	Treatment with ribavirin and slow release interferons (pegylated interferons)	Supportive care	Supportive care
Case report to local health authority	Yes	Yes	Yes	Yes	Yes

Modified from Grimes DE, Grimes KA, Zack CM Infectious diseases. In Thompson JM, McFarland GK, Hirsch JE, Tucker SM, editors: *Mosby's clinical nursing*, ed 5, St. Louis, 2002, Mosby. Data from Heymann DL, editor: *Control of communicable diseases manual*, ed 19, Washington, DC, 2008, APHA.

HAV, Hepatitis A virus; *HBV,* hepatitis B virus; *HCV,* hepatitis C virus; *HDV,* hepatitis delta virus; *HBIG,* hepatitis B immunoglobulin; *HBsAG,* hepatis B surface antigen; *HBcAG,* hepatitis B core antigen; *HBeAG,* hepatitis B early antigen.

TABLE 25-6 CHAIN OF TRANSMISSION AND CONTROL: TUBERCULOSIS

TUBERCULOSIS

Occurrence	Worldwide; TB cases declined in United States since 1993; drug-resistant cases continue to be reported; most newly reported cases in the United States are reactivation of a latent infection and occur in older age-groups, children, and immunosuppressed persons; in areas of world with high incidence of new transmission, cases are in working-age adults and among disadvantaged populations
Etiological agent	*Mycobacterium tuberculosis*; less often *M. bovis* or *M. africanum*
Reservoir	Humans; diseased cattle for *M. bovis*
Transmission	Inhalation of airborne droplets from the sputum of persons with active disease; children rarely transmit because they do not cough forcefully; infrequently by ingestion or skin penetration

	INFECTION	ACTIVE DISEASE (CASE)
Incubation period	2-10 wk	Anytime during one's lifetime
Communicability period	Not communicable unless there are viable bacilli in the sputum	As long as bacilli are in sputum; inadequately treated persons may be communicable for years
Susceptibility and resistance	Anyone, such as health care workers, family members, or the institutionalized, working or living in close contact with a person with active disease can become infected	Vulnerable persons such as children, persons over 65 years old, those with chronic diseases or compromised immune systems, people who are malnourished, etc.
Prevention and control	Skin test in high-risk groups, (e.g., health care workers), and treat those with new infections to prevent progression to active disease; routine skin testing, particularly of children, is no longer recommended in United States; Bacille Calmette-Guérin (BCG) vaccine is still used in some parts of the world	Promptly identify, diagnose, and treat those with active disease; ensure compliance with treatment; initiate respiratory isolation until sputum is clear of bacilli; have patient wear a mask; examine close contacts of TB cases and treat, if infected
Disease manifestations	Initial infection goes unnoticed; 5%-10% of infected persons will eventually develop active disease, 50% of those within the first 2 yr	Onset of active disease can occur immediately following an initial infection or after a variable period of latency for untreated persons; disease onset is usually insidious with fever, night sweats, and weight loss; cough with pulmonary disease; extrapulmonary symptoms correspond with the location of disseminated bacilli and lesions
Diagnosis	TB skin test reaction within 2-10 wk of infection; the immune suppressed may have a negative skin test due to anergy; skin test results: 5 mm induration = + for immune suppressed and close contacts with active cases; 10 mm induration = + for infections <2 yr and persons with high-risk conditions; 15 mm induration = + for all low-risk persons	10%-20% have a negative skin test; demonstration of acid-fast bacilli in stained smears of sputum or other body fluids; isolation of organism from cultured specimen; radiological evidence of TB in lungs or elsewhere
Treatment	Treat with isoniazid (INH) for 6-12 mo, or with other drug combinations for persons with HIV	Treat with combination of antimicrobial drugs, to which the strain of *Mycobacterium* is susceptible (INH, RIF, PZA, EMB) for 6-12 mo; monitor adherence carefully
Report to local health authority	No	Yes

Data from Heymann DL, editor: *Control of communicable diseases manual*, ed 19, Washington, DC, 2008, American Public Health Association.

Treatment for HIV and AIDS is complex and changes frequently. The Food and Drug Administration has approved many drugs for HIV infection and AIDS-related conditions. At present there are four classes of antiretroviral drugs, each corresponding to different mechanisms whereby HIV invades the cells of the immune system. It is beyond the scope of this chapter to review them all here. Current information on treatment is always available from the CDC. One source is the HIV/AIDS Treatment Information Service at www.aidsinfo.nih.gov.

Exposure of health care personnel to HIV, although rare, remains a concern for the CDC and health care workers. The CDC continues to update recommendations for postexposure prophylaxis (PEP) for occupational exposures. Although the principles of immediate treatment following exposure have not changed, the drugs and drug combinations have changed. These guidelines are among the many that can be downloaded from the website (www.cdc.gov/hiv/topics/treatment). Additional resources include a postexposure hotline for clinicians, the PEPline at 1-888-448-4911.

TABLE 25-7 CHAIN OF TRANSMISSION AND CONTROL: SEXUALLY TRANSMITTED DISEASES

	GONORRHEA	CHLAMYDIA TRACHOMATIS	SYPHILIS	GENITAL HERPES	WARTS, HUMAN PAPILLOMAVIRUS (HPV) INFECTION
Occurrence	Worldwide; highest in males and females 15-30 yr old	Worldwide; most prevalent STD	Worldwide and increasing; highest in males and females 20-30 yr old	Worldwide and increasing; highest in males and females 15-30 yr old	Worldwide
Etiological agent	Neisseria gonorrhoeae, the gonococcus	Chlamydia trachomatis	Treponema pallidum	Herpes simplex virus (HSV) type 2	Human papillomavirus (HPV); 70 types
Reservoir	Humans	Humans	Humans	Humans	Humans
Transmission	Contact with exudates from mucous membranes of infected persons; usually by direct sexual contact, although both pathogens can be transmitted during childbirth	Contact with exudates from mucous membranes of infected persons; usually by direct sexual contact, although both pathogens can be transmitted during childbirth	Direct sexual contact with infectious exudates from lesions; transplacentally; blood transfusion early in infection of donor	Direct contact with secretions from mucous membranes and lesions; transplacentally	Direct sexual contact; autoinoculation; during, childbirth
Incubation period	2-7 days	7-10 days	3 wk; range 10 days to 3 mo	2-12 days	2-3 mo; range 1-20 mo
Communicability period	Months if untreated	Unknown	When moist lesions are present during the primary and secondary stages, generally 1 yr	During and up to 7 wk after primary lesions; transient shedding of virus in absence of lesions for years	Unknown, probably as long as lesions persist
Susceptibility and resistance	General population is at risk; antibodies are not protective against reinfection	General population is at risk; no acquired immunity	General population is at risk; however, only 30% of exposures lead to infection; some immunity develops over time	General population is at risk; immune response does not prevent recurrence	General population is at risk; immunosuppressed persons are more susceptible
Prevention and control	Safer sexual practices; detect and treat cases and contacts; test pregnant women for infection and treat		Safer sexual practices; detect and treat cases and contacts; test pregnant women for infection and treat	Safer sexual practices; cesarean delivery if lesions are present during late pregnancy	Routinely immunize females aged 11 or 12 against HPV, with "catch up" vaccination for females 13-26; HPV vaccination may be recommended for some males aged 9-26 who are at high risk for genital warts; Safer sexual practices

Continued

TABLE 25-7   CHAIN OF TRANSMISSION AND CONTROL: SEXUALLY TRANSMITTED DISEASES—cont'd

	GONORRHEA	CHLAMYDIA TRACHOMATIS	SYPHILIS	GENITAL HERPES	WARTS, HUMAN PAPILLOMAVIRUS (HPV) INFECTION
Disease manifestations	Males: Urethritis with purulent discharge from anterior urethra; females: mucopurulent cervicitis, often asymptomatic; 20% progress to endometritis, salpingitis, and pelvic peritonitis; both genders may have pharyngeal or anorectal infections depending on their sexual practices; individuals are frequently co-infected with N. gonorrhoeae and C. trachomatis	Males: Urethritis with purulent discharge from anterior urethra; females: mucopurulent cervicitis, often asymptomatic; 20% progress to endometritis, salpingitis, and pelvic peritonitis; both genders may have pharyngeal or anorectal infections depending on their sexual practices; individuals are frequently co-infected with N. gonorrhoeae and C. trachomatis	Primary: moist lesion appearing within 3 wk at area of contact; secondary: symmetrical maculopapular rash in 4-6 wk; latency: indefinite time, no symptoms; tertiary: late lesions of bone, viscera, CNS, and cardiovascular system	Local, primary, vesicular lesions, period of latency and recurring; localized lesions; lesions start at area of contact but may spread to surrounding tissues or be disseminated in body, even to the CNS; other disease symptoms depend on extent of dissemination	Skin and mucous membrane lesions that are circumscribed, hyperkeratotic, and of varying sizes and shapes; certain types of HPV warts (16,18,31,33, and 45) have been found to be associated with cervical cancer
Diagnosis	Gram stain of discharges, bacteriological cultures or tests that detect gonococcal nucleic acid	Failure to detect N. gonorrhoeae in discharges from symptomatic persons; mononuclear antibody tests on discharges	Serological testing of blood and CSF, if indicated	Detection of cell changes in tissue scrapings or biopsy; isolation of virus from lesions or other affected tissue; serological tests	Visualization of the lesion; excision and histological examination of the lesion
Treatment	Treat with antibiotics, preferably with single dose, IM antibiotics, such as ceftriaxone; treatment depends on extent of the infection; follow-up testing is recommended	Treat with antibiotics such as single dose azithromycin or 7 days of doxycycline; advisable to treat for gonorrhea and chlamydia concurrently	Treat with antibiotics; treatment differs with stage of the disease	Treatment with antivirals; treatment varies depending on area of lesions and whether they are disseminated	Removal of the warts by freezing with liquid nitrogen or other chemical; removal reduces the risk of transmitting the virus
Report to local health authority	Yes	Yes	Yes, including congenital syphilis	No	No

Modified from Grimes DE, Grimes KA, Zack CM Infectious diseases, In Thompson JM et al, editors: Mosby's clinical nursing, ed 5, St. Louis, 2008, Mosby. Data from Heymann DL, editor: Control of communicable diseases manual, ed 19, Washington, DC, 2008, APHA; Centers for Disease Control and Prevention. HPV Vaccine, 2009, www.cdc.gov/vaccines/vpd-vac/hpv/default.htm#vacc.

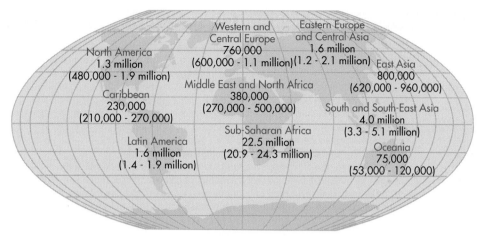

Total: 33.2 (30.6 - 36.1) million

FIGURE 25-4 HIV/AIDS worldwide, 2007. (From UNAIDS: *2007 report on the global AIDS epidemic,* Geneva, 2007, The Author: www.unaids.org/en/KnowledgeCentre/HIVData/GlobalReport/2008/2008_Global_report.asp.)

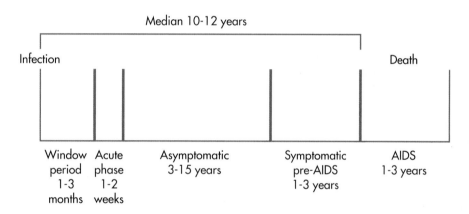

FIGURE 25-5 Usual course of HIV infection. (Modified from Grimes DE, Grimes RM: *AIDS and HIV infection,* St Louis, 1994, Mosby.)

Before the onset of effective antiretroviral therapies in the late 1990s, reported cases of AIDS provided a good indicator of the progression of the epidemic. With effective treatment, persons with HIV infection have taken longer to progress to AIDS, and the incidence of AIDS has declined. This has given the false impression that the epidemic was coming under control. Reporting cases of HIV infection has been incomplete and has varied by state. In 2009, all states reported AIDS cases by name and all but a few states reported HIV infection cases by name (CDC, 2009d).

Eradication of HIV/AIDS is dependent on development of a vaccine and the infrastructure necessary to vaccinate populations at risk worldwide. Neither possibility is foreseen in the near future. Given that reality, control of HIV/AIDS currently depends on preventing transmission of the virus. One current approach is to successfully treat those who are infected to lower their viral load, thus lowering their risk of transmitting the virus. Problems with adherence to the therapy are interfering with the "treatment as prevention" approach.

PREVENTION OF COMMUNICABLE DISEASES

All practicing nurses have a role in primary, secondary, and tertiary prevention of communicable diseases. Examples of appropriate interventions are reviewed here and in Table 25-9.

TABLE 25-8   CHAIN OF TRANSMISSION AND CONTROL: HIV/AIDS

HIV/AIDS

Occurrence	Worldwide; in 2004 about 40 million persons estimated to be living with human immunodeficiency virus (HIV), 62% reside in sub-Saharan Africa, 18% in south and south east Asia, 5% in Latin America, and 2.5% in the United States
Etiological agent	HIV, a retrovirus with two serologically and geographically distinct types (HIV-1 and HIV-2); HIV-1 makes up 90%-95% of the world's cases; it may be more pathogenic, lead to more rapid disease progression, and have higher mother-to-infant transmission than HIV-2 does; multiple subtypes (sometimes called clades) have been identified for both HIV-1 and HIV-2
Reservoir	Humans; HIV may have evolved from a chimpanzee virus
Transmission	Direct person to person through unprotected sexual contact, mother to fetus or mother to infant (during birth or by breastfeeding); indirect by contact of abraded skin or mucous membranes with infected blood or body fluids; injection of contaminated blood or fluids, or through use of contaminated needles; transplant of organs from infected person

	HIV INFECTION	AIDS
Incubation period	1-3 mo before antibodies are detectable	<1 yr to 15 yr; may be longer with effective antiretroviral therapy
Communicability period	Presumed to be <10 days after infection and lasting throughout life; may be highest in early infection when viral load is highest, and again later when clinical status worsens	
Susceptibility and resistance	General population is at risk; increased risk for infection with untreated ulcerative STDs and in uncircumcised males; evidence that some persons are less susceptible because of chemokine-receptor polymorphisms; very small percentage of infected persons do not progress to AIDS for an unknown reason	
Prevention and control	Practice universal precautions and safer sex; treat pregnant women with antiretrovirals to prevent transmission to fetus; teach infected women to avoid breastfeeding; treat drug users and provide needle exchange programs for injection drug users; treat STDs to decrease chance of acquiring HIV through sores on mucous membranes; maintain a safe blood supply; encourage autologous blood transfusions, when possible	Adherence to effective antiretroviral therapy delays progression to AIDS; prophylactic treatment for opportunistic infections delays onset of conditions associated with AIDS diagnosis
Disease manifestations	Acute, self-limiting illness lasting for 1-2 wk with symptoms that mimic other conditions (fever, rash, pharyngitis, myalgia, lymphadenopathy, and malaise); although immune deficiency may progress, the person may be without further symptoms for years	Progressive immune deficiency and increasing susceptibility to life-threatening infections and cancers
Diagnosis	*Early after infection:* The p24 and polymerase chain reaction blood tests identify the presence of viral nucleic acids; *within 1-3 months after infection:* Serologic tests (enzyme-linked immunosorbent assay, western blot) identify antibodies to HIV.	See Box 23-6 for case definition for AIDS
Treatment	Treatment with antiretroviral drugs to suppress the virus, not eradicate it; currently four classes of drugs are available: nucleoside reverse transcriptase inhibitors, nonnucleoside reverse transcriptase inhibitors, protease inhibitors, and fusion inhibitors; each attacks a different target in the reproduction process of the virus; current treatment strategies use at least 3 drugs from at least 2 classes; requires almost perfect adherence as development of drug-resistant HIV is common; treatment is very expensive and has many side effects; a person with AIDS will require additional treatment for infections and cancers that develop from impaired immune status	
Report to local health authority	Some states require reporting by name	Yes in all states

Data from Heymann DL, editor: *Control of communicable diseases manual,* ed 19, Washington, DC, APHA, 2008. UNAIDS: 2008 report on the global AIDS epidemic, Geneva, 2008 The Author.

Primary Prevention

Primary prevention of communicable diseases involves measures to prevent transmission of an infectious agent and to prevent pathology in the person exposed to an infection. All of the activities described in the section on breaking the chain of transmission are primary prevention activities. Immunization is primary prevention. Changing the behaviors that lead to exposure to a pathogen is primary prevention. See Tables 25-4 through 25-8 for primary preventions specific to the conditions in those tables.

Secondary Prevention

Secondary prevention includes activities to detect infections early and effectively treat persons who are infected.

TABLE 25-9	EXAMPLES OF PRIMARY, SECONDARY, AND TERTIARY PREVENTION ACTIVITIES FOR CONTROL OF INFECTIOUS DISEASES AT THE INDIVIDUAL AND POPULATION LEVELS	
INFECTIOUS DISEASE	**INDIVIDUAL**	**POPULATION**
Primary Prevention		
Sexually transmitted disease	Teach safe sex practices. IPV vaccine.	Place condom machines in accessible areas in places where young adults congregate.
Diseases caused by blood-borne pathogens	Teach barrier precautions to all health care workers. Teach injecting drug users about dangers of sharing needles.	Provide an adequate supply of gloves and sharps containers in patient care areas. Initiate citywide needle exchange programs and methadone programs.
Vaccine-preventable diseases	Ensure that all children who come to the clinic have age-appropriate immunizations.	Work with community groups to cosponsor immunization clinics where immunization rates are low.
Hepatitis A, gastrointestinal infections	Teach safe food-handling practices in the home.	Require, as part of the licensing of restaurants, that food handlers take a course in safe food handling.
Hepatitis A and B	Provide immune globulin after exposure to hepatitis A or B.	Mandate that health care workers are immunized for hepatitis A and B.
Secondary Prevention		
STDs	Screen and treat for all STDs.	STD partner notification program
Tuberculosis	Screen close contacts of persons with TB. Treat persons with a recent skin test conversion.	Initiate a program of yearly testing of health care workers for TB. Provide treatment to all recent converters free of charge at their workplace.
HIV/AIDS	Provide testing and treatment for HIV in local clinics.	Initiate reporting of HIV cases by name to the local health department to facilitate surveillance of HIV in population.
Meningitis	Immunize and provide chemoprophylaxis for person exposed to meningitis.	Provide immunization and chemoprophylaxis to all students in a school following an exposure.
Tertiary Prevention		
Tuberculosis	Provide therapy for person with active TB. Teach patients to take all doses of prescribed antibiotics and monitor adherence.	Initiate a directly observed therapy (DOT) program in the community shelters and jails. Initiate community education campaigns about the problem of drug resistance associated with incomplete antibiotic use.

Not only does this prevent progression of the infectious disease, but it also prevents transmission of the pathogen to others. Reporting infectious diseases, investigating contacts, notifying partners, finding new cases, and isolating cases are examples of secondary prevention.

Tertiary Prevention

Tertiary prevention includes activities involved in caring for persons with an infectious disease to ensure that they are cured or that their quality of life is maintained. Maybe the most important part of the treatment process is to ensure that the persons take their antimicrobials completely and effectively. In a time of increased resistance to pathogens, helping patients adhere to a drug regimen is critical. Additionally, caregivers should be taught to protect themselves and their environment by using appropriate precautions when caring for an infected family member.

SUMMARY

This chapter has presented the challenges of infectious diseases that face community health nurses everywhere. It has reviewed principles that are the foundation for the occurrence, transmission, and control of infectious diseases and applied those principles to infectious diseases that are emphasized in the *Healthy People 2020* objectives. Most important, because nurses will be impacted by infectious diseases wherever they practice, resources where any nurse can obtain up-to-date information on any infectious disease at any time have been included.

CASE STUDY

Assessment

Adrienne Zack is the Employee Health Nurse for a large city hospital. On a recent workday, she saw Beverly Yancy, a staff nurse in the newborn nursery of the hospital who presented to the employee health clinic with a productive cough, wheezing, low-grade fever, chills, and fatigue lasting over 1 month. Beverly stated that she had been treating her symptoms with over-the-counter antihistamines, cough suppressants, and antipyretics. When weighed in the clinic, Beverly was surprised that she had lost 10 lb since she weighed last. She told Adrienne that she has no history of asthma or lung disease.

Beverly's employee health record revealed that she had had a positive tuberculin skin test (TBST) of 15 mm induration when she was screened 11 years earlier for employment at the hospital. A chest radiograph at that time showed no evidence of tuberculosis (TB). Because Beverly was without TB symptoms at the time of employment and declined to take isoniazid (INH) for treatment of the latent tuberculosis infection (LTBT), she believed that the positive TBST was the result of having received bacille Calmette-Guérin (BCG) vaccination at birth in the Philippines. Further, she has been negative for symptoms during her annual symptom screen by the Employee Health Clinic.

A chest x-ray showed suspicious areas indicating that Beverly most likely had active, infectious pulmonary TB. The diagnosis was confirmed when a sputum smear was positive for acid-fast bacilli (AFB). On the basis of the timing of her symptoms, Adrienne determined that Beverly probably has been communicable for 3 months.

Diagnosis

Individual
- Active TB
- Potential for spread of TB to close contacts

Family
- Potential for undiagnosed TB

Community
- At risk for exposure to TB

Planning

Mycobacterium tuberculosis (MTB) is transmitted by airborne droplets of sputum from persons with active disease who cough or otherwise discharge respiratory droplets in the air. Health care workers are at risk for TB infection because of frequent exposure to patients with active TB disease. Beverly could not have been infected by the newborns in the nursery where she worked. Most likely she was exposed to TB before her screening 11 years previously. Her skin test of 15 mm induration suggested a latent TB infection rather than a BCG vaccination at birth. Latent TB infection can become active tuberculosis disease at any time. In this case, latency lasted more than 11 years.

Health care workers, like anyone with active TB, can transmit the infection to close contacts such as co-workers, high-risk patients, and personal contacts. Newborns and children under 2 years of age are at high risk for contracting TB infection and for progressing to TB disease. Such contacts must be found, screened, and treated as soon as possible. The incubation period for a detectable infection is 2 to 10 weeks following exposure. Recent contacts that are skin-test negative now should be retested in 2 to 3 months.

Goals

Individual

Short-Term Goals
- Beverly will begin her course of medications immediately.
- Beverly will take short-term disability and not return to work until cleared by the employee health clinic.

Long-Term Goals
- Beverly will complete her course of medications as directed.
- Beverly will provide sputum cultures and undergo chest x-ray examination at 3, 6, and 9 months and will be free of evidence of active TB.

Family

Short-Term Goals
- All of Beverly's family members will be tested for TB within 3 days.
- Any family member testing positive will be started on a course of medication as recommended by the health department and his or her health care provider.

Long-Term Goal
- All family members will be retested in 6 months.

Community (Hospital)

Short-Term Goals
- Beverly's co-workers will be tested for TB within 3 days.
- All of Beverly's patients from the past 3 months will be contacted to encourage them to be tested.
- Any contact or patient testing positive will be started on a course of medications as recommended by the local health department and his or her health care provider.

Long-Term Goal
- All contacts will be retested in 6 months.

Intervention

Tuberculosis must be reported to local public health authorities who are responsible for control of TB in the community. Control relies on identifying and adequately treating all active TB cases and those with latent infections. The public health department will investigate Beverly's contacts inside and outside the hospital during the previous 3 months. This will be done to identify and treat persons, including the discharged newborns, to whom Beverly might have transmitted MTB. Adrianne and the other health clinic employees may be asked to assist with screening hospital workers exposed to Beverly and providing education about treatment.

Tuberculin skin tests are determined to be positive under the following conditions:

1. Induration of 5 mm in persons with HIV infection, those in close personal contact with someone with active TB, or persons who have fibrotic chest radiographs
2. Induration of 10 mm in other high-risk persons, such as injecting drug users and persons with chronic disease or other causes of immune suppression and those from countries or communities where TB prevalence is high
3. Induration of 15 mm for anyone who does not meet the above criteria

All persons with a positive skin test should be tested for active disease. Those who have AFB in a stained smear of sputum, mycobacteria isolated from a cultured specimen, or radiological evidence of TB must be treated for active disease with a combination of drugs according to protocols established by the Centers for Disease Control and Prevention (CDC).

Multidrug-resistant TB (MDRTB) is an ever-increasing problem. Of active TB, 1% to 2% is now resistant to all available drugs. Patients must be helped to meticulously adhere to the prescribed regimen. Studies have demonstrated that health care workers are as poor as the general public at adhering to long-term drug therapy.

Persons with a recent conversion to a positive TBST should undergo treatment for latency according to CDC protocols. Such treatment reduces lifetime risk of a latent infection converting to active disease. Persons taking isoniazid should be taught symptoms of side effects to the drug, including hepatotoxicity, peripheral neuropathy, and central nervous system (CNS) changes.

Continued

CASE STUDY—cont'd

Teaching should include the following:
- The importance of isolating oneself from contact with others and wearing a mask in public until sputum is clear of bacilli—around 4 to 8 weeks with effective treatment.
- Proper discharge of sputum and materials contaminated with sputum.
- That drug therapy must be continued uninterrupted for designated time period even after sputum is negative for bacilli.
- That drug toxicity and side effects must be reported to physician immediately. These include, but are not limited to:
  - *Isoniazid (INH):* Hepatotoxicity, peripheral neuropathy, CNS changes
  - *Ethambutol:* Reduced visual acuity with inability to see the color green
  - *Streptomycin:* Rash, fever, malaise, vertigo, deafness, gastrointestinal disturbance, CNS changes
  - *Pyrazinamide:* Hypersensitivity, hepatotoxicity, gastrointestinal disturbances, renal failure
  - *Rifampin:* Red-orange urine, hepatotoxicity, CNS symptoms
  - *Ethionamide:* Gastrointestinal disturbance and symptoms of hepatotoxicity
  - *Cycloserine:* CNS effects
- Sputum must be reexamined monthly until negative for bacilli, then every 3 months for duration of therapy

Evaluation

Beverly and others with active TB can return to work when they have had three negative AFB sputum smear results collected 8 to 24 hours apart, with at least one being an early morning specimen. Adrienne will refer to the CDC's most recent guidelines for preventing transmission of tuberculosis in health care settings at www.cdc.gov/tb/topic/infectioncontrol/default.htm and update the hospital's infection control plan in accordance with the guidelines.

Levels of Prevention

Primary
- Educate health care workers and others about TB infection and disease.
- Educate staff on airborne precautions and the proper use of respiratory protection.
- Design and implement signage throughout the hospital to remind staff and patients about respiratory hygiene, cough etiquette, and hand hygiene.

Secondary
- Establish regular screening of health care workers for positive skin test conversions.
- Establish mechanisms for detection, referral, and treatment of staff with latent TB infections and with active TB.
- Implement procedures for rapid detection and treatment of patients with active TB.
- Coordinate efforts with the local health department.

Tertiary
- Monitor medication compliance and follow-up testing.

From Centers for Disease Control and Prevention: Guidelines for preventing the transmission of *Mycobacterium tuberculosis* in health-care settings, *MMWR Morb Mortal Wkly Rep* 54(RR17):1-141, 2005.

▌ LEARNING ACTIVITIES

1. Subscribe to the e-mail Listserv to receive *Morbidity and Mortality Weekly Report* (www.cdc.gov).
2. Attend an immunization clinic at your local health department to observe a nurse screening children for immunizations.
3. Obtain and evaluate health education materials regarding childhood immunizations from your local health department.
4. Log on to the website of an advocacy group against immunizations to understand the messages that they are communicating to the public.
5. Log on to your state health department website to learn about the process of reporting notifiable diseases in your state. Who is responsible for the reporting process? To whom do they report, what information is reported, and how often are diseases reported?
6. Log on to the CDC website to obtain the most recent guidelines for treating persons with HIV/AIDS, STDs, or tuberculosis.
7. Purchase a 1-year subscription to a public health nursing journal.

REFERENCES

Centers for Disease Control and Prevention: The principles of disease elimination and eradication, *MMWR Morb Mortal Wkly Rep* 48(SU01):23–27, 1999a.

Centers for Disease Control and Prevention: Recommendations of the advisory committee on immunization practices: revised recommendations for routine poliomyelitis vaccination, *MMWR Morb Mortal Wkly Rep* 48(27):590, 1999b.

Centers for Disease Control and Prevention: Summary of notifiable diseases: United States, 2007, *MMWR Morb Mortal Wkly Rep* 56(53):1–100, 2009a.

Centers for Disease Control and Prevention: *H1N1 flu (swine flu)*, 2009b. www.CDC.gov/h1n1flu. Accessed July 10, 2009.

Centers for Disease Control and Prevention: Trends in reportable sexually transmitted diseases in the United States, 2007, 2009c.

http://www.cdc.gov/std/stats07/trends.htm. Accessed September 9, 2009.

Centers for Disease Control and Prevention: Surveillance reports, cases of HIV infection and AIDS in the United States and dependent areas, 2007, 2009d. http://www.cdc.gov/hiv/topics/surveillance/resources/reports/2007report/table2.htm.

Heymann DL, editor: *Control of communicable diseases manual*, ed 19, Washington, DC, 2008, American Public Health Association.

Schneider M-J: *Introduction to public health*, ed 2, Boston, 2006, Jones and Bartlett.

UNAIDS: Report on the global AIDS epidemic: July 2008, 2008. http://data.unaids.org/pub/GlobalReport/2008/JC1511_GR08_ExecutiveSummary_en.pdf. Accessed August 31, 2009.

US Department of Health and Human Services: *Healthy People 2010*: immunization

and infectious diseases, 2000a, www.healthypeople.gov/document/html/volume1/14immunization.

US Department of Health and Human Services: *Healthy People 2010*: sexually transmitted diseases, 2000b, www.healthypeople.gov/document/html/volume2/25stds.

US Department of Health and Human Services: *Healthy People 2010*: HIV, 2000c, www.healthypeople.gov/document/html/volume1/13hiv.

US Department of Health and Human Services: *Healthy People 2010*: understanding and improving health, ed 2, Washington, DC, 2000d, US Government Printing Office.

World Health Organization: WHO report 2009 global tuberculosis control: Epidemiology, strategy, financing, 2009, www.who.int/tb/publications/global_report. Accessed July 10, 2009.

CHAPTER

26

Substance Abuse

*Marilyn R. Mouradjian**

Additional Material for Study, Review, and Further Exploration

evolve WEBSITE

http://evolve.elsevier.com/Nies
- Quiz
- Case Studies
- Glossary
- WebLinks

OBJECTIVES

Upon completion of this chapter, the reader will be able to do the following:

1. Discuss the historical trends and current conceptions of the cause and treatment of substance abuse.
2. Describe the current social, political, and economic aspects of substance abuse.
3. Describe the ethical and legal implications of substance abuse.
4. Detail the typical symptoms and consequences of substance abuse.
5. Identify issues related to substance abuse in various populations encountered in community health nursing practice.
6. Apply the nursing process to substance abuse problems.

KEY TERMS

addiction
dual diagnosis
harm reduction
initiation

intervention
mutual help groups
professional enablers
social consequences

substance abuse
war on drugs

OUTLINE

---

*The author would like to acknowledge the contributions of Joanne M. Hall and Josephine Wade, who wrote this chapter for the previous edition.

Perhaps no other health-related condition has as many far-reaching consequences in contemporary Western society as substance abuse. These consequences include a wide range of social, psychological, physical, economic, and political problems. Health problems and disability associated with substance abuse total approximately $276 billion annually. Each year, it costs an estimated $1000 per person for health care, law enforcement, accidents, treatment, and lost productivity. More deaths, illnesses, and disabilities are attributed to substance abuse than to any other preventable health condition in the United States (Substance Abuse and Mental Health Services Administration [SAMHSA], 2004c).

The social consequences of substance abuse include its role in crime (due to disinhibition), need for money to buy substances, and specific theft of drugs. Many offenders commit crimes while under the influence of drugs, alcohol, or both. Between 35% and 50% of inmates in correctional facilities reported that they had been under the influence of drugs when their crime was committed. Furthermore, almost 75% of inmates report prior drug use (Bureau of Justice Statistics [BJS], 2005).

All aggregates in society are potentially affected by substance abuse problems. Infants exposed in utero to alcohol, amphetamines, or opiates are at risk for withdrawal syndromes and later developmental problems. Indirect social effects of substance abuse include relationship conflicts, divorce, spousal and child abuse, and child neglect. Although well intended, many local and national efforts to fight substance abuse are often inadequate and ineffective (Drucker, 1999).

In the past, alcoholism and drug addiction were considered to be problems of the urban poor; society and most health professionals virtually ignored them. Substance abuse problems now pervade all levels of U.S. society, and awareness has increased. Community health nurses must be knowledgeable about substance abuse because it is a problem that frequently intertwines with other medical and social conditions.

This chapter focuses on helping community health nurses recognize substance abuse in their clients and in the larger community. The chapter reviews historical trends, the causes of substance abuse, the most common symptoms of these disorders, and treatment options. The author suggests nursing interventions appropriate for assisting those with substance-related problems, in a community context.

HISTORICAL OVERVIEW OF ALCOHOL AND ILLICIT DRUG USE

During the twentieth century, fluctuations in the use of alcohol and illicit drugs were influenced by shifts in public tolerance and political and economic trends. In general, alcohol use gained more social acceptance than other drug use. Alcohol consumption in the United States was higher during World Wars I and II and decreased during Prohibition and the Great Depression. Alcohol use was highest during the 1980s when states lowered the drinking age to 18 years of age. Lawmakers became alarmed at the increased rate of drinking and the increased number of alcohol-related deaths among 18- to 25-year-olds after lowering the drinking age and thereby reversed the decision. During the late 1980s, alcohol use declined after the minimum drinking age was reinstated to 21 years of age. The decline in alcohol consumption through the 1990s and into the twenty-first century is attributed to less-tolerant national attitudes toward drinking, increased societal and legal pressures and actions against drinking and driving, and increased health concerns among Americans. The identification of, and response to, driving under the influence is an example of a shift in thinking from addiction as the primary concern to other problems linked with, for example, alcohol use. These problems are thus termed *substance-related problems* and have become a significant community concern.

Public attitudes and governmental policies also have influenced the history of illicit drug use. Although nineteenth-century physicians prescribed morphine for a large variety of ailments, the discovery of the addictive properties of cocaine and opiates led to increased governmental regulation at the beginning of the twentieth century. The Harrison Narcotic Act of 1914, and subsequent laws, lessened the medical profession's control over the use of addictive drugs; the legislation specified that the physician could prescribe these drugs only in the course of general practice and not to maintain an addiction (Brecher, 1972). This limitation on the physician's power to prescribe and dispense addictive drugs, and restrictions on the importation of narcotics, limited the supply of these drugs until the 1950s and 1960s. At that time, an increase in illegal drug trafficking caused heroin use to proliferate, particularly in inner cities.

By the 1970s, drugs were increasingly available. During this period, a counterculture population, composed largely of young people, focused their efforts on enhancing social justice, ending the Vietnam War, and lessening "repressive" sexual mores; many conceptualized drug use as a way to liberate the mind. Marijuana use took place in communal, social settings; alcohol use was less favored because it was associated with the "establishment" they were critiquing. Consequently, the use of hallucinogens, cannabis, and heroin spread beyond urban drug subcultures to the general population. Alarmed by the social and personal problems inherent in this change, the public grew less tolerant of drug use, and prevention and treatment programs were given more attention and resources. After peaking in 1979, illicit drug use decreased among most segments of the population throughout the 1980s, reaching a low in the early 1990s. Between 1995 and 2000, it increased slightly before dropping again in recent years (SAMHSA, 2005).

To combat concerns of the physical, social, and psychological impact of drug abuse and dependence, federal drug policy has emphasized law enforcement and interdiction—the war on drugs—to reduce the supply. Despite the large amounts of money spent toward reaching this goal, this strategy has been only somewhat effective (Drucker, 1999). Trends have shown renewed interest in prevention and treatment efforts to decrease the amount of illicit drug use in society and to lessen its impact (SAMHSA, 2004c).

PREVALENCE, INCIDENCE, AND TRENDS

The increasing recognition of the widespread effects of substance abuse has initiated extensive collection of data by multiple agencies. This section describes selected statistics and current trends. The U.S. National Survey on Drug Use and Health is an annual survey conducted by SAMHSA, which estimates the prevalence of illicit drug and alcohol use in the United States. Findings from a 2008 report include the following (SAMHSA, 2008):

Alcohol

- Approximately 129 million Americans aged 12 years or older drink alcohol (51.6%). This compared with an estimate of 126.8 million users in 2007 (51.1%).
- Persons aged 12 years or older participated in binge drinking at least once in the 30 days prior to the 2008 SAMHSA survey (23.3%—no change from 2007).
- 17.3 million people reported heavy drinking in 2008 (6.9% of the population aged 12 years or older)—no significant change from 2007 data.
- Young adults aged 18 to 25 years had the highest prevalence of binge drinking and heavy drinking. Among older age groups, the prevalence of current alcohol use decreased with increasing age, from 67.4% among 26- to 29-year-olds to 50.3% among 60- to 64-year-olds and 39.7% among people aged 65 years or older (SAMHSA, 2008).

Illicit Drug Use

About 14.2% of the general U.S. population over age 12 years were drug users in 2008, compared with 7.1% in 2001 (SAMHSA, 2008). In 2008, marijuana was used by 75.7% of current illicit drug users and was the only drug used by 57.3% of them. Illicit drugs other than marijuana were used by 8.6 million persons, or 42.7% of illicit drug users aged 12 years or older. Current use of other drugs but not marijuana was reported by 24.3% of illicit drug users, and 18.4% used both marijuana and other drugs (SAMHSA, 2008).

In 2008, 9.3% of youths aged 12 to 17 years were current illicit drug users: 6.7% used marijuana, 2.9% engaged in nonmedical use of prescription-type psychotherapeutics, 1.1% used inhalants, 1.0% used hallucinogens, and 0.4% used cocaine (SAMHSA, 2008). Marijuana was the most commonly used illicit drug, especially among teens (15.2 million past month users). Interestingly, rates of current use among youths 12 to 17 years old declined significantly from 2002 to 2008 for several specific drugs including marijuana (from 8.2% to 6.7%), cocaine (from 0.6% to 0.4%), prescription-type drugs used nonmedically (from 4.0% to 2.9%), pain relievers (from 3.2% to 2.3%), stimulants (from 0.8% to 0.5%), and methamphetamine (from 0.3% to 0.1%).

Nonmedical Use of Prescription-Type Psychotherapeutics

There is a significant increase in the lifetime nonmedical use of pain relievers (20.8% of individuals aged 12 years and older) specifically Percocet, Percodan or Tylox, Vicodin, Lortab or Lorcet, Darvocet, Darvon or Tylenol with codeine, propoxyphene or codeine products, oxycodone, and hydrocodone (SAMHSA, 2008).

Hallucinogen, Inhalant, Needle, and Heroin Use

PCP, LSD, psilocybin, and ecstasy usage increase significantly after age 17 years (SAMHSA, 2008). Approximately 2% of individuals aged 12 to 25 years abuse inhalants. The inhalants of choice are amyl nitrite, "poppers," followed by glue, shoe polish, or toluene; correction fluid, degreaser, or cleaning fluid; gasoline or lighter fluid; and spray paints and other aerosols (SAMHSA, 2008).

Gender Differences

Female illicit drug use for ages 12 years and older is increasing while there is little change in male illicit drug utilization. According to SAMHSA in 2008, males were more likely to be current illicit drug users. The rate of current illicit drug use among females (12 years and older) increased from 5.8% (2007) to 6.3% (2008) while the rate for males, during the same period, did not change significantly (10.4% and 9.9% for 2007 and 2008, respectively). Current marijuana use among females also increased (3.8% to 4.4%) but did not change significantly for males (8% and 7.9%, respectively).

Demographics

Demographic correlates show some regional, racial, and gender differences and changes over the past few years. For example, people living in the West have the greatest percentage of past month drug use at 12.9%, compared with 9.7% for those in the Midwest, 9% for those in the Northeast, and 9% for those in the South. Additionally, rates of current illicit drug use vary significantly among major racial/ethnic groups. Rates were highest among American Indians or Alaska Natives (19.5%), followed by African Americans (16.9%), whites (14.4%), and Hispanics (12.3%). Asians had the lowest rate at 7.4% (SAMHSA, 2008). Visit the SAMHSA Office of Applied Studies website at www.oas.samhsa.gov/nhsda.htm for more information about substance abuse trends and statistics.

Trends in Substance Use

Research has revealed that problems associated with substance use may or may not relate to classically or clinically defined dependence or addiction. Many are turning to recovery before they have developed physiological dependence. Thus many in the field have begun to differentiate between use and misuse (misuse being interchangeable with abuse), and these terms now appear in the literature. This section describes significant trends in substances that are being abused and discusses substance abuse among special populations.

Healthy People 2020 and Substance Abuse

The U.S. Department of Health and Human Services (USDHHS, 2009) set goals and objectives related to substance abuse in *Healthy People 2020* (USDHHS, 2000). The objectives consist of norms and targets for the decade for health conditions for the U.S. population. The use of harmful substances is indirectly and directly related to all of the leading health indicators (i.e., tobacco use, alcohol and other drug abuse, physical activity, overweight and obesity, mental health, injury and violence, environmental quality, responsible sexual behavior, immunization, and access to health care). The *Healthy People 2020* table presents selected objectives and targets from *Healthy People 2020* related to substance abuse.

On review, there were mixed results related to progress toward the *Healthy People 2010* objectives. Whereas overall drug use, particularly among adolescents, declined, alcohol-related motor vehicle deaths remained steady, at about 30% of all fatalities (USDHHS, 2009). A disturbing trend is the large increase in the use of methamphetamines, steroids, and inhalants by young people.

Methamphetamine

Since 1997, methamphetamine (MA) has evolved as the most widely produced controlled substance in the United States. It is appearing in mass quantities, in part because of the ease in which the fertilizer anhydrous ammonia can be converted into MA; this has resulted in attracting more individuals into this clandestine business. Illegal street forms of the drug, often called crank, crystal, or meth, are available as a powder that can be injected, inhaled, or taken orally. In addition, a smokable form, known as ice or glass, is widely available. Currently, the preferred route of administration is by injection. This is possibly due to the undesirable physical difficulties related to smoking MA (e.g., damage to the nasal tract, coughing up blood, or difficulty breathing) (Cretzmeyer et al., 2003).

There is new attention being paid to MA manufacture and use because of the alarming increase in rates of abuse. The incidence of MA use rose steadily between 1990 (164,000 new users) and 2000 (344,000 new users). The new users during this time were approximately evenly split between 12- to 17-year-olds and 18- to 25-year-olds. This shift in age distribution from previous decades was reflected in the average age of new users, which fell from 22.3 years in 1990 to 18.4 years in 2000 (SAMHSA, 2004c). Hospital admissions for abuse of stimulants, mainly MA, increased from 1% to 7% between 1992 and 2002 (SAMHSA, 2003).

The pleasurable effects of MA are due to the release of high levels of dopamine in the brain, leading to increased energy, a sense of euphoria, and increased productivity. Short-term effects are increased heart rate, insomnia, excessive talking, excitation, and aggressive behavior. Prolonged use results in tolerance and physiological dependence. There are multiple negative effects for users of MA, their families, and communities. It appears to damage the brain in ways that are different from, and more severe than, damage from using other

 HEALTHY PEOPLE 2020

Selected Proposed Objectives for Substance Abuse

OBJECTIVE

HIV – HP2020–3: Reduce the number of new AIDS cases among adolescents and adults who inject drugs.

MICH HP2020–10: Increase abstinence from alcohol, cigarettes, and illicit drugs among pregnant women.

MHMD HP2020–14: Increase the proportion of persons with co-occurring substance abuse and mental disorders who receive treatment for both disorders.

SA HP2020–2: Reduce drug-induced deaths.

SA HP2020–4: Reduce the proportion of adolescents who report that they rode, during the previous 30 days, with a driver who had been drinking alcohol.

SA HP2020–5: Increase the age and proportion of adolescents who remain alcohol and drug free.

SA HP2020–7: Reduce the proportion of persons engaging in binge drinking of alcoholic beverages.

SA HP2020–15: Increase the proportion of persons who are referred for follow-up care for alcohol problems, drug problems after diagnosis, or treatment for one of these conditions in a hospital emergency department.

SA HP2020–19: Reduce the past-year nonmedical use of prescription drugs.

SA HP2020–20: Decrease the rate of alcohol-impaired driving (.08+ blood alcohol content [BAC]) fatalities.

From US Department of Health and Human Services: *Healthy People 2020*: 2009 draft objectives. Accessed from www.healthypeople.gov/HP2020/Objectives/TopicAreas.aspx.

drugs. Currently, there is rudimentary understanding of ways it affects the brain, but it is known that profound neurological changes occur even with first administration (Volm and de Araujo, 2004). Negative consequences range from anxiety, convulsions, and paranoia to brain damage (Block, Erwin, and Ghoneim, 2002). Use of MA is associated with an increased incidence of violence such as domestic abuse, homicide, and suicide, whether as a victim or as a perpetrator (Logan, Fligner, and Haddix, 1998).

MA is used predominantly by white young persons, with an overrepresentation of females. Thirty-six percent indicate that they were first introduced to the drug when they were under 16 years of age (SAMHSA, 2004a). Rates of admission for treatment of methamphetamine vary by region. The highest is Utah; however, most areas of the country are reporting an exponential rise of its manufacture and use.

The impact of MA abuse on communities, families, and social networks is considerable. Reported use is highest among 20- to 29-year-olds. This group often has young children, which puts these children at risk for abuse and neglect. The incidence of prenatal use is also rising, increasing the risk for children to be born with developmental problems, aggression, and attention disorders (Logan et al., 1998). Furthermore, exposure to combustible secondhand fumes puts children at risk for not only complications related to primary ingestion but also fatalities and injuries related to the highly combustible nature of the chemicals used in manufacture of the drug (Haight et al., 2005). Another pediatric issue is the growing number of teens recruited in the manufacture and selling of MA (Block et al., 2002).

Steroids

Evidence suggests that steroid use among adolescents is decreasing. In its annual survey used to assess drug use among our nation's teens in 2008, Monitoring the Future found that 0.9% of eighth graders, 0.9% of tenth graders, and 1.5% of twelfth graders had used anabolic steroids during the previous year. Steroid use is more commonly utilized in athletes and other individuals willing to risk potential and irreversible health consequences to build muscle (National Institute on Drug Abuse [NIDA], 2008). Data are scarce on the extent of steroid use by adults, but it has been estimated that hundreds of thousands of people aged 18 years and older use anabolic steroids at least once a year. Among both adolescents and adults, steroid use is higher among males than females (Gruber and Pope, 2000).

Use of steroids by popular sports figures may have influenced a generation of teenage athletes, girls as well as boys, to put themselves at risk. The health consequences of steroid use are well documented. Boys experience sexual changes, including decreased sperm count, impotence, shrinking of testicles, and difficulty urinating. In females, steroid use can manifest as masculinization, often producing increased facial hair and menstruation problems (Gruber and Pope, 2000). There are other more potentially fatal risks, including blood clots, liver damage, premature cardiovascular changes, and increased cholesterol (Sullivan, Martinez, Gennis et al.,

1998). Evidence also points at behavioral changes leading to an increased potential for suicide and aggressive and risky behaviors among steroid users (Pope, Kouri, and Hudson, 2000). Most negative effects are reversible on discontinuation of the drug. Collaborative treatment programs that monitor both psychological and physical issues, including consideration of the drug use route as injection, are necessary to combat steroid abuse.

Inhalants

Inhalants are defined by mode of administration (inhalation of fumes) and encompass a range of substances as diverse as glues, aerosols, butane, paint thinner, and nail polish remover. These products are inexpensive, legal, and easy to obtain, making them attractive to younger adolescents who have less access to illicit drugs.

Use of inhalants has consistently been highest among eighth graders, but a recent survey showed that inhalant use has increased among older teens as well. Further, studies monitoring drug- and alcohol-related emergency department admissions show that the largest increases in admission between 1995 and 2002 were for inhalants (186%) and amphetamines (166%) (NIDA, 2005).

ADOLESCENT SUBSTANCE ABUSE

Youth are a particularly susceptible aggregate for substance abuse. Individuals between 18 and 25 years of age have the highest prevalence of illicit drug use during their lifetime (65% of the population). One positive development is that teen use of cigarettes and smokeless tobacco has declined since the peak levels in the mid-1990s. Indeed, 30-day prevalence of smoking has declined by 56% in eighth grade, 47% in tenth, and 32% in twelfth. It is noteworthy, however, that this significant decline in adolescent smoking and use of smokeless tobacco has decelerated sharply and seems to be on the verge of halting among tenth graders (NIDA, 2005). Cigarettes continue to be highly available to the young, and concerned groups continue to monitor advertising that targets new potential smokers, such as youth and women.

Virtually all major theories of the origins of adolescent substance abuse agree that the perceived acceptance of problematic drug-using behavior among family, peers, and society is an important influence on an individual's decision to use or not use alcohol, tobacco, and drugs. The perception that alcohol use is socially acceptable correlates with the fact that more than 80% of American youth consume alcohol before their twenty-first birthday, and the lack of social acceptance of other drugs correlates with comparatively lower rates of use. Similarly, widespread societal expectations that young people will engage in binge drinking may encourage this highly dangerous form of alcohol consumption (USDHHS, 2000).

Trends in alcohol use by American teens are mixed. Throughout the early part of the century, there were drops in several indicators of alcohol use at all grade levels. In 2004, however, most drinking measures showed slight increases among twelfth graders (NIDA, 2005).

Most of the movement in teen substance use has been in a downward direction, but generally the declines have been marginal (Johnston et al., 2005). Between 1995 and 2002, there was no consistent increase or decline in marijuana users. However, the percentage of adolescents reporting that it is easy to obtain marijuana declined slightly, from 55% to 53.6% (SAMHSA, 2003). In addition, initiation of both LSD and ecstasy declined. Use of PCP, or phencyclidine, has been at low levels for some time, and use fell further in 2004. The resurgence of inhalant use among the eighth graders was one of the more troublesome recent findings, as was the continued rise in use of the highly addictive narcotic drug oxycodone (OxyContin) among high school seniors and eighth graders (NIDA, 2005).

In order to effectively plan for the present and future needs of the community, the community health nurse needs the most current overall perspective. Information on the prevalence, incidence, and trends in the amount and types of substance abuse at the general, state, and local levels is readily available on the Internet. As harmful, illicit substances come in and out of vogue, particularly among young people, the community health nurse needs a good understanding of drug culture, terminology, and differing signs and symptoms.

CONCEPTUALIZATIONS OF SUBSTANCE ABUSE

Conceptualizations of substance abuse and dependence have changed over the years, often for political and social reasons rather than for scientific reasons. Some conceptualizations focus on the phenomenon of addiction, which is manifested by compulsive use patterns and the onset of withdrawal symptoms when substance use is abruptly stopped. Other views focus on the problems resulting from the substance use itself, regardless of whether an addictive pattern is present. Problematic consequences of substance use include intoxication, psychological dependence, relational conflicts, employment or economic difficulties, legal difficulties, and health problems. For example, addiction need not be present for individuals to experience legal consequences of illicit drug use, such as driving while intoxicated, or alcohol- or drug-related domestic violence.

Drawing fine distinctions among ideas of dependence, addiction, and abuse concerning substance use may seem irrelevant if there is evidence that the substance use has become problematic. However, broadly labeling all habitual or compulsive behavior patterns as addiction or dependence may obscure the fact that interventions could precede the development of addiction, for example, in cases where use has become misuse and a problem is evident. It is also becoming increasingly evident that specific interventions may be needed for each separate addictive problem (e.g., overeating

and gambling). Moreover, in each specific group, there is wide individual diversity.

Definitions

The term substance abuse came into common usage in the 1970s. Earlier conceptualizations generally focused on either alcoholism or drug addiction as singular addictive disorders. Most substance abuse theories identify core commonalties that occur in regard to use of a variety of different substances or in relation to compulsive behavior syndromes (Leshner, 1997). There is also an emphasis on relapse prevention that may include moderate use goals and abstinence (Larimer and Marlatt, 1990).

There remains debate about how substance use and substance abuse should be defined and what substances should be included under each definition. Traditional conceptualizations of substance abuse focus solely on alcohol and illicit street drugs. Other conceptualizations include prescription medications such as tranquilizers or analgesics. In eating disorders such as bulimia and compulsive overeating food is viewed as the abused substance. Table 26-1 shows a classification scheme for commonly abused substances.

In addition to varying in their abuse potential, substances vary in their degree of potential harm to those who use them and to others in the immediate environment. Tobacco is an example of a substance that is unsafe to the smoker and to those who inhale secondhand smoke. Those who abuse alcohol may also harm others by driving under the influence, and lowering of inhibitions may foster violent activities in some (e.g., child or partner abuse).

Integrating the various opinions regarding the diagnosis of substance abuse, the American Psychiatric Association (APA) has classified substance use disorders as either "dependence" or "abuse" (APA, 2000). The APA focused on the following psychoactive substances that affect the nervous system: alcohol, amphetamines, caffeine, cannabis, cocaine, hallucinogens, inhalants, nicotine, opioids, phencyclidine, sedatives, and hypnotics or anxiolytics. Substance use disorders can also be categorized as being in partial or full remission. A diagnosis of substance abuse indicates a maladaptive pattern of substance use that is manifested by recurrent and significant adverse consequences related to repeated use of a substance. These adverse consequences include failure to fulfill major role obligations, repeated use in physically hazardous situations, multiple legal problems, and recurrent social and interpersonal problems.

The criteria for the diagnosis of dependence include a cluster of cognitive, behavioral, and physiological symptoms that indicate continued use of the substance despite significant substance-related problems. A pattern of repeated, self-administered use results in tolerance, withdrawal, and compulsive drug-taking behaviors, which are frequently accompanied by a craving or strong desire for the substance. This craving then motivates the user to be preoccupied with supply, money to purchase drugs, and getting through time between periods of use, all of which take up mental energy,

TABLE 26-1	CLASSIFICATION OF COMMONLY USED AND ABUSED SUBSTANCES	
SUBSTANCE	DESIRED EFFECT	POSSIBLE WITHDRAWAL SYMPTOMS
CNS Depressants		
Alcohol	Euphoria, disinhibition, and sedation	Anxiety, irritability, seizures, delusions,
Barbiturates	Retrograde amnesia	hallucinations, and paranoia
Sedative-hypnotics (e.g., benzodiazepines [Rohypnol])	Sedation and amnesia	
Tranquilizers (e.g., GHB, the "date rape" drug)		
CNS Stimulants		
Amphetamines (e.g., methamphetamine)	Euphoria, hyperactivity, omnipotence,	Depression, apathy, lethargy, and
Cocaine	insomnia, and anorexia	sleepiness
Nicotine		
Caffeine		
Narcotics-Opioids		
Codeine	Euphoria and sedation	Anxiety, irritability, agitation, runny
Meperidine and acetaminophen (e.g., Demerol)		nose, watery eyes, chills, sweating,
Hydromorphone (e.g., Dilaudid)		nausea and vomiting, diarrhea,
Fentanyl		tremors, and yawning
Heroin		
Methadone		
Morphine		
Opium		
Oxycodone (e.g., Percodan)		
Hallucinogens		
Mescaline	Hallucinations, illusions, and	Depression
LSD	heightened awareness	
PCP (e.g., ketamine)	PCP: violent dissociative and	
STP and MDMA (e.g., ecstasy)	anesthetic effect	
Psilocybin (e.g., mushrooms)		
Cannabis		
Marijuana	Relaxation, euphoria, and altered	Restlessness, insomnia, and anxiety
Hashish and THC	perceptions	
Inhalants		
Gasoline	Euphoria	Restlessness, anxiety, and irritability
Toluene acetate		
Cleaning fluids		
Airplane cement		
Amyl nitrate		

Modified from Faltz B, Rinaldi J: *AIDS and substance abuse: a training manual for health care professionals*, San Francisco, 1987, Regents of the University of California. Used with permission.
CNS, Central nervous system; *GHB*, gamma hydroxybutyrate; *MDMA*, methylenedioxymethamphetamine; *PCP*, phencyclidine; *STP*, 2,5-dimethoxy-4-methylamphetamine; *THC*, tetrahydrocannabinol.

effort that is diverted from work or school, and connectedness to significant others. This is how the use becomes problematic and how others around the user become confused and eventually often feel rejected, hurt, ignored, angry, or even responsible for the user's behavior.

Diagnostic Criteria for Substance Dependence

The APA has established the following criteria for substance dependence: the maladaptive pattern of *substance use*, leading to clinically significant impairment or distress. Three (or more) of the following criteria must be exhibited anytime within the same 12-month period:

1. Tolerance, as defined by either of the following:
   a. A need for markedly increased amounts of the substance to achieve intoxication or desired effect
   b. Markedly diminished effect with continued use of the same amount of the substance
2. Withdrawal, as manifested by either of the following:
   a. The characteristic withdrawal syndrome for the substance
   b. The same (or closely related) substance is taken to relieve or avoid withdrawal symptoms
3. The substance is often taken in larger amounts or over a longer period than intended.
4. There is a persistent desire or unsuccessful efforts to cut down or control substance use.
5. A great deal of time is spent in activities necessary to obtain the substance (e.g., visiting multiple doctors or driving long distances), use the substance (e.g., chain-smoking), or recover from its effects.

6. Important social, occupational, or recreational activities are given up or reduced.
7. The substance use is continued despite knowledge of having a persistent or recurrent physical or psychological problem that is likely to have been caused or exacerbated by the substance (e.g., current cocaine use despite the recognition of cocaine-induced depression, or continued drinking despite recognition that an ulcer was made worse by alcohol consumption).
8. Specify if with or without physiological dependence (e.g., tolerance or withdrawal) (APA, 2000).

Substance abuse must be understood and differentiated from substance dependence. The *Diagnostic and Statistical Manual of Mental Disorders*, fourth edition, text revision, uses the following criteria when diagnosing *substance abuse*, which is a maladaptive pattern of substance use leading to clinically significant impairment or distress, as manifested by one (or more) of the following, occurring with a 12-month period:

1. Recurrent substance use resulting in a failure to fulfill major role obligations at work, school, or home (e.g., repeated absences or poor work performance related to substance use; substance-related absences, suspensions, or expulsions from school; neglect or children or household).
2. Recurrent substance use in situations in which it is physically hazardous (e.g., driving a automobile or operating a machine when impaired by substance use).
3. Recurrent substance-related legal problems (e.g., arrests for substance-related disorderly conduct).
4. Continued substance use despite persistent or recurrent social or interpersonal problems caused or exacerbated by the effects of the substance (e.g., arguments with spouse about consequences of intoxication, physical fights).
5. The symptoms have never met the criteria for substance dependence for this class of substance (APA, 2000).

Etiology of Substance Abuse

Substance abuse has an impact on virtually every aspect of individual and communal life, and many institutions and academic fields have addressed it. Several theories attempt to explain the cause and scope of these problems and offer solutions. Some theories address individual, physiological, spiritual, and psychological factors. Others deal with social influences involving family, ethnicity, race, access to drugs, environmental stressors, economics, political status, culture, and sex roles. Most theories suggest that a combination of factors is the underlying impetus for substance abuse.

Although physiological, medical model theorists have defined alcoholism as a loss of control over drinking or an individual malfunction, the cause of alcoholism was ambiguous in the past (Brown, 1969; Keller, 1972). Although previous research studies have suggested a link between genetics and alcoholism, there is growing evidence that genetic variations may contribute to the nature of alcoholism within families (NIDA, 2006).

Individual and environmental factors also contribute to an increased risk for alcohol abuse. On the individual level, a person's inherited sensitivity to alcohol is a predictor for the development of alcohol abuse. Two broad personality dimensions are also associated with an increased risk for alcohol abuse. Impulsivity and ease of disinhibition add to risks for substance abuse. Proneness to anxiety and depression are also risks, and these comorbidities are not well understood. Alcohol expectancies (i.e., beliefs about anticipated consequences of drinking) are also a predictor of alcohol abuse. If one expects a certain effect, such as relief, one is more likely to feel it after use of a drug. The satisfied expectancies may set up neural pathways that are interpreted as pleasurable.

Medical models of alcoholism and other substance abuse conditions may not provide an understanding of commonalities among addictive behaviors (e.g., excessive drinking, gambling, eating, drug use, and sexual behavior). Crossaddiction, or multidrug use, is more prevalent now than in the past, and more studies point to the presence of both automatic and nonautomatic factors in physiological and psychological dependence. Specific biological medical models are giving way to multicausal models.

In the biopsychosocial model, risk factors interact with protective factors to develop a predisposition toward drug or alcohol use. This predisposition is then influenced by exposure to the substance, availability, and the experiential interpretation of the drug experience (e.g., pleasant or unpleasant). Continued availability of the substances and a social support system that enables or supports their use is also necessary. These factors combine to determine whether addiction develops and is maintained.

SOCIOCULTURAL AND POLITICAL ASPECTS OF SUBSTANCE ABUSE

Within community settings, substance-related problems are not always easy to identify. For example, the consequences of the sale and use of crack cocaine in an inner-city, African-American neighborhood may be apparent through media attention. The traffic of these drugs into the middle classes, on the other hand, is less easily recognized. The increasing tendencies of elderly persons to rely on alcohol and other, even illicit, drugs may be shocking to some nurses. It can be understood, however, contextually and may be the result of multiple factors such as isolation, fears, uncontrolled chronic pain, anxiety, and sleep disturbances. Nurses must incorporate sociocultural and political dimensions into caring for clients in the community. Nurses must also possess knowledge that is useful in countering media stereotypes and can model a more holistic, multifaceted approach to prevention and management of substance abuse.

Although there are subcultural and regional variations, drinking norms of the dominant culture in the United States are relatively permissive. Traditional ethnic ceremonial and symbolic substance use patterns vary significantly. As acculturation occurs, however, cultural definitions of "appropriate" use of alcohol and drugs have been dulled, leaving a void regarding social expectations. Subcultural groups such as gay, lesbian, bisexual, and transgender persons have often had a social center that was a bar, and alcohol use was historically a way of demonstrating and celebrating differentiation from a more repressive majority. These cultural conditions create ambiguity in clearly determining when a substance abuse problem exists. Furthermore, each subculture may define abuse differently. It can be theorized that stigmatized minorities might be under more stress, and perhaps more likely to use substances, but this cannot be assumed in any individual case.

A particular drug experience can be understood as an interaction between the individual's subjective mood and the actual pharmacological effects of the drug, but this interaction does not take place in a vacuum. Rather, the expectations of a drug's effect are shaped by the user's culture and involve the adoption of roles taught by more experienced users and reinforced by other social groups, including health care providers in some cases (Montagne and Scott, 1993).

Substances are also given economic value and are bought and sold as commodities in a variety of social arenas, both legal and illegal. The ways in which drugs, including nicotine, medications, and alcohol are produced and distributed among the various segments of the population are determined largely by economic, cultural, and political conditions. For example, the economic realities of poor Colombians and Peruvians who rely on the growth and production of the coca leaf for financial survival can be understood as a confluence of larger, society-level and individual-level factors. The drug trade is very lucrative for some; it raises their societal status, gives them access to material things, and provides an enhanced sense of power in that society. Among urban poor minority youth in the United States, the fact that drug trafficking often precedes drug use suggests that involvement in the drug trade satisfies a need for status and economic power (Greenberg and Schneider, 1994).

These changes in power can have other consequences as various subgroups attain and maintain status. A group without cultural values, or with competing cultural values, suffers from chaos and disorganization. Competing value systems lead to cultural disintegration and a sense of powerlessness and hopelessness. The group becomes susceptible to forces that further threaten the group's ability to survive. When they are unable to organize or determine a collective direction because of conflicting values, the group and its members are separated and disempowered. The history of cocaine abuse and dependence among people of color is an example of how these conditions are interrelated. Indeed, cocaine use was epidemic in the 1980s and early 1990s, with crack cocaine most prevalent in poor communities, but its use has declined markedly in recent years (SAMHSA, 2004c).

COURSE OF SUBSTANCE-RELATED PROBLEMS

There is no predictable course of addictive illness and no "addictive personality type." When habitual use is well established, behaviors may be clinically visible and similar; this has led to assumption of a singular, addiction-prone personality. However, not everyone who initiates drug or alcohol use will progress to dependency or display associated behaviors.

Because the path from initiation to dependency is multidimensional, the context of client and community experiences is key to understanding and responding to problems encountered. Nurses need to take a comprehensive health and substance use history and place this in a context of cultural, historical, family, and social factors. Neither addiction nor dependency is a unitary phenomenon with a single isolated cause; rather, it is the result of interactions among a host of variables.

The assessment process should include consideration of the triad: the person, the substance, and the context or environment. The person assessment includes demographic information, medical history, comorbidities, and known perceptions and meanings the individual displays. The drug assessment includes the qualities of the substance itself, physiopharmacological effects, pattern of use, availability, and toxicity. Context assessment should include family, social, employment, legal, cultural, and economic contingencies.

Hanson, Venturelli, and Fleckenstein (2002) categorize users of illicit substances as experimenters, compulsive users, or "floaters." Experimenters begin using substances largely because of peer pressure or curiosity; they are usually able to set limits. In contrast, compulsive users devote much of their time and energy to getting high and tend to immerse themselves in conversations and social interactions around drugs and alcohol. "Floaters" focus more on using other people's substances and generally have light to moderate use. This does not explain the meaning that substance use has for the individual, however, nor what kinds of experiences and perceptions are associated with use. The subjective experiences of using particular substances and other issues such as genetic predisposition, discrimination, past trauma, family strife, and economic status make each case of substance use or misuse as unique as one's fingerprint.

Genetic traits have been found to be associated with addiction to certain substances. For example, people of Chinese or Japanese extraction may become ill after ingestion of even small amounts of alcohol. A single nucleotide polymorphism (SNP) that encodes opiate receptors is more frequent among some heroin addicts, and an SNP that encodes dopamine receptors is more frequent in some alcoholics. Certainly there is a genetic and disease component to addiction, implying that prevention efforts can be more efficient when targeted at vulnerable individuals. As a result, prevention efforts should focus on children of addicts, who should be advised not to experiment (Goldstein, 2001).

The progression from initiation to continuation, transition to abuse, and, finally, addiction and dependency varies. Individuals often describe a progression that began with initiation through social interactions. For some, the substance and setting is reinforcing and primes the individual for a pattern of use. For others, the experience will be unpleasant enough to prevent further use. It cannot be assumed, however, that an unpleasant initiation will always be preventive. In the case of stimulants, such as MA, the drug produces such strong feelings of euphoria, alertness, control, and increased energy that future use is enticing, especially when the drug is easily accessible (Cretzmeyer et al., 2003).

The continuation stage of substance abuse is a subsequent period in which substance use persists but does not appear to be detrimental to the individual. In stimulant abuse, continued use often occurs in a binge pattern. Individuals are able to exercise some control over use, but use becomes more frequent. Neither the individual nor the social network views use during this stage as problematic.

A critical point is the transition stage from substance use to substance abuse. There may be evidence to both the users and their social networks that the use of the substance is having adverse effects. During this stage, users begin to use more often and in more varied settings. Rationalizations that deny the seriousness and consequences of the substance use are commonly constructed during this stage.

The research on correlates and antecedents of substance abuse points to a variety of personal and social motivations. For many young people, motivators are the attraction of a rebellious subculture, peer pressure, and nationwide fads. Considerable research exists on the self-medication aspects of individuals with comorbid mental illnesses. Once the addiction is established, unpleasant physical and emotional withdrawal symptoms are strong motivators to continue use. Abstinence in the stimulant abuser can result in symptoms such as depression, lethargy, and anhedonia (i.e., inability to feel pleasure). The depression experienced by the user when not using stimulants is contrasted with the recalled euphoria produced by the use of the drug. These factors, coupled with associated cues, help initiate the cycle of binge use, with increased craving and continued self-administration to relieve symptoms. Brain imaging techniques have demonstrated that abuse of drugs such as cocaine and amphetamine produce immediate and long-lasting physical changes that are likely to contribute to the maintenance of dependency (Obert, London, and Rawson, 2002).

The development of addiction or dependency is marked by changes in both behavior and cognition. There is an increasing focus on the substance and a narrowing of interests, social activities, and relationships. The process of becoming dependent or addicted requires the individual to deny or ignore evidence or information that may challenge their behavior or rationalization of their behavior. There is a preoccupation with the substance and its procurement during this stage, even in the face of negative consequences. Table 26-2 outlines the stages in the process of stimulant addiction.

LEGAL AND ETHICAL CONCERNS OF SUBSTANCE ABUSE

For the past 30 years, the United States has pursued a drug policy based on prohibition and the active application of criminal sanctions against the use and sale of illicit drugs. During this time, the number of criminal penalties for drug offenses has climbed to 1.5 million offenses. There has also been a tenfold increase in imprisonment for drug charges since 1979, despite an overall decline in drug prevalence (BJS, 2002).

This increase in drug-related imprisonment is a result of harsher enforcement policies and longer mandatory

TABLE 26-2	TYPICAL COURSE OF ADDICTIVE ILLNESS: STAGES IN CONTINUUM FROM INITIATION TO DEPENDENCY
STAGE	**CHARACTERISTICS**
Initiation	First use of the substance Exposure frequently through family or friends
Continuation	Continued, more frequent use of substance Usually social use only, with no detrimental effects
Transition	Beginning of change in total consumption, frequency, and occasions of use More than just social use, with beginning of loss of control
Abuse	Adverse effects and consequences to substance use Rationalizations for continued use and denial of adverse effects present in user and significant others Unsuccessful attempts at control of use
Dependency and addiction	Physical or psychological dependence, or both, on the substance; marked by behavioral and cognitive changes Preoccupation with the substance and its procurement, despite negative consequences Narrowing of interests, social activities, and relationships to only those related to the substance use

sentences for possession of smaller quantities of drugs. Although some individuals are in prison for violent crimes or major drug trafficking, many drug offenders are arrested for small-scale drug deals made to support their personal use (BJS, 2005).

Alcohol use and abuse are different issues because the possession and sale of alcoholic beverages is only illegal if the individual involved is a minor. Concerns arise when individuals are intoxicated during work, while driving, or in situations that may affect the welfare of others. Legal penalties have increased for driving under the influence of alcohol because groups such as Mothers Against Drunk Driving (MADD) influence legislation.

ETHICAL INSIGHTS
Ethical Issues Related to Substance Abuse

Ethical issues regarding substance use and abuse relate to behaviors that present a risk to self, co-workers, or the public. A health care worker diverting medication from a patient, thereby depriving the patient of pain relief, is both unethical and illegal. Other ethical areas of concern include property theft or damage and the general welfare of others.

Drug testing, as part of preemployment assessment and random testing during employment, has become commonplace. Beginning in 1986, federal legislation, such as the

Drug-Free Workplace Act and the Omnibus Transportation Employee Testing Act, has authorized drug and alcohol testing in specific job classifications. Although employees' attitudes toward workplace drug testing are mixed, it has been shown to have a positive effect, and currently about 90% of large U.S. companies have a drug screening policy in place (Levine and Rennie, 2004; Sweeney and Penner, 1997). There is evidence that the most effective deterrent to drug abuse in workers is a comprehensive program combining testing with an employee assistance program, supervisory training, employee education, and a clearly written substance use policy (Quazi, 1993). The legal conflict in testing is its opposition to rights of privacy; therefore testing is random rather than universal (Levine and Rennie, 2004).

One area that has also received the attention of the legal system is the use by pregnant women of substances known to increase risks to the fetus in terms of future long-term developmental and behavioral problems. Pregnant addicts have been imprisoned and forced into treatment, and their children have been removed from their custody after birth. Many treatment providers and patient advocates view this approach as punitive and counterproductive to assisting these women and their children. There is concern that such sanctions may prevent addicted women from seeking treatment, for fear of legal consequences (Chavkin et al., 1998; Paone and Alpern, 1998).

Heavy maternal use of alcohol during pregnancy can cause permanent birth defects, including fetal alcohol syndrome. Although alcohol-related defects are entirely preventable, the factors associated with maternal use of alcohol during pregnancy are complex and often resistant to change. The University of Washington has implemented a primary prevention and intervention program for those women identified as being at risk for producing children affected by prenatal alcohol exposure. Women identified as being at risk are referred to a multidisciplinary diagnostic clinic staffed by a physician, psychologist, language pathologist, occupational therapist, and social worker to facilitate diagnosis and comprehensive intervention for both the mother and affected children. This approach increases the potential for primary prevention of fetal alcohol syndrome by avoiding exposures and is a major protective factor in managing conditions among affected children (Astley, 2004; Cook, 2004).

MODES OF INTERVENTION

Correlating with the numerous theories about substance abuse is the wide variety of intervention strategies incorporating all levels of prevention. National, state, and local legislative measures have attempted to limit access to potentially addictive pharmaceuticals and illicit street drugs. The growing social demand for smoke-free environments in public buildings, restaurants, airplanes, and similar areas exemplifies how perceptions of tobacco and its risks have changed over the past 50 years. Alcohol taxes, zoning schemes for liquor outlets, a legal drinking age, and legal sanctions on driving while intoxicated are other examples of community efforts to prevent or contain substance abuse.

Media campaigns provide public service communications about the risks of substance abuse and the availability of treatment for these problems. However, these must include culturally relevant and realistic goals. Some have proved to be quite successful. For example, there was a long and substantial decline in the use of inhalants by adolescents after 1995, when the Partnership for a Drug-Free America conducted an anti-inhalant media campaign. This decline, however, has since reversed (Johnston et al., 2005).

One of the goals of *Healthy People 2020* (USDHHS, 2000) is to increase the proportion of middle, junior high, and senior high schools that provide school health education related to unintentional injury, violence, suicide, tobacco use and addiction, and alcohol and other drug use. Educational programs administered through schools and penal institutions have been developed, but evaluation and evidence of success or failure of the interventions have been sporadic.

The formation of national associations (e.g., the National Council on Alcoholism and Drug Dependence [NCADD]) and the establishment of federal research entities (e.g., the National Institute on Drug Abuse and the National Institute on Alcohol Abuse and Alcoholism) have facilitated centralized efforts in the areas of education, research, and treatment. At the state level, there have been legislative provisions to fund substance abuse treatment and rehabilitation. National organizations such as the Partnership for a Drug-Free America and the National Alliance on Mental Illness, which have local chapters, are also important forces for community education, research, and support.

NIDA released a report aimed at addressing the community-level disaster of the September 11, 2001, attack and extended the report to include the 2005 hurricanes, Katrina and Rita, which displaced hundreds of thousands, and killed at least 1000. In the report, the experience of stress resulted in a sharp increase in the corticotropin-releasing factor, setting in motion a host of biological changes related to posttraumatic stress and posttraumatic stress disorder. Stress may cause those with compulsive use patterns to relapse after a period of abstinence (NIDA, 2005) and may trigger those who have not previously misused substances to, at least temporarily, misuse them. These cases also delimit the efficacy of the "addictive personality" and the one-size-fits-all approach.

Prevention

The principles of prevention are paramount in community nursing practice. Primary prevention in the community includes working with other providers to perform a needs assessment. This will identify high-risk situations and potential problems that threaten the integrity of the community and its inhabitants—in particular, what factors in the community are encouraging initiation of substance abuse, how effective are school- and community-based programs, and what political issues in the community may be influencing resource allocation.

On the federal level, primary prevention efforts have been overshadowed by the ongoing "war on drugs." A significant amount of fiscal resources has been allocated to law enforcement, interdiction, crop eradication, and harsh, punitive laws to prosecute drug users and manufacturers. Debate continues at both the state and federal levels regarding the cost-benefit ratio of drug legalization or decriminalization. Supporters argue that legalization and decriminalization would lead to a reduction in crime and would move the drug problem out of the realm of the moral failure of individuals toward more humane treatment approaches.

Opponents argue that decriminalization and legalization of drugs would do little to abate crime related to drug manufacture, sale, and use and that problems associated with use (e.g., domestic violence and drunk driving) would potentially increase (Goldberg, 2004). There is no question that substance abuse is a costly medical, social, and legal problem and that until society can effectively deal with the serious effects of two lethal but legal drugs (i.e., alcohol and nicotine), the argument for adding additional sanctions is difficult to accept and justify. Other preventive efforts at government and private levels include community-based programs, training of health professionals, faith-based initiatives, volunteer consumer groups, organized sports programs, and employer programs.

The secondary prevention role of the community health nurse includes screening and finding resources and solutions specific to his or her particular community. It is important for the community health nurse to be aware of the evidence base for certain programs and modify or discard those programs that have not proved successful over time.

Screening tools such as the CAGE test (Box 26-1) are brief and simple and allow health providers to talk about substance abuse by incorporating relevant questions into the interview and history (Cherpitel, 1997; Ewing, 1984). A positive response to any of the CAGE questions does not constitute a diagnosis of alcohol or drug dependence, but it should raise suspicion and mandate further investigation. Prevention efforts should be specific to aggregates, rather than directed at the general public.

Prevention efforts focusing on minority groups such as African Americans have produced results that are only marginally successful (Straussner, 2003). Possible reasons are that treatment programs fail to incorporate culturally sensitive and appropriate interventions and strategies. The demand for a culturally specific approach is evidence that previous approaches, and the assumptions that underlie them, are insufficient for understanding and explaining the etiology of substance abuse among members of minority groups. Successful prevention efforts are usually not focused solely on alcohol and drug abuse but are community controlled and work toward improving individuals' general competencies, communication skills, and self-esteem.

Treatment

Substance abuse problems are socially defined and frequently attributed to sufferers who do not recognize their substance use as a problem. Furthermore, the substance abuse treatment system has increasingly taken on social welfare and criminal justice tasks. In this sense, substance abuse differs from many other health-related problems. Most states have laws pertaining to involuntary treatment of substance abusers. Employers and families are often enlisted to assist or coerce the identified client into accepting treatment. This aspect of substance abuse as a health concern raises some crucial questions for health care providers in terms of the encroachment of therapeutic intervention on individual rights to privacy, informed consent, and self-determination.

On the individual level, those providing substance abuse treatment should take into consideration cultural and educational background, the resources of the person, the attitudes of significant others, the degree of invasiveness of the effects of the substance use, and the existence of alternatives. Interventions have been developed to assist some individuals in achieving moderation. Additionally, some research has shown that a small percentage of individuals who recognize a harmful pattern of substance use are able to stop using the substance or to achieve a controlled, nonpathological pattern of use. There are those who, because they experience an important life change, such as graduating from college or getting married, appear to change from excessive use to social alcohol use.

Nevertheless, many people exhibit serious problems related to their use of substances and are usually not able to stop or control their use without outside intervention. Research on identified problem drinkers' ability to return to social alcohol use is still inconclusive. Consequently, most scientists and health care providers advocate abstinence as a cornerstone of recovery.

Abstinence is difficult to maintain on a long-term basis. Therefore, an important area of continuing research is relapse prevention (i.e., a behavioral approach that aims to prepare the client for the relapse situation in the hope of preventing it or minimizing its impact on recovery). Relapse prevention models can be applied to alcohol, drug, and behavioral addictive problems (e.g., overeating and compulsive gambling) and can have either controlled use or abstinence as their goal. In relapse prevention, relapses are reframed as learning opportunities, and the client makes plans for coping with negative mood states, meeting the challenge of craving, and stopping a relapse quickly if it should occur.

BOX 26-1 CAGE: AN ALCOHOLISM SCREENING TEST

C "Have you ever felt that you should **C**ut down on your drinking?"
A "Have people **A**nnoyed you by criticizing your drinking?"
G "Have you ever felt bad or **G**uilty about your drinking?"
E "Have you ever had a drink, or an **E**ye-opener, first thing in the morning to steady your nerves or get rid of a hangover?"
• Two positive responses to these questions are considered a positive test and indicate that further assessment is warranted.

Modified from Ewing JA: Detecting alcoholism: the CAGE questionnaire, *JAMA* 252:1905-1907, 1984.

Inpatient and outpatient are the two main types of treatment programs for substance abuse. Each of these programs may or may not include a detoxification component. Treatment programs also differ in the following ways: they may be voluntary versus compulsory and pharmacologically based versus drug free. In general, although treatment is intricately tied to the concept of recovery, disciplinary philosophy guides specific treatment approaches. There are a variety of treatment approaches and models, which are sometimes contradictory. The treatment models vary by such factors as the composition of staff and the philosophical approach (i.e., social vs. psychological vs. medical models) to substance abuse problems.

Inpatient treatment isolates individuals from the external world and provides an opportunity to focus only on substance abuse issues. Outpatient treatment is appropriate for those who do not require such structure and protection, those with strong supportive social networks and high levels of motivation, and those who need to continue working while in recovery.

The severity of the individual's alcohol or drug problems and pertinent cultural factors determine the necessity and type of treatment. Therefore the assessment process is of primary importance and begins with an accurate social and medical history. The history taking begins with more general questions about lifestyle, employment, relationships, and self-perception. This general line of questioning permits the development of a therapeutic relationship with the client.

A therapeutic relationship based on trust is essential to collecting information about sensitive issues such as drug and alcohol use. The assessment should then proceed to determining risky behavior patterns and stressors. The interviewer assesses dietary practices; prior health problems; allergies; hospitalizations, including psychiatric disorders; and family history of similar problems, including drug- and alcohol-related problems. This general line of questioning can be followed by more specific questions about harmful behaviors, such as smoking, drinking, and illicit drug use. This ordering of questions progresses from the more socially sanctioned behaviors to more "socially disapproved" behaviors and from the general to the more specific. Positive responses to questions about drug and alcohol use should be probed in a nonjudgmental, direct way and treated as "routine" in health care encounters.

A physical examination is another valuable tool in evaluating the client for potential or actual alcohol and drug problems. Although at-risk clients may not have physical signs of alcohol and drug problems and may even deny obvious consequences of such, certain physical findings warrant further investigation. Complaints such as vague, nonspecific abdominal pain, insomnia, depression, chronic fatigue, back pain, chronic anxiety, refractory hypertension, and night sweats require more intensive investigation. Spider angiomata on the thorax or face may be the result of long-term alcohol use. Consistent and heavy users of methamphetamine commonly experience extensive and rampant tooth decay, known as "Meth Mouth" due to the acidic nature of the drug. Although laboratory tests may not yield clues to drug or alcohol use, certain laboratory findings (e.g., abnormal liver function), in the absence of other etiological agents, may increase the index of suspicion.

Intervention strategies frequently begin with information about the effects of alcohol and drugs and a discussion of the solutions to substance abuse–related problems. This initial educational approach can defuse frequently encountered barriers to intervention such as shame, guilt, fear, and the client's erroneous perceptions regarding risks. Presenting information and solutions in a nonjudgmental and clear manner may help minimize defensiveness. Reframing interventions within the context of health maintenance or health promotion and education minimizes the sense of stigma.

Ambivalent clients may respond to education and decide to abstain from substances or seek treatment. Other clients, however, even when confronted with legal, financial, physical, and psychological consequences of substance abuse, may resist treatment offers. Therefore the clinician must continue to work with clients and involve important members of their social network to remove internal and environmental barriers and move clients toward readiness for change and treatment. Potential discrimination in group settings and logistical problems, such as lack of child care, may be barriers to treatment.

Much of the effort for substance abuse treatment has been invested in detoxification, residential, and outpatient treatment programs. Secondary problems related to drug and alcohol abuse are intoxication, overdose, and withdrawal. Overdose may be accidental or intentional and requires acute interventions to stabilize the client. As a client advocate, the community health nurse can be an important ally in ensuring that adequate follow-up is conducted for those admitted to emergency departments for overdose. Detoxification is best described as a short-term treatment intervention designed to manage acute withdrawal from the substance. It involves medical management to reduce the adverse side effects of the substance and help stabilize the client. This may be performed on an inpatient or outpatient basis, depending on the substance and severity of dependence.

Addressing acute withdrawal symptoms is of utmost importance in detoxification. The cocaine abuser may experience extreme depression with suicidal ideation. Withdrawal from central nervous system depressants, including alcohol, produces the most life-threatening medical consequences, including anxiety, tremors, delirium, convulsions, and possible death unless medically managed. Symptoms of withdrawal from narcotics, although less life threatening, are temporarily disabling and painful, including chills, sweating, cramps, and nausea. Such feelings may cause the individual who is withdrawing from treatment to begin the cycle of abuse again. Detoxification is one of the most crucial periods in the recovery process. Clinicians should be aware of the level of services offered in any detoxification program in order to make appropriate referrals.

Outpatient and inpatient treatment programs vary, but they usually include group and individual therapy and counseling, motivational interviewing, family counseling, education, and socialization into twelve-step mutual self-help groups. Many programs are integrating psychotherapy, such as cognitive-behavioral therapy, with pharmacotherapy. These medications are discussed more fully in the next section. Other strategies include hypnosis, occupational therapy, confrontation, assertiveness training, blood alcohol–level discrimination training, and other behavior modification approaches. Relapses are common; therefore the most effective treatment programs incorporate some form of relapse prevention as a part of the healing process.

Therapy that involves the family has proved to be most effective in aiding recovery. Family and social contacts can be helped to initiate change in the abuser, to aid in recovery, and to assist in maintenance of treatment gains. A well-known family involvement motivational technique is the Johnson Institute Intervention, involving a confrontation of the abuser with guidance from therapists. A less coercive version of this is called A Relational Sequence for Engagement (ARISE), where significant others are educated and coached over a period of time. Another effective strategy is Community Reinforcement and Family Training (CRAFT). With this approach, a concerned significant other is trained in techniques such as positive reinforcement, identification of dangerous situations, and stress reduction (Fals-Stewart, O'Farrell, and Birchler, 2003). NIDA (1999) published a research-based guide to drug addiction treatment. Important points from this publication are listed in Box 26-2.

Treatment programs have been unprepared for the influx and unique problems associated with MA. Prolonged use may lead to serious acute psychotic disorders with intensive physical and psychological withdrawal characterized by protracted anhedonia and dysphoria, accompanied by severe craving (Kuyper et al., 2004). Currently, there are no medications to reverse overdoses and no reliable drugs to treat the paranoia and psychosis associated with MA. Complications of treatment include high dropout rates, severe behavioral and psychotic states, and severe craving (Rawson, Gonzales, and Brethen, 2002).

Various treatments for MA abuse and addiction are being tried with mixed results. The effect of MA on brain functioning suggests a need for longer treatment plans. The most promising is a long-term comprehensive case study approach, using home visits and assisting with transportation and emergency fund provision (Cretzmeyer et al., 2003). Cognitive-behavioral therapy and contingency management are other promising approaches for treatment of MA abuse and dependence (Rawson et al., 2002). Treatments currently being studied include aversion therapy, medication therapy, and matrix treatment plans.

Studies show that clients respond favorably to treatment, but, because of the multiple dimensions, it is a very challenging problem. Women with MA problems who have young children require an increased level of care. Specific recommendations include a pretreatment and treatment safe place center for social and emotional support (Cretzmeyer et al., 2003). Because many abusers lack a supportive environment, the potential for relapse is increased. Also, because of MA

BOX 26-2 GUIDELINES FOR DRUG ABUSE TREATMENT

- A single treatment is not appropriate for all individuals. Treatment should be tailored to the specific needs of the individual because not all addicts and alcoholics are the same.
- Treatment must be readily available when people who are addicted are ready for treatment.
- Effective treatment attends to the multiple needs of the individual, not just his or her substance use. It must address associated medical, psychological, social, vocational, and legal problems. Treatment should stress the importance of interaction with family or significant others and attempt to engage important social network members in the process.
- An individual's treatment and services plan must be assessed continually and modified as necessary to ensure that the plan meets the individual's changing needs.
- Remaining in treatment for an adequate time is crucial for treatment effectiveness. For most patients, the threshold of significant improvement is reached in about 3 months.
- Individual or group counseling and other behavioral therapies are critical components of effective treatment for addiction.
- Medications are an important element of treatment for many patients, especially when combined with counseling and other behavioral therapies.
- Addicted or drug-abusing individuals with coexisting mental disorders should have both disorders treated in an integrated way.
- Medical detoxification is only the first stage of addiction treatment and does little to change long-term substance abuse.
- Treatment does not need to be voluntary to be effective.
- Possible drug use during treatment must be monitored continuously.
- Treatment programs should provide assessment for HIV and AIDS, hepatitis B and C, tuberculosis, and other infectious diseases and should provide counseling to help patients modify or change behaviors that place themselves or others at risk for infection.
- Recovery from drug addiction can be a long-term process and commonly requires multiple episodes of treatment. Relapses can occur, but participation in mutual help groups or self-help groups and ongoing support is helpful to maintain abstinence. Treatment is not recovery, but it is part of the recovery process and experience. Treatment programs must address the aftercare needs of the client to maintain the gains made in treatment.

From National Institute on Drug Abuse: *Principles of drug addiction treatment: a research-based guide*, NIH Pub No. 09-4180, Washington, DC, 2009, Government Printing Office.

---

addicts' typical inability to recognize the problematic nature of their use, combined drug court and outpatient treatment strategies are being developed.

Having a substance abuse problem does not mean that problems are always attributable to the addiction. Many substance-abusing clients also have other psychiatric problems (e.g., schizophrenia, depression, bipolar affective disorder, dissociative disorder, posttraumatic stress disorder). Likewise, many of these clients have chronic medical problems. In cases with compounding problems, specialized attention involving a case management approach is warranted.

Research demonstrates that treatment for substance abuse can be more effective than no treatment, but evaluation of treatment alternatives requires establishment of appropriate

BOX 26-3 CRITERIA FOR MEASURING EFFECTIVENESS OF SUBSTANCE ABUSE TREATMENT PROGRAMS

- Number of days abstinent
- Number of days without negative consequences of substance use
- Employability or work attendance
- Self-image improvement
- Spouse's assessment of client's functionality
- Regular attendance at twelve-step group meetings
- Compliance with follow-up appointments
- Absence of overt psychiatric symptoms such as depression or anxiety
- Self-reports of progress
- Evidence of personal satisfaction and growth

criteria to measure effectiveness (Simpson, 2004). Examples of criteria that have been used are shown in Box 26-3. It is clear that treatment programs vary and that certain programs will be more culturally appropriate and therefore more effective than others for particular aggregates of individuals.

Pharmacotherapies

In the search for successful treatment of those susceptible to drug and alcohol problems, several pharmacotherapeutic adjuncts to formalized treatment have been developed. Medications include drugs used to assist in the initiation and maintenance of abstinence, drugs used as a substitute for illegal drug use, or drugs used to treat comorbidities. This section discusses pharmacotherapies that providers currently use. Good clinical judgment and patient motivation should guide the use of any pharmacotherapy, and therapy should be combined with psychosocial support.

Pharmacotherapy is used in detoxification, stabilization, and maintenance; as antagonists; and as treatment for coexisting disorders. Clinically, it is considered better to prevent withdrawal symptoms with medication than to wait for symptoms to appear. Methadone is the treatment of choice in withdrawal from heroin or other opiates. As a detoxification agent, methadone is dispensed over an 8-day period in a tapering dose. Dosage is dependent on the degree of opiate withdrawal symptoms present. A widely used example of the use of medication for long-term stabilization is methadone maintenance. The client is prescribed daily administration of a long-acting opioid (methadone) as a substitute for the illicit use of opiates (typically heroin). A large body of research confirms its effectiveness in treatment retention and reduction of risks such as human immunodeficiency virus (HIV) (Carroll, 2003).

However, there are continuing varying philosophical opinions about abstinence versus sanctioned use in the debate over the use of methadone. Methadone maintenance is more controversial because the individual remains dependent on the drug. It is dispensed under medical supervision as part of a treatment program. Maintenance may minimize or abate illegal activity, eliminate the infection hazards of injection

drug use, reduce the social disruption typically seen with opiate use, and facilitate increased levels of functioning. A myth about maintenance programs is that methadone produces a euphoric "high" and is therefore merely a legal substitute for heroin.

Naltrexone is a long-acting narcotic antagonist traditionally used as an adjunct in the treatment of opiate dependence. It blocks the effects of opiates via competitive binding, but it does not block the effects of other substances such as benzodiazepines, cocaine, and alcohol (Carroll, 2003). Recent studies indicate that naltrexone is also effective in reducing craving, rates of relapse to alcohol, and severity of alcohol-related problems (Carmen, 2004).

Buprenorphine is an opioid agonist-antagonist that has been used in the treatment of opiate-dependent clients and those with concurrent cocaine dependence. Buprenorphine does not produce severe withdrawal on abrupt cessation, which is an advantage over methadone. Its antagonist component helps reduce the possibility of lethal overdose. Clinical studies support the use of buprenorphine in reducing the frequency of heroin and cocaine self-administration.

Use of disulfiram (Antabuse) to promote cessation of alcohol abuse is rare today because of serious safety issues. A select group (i.e., those who are relapse prone, those who have supportive networks, and those who have histories of abstinence) may benefit from short-term use. Requests for disulfiram should not be granted in the absence of treatment and supportive relationships. Disulfiram, when combined with alcohol, produces the classic disulfiram ethanol reaction (DER) (i.e., flushing, tachycardia, nausea, headache, chest tightness, and chest pain). The DER is thought to be the result of a disturbance in alcohol metabolism. The response, which typically begins within minutes after alcohol consumption, is dose dependent and highly variable. Significant risks of the DER are cardiovascular symptoms of tachycardia, hypotension, dysrhythmia, and shock. Preexisting cardiac disease is an absolute contraindication. Emergency treatment of the DER is symptomatic.

Benzodiazepines are considered effective tools for alcohol withdrawal because they decrease the likelihood of seizures and delirium (Naegle and D'Avanzo, 2001). Acamprosate (calcium acetyl homotaurinate) has been used successfully in Europe over the past decade and recently allowed for use in the United States. The main efficacy is with reducing drinking frequency and abstinence maintenance. Acamprosate (Campral) reduces glutamatergic transmission and neuronal hyperexcitability during withdrawal from alcohol. This drug has a low incidence of side effects but should be used under the care of a physician and prescribed cautiously in patients with liver or kidney problems. No withdrawal syndrome or abuse has been shown as yet (Mann, Lehert, and Morgan, 2004).

Mutual Help Groups

Mutual help groups are associations that are voluntarily formed, are not professionally dominated, and operate through face-to-face supportive interaction focusing on a mutual goal.

BOX 26-4 BASIC TENETS OF TWELVE-STEP PROGRAMS

- Admission of defeat and surrender to a higher power
- Inventory of past shortcomings and strengths
- Spiritual practices (e.g., prayer and meditation)
- Willingness to change
- Making amends
- Extension of this process into daily life

Many mutual help groups exist, and they are usually organized by recovering substance abusers or those recovering from compulsive behavior patterns. The first mutual help group was Alcoholics Anonymous (AA), founded in 1935. Initially, a small group of male alcoholics found a way to stay sober "one day at a time" through meeting regularly with others like themselves. The early AA members developed twelve steps to guide the recovery process (Kurtz, 1979). The process is summarized in Box 26-4.

As a nonprofessional ongoing source of assistance, AA is viewed as an invaluable resource to the community. However, not all of those with alcohol problems find AA comfortable, culturally relevant, and socially supportive. Because realities of social discrimination and regional variation in customs exist, AA should not be considered a universal form of assistance for alcohol problems. Predominantly in large cities, women and members of racial, ethnic, religious, or sexual preference minority groups with alcohol problems have formed their own AA groups and other mutual help organizations for support in recovery.

Other twelve-step programs have developed through the adaptation of AA's approach to similar addictive problems. Narcotics Anonymous, Gamblers Anonymous, Debtors Anonymous, Cocaine Anonymous, Overeaters Anonymous, and Sex and Love Addicts Anonymous are examples. Because they became organized more recently than AA, these groups may not be as well known or as widely available, and they may not exhibit as much diversity among their membership as AA. Children, partners, and close associates of substance abusers have also founded self-help groups, such as Al-Anon, Codependents Anonymous, and Adult Children of Alcoholics. Although these groups initially had a predominance of female members, the trend is moving toward participation by equal numbers of men and women.

AA meetings are not standardized. Customs shaping the actual format and sequence of the meeting vary according to region, group size, ethnic and sex composition, and other cultural variations of the members. In general, twelve-step meetings follow one of the following formats:

- Uninterrupted talks by one or more speakers about "what it was like, what happened, and what it is like now."
- Each person at the meeting has the opportunity to speak briefly during discussion.
- A combination of the first two options.
- Meetings may be either closed or open to the general public.

At least two mutual help groups have developed in response to their founders' negative experiences in AA or their failure to succeed in AA. Women for Sobriety was organized in 1976 to replace or augment AA for women; it addresses women's needs to overcome depression, guilt, and low self-esteem. Secular Sobriety Groups were organized to meet the needs of individuals who are unable to accept the concept of, or to depend on, a "higher power" in their recovery from alcohol problems.

Other mutual help groups that do not follow the twelve steps are available for a variety of addictive problems. AA does not require dues or fees, but some groups, such as Weight Watchers, require monetary commitment. Other groups, such as Recovery Incorporated, have more professional involvement. Any of these groups could be a resource for selected people with substance abuse problems.

To be effective, interventions for substance abuse must take place at multiple levels and involve a number of individuals, activities, policies, and substances. Table 26-3 summarizes some of the many interventions for substance abuse at various levels.

Harm Reduction

New approaches reflecting a changing view of drug and alcohol addiction have been proposed for substance use problems that

TABLE 26-3 MODES OF INTERVENTION FOR SUBSTANCE ABUSE

LEVEL	INTERVENTION
Individual and family levels	Education Treatment: detoxification, inpatient, outpatient, and residential Mutual help groups (e.g., AA, Narcotics Anonymous, Cocaine Anonymous, Al-Anon, and NarcAnon)
Community level	Law enforcement measures to limit access to and distribution of addictive substances (e.g., street drugs) Alcohol taxes and zoning schemes for liquor outlets Legal drinking age and legal sanctions on driving while intoxicated Educational programs at schools and penal institutions Television and radio public service communications concerning the risks of substance abuse and the availability of treatment
State and federal levels	Formation of national associations such as the National Council on Alcoholism and Drug Dependence Establishment of federal research entities such as the National Institute on Drug Abuse and the National Institute on Alcohol Abuse and Alcoholism to centralize research, education, and treatment efforts Legislative provisions at the state level to fund substance abuse treatment and rehabilitation

are not amenable to traditional approaches. Some of these have been grouped under the general term **harm reduction**. Harm reduction consists of individual and collective approaches to the treatment of substance use that are not primarily aimed at complete abstinence from all substances. Instead, incremental change is sought, which involves elimination of the more harmful effects of substance use through behavior and policy modifications. Harm reduction is a process rather than a static approach or an end in itself. It is used in various ways, depending on the context and the needs of individual clients (Erickson, 1999; MacCoun, 1998).

Harm reduction strategies remain controversial although some see them as a paradigm shift with the potential to significantly improve treatment results. They are often the only options that will preserve a therapeutic relationship when people continue to use or drink problematically. An early example of harm reduction is the substitution of methadone for heroin. Although they are still using an opiate, individuals taking methadone can be functional without getting high and without the need to engage in criminal activity for drugs. Harm reduction psychotherapy aims to support the process of self-transformation through empathetic resonance, raising awareness of harm, setting goals, and understanding the multiple meanings of the substance (Tatarsky, 2003). Harm reduction has been used in response to alcohol, illicit drugs, and tobacco. In the case of alcohol, harm reduction might involve decreasing the number of drinks, decreasing the number of days in which drinking occurs, or avoiding drinking when driving.

On a community level, harm reduction may include attempts to legislate for decreased access to alcohol or raising the legal age for drinking. More controversial public health projects aimed at harm reduction are legalization of some illicit drugs and needle exchange programs. Needle exchange programs have had some success, and although they may not lead the intravenous drug user to abstinence, they do, in fact, serve to break the link in the deadly chain of acquired immunodeficiency syndrome (AIDS) exposure and transmission (Des Jarlais, 2004).

Viewed from a community health perspective, harm reduction involves planned social and policy changes. The goal of these changes is to decrease health risks consequent to alcohol and other drug use among specific aggregates (Kearney, 1999; Wodak, 1995). Although harm reduction strategies are not usually sanctioned by lay support systems (e.g., twelve-step groups), they can have an important impact. Community health nurses using harm reduction strategies can help reduce drug- and alcohol-related social problems by advocating for programs that "bridge the gap" for those who cannot immediately reach the goal of abstinence.

People who drive while impaired by alcohol or other drugs are a public health hazard to themselves and others. During 2004, almost 16,700 deaths were due to alcohol- or drug-related motor vehicle accidents. Reduction in alcohol-involved motor vehicle–related fatalities requires a variety of interventions to change drinking and driving behaviors. These include altering drivers' perceptions of risk to themselves and to others riding with them, increasing efforts to screen for alcoholism among people convicted of driving while intoxicated, and changing public policy to deter adult drinking and driving (CDC, 2006).

SOCIAL NETWORK INVOLVEMENT

Family and Friends

The social network of the substance abuser can either be highly influential in helping the individual alter behavior or aid and abet the substance abuser in self-destruction. There is evidence for both positive and negative effects of social support in either mitigating or supporting the behaviors of substance abusers (Latimer, 2003). Particularly among adolescents and young adults, evidence suggests that substance use and abuse often occur in the context of social interactions. Adolescents may use alcohol and other substances as a social lubricant during an often-troubled developmental period (Stinchfield and Winters, 2003). Family treatment is considered essential because of the potential for enabling behavior. In addition, the family has suffered the effects of substance abuse emotionally, socially, economically, physically, and spiritually. The family's wounds must be acknowledged and treated in order for the substance abuser to return to an environment supportive of recovery.

A user's social network may play a role in allowing the substance abuse to continue. Spouses may call work to report that their partner is "sick" or remain silent when evidence of abuse is discovered. Complex community and family interactions that serve to promote certain behaviors are commonly known as *codependency* and *enabling*. The boundaries between the nonaddicted family members and addict waver with the result that the excessive substance-abusing behavior is covered up or excused (Hanson et al., 2002). Social network members may compensate for the fact that the student is absent from school, the car payment is late, or an important appointment is canceled or forgotten. These distress signals are common but often go unrecognized because periods of use are often interspersed with periods of abstinence. This reinforces the individual's, and often the significant other's, perceived sense of control over the substance use. There are mutual help groups for addressing codependency that are founded on the principles of AA and provide opportunities to discuss the issues germane to the alcoholic or addicted family system or network. Families participating in treatment should also be encouraged to participate in these mutual help groups.

Codependency cannot be concretely defined the same way in each culture. Cultural groups vary in the degree to which individuals are expected to anticipate the needs of others and care for them. The danger in applying a rigid definition of codependency in all cases is that it might unfairly and inappropriately label it as a disease in some cultures that value interdependency over individualism.

Through development of a therapeutic relationship and comprehensive assessment, the community nurse should identify the important members of the social network for each client and the ways in which these individuals provide support for the client. The nurse must also recognize that the concept of family refers not only to nuclear families but also to alternative family systems. Whatever the constellation of family, significant others should be included in the treatment and intervention. Substance abuse, addiction, and recovery do not occur in a vacuum, and many relapses are precipitated by interpersonal conflicts.

Effects on the Family

Substance abuse has been called a family disease because it affects the entire family system and holds potential adverse psychological and physical consequences for the family members in addition to the abuser. Family theorists view families, whether the traditional nuclear form or an alternative, as social systems that try to stay in balance (Friedmann, Bowden, and Jones, 2003). Professionals may see families as either functional or dysfunctional depending on how well they fulfill the social tasks expected of them by society. Substance-abusing families are frequently observed to be dysfunctional in clinical terms. However, cultural and political factors should also be considered because families may have developed these patterns for historical reasons rather than as the effects of substance abuse.

A functional family system is open and flexible and allows its members to be themselves. In the nuclear family model, the parents model intimacy for the children, differences are negotiated, boundaries are defined and maintained, and communication is consistent and clear. In functional family systems, whether the traditional nuclear family or other nontraditional forms, there is trust, individuality, and accountability among family members. All family members are able to have their needs met in a reasonable way.

On the other hand, dysfunctional families are closed systems with fixed, rigid roles. In the case of substance abuse, a major purpose of the system is to deny the substance abuse of the affected family member and keep it a "shameful" family secret. Generally, ego boundaries between the family members are weakened or nonexistent, with enmeshment of the members and an intolerance of individual differences. Rules are rigid and communication is unbalanced; the dynamics are either always conflicting or always superficially pleasant. Children may become involved in a "role reversal" in which they act as caretakers of their parents.

When one or more family members are substance abusers, family functions revolve around the substance abuser and accommodate or compensate the abuser's behavior (Naegle and D'Avanzo, 2001). The individual needs of other family members are often unmet. Denial is central to a "dysfunctional" family system. The spouse of the substance abuser may gradually take over that person's role, functions, and control of the family. The children are cast into various roles in their struggle for survival in this environment and to maintain the family.

The family role identification theory, which was developed by Wegscheider-Cruse (1981), showed the importance of four distinct family roles, the *Hero*, the *Scapegoat*, the *Lost Child*, and the *Mascot* that children will adopt.

The Hero role is exemplified by an overachieving individual, usually the eldest child, who receives validation through taking on responsibility and caretaking functions of the family. This individual excels in academic, sport, and/or other activities that will bring esteem to the family. However, to focus the family away from the main issue, the alcoholic, the Troublemaker or Scapegoat acts out in destructive manner. This child is blamed for the problems, or dysfunction, and is often in trouble at home, in school, or in the community. The Lost Child, usually the middle or third child, is disconnected from the family and finds intimacy outside of the immediate family. He or she avoids confrontation and is lonely. The Mascot role is usually fulfilled by the baby of the family who takes on the responsibility of levity and "clowning around" to deflect the negative consequences of the alcoholic's behavior. These roles are adopted to allow the dysfunctional alcoholic family to survive, but at the detriment of all family members. Each of these roles contributes to the stagnation of personal growth, self-sacrifice, low self-esteem, and unhappiness in order to preserve the "family."

Adult children from dysfunctional families often carry these roles and coping mechanisms into adult life, with many becoming substance abusers or partners of substance abusers. The children of alcoholics are four to nine times more likely to experience alcohol use disorders than are children of nonalcoholics (Anda, 2002). Frequently, they have difficulties with intimacy and parenting. Many have lifelong emotional problems such as depression and anxiety and physical illnesses often associated with these conditions (e.g., ulcers, colitis, migraine headaches, and eating disorders). However, some offspring exhibit thriving and resilient behavior. Using a strength-based approach, the community health nurse can work with resiliency factors (Mylant, 2002).

In addition to psychological burdens that substance abuse places on families, there are the financial burdens related to medical costs, loss of income from job difficulties or unemployment, and the financial losses attributable to divorce. Further, spousal violence and child abuse and neglect are strongly associated with substance abuse (Holtzworth-Munroe, 2004).

Professional Enablers

Health care professionals also can contribute to the initiation and continuation of substance abuse and dependency in various ways, becoming professional enablers. One obvious way is the physician's role in prescribing psychoactive medications. The medical model advocates the treatment of symptoms by medication. The relief of pain, anxiety, and insomnia is not an exception. The addictive potential of narcotic analgesics and antianxiety agents is often ignored if quick symptom relief is the main goal. Long-term goals for the treatment of medical problems and nonmedication management of pain and anxiety are more thoughtful approaches. However, undermedication or refusal to use "addictive" medicines can lead susceptible clients to self-medicate with illegal drugs or alcohol.

Physicians and nurses are often the first to see the physical effects of substance abuse and are in an excellent position to intervene. By focusing on the health consequences of substance abuse, they can form trusting relationships, provide information, and refer patients to the appropriate treatment. Too often, this opportunity is missed because the health care professional is reluctant to bring up this taboo subject. This reluctance may be based on professionals' inability to examine their own drinking or drug-taking behaviors, or those of significant others, or concerns of negative responses by clients.

In the past, many psychiatrists and psychotherapists have focused on the reasons their client uses substances rather than on the dependency itself. The assumption was that insight would lead to a change in behavior. This approach has usually not proved to be effective, especially if the psychiatrist is concurrently prescribing other potentially addictive antianxiety medications or hypnotics. Complete abstinence from all mood-altering medication is a model for preventing the cross-addiction common in substance abusers (i.e., substituting one substance for another such as a benzodiazepine for alcohol). Exceptions to this approach are patients with serious medical conditions requiring pain medication and those who also have a second psychiatric disorder that requires medication (i.e., schizophrenia, depression, bipolar affective disorder). Recovering substance abusers often need support when they must take medication for these psychiatric conditions because others may criticize the use of any medication and place the client in a difficult situation.

Caregivers have become more aware of signs of client substance abuse. Some providers are willing to begin therapy with a nonabstinent client under the stipulation that, if therapeutic gains are not made, the client will be referred for treatment or the caregiver will withdraw services. Clients who lack social support may succeed using this strategy, which allows the formation of a trusting relationship before taking the leap to abstinence. Clinical wisdom and research continue to point toward more tailored, individualized approaches to substance abuse.

VULNERABLE AGGREGATES

Substance abuse problems viewed from a community perspective clearly affect some populations more severely than others. Some groups are more susceptible to experiencing substance abuse problems, may tend to deteriorate more quickly in the process, or may have fewer sources of support for recovery. These groups are termed *vulnerable aggregates* and require special attention in terms of prevention, intervention, and rehabilitation strategies.

Current resources for prevention, treatment, and mutual support may not be flexible enough to meet the needs of various vulnerable aggregates who are at risk of experiencing substance abuse problems and are often excluded or alienated from services by policies, provider attitudes, economic con-

straints, and social isolation. This section describes the issues of substance abuse with several vulnerable aggregates, including adolescents, the elderly, women, and racial and ethnic minorities.

Preadolescents and Adolescents

Why do young people use drugs? It is clear that drug and alcohol use among adolescents is a pervasive problem with many devastating consequences. The trend data in some aspects are undoubtedly worse for adolescents than adults. The teenage years may be a turbulent time for some because of the necessary developmental tasks of discovering their own unique identity, learning how to form intimate relationships, and developing autonomy. Presently, this is accomplished in a confusing era when the cultural status of adolescents is undefined. Today's teenagers are an increasingly independent subculture with more money available than any time before, yet they have not attained full adult status.

The teenage years may be a time of experimentation, searching, confusion, rebellion, poor self-image, alienation, and insecurity. There is no such thing as the typical adolescent abuser, and there are multiple theories of causation. Researchers have concluded that adolescent drug use is a symptom and not the cause of maladjustment. Those with significant difficulty are usually using substances as coping mechanisms.

Studies have identified various predictors of adolescent substance abuse. For example, use of legal substances (e.g., tobacco, alcohol) almost always precedes use of illegal drugs. Poor school performance, a social setting where drug use is common, and drug use among peers are the strongest predictors of subsequent drug involvement, followed by strength of family bonds (Stinchfield and Winters, 2003). The younger the initiation, the greater the probability of prolonged and accelerated use. Other contributing factors are the feeling of powerlessness and selling drugs as a viable economic solution to poverty (Hanson et al., 2002). Subculture theory describes the status and power that charismatic leaders have to influence members of peer groups. In drug-using peer groups, such leaders have influence over inexperienced drug users and acculturate them into the drug scene. Thus it is crucial that communities work to maintain strong family and social bonds.

Some vulnerable adolescents may become victims of a vicious cycle. Labels used to describe people can have a profound influence on their self-perception. Labeling theory posits that when a person is judged by conventional society to be immoral, the person's perception of himself or herself will begin to mirror the accuser's perceptions (Hanson et al., 2002). For example, the teenager who experiments with marijuana and boasts about the amount may be perceived as a "stoner." In another example, teachers may find it difficult to have positive relationships with children with behavioral disorders. Research has shown that adolescents are at less risk for substance abuse if they have a positive relationship with their teachers (Stinchfield and Winters, 2003). Children with attention deficit disorder, traumatic brain injury, or psychiatric illness are known to be at increased risk because of impulsive behavior and difficulty gaining positive peer group acceptance (Ashman, 2004; Pelham, 2003). The community health nurse can play an important part in advocating for these vulnerable children and educating teachers on the vital importance of maintaining a validating, nonjudgmental attitude toward these students.

It is especially important that families are supported in the community. Substance abuse is less likely in families that give clear messages and have open communication and more likely in families where parents are alcoholic, condemning, overly demanding, or overly protective. Committed family involvement helps retain the adolescent in treatment. However, it must be remembered that many well-functioning families have children who succumb to substance abuse. These families also may experience significant community rejection and judgmental attitudes.

The preadolescent years are a particularly vulnerable time for initiation and subsequent problematic use. The number of teens between seventh and twelfth grades being offered drugs is increasing (NIDA, 2005). When drug use escalates in adolescents, it can have devastating long-lasting consequences. There is a strong relationship among adolescent behavior problems such as aggressiveness, delinquency, and criminal activity and heavy alcohol use between the ages of 12 and 17 years.

Use of marijuana has been acknowledged by 77% of teenagers (NIDA, 2005). One of the problems associated with this is that the strength of marijuana is much higher than it was in the mid-twentieth century. A phenomenon termed *amotivational syndrome* is marked by apathy and school failure and is thought to be the result of heavy marijuana use. However, there is some dissension about to whether this precedes or is the result of use of marijuana. Of much concern is the rising incidence of combining marijuana with more lethal substances, such as crack cocaine and MA (SAMHSA, 2003). Indeed, marijuana use is a strong precursor to use of more dangerous substances, such as MA and heroin (Hanson et al., 2002). Escalating use of substances enhances the risk of school and social failure, criminal activities, violent behavior, sexual risk taking, sexual violence (such as date rape), depression, suicide, and unintended injuries. Further, 50% of motor vehicle injuries in teenagers are related to drug or alcohol use (SAMHSA, 2003).

Primary prevention for adolescents is typically focused on education aimed toward complete abstinence, which some say is unrealistic. Education plays an important role. A striking feature is the strong adverse relationship between perceived risk and drug use. For all drugs, with no change in drug availability, when students perceive a drug as harmful, fewer students actually use it (SAMHSA, 2005). Large-scale media efforts can bring about change but only with accompanying parental and community efforts. Early detection of predisposing factors, such as underlying psychiatric illness, is important. Other strategies are providing structured clubs and organizations and facilitating school success, career skills, family communication skills, and conflict resolution. Secondary prevention is targeted at inpatient and outpatient treatment and harm reduction.

However, almost as important as intervention and treatment is recognizing when treatment is unnecessary. Not all drug use requires therapy, nor is it even desirable. Not all young drug users are antisocial or mentally unstable, nor should they be labeled as such. For the most part, most will develop a responsible philosophy concerning substance use if given support and opportunity.

The increasingly sophisticated technology used to prepare for athletic competition has been a significant factor in the self-administration of performance-enhancing substances and associated risky injection practices. These substances include steroids and over-the-counter stimulant drugs and herbs, with steroids the most common. Nonmedical use of steroids poses serious problems, because use is both illegal and dangerous. Behavioral and health problems that have been noted with steroid use include suicides, homicides, liver damage, and heart attacks.

Many substance abuse researchers believe that attempts to enhance athletic performance with steroids and other substances reduce the perceived negative consequences of substance abuse and increase the likelihood of using illicit drugs for other purposes. In addition, limited access to needles and other equipment results in a high rate of needle sharing among adolescent teammates who inject substances to enhance their performance (USDHHS, 2000).

Elderly

Elderly men and women are considered vulnerable to substance abuse problems because they have diminished physiological tolerance, increased use of medically prescribed drugs, and cultural and social isolation. Conservative estimates indicate that 6% to 11% of elderly patients admitted to hospitals exhibit symptoms of alcoholism, as do 20% of the elderly in psychiatric hospitals, and 14% of elderly patients in emergency departments (Adams and Cox, 1997).

Misuse of prescription drugs may be the most common form of drug abuse among the elderly. According to NIDA (1999), elderly persons use prescription medications approximately three times as frequently as the general population. In addition, data from the Veterans Affairs Hospital System suggest that elderly patients may be prescribed inappropriately high doses of benzodiazepines. Alcohol and prescription drug use, especially benzodiazepines, are significant factors in geriatric trauma (Zautcke et al., 2002).

Substance abuse in the elderly is commonly missed by health care providers (Beullens, 2004). An important part of early intervention efforts is thorough assessment and appropriate diagnosis. This can be difficult with the elderly because they do not manifest problems with substance abuse in the same ways as younger people. Thoughtful and routine use of assessment tools such as the MAST-G and the CAGE questionnaire can be valuable in determining the presence of substance abuse in the elderly (Beullens, 2004).

Women

Since the 1970s, much attention has been turned to substance abuse problems in women. Evidence is mounting that alcohol use and abuse affect women much differently than they affect men. Women absorb and metabolize alcohol differently than do men, partly because of body composition differences and the production of less gastric alcohol dehydrogenase by women (Cook, 2004). Specific aggregates of women may be more severely affected by substance abuse problems, including women from minority groups, low-income or no-income women, and working-class women. The increased risk stems from economic, social, and cultural factors.

Lesbians are another aggregate of women in whom substance abuse may be associated with marginalization and should be understood within the diversity of lesbians individually and culturally. This is especially heightened in periods when homosexuality is demonized through media, churches, and legislation linking homosexuality with pathology and when lesbians and gays are denied the right to marry (e.g., civil unions, partner benefits).

Women who were abused as children are more susceptible to substance abuse problems in adolescence and adulthood than are nonabused women. They also face many more distressing consequences in substance abuse treatment and recovery. Disclosure of abuse in group treatment contexts or twelve-step meetings is risky. In some cases, women are told to compartmentalize the abuse issues and only speak of addiction. In other cases, women are told that if they do not disclose in a group they will fail in their recovery program (Hall, 1996b). However, many current-day treatment programs designed for women now routinely address interpersonal violence in individual and group settings, leaving disclosure up to the client.

Drug-dependent women report frequent physical and medical problems, many related to their reproductive systems (Wetherington and Roman, 1998). Women tend to experience symptoms of alcoholic hepatitis and cirrhosis sooner than men because they metabolize alcohol at a different rate. They also have higher blood alcohol levels relative to body weight and higher mortality rates from heavy drinking (Cook, 2004).

Excessive alcohol use, especially binge drinking, during pregnancy continues to have long-term developmental consequences in the newborn (Cook, 2004). Cocaine use during pregnancy is associated with increased risk of spontaneous abortion, premature delivery, and abruptio placentae. Infants who have been addicted to cocaine in utero are hyperirritable, subject to seizures, and possibly at increased risk for sudden infant death syndrome. Long-term learning disabilities, behavioral problems, mental retardation, and physical handicaps are other potential consequences associated with children of cocaine-using mothers (Messinger, 2004).

Getting the pregnant woman into treatment and managing her withdrawal are frequently problematic. The woman's fear of punitive legal actions complicates the process. Additionally, the addiction itself often interferes with obtaining adequate prenatal care. If addiction is linked with risky sexual behavior, or sexual assault, there is an increased risk

of contracting HIV and hepatitis viruses that can infect the infant; testing should be recommended.

Ethnocultural Considerations

Community health nurses need to be culturally competent and aware of certain ethnocultural vulnerabilities and differing perspectives when considering treatments for individuals with substance abuse. Ethnocultural competency can be defined as "the ability of a clinician to function effectively in the context of ethnocultural differences" (Straussner, 2003, p. 7). Data on African Americans, Hispanics, and Native Americans suggest an increased risk for substance abuse. However, the usual ethnic/racial categories in research do not take into account the distinctions within each category. Consequently, there are limited data, especially about middle-class minorities. Creating another stereotype might undermine prevention and treatment strategies. However, it is true that, under the strain of poverty, underemployment, decreased job opportunities, macro-level and micro-level aggression, and ongoing racism, some members of these aggregates find the relief in using substances, as use numbs the "social pain" caused by their environments. Racial and ethnic minorities are overrepresented among the economically disenfranchised. Limited financial resources may limit alternatives to public treatment settings, which are often understaffed, underfunded, and filled to capacity and have long waiting lists. The privatization of treatment has further decreased access.

Theories of stress, social causation, and oppressed status support the belief that discrimination and racism are a factor in the generation of mental illness and alcohol and drug problems in members of racial and ethnic minorities. Socioeconomic, political, and historical realities have encouraged some minorities to enter into the illegal drug trade as a means of economic survival. In working with ethnic and racial minorities, health care professionals must recognize the sociopolitical and socioeconomic factors that form the context of substance use, abuse, and dependency. These same factors will have an impact on seeking help, treatment, and outcome. Traditional substance abuse treatment modalities, designed primarily for white working males, sometimes overlook ethnic and racial minority experiences (Straussner, 2003). Recovery for minority groups might be contextually and experientially different from that of whites, just as the environment that contributed to the initial abuse was different.

During periods of slavery, alcohol was used as a reward, and it was seen as a way to cope. The value themes for this aggregate are a oneness with nature and spirituality, the importance of extended family, a present orientation, and a spiral concept of time. Barriers to treating African Americans with substance abuse or addiction problems are listed in Box 26-5.

Myths about certain ethnicities must be critically examined. Native Americans, for example, fight the stereotype of the drunken, once-noble warrior. However, alcohol as the predominant drug of choice does pose a threat to this population,

BOX 26-5	BARRIERS TO TREATING SUBSTANCE ABUSE AND ADDICTION PROBLEMS IN AFRICAN AMERICANS

- Weekend drinking as a reward
- Ongoing sociocultural violence
- Use of substances to escape the emotional pain caused by racism
- Poverty, underemployment, and unemployment
- Prevalence of both drugs and liquor stores within the community
- Cultural and community disintegration, which has altered traditional values and behaviors
- Allure and economic rewards of selling drugs
- Inadequate social support system for recovery
- Internalized racism harming the self-concept, along with anger and frustration
- More likely to be arrested than treated (three to six times more than whites)
- Limited role models
- Unable to "change people and places" as advocated by twelve-step programs

BOX 26-6	INTERVENTION APPROACHES FOR WORKING WITH PEOPLE FROM DIVERSE CULTURES

- Recognize that interpersonal relationships affect motivation to change.
- Express genuine interest in cultural norms.
- Dispense with assumptions based on appearance.
- Be careful not to assume privilege by using client's first name prematurely.
- Show a willingness to understand the language of the client.
- Gradually request pertinent information.
- Be sensitive to words that might imply that the client is defective.
- Recognize the role of the elders and family.

Modified from Straussner SL: *Ethnocultural factors in substance abuse treatment*, New York, 2003, Guilford Press.

particularly among youth and young adults. Native-American adolescents use drugs and alcohol earlier and with more devastating consequences than other groups (NIDA, 2005). Evidence for a biological predisposition is conflicting, and many stop drinking when they reach adulthood and their sense of family and social responsibility increases. Interventions for this group must involve long-term outreach that gains respect from the community.

Mexican Americans come from a heritage of using hallucinogens, such as sacred mushrooms and peyote, in rituals. In addition, alcohol is woven into the fabric of family life. Sociocultural factors that the community nurse should understand when planning treatment for this group include the importance of religion, *familismo* (the significance of family), fatalism (things are inevitable, or meant to be), *machismo* (bravery, strength, being a good provider), and *personalismo* (one should be pleasant and engaging socially, with dignity and a sense of honor).

In contrast, among Chinese Americans there is an increased prevalence of narcotics and decreased use of alcohol (SAMHSA, 2003). This population has a very low use of treatment services. Individual counseling is preferred, as they have a strong desire for confidentiality. However, they are receptive of pharmacological treatment (Straussner, 2003).

Studies have identified that social support has a positive effect on treatment and outcome. Without this support, the individual completing treatment may return to the original social environment, undermining any gains made within the treatment setting. Environmental cues and conditioned reinforcement for continued drug and alcohol use may be extremely powerful. The individual may return to an environment of nonsupport, characterized by continued use by important members of the individual's social network. The individual needs a well-coordinated aftercare program that addresses these issues.

The treatment of ethnic and racial minority aggregates poses special challenges related to the individuals seeking treatment. Treatment providers must recognize that these vulnerable aggregates will encounter a host of barriers that will make treatment and long-term recovery extremely difficult. For example, providers should understand the effect of rituals, holidays, music, and customs and how they can hinder progress. Providers who work from the public health perspective of "thinking upstream" will examine larger macro-level issues that increase the susceptibility of people of color to alcohol and drug problems. Box 26-6 presents helpful information on working with people from diverse cultures.

Other Aggregates

Substance abuse is the most common psychopathological problem in the general population. Within this category is a smaller aggregate of people with one or more psychiatric diagnoses in addition to substance abuse; this is referred to as dual diagnosis. Nearly one third of adults with a mental disorder also experience a co-occurring substance abuse disorder (USDHHS, 2000). This may be less readily identified by health care providers, who may fail to recognize that both problems may coexist. Treatment of dual-diagnosis individuals is complicated when the individual must take prescribed psychotropic medications. It may be perceived as prescription drug abuse or as the substitution of one addiction for another. Special attention and flexibility are needed to meet the needs of the dual-diagnosis aggregate, and such strategies are still in the developmental phase.

Childhood maltreatment, including verbal, physical, emotional, and sexual abuse and neglect, frequently leads to the development of a wide array of difficulties in adulthood. Substance abuse is one of the most common aftereffects. Approximately one in four girls and one in six boys are sexually molested before age 18 years (Hall, 1996b; Van der Kolk, McFarlane, and Weisaeth, 1996). Therefore substance abuse prevention and treatment should address these issues. However, caution should be taken to avoid forcing the disclosure of a traumatizing event in a group setting (Hall, 1996a).

In assessing the risks for substance abuse and the extent of its impact on the community, nurses must be aware that there frequently are several bases for the vulnerability occurring in one individual or group. The adolescent, the low-income Hispanic male, the lesbian African-American mother receiving public assistance, and the Native-American family living on reservation land are all facing multiple sources of vulnerability that contribute to an increased potential for substance abuse.

Special attention must be paid to the impact of sexually transmitted diseases (STDs) (e.g., HIV, herpes, genital warts, and syphilis) and their relationship to substance abuse. Substance abusers are at increased risk of STDs, including HIV, in the following ways:

- Substances may cloud judgment, which leads to high-risk sexual practices involving the exchange of body fluids (e.g., sex without the use of appropriate barriers such as condoms).
- Intravenous drug use may involve the sharing of hypodermic needles.
- Chronic substance use (e.g., alcohol, heroin, amphetamines, nicotine, and cocaine) impairs the immune system and facilitates infection by HIV or other pathogens that increase the chances of HIV infection.
- Substance abuse may hasten physical and mental deterioration from the condition of seropositivity to an AIDS diagnosis and, eventually, the terminal phase of the disease.
- Chronic substance abusers generally have few supportive relationships available to them in the process of coping with the hardships that accompany severe and chronic illnesses.
- People facing a stigmatizing, terminal, debilitating illness, in themselves or in a significant other, are more prone to experience substance abuse problems in an attempt to cope with distress.

Finally, substance abuse among health care professionals cannot be ignored. Physicians, nurses, dentists, and pharmacists are vulnerable to substance abuse; alcohol or narcotic use is most common (Trinkoff and Storr, 1998). Health care professionals are assumed to be "immune" to dependency because they are knowledgeable about medications. However, their increased access to drugs, belief in pharmaceutical solutions, and work-related stress place them at increased risk for substance abuse. Typically, they gain access to drugs through their work settings by diverting medications for their own use or by abusing drugs obtained by prescription. State regulatory boards discover the abuse by these health care professionals following drug theft or when the effects of their substance abuse impair their professional functioning.

Community health nurses should be especially vigilant because colleagues are working in isolation and episodes of incompetence may not be easily observed. Most states have rehabilitation programs for health care professionals that consist of treatment and monitoring. They are allowed to retain their professional licenses during treatment. Despite their usually favorable recovery rate, it is difficult to get this population into treatment because they exhibit denial and shame related to their substance abuse. However, the threatened loss of their professional license to practice may be a good motivator to break through their denial of the problem and encourage them to seek treatment.

NURSING PERSPECTIVE ON SUBSTANCE ABUSE

Nurses have encountered substance abuse in clients whose health problems are clearly related to alcohol abuse, such as cirrhosis of the liver, heart disease, neurological syndromes, and nutritional deficits. Unfortunately, alcohol problems were often not addressed in these health encounters in the past because there is a stigma of alcoholism and a lack of effective treatments. The nursing literature did not clearly address substance abuse as a nursing problem until the late 1960s and did not address it as a significant problem until the 1970s. Before the 1970s, substance abuse was usually viewed as a moral problem or, if it involved illicit drugs, as a legal problem.

Since the 1970s, nursing has become more involved in the spectrum of compulsive behavior problems, including substance abuse. A specialized organization, the International Nurses Society on Addictions (IntNSA) has been established with the philosophy that alcohol abuse and other drug abuse; eating disorders; sexual and relational addiction; and compulsive gambling, working, and spending are closely related behavior patterns. Additionally, educational course work related to alcohol and drug abuse is now recommended for inclusion in general nursing school curricula (Naegle, 1994).

There is a tendency in society to deal with substance abusers in stigmatizing, devaluing, coercive, and punitive ways. Negative attitudes are ubiquitous in our culture. As part of the larger culture, nurses may reflect these attitudes and have difficulty providing care to these individuals. The moral view of substance abuse implies that individuals choose to become sick, injured, or addicted.

Strong negative feelings that conflict with nursing's humanistic stance may also stem from personal experiences. Being the emotionally or physically abused spouse or child of a substance abuser can have lasting effects on nurses' attitudes toward substance-abusing clients. If nurses use alcohol or drugs to relieve stress or self-medicate dysphoric states, they may overidentify with the patient and deny the severity of the client's substance abuse.

Frequently, substance abusers are difficult clients in health care settings. When intoxicated, they may be raucous, uncooperative, and antisocial. When not intoxicated, they may exhibit none of these negative behaviors, or they may be manipulative and demanding, using flattery or intimidation to hide drug-seeking behavior. Although nurses may initially be warm and understanding, once aware of manipulative attempts, they may have difficulty maintaining an accepting, nonjudgmental attitude. Realizing that recovery from substance abuse often comes very slowly can help nurses feel less pressured to get patients into treatment and be more able simply to raise consciousness by presenting the facts about addictive illness and leaving the decision making to the client.

Nursing Interventions in the Community

The problem of substance abuse is so widespread that it affects every community and its inhabitants in varying degrees. Hence, the community health nurse is often involved with substance abusers or their significant others. Substance abuse nursing interventions with clients and their caregivers are necessary to ensure the success of other health interventions. Ignoring substance abuse problems frequently leads to lack of progress and clients' inability to perform needed health practices. This is especially frustrating for the community health nurse and other professionals who have collaborated on a comprehensive plan to allow an individual with a serious health problem to remain at home and avoid placement in an institution.

There are many ways in which community health nurses can assist individuals, families, and groups experiencing substance abuse problems. Community health nurses may be the first to identify or suspect an alcohol or drug problem in the clients and families with whom they are working. Nurses in all care contexts should routinely assess substance use patterns when performing client histories. The client history is a critical assessment and screening tool that can identify those at risk. Using current knowledge and theories about substance abuse etiology and risk factors should help identify those individuals predisposed to alcohol and drug use.

The community health nurse can be alert to environmental cues in the home that indicate substance abuse, such as empty liquor and pill bottles. An indication of prescription medication abuse is the patient's involvement with several physicians from whom narcotic analgesics and tranquilizers are obtained. This type of assessment can help with case finding and treatment referral, although the individual may have denied the existence of a substance abuse problem initially.

Denial of substance abuse or dependence may range from completely blocked awareness of the problem to partial disavowal of the detrimental effects of the substance use and abuse. One of the primary tasks for intervention and treatment with the substance-dependent individual is to increase the individual's awareness of the problem. Family and significant others can assist with this process by being more honest and direct with the individual about the detrimental effects of the substance abuse. Before this occurs, the significant others must overcome their own denial of the problem and its associated shame and guilt. Referrals to community education programs on substance abuse and dependence and mutual help groups such as Al-Anon and NarcAnon are helpful interventions for families and significant others.

The community health nurse may also involve the social network in getting the client into treatment. Although individuals who are forced to enter treatment may not be willing to admit the severity of the abuse, they can still benefit from exposure to the treatment program and eventually begin recovery. Experiencing serious health consequences related to dependency may constitute "hitting bottom" for the individual. This may break through denial or collusion on the part of the family.

The trust that develops in a caring nursing relationship can support disclosure of substance abuse problems and decrease denial in the client or family members. A realistic and positive attitude toward the person with substance abuse can provide families with hope. Community health nurses must have knowledge of available community resources. One of the primary roles of the community health nurse in helping substance abusers is to facilitate contact with helping agencies such as local treatment programs or mutual help groups. Collaboration with the client's physician is helpful, should medical detoxification be necessary. Community health nurses should assume a validating, nonjudgmental position toward the whole family and should avoid being confrontational, as it fans the fires of resistance. It is imperative that nurses ascribe a noble intention to their substance-abusing clients and families and avoid negativity or preaching.

Other traditional community health nursing roles and interventions also are appropriate to use with substance abusers. Examples follow:

- Health teaching regarding addictive illness and addictive effects of different substances
- Providing direct care for abuse-related and dependence-related medical problems
- Counseling clients and families about problems related to substance abuse
- Collaborating with other disciplines to ensure continuity of care
- Coordinating health care services for the client to prevent prescription drug abuse and avoid fragmentation of care
- Providing consultation to nonmedical professionals and lay personnel
- Facilitating care through appropriate referrals and follow-up

CASE STUDY   APPLICATION OF THE NURSING PROCESS

Evelyn Weaver, a 72-year-old widow, was referred to the Visiting Nurses Association for follow-up after hospitalization for a seizure and fall she experienced in her home. Her hospital discharge diagnoses were ethyl alcohol abuse, seizure disorder, hypertension, and bruises and contusions on her left arm and leg. Her discharge medications were phenytoin sodium (Dilantin), 900 mg orally at bedtime; one multivitamin orally every day; hydrochlorothiazide, 50 mg orally every day; and methyldopa (Aldomet), 250 mg orally every day.

Mrs. Weaver lives alone in a two-bedroom house in a middle-class suburb. Her husband died 10 years earlier. Until 4 years previous, her daughter lived nearby with her two children and visited frequently. However, after a divorce, her daughter and grandchil-

dren moved several hundred miles away and visited only once or twice a year. Mrs. Weaver has a married son in the area. He pays her bills once or twice a month but otherwise has minimal contact. Mrs. Weaver's primary occupation was homemaker and mother. She stopped driving after her last automobile accident and is not involved in any local community organizations.

Assessment
Individual
The visiting nurse performed an in-home nursing assessment of the client and obtained information through the interview and physical assessment. Mrs. Weaver admitted to an alcohol abuse problem

but minimized its severity. She reported that she stopped drinking for 2 days on her own and had a seizure. She denied any past alcohol treatment, such as counseling or attendance at AA meetings, and said she was not interested in treatment. She has been abstinent from alcohol since her discharge from the hospital and thought she would remain that way. She admitted to some loneliness and social isolation. She also reported sleep disturbances (i.e., difficulty falling asleep and staying asleep) and decreased nutritional intake with loss of appetite. She denied using other psychoactive medication, such as hypnotics, narcotic analgesics, and tranquilizers, or benzodiazepines. She agreed to a social work referral to investigate attendant care and food delivery service for seniors (e.g., Meals on Wheels [MOW]) to help her.

Family
Telephone contact between the nurse and the client's daughter revealed that the daughter was very concerned about her mother. She denied that alcohol abuse was her mother's problem but thought poor nutrition and health practices were the cause of the hospitalization. She was anxious for the social work referral to obtain attendant care to assist her mother in the home. It took several calls and messages before the nurse was able to speak with the client's son. He said his mother was an alcoholic and that he tried unsuccessfully in the past to get her to stop drinking. He was unwilling to do more than visit her twice a month to pay her bills.

Community
The client's middle-class suburb did not have alcohol treatment services geared toward the elderly. AA meetings and private substance abuse counselors were available, but none of them was willing to make home visits and assist an elderly, homebound client. The local senior center did not have programs or education involving substance abuse and refused to allow AA meetings in its building because it feared its clients would be offended. The client's physician was aware of her alcohol abuse problem but did not know how to assist her. Referral to an inpatient program for substance abuse would not help because Mrs. Weaver refused to attend.

Diagnosis
Individual
- Altered cardiovascular status secondary to hypertension
- Altered neurological status secondary to alcohol withdrawal seizures
- Deficient knowledge about addictive disease and effects of alcohol abuse
- Disturbed sleep pattern
- Imbalanced nutrition: less than body requirements
- Social isolation
- Ineffective coping related to inability to adjust to role of widow and maintain involvement in community activities
- Deficient knowledge about the effects and side effects of all of her medicines

Family
- Deficient knowledge about addictive disease and effects of excessive alcohol intake
- Deficient knowledge of treatment approaches available for alcohol abuse and the recovery process
- Interrupted family processes secondary to poor communication and denial of alcohol abuse in client

Community
- Deficient knowledge in senior center staff regarding the prevalence of alcohol abuse problems in the elderly population and adverse health effects of alcohol consumption in the elderly

- Deficient knowledge in community agencies that assist alcohol abusers (e.g., local AA and counselors) regarding the need to make home visits and provide services geared to the elderly

Planning
Planning for Mrs. Weaver's care involved collaboration among her family, her physician, the agency's social worker, and the community alcohol treatment resources. Health teaching and counseling were the main approaches used to directly assist the client and her family. Indirect approaches involved networking with community agencies and supervising other caregivers.

Individual
Short-Term Goals
- Mrs. Weaver will follow her posthospitalization treatment regimen.
- Mrs. Weaver will correctly verbalize information related to all of her medications (e.g., rationale for taking the medication, when to take it, potential side effects).
- Mrs. Weaver will seek additional counseling/treatment (e.g., AA) to assist her in staying alcohol free.

Long-Term Goals
- Mrs. Weaver will continue to abstain from using alcohol.
- Mrs. Weaver's health will improve as indicated by increased weight, decreased hypertension, and reported improvement in sleep.
- Mrs. Weaver will become more involved in community/social activities.

Family
Short-Term Goals
- Mrs. Weaver's daughter will acknowledge that her mother has a problem with alcohol abuse.
- Communication will improve between Mrs. Weaver and her children.

Long-Term Goals
- Mrs. Weaver's son and daughter will become more active in her care.
- The family will seek counseling to resolve past issues.

Community
Long-Term Goals
- Health providers in area senior centers will become more knowledgeable about the problem of alcohol abuse among elders.
- Community agencies that assist alcohol abusers will recognize the need to enhance services to elders.

Intervention
Individual
- Nursing visits two to three times weekly initially to monitor the client's medication issues or problems as related to maintaining abstinence or medication dosing, cardiovascular status, neurological status, and nutritional status
- Social work referral to establish attendant assistance in the home and food delivery service for seniors
- Health teaching regarding addictive illness, effects of excessive alcohol intake on the body, alcohol withdrawal seizures, no-added-sodium diet, and effect of medications
- Health teaching about the client's medications, their effects and side effects, and the necessity of following recommended dosing schedules
- Referral for alcohol treatment counseling and AA meetings when the individual is receptive

Continued

Family

- Continued contact with the client's daughter and son to involve them in her care
- Health teaching to the family on the course and treatment of addictive illness and the adverse effects of alcohol abuse on the client and the family as related to functioning, cohesion, and communication
- Role modeling by the visiting nurse of the use of clear, direct, and nonjudgmental communication about the client's alcohol abuse problems

Community

- List of local and national referral resources for clients with substance abuse problems made available to physicians, with a particular focus on resources providing services for older or elderly substance abusers
- Health teaching to community groups (e.g., senior center, AA fellowship, and substance abuse counselors) regarding the prevalence of alcohol abuse in the elderly population and treatment and counseling approaches useful with this aggregate
- Collaboration with community organizations that provide outreach for homebound elderly to assist in identification and referral
- Establishment of a referral network (i.e., telephone hotline) of concerned older or elderly individuals recovering from alcohol abuse

Evaluation
Individual

Initially, interventions proceeded smoothly. Mrs. Weaver obtained attendant help for 2 hours per day, three times weekly, and also received food from MOW. The visiting nurse filled her medication-organizing container, or Mediset, weekly. The attendant made sure that the client took her medications and ate her meals and assisted Mrs. Weaver with personal care. Mrs. Weaver remained abstinent from alcohol during this time but refused any treatment or counseling for her alcohol abuse problem. However, after 3 weeks, she was rehospitalized after falling at home again. She was diagnosed with phenytoin toxicity; this occurred because she had secretly been taking extra phenytoin at night to help her sleep.

After a few days, Mrs. Weaver was discharged from the hospital, and the Visiting Nurses Association reopened the case. Private attendant care and MOW were also reinstated. This time, the physician discontinued the phenytoin and recommended that the client receive alcohol counseling. The client did follow up with the counseling referrals given to her by the visiting nurse, but her social situation did not change. She remained very isolated and refused involvement with AA.

Family

A third hospitalization occurred within a few weeks when Mrs. Weaver ingested an excessive amount of alcohol in combination with her hypertensive medications. She became physically ill and required treatment. After this hospitalization, her daughter decided to take action. She moved her mother into a retirement community

that provided meals and social activities. The visiting nurse continued to follow the case in the new setting.

Her daughter encouraged her to become involved with the social activities at the community. The visiting nurse continued to remain active in the client's care by arranging for aftercare, focusing on providing goal-specific social support for abstinence and general support for addressing the client's concerns and issues, particularly as related to feelings of isolating loss and transitions. The nurse also worked with Mrs. Weaver's daughter and encouraged both to attempt to involve Mrs. Weaver's son.

Community

Staff from the retirement community contacted an area AA group and other agencies who work with substance abusers. A social worker agreed to explore ways make all involved more aware of this problem and to set up potential interventions.

Levels of prevention
Primary

- Involves health teaching to individuals and groups on risk factors, early symptoms of substance abuse, adverse health and social consequences, addictive disease process, and available treatment services
- Need to gear educational approaches to the more vulnerable aggregates (e.g., adolescents, minorities, mentally ill, women, and elderly)

Secondary

- Involves screening and early treatment approaches aimed at minimizing health and social consequences of substance abuse
- Involvement of physicians, nurses, and other health care professionals in various health care settings in this process
- Use of various screening and assessment tools and referrals to treatment services and mutual help organizations

Tertiary

- Involves more direct approaches (e.g., detoxification and inpatient or outpatient treatment) to halt the physiologically damaging effects of the substance abuse (e.g., liver disease, organic mental deficits, and gastritis)
- Frequent use of medications to treat the symptoms of substance abuse–related disorders or as part of aversion therapy (e.g., disulfiram)
- Services provided by medical practitioners, treatment services, and mutual help organizations generally advocate abstinence from the substance and improving the individual's health status

This case study illustrates the possible complexity and frustration involved in helping the substance abuser. Significant others and the medical community must be involved to help the community health nurse provide care. Often, the social situation, living situation, or social acquaintances must also change to maintain long-term recovery. However, with patience, persistence, and a caring, nonjudgmental attitude, the nurse can often be effective in helping clients with substance abuse problems attain recovery and improve their health status.

SUMMARY

This chapter provides an overview of the complex, multifaceted phenomenon of substance abuse and its manifestations in the community. The focus is on social, economic, political, and health-related aspects of substance abuse. In addition, the concept of substance abuse is related to the more general

concept of addictive behaviors, not just those related to drug or alcohol abuse.

From the review of the various etiological theories, it is clear that there is not one causative factor in the development of substance abuse. Consequently, one treatment approach does not apply to all substance abusers. Recognition of multiple factors and issues specific to vulnerable aggregates, such as women, adolescents, the elderly, and people of color, must be considered when developing intervention plans and strategies and when evaluating outcomes. Resources for prevention and intervention at the individual, family, and community levels are outlined and should be familiar to nurses practicing in the community.

LEARNING ACTIVITIES

1. Attend a local AA, Narcotics Anonymous, or Cocaine Anonymous meeting, and share impressions with classmates.
2. Attend a local Al-Anon, NarcAnon, or Adult Children of Alcoholics meeting, and share impressions with classmates.

3. Visit a local treatment center that provides detoxification, inpatient, or outpatient treatment, and determine the center's treatment philosophy and the types of services it provides to patients and their families.
4. Visit a treatment program for women, and determine how the particular needs of this population are assessed and addressed.
5. Learn about the drug and alcohol education programs at a local community college or high school.
6. Contact mental health services or substance abuse treatment services at the county or city level, and obtain a list of local treatment and education resources.

REFERENCES

Adams WL, Cox N: Epidemiology of problem drinking among elderly people. In Gurnack AM, editor: *Older adults misuse of alcohol, medicines and other drugs: research and practice issues*, New York, 1997, Springer.

American Psychiatric Association: *Diagnostic and statistical manual of mental disorders, ed 4, text revision*, Washington, DC, 2000, The Author.

Anda R: Adverse childhood experiences, alcoholic parents, and later risk of alcoholism and depression, *Psychiatr Serv* 53(8):1001–1009, 2002.

Ashman TA: Screening for substance abuse in individuals with traumatic brain injury, *Brain Inj* 18(2):191–202, 2004.

Astley SJ: Fetal alcohol syndrome prevention in Washington State: evidence of success, *Paediatr Perinat Epidemiol* 18:344–351, 2004.

Beullens J: Screening for alcohol abuse and dependence in older people using DSM criteria: a review, *Aging Ment Health* 8(1):76–82, 2004.

Block RI, Erwin WJ, Ghoneim MM: Chronic drug use and cognitive impairments, *Pharmacol Biochem Behav* 73(3):491–504, 2002.

Brecher E: *Licit and illicit drugs*, Boston, 1972, Little, Brown.

Brown R: Vitamin deficiency and voluntary alcohol consumption, *Q J Stud Alcohol* 30:592–597, 1969.

Bureau of Justice Statistics: 2002: at a glance, Washington, DC, 2002, www.ojp.usdoj.gov/bjs/pub/pdf/bjsg02.pdf.

Bureau of Justice Statistics: Drug use and crime, 2005, www.ojp.usdoj.gov/bjs/dcf/duc.htm.

Carmen B: Efficacy and safety of naltrexone and acamprosate in the treatment of alcohol dependence: a systematic review, *Addiction* 99:811–828, 2004.

Carroll K: Integrating psychotherapy and pharmacotherapy in substance abuse treatment. In Rotgers F, Morgenstern J, Walters S, editors: *Treating substance abuse: theory and technique*, ed 2, New York, 2003, Guilford Press.

Centers for Disease Control and Prevention: Impaired driving fact sheet, 2006, www.cdc.gov/ncipc/factsheets/drving.htm.

Chavkin W, et al: National survey of the states: policies and practices regarding drug-using pregnant women, *Am J Public Health* 88(1):117, 1998.

Cherpitel CJ: Brief screening instruments for alcoholism, *Alcohol Health Res World* 21(4):348–351, 1997.

Cook LJ: Educating women about the hidden dangers of alcohol, *J Psychosoc Nurs Ment Health Serv* 42(6):24–31, 54–59, 2004.

Cretzmeyer M, et al: Treatment of methamphetamine abuse: research findings and clinical directions, *J Subst Abuse Treat* 24:267–277, 2003.

Des Jarlais DC: Assessing syringe exchange programs, *Addiction* 99(9):1081–1082, 2004.

Drucker E: Drug prohibition and public health: 25 years of evidence, *Public Health Rep* 114:15–29, 1999.

Erickson PG: Introduction: the three phases of harm reduction: an examination of emerging concepts, methodologies and critiques, *Subst Use Misuse* 34(1):1–7, 1999.

Ewing JA: Detecting alcoholism: the CAGE questionnaire, *JAMA* 252:1905–1907, 1984.

Fals-Stewart W, O'Farrell T, Birchler G: Family therapy techniques. In Rotgers F, Morgenstern J, Walters S, editors: *Treating substance abuse: theory and technique*, ed 2, New York, 2003, Guilford Press.

Friedmann MM, Bowden VR, Jones EG: *Family nursing: research, theory, and practice*, ed 5, Upper Saddle River, NJ, 2003, Prentice Hall.

Goldberg R: *Taking sides: clashing views on controversial issues in drugs and society*, ed 6, Guilford, CT, 2004, McGraw-Hill.

Goldstein A: *Addiction: from biology to drug policy*, ed 2, New York, 2001, Oxford University Press.

Greenberg M, Schneider D: Violence in American cities: young black males is the answer, but what is the question? *Soc Sci Med* 39:179–187, 1994.

Gruber AJ, Pope HG: Psychiatric and medical effects of anabolic-androgenic steroid use in women, *Psychother Psychosom* 69:19–26, 2000.

Haight W, et al: In these bleak days": parent methamphetamine abuse and child welfare in the rural Midwest, *Children Youth Serv Rev* 27(8):949–971, 2005.

Hall JM: Geography of childhood sexual abuse: women's narratives of their childhood environments, *ANS Adv Nurs Sci* 18:29–47, 1996a.

Hall JM: The pervasive effects of childhood sexual abuse in lesbians' recovery from alcohol problems, *Subst Use Misuse* 31:225–239, 1996b.

Hanson GR, Venturelli P, Fleckenstein A: *Drugs and society*, ed 9, Boston, 2002, Jones and Bartlett.

Holtzworth-Munroe A: Typologies of men who are maritally violent: scientific and clinical implications, *J Interpers Violence* 19(12):1369–1389, 2004.

Johnston LD, et al: *Monitoring the future: national results on adolescent drug use: overview of key findings, 2004*, NIH Pub No 05-5726, Bethesda, MD, 2005, National Institute on Drug Abuse.

Kearney MH: Drug treatment for women: traditional models and new directions, *J Obstet Gynecol Neonatal Nurs* 26(4):459–478, 1997.

Keller M: On the loss of control phenomenon in alcoholism, *Br J Addict* 67:153–166, 1972.

Kurtz E: *Not god: a history of alcoholics anonymous*, Center City, MN, 1979, Hazelden Educational Services.

Kuyper LM, et al: Factors associated with sex trade involvement among male participants in a prospective study of injection drug users, *Sex Transm Infect* 80(6):531–535, 2004.

Larimer ME, Marlatt GA: Applications of relapse prevention with moderation goals, *J Psychoactive Drugs* 22:189–195, 1990.

Latimer W: Integrated family and cognitive-behavioral therapy for adolescent substance abusers: a stage I efficacy study, *Drug Alcohol Depend* 71(3):303–317, 2003.

Leshner A: Addiction is a brain disease and it matters, *Science* 278:45–47, 1997.

Levine MR, Rennie WP: Pre-employment urine drug testing of hospital employees: future questions and review of current literature, *Occup Environ Med* 61:318–324, 2004.

Logan BK, Fligner CL, Haddix T: Cause and manner of death in fatalities involving methamphetamine, *J Forensic Sci* 43:28–34, 1998.

MacCoun RJ: Toward a psychology of harm reduction, *Am J Psychol* 53(11):1199–1208, 1998.

Mann K, Lehert P, Morgan M: The efficacy of acamprosate in the maintenance of abstinence in alcohol-dependent individuals: results of a meta-analysis, *Alcoholism* 28(1):51–63, 2004.

Messinger DS: The maternal lifestyle study: cognitive, motor, and behavioral outcomes of cocaine-exposed and opiate-exposed infants through three years of age, *Pediatrics* 113(6):1677–1685, 2004.

Montagne M, Scott DM: Prevention of substance abuse problems: models, factors and processes, *Int J Addict* 28:1177–1208, 1993.

Mylant M: Adolescent children of alcoholics: vulnerable or resilient? *J Am Psychiatr Nurses Assoc* 8(2):57–64, 2002.

Naegle M: The need for alcohol abuse-related education in nursing curricula, *Alcohol Health Res World* 18:154–157, 1994.

Naegle M, D'Avanzo C: *Addictions and substance abuse: strategies for advance nursing practice*, Upper Saddle River, NJ, 2001, Prentice Hall.

National Institute on Drug Abuse: Director, Dr. Nora D. Volkow, Published in December 2006 issue of the *Am J Med Genet B Neuropsychiatr Genet* 2006.

National Institute on Drug Abuse: *Principles of drug addiction treatment: a research-based guide*, NIH Pub No 99-4180, Washington, DC, 1999, Government Printing Office.

National Institute on Drug Abuse: *Monitoring the Future survey*, 2008, Department of Health and Human Services. Conducted by the University of Michigan's Institute for Social Research. www.drugabuse.gov.

Obert JL, London ED, Rawson RA: Incorporating brain research findings into standard treatment: an example using the Matrix model, *J Subst Abuse Treat* 7(4):107–113, 2002.

Paone D, Alpern J: Pregnancy policing: policy of harm, *Int J Drug Policy* 9:101, 1998.

Pelham M: Childhood predictors of adolescent substance use in a longitudinal study of children with ADHD, *J Abnorm Psychol* 112(3):497–507, 2003.

Pope HG Jr, Kouri EM, Hudson MD: Effects of supraphysiologic doses of testosterone on mood and aggression in normal men, *Arch Gen Psychiatry* 57(2):133–140, 2000.

Quazi M: Effective drug-free workplace plan uses worker testing as a deterrent, *Occup Health Saf* 6:26–32, 1993.

Rawson R, Gonzales R, Brethen P: Treatment of methamphetamine use disorders: an update, *J Subst Abuse Treat* 23:145–150, 2002.

Simpson D: A conceptual framework for drug treatment process and outcomes, *J Subst Abuse Treat* 27(2):99–121, 2004.

Stinchfield R, Winters K: Predicting adolescent drug abuse treatment outcome with the Personal Experience Inventory (PEI), *J Child Adolesc Subst Abuse* 13(2):103–120, 2003.

Straussner SL: *Ethnocultural factors in substance abuse treatment*, New York, 2003, Guilford Press.

Sullivan ML, Martinez CM, Gennis P, Gallagher EJ: The cardiac toxicity of anabolic steroids, *Prog Cardiovasc Dis* 41(1):1–15, 1998.

Substance Abuse and Mental Health Services Administration: *Overview of findings from the 2002 National Survey on Drug Use and Health*, NHSDA Series H-21, USDHHS Pub No SMA 03-3774, Rockville, MD, 2003, The Author.

Substance Abuse and Mental Health Services Administration: *Drug Abuse Warning Network, 2003: interim national estimates of drug-related emergency department visits*, DAWN Series D-26, USDHHS Pub No SMA 04-3972, Rockville, MD, 2004a, The Author.

Substance Abuse and Mental Health Services Administration: *Mortality data from the Drug Abuse Warning Network, 2004*, DAWN Series D-25, USDHHS Pub No SMA 04-3875, Rockville, MD, 2004b, The Author.

Substance Abuse and Mental Health Services Administration: *Results from the 2003 National Survey on Drug Use and Health: national findings*, NSDUH Series H-25, USDHHS Pub No SMA 04-3964, Rockville, MD, 2004c, The Author.

Substance Abuse and Mental Health Service Administration: *Overview of findings from the 2004 National Survey on Drug Use and Health*, NSDUH Series H-27, USDHHS Pub No SMA 05-4061, Rockville, MD, 2005, The Author.

Sweeney M, Penner S: A study of employees' attitudes toward workplace drug testing: nursing implications, *J Addict Nurs* 9(4): 156–163, 1997.

Tatarsky A: Harm reduction psychotherapy: extending the reach of traditional substance abuse treatment, *J Subst Abuse Treat* 25(4):249–256, 2003.

Trinkoff A, Storr C: Substance abuse among nurses: differences between specialties, *Am J Public Health* 88(4):581–585, 1998.

U.S. Department of Health and Human Resources: Substance Abuse and Mental Health Services (SAMHSA), www.samhsa.gov, 2008.

U.S. Department of Health and Human Services: *Healthy People 2010*, ed 2, Washington, DC, 2000, The Author.

U.S. Department of Health and Human Services: *Healthy People 2020*, Draft Objectives, 2009. http://www.healthypeople.gov/hp2020/Objectives/files/Draft2009Objectives.pdf.

Van der Kolk BA, McFarlane AC, Weisaeth L, editors: *Traumatic stress: the effects of overwhelming experience on mind, body and society*, New York, 1996, Guilford Press.

Volm BA, de Araujo IE: Methamphetamine activates reward circuitry in drug naïve human subjects, *Neuropsychopharmacology* 29(9):1715–1722, 2004.

Wegscheider-Cruse S: *Developed family role identification theory*, 1981.

Wetherington C, Roman S: *Drug addiction research and the health of women*, NIH Pub No 98-4289, 1998, National Institute on Drug Abuse, www.health.org.

Wodak A: Harm reduction: Australia as a case study, *Bull N Y Acad Med* 72(2):339–347, 1995.

Zautcke JL, et al: Geriatric trauma in the state of Illinois: substance use and injury patterns, *Am J Emerg Med* 20(1):14–17, 2002.

CHAPTER

27

Violence

Catherine A. Pourciau, Elaine C. Vallette*

Additional Material for Study, Review, and Further Exploration

evolve WEBSITE

http://evolve.elsevier.com/Nies

- Quiz
- Case Studies
- Glossary

- WebLinks
- Resource Tool
  - 27A: Planning for Safety

OBJECTIVES

Upon completion of this chapter, the reader will be able to do the following:

1. Describe the concepts of interpersonal and community violence.
2. Identify factors that influence violence.
3. Identify at-risk populations for violence and the role of public health in dealing with the epidemic of violence.
4. Describe the role of the nurse in primary, secondary, and tertiary prevention of violence.

KEY TERMS

child abuse	intentional injuries	shaken baby syndrome
date rape drugs	interpersonal violence	stalking
dating violence	intimate partner violence (IPV)	terrorism
elder abuse	physical abuse	violence
emotional abuse	physical neglect	workplace violence
emotional neglect	prison violence	youth-related violence
hate crimes	sexual abuse	

OUTLINE

Overview of Violence
History of Violence
Interpersonal Violence
    Homicide and Suicide
    Intimate Partner Violence
    Child Abuse
    Elder Abuse
Community Violence
    Workplace Violence
    Youth-Related Violence
    Gangs
    Prison Violence

    Hate Crimes
    Terrorism
Factors Influencing Violence
    Firearms
    Media
Violence from a Public Health Perspective
    Healthy People 2020 and Violence
Prevention of Violence
    Primary Prevention
    Secondary Prevention
    Tertiary Prevention

*The authors would like to acknowledge the contributions of Linda Stevenson and Alice Pappas, who wrote this chapter for the previous edition.

A mentally unstable young man killed thirty-two people, wounded many others, and committed suicide on a college campus. A young woman who complained to the police about being stalked was killed when she opened a package delivered to her apartment. A heavily armed truck driver killed five girls in an Amish schoolhouse before killing himself. A mentally ill mother drowned her five children in the bathtub. A young male tracked down a former girlfriend through the Internet and sent hundreds of violent and threatening e-mails.

Two adolescent males ambushed their high school classmates with guns, killing thirteen and wounding many others before they killed themselves. A black male was dragged to death by five white supremacists. Two men bombed a federal building to retaliate for perceived governmental injustices. Nineteen terrorists hijacked four planes, intentionally crashing two of them into the World Trade Center's twin towers, a third into the Pentagon, and the fourth into an empty field in Pennsylvania, killing a total of 2974 people from 90 different countries.

Violence is a national public health problem. The purpose of this chapter is to explore the influence of violence from a public health perspective as it relates to individuals and communities. Included in this chapter are discussions of the effects of violence in terms of homicides and suicides; death and injury from use of firearms; the direct influence of violence on individuals and communities; public health interventions to reduce violence; the roles and responsibilities of the community health nurse in dealing with those experiencing violence; and measures to increase awareness of violence in the workplace. An in-depth look at the causes, effects, interventions, and measures to increase awareness of violence is presented.

OVERVIEW OF VIOLENCE

Violence is the intentional use of physical force against another person or against oneself, which results in or has a high likelihood of injury or death. In public health, injuries from violence are referred to as intentional injuries. Violence threatens the health and well-being of people of all ages across the globe. Worldwide, 1.6 million people lose their lives as a result of violence, and it is among the leading causes of death among people aged 15 to 44 years (World Health Organization, 2009). In 2005, in the United States, more than 18,000 people were victims of homicide and more than 32,000 people committed suicide. Many more people survive acts of violence and are left with emotional and/or physical scars (Centers for Disease Control and Prevention [CDC], National Center for Injury Prevention and Control, 2009).

The reasons for the high rate of violence in society are highly complex. Universally recognized factors that contribute to violence include:
1. Poverty, unemployment, economic dependency
2. Polydrug and alcohol abuse
3. Dysfunctional family and/or social environment and lack of emotional support

4. Media influence (e.g., violent video games, television shows, and movies)
5. Access to firearms
6. Political and/or religious ideology
7. Intolerance and ignorance

HISTORY OF VIOLENCE

Violence is not limited to present day or to the United States. Since the beginning of time, humans have dealt violently with other humans. In the Bible, Cain killed his brother Abel out of jealousy and anger. Throughout history, sporting events often resulted in death for the audience's pleasure, such as the gladiators in Rome. Infanticide, or the killing of unwanted newborn children, has been practiced throughout history. For example, children were left to die of exposure when they were born a female, a twin, sickly, or deformed. Children, especially firstborn children, were often sacrificed for religious reasons. Infanticide was not condemned until early in the fifth century; however, this did not protect children in many societies. Children were considered to be the property of the father, and he could do whatever he wanted with them (Campbell and Humphreys, 1993).

Throughout the ages, corporal punishment has been used as a means of controlling children. Biblical reference to corporal punishment has often been used as justification for some types of child abuse. To some parents, "spare the rod and spoil the child" (Proverbs 13:24) implies an imperative to abusively discipline an errant child. The idea of "beating some sense into him" was considered necessary to ensure that a lesson was learned. In 1874, the first legal protection against child abuse in the United States occurred when the Society for the Prevention of Cruelty to Animals intervened to protect an 8-year-old girl. As a result of the notoriety associated with this case, the New York Society for the Prevention of Cruelty to Children was organized later that year (Campbell and Humphreys, 1993).

Even nursery rhymes that adults read to small children seem to condone violence against them. Consider the following Mother Goose nursery rhyme:

> There was an old woman who lived in a shoe,
> She had so many children she didn't know what to do,
> She gave them some broth without any bread,
> And whipped them all soundly and sent them to bed.
> (Mother Goose Nursery Rhymes, 2000, pp. 195-196)

Wife beating was legal in the United States until 1824. Wives were seen as their husbands' chattel and could be beaten for such offenses as "nagging too much." In fact, the common phrase "rule of thumb" was derived from English law that allowed a man to beat his wife with a cane no wider than his thumb. Biblical interpretation of "wives be subject to your husband" (Ephesians 5:22) still provides some males with a faulty rationalization for wife beating. Some cultures and religions still allow, and even support, abuse of wives.

The silence that long surrounded domestic violence is derived from a historical perspective of women as their husbands' property. The problem of assault against women was not explored in America until the Civil Rights Movement of the 1960s. In fact, marital rape was not considered an offense in the United States until 1980. In the last two decades, additional cultural issues have surfaced in the United States regarding domestic abuse that includes female circumcision and genital mutilation, abuse between gay partners, and the realization that men are also victims of domestic violence.

Elder abuse is also a problem that is not new. The problem is of greater magnitude now because people are living longer, resulting in increased numbers of dependent and vulnerable adults. Elder abuse frequently goes undetected because of a lack of awareness on the part of health care professionals and society. The exact prevalence of elder abuse is unknown because reporting is not mandatory in all states.

INTERPERSONAL VIOLENCE

Homicide and Suicide

In the United States, homicide claimed the lives of 18,124 individuals in 2005, making it the fifteenth leading cause of death. Sixty-eight percent of these were firearm-related homicide deaths (CDC, 2009a). Young people, women, and black and Hispanic males are at higher risk than the general population. Further, in 2005, blacks were seven times more likely to commit homicide than whites and six times more likely to be victims of homicides than whites. Most murders are intraracial with 86% of white victims being killed by whites and 94% of blacks being killed by blacks (U.S. Department of Justice [USDOJ], Bureau of Justice Statistics, 2007a).

Homicide is the third leading cause of death among females in the age groups of 1 to 4 and 15 to 24 years, is the fourth leading cause of death in the 10- to 14-year age group, and ranks fifth in both the 5- to 9-year and 25- to 34-year age groups. Black females are more likely to be victims than white females, but among all females, homicide ranks in the top five causes of death among ages 1 to 34 years. Notably, approximately 30% of female murder victims are killed by an intimate partner, whereas only 5% of male murder victims were killed by an intimate partner (USDOJ, Bureau of Justice Statistics, 2007b).

Homicide is the second leading cause of death among Americans aged 15 to 24 years and the fourth leading cause of death among ages 5 to 14 years. For black males aged 15 to 34 years, it is the leading cause of death and the second leading cause of death among black males aged 1 to 4 and 10 to 14 years, compared with white males, where homicide is the third leading cause of death in ages 15 to 34 years (CDC, 2005). In the past several decades, the only major cause of childhood death that has significantly increased is homicide (Finkelhor and Ormrod, 2001).

Often ignored or overlooked, suicide is the eleventh leading cause of death for all Americans. More people die of suicide than of homicide in the United States; suicide took the lives of 32,637 people in 2005. It affects virtually all ages. For people between the ages of 15 and 34 years, suicide is the second leading cause of death, and it is the third leading cause of

death in people aged 10 to 24 years. White males commit suicide at a rate almost double that of black males and more frequently than black or white females. In Native Americans and Alaska Natives, suicide is the second leading cause of death in ages 10 to 34 years and ranks eighth in all age groups. People of Asian or Pacific Island descent also have a high suicide rate in ages 10 to 44 years, with an overall suicide ranking of nine. Among men, 58% of all suicides in 2005 were committed with a firearm.

In women, the leading method of suicide was poisoning (39%) followed by the use of firearms (31%) (CDC, 2005). Not surprisingly, research indicates that suicidal individuals are more likely to kill themselves if a gun is in the home (Kellerman et al., 1992). Women with a history of sexual assault are more likely to attempt or commit suicide than other women. Studies show that women who attempt suicide are more likely to have been physically abused by intimate partners and are more likely to have posttraumatic stress disorder.

Intimate Partner Violence

Intimate partner violence (IPV), formerly known as domestic violence, is a pattern of coercive behaviors perpetrated by someone who is or was in an intimate relationship with the victim, such as a spouse, ex-spouse, boyfriend or girlfriend, ex-boyfriend or ex-girlfriend, or date. These behaviors may include battering resulting in physical injury, psychological abuse, and sexual assault that contributes to progressive social isolation and intimidation of the victim. Abuse is typically repetitive and often escalates in frequency and severity. IPV is the single greatest cause of injury to women between the ages of 15 to 24 years in the United States.

RESEARCH HIGHLIGHTS
Sexual and Physical Dating Violence

In a 2006-2007 study, 1312 youth were surveyed in four public high schools in New York City. Of these, 10.1% reported nonpartner sexual violence while 14.1% reported dating partner sexual violence. Adverse health outcomes associated with sexual dating violence included low self-esteem (20%), high physical discomfort (31%), and high emotional discomfort (28%). This is compared with victims of physical dating violence who reported low self-esteem (25%), high physical discomfort (30%), and high emotional discomfort (25%).

From New York City Alliance Against Sexual Assault, Partner and Peers: *Sexual and dating violence in the lives of NYC youth*, 2009: www.nycagainstrape.org/research_par_3.html.

More than 4.5 million incidents of IPV occur each year. In 2004, there were 1544 deaths as a result of IPV, and 75% of these were female (CDC, National Center for Injury Prevention and Control, 2006). Violence may also be directed by women against women in lesbian relationships, by men against men in homosexual relationships, and by women against men.

IPV crosses all ethnic, racial, socioeconomic, and educational lines. About 22% of women and 7% of men report experiencing physical forms of IPV at some point in their lives (CDC, 2008). The following are risk factors for victims of IPV (CDC, National Center for Injury Prevention and Control, 2006):

- Low self-esteem
- Poverty
- Risky sexual behavior
- Eating disorders and/or depression
- Smoking, alcohol or drug abuse
- Trust and relationship issues

Victims of IPV frequently suffer in silence and accept abuse as a transgenerational pattern of normative behavior. When children witness abuse between parents they learn that violence is a means of control.

Greater than 17 million women in the United States have been victims of attempted or completed rape, while 3% of men have been victims. In 55% of reported rapes, the women knew the perpetrator (Rape, Abuse, & Incest National Network, 2008). Women may report that they were subjected to forced intercourse when they were ill or had recently given birth. They also report forced anal intercourse and other violent sexual acts. Box 27-1 presents considerations for working with victims of violence.

BOX 27-1 CONSIDERATIONS FOR WORKING WITH VICTIMS OF VIOLENCE

1. Working with victims of intimate partner violence (IPV):
   - Establish rapport and trust.
   - Deal with issues of confidentiality honestly.
   - Provide current information regarding shelters and sources of support.
   - Recognize and accept that clients may "choose" to stay in an abusive relationship.
2. Working with victims of child abuse:
   - Protect the well-being of the child; this is the primary obligation of health care providers.
   - Report child abuse; it is a legal and ethical obligation in all states.
   - Establish rapport and trust; this may take time.
   - Remain objective when dealing with suspected family members.
3. Working with victims of elder abuse:
   - Establish rapport and trust; this may take time.
   - Report elder abuse; it is a legal and ethical obligation in all states.
   - Remember that competent adults have the right to make decisions about their own care, even if it means staying in an abusive situation.
   - Support efforts to create respite programs and support groups for caregivers.
4. Advocating for the rights of vulnerable populations is the responsibility of all health care professionals:
   - Support research on effective interventions for violence prevention and reduction.
   - Lobby for a decrease in media violence.
   - Support community efforts to increase resources for victims of violence.
   - Lobby for effective regulation of firearms and cyberstalking.

Pregnancy does not exclude women from the danger of abuse. Indeed, pregnancy may increase stress within the family and provoke the first instances of battering. It is believed that during the first 4 months of pregnancy, approximately 15% of women are assaulted by their partner, and 17% of women are assaulted during the fifth through ninth months of pregnancy.

Homicide is the leading cause of death in pregnant women. Societal awareness of IPV during pregnancy is a relatively recent phenomenon; the mention of abuse during pregnancy began to appear in the literature in the 1980s. The image of a woman being battered during pregnancy shatters the idealized image of pregnancy as a time of nurturing and protection. All pregnant women should be routinely screened for abuse. Common signs of IPV in pregnancy are delay in seeking prenatal care, unexplained bruising or damage to breasts or abdomen, use of harmful substances (cigarettes, alcohol, drugs), recurring psychosomatic illnesses, and lack of participation in prenatal education (University of Michigan Health System, 2005). Violence during pregnancy can result in hemorrhage, spontaneous abortion, stillbirths, preterm deliveries, and fetal fractures (U.S. Department of Health and Human Services [USDHHS], 2007).

Dating violence has become a national concern. Dating violence refers to abusive, controlling, or aggressive behavior in an intimate relationship that can take the form of emotional, verbal, physical, or sexual abuse. It happens in straight or gay relationships. Research indicates that one in eleven adolescents has been a victim of physical dating violence and that it occurs more frequently among black students than Hispanics or whites (CDC, 2006). A national study of college students found that 2.8% of women reported a completed or attempted rape within a 7-month period, and approximately 90% were committed by someone the victim knew. Furthermore, almost 16% of college women reported some form of sexual abuse during the academic year and that most of these occurred in their own living quarters (Wasserman, 2004).

Victims of dating violence are typically women aged 16 to 24 years with female peers who have been sexually victimized, show acceptance of dating violence, and have experienced a previous sexual assault. Perpetrators of dating violence are usually males with sexually aggressive peers, heavy drug or alcohol users, accepting of dating violence, prefer impersonal sex, and exhibit impulsive and antisocial tendencies (CDC, 2009b).

Dating violence can involve the use of date rape drugs, such as gamma hydroxybutyrate (GHB), Rohypnol, and ketamine, to reduce inhibitions and promote anesthesia or amnesia in the victim. GHB is odorless and colorless and can easily be made at home. Instructions are available in libraries and on the Internet, which may explain the drug's rapid rise in popularity. Although illegal in the United States, it has become popular in many nightclubs where it is available in clear liquid form. GHB has been touted as an aphrodisiac and an anesthetic. It is actually a depressant that slows down the respiratory system and has been responsible for numerous overdoses and multiple deaths. When mixed with alcohol, in particular, it can be deadly.

Rohypnol (flunitrazepam), classified as a benzodiazepine, has been compared to Quaalude, the "love drug" of the 1960s and 1970s. Like GHB, Rohypnol is not legal in the United States, but many reports have been received of its use at fraternity parties, at college gatherings, and in gay bars on both coasts. The ability to provide a quick, cheap high with long-lasting effects may explain its popularity. Combined with alcohol, serious side effects including death have been reported. Ketamine (ketamine hydrochloride) is an anesthetic used primarily in veterinary practice. It causes a lost sense of time and problems with memory. Another drug that is becoming more common as a date rape drug is Soma. It is a prescription muscle relaxant and central nervous system depressant.

Recent studies have linked alcohol, "a hallmark of college campus social life," with dating violence. Substance abuse was implicated in 74% of sexual assaults on college campuses (Wasserman, 2004). Alcohol contributes to sexual assault because it impairs the ability to think clearly, lowers inhibitions, and impairs ability to evaluate an unsafe situation.

Stalking is a pattern of repeated and unwanted attention, contact, harassment, or any type of conduct directed at a person that instills fear. Types of stalking include messaging through the Internet or cell phone, damaging the victim's property, following the victim, obtaining personal information about the victim, and making direct or indirect threats to the victim's family or friends. Females are three times more likely to be stalked than males. In one 12-month period, approximately 3.4 million people reported being stalked (USDOJ, Office of Violence Against Women, 2009).

IPV is about control, not anger. The objective of abuse is to exert power and control over the victim. Victims may have been exposed to violence as a child. In these cases, the learned response is often one of helplessness that implies passivity and acceptance of abuse. Box 27-2 presents commonly held myths associated with IPV.

The Domestic Abuse Intervention Project in Duluth, Minnesota, has developed a wheel of violence that depicts the types of power and control that are used. These include emotional abuse and intimidation, minimization, denial and blaming, coercion and threats, isolation, economic abuse, use of children, and male privilege. Figure 27-1 depicts the power and control wheel.

Chronic stress characterizes the lives of people in relationships with violent partners. When subjected to repeated abuse, the abuse victim may experience a variety of responses including shock, denial, confusion, withdrawal, psychological numbing, and fear. Victims live in anticipatory terror and often have chronic fatigue and tension, disturbed sleeping and eating patterns, and vague gastrointestinal and genitourinary complaints. Health care providers frequently overlook or misdiagnose these obscure symptoms. In many instances, providers may label the abuse victim as hypochondriacal or clinically depressed. Few victims spontaneously disclose that they are being abused, and the failure of health care professionals to routinely assess for abuse significantly contributes to a missed diagnosis.

Fear, helplessness, and lack of knowledge regarding resources are primary reasons that many victims do not readily leave an abusive situation. The legal system is cumbersome and often inadequate. Victims who seek help through restraining orders or other judicial means find that such methods do not provide real safety or solutions. For example, after reporting abuse to the police, the partner may be jailed and given bail within 24 hours only to return home, unannounced, to deliver another beating. After attempting to use the judicial system as a solution and experiencing its failure, the victim is unlikely to consider the legal system as a source of safety. Victims may also fear that legal intervention might be a threat to custody of their children.

Other factors that keep a victim in an abusive situation are culture, religion, and economics. For example, victims with few marketable skills who leave an abusive situation face serious economic problems and may fall into poverty. When children are involved in such economically dependent relationships, the victim may choose to remain in the setting as a means of economic survival for the children. Health care providers, including nurses, often ask the victim, "Why don't you just leave?" or "What did you do to deserve this?" These misdirected questions often reinforce the victim's sense of helplessness and guilt regarding the abusive situation. These questions reflect a lack of understanding regarding the dynamics of abuse and a lack of sensitivity toward the victim.

Victims who are most likely to leave a battering situation include the following (Campbell and Humphreys, 1993):

1. Those who have resources, such as money, friends, family, and support
2. Those who have power (e.g., a job, credit cards, and status outside the family)
3. Those without children
4. Those who were not abused as children
5. Those who did not see their mothers beaten
6. Those involved in battering situations that are frequent or severe
7. Those whose partner begins to beat children in the family

The most dangerous time for victims is when they leave or attempt to leave the relationship, because it is seen as an erosion of the abuser's control. The victim is more likely to be killed at this time than at any other time in the relationship (Campbell and Humphreys, 1993).

BOX 27-2   COMMON MYTHS ASSOCIATED WITH IPV

- It occurs only in poor, uneducated, minority households.
- It is a private family matter (vs. a societal problem).
- It only occurs in heterosexual relationships.
- Victims deserve the abuse.
- Victims can change the abuser's behavior.
- Abusers will stop the abuse on their own without professional intervention.

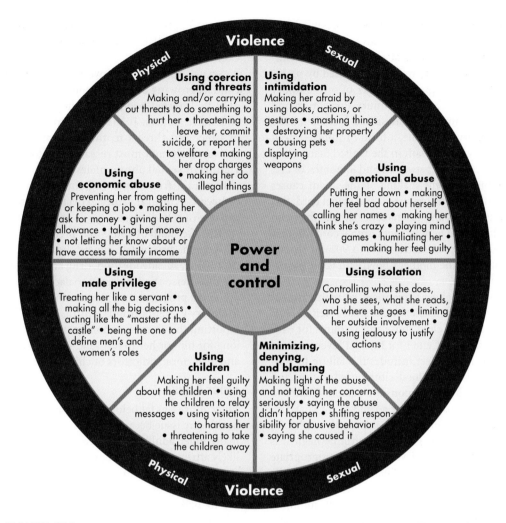

FIGURE 27-1 Power and control wheel developed by the Domestic Abuse Intervention Project (206 West Fourth Street, Duluth, MN 55806).

Child Abuse

Most child abuse occurs within the family. Parents and relatives who were abused themselves are most often the perpetrators. Abuse of children is more commonly seen in families living in poverty, by teenage parents, or by parents who are drug or alcohol abusers. In some families all children are equal targets of abuse, whereas in other families a particular child may be selected as the designated recipient of abuse. The child may be singled out by a particular physical characteristic such as hair color or resemblance to another family member who evokes negative emotions in the abusive parent. Child abuse, like domestic violence, is often a learned transgenerational behavior. Although statistical reporting of child abuse is mandatory throughout the country, reported numbers are probably an underestimation. Children are not likely to report the abuse because they fear reprisal.

There were more than 900,000 (or twelve per 1000) cases of child abuse reported in the United States in 2006. Girls are more likely to be victims than boys, and women are more likely to be the perpetrator. More than 1500 children died in

the United States of abuse and neglect in 2006 (CDC, National Center for Injury Prevention and Control, 2008). The four types of child abuse are as follows:

1. Physical abuse
2. Physical and emotional neglect
3. Emotional abuse
4. Sexual abuse

Physical abuse is an intentional injury inflicted on a child by another person and accounts for 16% of child abuse cases (CDC, National Center for Injury Prevention and Control, 2008). Parents who abuse often have unreasonable expectations of their children and may misinterpret the child's behavior as threats to their parental self-esteem and need to control. Physical abuse includes beating, burning, biting, bruising, and head and internal injuries. The type of physical injury varies only with the adult's imagination. Patterned injuries may give some clue as to how the child was injured. A child who touches a light cord or light plug might be beaten with it, producing a looped or linear pattern. A child who plays with matches or the stove might have his or her hand placed in the flame. A crying child or a child who talks back might have hot pepper or Tabasco sauce poured into his or her mouth or might be suffocated with a pillow.

Young children under the age of 1 year, followed by children aged 1 to 3 years, are most frequently injured by physical abuse. Infants are in the greatest danger of severe injury or death (CDC, National Center for Injury Prevention and Control, 2008). One example of infant abuse is shaken baby syndrome. Shaken baby syndrome, a form of inflicted head trauma, is a leading cause of death in the United States from child abuse. Most victims are between 3 and 8 months of age. In this form of abuse, violent shaking of the infant causes trauma at the junction of the brainstem and spinal cord; this can lead to death. Serious and permanent damage may also occur; this includes retinal hemorrhages, spinal cord injuries, and brain injuries. In approximately 65% to 90% of shaken baby cases, the father or the mother's boyfriend is the perpetrator (KidsHealth, 2009).

Physical neglect is negligent treatment or maltreatment of a child by a person responsible for the child's welfare. It is the most common form of child abuse and accounts for 64% of all cases (CDC, National Center for Injury Prevention and Control, 2008). Physical neglect includes the failure to provide basic needs such as shelter, food, clothing, education, and access to medical care by the responsible person. Failure to provide a nurturing environment for a child to thrive, learn, and develop and failure to provide for the health needs of a child can also be construed as neglect. Emotional neglect is the failure to nurture a child in developmentally appropriate ways. Examples of emotional neglect include failure to cuddle and/or physically stimulate a newborn, failure to give positive feedback, failure to pay attention to the overall emotional needs of a child, or failure to show affection.

Emotional abuse accounts for approximately 7% of all child abuse cases and is the behavior that may damage a child's self-worth or emotional well-being (CDC, National Center for Injury Prevention and Control, 2008). The child may demonstrate a substantial impairment in behavior such as an overly compliant or passive child, a very aggressive child, or a child who is inappropriately adult or infantile. Emotionally abused children frequently do not progress at a normal rate of physical, intellectual, or emotional development. They also have an increased risk for suicide. Emotional abuse usually occurs in the home, unwitnessed by others. Emotional abuse might include name calling, such as "you're stupid," "you're a slut," "you're bad," or "you're evil," shaming, withholding love, rejection, or threatening behavior. Impairment in behavior may also occur in children who are not abused; therefore, identification is difficult.

Sexual abuse is any sexual activity between an adult and a child, including use of a child for sexual exploitation, prostitution, or pornography. Sexual abuse can also involve an older child with a younger child, usually defined as a difference of 5 or more years of age between the two. Incest is the term used for sexual relations between close family members, such as father and daughter, mother and son, or siblings. Approximately 9% of child abuse cases are sexual abuse (CDC, National Center for Injury Prevention and Control, 2008).

Sexual abuse often involves a person known to the child. A growing concern is the sexual exploitation of children by Internet pedophiles who prey upon unsuspecting and naive targets. It may occur over a prolonged period of time, and threats to the child may be used to ensure secrecy. Although most research has focused on females as victims of sexual abuse, males are also targets. The victim may refrain from reporting abuse because he is ashamed or because cultural values expect males to be assertive and capable of self-defense.

The aftermath of abuse may predispose the victims to low self-esteem, psychiatric illness, health problems as adults, depression, suicide ideation, drug and alcohol addiction, eating disorders, obesity, sexual maladjustment, delayed developmental processes, and prostitution (CDC, National Center for Injury Prevention and Control, 2008). The child may delay reporting the abuse for months or years, as it may take that long for him or her to feel safe. Table 27-1 describes physical and behavioral indicators of child abuse and neglect.

Elder Abuse

Elder abuse lags far behind child abuse and IPV as a social and health care issue because society fails to recognize the cruelty many older adults experience. Failure to recognize abuse is likely attributable to perception of elders as an "invisible" segment of the population. The exact number of abused elders is unknown because of underreporting. Estimates indicate that 2% to 10% of the older adult population suffer some form of maltreatment. Reasons for underreporting include shame on the part of the victim, social and physical isolation from resources, and the failure of health care providers to routinely assess for abuse and neglect during points of contact. The most likely victims are those in poor physical or mental health, dependent on others for physical or financial support, confused, depressed, or who are socially isolated (National Center on Elder Abuse, 2005).

Commonly described types of abuse and neglect of older adults are as follows:

- Physical abuse (purposeful infliction of physical pain or injury or unnecessary physical or drug-induced restraints)
- Psychological-emotional abuse (verbal assault, threats, provoking fear, or isolation)
- Sexual abuse (unwanted sexual contact or pornography)
- Neglect (withholding of personal care, food, or medications, intimidation, humiliation, abandonment)
- Financial exploitation (theft or misuse of money or property)
- Health care fraud and abuse (charging for services not delivered, or Medicaid fraud)

Elder abuse tends to escalate in incidence and severity. When an older adult cannot provide self-care because of the physical or mental infirmities of age, what happens to that person may depend on whether relatives can provide care,

TABLE 27-1   PHYSICAL AND BEHAVIORAL INDICATORS OF CHILD ABUSE AND NEGLECT

PHYSICAL INDICATORS	BEHAVIORAL INDICATORS
Physical Abuse	
Unexplained bruises and welts in various stages of healing that may form patterns	Wary of adult contact
Unexplained burns by cigars or cigarettes or immersion burns (e.g., socklike, glovelike, or on buttocks or genitalia)	Apprehensive when other children cry
Burns in the shape of objects	Constantly on alert
Rope burns	Exhibiting extremes of behavior; aggressive or passive and withdrawn, or overly friendly to strangers
Unexplained lacerations or abrasions	Frightened of parents
Unexplained fractures in various stages of healing; multiple or spiral fractures	Afraid to go home
Unexplained injuries to mouth, lips, gums, eyes, or external genitalia	
Physical and Emotional Neglect	
Hunger	Begging or stealing food
Poor hygiene	Alone at inappropriate times or for prolonged periods
Poor or inappropriate dress	Delinquent
Lack of supervision for prolonged periods of time	Stealing
Lack of medical or dental care	Arriving early to and departing late from school
Constant fatigue, listlessness, or falling asleep in class	Lack of affection
Sexual Abuse	
Difficulty in walking or sitting	Exhibiting negative self-esteem
Torn, stained, or bloody underwear	Exhibiting inability to trust and function in intimate relationships
Genital pain or itching	Exhibiting cognitive and motor dysfunctions
Bruises or bleeding from the external genitalia, vaginal, or anal areas	Exhibiting deficits in personal and social skills
Sexually transmitted disease	Exhibiting bizarre, sophisticated, or unusual sexual behavior or knowledge
Drug and alcohol abuse	Delinquent or a runaway
Developmental delays	Exhibiting suicide ideation
	Reporting sexual assault
Emotional Abuse	
Failure to thrive	Exhibiting behavior extremes from passivity to aggression
Lags in physical development	Exhibiting habit and conduct disorders (e.g., antisocial behavior and destructiveness)
Speech disorders	Exhibiting neurotic traits
Developmental delays	Attempting suicide

or whether the person has financial resources to obtain care in his or her own home, a retirement home, or a residential care facility. Caregivers are often adult children or other relatives. This generation of individuals in their 40s, 50s, and 60s is often called the sandwich generation because they are caring for their children at the same time they are providing care for their aging parents. As parents age, the role reversal is often painful and demanding for both the elder and the caregiver.

Care of an aging parent requires sacrifice and commitment. As parents age, they may become more physically and cognitively impaired, increasing the likelihood of abuse. Elders who were themselves abusers are more likely to be abused by their caregivers. Older adults may have changes in personality that make it difficult for their adult children to care for them. They may need to be lifted, which may be difficult for someone with limited strength. They may need assistance walking, toileting, or eating that requires time the caregiver may not have. There is also an intimacy in caring for a parent that the caregiver may not be comfortable with.

All of these factors cause stress, which can be associated with abuse. This is especially true in families in which violence is a response to stress. The needs of the older adult may exceed the family's ability to meet them.

In many ways, helpless older adults are in the same vulnerable position as a child because they are dependent on others to care for them. The population of the United States is aging, and the number of frail older adults over 85 years of age is the fastest growing demographic segment with increasing dependency needs. Recognition of physical and behavioral indicators helps the professional become aware of possible abusive situations. None is conclusive in itself; however, they alert the professional to the need for careful and complete assessment. Table 27-2 lists the indicators of possible abuse of older adults.

COMMUNITY VIOLENCE

The United States is one of the most violent countries in the industrialized world. Not a day passes that one does not hear about some community, region, or country that has been

TABLE 27-2   INDICATORS OF POSSIBLE ELDER ABUSE

PHYSICAL INDICATORS	EMOTIONAL/BEHAVIORAL INDICATORS
Bruises, black eyes, welts, lacerations, and rope marks	Being emotionally upset or agitated
Bone fractures, broken bones, and skull fractures	Being extremely withdrawn and noncommunicative or nonresponsive
Open wounds, cuts, punctures, untreated injuries in various stages of healing	Unusual behavior usually attributed to dementia (e.g., sucking, biting, rocking)
Sprains, dislocations, and internal injuries/bleeding	Sudden change in behavior
Signs of being subjected to punishment and signs of being restrained	Report of being verbally or emotionally mistreated
Laboratory findings of medication overdose or underutilization of prescribed drugs	
Report of being hit, slapped, kicked, or mistreated	
The caregiver's refusal to allow visitors to see an elder alone	
NEGLECT	**FINANCIAL INDICATORS (MATERIAL EXPLOITATION)**
Dehydration, malnutrition, untreated bedsores, and poor personal hygiene	Sudden changes in bank account or banking practice (e.g., unexplained withdrawal of large sums of money, inclusion of additional names on an elder's bank signature card)
Unattended or untreated health problems	Unauthorized withdrawal of the elder's funds using the elder's ATM card
Hazardous or unsafe living conditions/arrangements (e.g., improper wiring, no heat, or no running water)	Abrupt changes in a will or other financial documents (e.g., power of attorney)
Unsanitary and unclean living conditions (e.g., dirt, fleas, soiled bedding, fecal/urine smell, inadequate clothing)	Unexplained disappearance of funds or valuables
Report of being mistreated or neglected	Bills unpaid despite the availability of adequate financial resources
	Elder's signature being forged for financial transactions or for the titles of his/her possessions
	Sudden appearance of previously uninvolved relatives interested in the elder's affairs and possessions
	Unexplained sudden transfer of assets to a family member or someone outside the family
	The provision of services that are not necessary
	Report of financial exploitation

Modified from Administration on Aging/National Center on Elder Abuse: *Signs and symptoms of elder abuse,* September 2007, www.ncea.aoa.gov/NCEAroot/Main_Site/FAQ/Basics/Types_Of_Abuse.aspx.

affected by violent crime. Community violence may not affect everyone directly, but it affects all indirectly. In contrast to inter-personal violence that affects only one or two individuals, community violence usually occurs suddenly and without warning and can potentially destroy entire segments of the population. Community violence includes workplace violence, youth violence, gang-related violence, hate crimes, and terrorism.

Workplace Violence

Workplace violence is a serious safety and health issue. Violence in the workplace includes physical assaults such as rape and homicide, muggings, and verbal and written threats. According to the Occupational Safety and Health Association (OSHA) (2007), homicide, the most extreme form of workplace violence, is the fourth leading cause of death in the occupational setting. In 2005, there were 564 workplace homicides out of a total of 5702 fatal work injuries in the United States. Workplace violence tends to be higher in some service-oriented work environments including health care. Such violence is widely believed to be underreported, perhaps in part because of beliefs that it is an expected part of certain jobs. In the health care field, the most frequent areas for the occurrence of violence are the emergency departments, psychiatric units, geriatric units, and waiting rooms. Nurses and nursing assistants who work directly with patients are at higher risk (CDC, National Institute for Occupational Safety and Health, 2002). Nurses

who work in public health roles are not immune to violence because their work may bring them in direct contact with individuals prone to violent behavior. Identification of risk factors may offer some protection to the worker whether in the hospital or in the home care or public health setting. Examples of risk factors include:

- Increasing number of acute and chronic mentally ill patients
- Working alone
- Availability of drugs at hospitals, clinics, or pharmacies
- Low staffing levels
- Poorly lit parking levels, corridors
- Long waits for service
- Increasing use of hospitals for holding criminals
- Inadequate security
- Increasing number of gang members and drug or alcohol abusers
- Access to firearms

Violence also negatively impacts the workplace causing low worker morale, increased job stress, increased turnover, reduced trust of management and/or co-workers, and hostile work environments (OSHA, 2002).

Youth-Related Violence

Violence is taking a toll on American youth. More than 2 million arrests were made involving people under the age of 18 years in 2006, and 17% of those were for

TABLE 27-3	RISK FACTORS FOR YOUTH-RELATED VIOLENCE
INDIVIDUAL RISK FACTORS	**COMMUNITY RISK FACTORS**
Involvement with drugs and alcohol	Diminished economic opportunities
Antisocial behavior and attitudes	High concentration of poor residents
Low IQ and/or learning disabilities	High concentration of family disruption
History of violent victimization	Low levels of community participation
History of early aggressive behavior	Socially disorganized neighborhoods
Low parental involvement/attachment	
Parental substance abuse or criminality	
Low parental education and income	
Harsh, lax, or inconsistent disciplinary practices	
Involvement in gangs	
Poor academic performance	
Rejection by peers	
Lack of involvement in conventional activities	
Poor family functioning	

From Centers for Disease Control and Prevention, National Center for Injury Prevention and Control, Division of Violence Prevention: 2008: Youth Violence Risk and Protective Factors, www.cdc.gov/ViolencePrevention/youthviolence/riskprotectivefactors.html.

violent crimes. Racial disparities are evident in youth crimes as white juveniles are arrested more often for property crimes and black juveniles for violent crimes. Most of the increased homicide rates among American youth are attributable to death caused by firearms (USDOJ, Office of Justice Programs, 2008). Table 27-3 lists risk factors for youth-related violence.

Youth-related violence is more concentrated in minority communities and inner cities, causing a disproportionate burden on these communities. Shooting or killing someone has become the symbol of a new rite of passage and the bestowing of manhood among some segments of society. Minority youth are particularly influenced, and violence among them is a complex problem.

Adolescents and children increasingly use violence to handle disputes. Children are often not taught peaceful ways of resolving differences and learn by default from what they observe on television and in movies. Consequently, schools have become a common site for violence (see Chapter 29 for more information on violence in schools).

Gangs

Gangs are increasingly responsible for crimes and violence throughout the United States. Although gang problems declined in the 1990s, they have steadily increased since that time. In 2007, there were an estimated 788,000 youth gang members in 27,000 active gangs in the United States. Urban and suburban areas continue to be the primary location for

gangs and gang members with one in five large cities reporting increases in gang-related homicides (Egley and O'Donnell, 2009).

Reasons that young people give for joining gangs include the belief that gangs will protect them, peer pressure, the need for respect, and a sense of belonging. According to the National Gang Intelligence Center (2009), gangs exist in all fifty states, and it appears that gangs are responsible for as much as 80% of all crime in many communities. These crimes include illegal alien smuggling, armed robbery, assault, auto theft, drug and weapon trafficking, identity theft, and murder.

Prison Violence

The United States has the world's highest incarceration rate; with only 5% of the world's population, the United States houses nearly 25% of the world's prisoners, a rate nearly five times the average worldwide (Webb, 2009). Inmates are both victims and perpetrators of violence. With more than 2 million prisoners in federal and state prisons or local jails, the rate of prison violence has increased and includes allegations of physical abuse, as well as reports of rape by both corrections officers and inmates (USDOJ, Bureau of Justice Statistics, 2009). The public and the judicial system have expressed little sympathy for this population for a variety of reasons including indifference, disbelief, and denial. Little research exists to reflect the long-term effects on these victims or society when they are released. See Chapter 31 for more information on forensic and correctional nursing.

Hate Crimes

Hate crimes are crimes based on an individual's race, sexual orientation, religious beliefs, ethnic background, or national origin. Hate crimes may include rape, sexual or physical assault, harassment, attacks on homes or on places of worship, and vandalism. Because hate crimes attack an individual's identity, the emotional effects are compounded. In 2007, there were 7624 hate crimes reported in the United States. The most commonly reported hate crimes were racially motivated, followed by religious and sexual orientation bias (Federal Bureau of Investigation, 2008).

Terrorism

Terrorism has been present throughout history and is difficult to define. Terrorism has been described as a tactic and a strategy, a crime, a holy duty, a justified reaction to oppression, and an inexcusable abomination. The Department of Defense defines terrorism as "the calculated use of unlawful violence or threat of unlawful violence to inculcate fear; intended to coerce or intimidate governments or societies in the pursuit of goals that are generally political, religious, or ideological." All terrorist acts include three key elements—violence, fear, and intimidation. Nurses need to be prepared for terrorism in whatever form it takes from an act in the local community, such as an explosion, to a larger act that affects an entire region or country, such as biological, chemical, or nuclear incidents. Mental and physical health issues remain a nursing concern for the victims, responders, and the community long after the act has occurred. See Chapter 28 for a more detailed discussion on terrorism.

FACTORS INFLUENCING VIOLENCE

Controversy surrounds the factors that influence violence in today's society. Two of these are easy access to firearms and the impact of media. Firearms are readily available, and even children are carrying guns to school. The influence of media is pervasive in our society, especially among adolescents and young adults.

Firearms

Approximately 250 million privately owned firearms exist in the United States, and more than 1 million new handguns are sold in the United States annually (National Rifle Association, 2008). Statistics indicate that firearms are the number one weapon of choice in homicides in the United States. In 2005, 18,124 people were murdered in the United States; firearms were used in 12,352 of those murders (CDC, 2005).

Concern about firearms arises when it has been shown that guns kept in the home for self-protection are forty-three times more likely to kill a family member or a friend than an attacker. Furthermore, the presence of a gun in the home triples the risk of homicide in the home and increases the risk of suicide fivefold (CDC, 1999). The cost of violence from guns is staggering. Violence related to firearms costs the United States millions of dollars annually in direct cost. Indirect costs, including loss of productivity, mental health treatment, rehabilitation, and legal and judicial costs, add more than $100 billion to the cost of violence (Ludwig and Cook, 2003).

Discussion regarding firearms often evokes a heated response from opponents of gun control who see violence as the work of aberrant individuals. According to their view, the focus on guns as a major public health threat is misdirected in comparison with other health issues. Many opponents of gun control cite their constitutional "right to bear arms" and interpret efforts to control guns as an assault on their personal freedom. They believe that "law-abiding citizens" have a right to protect themselves despite the hazards of private gun ownership.

Media

Media violence has reached epidemic proportions because it is prevalent and accessible to all age groups. Media violence includes the exposure to and participation in violent video games, music and music videos that advocate date rape or violence, and virtual violence that allows subscribers to harm or kill victims. Television and movies often depict people being tortured or killed in graphic detail that makes it hard for children and adults to distinguish between reality and fantasy. Media violence has become more violent, graphic in nature, and sadistic. The public health community believes that repeated exposure to media violence leads to emotional desensitization to real-life violence.

VIOLENCE FROM A PUBLIC HEALTH PERSPECTIVE

Dealing with violence has traditionally been the U.S. criminal justice system's responsibility. However, since violence is also a *public health epidemic*, efforts are being made to prevent and manage it using public health strategies. Violence has a tremendous influence on morbidity and mortality rates, quality of life indicators, and health care resources. The public health system has been challenged to go beyond its traditional programs to include prevention and management of violence. Many public health problems are interrelated, and thus a coordinated approach should be used to address the issues.

Healthy People 2020 and Violence

Violence was one of the areas addressed by *Healthy People 2000* and again in *Healthy People 2010* and *Healthy People 2020*. Several objectives regarding violence and abuse prevention have been established. The *Healthy People 2020* table lists a few of these (USDHHS, 2009). These objectives are intended to target causes of violence and abuse, improve national data collection and analysis, provide input for legislative funding, facilitate research efforts, and concentrate public health efforts on models that demonstrate effectiveness.

Many of the *Healthy People 2020* objectives are difficult to achieve because there are complex barriers. These barriers include lack of comparable data sources, standardized

---

♥ HEALTHY PEOPLE 2020

Selected Proposed Objectives Related to Violence

OBJECTIVE
IVP HP2020–12: Reduce physical assaults.
IVP HP2020–13: Reduce physical fighting among adolescents.
IVP HP2020–14: Reduce weapon carrying by adolescents on school property.
IVP HP2020–29: Reduce nonfatal child maltreatment.
IVP HP2020–30: Reduce child maltreatment deaths.
IVP HP2020–31: Reduce violence by current or former intimate partners.
IVP HP2020–32: Reduce sexual violence.
IVP HP2020–35: Increase the number of states and the District of Columbia where 90 percent of sudden and unexpected deaths of infants are reviewed by a child fatality review team.
IVP HP2020–41: Reduce bullying among adolescents.

USDHHS Healthy People 2020 Draft Objectives. 2009. http://www.healthypeople.gov/hp2020/Objectives/files/Draft2009Objectives.pdf

definitions, resources to adequately establish consistent tracking systems, and resources to fund promising prevention programs. The achievement of positive change in thirteen of the original nineteen objectives indicates that coordinated national efforts can bring about progress.

PREVENTION OF VIOLENCE

The nurse who cares for people experiencing violence must be a skilled clinician who is knowledgeable about both the problem and the available community resources. Box 27-3 presents tips regarding safety issues for a community health nurse. Over the last 25 years, a considerable body of knowledge has been developed regarding the trends in violence. Table 27-4 provides the current components of a comprehensive program to reduce violence in individuals and the community.

Primary Prevention

The goal of primary prevention is to stop violence, abuse, or neglect before it occurs. Education plays a major part in primary prevention and may include parenting and family wellness and anger management or conflict resolution. Professionals should increase their awareness of violence, identification of cases, and provision of early treatment. The nurse can work in or with the community to educate citizens about the problem of violence, potential causes of violence, and available community services.

Primary prevention must begin at a community level, helping to change attitudes about abuse and violence. Primary prevention must focus on stopping the transgenerational aspect of abuse, starting with young children and continuing across the life span. For example, parenting is the most difficult job

that most individuals will undertake, yet there is a widespread myth that parenting "comes naturally." Classes for parents should focus on physical care of the infant including ways to soothe and manage a "fussy" baby, the effect of fatigue on new parents, the need for support, and fears and questions of new parents. Nurses in the hospital have little time to help new parents learn basic newborn care before discharge. Some hospitals and public health agencies provide follow-up to new parents to ensure that they can adequately care for their newborn. This is especially true of any person deemed to be high risk including teenage mothers, mothers without support, or women with a history of spousal abuse.

Secondary Prevention

The goal of secondary prevention is to assess, diagnose, and treat victims and perpetrators of violence. Consideration of the safety of the potential victim is critical.

Secondary prevention begins with assessment. For example, consistent assessment of women during health care visits will increase case finding and provide opportunities for early intervention that is particularly crucial during pregnancy. Women should be interviewed in private when asked about abuse. Questions should be asked in a matter-of-fact way, and the health care provider should not show shock or dismay at the response. The Nursing Research Consortium on Violence and Abuse has developed a simple three-question abuse assessment screen (Figure 27-2). These three questions should be asked of all women at each visit, and careful and detailed documentation should be done.

Victims, once identified, must be offered resources to increase their safety. However, all victims may not be ready or able to leave the situation, and available options must be

---

BOX 27-3 SAFETY ISSUES FOR THE COMMUNITY HEALTH NURSE

Plan Ahead
- Know the area you are visiting.
- Schedule the visit ahead of time, and get the correct address, directions, and information about who will be in the home.
- Tell the office where you will be, and check in regularly.
- Carry a cell phone, possibly a pager, and a small amount of money.
- Dress for function and mobility and wear a name tag. Avoid any provocative clothing.
- Ensure that the vehicle you drive is in good repair, has a full gas tank, and has emergency equipment. Always carry two sets of car keys.

Approaching the Home
- Notice the environment, animals, fences, activity, possible indicators of crime, and places you could go for assistance if necessary.
- Walk with confidence, and maintain a professional attitude.
- Listen for signs of fighting before knocking. If you hear sounds of fighting, leave!
- Do not enter a home if you suspect an unsafe situation.

In the Home
- Be aware of who is in the home and what is going on. If angry people are in the home, use your professional and social skills. Do not expect the client to protect you.
- Note the exits, and sit between the client and an exit of the home. Be prepared to leave quickly if the situation changes suddenly.
- If someone in the home is violent, leave and call 911.

Handling a Tight Situation
- Do not show fear; control your breathing.
- Speak calmly and in a soothing manner. Be assertive but not aggressive.
- Repeat the reason for your visit, and find a reason to leave.

Leaving the Home
- Take all of your belongings, and keep your car keys in your hand.
- Watch for cars following you when you leave. Do not stop. If you feel that you are in danger, go to the nearest police station or well-lighted business and ask for help.
- Trust your instincts. Never forget your own safety.

Modified from Oregon Public Health Association, Public Health Nursing Section, Seattle–King County Department of Public Health, Washington State Public Health Association: *Public health nursing domestic violence protocol* (booklet), Seattle, WA, and Salem, OR, 1993, The Authors.

TABLE 27-4	COMPONENTS OF A COMPREHENSIVE PROGRAM TO REDUCE VIOLENCE FOR INDIVIDUALS AND COMMUNITIES
INDIVIDUALS	**COMMUNITY**
Primary Prevention—Goal: Promotion of Optimal Parenting and Family Wellness	
Family life education in schools, churches, and communities	Community education concerning violence
Education of children and adults on methods of conflict resolution	Reduction of media violence
Parenting classes in hospitals, schools, and other community agencies	Development of community support services such as crisis lines, respite care for families with dependent members, shelters for battered women and their children, and development and vigorous enforcement of antistalking measures, including cyberstalking
Preventive mental health services for adults and children	Handgun control
Training for professionals in early detection of violence	
Secondary Prevention—Goal: Diagnosis of and Service for Families in Stress	
Nursing assessment for evidence of violence in all health care settings	All health professionals should be educated in assessment of violence and possible protocols for dealing with victims
A safety plan for victims	Hospital emergency departments and trauma centers with 24-hour response, reporting, case intake, coordination with legal and medical authorities, coordination with voluntary agencies that have services, coordination with social services departments for provision of services
Knowledge of legal options	
Shelter or foster home placement for victims	
Social services for individuals or families	Death review teams to review deaths from injury, especially for infants and children
Referral to self-help groups in the community	Public authority involvement by police, district attorneys, and courts
Referral to appropriate community agencies	Epidemiological tracking and evaluation of violence
	Handgun control
Tertiary Prevention—Goal: Reeducation and Rehabilitation of Violent Families	
Empowerment strategies for battered women	Foster homes, shelters, and care for dependents
Professional counseling services for individuals	Public authority involvement
Parenting reeducation (i.e., formal training in child rearing)	Follow-up care for known cases of abuse, neglect, or violence
Counseling services for individuals and families	Handgun control
Self-help groups	

explored. All victims should have knowledge of legal options and how to access them. The nurse must be ready to intervene when the abuse involves a child or someone who is cognitively impaired. Some states have developed protocols for nurses who deal with victims of violence. Review of these protocols can help the nurse become familiar with the questions to ask and suggestions that should be made to help the victim develop a safety plan. Visit the book's website at http://elsevier.com/Nies, and see **Resource Tool 27A** for a sample of a safety plan.

Another example of secondary prevention involves screening for abuse in the elderly that should occur at every health care visit. Elder abuse remains underreported across the United States; therefore routine screening can facilitate early intervention. Nurses can help raise professional and community consciousness of elder abuse by participating in political activities to create or strengthen mandatory reporting laws and funding of support groups.

The nurse should work with family members or caregivers who provide care for the elderly to promote healthier relationships. Assisting the caregiver to deal with stress by finding respite care, a home health aide, or counseling may help. Documentation is crucial in meeting medical-legal requirements. The nurse should record observations accurately and refrain from opinions and interpretations. This is especially important because court proceedings may use this documentation that has direct bearing on the victim's welfare.

The problem of violence cannot be managed by nursing alone, but rather in combination with other disciplines that include physicians, child and adult protective services, social workers, probation officers, chaplains, and police. This interdisciplinary approach leads to optimal outcomes. Public health surveillance is important in obtaining accurate numbers of intentional injuries for individuals. Death review teams can analyze records to determine whether the injury was intentional or unintentional.

Tertiary Prevention

Tertiary prevention is aimed at rehabilitation of individuals, families, groups, or communities and includes both victims and perpetrators of violence. Rehabilitation may take months or even years depending on the situation. For example, the September 11, 2001, attack on the United States disrupted thousands of lives and changed the country's sense of security. This attack affected everyone in the country, not just those in the immediate vicinity. Even after all these years, the effects continue. The nurse must be able to work in conjunction with a variety of mental health professionals and social service agencies to provide coordinated care. The nurse may have also been a victim and may be experiencing many of the same problems as those he or she is trying to help. Self-care and recognition of the nurse's own limitations or needs are critical.

1. WITHIN THE LAST YEAR, have you been hit, slapped, kicked, or otherwise physically hurt by someone?	YES	NO
If YES, by whom? _____		
Total number of times _____		
2. SINCE YOU'VE BEEN PREGNANT, have you been hit, slapped, kicked, or otherwise physically hurt by someone?	YES	NO
If YES, by whom? _____		
Total number of times _____		
MARK THE AREA OF INJURY ON THE BODY MAP. SCORE EACH INCIDENT ACCORDING TO THE FOLLOWING SCALE:		SCORE
1 = Threats of abuse including use of a weapon		_____
2 = Slapping, pushing; no injuries and/or lasting pain		_____
3 = Punching, kicking, bruises, cuts, and/or continuing pain		_____
4 = Beating up, severe contusions, burns, broken bones		_____
5 = Head injury, internal injury, permanent injury		_____
6 = Use of weapon; wound from weapon		_____
If any of the descriptions for the higher number apply, use the higher number.		
3. WITHIN THE LAST YEAR, has anyone forced you to have sexual activities?	YES	NO
If YES, by whom? _____		
Total number of times _____		

FIGURE 27-2 Abuse assessment screen. (From McFarlane J, Parker B: Preventing abuse during pregnancy: an assessment and intervention protocol, *MCN Am J Matern Child Nurs* 19[6]:321-324, 1994. [Developed by the Nursing Research Consortium on Violence and Abuse. Readers are encouraged to reproduce and use this assessment tool.])

SUMMARY

Violence is a major public health issue in the United States and affects individuals across the life cycle. Morbidity and mortality statistics indicate that violence is epidemic in many communities. Whether at home, in the neighborhood, or at school, violence affects countless numbers of individuals. The influence of media and easy access to and proliferation of handguns in the United States are considered major contributing factors to violence. The cycle of violence can become transgenerational if not broken. The abuser is also a victim, and the ultimate victim is society, which must care and pay for the results of violent acts.

Violence is a public health epidemic, and national objectives for reducing violence have been identified. The core public health functions of needs assessment and surveillance, policy development, and assurance are useful methods of combating this epidemic. The literature describes interventions that focus on the three levels of prevention. The need for continued research in violence should be a funding priority at the local, state, and national levels. The disheartening reality of violence has been validated. Everyone is affected.

CASE STUDY   APPLICATION OF THE NURSING PROCESS

Caryn is a 23-year-old mother of two, ages 3 years and 2 months. She was separated from her husband of 4 years for a few months, but they recently reconciled. He works as a computer programmer and is the sole support of the family. Both her parents and his live 2 to 3 hours away and are in ill health. She is a patient at the local Planned Parenthood clinic for a postpartum examination and contraceptive counseling. During the exam, the nurse notes that she has numerous bruises on her external genitalia and upper torso along with a black eye. When asked about possible abuse, she avoids eye contact and is reluctant to answer questions. Looking over her history, the clinic nurse notes that Caryn has completed high school but has not worked outside the home for the past 3 years. This is Caryn's fourth visit to the clinic, and the same nurse has seen her each time. The clinic is located in a small town where "everyone knows each other." Caryn refuses to leave her husband, stating, "I have no place to go and he loves me." She also states that he has a bad temper. Caryn is given a card with the phone number of the domestic violence hotline. She agrees to take the card but declines any further conversation about abuse. Caryn is fitted with a diaphragm and given spermicidal gel. She is able to effectively perform a return demonstration indicating appropriate insertion and removal and is scheduled to return in 6 months for a follow-up appointment.

Seen in the clinic 3 months later for amenorrhea and pregnancy testing, Caryn denies any further injuries stating that things are going very well at home. An exam reveals that Caryn is 6 weeks' pregnant. She states that her husband refused to allow her to use the diaphragm because it interfered with spontaneity. Although unplanned, she expresses acceptance of the pregnancy and says that things will work out for the best. The clinic nurse is frustrated with Caryn's situation and the patient's refusal to take control of her life. She struggles to maintain objectivity in her conversations with Caryn and offers information regarding safe shelters for abused women with children even though Caryn denies a need for the service.

Caryn misses two consecutive prenatal visits, and a follow-up phone call is made to arrange a home visit. The community health nurse notes a very clean apartment and two quiet children who appear well cared for. She also notes facial bruising on Caryn. Caryn's husband questions the necessity for the visit stating, "You should have better things to do than snoop into people's homes." He refuses to leave the room when the public health nurse asks to speak with Caryn alone. Caryn explains her bruising by stating, "I am so clumsy. I walked into the door when I was getting up to go to the bathroom." She promises to keep her next clinic visit that is scheduled for the following week.

When Caryn comes to the clinic she reveals that her husband is reluctant for her go out alone, saying that she might be seeing other men when he is at work. She also says that she is starting to fear his unprovoked temper outbursts during which he hits her. His drinking on the weekends seems to make things worse. She makes a point of saying that he always apologizes for what he does and asks her forgiveness. She feels that she can handle the situation because of her deep faith in God. Caryn does acknowledge that she has held onto the abuse hotline card.

Caryn delivers her third child at 36 weeks' gestation after "falling down the stairs" in her apartment. Both mom and baby are physically well at her 6 weeks' postpartum visit, though Caryn reports fatigue in keeping up with the three children and the apartment. She is breastfeeding but reports that this baby is an additional challenge because he has colic. Her husband is disappointed that she does not always have dinner ready when he gets home and that she seems preoccupied with the children. The baby's crying "gets on his nerves because he is under a lot of pressure at work and needs to relax when he gets home." Caryn asks for information about sterilization, stating that "three kids are probably all that I can handle. I am tired all the time." She takes information regarding both tubal ligation and vasectomy stating that she wants to discuss them with her husband. Caryn calls the clinic the following week sobbing and stating that her husband has beaten her. He accused her of infidelity after she brought up the subject of sterilization.

Assessment
The following are the summary assessment points:
- Family has a history of suspected IPV.
- Caryn is a stay-at-home mom, with three children under the age of 5 years.
- Caryn reports loss of friends due to husband's disapproval.
- Caryn's deep faith in God is a source of strength.
- The husband has a strong need for control.
- Caryn believes she lacks employable skills.
- Both sets of grandparents live 2 to 3 hours away and are unable to assist because of health issues.
- The husband's abuse is aggravated by drinking.

Diagnoses
- Risk for severe injury or death related to spousal abuse
- High risk for emotional trauma from dysfunctional family dynamics
- High risk for isolation from fear and shame
- Potential risk for physical abuse of children

Planning
Long-Term Goals
- Caryn and her family will be free of IPV.
- Caryn will enter individual counseling.
- Family will demonstrate appropriate coping skills.
- Family will enter counseling.

Short-Term Goals
- Caryn and her children will be assessed for possible injury.
- Husband will be referred for anger management classes.
- Support will be identified to help Caryn with the children.
- A safe setting will be identified for Caryn and the children.

Intervention
Individual
Since Caryn's phone call indicates a possible life-threatening situation, the immediate action is to call the police. Caryn was treated in the emergency department and released with a referral for nursing services for facial and head wound care. She decided to press charges, and her husband was arrested.

Caryn agreed to enter counseling, moved to a battered women's shelter, and sought legal assistance to have a restraining order issued against her spouse. Over the next 2 weeks, the community health nurse visited Caryn three times weekly because of her need for dressing changes. The nurse's goals were centered on Caryn's ongoing physical and emotional well-being.

During these visits, the nurse was able to engage Caryn in conversation regarding her future and that of her children. Caryn indicated that this most recent episode of violence had frightened her and caused her to question the wisdom of her decision to stay with her husband in the past. Her husband was found guilty of assault and battery and was sentenced to 2 years probation and mandatory anger management classes.

Community
The community health nurse arranged to speak at the monthly breakfast meeting of community pastors where she offered to present an informational program on IPV to area churches. Within 3 weeks she received invitations from four of the nine churches represented at the meeting. The first of the programs will take place in the next month. Two of the churches have mother's day out available to church members. After an appeal from the community health nurse, one of the churches has expressed a willingness to open their program to non–church members.

Evaluation
Individual and Community
The clinic and community health nurses jointly focused on safety as a priority of care for both Caryn and her children. The call to the police started the chain of events that resulted in Caryn's emergency department visit. Caryn's injuries created an opportunity for the community health nurse to maintain contact and provide psychosocial support. Caryn's social isolation that had been created by her husband was lessened by the restraining order. During the nurse's visits she was able to speak openly with Caryn and offer options to enhance her coping skills. Caryn reported receiving parental support on the phone for her decisions. One of the local pastors has encouraged her to focus on her children and her own future.

Continued

CASE STUDY   APPLICATION OF THE NURSING PROCESS—cont'd

During her 6-week stay at the women's shelter, Caryn received intensive counseling and job skill training to prepare for beginning job placement. Paperwork was initiated to begin divorce proceedings.

Six months after Caryn's return to the community she visited Planned Parenthood for an annual exam. The two older children have received counseling. Caryn is now working full-time as a receptionist at a law firm. Her children are attending day care at one of the local churches where Caryn has made friends and is considering joining. The divorce proceedings are on hold as she and her husband are discussing a possible reconciliation. Caryn's husband continues to fulfill the requirements of his probation. Caryn stated that her husband's remorse includes the fact that he wants to break the cycle that began with his father's abuse of him and his mother. He acknowledges that this will be an ongoing recovery process.

Levels of Prevention
Primary
Goal: Promote safety and prevent violence.
- Encourage contact with friends in the neighborhood and at church.
- Provide services of the community health nurse.
- Provide community education programs on anger management.
- Provide community education programs about IPV.

Secondary
Goal: Assess for signs of IPV and possible child abuse.
- Facilitate health care for treatment of injuries.
- Provide both physical and psychosocial support.
- Provide referral for anger management.
- Provide individual and family counseling.
- Provide a 24-hour abuse hotline number.

Tertiary
Goal: Promote development of healthy family dynamics.
- Encourage continued use of community resources.
- Provide information regarding local women's shelters.
- Encourage community involvement with other young families.
- Encourage establishment of mother's day out programs at area churches.
- Provide community education programs on the cycle of violence.

LEARNING ACTIVITIES

1. Investigate professional responsibilities relative to reporting abuse, neglect, or violence in your state. Share findings with classmates.
2. Using the telephone directory or computer search engine, find three public or private agencies in the community that provide help for victims of violence. Make a list of the telephone numbers and post in public areas.
3. Call a child abuse center in the community, and ask what services they provide.
4. Call a battered women's shelter, and determine the procedure for securing shelter placement for a battered victim and children.
5. Visit a respite center for the elderly, and observe the clients and the activities that are provided. Observe behaviors that would contribute to stress in the caregiver.
6. Find out what support groups exist in the community for older adult caregivers.
7. Read your local newspaper for 1 month, and clip articles that deal with violence. Determine how many individuals were killed or injured during that period. How many of them were gun related?

REFERENCES

Campbell J, Humphreys J: *Nursing care of survivors of family violence*, St. Louis, 1993, Mosby.

Centers for Disease Control and Prevention: Nonfatal and fatal firearm-related injuries: United States, 1993-1997, *MMWR Morb Mortal Wkly Rep* 48(45):1029–1034, 1999.

Centers for Disease Control and Prevention: *Health statistics (NCHS) National vital statistics system*, 2005, webappa.cdc.gov/.

Centers for Disease Control and Prevention: Physical dating violence among high school students—United States, 2003, *MMWR Morb Mortal Wkly Rep* 55:532–535, 2006, www.cdc.gov/mmwr/preview/mmwr.html/mm5519a3.htm.

Centers for Disease Control and Prevention: *Intimate partner violence can lead to serious injury: fact sheet on dating violence*, October 13, 2008, www.cdc.gov/Features/IntimatePartnerViolence/.

Centers for Disease Control and Prevention: *FastStats, assault or homicide*, April 2, 2009a. http://www.cdc.gov/nchs/fastats/homicide.htm.

Centers for Disease Control and Prevention: *Violence prevention: sexual violence*, January 27, 2009b, www.cdc.gov/ViolencePrevention/sexualviolence/riskprotectivefactors.html.

Centers for Disease Control and Prevention, National Center for Injury Prevention and Control: *Intimate partner violence: fact sheet*, 2006, www.cdc.gov/injury.

Centers for Disease Control and Prevention, National Center for Injury Prevention and Control: *Child maltreatment facts at a glance*, Spring 2008, www.cdc.gov/injury.

Centers for Disease Control and Prevention: National Center for Injury Prevention and Control: Division of violence prevention, January 27, 2009, www.cdc.gov/ViolencePrevention/index.html.

Centers for Disease Control and Prevention: National Institute for Occupational Safety and Health, 2002, www.cdc.gov/niosh/docs/2002-101/.

Egley A, O'Donnell C: *United States Department of Justice: Highlights of the 2007 National Youth Gang Survey*, April 2009, www.ojp.usdoj.gov.

Federal Bureau of Investigation: *Hate crime statistics, 2007*, 2008, www.fbi.gov/ucr/hc2007/incidents.htm.

Finkelhor D, Ormord R: *US Department of Justice, Juvenile Justice Bulletin, homicides of children and youth*, 2001.

Kellerman AL, et al: Suicide in the home in relation to gun ownership, *N Engl J Med* 327:467–472, 1992.

KidsHealth: *Abusive head trauma (shakenbaby-syndrome)*, 2009, www./kidshealth.org/parent/medical/brain/shaken.html.

Ludwig J, Cook P: *Evaluating gun policy: effects on crime and violence*, Washington, DC, 2003, Brookings Institution Press.

Mother Goose nursery rhymes, Bath, England, 2000, Robert Frederick Publishing.

National Center on Elder Abuse: *Elder abuse prevalence and incidence: FactSheet*,

Washington, DC, 2005, US Department on Aging, Department of Health and Human Services. Grant No 1 90-AM-2792. National Gang Intelligence Center: National Gang Threat Assessment, 2009: Product No 2009-M0335-001.

National Rifle Association, Institute for Legislative Action: *Handgun: summary*, 2008, www.nraila.org/Issues/FactSheets/read.aspx.

Occupational Safety and Health Administration: *Workplace violence*, 2007, www.osha.gov/SLTC/workplaceviolence/index.html.

Rape, Abuse, & Incest National Network: *Statistics*, 2008, www.rainn.org/statistics.

University of Michigan Health System: *Abuse during pregnancy*, 2005, www.med.umich.edu./1libr/wha/wha_batpreg_bha.htm.

U.S. Department of Health and Human Services: *Healthy People 2010*, Washington, DC, 2000, The Author.

U.S. Department of Health and Human Services: *Domestic violence fact sheet*, January 11, 2007, www.atahealth.com/Consumer/Disorders/Dom/ViolFacts.html.

U.S. Department of Justice, Bureau of Justice Statistics: *Homicide trends in the United States*, July 11, 2007a, The Author, www.ojp.usdoj.gov/bjs/homicide/race.htm.

U.S. Department of Justice, Bureau of Justice Statistics: *Intimate partner violence in the US*, December 19, 2007b, www.ojp.usdoj.gov/bjs/intimate/victims.htm.

U.S. Department of Justice, Bureau of Justice Statistics: *Prison statistics*, 2009, www.ojp.usdoj.gov/bjs/prisons.htm.

U.S. Department of Justice, Office of Justice Programs: *Juvenile arrests, 2006*, 2008, www.ojp.usdoj.gov/ojj2p.

U.S. Department of Justice, Office on Violence Against Women: *About stalking*, 2009, www.ovw.usdoj.gov/aboutstalking.htm.

Wasserman C: *Dating violence on campus: a fact of life*, National Center for Victims of Crime, Winter 2004, cwasserman@ncvc.org.

Webb J: Why we must fix our prisons, *Parade* March 29, 2009.

World Health Organization: *Violence and injury prevention and disability (VIP)*, 2009, www.who.int/violence:injury_prevention/violence/en/.

Natural and Man-Made Disasters

Edith B. Summerlin

Additional Material for Study, Review, and Further Exploration

evolve WEBSITE

http://evolve.elsevier.com/Nies

- Quiz
- Case Studies
- Glossary
- WebLinks

OBJECTIVES

Upon completion of this chapter, the reader will be able to do the following:

1. Identify the types of disasters.
2. Discuss the characteristics of disasters.
3. Describe the stages of a disaster.
4. Discuss the stages of disaster management.
5. Describe the role of federal, state, local, and volunteer agencies involved in disaster management.
6. Identify potential bioterrorist chemical and biological agents.
7. Discuss the impact of disasters on a community.
8. Describe the role and responsibilities of nurses in relation to disasters.

KEY TERMS

American Red Cross
direct victim
disaster
disaster triage
displaced persons
Federal Emergency Management
   Agency (FEMA)
first responders
frequency

imminence
indirect victim
mass casualty
multiple casualty
NA-TECH (natural-technological)
   disaster
National Incident Management System
Office of Emergency Management
predictability

preventability
refugees
resource map
risk map
shelter in place
terrorism
U.S. Department of Homeland
   Security
weapons of mass destruction

OUTLINE

Disaster Definitions
Types of Disasters
Characteristics of Disasters
   Frequency
   Predictability
   Preventability
   Imminence
   Scope and Number of Casualties
   Intensity

Disaster Management
   Local, State, and Federal Governmental Responsibilities
   Public Health System
   American Red Cross
Disaster Management Stages
   Prevention Stage
   Preparedness and Planning Stage
   Response Stage
   Recovery Stage

Communities throughout the world experience an emergency or disaster incident of one kind or another almost daily. The media may only mention these events or may report on them in great detail, depending on the number of dead or injured, the amount of devastation or damage to the area involved, and how much the event has disrupted normal activities within the community.

The health of a community can be affected significantly by disasters. Hurricane Katrina and Hurricane Rita, which hit the same geographic area (U.S. Gulf Coast between Houston, Texas, and Biloxi, Mississippi) within a few weeks (September 2005), are examples of how communities and their hospitals, clinics, nursing homes, and other health care facilities are directly affected as a result of a disaster. During these hurricanes, access to health care was impeded by physical barriers, such as road closures due to flooding, inadequate numbers of first responders, and limited transportation for search and rescue. Patients were evacuated from one hospital to another, sometimes more than once. Medical and nursing personnel, medicines, and needed supplies were unavailable, scarce, or depleted because of the increased demand. Temporary shelters and health care services were established in schools, churches, and a variety of other facilities throughout the area. The wind damage and extensive flooding from Hurricane Katrina resulted in panic for food, water, and rescue in the Gulf Coast regions between New Orleans, Louisiana, and Biloxi, Mississippi. First responders and rescue teams were overwhelmed in their attempts to reach the victims.

The evacuation of Houston, Texas, and the surrounding coastal area due to Hurricane Rita created severe traffic jams, many lasting 18 to 20 hours, and resulted in travelers needing water, food, and gasoline before they reached shelter. As a result, many people suffered from dehydration and urinary tract infections. In addition, Hurricane Rita occurred during a period of record heat, and many travelers became victims of heat exhaustion caused by the high temperature and humidity. The lessons learned from these events resulted in changes in disaster plans that made a significant difference in how the next major hurricane—Ike in September 2008—was managed.

Hurricanes, tornadoes, floods, wildfires, and industrial accidents occur yearly in some parts of the United States. Further, in recent years, terrorist attacks have become more common. The bombing of the World Trade Center in New York City in 1991 and the bombing of the Alfred P. Murrah Federal Building in 1995 occurred more than a decade ago, but the combined terrorist attacks on the twin towers of the World Trade Center in New York City, the Pentagon in Washington, DC, and the plane hijacking and crash in Pennsylvania in 2001 indicate that the potential is ever present. Additionally, terrorist attacks occur all over the world on an almost daily basis, and concerns about potential terrorist attacks have increased the focus on what needs to be done in terms of prevention, preparedness, response, and recovery—not only in the event of terrorist attacks but also in the event of disasters of all kinds.

Because of the recognition of the need to be prepared, programs have been created to address the national, state, and local management of disasters. In March 2003, President G. W. Bush established the U.S. Department of Homeland Security and put into place the National Incident Management System (NIMS) the following year. The NIMS provides a systematic, proactive approach for all levels of governmental and nongovernmental agencies to work seamlessly to prevent, protect against, respond to, recover from, and prevent the effects of disasters (Federal Emergency Management Agency [FEMA], 2009). Local Citizen Corps Councils have been established throughout the country to provide volunteers an opportunity to support local fire, law enforcement, emergency medical services, and community public health efforts and to contribute to the four stages of emergency management: prevention, preparedness, response, and recovery (Texas Association of Regional Councils, 2009).

Efforts to prepare for disasters have also been significantly enhanced at the state level. In Texas, for example, the Texas Legislature passed a bill requiring nurses to attend a continuing education program related to bioterrorism (Board of Nurse Examiners for the State of Texas, 2005). Further, the Ready Texas Nurses Emergency Response System (Ready Texas Nurses) was created to provide mobilization of volunteer nurses to support communities in times of crisis or disaster (Texas Department of Health and Texas Nurses Association, 2004). Similar actions are occurring throughout the country.

Nurses are uniquely positioned to provide valuable information for the development of plans for disaster prevention, preparedness, response, and recovery for communities. Nurses, as team members, can cooperate with health and social representatives, government bodies, community groups, and volunteer agencies in disaster planning and preparedness programs (i.e., drills). Nurses using their knowledge of nursing, public health, and cultural-familial structures, as well as their clinical skills and abilities, can actively assist or participate in all aspects and stages of an emergency or disaster, regardless of the setting in which the event may occur. Nurses have a significant role in meeting the health care needs of the community, not only on a day-to-day basis, but also in relation to disasters.

DISASTER DEFINITIONS

A disaster is any event that causes a level of destruction, death, or injury that affects the abilities of the community to respond to the incident using available resources. Emergencies differ from disasters in that the agency, community, family, or individual can manage an emergency using their own resources. But a disaster event, depending on the characteristics of the disaster, may be beyond the ability of the community to respond and recover from the incident using their own resources. Disasters frequently require assistance from outside the immediate community, both to manage resulting issues and to recover.

Some disasters (e.g., a house fire) may affect only a few persons, whereas others (e.g., a hurricane) can impact thousands. A mass casualty event is one in which 100 or more individuals are involved; a multiple casualty event is one in which more than two but fewer than 100 individuals are involved. Casualties can be classified as a direct victim, an indirect victim, a displaced person, or a refugee. A direct victim is an individual who is immediately affected by the event; the indirect victim may be a family member or friend of the victim or a first responder. Displaced persons and refugees are special categories of direct victims. Displaced persons are those who have to evacuate their home, school, or business as a result of a disaster; refugees are a group of people who have fled their home or even their country as a result of famine, drought, natural disaster, war, or civil unrest.

TYPES OF DISASTERS

Disasters are identified as natural, man-made, or a combination of both. A NA-TECH (natural-technological) disaster is a natural disaster that creates or results in a widespread technological problem. An example of a NA-TECH disaster is an earthquake that causes structural collapse of roadways or bridges that, in turn, causes downed electrical wires and subsequent fires. Another example is a chemical spill resulting from a flood. Types of natural disasters and man-made disasters are listed in Box 28-1.

The American Public Health Association (2005) identified types of disasters and their consequences. Types of disasters include blizzards, cold waves, heavy snowfalls, cyclones, tornadoes, drought, earthquakes, floods, heat waves, thunderstorms, volcanic eruptions, wildfires, man-made and technological events, explosions or blasts, and epidemics. It was noted in the report that injury or death from the disaster in question may be direct or indirect. For example, injuries from hurricanes occur because people fail to evacuate or take shelter, do not take precautions in securing their property despite adequate warning, and do not follow guidelines on food and water safety or injury prevention during recovery. Drowning, electrocution, lacerations or punctures from flying debris, and blunt trauma from falling trees or other objects are some of the morbidity concerns. Heart attacks and stress-related disorders also occur. Injuries also may occur from activities in the recovery phase, for example, from use of chain saws or other power equipment or from bites from animals, snakes, or insects.

Americans are familiar with most of the disasters listed in Box 28-1, but terrorism was largely unknown or unheeded prior to the bombing of the Alfred P. Murrah Federal Building in Oklahoma City in 1995. The U.S. Code of Federal Regulations defines terrorism as "the unlawful use of force and violence against persons or property to intimidate or coerce a government, the civilian population, or any segment thereof, in furtherance of political or social objectives" (FBI, 2004). The Federal Emergency Management Agency (FEMA) defines terrorism as "the use of force or violence against persons or property in violation of the criminal laws of the United States for purposes of intimidation, coercion, or ransom" (FEMA, 2005b). The Central Intelligence Agency (2007) states that terrorism "is premeditated, politically motivated violence perpetrated against noncombatant targets by sub-national groups or clandestine agents, usually intended to influence an audience" (p. 2). In short, terrorists often use threats of violence, as well as acts of mass destruction, to create fear among the public, to try to convince citizens that their government is powerless, and to seek immediate publicity (FEMA, 2005b).

Acts of terrorism include threats of terrorism, assassinations, kidnappings, hijackings, bomb scares and bombings, computer-based attacks, and the use of chemical, biological, nuclear, and radiological weapons. In addition to those mentioned earlier (i.e., September 11, 2001; bombing of the Alfred P. Murrah Federal Building, 1995), other examples of terrorist acts include the nerve gas (sarin) attack in the Tokyo subway in March 1995, which killed 12 and injured more than 6000 people; the bombing of the commuter train in Spain in March 2004, which killed 191 people; the suicide bombing in the London subway in July 2005, which killed 52 commuters and four terrorists; and the shooting and bombing attacks in Mumbai's financial district in November 2008, which killed more than 170.

Concerns now are increasingly focused on weapons of mass destruction. Weapons of mass destruction refer to any weapon that is designed or intended to cause death or serious bodily injury through release, dissemination, or impact of toxic or poisonous chemicals, or their precursors; any weapon involving a disease organism; or any weapon that is designed to release radiation or radioactivity at a level dangerous to human life. Biological organisms considered to be potential weapons of mass destruction are found in Table 28-1, and chemicals that are potential weapons of mass destruction are listed in Table 28-2. Chemical warfare agents are classified as nerve agents, vesicants, pulmonary agents, and cyanides (formerly "blood agents"). These tables also include information about the lethality, treatment, and impact related to each.

CHARACTERISTICS OF DISASTERS

Several characteristics have been used to describe disasters (Box 28-2). These characteristics are interdependent and therefore important to consider in plans for managing any disaster event. Each is discussed briefly.

BOX 28-1 TYPES OF DISASTERS	
NATURAL DISASTERS	**MAN-MADE DISASTERS**
Avalanches	Terrorism
Blizzards	Civil unrest (riots)
Communicable disease epidemics	Explosions, bombings
Droughts, wildfires	Fires
Earthquakes, tsunamis	Structural collapse (bridges)
Hailstorms	Floods, mudslides
Heat waves	Toxic or hazardous spills
Hurricanes	Mass transit accidents
Tornadoes, cyclones	Pollution
Volcanic eruptions	Wars

TABLE 28-1 BIOLOGICAL WEAPONS OF MASS DESTRUCTION

BIOLOGICAL ORGANISM	LETHALITY	PREVENTION	TREATMENT	POTENTIAL FOR USE
Smallpox (incubation 1-5 days)	High	Vaccine	Symptomatic; secondary infections	One person could possibly cause a national epidemic
Anthrax (incubation 2-60 days)	Very high	Vaccine	Antibiotics early; if late, nothing	Likely agent; resistant to weather; can be stored
Plague *(Yersinia pestis)* (incubation 1-3 days)	Very high; 100% if untreated	No vaccine	Antibiotics	Not considered a likely agent; difficult to turn into a weapon
Botulism	High	Vaccine being tested	Antitoxin; requires intensive supportive care	Not considered a likely weapon
Tularemia	Moderate	Vaccine being studied	Antibiotics	Difficult to stabilize for use as a weapon
Ebola	Very high	No vaccine	Minimal	Not considered a likely weapon; difficult to acquire; poorly understood
Brucellosis (incubation 5-21 days)	Low	No vaccine	Antibiotics; begin upon suspicion of disease	Not considered a likely weapon; low lethality
Q fever *(Coxiella burnetii)* (incubation 14-26 days)	Low	Vaccine	Antibiotics; begin in incubation period	Not considered a likely weapon; low lethality
Other potentials: Viral Venezuelan equine encephalitis, cholera, salmonella, influenza, and staphylococcal enterotoxin B				

From Cieslak TJ, Eitzen EM: Bioterrorism: agents of concern, *J Public Health Manag Pract* 6(4):19-29, 2000.

TABLE 28-2 CHEMICAL AGENTS OF MASS DESTRUCTION

CHEMICAL AGENT	LETHALITY	TREATMENT	IMPACT
Sarin (nerve agent)	High	Move to fresh air; wash skin; drugs limited effectiveness	Likely nerve agent; chemicals needed to produce are banned by International Chemical Weapons Convention
VX (nerve agent)	Very high	Move to fresh air; wash skin; drugs limited effectiveness	Not likely weapon; difficult to manufacture
Tabun (nerve agent)	High	Move to fresh air; wash skin; drugs limited effectiveness	Easy to manufacture nerve agent; likely agent to be used
Chlorine (pulmonary agent)	Low	Move to fresh air; wash skin; no antidote	Readily available; likely agent because of availability; breaks down with water
Hydrogen cyanide (blood agent)	Low to moderate	Move to fresh air; wash skin; some drugs mitigate effects	Industrial product; some chemicals used to produce are banned; likely agent because of availability

From Cieslak TJ, Eitzen EM: Bioterrorism: agents of concern, *J Public Health Manag Pract* 6(4):19-29, 2000.

BOX 28-2 CHARACTERISTICS OF DISASTERS

Frequency
Predictability
Preventability
Imminence
Scope and number of casualties
Intensity

Frequency

Frequency refers to how often a disaster occurs. Some disasters occur relatively often in certain parts of the world. Terrorist activities are occurring on an almost daily basis in Iraq and elsewhere in the world. Other examples are hurricanes, which occur with variable frequency between the months of June and November, and earthquakes, which occur periodically throughout the world. In the United States, earthquakes are generally considered to be a West Coast problem, but forty-five states and territories are at moderate to high risk for an earthquake, and earthquakes have occurred in every region of the country (U.S. Department of Homeland Security, 2004). Other disasters, such as volcanic eruptions, are far less frequent and are geographically limited to certain regions.

Predictability

Predictability relates to the ability to tell when and if a disaster event will occur. Some disasters, such as floods, may be predicted in the spring by monitoring the snowmelt. Weather forecasters can predict when conditions are right for the development of tornadoes; these generally occur between April and June, but they may occur at any time of the year or occur as a secondary result of hurricanes. Weather forecasters can predict hurricanes with increasing accuracy. Other disasters (e.g., fires and industrial explosions) may not be predictable at all.

Preventability

Preventability refers to actions taken to avoid a disaster. Some disasters (e.g., hurricanes, tornadoes, and earthquakes) are not preventable, whereas others can be easily controlled if not prevented entirely. For example, flooding can be controlled or prevented through construction of dams or levees or deepening bayous.

Primary prevention is aimed at preventing the occurrence of a disaster or limiting consequences when the event itself cannot be prevented. Primary prevention occurs in the nondisaster and predisaster stages. The nondisaster stage is the period before a disaster occurs, and the predisaster stage refers to action(s) taken when a disaster is pending. Preventive actions during the nondisaster stage include assessing communities to determine potential disaster hazards; developing disaster plans at local, state, and federal levels; conducting

drills to test the plan; training volunteers and health care providers; and providing educational programs of all kinds.

Risk maps and resource maps are developed to aid in planning. A risk map is a geographic map of an area that is analyzed for the impact of a potential disaster on the population and buildings in the area that would be involved (e.g., an area in a flood plain, an area covered if a nuclear explosion would occur, an area involved in an explosion of an industrial site) (Figure 28-1). A resource map is a geographic map that outlines the resources that would be available in or near the area affected by a potential disaster (e.g., potential shelter sites, potential medical sources, and location of equipment that might be needed) (Figure 28-2).

The disaster plan is initiated predisaster or when a disaster is imminent. Primary prevention actions during this stage include notification of the appropriate officials, warning the population, and advising what response to take (e.g., shelter in place or evacuate).

Secondary prevention strategies are implemented once the disaster occurs. Secondary prevention actions include search,

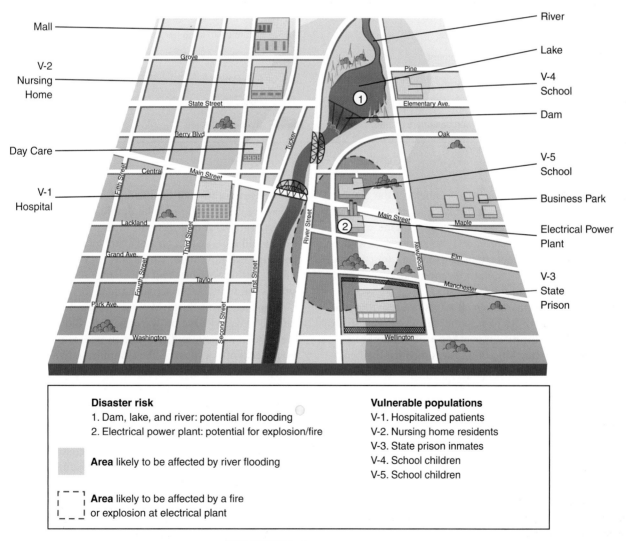

Disaster risk
1. Dam, lake, and river: potential for flooding
2. Electrical power plant: potential for explosion/fire

Area likely to be affected by river flooding

Area likely to be affected by a fire or explosion at electrical plant

Vulnerable populations
V-1. Hospitalized patients
V-2. Nursing home residents
V-3. State prison inmates
V-4. School children
V-5. School children

FIGURE 28-1 Community risk map.

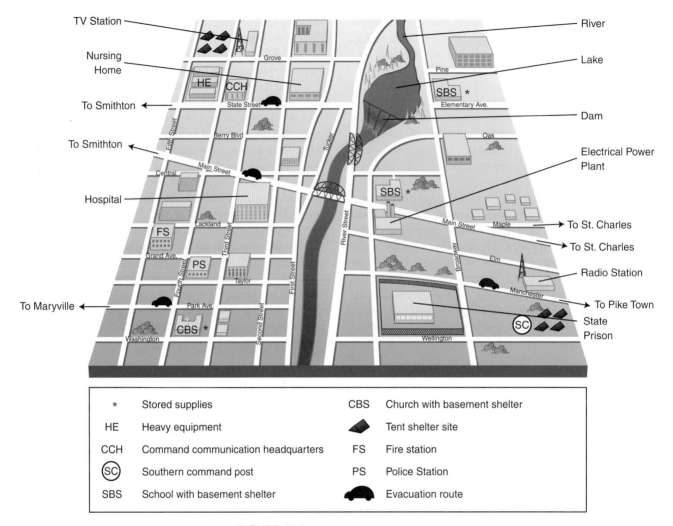

*	Stored supplies	CBS	Church with basement shelter
HE	Heavy equipment	◣	Tent shelter site
CCH	Command communication headquarters	FS	Fire station
SC	Southern command post	PS	Police Station
SBS	School with basement shelter	🚗	Evacuation route

FIGURE 28-2 Community resource map.

rescue, and triage of victims and assessment of the destruction and devastation of the area involved.

Tertiary prevention focuses on recovery of the community, that is, restoring the community to its previous level of functioning and its residents to their maximum functioning. Tertiary prevention is aimed at preventing a recurrence or minimizing the effects of future disasters.

Nurses should be involved in all stages of prevention and related activities. In order to respond effectively, personally, and professionally during different types of disasters, nurses need to know: (1) what kind of disasters threaten their communities, (2) what injuries to expect from different disaster scenarios, (3) evacuation routes, (4) location of shelters, and (5) warning systems. They must be able to educate others about disasters and how to prepare for and respond to them. Finally, nurses need to keep up-to-date on the latest recommendations and advances in lifesaving measures (e.g., basic first aid, cardiopulmonary resuscitation [CPR], and use of automated external defibrillators).

Imminence

Imminence is the speed of onset of an impending disaster and relates to the extent of forewarning possible and the anticipated duration of the incident. Weather forecasters can tell when a hurricane may be developing days ahead of its expected arrival and can give the time of arrival, general direction it will take, and an approximate location for its landing and forward movement. Hurricanes, however, are subject to other weather variables and can change direction and intensity several times before actual landfall.

Some disastrous incidents (e.g., wildfires, explosions, and terrorist attacks) have no warning time. Bioterrorist attacks are generally silent, and the first awareness may be days or even weeks after exposure. For example, individuals exposed to a pathologic agent (e.g., anthrax, smallpox) may arrive at health care facilities at various times and to various providers, making diagnosis and early treatment difficult. Nurses and medical personnel need to know the signs and symptoms of biological, chemical, radiation, and nuclear exposure in order to identify the nature of the threat and then to treat and control the spread of both biological and chemical agents (see Table 28-1 and Table 28-2).

Scope and Number of Casualties

The scope of a disaster indicates the range of its effect. The scope is described in terms of the geographic area involved and in terms of the number of individuals affected, injured, or killed. From a health care perspective, the location, type, and timing of a disaster event are predictors of the types of injuries and illnesses that might occur. For example, the October 1989 earthquake in San Francisco occurred while people were on their way to work. Overall, more than 60 people died from a multitude of causes, including a motorcycle officer who was killed following the collapse of a freeway, sixteen people who were killed from building collapses, five who died as a result of falls, and nine who died of heart attacks.

In contrast, the earthquake and tsunami in October 2004 killed more than 174,000 people in South Asia, Southeast Asia, and East Africa; most died of drowning (Centers for Disease Control and Prevention [CDC], 2005). Another example of the horribly destructive power of earthquakes occurred in Pakistan in October 2005. That quake resulted in landslides that killed more than 73,000 people; many of the dead were children whose schools were buried from the mudslides.

Hurricanes generally affect a large geographic area. Despite this, they may cause few if any deaths if sufficient preventive measures are taken. The scope of Hurricane Katrina in September 2005 covered all of New Orleans, most of south Louisiana, and parts of Florida, Alabama, and Mississippi. Hurricane Rita, only a few days later, struck New Orleans again, as well as south Louisiana and much of eastern Texas. Remarkably, despite the widespread destruction caused by these storms, the number of dead from Katrina was more than 1300, and the number of dead from Hurricane Rita was 58, including 23 elders who were killed in a bus accident while evacuating.

Intensity

Intensity is the characteristic describing the level of destruction and devastation of the disaster event. Factors contributing to the amount of damage from a disaster event such as a hurricane are the distance from the zone of maximum winds, how exposed the location is, building standards, vegetation type, and resultant flooding. Parts of New Orleans were under water from the primary effects (storm surge and rain) and secondary effects (levee failure) from Hurricane Katrina. Some buildings and homes were completely destroyed, and others were left in terrible conditions because of flooding and wind damage.

Various hurricane and tornado scales have been developed based on wind intensity and predicted level of destruction. The Fujita Tornado Intensity Scale developed in 1971 categorized each tornado by its intensity and the area involved. In 1992, Fujita updated the scale to include an estimate of F-scale damage. The new scale, the Enhanced Fujita Scale (EF Scale), implemented in the United States on February 1, 2007, is still a set of wind estimates (not measurements) based on types of structural damage. The estimates vary with height of apparent damage above the ground and exposure (National Oceanic and Atmospheric Administration, 2009).

BOX 28-3 THE SAFFIR-SIMPSON HURRICANE WIND SCALE

Category 1 (74-95 mph): Damaging winds are expected.
Category 2 (96-110 mph): Very strong winds will produce widespread damage.
Category 3 (111-130 mph): Dangerous winds will cause extensive damage.
Category 4 (131-155 mph): Extremely dangerous winds causing devastating damage are expected.
Category 5 (Sustained winds greater than 155 mph): Catastrophic damage is expected.

Hurricanes have been categorized since 1975 with use of the Saffir-Simpson Hurricane Scale, which includes sustained wind intensity, storm surge ranges, and flooding references. On an experimental basis for the 2009 tropical cyclone season, the storm surge ranges and flooding references were removed for each of the five categories (Box 28-3) because storm surge information is inaccurate. For example, Hurricane Ike in 2008 was a category 2 hurricane but had a storm surge at Galveston, Texas, equivalent to a category 4–5 storm surge, and Hurricane Katrina in 2007 was a category 3 hurricane with a storm surge equivalent to a category 5. The revised scale is called the Saffir-Simpson Hurricane Wind Scale. The new scale does not include storm surge, rainfall-induced floods, and tornadoes. The National Weather Service is currently debating whether or not to make the change (National Weather Service, 2009).

DISASTER MANAGEMENT

When one is aware of the types and characteristics of disasters, the question then becomes: What can be done to prevent, prepare for, respond to, and recover from disasters? Disaster management requires an interdisciplinary, collaborative team effort and involves a network of agencies and individuals to develop a disaster plan that covers the multiple elements necessary for an effective plan. Communities can respond more quickly, more effectively, and with less confusion if the efforts needed in the event of a disaster have been anticipated and plans for meeting them identified. The result of planning is that more lives are saved and less property is damaged. Planning ensures that resources are available and that roles and responsibilities of all personnel and agencies, both official and unofficial, are delineated.

Nurses need to know their personal, professional, and community responsibilities. They should realize that conflicts may arise between their personal and professional responsibilities if these have not been considered and planned for in advance (Ethical Insights box). Also, nurses may be direct or indirect victims and may even be displaced persons as a result of a disaster event. Recognizing this possibility, nurses need to plan, prepare, practice, and teach their family and significant others how to respond.

⚖ ETHICAL INSIGHTS

Deciding Whether to Care for Family or Care for Patients

During a disaster, a nurse might face an ethical dilemma because of competing responsibilities to family, employer, and patients. For example, a nurse who is a single parent with young children and has a limited support system may be forced to decide between her responsibility to care for her children or a mandate to report to work to care for patients. Choosing may result in loss of employment or danger to the children. Potential conflicts such as this should be considered, discussed, and decisions made in conjunction with the employer before a disaster event.

BOX 28-4   GUIDELINES FOR EARLY DETECTION FOR BIOCHEMICAL TERRORIST INCIDENTS

- A rapidly increasing disease incidence (within hours or days) in a normally healthy population.
- An unusual increase in the number of people seeking care, especially with fever, respiratory, or gastrointestinal complaints.
- An endemic disease rapidly emerging at an uncharacteristic time or in an unusual pattern.
- Clusters of patients arriving from a single locale.
- Large numbers of rapidly fatal cases—patients who die within 72 hours after admission to the hospital.
- Any patient presenting with a disease that is relatively uncommon and has bioterrorism potential (e.g., pulmonary anthrax, smallpox, or plague).

From Chettle C: Recognizing bioterrorism: nurses on the frontline, *NurseWeek* 6:29-30, Nov 12, 2001.

Local, State, and Federal Governmental Responsibilities

Local Government

The local government is responsible for the safety and welfare of its citizens. Emergencies and disaster incidents are handled at the lowest possible organizational and jurisdictional level. Police, fire, public health, public works, and medical emergency services are the first responders responsible for incident management at the local level. Local officials and agencies are responsible for preparing their citizens for all kinds of emergencies and disasters and for testing disaster plans with mock drills. They manage events during an incident by carrying out evacuation, search, and rescue and maintaining public health and public works responsibilities. Local communities should have contingency operation plans for multiple disaster situations and for various aspects of the plan. For example, land-line telephone service and cell phone service may not work because of being restricted for emergency use only or damage to the infrastructure, so other forms of communication need to be available.

In an incident other than a biological, chemical, radiation, or nuclear event, in most cases, it is the 911 communication center or the fire or police department that gets the initial message. The emergency communication center then communicates the incident to the other first responders and the director of the Office of Emergency Management, who determines others who may be needed (e.g., ambulances, other officials, and voluntary group representatives). Local hospitals are notified of the incident and the predicted nature of impending casualties. The hospitals may begin to receive victims via private automobiles who have not been triaged at the site of the incident. According to the CDC, a hospital can assess the expected number of victims that it may receive by counting the number that arrive within the first hour and doubling that number.

For a biological or chemical terrorist incident, the process is very different. First responders generally are not involved. Rather, nurses and doctors in health care facilities may be the first to suspect that a biological or chemical agent has been released into the community. Box 28-4 lists the guidelines for detecting biochemical incidents. If any of these instances occurs in a health care provider setting, the suspicion should be immediately reported to the infection control department,

the administration of the facility, or both. Each setting should post, near the telephone, the numbers to be called if a biochemical incident (whether internal or external) is suspected. These numbers should include those of the CDC Bioterrorism Emergency Response, the CDC Hospital Infections program, and the U.S. Army Medical Research Institute of Infectious Diseases (Chettle, 2001).

The Office of Emergency Management involves representatives from all official and unofficial agencies in developing the community disaster plan, developing scenarios to test the plan through drills, and assessing the scope, intensity, and number of casualties (once an incident has occurred) in order to initiate the proper response. For those events that are not within the abilities of the local community or in the event of a terrorist-type incident, higher-level agencies and resources must be requested and will become involved.

State Government

When a disaster overwhelms the local community's resources, then the state's Department or Office of Emergency Management is called for assistance. Prior to an event, state officials provide technical support for prevention, preparedness, response, and recovery. State officials visit local officials to assist and assess local emergency management plans, promote and conduct workshops and training courses, assist with training exercises, advise and support local government officials, and are on scene at disaster events to facilitate coordination of state resources and to disseminate information. In some cases, the National Guard may be called in to aid the community. When the scope of the event is so great that local and state resources are not adequate to meet the needs, the state calls on the federal government; at that point, the President may declare the incident a "national disaster." Once the President declares a national disaster, federal aid is made available. At that point, the National Response Plan, the core operational plan for domestic incident management, would be initiated.

Federal Government

The policy of the federal government is to have a comprehensive and effective program in place to ensure continuity of essential federal functions across a wide array of incidents. The national strategy is to develop a system connecting all levels of government without duplicating efforts. More than 87,000 governmental jurisdictions at the federal, state, and local level have security responsibilities. All federal agencies are required to have in place a viable Continuity of Operations capability plan that ensures the performance of their essential functions during any incident that disrupts normal operations (FEMA, 2005d).

U.S. Department of Homeland Security. As explained previously, the U.S. Department of Homeland Security (DHS) was established in March 2003 to realign the existing agencies, groups, and organizations into a single department, focusing on protecting the American people and their homeland. The DHS consolidated 22 agencies and their 180,000 employees into a single agency (The White House, 2005).

The mission of DHS is to: (1) lead the unified national effort to secure America, (2) prevent and deter terrorist attacks, and (3) protect against and respond to threats and hazards to the nation (DHS, 2009a). The organizational structure of the DHS contains several divisions: the Office of the Secretary, Border and Transportation Security, Emergency Preparedness and Response Directorate, Information Analysis and Infrastructure Protection, Science and Technology, Office of Management, U.S. Citizenship and Immigration Services, U.S. Coast Guard, and the U.S. Secret Service. Within each of these divisions are multiple offices and centers (DHS, 2009b).

The DHS established its Homeland Security Advisory System to build a comprehensive and effective communication structure for disseminating threat information to public safety officials and the public at large. The color-coded threat level system communicates using a threat-based system of low risk to severe risk so that protective measures can be implemented to reduce the likelihood or impact of an attack. Figure 28-3 shows the five different risk levels. The actions to take build on what is done at the low-risk or green level (e.g., develop a family emergency plan) to monitoring local emergency management officials and the media for specific measures to take at the severe-risk or red level (e.g., evacuate).

Preparation for a terrorist incident is similar to preparation for other crisis events. General guidelines from FEMA are to be aware of surroundings; move or leave if you feel uncomfortable; take precautions when traveling; do not accept packages from strangers; report unusual behavior; learn where emergency exits are located in buildings; plan how to get out of buildings in the event of an emergency; be prepared to do without services you are normally dependent on (i.e., electricity, telephone, natural gas, gasoline pumps, cash ATMs, and Internet transactions). An additional guideline is to ensure the following items are available: a portable, battery-operated radio with extra batteries; several flashlights with extra batteries; a first aid kit and manual; hard hats and dust masks; and fluorescent tape to rope off dangerous areas (FEMA, 2005b).

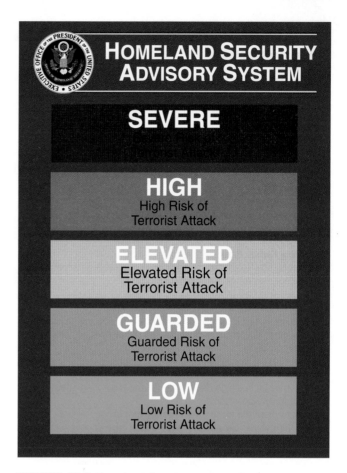

FIGURE 28-3 Homeland Security Advisory System. (From US Department of Homeland Security: *Homeland Security Advisory System: current threat level,* 2009c: www.dhs.gov/dhspublic/display?theme=29&content=3927&print=true.)

In addition to the Homeland Security Advisory System, DHS has published other information for public use. The DHS pamphlet *Preparing Makes Sense: Get Ready Now* (DHS, 2009d) gives advice as to what plans need to be in place to survive without help for a period of time. Other publications are *Homeland Security Advice* and *What To Do in Different Types of Emergencies* (Boxes 28-5 and 28-6).

The National Response Plan and National Response Framework. The National Response Plan (NRP) was part of the reorganization of DHS in 2003 and was updated as the National Response Framework (NRF) in 2008. The NRF explains how all of the agencies work together to coordinate national response, describes specific authorities and best practices for managing incidents, and builds upon the NIMS. The NRF establishes a comprehensive, national all-hazards approach to domestic incidents response (DHS, 2009c).

The DHS Emergency Preparedness and Response Directorate and FEMA, in conjunction with the DHS Office of the Secretary, function as the executive agent for NRP management and maintenance. The Secretary of DHS developed the NIMS, which integrates practices in disaster preparedness and response into a comprehensive national framework for incident management. The NIMS enables responders at

BOX 28-5   HOMELAND SECURITY ADVICE

Emergency Supplies

Food
- Store at least a 3-day supply of nonperishable food.
- Have a manual can opener.
- Keep disposable plates/cups and utensils.

Clean Air
- Store snugly fitting face masks.
- Store plastic sheeting, duct tape, and scissors to seal off a room.

First Aid Kit
- Sterile gloves, dressings, soap, antibiotic ointment, bandages, eye wash, nonprescription medications (e.g., aspirin).

Make a Plan

Create a Family Plan
- Plan on how to contact one another if the family is separated.
- Review plan for different situations.

At Work and School
- Schools, day care providers, workplaces, apartment buildings, and neighborhoods should all have site-specific emergency plans.

In a High-Rise Building
- You may be in a high-rise building at the time of an attack.
- Plan for the possibility.
- Note where the closest **emergency exit** is.
- Be sure you know **another way out** in case your first choice is blocked.

- **Take cover** against a desk or table if things are falling.
- **Face away** from windows and glass.
- **Move away** from exterior walls.
- **Do not use elevators**.
- **Stay to the right** while going down stairwells to allow emergency workers to come up.

Water
- Store at least a 3-day supply; 1 gallon per day per person.
- Store water in clean plastic bottles.

Supply Checklist
- Basic supplies include flashlight, batteries, radio, garbage bags, map, moist towelettes, whistle, clothing, bedding, and tools.

Special Needs Items
- Prescription medications; special items for infants (diapers, formula), elders, or persons with disabilities.

In a Moving Vehicle
- If the vehicle becomes difficult to control, pull over.
- Avoid road hazards.
- Obey barriers and signs.

Deciding to Stay or Go
- Depending on your circumstances and the nature of the attack, the first important decision is whether you stay put or get away.
- You should understand and plan for both possibilities.

From Department of Homeland Security: 2005, www.Ready.gov.

BOX 28-6   WHAT TO DO IN DIFFERENT TYPES OF EMERGENCIES

Biological Attack
- Quickly get away.
- Cover your mouth and nose to filter air.
- Wash with soap and water.

Nuclear Blast
- Take cover quickly.
- Limit amount of radiation exposure by shielding, getting away from blast, and minimizing time exposed.

Chemical Attack
- Quickly get away.
- If exposed, strip immediately and wash.
- Seek medical attention.

Radiation Threat
- "Dirty bomb" uses common explosives to spread radioactive material.
- Limit exposure same as for nuclear blast.

Explosions
- Take shelter against a desk or sturdy table.
- Quickly exit building.
- Crawl if there is fire.

Trapped in Debris
- Use flashlight, whistle, or tap on pipe or wall to signal rescuers.
- Unnecessary movement and shouting risk breathing unsafe dust.

From US Department of Homeland Security: 2005, www.Ready.gov.

all levels to work together effectively in managing domestic incidents, no matter what the cause, size, or complexity (FEMA, 2005c).

The Federal Emergency Management Agency. FEMA became part of DHS in 2003. FEMA's mission is "to lead the efforts to prepare the nation for all hazards and effectively manage federal response and recovery efforts following any national incident (FEMA, 2005a). FEMA also initiates proactive mitigation activities, trains first responders, and manages the National Flood Insurance Program and the U.S. Fire Administration.

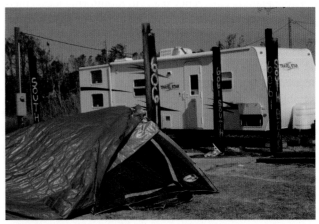

A FEMA trailer sits on the home site of Regina Fowler who lost her home during Hurricane Katrina in Waveland, Mississippi. (Photo by Patsy Lynch/FEMA.)

Department of Health and Human Services/Centers for Disease Control and Prevention. After the rescue of survivors has been accomplished, the Department of Health and Human Services, CDC steps in to ensure that clean drinking water, food, shelter, and medical care are available for those affected. Its involvement may be necessary depending on the type of disaster. For example, floods pose risks of contaminated water (e.g., cholera) and food supplies (e.g., *Escherichia coli*); loss of shelter leaves people vulnerable to heat or cold and other environmental hazards (e.g., insects); and earthquakes create traumatic injuries (e.g., broken bones, head injuries) that will need to be addressed.

Public Health System

The public health system's mission is the promotion of health, prevention of disease, and protection from threats to health. The *public health system* is a broad term used to describe all of the governmental and nongovernmental organizations and agencies that contribute to the improvement of the health of populations. Public health agencies are the primary agencies for the health and medical response to disaster incidents and therefore are a part of the initial response activities.

Public health officials provide advice and assistance to other public officials related to environmental and health matters. Preparedness includes vigilance and reporting of suspicious illnesses (e.g., signs and symptoms of biological agents, food-borne diseases, and communicable diseases) in the community by physicians and nurses in local health care facilities or private offices and clinics. Public health officials then have the responsibility of detecting outbreaks, determining the cause of illness, identifying the risk factors for the population, implementing interventions to control the outbreak, and informing the public of the health risks and preventive measures that need to be taken. These relate both directly and indirectly to the ten essential public health services.

American Red Cross

The American Red Cross (ARC) is not a governmental agency. The ARC, however, is chartered by Congress to provide disaster relief. It works in partnership with FEMA, DHS, the CDC, and other federal agencies to provide and manage needed services.

The ARC is primarily a volunteer organization with chapters in all 50 states, Puerto Rico, the Virgin Islands, and the Pacific Rim; the national headquarters is in Washington, DC. Disaster Services is only one of the programs that the ARC provides. Other program services provided are International Services; Biomedical Services; Armed Forces Emergency Services; and Health, Safety, and Community Services.

The ARC places great emphasis on preparedness and participates with communities in developing and testing their disaster plans, maintaining and training personnel for disaster response, and responding during an actual emergency or disaster. The ARC publishes many pamphlets and educational materials to help individuals, families, neighborhoods, schools, and businesses prepare for potential disasters. The key actions they recommend are: (1) identify potential disaster

events, (2) create a disaster plan for sheltering in place or for evacuation, (3) assemble a disaster supplies kit, and (4) practice and maintain the plan. The disaster plan should include an emergency communications plan, a predetermined meeting place for family members or significant others, and plans for care of pets in the event that evacuation is required.

If local authorities issue a shelter-in-place communication, instructions that address what actions to take if at home, at work, at school, or in a vehicle should be followed (see Table 28-4). For example, during a disaster, such as hazardous gas emission from an industrial plant, if someone is at home, a business, or public building, he or she may be instructed to go inside and follow home or work shelter-in-place recommendations (e.g., close doors, turn off fans and air-conditioning, bring children and pets inside, and stay inside until "all clear" has been called).

RESEARCH HIGHLIGHTS
School Nurses and Emergency Preparedness

A survey of 193 school nurses was recently conducted to assess knowledge of bioterrorism and educational needs for emergency preparedness (Evers and Puzniak, 2005). The researchers reported that although 80% of the respondents stated that their school had an emergency plan and an evacuation plan, only about half (48.5%) had a shelter-in-place plan. Further, although most (62%) stated that their school was "somewhat prepared" for a disaster, only 6.2% rated their school as "very prepared." Knowledge of specific information on bioterrorism was only fair. For example, it was noted that only 55% of survey respondents could distinguish between signs and symptoms of anthrax and influenza. Finally, slightly more than half of respondents believed that a biological or chemical attack was "somewhat likely," and nearly 40% believed that a nuclear attack was "somewhat likely." The researchers concluded that school nurses need more training and preparation to be able to respond appropriately to an emergency or disaster situation.

From Evers S, Puzniak L: Bioterrorism knowledge and emergency preparedness among school nurses, *J School Health* 75(6):232-237, 2005.

The Red Cross disaster response efforts focus on meeting the immediate disaster-related needs of affected people and providing support services to the emergency rescue and recovery workers (ARC, 2003). The disaster response functions are to provide health services, mental health services, family services, and mass care, and to inquire about family well-being. Mass care includes feeding, sheltering, providing basic first aid, bulk distribution, and a Disaster Welfare Information system (ARC, 2005). Table 28-3 shows the breadth of services that the ARC provided for hurricane disaster relief in 2004.

DISASTER MANAGEMENT STAGES
Prevention Stage

The first stage in disaster management occurs before a disaster is imminent and is known as the *nondisaster stage*. Potential disaster risks should be identified and risk maps created (see Figure 28-1). The population demographics and vulnerabilities, as well

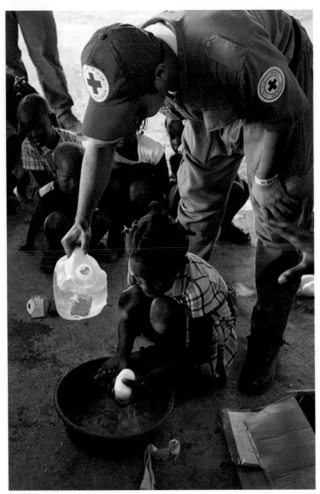

Red Cross volunteers share health and hygiene messages with young earthquake survivors. (Photo by Bonnie Gillespie/American Red Cross.)

TABLE 28-3	AMERICAN RED CROSS DISASTER SERVICES FOLLOWING HURRICANES KATRINA, RITA, AND WILMA
TYPE OF ASSISTANCE	**NUMBER**
Shelters and evacuation centers opened	1400 in 27 states and DC 3.8 million overnight stays
Shelter population	450,000 evacuees
Emergency assistance	1.4 million families and 4 million people
Meals and snacks served	68 million to evacuees and responders

as the community's capabilities, should be analyzed. Primary prevention measures include educating the public regarding what actions to take to prepare for disasters at the individual, family, and community levels. Further, based on the assessment of potential risks, the community must develop a plan for meeting the potential disasters identified.

With regard to bioterrorist attacks, prevention means that health care providers need to be knowledgeable about the biological and chemical agents that might be used. In addition, health care providers need to know the signs and symptoms of the various biological and chemical agents that have been recognized as potential threats. As mentioned, unlike other disasters, biochemical terrorist threats may be identified only when events raise suspicions of health care providers, rather than first responders at a particular site.

Early identification of ill or exposed persons, rapid implementation of preventive therapy, special infection control considerations, and collaboration or communication with the public are essential in controlling the spread of cases. Hospitals need to identify rooms that can be converted into isolation units to meet the demand. Nurses need to be instructed in decontamination and reminded of isolation techniques that might be needed, depending on the biological agent. Volunteers and professionals must remain current in first aid, CPR, and advanced lifesaving procedures.

Preparedness and Planning Stage

Individual and family preparedness includes training in first aid, assembling a disaster emergency kit, establishing a predetermined meeting place away from home, and making a family communication plan. Recommendations for what needs to be included in each of these are available from many sources (e.g., ARC, DHS, and FEMA). These are guidelines, and each individual and each family needs to modify the preparations to meet their personal needs.

Although there will be some variation according to the individual community's needs, all community disaster plans should address the following elements: authority, communication, control, logistical coordination of personnel, supplies and equipment, evacuation, rescue, and care of the dead. The plan should indicate who has the power to declare that there is a disaster and who has the power to initiate the disaster plan.

Authority should be designated by the title of the person; it should not specify a person by name. There should also be backup positions identified in the event the first individual is not available. Every individual should be equally informed about the role and responsibilities that go with this authority. A clear chain of authority for carrying out the plan is critical for successful implementation of the plan. Authority may change, depending on whether the disaster is natural or man-made as a result of some criminal action, and change of authority should be addressed in the plan.

Communication is recognized as a very significant problem during disasters. Misinformation and misinterpretation can occur when communication is ineffective. Reliance on telephone systems or cell phones should not be the sole planned means of communicating because these may not work or the systems might be overwhelmed. The communication section of the disaster plan should address how the authority figure will be notified of the disaster, how the emergency management team members will be notified, how the community residents will be warned about the incident, and what actions to take. This section needs to address how communication between relief workers and authorities will be maintained. Also, it should include information on the role of the media in keeping people informed and in letting people know what assistance and supplies are needed.

The analysis of the population that was completed during the nondisaster stage should identify groups that need special attention as to how they will be notified. These people include those who speak different languages, are homeless or poor, are without television or other means of communication, and are in institutions such as prisons, nursing homes, day care settings, or schools. Effective communication during a disaster must be credible, current, and authoritative and give some indication of future events.

The *logistical* section should specify where supplies and equipment are located or where additional supplies and equipment can be obtained, where these will be stored or found, and how they will be transported to the disaster site (see Figure 28-2). Essential *human resources* (e.g., emergency and disaster specialists, officials of governmental and voluntary agencies, engineers, weather specialists, and community leaders) should be identified and where they will be located together determined. The plan should include information about transportation for *evacuation and rescue* (particularly taking into account vulnerable groups), documentation and record keeping, and plans for evaluation of the success or failure of the plan.

A disaster plan is a dynamic entity. Planning is a continuous process, and plans change with circumstances and when gaps are identified during drills or from actual disaster incidents. The plan should set realistic expectations of effects and needs, should be brief and concise, and should establish priorities and timelines for actions. Plans should follow the disaster planning principles discussed in Box 28-7.

For a plan to be effective, it must be tested by having different disaster scenario drills. The more times realistic scenarios are created to test the plan in actual practice sessions, and not just table top or paper drills, the more problems with the plan will be identified and solutions for those problems can be found. Without practice drills, plans may have many unrecognized faults and, as a result, many more individuals may be harmed and communities damaged when an actual disaster occurs.

Response Stage

This stage begins immediately after the disaster incident occurs. The community preparedness plans that have been developed are initiated. If a disaster occurs, people should remain calm and exert patience, follow the advice of local emergency officials, and listen to the radio or television for news and instructions. If people nearby are injured, one should give first aid, seek help, and check the area for dangerous hazards. Those at home should shut off any damaged utilities, confine or secure pets, call family contact(s), and check on neighbors, especially the elderly or disabled.

The plan may call for people to shelter in place or to evacuate, or for search and rescue to begin. If the only response

BOX 28-7　DISASTER PLANNING PRINCIPLES

1. Measures usually taken are not sufficient for major disasters.
2. Plans should be adjusted to people's needs.
3. Planning does not stop with development of a written plan.
4. Lack of information causes inappropriate responses by community members.
5. People should be able to respond with or without direction.
6. Plans should coordinate efforts of the entire community, so large segments of the citizenry should be involved in the planning.
7. Plans should be linked to surrounding areas.
8. Plans should be general enough to cover all potential disaster events.
9. As much as possible, plans should be based on everyday work methods and procedures.
10. Plans should specify a person's responsibility for implementing segments by position or title rather than by name.
11. Plans should develop a record-keeping system before a disaster occurs, regarding:
    * Supplies and equipment
    * Records of all present at any given time (to account for everyone and to identify the missing)
    * Identification of victims and deceased, conditions and treatment documented, and to which facility victims are sent
12. Backup plans need to be in place for the following:
    * Disruption of telephone and cell phone lines
    * Disruption of computer data (should be downloaded weekly and stored off-site)
    * Protecting essential public health functions (e.g., vital records and communicable disease data)

needed is shelter in place, then people need to know what to do if they are at home, at work, at school, or in their vehicle.

Shelter in Place

The ARC has provided explicit instructions for individuals and families to be followed when told by authorities to "shelter in place" in the event of a disaster. Table 28-4 shows these guidelines.

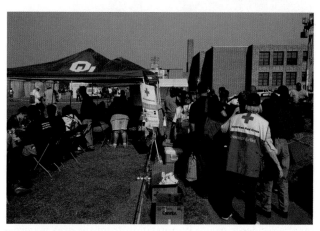

Bus loads of Galveston, Texas residents returned from temporary shelter in San Antonio after the hurricane in September 2008. (Photo by Mike Moore/FEMA.)

TABLE 28-4	SHELTER-IN-PLACE INSTRUCTIONS
LOCATION	**INSTRUCTIONS**
Home	Bring children and pets indoors immediately; close and lock all outside doors and windows; close the window shades, blinds, or curtains; turn off fans, heating, ventilation, or air conditioning system, and close the fireplace or woodstove damper; get the disaster supplies and make sure the radio is working; take everyone, including pets, into an interior room with no or few windows and shut the door; if instructed to seal the room, use duct tape and plastic sheeting (e.g., heavy-duty plastic garbage bags) to seal all cracks around the door into the room; keep the phone handy in case it is needed to report a life-threatening condition; keep listening to the radio or television until told all is safe or told to evacuate (do not evacuate unless instructed to do so).
Daycare centers and schools	Close the school; activate the school's emergency plan and follow reverse evacuation procedures to bring students, faculty, visitors, and staff indoors; have all children, staff, and visitors take shelter in preselected rooms that have phone access and stored disaster supply kits and, preferably, access to a bathroom; shut the doors and lock all windows and doors; if it is not possible for a person to monitor the telephone and the school has voice mail or an automated attendant, change the recording to indicate that the school is closed and that students and staff are remaining in the building until authorities say it is safe to leave; turn off heating, ventilating, and air conditioning systems; if children have cell phones, allow them to use them to call a parent or guardian to let them know that they have been asked to remain in school until further notice and that they are safe; one teacher or staff member in each room should write down the names of everyone in the room and call the designated contact to report who is in that room; everyone should stay in the room until school officials announce that all is safe or say everyone must evacuate.
Work	Close the office or business, making any customers, clients, or visitors in the building aware that they need to stay until the emergency is over; close and lock all windows, exterior doors, and any other openings to the outside; a knowledgeable person should use the building's mechanical systems to turn off all heating, ventilating, and air conditioning systems (systems that automatically provide for exchange of inside air with outside air, in particular, need to be turned off, sealed, or disabled); turn on call-forwarding or alternative telephone answering systems or services; if there is danger of explosion, close any window shades, blinds, or curtains; go to a predetermined sheltering room(s), and when everyone is in, shut and lock the doors; monitor radios or TVs for updates until you are told all is safe or you are told to evacuate.
Vehicle	If close to home, workplace, or a public building, go there immediately and go inside. If unable to get indoors quickly and safely, stop the vehicle in the safest place possible (e.g., stop under a bridge or in a shady spot to avoid being overheated); turn off the engine and close windows and vents; if possible, seal the heating, ventilating, and air conditioning vents with duct tape or anything else you may have available; listen to the radio periodically for updated advice and instructions; stay in place until you are told it is safe to get back on the road, and follow the directions of law enforcement officials.

Modified from American Red Cross: *Shelter-in-place during a chemical or radiation emergency:* February 2006, www.redcross.org/preparedness/cdc_english/Sheltering.asp#howdo.

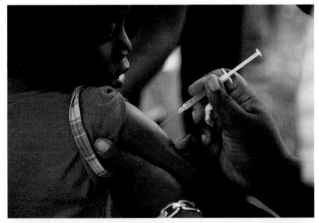

Between February 8 and March 9, 2010, 125,000 earthquake survivors in Port-au-Prince were vaccinated against measles, diphtheria, pertussis, and tetanus. (Photo by Bonnie Gillespie/American Red Cross.)

Evacuation

Each community should have established evacuation routes for the residents to use if evacuation from the area is necessary. In some instances, mandatory evacuation may be implemented. However, there are always some individuals who will not leave their home for any numbers of reasons (e.g., fear of vandalism, denial of the potential extent of the disaster, pride in their home and belongings). Education of residents as to the potential damage, deaths, and injuries that will be incurred from the potential disasters that may affect their community needs to be done in the preparedness stage and not when evacuation is ordered. In some extreme cases, it may be necessary for hospitals and other facilities, such as nursing homes, to evacuate patients. This requires significant advance planning, as health practitioners must determine how to move seriously, and even critically, ill people and coordinate transportation and placement for their disposition to safe facilities.

Search and Rescue

Before search and rescue should begin, safety must be considered. In some instances, if a criminal action is suspected, law officials will be among the first to respond in order to secure the area and possibly gather evidence. While the area is being checked and then cleared of potential threats, a staging area can be set up at or near the site of the incident to direct on-site activities. Search and rescue of victims can begin once

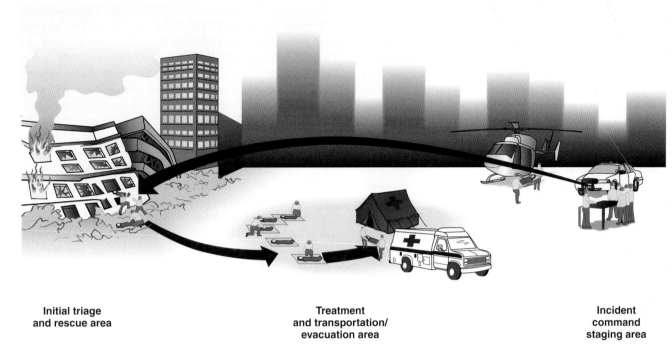

| Initial triage and rescue area | Treatment and transportation/ evacuation area | Incident command staging area |

FIGURE 28-4 Areas of operation of disaster response.

clearance is given, a disaster triage area is established, and an emergency treatment area is set up to provide first aid until transportation for victims to hospitals or health care facilities for treatment can be coordinated (Figure 28-4).

Staging Area

The staging area is the on-site incident command station. Disaster responders should report to this area to "check in" so that everyone is accounted for and can be given an assignment. This will allow for the most effective use of the skills and abilities of those responding. No one should go to the disaster site unless directed to do so by the staging area commander. The staging area is also where the authority rests for decisions as to additional resources to be called to the area to manage the disaster incident. Resources may be construction equipment to move building materials, rescue dogs to locate humans who are buried in the debris, or more fire, police, or medical personnel.

Disaster Triage

Triage at the site and again at the treatment area is very different from triage that is routinely conducted in the emergency department. The focus of disaster triage is to do as little as possible, for the greatest number, in the shortest period of time. One triage system that is used by first responders is the SMART triage system. SMART stands for "simple triage and rapid treatment." This system describes what to do when first arriving at a multicasualty or mass casualty incident. Disaster triage of an injured person should occur in less than 1 minute. This system also describes how to use people with minor injuries to assist. As a decision is made regarding the status of an individual, the person is tagged with a colored triage tag (Figure 28-5).

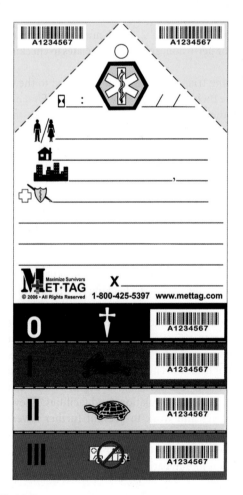

FIGURE 28-5 Disaster triage tag. (Source: http://www.mettag.com.)

Green on the triage tag is for the walking wounded or those with minor injuries (e.g., cuts and abrasions) who can wait several hours before they receive treatment; yellow is for those with systemic but not yet life-threatening complications who can wait 45 to 60 minutes (e.g., simple fractures); red is considered top priority or immediate and is for those with life-threatening conditions but who can be stabilized and have a high probability of survival (e.g., amputations); black is for the deceased or for those whose injuries are is so extensive that nothing can be done to save them (e.g., multiple severe injuries).

A new classification of victim, those who are contaminated, will require a hazmat (for "hazardous materials") tag. To assess an individual within the 1-minute guideline, the system uses three characteristics. First, respirations are checked; if they are over 30 per minute, the individual is tagged red or immediate. If the individual has fewer than 30 respirations, then the assessor moves to the second step—perfusion. Pinching the nail bed and observing the reaction are done to check perfusion; color should return to normal within 2 seconds. The third step is checking mental status. The assessor should ask the individual simple questions (e.g., Who are you?). By doing these steps, the individual responsible for triage can very quickly assess an individual and decide which color tag fits his or her condition. Further, the steps are easy to remember by thinking "30—2—can do," where "30" is the number of respirations, "2" is the number of seconds needed to check for perfusion, and "can do" relates to checking mental status.

Following triage, victims are then moved to the treatment area where their condition is checked again. First aid may be provided there, until transportation is available. Ambulances, helicopters, busses, or all three may be used to transport the victims to various hospitals or health care facilities. Some victims, such as those in the surrounding area that may have been affected by the incident, may even go by private vehicle to a hospital or medical facility. This process may go on for days as it did in the September 11 incidents, the 2005 tsunami in South Asia, and Hurricanes Katrina and Rita. Search and rescue eventually will be called off, and the recovery stage will begin.

While search and rescue is going on, other agencies (e.g., public health agencies) are checking for threats such as contaminated water, vectors, and air quality. They also disseminate data on what has been found and relate health information to officials, the media, and the public as appropriate. Designated agencies measure the occurrence and distribution of health-related events associated with the disaster, describe factors contributing to health-related effects, and assess the needs of populations and facilities. They will allocate resources and work to prevent further adverse health problems that may result from the disaster. For example, following Hurricane Katrina, public health officials administered tetanus and hepatitis A immunizations to rescuers and victims.

Although triage of individuals exposed to chemical warfare agents is basically the same as for any multiple or mass casualty incident, it poses special challenges. For these events, the triage area is set up in the "hot zone" to assist in determining priorities for resuscitation, decontamination, pharmacological therapy, and site evacuation. Only specially trained emergency personnel who are familiar with chemical agents and the use of personal protection equipment should triage chemical agent victims. The same triage categories can be assigned to these victims.

Psychological triage presents the challenge of determining who most needs help and deciding what interventions will help. Mental health disorders related to disasters can include anxiety disorders, exacerbation of existing substance abuse problems, somatic complaints, depression, and later, post-traumatic stress disorder (PTSD). Research has identified four keys to gauging the mental health impact of such events, any two of which may result in severe, lasting, and pervasive psychological effects. The key factors are: (1) extreme and widespread property damage; (2) serious and ongoing financial problems; (3) high prevalence of trauma in the form of injuries, threat to life, and loss of life; and (4) when human intent caused the disaster. In addition, panic during the disaster, horror, separation from family, and relocation or displacement are factors that may play a part in psychological impairment. Nurses need to evaluate an individual's danger to self or others. Nurses need to know the symptoms to look for and know what resources are available for people who need help (Patterson, 2005).

Community Responses to a Disaster

Heroic phase. The classic four phases of a community's reaction to a disaster are the heroic phase, honeymoon phase, disillusionment phase, and reconstruction phase. During the heroic phase, nearly everyone feels the need to rush to help people survive the disaster. Medical personnel may work hours without sleep, under very dangerous and life-threatening conditions, in order to take care of their patients. Medical personnel may help out in areas in which they are not familiar and have no experience. Disaster Medical Assistance Teams, consisting of professionals and paraprofessional medical personnel, provide emergency relief during a disaster and may travel long distances to help out in a disaster. This was illustrated by the thousands of people who volunteered to help in the immediate aftermaths of September 11 and Hurricanes Katrina and Rita.

Honeymoon phase. Individuals who have survived the disaster gather together with others who have simultaneously experienced the same event; this is known as the honeymoon phase. People begin to tell their stories and review over and over again what has occurred. Bonds are formed among victims and health care workers. Gratitude is expressed for being alive.

Disillusionment phase. When time has elapsed and a delay in receiving help or failure to receive the promised aid has not occurred, feelings of despair arise. Medical personnel and other first responders may begin to experience depression due to exhaustion from many long days of long hours. Depression may set in as a result of knowledge of what has happened to the community, friends, and family. People realize the way

NATURAL AND MAN-MADE DISASTERS

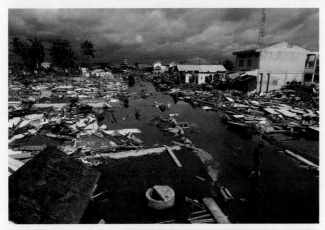

The devastation of the tsunami that occurred in Indonesia in December 2004. (Copyright Associated Press.)

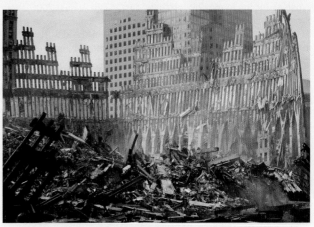

The remaining section of the World Trade Center is surrounded by a mountain of rubble following the September 11 terrorist attacks. (Photo by Bri Rodriguez/FEMA News Photo.)

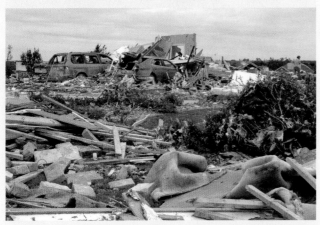

Only an interior wall remains after an F-4 tornado ripped through Manhattan, Kansas in June 2008. (Photo by Anita Westervelt/FEMA.)

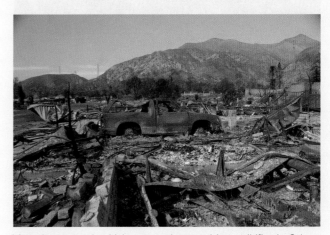

Many homes and vehicles were destroyed in a wildfire in Sylmar, California in November 2008. (Photo by Michael Mancino/FEMA.)

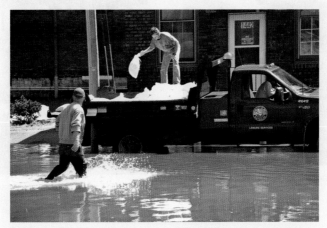

Waterloo and other towns in Iowa experienced record flooding in June 2008. (Photo by Patsy Lynch/FEMA.)

DISASTER RELIEF: HURRICANE KATRINA, SEPTEMBER 2005

When Hurricane Katrina hit the Gulf Coast in late August 2005, thousands of evacuees from New Orleans and south Louisiana were sent to Houston. Two huge shelters were set up in the city to accommodate those displaced, and the needs, as was documented in the media, were massive.

Faculty, staff, and students from the University of Texas Health Science Center at Houston (UT-Houston), personnel from the city and county health departments, and local EMS personnel were joined by thousands of volunteers to care for these disaster victims. Indeed, doctors, nurses, and other health care providers came from across Texas and the Gulf Coast area and from as far away as California, Arizona, Illinois, and New York to help.

To care for the health needs of the evacuees, a clinic was established in the George R. Brown Convention Center. According to one of the officials at UT-Houston, "We got the call at 9 AM Friday [to create the clinic], and by 5 PM it was all set up." The clinic was modeled after army field hospitals, with a command center, triage areas, and various clinics. There were sections for trauma and acute care, adult medical care, women's/gynecological care, pediatric care, and an area for persons with mental health concerns. A full-service pharmacy was also set up.

During the next 17 days, more than 10,000 patient visits were logged, and there were more than 6000 volunteers. These photos depict how care was organized and show the efforts of the many volunteers.

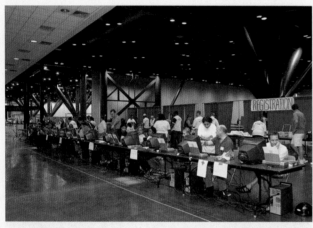

Setting up the registration area to check in clinic clients.

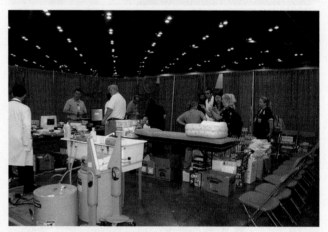

Organizing medical supplies.

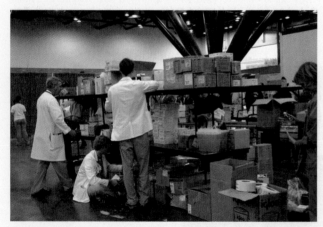

Setting up one of the client care areas (note the portable water supply).

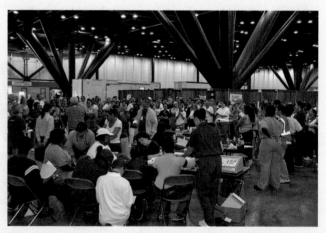

Registration and triage area as clients are being seen.

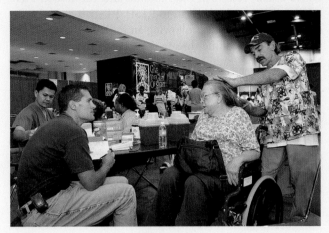

Triage area.

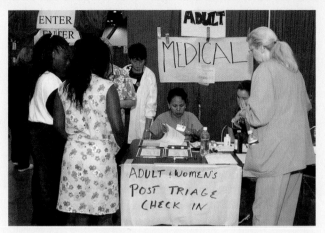

Check-in for the adult clinic.

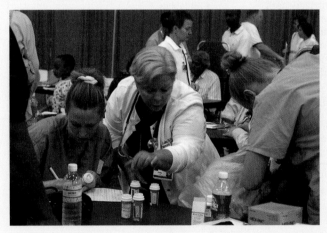

Nurses organizing client medications.

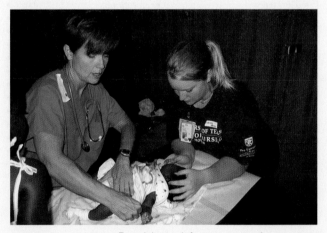

Examining an infant.

Photos courtesy the University of Texas Health Science Center, Houston, Texas.

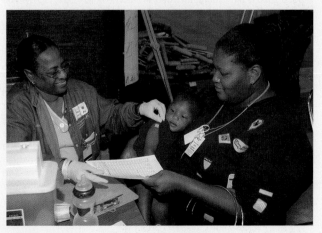

Immunizing a small child.

things were before the disaster is not the way things are now and may never be the same again. They recognize that many things are different and much needs to be done to adjust to the current situation.

Reconstruction phase. Once the community has restored some of the buildings, businesses, homes, and services, and some sense of normalcy is returning, feelings of despair will subside. Counseling support for victims and helpers may need to be initiated to help people to recover more fully. During this phase, people begin to look to the future.

Common Reactions to a Disaster

The reactions by individuals to a disaster vary. Table 28-5 lists some of the more commonly encountered emotional, cognitive, physical, and interpersonal reactions to a disaster that may be experienced.

Posttraumatic stress disorder (PTSD). The reactions mentioned usually resolve in 1 to 3 months after the disaster event but, in some cases, may lead to PTSD. PTSD is a psychiatric disorder that can occur following an individual's experiencing or witnessing a life-threatening event, such as a disaster. Men and women, adults and children, and all socioeconomic groups can experience PTSD. People who have PTSD often relive the experience through nightmares and flashbacks. The social and psychological symptoms mentioned in Table 28-5 can be severe enough, and last long enough, to significantly impair a person's daily life. If PTSD occurs in conjunction with related disorders (e.g., depression, substance abuse, and other problems of physical and mental health), the situation becomes more complicated. Individuals experiencing PTSD require medical attention (National Center for Posttraumatic Stress Disorder, 2005).

TABLE 28-5	COMMON RESPONSES TO A TRAUMATIC EVENT		
COGNITIVE	**EMOTIONAL**	**PHYSICAL**	**BEHAVIORAL**
• Poor concentration • Confusion • Disorientation • Indecisiveness • Shortened attention span • Memory loss • Unwanted memories • Difficulty making decisions	• Shock • Numbness • Feeling overwhelmed • Depression • Feeling lost • Fear of harm to self and/or loved ones • Feeling nothing • Feeling abandoned • Uncertainty of feelings • Volatile emotions	• Nausea • Lightheadedness • Dizziness • Gastrointestinal problems • Rapid heart rate • Tremors • Headaches • Grinding of teeth • Fatigue • Poor sleep • Pain • Hyperarousal • Jumpiness	• Suspicion • Irritability • Arguments with friends and loved ones • Withdrawal • Excessive silence • Inappropriate humor • Increased/decreased eating • Change in sexual desire or functioning • Increased smoking • Increased substance use or abuse

From Centers for Disease Control and Prevention: *Coping with a traumatic event: information for health professionals*, July 2005, http://emergency.cdc.gov/masscasualties/copingpro.asp.

CASE STUDY   APPLICATION OF THE COMMUNITY ASSESSMENT PROCESS

Assessment
Deer Park, Texas, is a city 20 miles east of Houston, Texas. The population is approximately 30,000 people. The majority of the people are white (80.8%) and Hispanic (15.2%). The median age of the population is 34.7 years; the median income is $61,334. Eighty-nine percent of the population over 25 years of age has a high school diploma or higher education degree. The unemployment rate is 5.6%. The city consists of residential homes, apartment complexes, and retail and service businesses. There are nine schools and several churches of all denominations. Many AM and FM radio stations and TV broadcast stations are available to the Deer Park area.

The Federal Communications Commission (FCC) has developed the Emergency Alert System to warn of any emergency (nuclear attack, hurricane, tornado, flood, or chemical release). The FCC has designated KTRH 740 AM as the station for the Houston area. The city has a volunteer fire department (five full-time employees) and a city police department (fifty-five full-time employees). The city government consists of a mayor, city council, and city manager. The city has two emergency committees: the Community Awareness and Emergency Response Committee and the Local Emergency Planning Committee.

There are no hospitals in Deer Park. The closest hospitals are 6 to 7 miles away and take 20 minutes to reach. The closest level 1 trauma center is 15 miles away, and the nearest adult care burn center is 20 miles away; the pediatric burn center is in Galveston, Texas, which is about 45 miles away.

The city is also the home of the Shell Deer Park Chemical Plant and the Shell Deer Park Refining Company. The company processes 3% of the nation's oil supply into gasoline. The Shell plants are located on 1500 acres in the Houston Ship Channel. Shell employs approximately 1100 people and 2200 contract workers. The chemical plant and the refining company have their own fire stations, an internal railroad, docks and transportation networks, small medical facilities (one physician and four nurses, 7 days a week, 24 hours a day), first responder teams, two ambulances, and a vehicle that can handle 30 casualties.

Diagnosis
Individual
Because of Deer Park's location on the Gulf Coast and the presence of the Shell Deer Park Refining Company and Shell Deer Park Chemical Plant, the residents are at risk for injury or death due to

Continued

hurricane disasters and potential industrial accidents from either accidental or terrorist causes.

Family

The families of Deer Park are at risk for losing their homes, separation from family members, and having to evacuate from their homes either temporarily or permanently due to hurricane damages or industrial accidents.

Community

The community of Deer Park is at risk for destruction of buildings and city public works due to hurricane disasters and potential explosions from either accidental or terrorist causes.

Planning
Disaster Management

Deer Park is in the storm surge zone that requires its residents to evacuate when a category 1 hurricane is predicted to land in, or within a 100-mile radius of, the Deer Park area. The media sources available to the Deer Park area or the city officials are to give instructions about supplies and equipment to have ready and when to leave. There is only one evacuation route available to the community.

A survey was conducted during the nondisaster stage to identify vulnerable groups that would need help in evacuating.

Individual

Vulnerable individuals that would need to have special consideration for evacuation are the very young (4000 individuals between birth and 10 years), the elderly (2110 individuals aged 65 years and over), and families below the poverty level (1200). It was determined that more than 7000 individuals might need some form of transportation in order for them to evacuate.

Long-Term Goal
- Residents will have a disaster kit prepared according to ARC and FEMA guidelines.

Short-Term Goals
- Residents will follow officials' instructions for sheltering in place or evacuation.
- Vulnerable individuals will know what to do in the event of an evacuation order or shelter-in- place announcement.

Family
Long-Term Goal
- Family members will continually update the family disaster plan according to family dynamics.

Short-Term Goals
- Families will have in place a disaster plan for communicating.
- Families will have a disaster kit in place to accommodate each family member for a period of at least 3 days.

Community
Long-Term Goals
- Additional evacuation routes will be identified for area residents.
- Central meeting locations will be identified for those needing transportation assistance for evacuation.

Short-Term Goal
- School buses will be used for evacuation of vulnerable individuals and families who need transportation.
- Identify other sources that could be called upon to provide transportation.

- Allow school bus drivers to include their family members on the bus with others being evacuated, so they will not have to worry about their families.

If all individuals follow instructions, there should be no injuries to, or deaths of, Deer Park residents from a hurricane or related storm surge. Homes may be damaged or destroyed, but no lives should be lost. With the help of local, state, and possibly federal agencies, the community should recover.

Long-Term Goal
- City officials will continually update the community disaster plan as gaps are identified and keep the residents informed as plans change.

Onsite Management

The figure below summarizes the disaster plan in place for the Deer Park Shell plants for handling any industrial accident that occurs on their property.

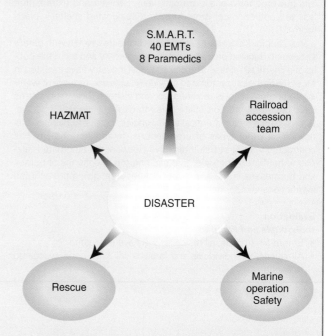

Shell has annual drills with the Harris County's Emergency Management and Channel Industries Mutual Aid organization to evaluate emergency response. This group is Shell's direct link to support in the event of a disaster. Many buildings on Shell property can serve as shelters, and no visitor or employee is allowed on the property without having a "safe shelter map" in his or her possession. If an explosion occurs that is confined to the property, and only minor casualties result, the resources available should be sufficient to manage the disaster.

Shell has developed a buffer zone between the plants and the city of Deer Park. However, if fumes escape as a result of the explosion, a shelter-in-place warning would be issued for Deer Park residents through a specific six sounding message system. Chemical products that are used and that might potentially escape are benzene, toluene, solvent xylene, isoprene butadiene, sulfur, phenol, hydrogen sulfide, and asbestos. Citizens would be advised about actions to take according to the chemical released. Most plants have also installed dedicated, fiber optic telephone lines so that the city and industry can stay in touch, even when normal phone circuits are overloaded or out of service.

CASE STUDY   APPLICATION OF THE COMMUNITY ASSESSMENT PROCESS—cont'd

Community and Local Response Preparedness

Deer Park's police and fire dispatchers have been trained on how to handle calls from industries about a chemical release and how to quickly activate the city's emergency warning systems. The Local Emergency Planning Committee has adopted a three-level Community Awareness and Emergency Response system to categorize the severity of each chemical release. Level 1 is information only, level 2 is standby alert, and level 3 is full emergency condition, with shelter-in-place required. The final level is "all clear." Deer Park has a website featuring Wally Wise Guy who gives instructions to the citizens about what to do if a shelter-in-place emergency is issued.

The Local Emergency Planning Committee hired a consulting group to study the impact of toxic substances on the community to ensure that shelter-in-place procedures are adequate for protecting the residents. They recommended that each home in the region have a shelter-in-place kit containing 2- to 3-inch wide masking tape, plastic film or sheets, towels or sheets for sealing under doors, battery-powered radio and extra batteries, flashlight and extra batteries, and bottled water stored inside a designated shelter-in-place room.

The Deer Park Communications Subcommittee works with others to develop detailed procedures on how to notify and warn the public of a chemical release. The city and local industry have invested in six state-of-the-art systems to provide reliable and redundant warning to homes, schools, businesses, and visitors. Siren-type alarms have been mounted on utility poles throughout the city. This system is used only for chemical emergencies, not for tornadoes, hurricanes, or other types of emergencies. In addition, the city has contracted with First Call Interactive Network, an automated telephone notification network that can ring the telephones of homes and businesses in the immediate danger area, giving prerecorded instructions about what to do.

Evaluation
Individuals and Families
- Before a hurricane, all residents will have evacuated.
- All vulnerable individuals and families will have been evacuated to shelters.
- All residents will know and respond to shelter-in-place warnings as indicated by the siren-type alarm system in place.

Community
- City officials will evaluate and continually update the community disaster plan as gaps are identified.
- Community residents will remain informed and prepared.

The City of Deer Park and the Deer Park Shell plants have detailed plans for prevention, preparedness, and response in the event of an industrial accident. In the event of an accident, evaluation of the plan will take place to identify gaps and make appropriate changes. A plan needs to be in place for hurricane preparedness of the plants to avoid industrial accidents and the plan evaluated for effectiveness. Drills are conducted to test their industrial accident plans; they provide training of personnel; they have identified sites for shelters both on Shell property and in the city; and they have elaborate notification and warning systems in place.

Areas that need to be enhanced include city health resources readily available (lack of a nearby trauma hospital or burn center to care for the type of injuries that would occur). Plans for preparing the plants for hurricanes and evacuation need to be developed and made available to the workers.

Prevention
Primary
- Perform periodic education of area residents regarding warning systems in place and appropriate response to take should they be implemented.
- Perform periodic review of plans in response to changing demographics.

Secondary
- Check credentials of first responders for currency.
- Screen first responders for training needs and preparedness to take action during disasters.

Tertiary
- Institute building codes that will reduce amount of damage to infrastructures.

Recovery Stage

The recovery stage begins when the danger from the disaster has passed and all local, state, and federal agencies are present in the area to help victims rebuild their lives and help the community restore public services. Cleanup of the damage and repair of homes and businesses begin. Evaluation and revision of the disaster plans based on lessons learned from the experience are made. Understanding the financial impact on the community and agencies involved is essential in developing future public health policy.

Research is needed on all aspects of prevention, preparedness, response, and recovery stages of disasters. Research is also needed on the education and training needs of first responders, health care providers, and community populations. Nurse researchers, in partnership with researchers from other disciplines, can play a significant role in conducting research on disaster management.

SUMMARY

Communities, now more than ever, need to be aware of potential disasters that may affect their community. Comprehensive disaster plans at all levels of government and by all communities, families, and individuals need to be developed. Having disaster plans in place increases the likelihood of an effective response, resulting in saved lives and minimized destruction to the community.

Nurses have a role and contribution to make at every stage of disaster management. Nurses need to have personal and professional plans in place for any disaster. All medical personnel must keep their credentials current and must learn the signs and symptoms of the weapons of mass destruction so that they will recognize people who may have been exposed. They should learn what injuries may be sustained from various disasters and know which types of disasters are most likely to affect their communities, so that disaster triage and treatment can save lives. Finally, they must take drills in their respective health care facilities seriously. The more prepared the population and health care providers are for all kinds of disasters, the fewer lives will be lost.

LEARNING ACTIVITIES

1. Assess the community where you live for potential disasters that could result in mass casualties. What disasters are predictable? Are there measures that can be taken to prevent or minimize injuries, death, or destruction?
2. Find out who is responsible for disaster management in your community. What plans are in place for warning people and for communicating which actions to take in the event of a disaster? Are the people aware of these plans?
3. What social and cultural factors need to be considered in disaster planning in your community? Are there vulnerable populations with special needs (e.g., homeless, prisoners, mobility impaired)? If evacuation of the community is mandated, have plans for evacuation of these groups been made?
4. Create an emergency plan for yourself, your family, or both. What factors would you consider in deciding whether to stay or leave your home? If evacuation were mandated, what important documents and mementos would you need to take with you?
5. Interview the person or persons in the ARC responsible for disaster services in your area. What is the role of their disaster nurses? What are the requirements to become a disaster nurse for the ARC?
6. Speak with police and fire department personnel about their responsibilities during a disaster. Do their roles during a disaster differ from their roles on a day-to-day basis? Do they have special teams and plans for biological, chemical, nuclear, or radiological incidents?
7. What emergency supplies does your health care facility have available in the event of a disaster? What provisions have been made available for vulnerable patients when there is no electricity? How would patients be evacuated from your facility to safe shelters?

REFERENCES

American Public Health Association: *Types of disasters and their consequences*, 2005. www.medscape.com/viewarticle/513258_print.

American Red Cross: *Disaster service*, 2005. www.redcross.org/services/disaster/0,1082,0_319_,00.html.

American Red Cross: *Disaster services: terrorism—preparing for the unexpected*, 2003b. www.seattleredcross.org/prepare/unexpected.htm.

Board of Nurse Examiners for the State of Texas: Legislative report: 78th Regular Texas Legislative Session, *RN Update* 34(5):1, 2005.

Centers for Disease Control and Prevention: *Tsunami disaster: health information for humanitarian workers*, Washington, DC, 2005, US Department of Health and Human Services.

Central Intelligence Agency: *The war on terrorism: terrorism FAQs*, 2007. www.cia.gov/terrorism/faqs.html.

Chettle C: Recognizing bioterrorism: nurses on the frontline, *Nurse Week* 6:29–30, 2001.

Federal Bureau of Investigation: *Terrorism 2000/2001* (Fed Publication # 0308), Washington, DC, 2004, US Government Printing Office. www//fbi.gov/publications/terror99.pdf

Federal Emergency Management Agency: *About FEMA: what we do*, 2005a. www.fema.gov/about/.

Federal Emergency Management Agency: *Are you ready? General information about terrorism*, 2005b. www.fema.gov/areyouready/terrorism_general_info.shtm.

Federal Emergency Management Agency: *National Incident Management System*, 2005c. http://www.fema.gov/nims/.

Federal Emergency Management Agency: *Office of National Security Coordinating Agency*, 2005d. http://www.fema.gov/onsc/.

Federal Emergency Management Agency: *Make a plan: Family emergency plan*, 2010. www.ready.gov/america/makeaplan/index.html.

James DC, Langan JC: *Nurses as heroes*. www.Advanceweb.com. Accessed July 6, 2009.

National Center for Post-Traumatic Stress Disorder: *What is posttraumatic stress disorder?* 2005. www.ncptsd.va.gov/facts/general/fs_what_is_ptsd.html.

National Oceanic and Atmospheric Administration, National Weather Service, Storm Prediction Center: *The Enhanced Fujita Scale (EF Scale)*. www.spc.noaa.gov/efscale. Accessed June 27, 2009.

National Weather Service, National Hurricane Center: *The Saffir-Simpson Hurricane Wind Scale (Experimental)*. www.nhc.noaa.govaboutsshs.shtml. Accessed June 16, 2009.

Patterson K: *Psychological triage: in Katrina's wake, sorting out who will need mental health care the most won't be easy*, 2005. www.nursingspectrum.com/Katrina/PsychTriage.cfm.

Texas Association of Regional Councils: *Texas Citizen Corps: what is Citizen Corps?* 2009. www.txregionalcouncil.org/cc_cert/.

Texas Department of Health and Texas Nurses Association: Strategic National Stockpile (SNS) volunteer nurses needed for Ready Texas Nurses Emergency Response System, *Texas Board Nurs Bull* 35(4):2004.

U.S. Department of Homeland Security: *National response plan*, December 2004. www.dhs.gov/dhspublic/display?theme=14&content=4264&print=true.

U.S. Department of Homeland Security: *DHS organization: department subcomponents and agencies*, 2009a. www.dhs.gov/xabout/structure/#1.

U.S. Department of Homeland Security: *DHS organization: the DHS transition*, 2009b. www.dhs.gov/files/unified-dhs.shtm.

U.S. Department of Homeland Security: *Homeland Security Advisory System: current threat level*, 2009c. www.dhs.gov/files/programs/Copy_of_press_release_0046.shtm.

U.S. Department of Homeland Security: *Preparing makes sense: get ready now*, 2009d. www.ready.gov./america/_downloads/Ready_Brochure_Screen_EN_20040129.pdf.

The White House: *Improving homeland security*, 2009. www.whitehouse.gov/infocus/homeland/index.html.

School Health

Catherine A. Pourciau, Elaine C. Vallette

Additional Material for Study, Review, and Further Exploration

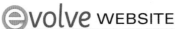 WEBSITE

http://evolve.elsevier.com/Nies

- Quiz
- Case Studies
- Glossary

- WebLinks
- Resource Tool
  - 29A: 2007 United States Youth Risk Behavior Survey Data

OBJECTIVES

Upon completion of this chapter, the reader will be able to do the following:

1. Discuss how *Healthy People 2020* can be used to shape the care given in a school health setting.
2. Identify and discuss the eight components of a comprehensive school health program.
3. Recognize the major stressors that can negatively affect an adolescent's mental and physical health.
4. Identify common health concerns of school-aged children and associated health interventions.
5. Explore the various roles of the nurse in the school setting.
6. Be familiar with the standards under which school nurses practice.
7. Cite several resources available to the school nurse.

KEY TERMS

Early and Periodic Screening, Diagnostic, and Treatment (EPSDT)
Family Educational Rights and Privacy Act (FERPA)
Health Insurance Portability and Accountability Act of 1996 (HIPAA)

Individuals With Disabilities Education Act (IDEA) of 1990
Public Law 99-142
school health
school nurse
school-based health centers

Youth Risk Behavior Surveillance System (YRBSS)

OUTLINE

History of School Health
School Health Services
  Health Education
  Physical Education
  Health Services
  Nutrition
  Counseling, Psychological, and Social Services

Healthy School Environment
Health Promotion for School Staff
Family and Community Involvement
School Nursing Practice
School-Based Health Centers
Future Issues Affecting the School Nurse

Schools could do more than perhaps any other single institution in society to help young people, and the adults they will become, to live healthier, longer, more satisfying, and more productive lives. (Carnegie Council on Adolescent Development, Centers for Disease Control and Prevention [CDC], 2006, p. 1)

School-aged children and adolescents face increasingly difficult challenges related to health. Many of today's health challenges are different from those of the past and include behaviors and risks linked to the majority of the leading causes of death, such as heart disease, injuries, and cancer. The use of tobacco, alcohol, and drugs; poor nutritional habits; inadequate physical activity; irresponsible sexual behavior; violence; suicide; and reckless driving are examples of behaviors that often begin during youth and increase the risk for serious health problems (Box 29-1).

In the United States, approximately 50 million children attend school every day. This creates a unique opportunity for the school nurse to make a positive impact on the nation's youth. The primary providers of health services in schools are school nurses, and there are approximately 60,000 registered nurses working in schools in the United States (National Association of School Nurses [NASN], 2003a). Although the NASN recommends one school nurse for every 750 students in the general population, one for every 225 students in mainstreamed special education populations, and one for every 125 severely chronically ill or developmentally disabled students, caseloads vary widely depending on mandated functions, socioeconomic status of the community, and service delivery model (NASN, 2006a).

On a daily basis, school nurses see students with a variety of complaints. Increasing numbers of children are being seen in the school setting because they lack a source of regular medical care. According to the Children's Defense Fund (2008), in the United States there are 9 million children, or one in nine children, who do not have health insurance. This is a decrease from the nearly 12 million in previous years. Table 29-1 illustrates the racial and ethnic breakdown of uninsured children in the United States in the year 2007. Through education, counseling, advocacy, and direct care across all levels of prevention, the nurse can improve the immediate and long-term health of this population.

Seventeen percent of the nation's children are living in poverty and are less likely to have access to primary and preventive care (Annie E. Casey Foundation, 2007). Decreased or inferior medical care has been linked to serious health

TABLE 29-1	RACIAL AND ETHNIC BREAKDOWN OF UNINSURED CHILDREN IN THE UNITED STATES IN THE YEAR 2007	
RACE	NUMBER	PERCENTAGE
White	3.4 million	7.5
Hispanic	3.4 million	20.7
Black	1.5 million	12.8
Asian and Pacific Islander	379,000	11.6
American Indian	103,000	18.9
Other (multiracial)	154,000	7.4

From Children's Defense Fund: *State of America's children*, 2008, www.childrensdefense.org/child-research-data-publications/data/state-of-americas-children-2008-report.html.

problems resulting in an increase in absenteeism that may be correlated with failure in school. The school nurse can effectively manage many complaints and illnesses, allowing these children to return to or remain in class.

There is a need for mental and physical health services for students of all ages in an effort to improve both their academic performance and their sense of well-being. This chapter provides an overview of school health and the role of the nurse in the provision of health services and health education. An in-depth look at the components of a successful school health program related to the major problems of today's youth is included.

HISTORY OF SCHOOL HEALTH

Before 1840, education of children in the United States did not exist or was uncoordinated and sparse. In 1840, Rhode Island passed legislation that made education mandatory, and other states soon followed. In 1850, a teacher and school committee member, Lemuel Shattuck, spearheaded the legendary report that has become a public health classic. This report, known as the Shattuck Report, has had a profound impact on school health because it proposed that health education was a vital component in the prevention of disease.

Public health officials and others soon realized that schools played an important part in the prevention of communicable disease. When smallpox broke out in New York City in the 1860s, health officials were faced with trying to implement a widespread prevention program. They chose to target the schools and began vaccinating children. In 1870, this led to the requirement that all children be vaccinated against smallpox before entering school (Allensworth et al., 1997).

At that time, schools were poorly ventilated and lacked fresh air, effectively spreading diseases among the children. Late in the nineteenth century, a practice of inspecting schools began to identify children who were ill and exclude them until it was deemed they were no longer infectious. Soon thereafter, compulsory vision examinations became a requirement to identify children who might have difficulty in school. In 1902, New York City hired the first nurses to help inspect children, educate families, and ensure follow-up

BOX 29-1   YOUTH AT RISK

- Every day, nearly 4000 young people start smoking.
- Daily participation in high school physical education classes dropped from 42% in 1991 to 30% in 2007.
- Seventy-eight percent of young people do not eat the recommended number of servings of fruits and vegetables.
- Marijuana use among young people increased from 15% in 1991 to 20% in 2007 (CDC, 2007a,b).

treatment. Within a few years the renowned nurse Lillian Wald was able to show that the presence of school nurses could reduce absenteeism by 50%. By 1911, slightly more than 100 cities were using school nurses; in 1913, New York City employed 176 school nurses (Allensworth et al., 1997).

As they became more comfortable in their positions, early school nurses began to take on a more active role in the assessment of children, treatment of minor conditions, and referral for more serious problems. In addition to identification, treatment, and exclusion for communicable diseases and screening for problems that might affect learning, other issues quickly became part of school nurse practice. In the early part of the twentieth century the temperance movement led schools to teach about the effects of alcohol and tobacco. Also, early in the twentieth century "gymnastics" was introduced in schools in an effort to promote physical activity.

World War I was a pivotal point for school health services, and the call for a national effort to improve the health of schoolchildren emerged. In 1918 the National Education Association joined forces with the American Medical Association (AMA) to form the Joint Committee on Health Problems and publish the report *Minimum Health Requirements for Rural Schools.* This group also called for the coordination of health education programs, medical supervision, and physical education that some authorities contend is still lacking. By 1921 nearly every state had laws that required physical and health education in schools. Additionally, fire drills became part of safety education programs introduced during and after World War I (Allensworth et al., 1997).

Even though emphasis was placed on health services in schools, barriers still existed. Many schools and cities were unwilling to take on the task of providing primary health care for all children. The idea that schools should simply identify and refer problems to physicians was a common practice that the AMA backed. By the 1920s, medical services and preventive health services were clearly separated in the public health arena and in the schools. Not surprisingly, school health became known as school health education. The federal government did not get involved with school health until the passage of the National School Lunch Program in 1946. The School Breakfast Program was implemented 30 years later (Allensworth et al., 1997).

There was no impetus to change the direction of school health programs until the 1960s and 1970s. During these decades there was increasing publicity about children living in poverty and the move to mainstream children with disabilities. These two issues, with an increase in the number of children of immigrants, contributed to changes in school health programs.

During the 1960s the first nurse practitioner training programs opened and made the inclusion of primary care services in schools possible. In 1976 the first National School Conference, supported by the Robert Wood Johnson Foundation, was held in Galveston, Texas. Following this conference a variety of school health service models began to emerge with new partnerships and ideas created to provide the most comprehensive health care services for school-aged

children. In addition, the Education for the Handicapped Act in 1975 mandated that all children, regardless of disabilities, have access to educational services.

The 1980s and 1990s saw several measures aimed at improving the health of schoolchildren. The Drug-Free Schools and Community Act was implemented in 1986 to fight substance abuse through education and was expanded in 1994 to include violence prevention measures. The Centers for Disease Control and Prevention (CDC), Division of Adolescent and School Health, began funding state education agencies to develop and implement programs aimed at alcohol and tobacco use, physical education, and the reduction of sexually transmitted diseases (STDs) and human immunodeficiency virus (HIV) infection among the nation's youth. Also, the federal government encouraged states to use part of their maternal and child block grant monies to fund school-based health centers.

School health services vary widely among states and school districts. There continues to be a lack of coordination among providers, and no single agency is responsible for tracking services. Recognizing that there are differences among schools in the United States and that important health information must be delivered to children and adolescents, the U.S. Department of Health and Human Services (USDHHS) addressed many related issues in *Healthy People 2020*. Objectives targeting children and adolescents are written for diverse areas, including physical activity, sex education and HIV prevention, nutrition, smoking prevention, school absences related to asthma, and many others. The *Healthy People 2020* table lists a few of the objectives of *Healthy People 2020* related to school health.

SCHOOL HEALTH SERVICES

The School Health Policies and Programs Study (SHPPS) describes school health services as a "coordinated system that ensures a continuum of care from school to home to community health care provider and back" (Allensworth et al., 1997, p. 153). School health services goals and objectives vary from state to state, community to community, and school to school. These differences reflect wide variations in student needs, community resources, funding sources, and school leadership preferences. Many organizations, such as the American School Health Association and NASN, are involved in the care and welfare of school-aged children and have compiled and adopted definitions, standards, and statistics related to school health.

According to SHPPS (CDC, 2000), 89% of states have at least one school-based health center. The percentage with a full-time nurse was 36% in 2006, and 51% of schools had a part-time nurse who provides health services that might include vision, hearing, and scoliosis screening; first aid care; and medication administration. Nearly all schools maintain a health record on every student and, at a minimum, monitor immunization status. Most authorities agree that comprehensive school health programs should include the following eight components (Figure 29-1): health education; physical education; health services; nutrition services; counseling, psychological and social services; healthy school environment; health promotion for staff; and family and community involvement.

♥ HEALTHY PEOPLE 2020

Selected Proposed Objectives for School Health

OBJECTIVE

AH HP2020 – If: Decrease the number of whole school days missed because of illness or injury.

AH HP2020 – 6: Decrease the percentage of adolescents who did not go to school at least once in the past month because of safety concerns.

DSC HP2020 – 6: Increase the proportion of children and youth with disabilities who spend at least 80 percent of their time in regular education programs.

EMC HP2020 – 2: Increase the proportion of children who are ready for school in all five domains of healthy development.

EMC HP2020 – 3: Increase the proportion of elementary, middle, and senior high schools that require school health education.

ECBP HP2020 – 1: Increase high school completion.

ECBP HP2020 – 4: Increase the proportion of the Nation's elementary, middle, and senior high schools that have a nurse-to-student ratio of at least 1:750.

EH HP2020 – 19: Increase the proportion of the Nation's elementary, middle, and high schools that have official school policies and engage in practices that promote a healthy and safe physical school environment.

EH HP2020 – 25: Decrease the number of new schools sited within 500 feet of a freeway or other busy traffic corridors.

FP HP2020 – 11: Increase the proportion of adolescents who received formal instruction on reproductive health topics before they were 18 years old.

ENT-VSL HP2020 – 21: Increase the proportion of young children with phonological disorders, language delay, or other developmental language problems who have participated in speech-language or other intervention services.

IID HP2020 – 19: Maintain vaccination coverage levels for children in kindergarten.

IVP HP2020 – 28: Increase the proportion of public and private schools that require students to wear appropriate protective gear when engaged in school-sponsored physical activities.

MHMD HP2020 – 6: Increase the proportion of children with mental health problems who receive treatment.

NWS HP2020 – 5: Reduce the proportion of children and adolescents who are overweight or obese.

NWS HP2020 – 20: Increase the percentage of schools that offer nutritious foods and beverages outside of school meals.

OH HP2020 – 4: Increase the proportion of low-income children and adolescents who received any preventive dental service during the past year.

PAF HP2020 – 2: Increase the proportion of the Nation's public and private schools that require daily physical education for all students.

RD HP2020 – 7a: Reduce the number of school days missed among children (aged 5 to 17 years) with current asthma.

SA HP2020 – 5: Increase the age and proportion of adolescents who remain alcohol and drug free.

TU HP2020 – 7: Reduce the initiation of tobacco use among children, adolescents, and young adults.

V HP2020 – 2: Reduce uncorrected visual impairment due to refractive errors.

USDHHS Healthy People 2020 Draft Objectives. 2009. http://www.healthypeople.gov/hp2020/Objectives/files/Draft2009Objectives.pdf

Health Education

An objective of *Healthy People 2020* sets a goal that 70% of middle, junior, and senior high schools provide health education courses in priority areas. The six behavioral categories or topics identified by the CDC (2007a) include the following negative behaviors that often start in childhood or adolescence and persist into adulthood:

1. Alcohol and drug use
2. Injury and violence (including suicide)
3. Tobacco use
4. Poor nutrition
5. Lack of physical activity
6. Sexual behavior that results in STDs or unwanted pregnancies

These problems and behaviors are preventable and often coexist. They also lead to both social and educational problems that contribute to our nation's high dropout and unemployment rates and crime statistics.

In a comprehensive health education program, students should be given the opportunity to practice decision-making and communication skills. To learn more about high-risk behaviors among youth, the CDC conducted the Youth Risk Behavior Survey (YRBS) (CDC, 2007a). This survey is conducted every 2 years among selected high school students throughout the United States. Box 29-2 lists the purposes of the YRBS. Reports from this study provide valuable information that can help improve health education programs in schools. See **Resource Tool 29A** on the book's website at http://evolve. elsevier.com/Nies/ for a summary of selected YRBS data.

Injury Prevention

Injury prevention should be taught very early in schools, and the information should be age appropriate. For example, bicycle safety, including the importance of wearing a helmet, as well as the proper use of backpacks, must be stressed

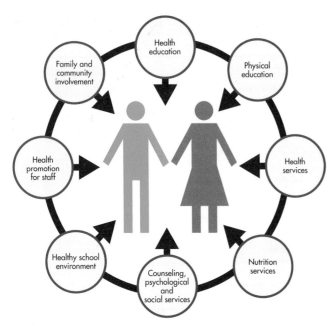

FIGURE 29-1 The eight components of school health programs.

BOX 29-2 **PURPOSES OF THE YOUTH RISK BEHAVIOR SURVEY**

- Determine the prevalence of health risk behaviors.
- Assess whether health risk behaviors increase, decrease, or remain the same over time.
- Examine the co-occurrence of health risk behaviors.
- Provide comparable data among subpopulations of youth.
- Provide comparable national, state, territorial, tribal, and local data.
- Monitor progress toward achieving the *Healthy People 2020* objectives and other program indicators.

From Centers for Disease Control and Prevention: Youth Risk Behavior Surveillance System, 2007, *MMWR Morb Mortal Wkly Rep* 57(SS04),1-131, 2007a, www.cdc.gov/mmwr.

beginning in elementary schools. Safety on the schoolyard and playground is also important for this age group because approximately 200,000 children per year are injured on playgrounds in the United States. According to the National Program for Playground Safety (Tinsworth and McDonald, 2001), approximately 45% of these injuries occurred on school property. Motor vehicle safety should be included in programs for adolescents who are beginning to drive.

Sports safety is particularly important among adolescents because participation in sports continues to grow, especially among girls. Greater than 3.5 million children under the age of 14 years receive medical treatment each year for sports-related injuries (SAFE KIDS Worldwide [SKW], 2007a). Males are injured more frequently than females. Injury rates occur most commonly on playgrounds, athletic fields, and gymnasiums (SKW, 2007b). Injuries include orthopedic injuries (e.g., strains, sprains, fractures, and dislocations), dental injuries, neurological problems (e.g., head injury), ophthalmic injuries, cuts, abrasions, and bruises.

Use of proper equipment should be mandatory for children and adolescents. Fitted mouth guards, shin guards, pads,

helmets, and other protective gear should be required to prevent injury. Regular hydration and frequent rest periods should be required to prevent heat-related illnesses, especially during hot weather. Effective warm-up and cool-down exercises should be encouraged to prevent muscle strain. Schools that participate in aquatic sports should include pool safety.

The sports physical is a good time for the school nurse to talk with and counsel the student about the risk of developing health problems related to physical activity. This is a perfect setting for the nurse to question girls about menstrual irregularities and to ask all students about their eating behaviors, feelings about their weight, and history of musculoskeletal injuries. It is also a good time for the nurse to stress the importance of stretching exercises to help prevent injuries. This also presents an opportunity for the nurse to work with the coaching staff to promote positive health outcomes.

Many school districts have school safety committees that make recommendations for sports-related safety. These committees collect data on injuries, develop safety inspection policies, and plan staff training and student education related to school environmental factors. These committees should include school nurses.

Tobacco Use

For the past several decades, major concerns have been raised about long-term health problems associated with adolescents' use of tobacco, alcohol, and illegal substances. There is an increased likelihood that these youthful abusers will ultimately engage in other high-risk behaviors.

Smoking is a major problem in this country and is the single leading preventable cause of death in the United States. Prevention should be emphasized in young people because an estimated 90% of adults who use tobacco began before the age of 19 years (American Cancer Society, 2008). Although the overall percentage of high school students who report smoking has declined in recent years, rates remain high at about 20%. An estimated 4000 youths, aged 12 to 17 years, try their first cigarette each day. Smoking by young people can cause serious health problems such as heart disease, chronic lung disease, or cancers of the lung, pharynx, esophagus, and bladder. Prevalence of smoking increases as the student progresses through the grade levels. White students have the highest rate of current cigarette use at 23%, followed by Hispanics at 17%, and blacks at 12% (CDC, 2007b).

Eight percent of youth currently report using smokeless tobacco, and studies show that adolescents who use smokeless tobacco are likely to become cigarette smokers. The use of smokeless tobacco can cause cancers of the mouth, esophagus, and pharynx and can increase the risk of development of heart disease and stroke. Of particular interest is that 14% of students surveyed report having smoked cigars, cigarillos, or little cigars within the past month (CDC, 2007b).

Risk factors for development of oral cancer include the use of tobacco in all forms, and, when combined with alcohol, the risk increases (CDC, Division of Oral Health, 2006). Therefore all adolescents should be queried as to their use of both tobacco and alcohol. Education and counseling should be offered to students who use tobacco products. Limiting adolescents' exposure to tobacco advertising and teaching them the negative consequences associated with tobacco are essential in preventing its use.

Substance Abuse

The use of alcohol and other drugs is associated with problems in school, injuries, violence, and motor vehicle deaths. All 50 states and the District of Columbia have outlawed the sale of alcohol to anyone under the age of 21 years, yet it is still the most commonly used drug among children and adolescents. In 2007 statistics show that 39% of eighth graders tried alcohol with increasing frequency as they progressed in school (CDC, 2008a). Additionally, alcohol use, defined as five or more drinks in a row on one or more of the past 30 days, is more prevalent among Hispanics (48%) and whites (47%) than blacks (35%). The reported use of alcohol on school property remains relatively unchanged at 4.3%. Research shows a direct correlation between alcohol abuse and liver disease, cancer, cardiovascular disease, as well as neurological and psychiatric problems.

The use of illicit drugs, except for the use of illegal steroids, remains essentially unchanged over the past 14 years. The use of illegal steroids actually increased from 2.7% in 1991 to 4% in 2005. Most anabolic steroid users are athletes who believe that these drugs will produce an increase in strength and muscle mass. Approximately 5% of ninth-grade students reported using these drugs in 2007, and use was higher among males than females (CDC, 2007a). Part of the problem is that students are trying to emulate professional sports figures, some of whom purportedly have used these drugs to enhance performance. There are more than 100 different types of anabolic steroids, and each one requires a prescription. Abuse or improper use of anabolic steroids can result in severe problems including liver cancer, jaundice, high blood pressure, elevated cholesterol levels, stunted growth patterns, and accelerated puberty changes (National Institute on Drug Abuse, 2007).

The most commonly used illicit drug among youth in the United States is marijuana. In 2005, 38% of young people reported using marijuana one or more times in their life. The percentage of students who report the use of marijuana on high school property was 4.5%, and 25.4% of students were offered, sold, or given marijuana (CDC, 2007a). Marijuana use has been linked to the same health problems as tobacco.

Sex Education

A number of objectives of *Healthy People 2020* address issues of human sexuality and prevention of pregnancy, STDs, and HIV. These issues are important when working with older children and adolescents.

Teens are becoming sexually active at earlier ages, and, despite recent declines, pregnancy rates continue to be high (Box 29-3). Data obtained from the Youth Risk Behavior Surveillance System (YRBSS) reveal a decrease from 48.4% in 1997 to 47.8% in 2007 of adolescents in grades 9 through 12 who have had sexual intercourse (CDC, 2007a). Even though

---

BOX 29-3   TEEN PREGNANCY

- The U.S. teen pregnancy rate is one of the highest among developed countries, with one of the highest teen birth rates.
- More than 750,000 teenagers become pregnant each year.
- Black and Hispanic youth are disproportionately affected by teen pregnancy.
- Teen mothers are less likely to complete high school.
- Teen mothers are more likely to be single parents and live in poverty.
- Birth rates among teenagers vary substantially from state to state (MacKay and Duran, 2007; CDC, Adolescent Reproductive Health, 2007).

89.5% of students have been given HIV/AIDS education in school, HIV transmission remains high among adolescents and young adults. In 2005, AIDS was the seventeenth leading cause of death among people aged 10 to 14 years and the eleventh cause of death in people aged 15 to 24 years (CDC, National Center for Health Statistics, 2008). Research shows that HIV transmission is at least two to five times higher in the presence of a coexisting STD (USDHHS, 2000). Therefore it is imperative that older children and adolescents have age-appropriate information on sexuality issues, including prevention of pregnancy and STDs, before becoming sexually active.

According to the CDC, 982,498 cases of AIDS had been reported in the United States through the end of 2006. Of these, 9144 were reported in children under age 13 years. During this same time there were 540,436 AIDS deaths, and, of these, 5369 occurred in children under age 13 years (CDC, 2009a). It is important to note that HIV reporting is not mandatory in all states and may underestimate the devastation of this illness on school-aged children.

School-based education related to sexual orientation is a controversial topic. Children with gender identity confusion must also face the same growth and developmental issues as other adolescents. However, there are unique health problems and risks for these children both emotionally and physically. The school nurse needs to be aware of these students and be sensitive and understanding.

Sex education in the school setting is another controversial topic. Opponents of sex education in the schools believe that parents have the responsibility for teaching this content to their children. Laws in certain states prohibit or dramatically limit sex education in public schools. Proponents argue that for many children sex education will not be addressed in the home. If this information is not taught in schools, children may receive inadequate or incorrect information from peers, media, or other sources. School nurses have been caught in the center of this controversy but historically have advocated for education on normal human sexuality, encouraging discussion in an objective, nonjudgmental manner in which students are free to ask questions and receive correct answers.

Tattoos and Body Piercings

Tattoos and body piercings are a form of self-expression and attention-seeking behavior. This practice has risen dramatically in the last several years. Unfortunately, these procedures are often done at home, on the streets, or in parlors where sterile technique and safety precautions are not practiced. Both hepatitis C and methicillin-resistant *Staphylococcus aureus* have been linked to tattoos and body piercings. This presents a unique opportunity for the school nurse to educate students on the importance of making healthy decisions on whether to have this done and, if so, where and under what conditions it is performed.

Dental Health

One of the most frequent complaints of school-aged children is dental caries. There are numerous contributing factors, including poor oral hygiene, lack of fluoridated water, and lack of funds or insurance for dental care. Half of children aged 12 to 15 years will have dental caries. This is more common in lower-income children, and approximately 75% of those between the ages of 12 and 19 years have had tooth decay. Untreated cavities can greatly affect a child's quality of life and cause pain, absence from school, and decreased self-worth (CDC, 2008b). Proper brushing of teeth should be taught along with good nutritional habits and the importance of regular dental checkups. Children should also be taught the relationship between high-sugar foods and dental caries. All children should be encouraged to see a dentist regularly.

Physical Education

One of the major objectives of *Healthy People 2020* is improvement of health and fitness through regular daily physical activity. Children today are less active than children in the past. Daily enrollment among high school students in physical education classes dropped from 42% in 1991 to 30% in 2007. With the advent of computers and television and the decreasing requirement of physical education in schools, children are becoming more sedentary. It was reported in 2007 that the proportion of children in grades 11 and 12 who engaged in strenuous physical activity was lower than in previous grades (CDC, 2007a).

A sedentary lifestyle is associated with obesity, hypertension, heart disease, and diabetes. Studies show that people who are active outlive those who are inactive and that those who are active have a better quality of life. Habits in childhood are likely to continue into adulthood, making it imperative that children are taught the importance of being physically active at a young age. Studies also show that children and adolescents who are physically active have increased self-confidence and self-esteem and decreased anxiety, stress, and depression. Regular physical activity helps build and maintain healthy bones and muscles.

Physical education should focus on activities that children can continue into their adult years, such as walking, swimming, biking, and jogging. The educational content may change as the child ages. For example, what may appeal to a young child such as playing on the playground with friends is different from what motivates an adolescent, such as competitive sports or weight control. The CDC has made ten recommendations for the promotion of lifelong physical activity (Box 29-4).

BOX 29-4   GUIDELINES FOR SCHOOL AND COMMUNITY PROGRAMS: PROMOTING LIFELONG PHYSICAL ACTIVITY

1. Establish policies that promote enjoyable, lifelong physical activity.
2. Provide physical and social environments that encourage and enable young people to engage in safe and enjoyable physical activity.
3. Implement sequential physical activity education curricula and instruction in grades K to 12.
4. Implement health education curricula.
5. Provide extracurricular physical activity programs that offer diverse, developmentally appropriate activities—both noncompetitive and competitive—for all students.
6. Encourage parents and guardians to support their children's participation in physical activity, to be physically active role models, and to include physical activity in family events.
7. Provide training to enable teachers, coaches, recreation and health care staff, and other school and community personnel to promote enjoyable, lifelong physical activity to young people.
8. Assess the physical activity patterns of young people, refer them to appropriate physical activity programs, and advocate for physical activity instruction and programs for young people.
9. Provide a range of developmentally appropriate community sports and recreation programs that are attractive to all young people.
10. Regularly evaluate physical activity instruction, programs, and facilities.

From Centers for Disease Control and Prevention: *Physical activity: school and community guidelines—recommendations for ensuring quality physical activity programs,* 2006, www.cdc.gov/healthyyouth/physicalactivity/guidelines/summary.htm.

Health Services

Health care provided in schools includes such preventive services as immunizations and screenings. This component of a comprehensive school health program may include emergency care, management of acute and chronic health conditions, appropriate referrals, health counseling, education about healthy lifestyles, and medication administration. Care of children with special health needs is also included.

Immunizations

Immunizations are a vital component of routine health care. They provide long-lasting protection against many diseases. Vaccine-preventable deaths (VPD) are at or near record-low levels. According to the CDC (2005) many communicable diseases have been reduced by greater than 95% as a result of immunizations. Undervaccination of children, especially those in large urban areas, is causing concern because of the potential for disease outbreaks.

All states now require proof of current immunization status or evidence of immunity before school entrance. Certain exceptions may apply based on religious and philosophical beliefs, or medical contraindications. The school nurse plays an important role in verifying compliance with immunization requirements and in educating children and parents about the benefits of immunization. School nurses play a vital role in coordinating school immunization programs and teaching families about both infant and adult immunizations. See the CDC website (http://www.cdc.gov) for current immunization schedules.

Health Screenings

Unfortunately, many children in the United States are not appropriately screened for treatable conditions that then remain undetected. Impaired vision and hearing can result in poor academic performance, slowed emotional development, and stress-related disorders. Children are exposed to a variety of potentially harmful noises in school and at home. Identifying and treating these problems early are highly effective and less costly in the long run. Height, weight, vision, and hearing screenings are provided at most schools according to a schedule set by the state or school district. These screenings usually occur at least upon initial entry to school and at least once during elementary, middle, and high school. Children and adolescents may need to be screened more often based on family history, developmental delays, recurrent ear infections, or exposure to loud noise.

Vision screening is required in most states with referrals as needed. The standard Snellen vision chart is the usual screening tool. Screening for strabismus is a nursing responsibility, and this condition must be identified and treated early to prevent amblyopia. If left untreated, amblyopia may result in loss of vision. Referral to an eye specialist is a critical component of all abnormal eye examinations.

Scoliosis or postural screening should be done to identify spinal deviations and intervene early to prevent related secondary problems. Spinal problems may lead to deformities that are cosmetic, functional, or both. Scoliosis screening in the school setting consists primarily of a visual inspection of the back. The American Academy of Pediatrics and the American Academy of Orthopedic Surgeons (2007) recommends screening of all girls twice, at ages 10 and 12 years, and boys once at either age 13 or 14 years.

The detection of high blood pressure during childhood is important in identifying children who have hypertension and who will benefit from early intervention and follow-up. Vascular and end-organ damage can begin in childhood. Periodic blood pressure measurements are inexpensive and should be performed routinely for all children.

The Children's Health Insurance Program (CHIP) is a national program designed for children of families who earn too much money to qualify for Medicaid but cannot afford the high cost of health insurance. Medicaid-eligible children are guaranteed access to comprehensive health care services and routine dental examinations. Medicaid created the Early and Periodic Screening, Diagnostic, and Treatment (EPSDT) service because of the large number of uninsured children. EPSDT is a comprehensive child health program for uninsured people under the age of 21 years and includes health education and periodic screening. Services provided under the EPSDT program are often performed through the public health offices in each state but may occur in community health clinics and schools. Screening services must include a comprehensive health and developmental history, an unclothed physical examination, plus immunizations and laboratory testing that are age appropriate, as well as lead toxicity screenings (Centers for Medicare & Medicaid Services, 2006).

Emergency Care

Schools are a frequent site for student injuries that range from minor scrapes and bruises to serious injuries, such as fractures and seizures, to severe and life-threatening injuries, such as head injuries and severe asthma attacks. Injuries may occur in school buildings, classrooms, physical education classes, or during athletic events. Emergencies can include natural events such as hurricanes, tornadoes, and earthquakes, or man-made disasters, such as hazardous material spills, fires, and civil disobedience. Basic first aid equipment should be available in all schools. The school nurse must be knowledgeable about standard first aid and certified in cardiopulmonary resuscitation. Additionally, a procedure for activating an emergency management system should be in place.

Care of the Ill Child

The school nurse is responsible for monitoring the health of all students. For students with acute or chronic illnesses, administration of medications or treatments may be necessary. The nurse is often required to assess an ill child to determine the type of illness or health problem, identify the source of the illness, and determine how to manage the illness (i.e., contact the parent or send the child back to class).

In 2007 it was reported that 6.7 million children (9%) under the age of 18 years had asthma. Asthma is one of the most common chronic childhood conditions and accounts for some 14 million lost school days every year (CDC, 2009b). Because asthma is so prevalent, it is recommended that school-based support exists. Actions undertaken by some schools across the country include immediate access to asthma medications, development and implementation of asthma action plans, and student and staff education on asthma. An assessment tool (Box 29-5) has been developed to determine how well schools assist children with asthma. Answers to all the questions in the assessment tool should be "yes." "No" answers indicate that students may not be in an environment conducive to asthma control.

Diabetes is also prevalent in the school-aged child and affects 186,300 young people less than 20 years of age. Two million adolescents aged 12 to 19 years have prediabetes. Type 2 diabetes is now being diagnosed in children, a condition that has historically been diagnosed only in adults. Childhood obesity and the decline in physical activity are thought to be major factors in this development. In general, teachers are inadequately prepared to care for children with diabetes and must rely on the nurse. According to the American Diabetes Association (ADA) (2009), children should be able to participate in their care to the extent that they are able. The ADA has specific recommendations based on age, as shown in Box 29-6.

BOX 29-5 HOW ASTHMA-FRIENDLY IS YOUR SCHOOL? CHECKLIST

Children with asthma need proper support at school to keep their asthma under control and be fully active. Use the questions below to find out how well your school assists children with asthma:

☐ Yes ☐ No 1. Is your school free of tobacco smoke at all times, including during school-sponsored events?

☐ Yes ☐ No 2. Does the school maintain good indoor air quality? Does it reduce or eliminate allergens and irritants that can make asthma worse? Check if any of the following are present:
    ☐ Cockroaches
    ☐ Dust mites (commonly found in humid climates in pillows, carpets, upholstery, and stuffed toys)
    ☐ Mold
    ☐ Pets with fur or feathers
    ☐ Strong odors or fumes from art and craft supplies, pesticides, paint, perfumes, air fresheners, and cleaning chemicals

☐ Yes ☐ No 3. Is there a school nurse in your school all day, every day? If not, is a nurse regularly available to help the school write plans and give the school guidance on medicines, physical education, and field trips for students with asthma?

☐ Yes ☐ No 4. Can children take medicines at school as recommended by their doctor and parents? May children carry their own asthma medicines?

☐ Yes ☐ No 5. Does your school have a written, individualized emergency plan for each child in case of a severe asthma episode (attack)? Does the plan make clear what action to take? Whom to call? When to call?

☐ Yes ☐ No 6. Does someone teach school staff about asthma, asthma management plans, and asthma medicines? Does someone teach all students about asthma and how to help a classmate who has it?

☐ Yes ☐ No 7. Do students have good options for fully and safely participating in physical education class and recess? (For example, do students have access to their medicine before exercise? Can they choose modified or alternative activities when medically necessary?)

If the answer to any question is "no," students in your school may be facing obstacles to asthma control. Uncontrolled asthma can hinder a student's attendance, participation, and progress in school. School staff, health professionals, and parents can work together to remove obstacles and promote students' health and education.

From National Heart, Lung, and Blood Institute, National Asthma Education and Prevention Program, School Asthma Education Subcommittee: How asthma friendly is your school? Checklist, *J Sch Health* 68(4):167-168, 1998, www.nhlbi.nih.gov/health/public/lung/asthma/sch_chk.htm.

BOX 29-6 EXPECTATIONS OF THE CHILD WITH DIABETES

Elementary School
- The child should be able to assist in all diabetes tasks at school.
- By the age of 8 years, the child is usually able to perform his or her own finger-stick glucose monitoring.
- By the age of 10 years, some children can administer their own insulin with supervision.

Middle School and Junior High School
- The child should be able to perform self-monitoring of blood glucose.
- Most children should be able to administer their own insulin with supervision.

High School
- The child should be able to perform self-monitoring of blood glucose.
- Adolescents should be able to administer insulin without supervision.
- All children may need assistance with blood glucose testing when the glucose level is low.

From American Diabetes Association: Position statement: care of children with diabetes in the school and day care setting, *Diabetes Care* 31:S79-S86, 2008.

Medication Administration

Administration of medications is a service provided almost universally by school districts across the country. The use of medications by school-aged children has increased over the last several years. This has allowed many children to attend school despite serious health problems.

Medication administration in the schools is a serious undertaking. Issues facing the school nurse include safety, monitoring of both therapeutic and side effects, proper documentation, confidentiality, and ongoing communication with the student and family. The nurse must comply with all legal regulations and school policies. Only those medications considered necessary are administered at school.

The following guidelines from NASN (2003b) indicate that medications should be:
- In containers that are properly labeled with all appropriate student and medication information
- Accompanied by a written request from the health care provider and parent or guardian
- Administered without violating standing orders or nursing protocols
- Kept in locked containers

Also, school nurses must monitor self-administration of medications and provide education as needed to both children and parents. Rescue medications such as albuterol must be available to the child with asthma, and the nurse must be familiar with its expected effects to properly assist the child. With the increasing number of children with diabetes, it is imperative that the nurse recognize the signs and symptoms of hypoglycemia and hyperglycemia in order to assist the child in the monitoring of glucose levels and insulin administration.

Medications commonly given in schools include analgesics and antipyretics (e.g., Tylenol or Advil), antacids, antitussives, anticonvulsants, antiemetics and antidiarrheals, antifungals, antihistamines, and antibiotics. Medications used to treat attention deficit hyperactivity disorder are the most commonly administered, followed by nonprescription medications and medications used in the treatment of asthma (McCarthy, Kelly, and Reed, 2000).

Alternative and complementary medicine includes practices and products outside the realm of conventional medicine. The NASN recommends that an advisory committee be formed in the community to address the administration of these products. NASN also recommends that the school not allow the child to carry or self-administer any products that could be considered a drug, without written orders from a health care provider, a written request from the parent, and verification that the product and dosage are safe. The request for the administration of any of these medications provides the nurse with an excellent health teaching opportunity (NASN, 2006b).

Children With Special Health Needs

In 1976 Public Law 99-142 was enacted, giving all students, including those who are severely handicapped, the right to public education in the least restrictive environment possible, regardless of mental or physical disabilities. The Education for All Handicapped Children Act of 1973 and the subsequent Individuals With Disabilities Education Act (IDEA) of 1990 enhanced the opportunities for children previously served in acute-care and long-term-care settings to have access to public education (Duncan and Igoe, 1998). President George W. Bush signed the reauthorized IDEA into law on December 3, 2004, to support more than 6 million children with disabilities in the U.S. school systems. Children affected by these laws include those who are hearing impaired, mentally challenged, multihandicapped, orthopedically impaired, "other" health impaired (e.g., chronic or acute health problems such as heart condition or epilepsy), seriously emotionally disturbed, speech impaired, visually handicapped, or have a specific learning disability.

The rapid development of medical technology has enabled students to attend public school when their conditions may have prevented them from leaving an institution or controlled environment in the past. These children need nursing services of varied types to continue their progression in school. Public Law 94-142 requires school nurses to screen or identify children in need of special education and related services, and complete an Individualized Education Program that is developed by an interdisciplinary team and includes educational goals and specific services to be provided. It also requires provision of "designated instruction and services," which outlines services, including nursing care, required to help the child benefit from education. The nurse is responsible for the development of an individualized health plan for all students requiring continuous nursing management while at school. Table 29-2 gives an overview of the increase in the number of students with disabilities.

Student Records

Health records should be maintained for all students according to individual school district policy. At a minimum, student health records should include immunization status, pertinent health concerns, results of screenings and examinations, health history, and individualized plans of care. The Family Educational Rights and Privacy Act (FERPA), a strong privacy protection act, protects student education records, including the health record. Student health records should be afforded the same level of confidentiality as that given to clients and patients in other settings (i.e., sharing confidential information with others without approval is considered unethical and improper except in emergency situations).

The Health Insurance Portability and Accountability Act of 1996 (HIPAA) was published in 2002 and instituted nationwide in 2003. A major component of HIPAA is ensuring confidentiality of personal health information. Public schools that provide health care services fall under HIPAA regulations. Private schools that do not receive federal funding but engage in HIPAA-related activities are also governed by this act.

Delegation of Tasks

Not every school has a full-time nurse available on-site. Often, a nurse is assigned to three or four schools, resulting

TABLE 29-2 OVERVIEW OF INCREASE IN NUMBER OF STUDENTS WITH DISABILITIES

TYPE OF DISABILITY	1976 TO 1977	1990 TO 1991	1996 TO 1997	2003 TO 2004
All disabilities	8.3	11.4	12.9	13.7
Specific learning disabilities	1.8	5.2	5.9	5.8
Speech or language impairments	2.9	2.4	2.3	3.0
Mental retardation	2.2	1.3	1.3	1.2
Serious emotional disturbance	0.6	0.9	0.9	1.0
Hearing impairment	0.2	0.1	0.2	0.2
Orthopedic impairments	0.2	0.1	0.1	0.2
Other health impairments	0.3	0.1	0.4	1.0
Visual impairments	0.1	0.1	0.1	0.1
Multiple disabilities	—	0.2	0.2	0.3
Autism and related disorders	—	—	0.1	0.4

From National Center for Education Statistics: *NCES fast facts: students with disabilities,* 2006, www.nces.ed.gov/fastfacts/display.asp?id=64.
Children from birth to age 21 years who were served by federally supported programs for students with disabilities, as a percentage of total public K to 12 enrollment; 1976 to 1977 to 2003 to 2004.

in delegation of certain tasks to unlicensed personnel. Each state's nurse practice act stipulates which procedures may be delegated. The responsibility for assessment, diagnosis, goal setting, and evaluation may never be delegated. When tasks are delegated, the nurse must provide appropriate education, written procedures, and ongoing supervision and evaluation of the caregivers.

Nutrition

School-aged children are undergoing periods of rapid growth and development and consequently have high nutritional needs. A variety of foods must be ingested to meet their daily requirements. Diets should include a proper balance of carbohydrates, protein, and fat, with sufficient intake of vitamins and minerals. However, children and adolescents share a well-known preference for junk food. Their diet is often high in fat and sugar and frequently consists of fast-food items, such as hamburgers and French fries, instead of fruits and vegetables. Skipping meals, especially breakfast, and eating unhealthy snacks contribute to poor childhood nutrition. Identifying nutritional problems, counseling, and making appropriate referrals are important in the school setting.

Poor nutritional status is closely associated with poverty. Federally funded programs such as the School Breakfast Program and National School Lunch Program were initiated to ensure that all children have access to these meals during the school day.

VENDING MACHINE FOOD CHOICES

In 2004, the NASN addressed the issue of unhealthy foods found in school vending machines and sold in school fund-raising projects. They specifically resolved that schools should provide healthy food choices in school vending machines and for sale in fund-raising projects (NASN, 2004).

Eating Disorders

Statistics have shown that few adolescents feel good about their bodies. Of those surveyed, 24% of boys and 35% of girls describe themselves as being overweight, and as many as 30% of boys and 60% of girls are dieting at any one time. It has been reported that 6% of girls in high school take laxatives or vomit to lose weight or keep from gaining weight, and approximately 8% take diet pills. These kinds of harmful practices have been reported in girls as young as 11 years old (CDC, 2007a).

It is imperative that the school nurse recognize the association between feelings of inadequacy (e.g., low self-esteem, anger, anxiety, and depression) and unhealthy eating practices in adolescents and young people. These self-perceptions begin early in life; therefore education and counseling must begin in elementary school. Prevention should concentrate on eliminating misconceptions surrounding nutrition, dieting, and body composition and should stress optimal health and personal performance. Unfortunately, outside influences such as commercials and advertisements make this a serious problem; adolescents and young children are bombarded with such messages as "you can never be too thin" and "life will be wonderful if you look and dress like a model."

Nurses must also be aware of eating disorders, as they frequently co-occur with other mental disorders. Anorexia, bulimia, and binge eating have been shown to be the three most common eating disorders. *Binge eating* is defined as recurrent, out-of-control eating of large amounts of food whether a person is hungry or not. Anorexia is a severely restricted intake of food based on an extreme fear of weight gain. Literature has shown that anorexia is multifactorial, seen primarily in females, and often correlated with family dysfunction or a history of sexual abuse. Bulimia is a form of anorexia characterized by a chaotic eating pattern with recurrent episodes of binge eating followed by purging. Health consequences of eating disorders may include reduction of bone density, severe dehydration, tooth decay, and potentially fatal electrolyte imbalances.

FEMALE ATHLETE TRIAD

The "female athlete triad" is a syndrome consisting of eating disorders, amenorrhea, and osteoporosis. Pressure to attain a particular body shape or weight considered desirable in a selected sport may place the female athlete in danger of developing this disorder. It is a complex problem with psychological and physiological factors. It can result in menstrual irregularities, premature osteoporosis, and decreased bone mineral density; if taken to the extreme, it can become life threatening (Sherman and Thompson, 2004).

Obesity

Obesity is not considered an eating disorder, and therefore many professionals, including nurses, overlook it. Obesity is the fastest-rising public health concern in the nation and may overtake tobacco use as the single leading preventable cause of death. The childhood obesity rate has more than doubled in children aged 2 to 5 years and adolescents aged 12 to 19 years over the past 3 decades. It has more than tripled in children aged 6 to 11 years (Institute of Medicine, 2004). Obesity and its prevention or treatment must be of concern to the school nurse. Statistics show that obese children and adolescents are more likely to become obese adults.

Although many of the underlying causes of obesity are not well understood, several contributing factors have been identified that include reduced access and affordability of nutritious foods, decreased physical activity, and cultural and genetic influences. Obesity is associated with development of diabetes, dyslipidemia, hypertension, and other disorders, such as osteoarthritis, sleep apnea, and cholelithiasis. In addition, obesity may result in social and quality-of-life impairments related to physical endurance, and these children are often labeled by their peers and ridiculed. Guidelines for Adolescent Preventive Services recommend the determination of body mass index (BMI) for all adolescents. A BMI greater than the 85th percentile for age and gender indicates the need for further assessment and referral. To be successful, the treatment of obesity must begin early and be multifaceted (Montalto, 1998).

Nutritional Education Programs

Nutritional education is essential and must include parents, teachers, and the child. Children need to know and understand the food pyramid, how to make healthy snack choices, and the importance of balancing physical activity with food intake. Obesity, dental caries, anemia, and heart disease can be reduced or prevented with proper education and lifestyle changes. In addition, all adolescents and school-aged children should receive counseling regarding intake of saturated fat.

Congress enacted the Nutritional Education and Training (NET) Program in 1977. NET focuses on healthy nutritional choices and health promotion and disease prevention topics in school and child care settings. In addition, the American Dietetic Association, the American School Food Service Association, and the Society for Nutrition Education take the position that comprehensive school-based nutrition programs and services should be provided to all elementary and secondary students. The ultimate goal of these efforts is that children will make healthy nutritional choices in and out of the school setting.

Counseling, Psychological, and Social Services

The mental health of a child or adolescent is affected by physical, economic, social, psychological, and environmental factors. Children, like adults, often hide problems from themselves and from others. They may see problems as a sign of weakness or as a lack of control. Children may also be trying to protect themselves or someone they love and not seek help. This can have tragic results. Promotion of mental health and reduction or removal of threats to mental health are important to children and adolescents. Mental health is often difficult, yet essential, to assess.

Children and teens often struggle with depression, substance abuse, conduct disorders, self-esteem, suicide ideation, eating disorders, and under- or overachievement. They may also have to cope with physical or mental abuse, pregnancy, and STDs. Common warning signs of stress in children are presented in Box 29-7. Drugs and alcohol can enter a child's life as early as elementary school. Many children live in single-parent households with little social or economic support. They may not have enough to eat or a safe, warm place to sleep, yet they are expected to come to school each day ready to learn. Services aimed at helping children cope with these problems are often lacking or are too costly for many families.

The nurse or teacher may be the only stable adult in the child's life who will listen without being judgmental. Therefore, one of the most important roles of the school nurse is to act as counselor and confidante. Children may come to the school nurse with various vague complaints, such as recurrent stomachaches, headaches, or sexually promiscuous behavior, and the nurse must look beyond the initial complaint to identify underlying problems.

Major depressive disorders often have their onset in adolescence and are associated with an increased risk of suicide. Early detection and treatment may prevent untoward consequences. In 2005 the third leading cause of death among 10- to 24-year-olds was suicide, whereas homicide was the second leading cause of death in 15- to 24-year-olds and the fourth leading cause of death in 10- to 14-year-olds (CDC, National Center for Health Statistics, 2008). It is well known that suicide attempts are more common than completed suicides. A survey of students in grades 9 through 12 in 2007 showed that 7% attempted suicide in the preceding year and 17% reported having seriously considered suicide. Attempted suicide rates were higher among female students than male students, but the rate of successful suicides was higher in males (CDC, 2007a). The nurse and other school personnel must be on the alert for suicide clusters that are often known to follow a successful suicide. Adolescents often approach school nurses and other school professionals for help before a suicide attempt. Therefore, it is important for the school nurse to be cognizant of the warning signs associated with suicide and to recognize and refer at-risk adolescents to appropriate mental health professionals (Box 29-8).

Unfortunately, a large number of children are abused daily in this country. Physical and psychological abuse and neglect

---

BOX 29-7   WARNING SIGNS OF STRESS

- Problems eating or sleeping
- Use of alcohol or other substances (e.g., sedatives, sleep enhancers)
- Problems making decisions
- Persistent angry or hostile feelings
- Inability to concentrate
- Increased boredom
- Frequent headaches and ailments
- Inconsistent school attendance

BOX 29-8   TRUTHS ABOUT ADOLESCENT SUICIDES

1. Most adolescents who attempt suicide are ambivalent and torn between wanting to die and wanting to live.
2. Any threat of suicide should be taken seriously.
3. There are usually warning signs preceding a suicide attempt, and these may include depression, substance abuse, decreased activity, isolation, and appetite and sleep changes.
4. Suicide is more common in adolescents than homicide.
5. Education concerning suicide does not lead to an increased number of attempts.
6. Females are more likely to consider or attempt suicide, and males are more likely to complete a suicide attempt.
7. One suicide attempt is more likely to result in a subsequent attempt.
8. Firearms and strangulation are the predominant modalities of completed suicides in children and adolescents.
9. Most adolescents who have attempted or completed suicide have not been diagnosed as having a mental disorder.
10. All socioeconomic groups are affected by suicide.

BOX 29-9   POSSIBLE SIGNS OF ABUSE

Physical Abuse
- Has unexplained burns, bites, bruises, black eyes, or broken bones
- Shrinks at the approach of adults
- Appears frightened of parents or other relatives and cries when it is time to go home

Neglect
- Is frequently absent from school
- Steals food or money
- Lacks adequate medical or dental care
- Appears dirty or disheveled or is underweight
- Does not have proper seasonal clothing

Sexual Abuse
- Has difficulty walking or sitting
- Reports new onset of nightmares or bedwetting
- Refuses to change into gym attire or participate in physical activities
- Runs away from home
- Becomes pregnant or has an STD develop

Emotional Abuse
- Exhibits changes in behavior, such as acting out or extreme passivity
- Exhibits delay in either physical or emotional development
- Has attempted suicide
- Exhibits inappropriate adult or infantile behavior

From Child Welfare Information Gateway: *Recognizing child abuse and neglect: signs and symptoms,* 2007, www.childwelfare.gov/factsheets/signs.cfm.

are usually a result of many interacting factors such as poverty, social isolation, and drug and alcohol abuse. School nurses and other school personnel are mandated to report cases of child abuse and neglect. The nurse must be alert to subtle changes in behavior or physical appearance that may point to abuse. Box 29-9 outlines some of the signs and symptoms of different types of child abuse.

The school nurse may help the child learn how to solve problems, how to cope, and how to build self-esteem. The role of the nurse often extends outside the school campus. The family is an integral part of a child's well-being, and the nurse may need to work closely with families to develop an appropriate health plan for a particular child.

Healthy School Environment

A healthy school environment is one in which distractions are minimized and free of physical hazards and psychological threats. NASN believes that all students and staff have an inherent right to learn and work in a school environment that is healthy and that school nurses "have the expertise and responsibility to promote a healthy physical environment for all members of the school community" (NASN, 2005).

Violence

Violence is a major public health problem because it threatens the health and well-being, both physical and psychological,

of many children and adolescents. According to the U.S. Department of Justice/Bureau of Labor Statistics (2009), during the 2007–2008 school year, 85% of public schools recorded one or more occurrences of violence, theft, or other signifcant incidents, totaling an estimated 2 million crimes. In 2004, there were 309,000 instances of serious violence to students aged 12 to 18 years away from school, compared with approximately 88,000 instances at school (U.S. Department of Justice, 2004).

The CDC (2007a) reports that 27% of students had property stolen or deliberately damaged on school grounds. The percentage of high school students who reported being in a fight on school property declined from 16.2% in 1993 to 12% in 2007. This decline has been overshadowed by the increase in truly violent crimes such as school shootings.

In recent years there have been a number of shootings and other acts of serious violence in schools. The YRBSS data reveal that 8% of students in this country were either threatened or injured with a weapon while on school property in 2007 (CDC, 2007a). Serious violent behavior at school includes gang activity, bullying and intimidation, gun use, and assault. The school shooting at Columbine High School in Littleton, Colorado in 1999 shocked the nation and was probably the first time that people in this country realized how unsafe schools could be. In that incident, two students attending Columbine killed twelve classmates, a teacher, and then themselves, making this the nation's worst school shooting. As of fall 2008, there had been at least twenty-eight other school shootings in the United States.

School nurses and other school personnel should be aware of risk factors and signs that could indicate a tendency toward violence. Factors common in those who commit violent acts in school include being a male, coming from a disadvantaged or poor socioeconomic background, and having a history of abuse. Media influences that desensitize the impact of violence are being studied more closely as another cause of increased violence among children and adolescents. These children often have a need for instant gratification, have easy access to guns, and may have a history of discipline problems. Most events occurred at either the beginning or the end of the school day or during the lunch period (Anderson et al., 2001).

Although the number of students who commit violent acts is small, these random acts are frightening, and school officials are struggling with ways to prevent their occurrence and to recognize the signs of troubled youth early. Violence prevention programs should begin in elementary schools. Children who exhibit aggressive behavior in elementary school are more likely to exhibit antisocial and violent behavior as adolescents and adults. Programs should target stress management, conflict and anger resolution, and personal and self-esteem development. Nurses should use data collected through the YRBSS and other local data as a means of assessment when developing violence policy and prevention programs in the school and community. Additionally, nurses should initiate and participate in research that examines the complex developmental, social, and psychological factors surrounding violence.

Terrorism

Even though schools may not be the primary target in an act of terrorism, they will be affected by terrorism. Events following the September 11, 2001, attack illustrated potential problems that face schools when an act of terrorism has occurred. These problems included direct or near exposure of students to the incident; fear and panic among students, teachers, and parents; and anxiety among those directly affected.

Every school is encouraged to develop an emergency management plan. In fact, many states mandate that schools develop plans to address the potential threat of another terrorist attack or a natural or man-made disaster. School nurses must be prepared to act after any form of terrorism has occurred, including a bioterrorist attack. The school nurse has an important role as a potential first responder in any emergency situation and should be an active participant in planning and policy development with local governments and health departments.

Health Promotion for School Staff

According to the National Center for Education Statistics (2007), schools in the United States employ more than 5.5 million teachers and other employees. Health promotion programs at the work site produce beneficial results including positive effects on blood pressure control, daily physical activity, smoking cessation, and weight control. Staff that participate in health promotion programs increase their health knowledge and positively change their attitudes and behaviors relative to smoking practices, nutrition, physical activity, stress, and emotional health. Other studies show that health promotion programs improve morale, reduce job stress and absenteeism, and heighten interest in teaching health-related topics to students. School nurses play an important role in all levels of prevention through assessment, planning, intervention, and evaluation. The school nurse can assist the faculty and staff by giving workshops on exercise and nutrition, screening for increased blood pressure, and establishing weight management programs.

Family and Community Involvement

School nurses are often asked to provide health content to family, parents, and the community on a variety of topics, such as sexuality, STDs, HIV, communicable diseases, and substance abuse. Health education in the community should consist of programs that are designed to positively influence parents, staff, and others in matters related to health. School nurses are a ready resource to the community whenever health-related problems arise. They must step forward and volunteer their services and expertise in a way that can positively affect their community. Programs such as smoking cessation can include the entire community. School nurses should be aware of the existence of these programs; they may also serve as a consultant during implementation and as an advocate for programs to remain in place.

FAMILY RISK INDEX

Children living in families with four or more of the following characteristics are considered "high risk" (Annie E. Casey Foundation, 2002):

- Child is not living with two parents.
- Household head is a high school dropout.
- Family income is below the poverty line.
- Child is living with parent(s) who does not have steady, full-time employment.
- Family is receiving welfare benefits.
- Child does not have health insurance.
- Percentage of children living in "high-risk" families, based on the definition above, is 10%.

Programs aimed at adolescent weight control may also need to be targeted to the parents. Parents may not be aware of the important role they play in helping to prevent obesity in their children. School nurses can help parents develop healthier eating habits in the home that will directly affect their families. The nurse can also help develop physical activity programs in the community that include both the child and the family.

Nurses should become adept at working in the public sphere by increasing their visibility and becoming skilled in working with the media and legislators. The media can be a useful tool in assisting school nurses with health education advocacy.

SCHOOL NURSING PRACTICE

School nursing is a specialty unto itself. School nurses need education in specific areas, such as growth and development, public health, mental health nursing, case management, program management, family theory, leadership, and cultural sensitivity, to effectively perform their roles. They must be prepared to work with children of different ages and under highly variable circumstances. The nurse must also keep abreast of issues affecting children and participate in research that explores and expands the role. The school nurse's practice is relatively independent and autonomous, even though the school nurse functions as a member of an interdisciplinary team. For entry into school nursing, it is recommended that nurses hold a minimum of a bachelor's degree. Some universities are now preparing school nurses at the master's level. The school nurse must be able to identify and access professional development in order to maintain competency in the care of children and adolescents.

DEFINITION OF SCHOOL NURSING

School nursing is a specialized practice of professional nursing that advances the well-being, academic success, and lifelong achievement of students. To that end, school nurses facilitate positive student responses to normal development; promote health and safety; intervene with actual and potential health problems; provide case management services; and actively collaborate with others to build student and family capacity for adaptation, self-management, self-advocacy, and learning (NASN, 2000).

TABLE 29-3   STANDARDS OF SCHOOL NURSING PRACTICE

Standards of Practice

Standard 1. Assessment	The school nurse collects comprehensive data pertinent to the client's health or the situation.
Standard 2. Diagnosis	The school nurse analyzes the assessment data to determine the diagnoses or issues.
Standard 3. Outcomes identification	The school nurse identifies expected outcomes for a plan individualized to the client or the situation.
Standard 4. Planning	The school nurse develops a plan that prescribes strategies and alternatives to attain expected outcomes.
Standard 5. Implementation	The school nurse implements the identified plan.
Standard 5A: Coordination of care	The school coordinates care delivery.
Standard 5B: Health teaching and health promotion	The school nurse provides health education and employs strategies to promote health and a safe environment.
Standard 6. Evaluation	The school nurse evaluates the client's progress towards attainment of outcomes.

Standards of Professional Performance

Standard 7. Quality of practice	The school nurse systematically enhances the quality and effectiveness of nursing practice.
Standard 8. Education	The school nurse attains knowledge and competency that reflects current school nursing practice.
Standard 9. Profession practice evaluation	The school nurse evaluates one's own nursing practice in relation to professional standards and guidelines, relevant statutes, rules, and regulations.
Standard 10. Collegiality	The school nurse interacts with, and contributes to the professional development of, peers and school personnel as colleagues.
Standard 11. Collaboration	The school collaborates with the client, family, school staff, and others in the conduct of school nursing practice.
Standard 12. Ethics	The school nurse integrates ethical provisions in all areas of practice.
Standard 13. Research	The school nurse integrates research findings into practice.
Standard 14. Resource utilization	The school nurse considers factors related to safety, effectiveness, cost, and impact on practice in the planning and delivery of school nursing services.
Standard 15. Leadership	The school nurse provides leadership in the professional practice setting and the profession.
Standard 16. Program management	The school nurse manages school health services.

From American Nurses Association and National Association of School Nurses: *School nursing: scope & standards of practice,* Silver Spring, MD, 2005, nursesbooks.org.

School nurses function in many roles. Among these are care provider, student advocate, educator, community liaison, and case manager. Additional skills needed by school nurses include the ability to supervise others, to practice independently, and to delegate care. Table 29-3 presents the standards of school nursing practice.

The school setting is a perfect place to conduct research on how children adapt to life transitions such as divorce, illness or death of a loved one, illness of either themselves or a peer, domestic violence, and health-related behaviors of the young. Edwards (2002) reported on the establishment of research priorities for school nursing through the use of the Delphi technique. The study resulted in the identification of the top ten–ranked research priorities for school nursing.

RESEARCH HIGHLIGHTS

Research Priorities in School Nursing

Gordon and Barry (2006) surveyed 263 school nurses to identify what the nurses believed to be the top research priorities for the specialty. Ten areas were identified as being priority research topics. These priority areas, and examples for each, are presented below.

- *Obesity/nutrition*—nutrition and weight-loss counseling programs, eating disorders, obesity in children and teens, importance of exercise
- *Role of the school nurse*—correlation of the school nurse and better academic outcomes, case management, role of the school nurse as health consultant, delegation to nonnursing personnel, mental health support
- *Legal/ethical issues*—legal liability when delegating to nonmedical personnel, ethical issues related to children with Do Not Resuscitate orders, confidentiality, HIPAA mandates
- *Emergencies*—emergency preparedness, administering Diastat and EpiPens in school, standing orders for emergencies

- *Health education*—effective curricula for health promotion on hot topics (drugs, sexual activity, nutrition, exercise)
- *Absenteeism/attendance*—the school nurse's impact on student attendance, impact of absenteeism on educational success, strategies to decrease absenteeism
- *Diabetes/insulin*—diabetes management and safe delegation to nonlicensed personnel, managing insulin pumps at school
- *Injuries*—playground safety, sports injuries
- *Health services*—funding of school health services by using matching reimbursement (Medicaid), access to health services for students and their families, benefits and cost-effectiveness of school health services
- *Asthma*—environmentally unsafe schools, asthma education, asthma prevalence, use of peak flow meters

From Gordon SC, Barry CD: Development of a school nursing research agenda in Florida: a Delphi study, *J Sch Nurs* 22(2):114-119, 2006.

SCHOOL-BASED HEALTH CENTERS

School-based health centers are one of the best ways to offer comprehensive health care services to school-aged children and adolescents. The center or clinic works in collaboration with, but does not take the place of, the school nurse. The collaboration between the school nurse and the school-based health center staff prevents fragmented care and duplication of services. School-based health centers provide an interdisciplinary team approach with personnel such as nurse practitioners, social workers, psychologists, and physicians who provide services; they are usually employed by one or more local agencies, such as health departments, hospitals, or medical schools. Some of the services provided in these centers include nutrition education, injury treatment, general and sports physicals, prescriptions, pregnancy testing, laboratory services, immunizations, gynecological examinations, medication dispensing, social work services, and management of chronic illnesses. Close collaboration must exist within and among the community, the educational board, and the families for such a center to develop and flourish. The National Assembly on School-Based Health Care (2009) outlined the core values for school-based health care programs. They believe that all children should have access to high-quality health care; that the school setting is the appropriate place to deliver health care; that all services should be provided directly; that health care inequities can be reduced; and that fair reimbursement should be provided.

FUTURE ISSUES AFFECTING THE SCHOOL NURSE

Our nation's youth are our greatest asset and hope for the future. The school nurse's role must be constantly evolving to meet the demands of the future. Issues that will face the school nurse of tomorrow include ethical dilemmas, use of telehealth, threat of bioterrorism, new and emerging infectious diseases, and increase in antibiotic-resistant diseases. The school nurse will need to understand and appreciate the multicultural community in which he or she will practice.

SUMMARY

Components of a comprehensive school health program have been clearly identified and discussed. Many of the *Healthy People 2020* objectives specifically relate to issues that can be addressed in the school setting. The role of the school nurse has changed dramatically since its inception and continues to evolve to meet the demands of school-aged children, their parents, and the communities in which they live. School nurses continue to reduce the number of days and the frequency with which students miss school related to illness. They have become child advocates, counselors, health promoters and collaborators, educators, researchers, and resources, in both the school and the community.

⚖ ETHICAL INSIGHTS

An Ethical Dilemma: What Would You Do?

You are working as the school nurse in a rural high school when Grace, a 15-year-old female student, enters the clinic. Grace appears very worried, and, after several hesitant starts, she begins to cry and tells you that she is sexually active with a 17-year-old senior. She goes on to tell you that she has missed her last period and that her home pregnancy test is positive. She states that she is afraid to tell her parents because she feels that they will be very disappointed in her and because she is afraid of what her father will do. She asks you where she can go to get an abortion. You speak with Grace for quite a while and encourage her to speak with her parents. She leaves the clinic a little more composed and promises you that she will think about what you have said. The next day Jenny, Grace's mother, comes into the clinic and asks to speak with you. She confides that she is worried about Grace and asks if you know what is going on with her child. What would you do in this situation?

Although maintaining confidentiality and a professional relationship respectful of the student's wishes is vital, state laws and school district policies will determine what a school nurse may do, and in some cases is required to do, when providing care to minor children. When dealing with personal and sensitive information such as is described above, the school nurse should be well-versed in relevant laws and policies and follow them. When in doubt, contact a supervisor.

■ LEARNING ACTIVITIES

1. Explain how the *Healthy People 2020* objectives can be used to shape school-based health care.
2. Attend a meeting of the school nurse association in the area. Identify the major pros and cons of being a school nurse. Look at factors such as working conditions, number of children assigned to each nurse, job functions, and job satisfaction.
3. Visit a comprehensive school-based clinic in the area. Discuss how the care given in this type of clinic differs from the care that a school nurse can provide. Review the protocols of both settings and see how they differ.
4. Purchase a 1-year subscription to a school health journal.
5. Interview a member of the local school board about controversial subjects in health education in the local school system (e.g., sex education).
6. Review the most common diseases and reported injuries in school-aged children in the area. Develop a plan for how the school and the community can work together to decrease their incidence.
7. Interview the parents of several school-aged children. Ask what health services they would like to see provided in the school setting.
8. Arrange with the principal of a local school to have a discussion session with children in a particular grade level. Ascertain what their eating habits are and then develop a class that can enhance healthy eating.

APPLICATION OF THE NURSING PROCESS

The nursing process is a systematic, organized approach to problem solving that nurses use when working with clients. It is neither fixed nor stagnant. It is a flexible process that allows for ongoing changes. This case study illustrates the use of the nursing process in a school setting.

Sandra Baker is a nurse at an elementary school in a small town. A second-grade teacher brought Carrie Broussard to the clinic and told Sandra that Carrie had been scratching her head all day and she was worried that Carrie might have an infection.

Assessment

Carrie is 7 years old. Her shoulder-length blond hair appeared neat and clean. When questioned by Sandra, Carrie replied that her head had been itching for 2 or 3 days, but she denied any pain or trauma. Sandra noted that Carrie did not have a fever or swollen lymph nodes, but examination of her scalp revealed multiple excoriated areas. Carrie's hair was examined with a Wood's light, and Sandra saw adult lice at the base of her hair follicles on the back of her head near the nape of the neck. Multiple nits were also noted. Sandra learned that Carrie had two brothers in the school and one sister who was a toddler at home.

On Carrie's initial visit to the clinic, Sandra assessed the following:
* Temperature
* Lymph nodes
* Scalp for any abnormal findings

Diagnosis
Individual
* Head lice

Family and Community (School)
* Potential for spread of infestation in both family and school
* Potential deficient knowledge related to spread and treatment of lice by teachers and family members

Planning

Sandra is familiar with the school district's policy that covers head lice in schoolchildren. According to the policy, the nurse must do the following:

Individual
Long-Term Goal
* Carrie's return to school after successful treatment

Short-Term Goals
* Contact Carrie's parents to tell them about the lice.
* Inform Carrie's parents that she must be picked up from school.
* Recommend treatment based on school protocol.
* Provide guidelines for returning to school.

Family and Community
Long-Term Goal
* Ensure that the teachers, staff, and family members have the necessary education relative to prevention and treatment of head lice.

Short-Term Goals
* Examine the hair of all other children in Carrie's class for lice, and treat each according to the school protocol.
* Check the hair of all siblings who attend the school for lice.

* Check the hair of all students in the siblings' classes if lice are identified.

Intervention
Family

Carrie's brothers, David and Paul, are brought to the clinic for examination. Both brothers have lice. Sandra contacted Mrs. Broussard, explained the situation to her, and requested that she come to the school to pick up her children. When Mrs. Broussard arrived at the school, Sandra gave her written information on treatment and prevention of lice and showed her what nits and lice look like. Mrs. Broussard was also instructed to check other members of the family not attending this school, especially those who share hairbrushes, pillowcases, and towels, because all family members with lice must be treated or the lice would continue to be passed from member to member. Sandra also explained procedures for cleaning combs, brushes, bedding, and potentially contaminated clothing and toys. Finally, Mrs. Broussard was informed that the children could return to school the day after treatment.

It was obvious to Sandra that Mrs. Broussard was embarrassed. To ease her mind, Sandra carefully explained that head lice are highly contagious, are easily passed from child to child, and are not an indication of poor hygiene. Mrs. Broussard repeated the instructions and left with her three children.

Community

Sandra examined all of the students from each of the Broussard children's classes for head lice. From the three classes, she identified five more children with head lice and notified their parents. Those children had siblings in three additional classrooms and she repeated the procedure for each of them. At the end of the day, she had identified a total of 15 children with head lice and contacted all parents.

Sandra investigated whether the teachers and staff desired an information session on the transmission and spread of head lice because so many students had lice. She discovered that it had been 2 years since this was done and arranged a class for the coming week for the teachers and teachers' aides to learn how to identify and treat head lice.

Evaluation
Individual and Family

Mrs. Broussard brought Carrie, David, and Paul to school the following day, and on examination Sandra found their hair to be free of lice and nits. Mrs. Broussard expressed her appreciation for the nurse's help and nonjudgmental approach to the problem.

Community

Over the next 2 days, Sandra reexamined all of the children in the affected classrooms and found that the infected children had been successfully treated and that there were not any new cases. New cases were not identified during the remainder of the semester. The teachers and staff gave her positive feedback about the head lice education class and asked for it to be repeated at the beginning of each school year.

Levels of Prevention and School Health

School nursing encompasses all three levels of prevention (i.e., primary, secondary, and tertiary), and all three may be practiced individually or concurrently. Table 29-4 lists examples of school nursing interventions for each of the three levels of prevention.

TABLE 29-4 EXAMPLES OF PREVENTION AND THE ROLE OF THE NURSE IN THE SCHOOL SETTING

EXAMPLE	NURSE'S ROLE
Primary Prevention	
Nutrition education	Provide education to children and parent; consult with dietary staff
Immunizations	Provide for or refer to source(s) for immunizations; offer consultation for immunization in special circumstances
Safety	Provide safety education; inspect playgrounds and buildings for safety hazards
Health education	Teach healthy lifestyle education; develop health education curriculum for appropriate grade levels; provide health education to parents, faculty, and staff; develop suicide prevention programs and sex education materials
Secondary Prevention	
Screenings	Schedule routine screenings for scoliosis, vision and hearing problems, eating disorders, obesity, depression, anger, dental problems, abuse, and Early and Periodic Screening Diagnostic and Treatment (EPSDT) program
Case finding	Identify at-risk students
Treatment	Administer medications; develop individualized health plan; implement procedures and tasks necessary for student with special health needs; administer first aid
Home visits	Assist with family counseling and assess special and at-risk students
Tertiary Prevention	
Referral of student for substance abuse or behavior problems	Serve as an advocate; assist with resource referrals; assist parent, faculty, and staff; consult with neighborhood and law enforcement officials; initiate outreach programs
Prevention of complications and adverse effects	Follow-up and referral for student with eating disorders and obesity; participate with faculty and staff to reduce recurrence and risk factors; serve as a case manager
Faculty and staff monitoring	Follow-up for faculty and staff experiencing chronic or serious illness; follow-up of work-related injuries and accidents

REFERENCES

Allensworth D, et al, editors: *Schools and health: our nation's investment*, 1997, Institute of Medicine, Division of Medicine.

American Academy of Orthopedic Surgeons-AAOS-SRS-POSNA-AAP Information Statement: *Screening for idiopathic scoliosis in adolescents*, September 2007, www.aaos.org/about/papers/position/112.asp.

American Cancer Society: *Child and teen tobacco use: understanding the problem*, 2008, www.cancer.org.

American Diabetes Association: *Total prevalence of diabetes & pre-diabetes*, 2009, www.diabetes.org/diabetes-statistics/prevalence.jsp.

Anderson M, et al: School-associated violent deaths in the United States: 1994-1999, *JAMA* 286(21):2695–2702, 2001.

Annie E: *Casey Foundation: Children at risk: state trends 1990–2000*, 2002, www.aecf.org/kidscount/c2ss/.

Annie E: *Casey Foundation: Kids Count data center*, 2007, www.kidscount.org/datacenter/compare_results.jsp?i=800.

Centers for Disease Control and Prevention: *School health policies and program study 2000: fact sheet—school based health centers and services provided at other sites*, www.cdc.gov/healthyyouth/shpps/factsheets/school_based_health.htm.

Centers for Disease Control: Summary of notifiable diseases: United States, 2003, *MMWR Morb Mortal Wkly Rep* 52(54):1–95, 2005, www.cdc.gov/mmwr/preview/mmwrhtml/mm5254a1.htm.

Centers for Disease Control and Prevention: Youth risk behavior surveillance: United States—2007, *MMWR Morb Mortal Wkly Rep* 57(SS04):1–131, 2007a, www.cdc.gov/mmwr.

Centers for Disease Control and Prevention: *Tobacco use and the health of young people*, 2007b, www.cdc.gov/HealthyYouth/tobacco/facts.htm.

Centers for Disease Control and Prevention: *Quick stats: underage drinking*, 2008a, www.cdc.gov/alcohol/quikstats/underage-drinking.htm.

Centers for Disease Control and Prevention: *Oral health: preventing cavities, gum disease, and tooth loss*, 2008b, www.cdc.gov/needphp/publications/aag/doh/htm.

Centers for Disease Control and Prevention: *HIV/AIDS statistics and surveillance*, 2009a, www.cdc.gov/hiv/topics/surveillance/basic.htm.

Centers for Disease Control and Prevention: *Vital and summary health statistics for U.S. children: National Health Interview Survey, 2007*, 2009b. www.cdc.gov.

Centers for Disease Control and Prevention, Adolescent Reproductive Health: *Home-teen pregnancy*, 2007, www.cdc.gov/reproductivehealth/AdolescentRepro Health/.

Centers for Disease Control and Prevention, Division of Oral Health: *Oral health for adults*, 2006, www.cdc.gov/OralHealth/publications/factsheets/adult.htm.

Centers for Disease Control and Prevention, National Center for Health Statistics: *National Vital Statistics System*, 2008, http://webappa.cdc.gov/cgi-bin/broker.exe.

Centers for Medicare & Medicaid Services: *Early and periodic screening diagnostic and treatment program (EPSDT): overview*, 2006, www.cms.hhs.gov/MedicaidEarly PeriodicScrn/01_Overview.asp#TopOf Page.

Children's Defense Fund: *State of America's children*, 2008, www.childrensdefense.org/child-research-data-publications/data/state-of-americas-children-2008-report.html.

Duncan P, Igoe J: School health services. In Marx E, Wooley SF, Northrop D, editors: *Health is academic: a guide to coordinated school health programs*, New York, 1998, Teachers College Press.

Edwards L: Research priorities in school nursing: a Delphi process, *J Sch Health* 72(5):173–178, 2002.

Institute of Medicine: *Childhood obesity in the United States: facts and figures—fact sheet*, 2004, www.iom.edu/Object.File/Master/22/606/0.pdf#search='childhood%20obesity%20in%20the%20United%20States%3A%20Facts%20and%20Figures'.

MacKay AP, Duran C: *Adolescent health in the United States*, Hyattsville, MD, 2007, National Center for Health Statistics.

McCarthy A, Kelly M, Reed D: Medication administration practices of school nurses, *J Sch Health* 70(9):371–376, 2000.

Montalto N: Implementing the guidelines for adolescent preventive services, *Am Fam Physician* 57(9):2181–2190, 1998.

National Assembly on School-Based Health Care: *Core values*, 2009, www.nasbhc.org/site/c.jsJPKWPFJrH/b.2663979/k.7566/Vision_Mission_Core_Value.

National Association of School Nurses: NASN board of directors meeting, Providence, Rhode Island, June 1999, Definition of school nursing, *J Sch Nurs* 16(1):5, 2000.

National Association of School Nurses: Access to a school nurse: *NASN position statement*, 2003a, www.nasn.org/Portals/0/statements/resolutionaccess.pdf.

National Association of School Nurses: *Medication administration in the school setting: NASN position statement*, 2003b, www.nasn.org/Default.aspx?tabid=230.

National Association of School Nurses: *Resolution: vending machines and healthy food choices in schools*, 2004, www.nasn.org.

National Association of School Nurses: *Environmental impact concerns in the school setting*, 2005, www.nasn.org/Default.aspx?tabid=293.

National Association of School Nurses: Caseload assignments: *NASN position statement*, June 2006a, www.nasn.org/Default.aspx?tabid=209.

National Association of School Nurses: Alternative medicine use in the school setting: *NASN position statement*, 2006b, www.nasn.org/Default.aspx?tabid=199.

National Center for Education Statistics: *Context of elementary and secondary education*, 2007, www.nces.ed.gov/programs/coe/2008/section4/table.asp?tableID=920.

National Institute on Drug Abuse: *Infofacts: steroids*, 2007. http://www.drugabuse.gov.

Safe Kids Worldwide: *Sports and recreation safety*, Washington, DC, 2007a, The Author.

Safe Kids Worldwide: *School safety*, Washington, DC, 2007b, The Author.

Sherman R, Thompson R: The female athlete triad, *J Sch Nurs* 20(4):197–202, 2004.

Tinsworth D, McDonald J: *Special study: injuries and death associated with children's playground equipment*, Washington, DC, 2001, US Consumer Product Safety Commission.

U.S. Department of Health and Human Services: *Healthy People 2010*, Washington, DC, 2000, Public Health Service.

U.S. Department of Justice, Bureau of Justice Statistics: *Criminal victimization in the United States*, 2002, www.ojp.usdoj.gov/bjs/pub/pdf/cvus02.pdf.

U.S. Department of Justice: *Indicators of school crime and safety*, 2004, www.ojp.usdoj.gov/bjs/pub/pdf/iscs04.pdf.

U.S. Department of Justice/Bureau of Justice Statistics: *Indicators of school crime and safety*, 2009, http://nces.ed.gov/pubs2010/2010012.pdf.

Occupational Health

Bonnie Rogers

Additional Material for Study, Review, and Further Exploration

evolve WEBSITE

http://evolve.elsevier.com/Nies

- Quiz
- Case Studies
- Glossary
- WebLinks

- Resource Tools
  - 30A: Preplacement Health Evaluation
  - 30B: Occupational Health History
  - 30C: Example of Screening and Surveillance: Guide to OSHA Standard for Benzene
  - 30D: Physical Demands Analysis

OBJECTIVES

Upon completion of this chapter, the reader will be able to do the following:

1. Describe the historical perspective of occupational health nursing.
2. Discuss emerging demographic trends that will influence occupational health nursing practice.
3. Identify the skills and competencies germane to occupational health nursing.
4. Apply the nursing process and public health principles to worker and workplace health issues.
5. Discuss federal and state regulations that affect occupational health.
6. Describe a multidisciplinary approach for resolution of occupational health issues.

KEY TERMS

Ada Mayo Stewart
Americans With Disabilities Act (ADA)
disability syndrome
ergonomics

industrial hygiene
occupational health nursing
Occupational Safety and Health
   Administration (OSHA)

safety
toxicology
Workers' Compensation Acts

OUTLINE

Evolution of Occupational Health Nursing
Demographic Trends and Access Issues Related to Occupational Health Care
Occupational Health Nursing Practice and Professionalism
Occupational Health and Prevention Strategies
   Healthy People 2020 and Occupational Health
   Prevention of Exposure to Potential Hazards
   Levels of Prevention and Occupational Health Nursing
Skills and Competencies of the Occupational Health Nurse
   Competent
   Proficient

Expert
Examples of Skills and Competencies for Occupational
   Health Nursing
Impact of Federal Legislation on Occupational Health
   Occupational Safety and Health Act
   Workers' Compensation Acts
   Americans With Disabilities Act
Legal Issues in Occupational Health
Multidisciplinary Teamwork

Occupational health nursing, a subspecialty of public health nursing, is defined by the American Association of Occupational Health Nurses (AAOHN) as the following:

> The specialty practice that focuses on the promotion, prevention, and restoration of health within the context of a safe and healthy environment. It includes the prevention of adverse health effects from occupational and environmental hazards. It provides for and delivers occupational and environmental health and safety programs and services to clients. Occupational and environmental health nursing is an autonomous specialty and nurses make independent nursing judgments in providing health care services (AAOHN, 2004, p. 2).

As depicted in Figure 30-1, occupational health nursing derives its theoretical, conceptual, and factual framework from a multidisciplinary base. Elements of this multidisciplinary base include the following (Rogers, 1998, 2003b):

- *Nursing science,* which provides the context for health care delivery and recognizes the needs of individuals, groups, and populations within the framework of prevention, health promotion, and illness and injury care management, including risk assessment, risk management, and risk communication
- *Medical science* specific to treatment and management of occupational health illness and injury, integrated with nursing health surveillance activities
- *Occupational health sciences,* including toxicology, to recognize routes of exposure, examine relationships between chemical exposures in the workplace and acute and latent health effects such as burns or cancer, and understand dose-response relationships; industrial hygiene, to identify and evaluate workplace hazards so control mechanisms can be implemented for exposure reduction; safety, to identify and control workplace injuries through active safeguards and worker training

and education programs about job safety; and ergonomics, to match the job to the worker, emphasizing capabilities and minimizing limitations

- *Epidemiology,* to study health and illness trends and characteristics of the worker population, investigate work-related illness and injury episodes, and apply epidemiological methods to analyze and interpret risk data to determine causal relationships and to participate in epidemiological research
- *Business and economic theories, concepts, and principles* for strategic and operational planning, for valuing quality and cost-effective services, and for management of occupational health and safety programs
- *Social and behavioral sciences,* to explore influences of various environments (e.g., work and home), relationships, and lifestyle factors on worker health and determine the interactions affecting worker health
- *Environmental health,* to systematically examine interrelationships between the worker and the extended environment as a basis for the development of prevention and control strategies
- *Legal and ethical issues,* to ensure compliance with regulatory mandates and contend with ethical concerns that may arise in competitive environments

EVOLUTION OF OCCUPATIONAL HEALTH NURSING

The evolution of occupational health nursing in the United States has mirrored the societal changes in moving from an agrarian-based to an industrial-based economy and, entering the twenty-first century, a continuing move to a service-based economy. Occupational health nursing dates to the late 1800s with the employment of Betty Moulder and Ada Mayo Stewart (Parker-Conrad, 2002; Rogers, 2003b).

A group of coal-mining companies hired Betty Moulder in 1888 to care for coal miners and their families (American Association of Industrial Nurses [AAIN], 1976). Seven years later, the Vermont Marble Company hired Ada Mayo Stewart to care for workers and their families. Stewart is often referred to as the first "industrial nurse," and her activities are well documented (Parker-Conrad, 1988). In 1897, Anna B. Duncan was employed by the John Wanamaker Company to visit sick employees at home; then, in 1899, a nursing service was established for employees of the Frederick Loeser department store in Brooklyn, New York (AAIN, 1976).

At the turn of the twentieth century, the industrial revolution was well under way, and the concept of health care for employees spread rapidly. Companies hiring industrial nurses in the early 1900s included the Emporium in San Francisco; Plymouth Cordage Company in Massachusetts; Anaconda Mining Company in Montana; Broadway Store in Los Angeles; Chase Metal Works in Connecticut; Hale Brothers in San Francisco; Filene's in Boston; Carson, Pirie, Scott in Chicago; Fulton Cotton Mills in Georgia; and Bullock's in Los Angeles (McGrath, 1946; Parker-Conrad, 1988). The

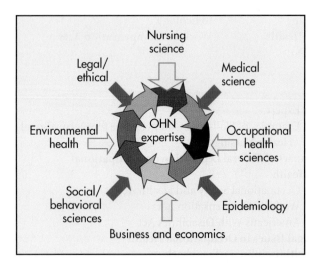

FIGURE 30-1 Occupational health nursing knowledge domains. (From Rogers B: Occupational health nursing expertise, *AAOHN J* 46:477-483, 1998. Copyright Bonnie Rogers, 1998.)

cost-effectiveness of providing health care to employees was achieving increased recognition, and by 1912, after workers' compensation legislation had been instituted, 38 nurses were employed by business firms (McGrath, 1946; Parker-Conrad, 1988). The following year, a registry of industrial nurses was initiated, and in 1915 the Boston Industrial Nurses Club was formed, later evolving into the Massachusetts Industrial Nurses Organization.

In 1916, the Factory Nurses Conference was organized. This group was open only to graduate, state-registered nurses affiliated with the American Nurses Association (ANA), and their efforts identified the industrial nurses' need to explore the uniqueness of this evolving specialty area (AAIN, 1976). More important, industrial nurses were practicing in single-nurse settings and recognized the benefit of uniting as a group for the purpose of sharing ideas with peers practicing in the same nursing arena. In 1917, the first educational course for industrial nurses was offered at Boston University's College of Business Administration.

During and after the Great Depression, many nurses lost jobs because employers and business managers viewed industrial nursing as a nonessential aspect of business (Felton, 1985, 1986). The focus of health care for employees again changed as a result of many factors, including the impact of the two world wars. During World War I, the government demanded health services for workers at factories and shipyards holding defense contracts. Demographics in the workplace were also dramatically different during World War II because increased numbers of women entered the workforce. In 1942, the U.S. Surgeon General told an audience of nurses that the health conservation of the "industrial army" was the most urgent civilian need during the war (Felton, 1985).

From 1938 to 1943, the number of occupational health nurses increased by more than 10,000. In 1942, some 300 nurses from sixteen states voted to create a national association for the specialty. Catherine R. Dempsey, a nurse at Simplex Wire and Cable Company in Cambridge, Massachusetts, was elected president of the national association. By 1943, approximately 11,000 nurses were employed in industry (AAIN, 1976).

Nine years later, members of AAIN voted to remain an independent, autonomous association rather than merge with the National League for Nursing or the ANA. In 1953, another important step was taken toward formalizing this specialty area of nursing practice when the *Industrial Nurses Journal* (i.e., now the *AAOHN Journal*) was published. In 1977, the organization changed its name to the AAOHN, reflecting a broader, more diverse scope of practice.

In the 1980s and 1990s, occupational health nursing moved rapidly into increased role expansion in health promotion, policy development, management, and research and maintained traditional occupational health nursing practice. In 1989, AAOHN developed its first research agenda, and in 1993 the Occupational Safety and Health Administration (OSHA) established the Office of Occupational Health Nursing, reenergizing the concept of occupational health into practice. In 1999, the AAOHN Foundation was established,

and competencies in the specialty were delineated. In the twenty-first century, the AAOHN continues to expand specialty borders, emphasizing the importance of occupational health concepts and population-based practice.

DEMOGRAPHIC TRENDS AND ACCESS ISSUES RELATED TO OCCUPATIONAL HEALTH CARE

At the beginning of the twenty-first century, sweeping transformations in industry are influencing the direction of occupational health nursing. These transformations include changing workforce demographics, rising health care costs, diversity of health care systems with the integration of managed care, influence of the world economy, shift in production from goods to services, and proliferation of advanced technologies. The focus of U.S. industry is moving away from large manufacturing facilities to smaller, service-based businesses, and other changes are anticipated (Hecker, 2001). Work may be performed where and when the customer requires, which will force employers to make different demands on their employees. Flexible and varying work schedules and worksites have become more common than the daily trek to the same building for the 40-hour, 9-to-5 routine that has been the standard for decades. Of major importance will be the demand for an increase in skill level of all employees. The ability to read, follow directions, perform mathematical calculations, and be computer literate will be core skills for workers. The increasing availability of older workers, women, minorities, and immigrants will have far-reaching implications for employers and pose specific challenges for occupational health professionals.

In 2006, most U.S. workers (68%) fell within the prime working ages of 25 to 54 years; 15% were younger than 25 years, and 17% were 55 years old or older. By 2010, the baby boom generation will reach the ages of 45 to 64 years, and middle and older age groups in the labor force will outnumber younger workers. Data for 2006 indicate that the occupational groups of managerial and professional specialty; technical, sales, and administrative support; and services account for more than 50% of employed persons in the United States. Among industry sectors, services employed the most workers (37.4% of the labor force, or 50.5 million workers), followed by retail trade (16.7%), and manufacturing (14%). The Bureau of Labor Statistics estimates that the service sector will have the greatest growth by 2016. Employment will increase to 52.2 million for the service sector and to 34.2 million for wholesale and retail trade (Bureau of Labor Statistics, 2006; National Institute for Occupational Safety and Health [NIOSH], 2004). These trends are important to understand because they have a direct impact on the national rate of economic growth, especially in the area of population-sensitive products such as food, automobiles, housing units, household goods, and services such as health care, education, and transportation. With expansion of each of these sectors, there are concomitant hazards.

Within the context of these evolving organizational trends, key characteristics include a focus on a shared vision, strategy, and long-term objectives within an environment composed of individuals working in teams. In contrast to the past, occupational health nurses have opportunities to work on cross-functional teams to shape decisions in areas such as benefits, research, safety, and legal matters. Specifically, occupational health nurses have opportunities to positively affect the transformation of the health care delivery system, establish policies within the managed care environment and within corporations, and assume leadership positions on legislative staffs and in governmental agencies.

Corporations have become driving forces in shaping the development of alternative approaches to health care. Rapidly increasing health care costs have spawned a number of alternative approaches to providing health care, such as preferred provider organizations.

It is important that the occupational health nurse remains informed about the various health care options available to the workforce as rapid changes occur regarding corporate benefits. This is of particular importance when considering the referral of an employee to a health resource. Participation in one of the managed care plans requires that treatment take place according to the organization's guidelines and within its health service delivery system. Managed care plans have nearly replaced traditional indemnity plans. Access to care is closely managed and often limited. As this trend continues, the role of the occupational health nurse will take on added importance. The nurse must be prepared to accept increasing responsibilities as a primary care provider, as well as tertiary care coordinator/case manager.

As businesses seek ways to maximize the value of their dollars spent on health care services, occupational health nurses and other health professionals face both an opportunity and a threat. The opportunity comes from being able to demonstrate that cost-effective, quality health programs do improve the health of employees and their dependents, positively influencing their company's attempts to control rising health care costs. The threat is that if health professionals cannot prove cost-effectiveness and value to companies, their functions may be eliminated or replaced by contract services (Intili and Laws, 2003).

OCCUPATIONAL HEALTH NURSING PRACTICE AND PROFESSIONALISM

As workplaces have continued to change over the past few decades, the role of the occupational health nurse has become even more diversified and complex. Often working as the only on-site health care professional, the occupational health nurse collaborates with workers, employers, and other professionals to identify health problems or needs, prioritize interventions, develop and implement programs, and evaluate services delivered. The occupational health nurse is in a unique and critical position to coordinate a holistic approach to the delivery of quality, comprehensive occupational health services. The Standards of Occupational and Environmental Health Nursing, the Code of Ethics, and AAOHN practice competencies guide the nurse.

AAOHN's Standards of Occupational and Environmental Health Nursing Practice (AAOHN, 2004) form the basis by which the profession describes its responsibilities and accountabilities. The eleven standard statements are listed in Table 30-1. For each standard, identifiable criteria are detailed that can be used to evaluate practice relative to the specific standard. Refer to the complete standards document from the AAOHN for this information.

TABLE 30-1   STANDARDS OF OCCUPATIONAL AND ENVIRONMENTAL HEALTH NURSING

Standard	Statement
Standard I: Assessment	The occupational and environmental health nurse systematically assesses the health status of the client(s).
Standard II: Diagnosis	The occupational and environmental health nurse analyzes assessment data to formulate diagnoses.
Standard III: Outcome identification	The occupational and environmental health nurse identifies outcomes specific to the client(s).
Standard IV: Planning	The occupational and environmental health nurse develops a goal-directed plan that is comprehensive and formulates interventions to attain expected outcomes.
Standard V: Implementation	The occupational and environmental health nurse implements interventions to attain desired outcomes identified in the plan.
Standard VI: Evaluation	The occupational and environmental health nurse systematically and continuously evaluates responses to interventions and progress toward the achievement of desired outcomes.
Standard VII: Resource	The occupational and environmental health nurse secures and manages the resources that support occupational health and safety programs and services.
Standard VIII: Professional	The occupational and environmental health nurse assumes accountability for professional development to enhance professional growth and maintain competency.
Standard IX: Collaboration	The occupational and environmental health nurse collaborates with the client(s) for the promotion, prevention, and restoration of health within the conduct of a safe and healthy environment.
Standard X: Research	The occupational and environmental health nurse uses research findings in practice and contributes to the scientific base in occupational and environmental health nursing to improve practice and advance the profession.
Standard XI: Ethics	The occupational and environmental health nurse uses an ethical framework for decision making in practice.

From American Association of Occupational Health Nurses: Standards of occupational and environmental health nursing, *AAOHN J* 52:270-274, 2004. Copyright American Association of Occupational Health Nurses, http://www.aaohn.org.

BOX 30-1 AAOHN CODE OF ETHICS

- Occupational and environmental health nurses provide health, wellness, safety, and other related services to clients with regard for human dignity and rights, unrestricted by consideration of social or economic status, personal attributes or the nature of the health status.
- Occupational and environmental health nurses, as licensed health care professionals, accept obligations to society as professional and responsible members of the community.
- Occupational and environmental health nurses strive to safeguard clients' rights to privacy by protecting confidential information and releasing information only as required or permitted by law.
- Occupational and environmental health nurses promote collaboration with other professionals, community agencies, and stakeholders in order to meet the health, wellness, safety, and other related needs of the client.
- Occupational and environmental health nurses maintain individual competence in nursing practice, based on scientific knowledge, and recognize and accept responsibility for individual judgments and actions, while complying with appropriate laws and regulations.

From American Association of Occupational Health Nurses: Standards of occupational and environmental health nursing, *AAOHN J* 52:140-142, 2004.

Guided by an ethical framework made explicit in the AAOHN Code of Ethics (AAOHN, 2009), occupational health nurses encourage and enable individuals to make informed decisions about health care concerns (Box 30-1). The occupational health nurse is a worker advocate and has the responsibility to uphold professional standards and codes. The occupational health nurse is also responsible to management, is usually compensated by management, and must practice within a framework of company policies and guidelines (Rogers, 2003a). Ethical dilemmas arise because the nurse is loyal to both workers and management. Issues such as screening, drug testing, informing employees regarding hazardous exposures, and confidentiality of health information, which is integral and central to the practice base, often create ethical debates. As advocates for workers, occupational health nurses foster equitable and quality health care services and safe and healthy work environments.

Occupational health nurses make up the largest professional group providing health care services to employees in highly complex work environments. The roles of occupational health nurses are changing as a result of many factors, including rising health care costs, increased recognition of health effects associated with various exposures, emphasis on health promotion and wellness, health surveillance, women's issues, ergonomics, reproductive issues, downsizing, trends in managed care, and multicultural workforces. Box 30-2 reflects this growth in scope of practice and outlines occupational health nursing services currently mandated by state and federal regulations and occupational health nursing services generally mandated by company policies.

BOX 30-2 OCCUPATIONAL HEALTH NURSING SERVICES

Services Mandated by Federal and State Regulations
Safe and healthful workplace
Emergency medical response
First aid responder selection and training
First aid space, supplies, protocols, and records
Designated medical resources for incident response
Workers' compensation
Confidentiality of medical records
Compliance with medical record retention requirements
OSHA compliance
Medical personnel requirement (29 CFR 1910.15)
Injury and illness reporting and recording
Accident and injury investigation
Cumulative trauma disorder prevention
Employee access to medical and exposure records
Medical surveillance and hazardous work qualification
Personal protective equipment evaluation and training
Infection control
Employee Right-to-Know Act notification and training
Community Right-to-Know Act compliance
ADA compliance
Rehabilitation Act: handicap, preplacement, fitness for duty evaluations, accommodations
Department of Defense, Department of Transportation, Nuclear Regulatory Commission, and Drug-Free Workplace Act compliance
Policy development
Drug awareness education
Drug testing and technical support
Employee Assistance Program services
Threat of violence and duty to warn
Video display terminal (VDT) local regulations

State and local public health regulations
Nursing practice acts
Board of Pharmacy and Drug Enforcement Agency regulations
Continuing professional education required for licensure

Services Often Mandated by Company Policy
Clinical supervision of on-site health services
Health strategy development
Health services standards
Space, staffing, and operational standards
Occupational illness and injury assessment, diagnosis, treatment, and referral
Nonoccupational illness and injury assessment, diagnosis, treatment, and referral
Disability and return-to-work evaluations and accommodations
Impaired employee fitness for duty evaluation
Preplacement evaluation and medical accommodation
Handicap evaluation, placement, and accommodation
Employee Assistance Program standards
International health: travel, medical advisory, and immunizations
Data collection and analysis
Medical consultation
Pregnancy placement in hazardous environments
Professional education and development
Audit and quality assurance

Optional Services
Health education and health promotion
Medical screening for early detection and disease prevention
Physical fitness programs
Allergy injection programs

ADA, Americans With Disabilities Act; *OSHA,* Occupational Safety and Health Administration.

⚖ ETHICAL INSIGHTS
Confidentiality of Employee Health Information

Occupational health nurses sometimes experience ethical dilemmas because of dual responsibility to both their employer and employees. In dealing with health information, the employee has a right to privacy and should "be protected from unauthorized and inappropriate disclosure of personal information" (AAOHN, 2004, p. 1). Exceptions can, and in some situations must, be made, however. These include (1) life-threatening emergencies, (2) authorization by the employee to release information to others (e.g., insurance company, health care provider), (3) workers' compensation information, and (4) compliance with government laws and regulations.

The AAOHN identifies three "levels of confidentiality" of health information. Level I relates to information required by law (e.g., data on occupational illness and injuries, exposure data, and information derived from special examinations [i.e., tests given to food handlers]). Level II covers information that will assist in management of human resources (e.g., information obtained from job placement and other health examinations to determine "workability status" of the employee). Finally, Level III focuses on "personal health information." This includes non–job-related health problems or health counseling.

Disclosure of Levels I and II information to management should be allowed only on a "need-to-know" basis, generally with reference to workability status and regulatory compliance. Disclosure of Level III information to management and regulatory agencies should only be allowed as required by law. Finally, disclosure of Level III information health insurance providers should be made only with appropriate written authorization of the employee.

From American Association of Occupational Health Nurses: *Position statement: confidentiality of employee health information,* 2004, www.aaohn.org/practice/positions/upload/Confidentiality_of_Emp_Health_Info.pdf.

Approximately 35,000 nurses are practicing in the occupational health field in the United States (1.5% to 2% of the total nursing population). Approximately 60% of these 35,000 nurses work alone, making decisions regarding health and safety issues, influencing policy in health and safety, and planning and implementing myriad health programs. More than 65% of nurses practicing in occupational health are prepared at the baccalaureate level or higher and have been practicing in the field of occupational health for at least 10 years (AAOHN, 2007).

Meeting the needs of employees in smaller businesses is another important practice priority. The integration of occupational health and safety principles into the curricula of schools of nursing, engineering, and management is critical. Community health nurses may assume occupational health nursing roles; therefore community health nurses must be knowledgeable about the specialty area of occupational health nursing. Municipalities, smaller companies, visiting nurse associations, and home care agencies may provide opportunities for community health nurses to be involved in screening programs, health education activities, workplace hazard evaluations, and other occupational health–related activities.

The occupational health nurse's strengths are embedded in assessing, planning, implementing, and evaluating health programs for populations, care plans for individuals, and health education activities for worker aggregates. Often, lack of understanding or misconceptions about the occupational health nurse's role have fostered the invisibility of the nurse, both within the nursing profession itself and within the business environment, thereby exacerbating the difficulties faced in being the sole guardian of health for workers in many companies. Empowered, well-trained, educated occupational and environmental health nurses can help bring about crucial changes in the areas of primary, secondary, and tertiary prevention in occupational health.

In response to societal changes and historical events, the practice of occupational health nursing has changed dramatically, demanding a sophisticated knowledge base and problem-solving skills that are empirically grounded and multidisciplinary in nature (Rogers, 2003b). The roles and responsibilities of the occupational health nurse must be clearly articulated to lay people; managers; workers; union representatives; and colleagues in occupational health, nursing, and medicine to ensure that occupational health nursing can continue to positively affect workers' health, contribute to decreasing health care costs, and foster reduction in health risks. Occupational health nurses must seize opportunities in areas such as program planning, research, and policy making during this era fraught with a health care system in crisis. Issues to be addressed and managed include nursing shortages in many areas of the country, dramatic changes in the business environment, employees' increasing awareness of workplace hazards, and the ever-increasing need to demonstrate the cost-effectiveness of occupational health nursing care and services (Richlin, 2003).

Research is an integral component of occupational and environmental health nursing practice because it provides the basis for scientific discovery that improves practice. In 1989, research priorities in occupational health nursing were first identified and published (Rogers, 1989). They have been updated periodically to serve as the scientific basis to continue to build the body of knowledge in occupational and environmental health nursing for practice improvement and expansion (Box 30-3).

BOX 30-3   RESEARCH PRIORITIES IN OCCUPATIONAL HEALTH NURSING

- Effectiveness of primary health care delivery at the worksite
- Effectiveness of health promotion nursing intervention strategies
- Methods for handling complex ethical issues related to occupational health
- Strategies that minimize work-related health outcomes (e.g., respiratory disease)
- Health effects resulting from chemical exposures in the workplace
- Occupational hazards of health care workers (e.g., latex allergy and blood-borne pathogens)
- Factors that influence workers' rehabilitation and return to work
- Effectiveness of ergonomic strategies to reduce worker injury and illness
- Effectiveness of case management approaches in occupational illness and injury
- Evaluation of critical pathways to effectively improve worker health and safety and enhance maximum recovery and safe return to work
- Effects of shift work on worker health and safety
- Strategies for increasing compliance with or motivating workers to use personal protective equipment

From American Association of Occupational Health Nurses: *Research priorities in occupational and environmental health nursing,* 2009, www.aaohn.org/practice/priorities.cfm.

OCCUPATIONAL HEALTH AND PREVENTION STRATEGIES

Like the practice of all community health professionals, the occupational health nurse's practice is based on the concept of prevention. Promotion, protection, maintenance, and restoration of worker health are priority goals set forth in the definition of occupational health nursing. Prevention of exposure to occupational and environmental safety hazards and specific strategies for each level of prevention are described along with objectives from *Healthy People 2020*.

Healthy People 2020 and Occupational Health

Healthy People 2020 is the federal government initiative that focuses on health promotion and illness prevention. One topic area of *Healthy People 2020* concentrates on Occupational Safety and Health (US Department of Health and Human Services [USDHHS], 2009). Objectives from this priority area cover work-related injuries and deaths, repetitive motion injuries, homicide, assault, lead exposure, skin disorders, stress, and hearing loss. In addition, objectives from other topic areas also address issues related to occupational health and safety. The *Healthy People 2020* table lists objectives that deal with occupational health.

Prevention of Exposure to Potential Hazards

To prevent occupational and environmental safety hazards in the work environment, it is important to identify work-related agents and exposures that are potentially hazardous. These can be categorized as follows:

1. *Biological-infectious hazards:* Infectious-biological agents such as bacteria, viruses, fungi, or parasites that may be transmitted via contact with infected clients or contaminated objects or substances
2. *Chemical hazards:* Various forms of chemical agents, including medications, solutions, and gases, that interact with body tissues and cells and are potentially toxic or irritating to body systems
3. *Enviromechanical hazards:* Factors encountered in work environments that cause accidents, injuries, strain, or discomfort (e.g., poor equipment or lifting devices and slippery floors)
4. *Physical hazards:* Agents within work environments such as radiation, electricity, extreme temperatures, and noise that can cause tissue trauma through transfer of energy from these sources
5. *Psychosocial hazards:* Factors and situations encountered or associated with the job or work environment that create stress, emotional strain, or interpersonal problems

---

 HEALTHY PEOPLE 2020

Proposed Objectives for Some Areas of Occupational Health

OBJECTIVE

DSC HP2020-4: Eliminate disparities in employment rates between working-aged adults with and without disabilities.

ECBP HP2020-5: Increase the proportion of worksites that offer a comprehensive employee health promotion program to their employees.

FP HP2020-4: Increase the proportion of health insurance plans that cover contraceptive supplies and services.

ENT-VSL HP2020-5: Increase the use of ear protection devices.

HDS HP2020-10: Increase the proportion of out-of-hospital cardiac arrests in which appropriate bystander and emergency medical services (EMS) were administered.

IID HP2020-15e: Reduce hepatitis B among occupationally exposed workers.

NWSS HP2020-12: Increase the proportion of worksites that offer nutrition or weight management classes or counseling.

OSH HP2020-1: Reduce the rate of injury and illness cases involving days away from work due to overexertion or repetitive motion.

OSH HP2020-3: Reduce deaths from work-related homicides.

OSH HP2020: Reduce occupational skin diseases or disorders among full-time workers.

OSH HP2020-6: Reduce new cases of work-related, noise-induced hearing loss.

OHS HP2020-7: Reduce deaths from work-related injuries.

OHS HP2020-8: Reduce nonfatal work-related injuries.

OSH HP2020-10: Increase the proportion of employees who have access to workplace programs that prevent or reduce employee stress.

PAF HP2020-9: Increase the proportion of employed adults who have access to and participate in employer-based exercise facilities and exercise programs.

RD HP2020-7b: Reduce the number of workdays missed among adults (aged 18–64 years) with current asthma.

TU HP2020-2: Increase the proportion of persons covered by indoor worksite policies that prohibit smoking.

TU-HP2020-10: Increase insurance coverage of evidence-based treatment for nicotine dependency.

V HP2020-3: Reduce occupational eye injuries.

USDHHS Healthy People 2020 Draft Objectives. 2009. http://www.healthypeople.gov/hp2020/Objectives/files/Draft2009Objectives.pdf.

TABLE 30-2	TYPES OF OCCUPATIONAL HAZARDS AND ASSOCIATED HEALTH EFFECTS	
CATEGORY	**EXPOSURES**	**HEALTH EFFECTS**
Biological	Blood or body fluids	Bacterial, fungal, and viral infections (e.g., hepatitis B)
Chemical	Solvents	Headache and central nervous system dysfunction
	Lead	Central nervous system disturbances
	Asbestos	Asbestosis
	Acids	Burns
	Glycol ethers	Reproductive effects
	Mercury	Ataxia
	Arsenic	Peripheral neuropathy
Enviromechanical	Static or nonneutral postures	Musculoskeletal disorders
	Repetitive or forceful exertions	Back injuries
	Lighting	Headache and eye strain
	Shift work	Sleep disorders
	Electrical	Electrocution
	Slips and falls	Musculoskeletal conditions
	Struck by or against object	Injury
Physical	Noise	Hearing loss
	Radiation	Reproductive effects and cancer
	Vibration	Raynaud's disease
	Heat	Heat exhaustion and heat stroke
Psychosocial	Stress	Anxiety reactions and a variety of physical symptoms
	Work-home balance	

Table 30-2 provides examples of work-related exposures in each of these areas. Having a good understanding of the nature of these hazards will allow for the development of health promotion and prevention strategies to mitigate exposure risk.

Levels of Prevention and Occupational Health Nursing

As occupational health nurses usually practice autonomously in their role as health care providers, the occupational health nurse's activities in primary, secondary, and tertiary prevention strategies are expected to assume an even more important role in the prevention and treatment of illness, injury, and chronic disease in the future (Rogers and Lawhorn, 2000). For example, a study by Rogers and Livsey (2000) examined the scope of independent and interdependent practice by occupational health nurses related to these activities and found that 71% of occupational health nurses had overall responsibility for program management, and the majority performed surveillance, screening, and prevention functions as independent practice. Physician supervision for any of these activities ranged from only 0% to 8% in reporting. The results of this study validate the independent functioning in scope of occupational health nursing practice related to surveillance, screening, and prevention activities while recognizing the contributions all providers make to a healthy workforce.

Primary Prevention

In the area of primary prevention, the occupational health nurse is involved in both health promotion and disease prevention. O'Donnell (2009) describes health promotion as the following:

The art and science of helping people discover the synergies between their core passions and optimal health, enhancing their motivation to strive for optimal health, and supporting them in changing lifestyle to move toward a state of optimal health. Optimal health is a dynamic balance of physical, emotional, social, spiritual and intellectual health. Lifestyle change can be facilitated through a combination of learning experiences that enhance awareness, increase motivation, and build skills and most importantly, through creating opportunities that open access to environments that make positive health practices the easiest choice (p. iv).

Disease prevention begins with recognition of a health risk, a disease, or an environmental hazard and is followed by measures to protect as many people as possible from harmful consequences of that risk.

The occupational health nurse uses a variety of primary prevention methods, with one-on-one interaction as an important strategy for evaluating risk reduction behavior for individuals. The occupational health nurse has daily contact with numerous employees for many reasons (e.g., assessment and treatment of episodic illness or injury and health surveillance); therefore this is an important method of promoting health. The phrase "seize the moment" aptly describes the opportunity that exists with every employee encounter.

Occupational health nurses plan, develop, implement, and evaluate aggregate-focused intervention strategies. The occupational health nurse plans and implements programs such as weight and cholesterol reduction, acquired immunodeficiency syndrome (AIDS) awareness, ergonomics training, and smoking cessation. Performing "walk-throughs" in the workplace on a regular basis, recognizing potential and existing hazards, and maintaining communications with safety and industrial hygiene resources to prevent illness and injury from occurring will continue to be critical work for the occupational health nurse (Levy et al., 2005).

For overall *health promotion*, the nurse may plan, implement, and evaluate a health fair, which is a multifaceted health promotion strategy that usually includes a number of community health resources to provide expertise on a wide range of health issues and community services. As part of an overall health and wellness strategy, the occupational health nurse may negotiate with the employer for an on-site fitness center or area with fitness equipment; if cost or space is prohibitive, the employer may choose to partially subsidize membership at a local fitness center (Rogers, Randolph, and Mastrianno, 2009).

Types of *nonoccupational programs* included in the area of primary prevention are cardiovascular health, cancer awareness, personal safety, immunization, prenatal and postpartum health, accident prevention, retirement health, stress management, and relaxation techniques. Occupational health programs could include topics such as emergency response, first aid and cardiopulmonary resuscitation training, right-to-know training, immunization programs for international business travelers, prevention of back injury through knowledge of proper lifting techniques, ergonomics, and other programs targeted to the specific hazards identified in the workplace (Walz and Wehse, 2002; Rogers, Randolph, and Mastrianno, 2009).

Women's health and safety issues such as maternal-child health, reproductive health, breast cancer education and early detection, stress management, and work-home balance issues will achieve heightened significance as more women enter the workforce. Thirty percent of women currently in the workforce are between ages 16 and 44 years, and each year approximately 1 million infants are born to these women. Interest in workplace safety and the relationship to reproductive outcomes continues to grow as women of childbearing age enter the workplace in greater proportions than ever before.

The occupational health nurse can play a key role in the development and delivery of prenatal, postpartum, and childhood programs in the workplace. Of primary importance will be the ability to serve as a change agent to initiate needed programs in the work environment. Employers must be educated regarding strategies not only to reduce health care costs for women and infants but also to improve the work environment for mothers (Wyatt, 2002). Women who believe their employers are interested in the well-being of themselves and their families are more apt to be productive and satisfied employees. The occupational health nurse can play a critical role in the shaping of supportive policies and practices to accommodate the needs of families, including flexible working hours, parental leave, and on-site child care (Rogers, Franke, Jeras, et al., 2009).

Members of *racial and ethnic minority* groups make up a large share of the labor force, and as the number of minority and ethnic workers in the workforce increases, so will the illnesses traditionally associated with these groups of workers

TABLE 30-3	WORK-RELATED DISEASES AND INJURIES	
WORK-RELATED DISEASE OR INJURY	**EXAMPLES OF EFFECT**
Occupational lung disease	Cancer and asthma
Musculoskeletal injuries	Back, upper extremity, and musculoskeletal disorders
Occupational cancers	Leukemia, bladder, and skin
Trauma	Death, amputation, and fracture
Cardiovascular diseases	Hypertension and heart disease
Reproductive disorders	Infertility and miscarriage
Neurotoxic disorders	Neuropathy and toxic psychosis
Noise-induced hearing loss	Loss of hearing
Dermatological conditions	Chemical burns and allergies
Psychological disorders	Neurosis; alcohol or substance abuse

(e.g., heart disease and stroke, hypertension, cancer, cirrhosis, and diabetes) (NIOSH, 2004). In addition to basic health concerns for this population, available statistics indicate that minority workers have been disproportionately concentrated in some of the most dangerous work, and they are at greater risk for experiencing many of the leading occupationally related diseases and injuries. Table 30-3 illustrates examples of common occupational diseases and injuries.

The occupational health nurse may face challenges in developing programs that are culturally and linguistically appropriate. The occupational health nurse may be in an advocacy role to negotiate with the employer for changes in the work environment that will reduce or eliminate existing or potential occupational exposure to risk factors.

Secondary Prevention

Secondary prevention strategies are aimed at early diagnosis, early treatment interventions, and attempts to limit disability. The focus at this level of prevention is on identification of health needs, health problems, and employees at risk.

As with primary prevention, the occupational health nurse uses a number of different secondary prevention strategies (Rogers, 2003b). By providing direct care for episodic illness and injury, the occupational health nurse is afforded the opportunity to conduct assessments and provide treatment and referrals for a variety of physical and psychological conditions. The occupational health nurse can offer health screenings, which are designed for early detection of disease, at the worksite with relative ease and at minimal cost. Screenings may focus on vision, cancer, cholesterol, hypertension, diabetes, tuberculosis, and pulmonary function. Other types of screening, such as mammography, may be contracted with a vendor who uses mobile equipment.

Secondary prevention efforts provided by the occupational health nurse include *preplacement, periodic,* and *job transfer evaluations* to ensure that the worker is being placed or is continuing to work in a job that is safe for that worker (Rogers, 2003b). The preplacement evaluation is performed before the worker begins employment in a new company or is placed in a different job. The evaluation is a baseline examination that consists of a medical history, an occupational health history, and a physical assessment that should target the type of work that the employee will be performing. For example, if the employee is going to be lifting materials in a warehouse, special attention should be paid to any history of musculoskeletal problems. Strength testing and range of motion should be performed for all muscle groups. (See **Resource Tool 30A**, Preplacement Health Evaluation, and **Resource Tool 30B**, Occupational Health History, on the book's website at http://evolve.elsevier.com/Nies/).

The preplacement examination may also include medical tests to determine specific organ functions that may be affected by exposure to existing agents in the employee's workplace. For example, if the employee is working with a chemical that is a known liver toxin, baseline liver function tests may be appropriate to determine the current health status of the liver and its ability to handle this specific chemical exposure. However, the preplacement examination must be carefully evaluated to ensure compliance with the Americans With Disabilities Act (ADA), which is discussed later in the chapter.

Periodic assessments usually occur at regular intervals (e.g., annual and biannual) and are based on specific protocols for those exposed to substances or irritants such as lead, asbestos, noise, or various chemicals. Examinations of individuals transferring to other jobs are critical to document any changes in health that may have occurred while the employee was working in a specific area or with a specific process. This is usually done to comply with OSHA regulations or NIOSH recommendations. (See **Resource Tool 30C** on the book's website at http://evolve.elsevier.com/Nies/ for an example of an OSHA screening and surveillance guide.) For full details of compliance requirements, OSHA standards must be consulted.

Activities must continue to focus on prevention and early detection by increasing awareness of the incidence of commonly occurring health conditions such as breast cancer and providing accessible and affordable screening programs. For example, it is estimated that invasive breast cancer will be diagnosed in almost 200,000 women and that about 40,000 women will die of the disease each year, making breast cancer one of the most commonly diagnosed malignancies among women in the United States and the second leading cause of cancer death (after lung cancer). Further, breast cancer accounts for about 15% of cancer deaths among women (American Cancer Society, 2009). By detecting early malignancies, breast cancer screening reduces the mortality rate in women between ages 50 and 69 years. Mammography is the most effective method for detecting these early malignancies. The occupational health nurse is in an excellent position to play a key role in reducing morbidity and mortality associated with breast cancer. Increasingly, the occupational health nurse will be expected to document the return on investment for these and other related activities in the workplace.

Tertiary Prevention

On a tertiary level, the occupational health nurse plays a key role in the rehabilitation cand restoration of the worker to an optimal level of functioning. Strategies include case management, negotiation of workplace accommodations, and counseling and support for workers who will continue to be affected by chronic disease (Rogers, 2003b; Rogers, Randolph, and Mastrianno, 2009).

In industry, disability costs average 8.4% of payroll. Four percent of the gross national product, or $170 billion, is the figure cited for costs associated with total disability (Boden, Biddle, and Spieler, 2001). In the United States, it is estimated that more than 500,000 workers take an estimated 5 months of leave from work each year because of a physical disability; only 48% return to work (Fletcher, 2003). Research findings indicate the importance of developing strategies to reinforce the behavioral change of the individual to avoid what is often referred to as the disability syndrome, a state in which an individual chooses not to work when medical clearance has been granted (Curtis and Scott, 2004).

Knowledge of the workplace, the ability to negotiate with the employer for appropriate accommodations, early intervention, and comprehensive case management skills have been and will continue to be essential to the disabled employee's successful return to work. The process of returning an individual to work begins with the onset of injury or illness (Rogers, 2003b; Rogers, Randolph, and Mastrianno, 2009). Regardless of whether this involves an occupational or a nonoccupational condition, the occupational health nurse is the center of case management (Kalina, Haag, and Tourigan, 2004). The nurse works closely with the primary care provider to monitor the progress of the ill or injured worker and to identify and eliminate potential barriers in the return-to-work process. The nurse has a comprehensive understanding of the workplace and of the physical requirements necessary for the employee to work. The physical demands analysis (Randolph and Dalton, 1989) is a useful tool in objectively assessing the physical demands of any job. (See **Resource Tool** **30D**, Physical Demands Analysis, on the book's website at http://evolve.elsevier.com/Nies/.) Once the assessment is completed, the occupational health nurse can relay this information to community health professionals caring for the employee.

For workers needing special accommodations, the occupational health nurse can negotiate and facilitate those appropriate to the employee's health limitations (Kalina et al., 2004). The nurse is often the driving force behind the employer's creating a transitional duty pool. The goal of this type of program is to provide temporary work that is less physically demanding in nature than the employee's regular work. This facilitates the employee's return to the workplace earlier than if required to wait until full strength is regained.

The occupational health nurse can monitor and support the health of employees returning to work who continue to experience adverse health effects of chronic disease. For example, the employee who is returning to work after sustaining a myocardial infarction may have blood pressure monitored on a routine basis. Counseling regarding adjustment to normal work life and support for behavior modification (e.g., smoking cessation) also may be provided (Byczek et al., 2004).

In addition, because the workforce is aging and because older workers are more prone to chronic disease, the occupational health nurse can implement and monitor treatment protocols and assist workers to live and work at their optimum comfort level while managing their disease. Responsibilities for the care of elderly parents or significant others will influence the balance of work and home for older workers. The occupational health nurse's role as counselor, referral resource for workers, and consultant to management can influence future beneficial changes.

SKILLS AND COMPETENCIES OF THE OCCUPATIONAL HEALTH NURSE

Although clinical and emergency care remains an important tenet of occupational health nursing, the current and future practice must focus on a proactive approach with the goal of preventing illness and injury and promoting health. Therefore the occupational health nurse must possess competencies necessary to recognize and evaluate potential and existing health hazards in the workplace. Management and budgeting skills and knowledge of legal and regulatory requirements, toxicology, ergonomics, epidemiology, environmental health, safety, counseling, and health promotion and education are essential to meet the present and future demands of occupational health nursing practice.

Competencies in occupational and environmental health nursing have been delineated in nine categories by AAOHN (Box 30-4) (AAOHN, 2007). Each competency delineates comprehensive performance criteria at the competent, proficient, and expert levels. Each level is described, followed by an example of occupational health nursing practice at that level.

Competent

At the "competent" level of practice, the nurse has gained confidence and his or her perception of the role is one of mastery and an ability to cope with specific situations. There is less of a need to rely on the judgments of peers and other professionals. Work habits tend to stress consistency rather than routinely tailoring care to encompass individual differences (Benner, 1984).

BOX 30-4 **COMPETENCY CATEGORIES IN OCCUPATIONAL AND ENVIRONMENTAL HEALTH NURSING**

1. Clinical and primary care
2. Case management
3. Workforce, workplace, and environmental issues
4. Regulatory and legislative
5. Management
6. Health promotion and disease prevention
7. Occupational and environmental health and safety education and training
8. Research
9. Professionalism

From American Association of Occupational Health Nurses: Competencies in occupational and environmental health nursing, *AAOHN J* 51:290-302, 2007.

Occupational and environmental health nursing example: The competent nurse is an occupational and environmental health nurse with sufficient experience to recognize a range of practice issues and function comfortably in such roles as clinician, occupational health services coordinator, and case manager. This nurse follows company procedures and relies on assessment checklists and clinical protocols to provide treatment.

Proficient

The "proficient" nurse has an increased ability to perceive client situations as a whole on the basis of past experiences, focusing on the relevant aspects of the situation. The nurse is able to predict the events to expect in a particular situation and can recognize that protocols sometimes must be altered to meet the needs of the client (Benner, 1984).

Occupational and environmental health nursing example: A proficient occupational and environmental health nurse is able to quickly obtain the information needed for accurate assessment and move rapidly to the critical aspects of the problem. Structured goals are replaced by priority setting in response to the situation. This nurse usually possesses sophisticated clinical or managerial skills in the occupational health setting.

Expert

The "expert" nurse has extensive experience and a broad knowledge base and is able to grasp a situation quickly and initiate appropriate action. The nurse has a sense of salience grounded in practice guiding actions and priorities (Benner, 1984).

Occupational and environmental health nursing example: Occupational and environmental health nurses at the expert level include those providing leadership in developing occupational and environmental health policy within an organization, those functioning in upper executive or management roles, those serving as consultants to business and government, and those designing and conducting significant research in the field.

Examples of Skills and Competencies for Occupational Health Nursing

As described, numerous skills and competencies are necessary for occupational health nursing practice. Examples of some of these are outlined here, according to the nine defined areas of competence.

Clinical and Primary Care

- Applying the nursing process in delivery of care
- Providing first aid and primary care according to treatment protocols
- Conducting a physical assessment
- Taking an occupational and environmental health history
- Diagnosing and treating
- Being knowledgeable about immunization protocols
- Identifying employees' emotional needs and providing support and counseling

- Using a multidisciplinary problem-solving approach to occupational health illness and injury
- Maintaining records
- Clinical testing and monitoring
- Responding to medical emergencies
- Being knowledgeable about trends in health-related issues

Case Management

- Identifying the need for case management services
- Conducting case management assessments using a multidisciplinary framework
- Developing case management care plans
- Evaluating resources and vendors for case management
- Implementing early return-to-work programs
- Monitoring and evaluating outcomes
- Developing policies and programs for case management
- Analyzing trends for case management services
- Designing disability management systems
- Conducting case management outcomes-based research

Workforce, Workplace, and Environmental Issues

- Having knowledge of worksite operations, manufacturing processes, and job tasks
- Identifying and monitoring potential and existing workplace exposures
- Influencing appropriate and targeted recommendations for control of workplace hazards
- Having knowledge of toxicological, epidemiological, and ergonomic principles
- Understanding appropriate engineering and administrative controls and personal protective equipment specific to preventing workplace health hazard exposures
- Understanding roles and collaboration with other cross-functional groups as an integral part of a core multidisciplinary team
- Performing risk assessments
- Managing health surveillance programs

Legal and Ethical Responsibilities

- Being knowledgeable of state nursing practice acts and ability to practice occupational health nursing within state guidelines
- Being knowledgeable of federal, state, and municipal regulations pertaining to occupational and environmental health
- Being knowledgeable of the ADA, associated guidelines, and other relevant occupational and environmental health laws
- Being knowledgeable of all aspects of medical record-keeping practices in compliance with nursing practice, state law, and standards of practice
- Being knowledgeable of current legal trends related to negligence and malpractice cases in professional nursing and in the occupational health setting
- Being knowledgeable of confidentiality parameters
- Influencing regulatory and legal processes related to occupational and environmental health

Management and Administration

- Managing budgets
- Hiring staff and management of staff performance
- Fostering professional development plans
- Developing program goals and objectives
- Developing business plans through knowledge of internal and external resources
- Providing comprehensive on-site services and programs
- Knowing needs of business and employees
- Writing reports
- Performing audits and quality assurance
- Handling workers' compensation and disability
- Performing cost-benefit analyses, cost-effectiveness analyses, and outcomes monitoring
- Allocating appropriate staff resources
- Providing leadership in health-related issues
- Negotiating
- Facilitating work accommodations and return-to-work processes
- Coordinating medical response activities and site disaster planning
- Being a resource expert on health issues for employees and management
- Participating in strategic operations planning

Health Promotion and Disease Prevention

- Conducting needs assessments
- Recognizing cultural differences and their relationship to health issues
- Using effective communication styles to match diverse employee and management audiences
- Making effective presentations
- Planning, developing, implementing, and evaluating health programs designed to meet the needs of specific employee groups or organizations
- Evaluating health promotion outcomes
- Applying adult learning theory and principles to health education programs
- Integrating all levels of prevention into company culture

Occupational and Environmental Health and Safety Education

- Creating effective professional and technical support networks both functionally and cross-functionally
- Developing and implementing training programs for workers and professionals

Research

- Identifying researchable problems
- Systematically collecting, analyzing, and interpreting data from different sources
- Recognizing trends in health outcomes by department, work area, or work process
- Planning, developing, and conducting research
- Developing and testing models and theories relative to occupational and environmental health nursing practice

Professionalism
- Engaging in a lifelong learning plan
- Being knowledgeable of AAOHN Standards of Occupational and Environmental Health Nursing and Code of Ethics
- Maintaining currency in practice
- Acting as a professional role model for students and colleagues
- Advancing the specialty through knowledge and science

IMPACT OF FEDERAL LEGISLATION ON OCCUPATIONAL HEALTH

Legislation and associated activities have influenced the practice of occupational health in the United States. Table 30-4 presents a historical perspective of some of the major pieces of legislation that have had, and will continue to have, a direct impact on the general practice of occupational and environmental health nursing. The Occupational Safety and Health Act, Workers' Compensation Acts, and the ADA are highlighted below.

Occupational Safety and Health Act

The Occupational Safety and Health Act of 1970 was enacted 2 years after a major coal-mining disaster in West Virginia. The passage of this legislation came about

because there were concerns for workers' health, a burgeoning environmental awareness, union activities, and an increased knowledge about workplace hazards. The general duty clause of the act states that employers must "furnish a place of employment free from recognized hazards that are causing or likely to cause death or serious physical harm to employees." The act also identifies the roles of the various governmental agencies, provides for the establishment of federal occupational safety and health standards, and identifies a structure of penalties, fines, and sentences for violations of regulations. Under the act, any state has the right to implement its own occupational safety and health administration. The only requirement is that the state standards meet or exceed federal standards. Currently, twenty-five states and the Virgin Islands operate state occupational safety and health administrations. The following organizations were formed under the provisions of the Act:

- Under the jurisdiction of the Department of Labor, the Occupational Health and Safety Administration (OSHA) is responsible for promulgating and enforcing occupational safety and health standards.
- Under the jurisdiction of the USDHHS, NIOSH is responsible for funding and conducting research, making recommendations for occupational safety and health standards to OSHA, and funding

TABLE 30-4 HISTORICAL PERSPECTIVE OF LEGISLATION AFFECTING OCCUPATIONAL HEALTH IN THE UNITED STATES

YEAR	LEGISLATION
1836	First restrictive child labor law enacted (Massachusetts)
1877	State legislation passed requiring factory safeguards (Massachusetts)
1879	State legislation passed requiring factory inspections (Massachusetts)
1886	State legislation passed requiring reporting of industrial accidents (Massachusetts)
1910	State legislation passed requiring formation of an Occupational Disease Commission (Illinois)
1911	Workmen's Compensation Act passed (New Jersey)
1935	Social Security Act passed (state and federal unemployment insurance program)
1936	Walsh-Healey Act (federal legislation setting occupational safety and health standards for certain government contract workers)
1938	Fair Labor Standards Act (setting minimum age for child labor)
1948	All states have workers' compensation acts
1964	Civil Rights Act
1965	McNamara-O'Hara Act (extends protection of the Walsh-Healey Act to include suppliers of government services)
1966	Mine Safety Act (mandatory inspections and health and safety standards in mining industry)
1969	Coal Mine Health and Safety Act (mandatory health and safety standards for underground mines)
1970	Occupational Safety and Health Act
1970	Environmental Protection Agency established
1970	Consumer Protection Agency established
1972	Equal Employment Opportunity Act
1972	Noise Control Act
1972	Clean Water Act
1973	HMO Act
1973	Rehabilitation Act
1976	Toxic Substances Control Act
1976	Resources Conservation and Recovery Act
1977	Federal Mine Safety and Health Act
1990	Americans With Disabilities Act
1991	Bloodborne Pathogens Standard
1993	Family Medical Leave Act
2001	Needlestick Safety and Prevention Act
2002	Recordkeeping Rule Amended

Occupational Safety and Health Education and Research Centers for the training of occupational health professionals.

- The Occupational Safety and Health Review Commission, which is appointed by the president, is responsible for advising OSHA and NIOSH regarding the legal implications of decisions or actions in the course of performing their duties.
- The National Advisory Committee on Occupational Safety and Health, which is appointed by the president, is a group of consumers and professionals who are responsible for making recommendations to OSHA and NIOSH regarding occupational health and safety.
- The National Commission on State Workers' Compensation Laws, appointed by the president, studied the adequacy of state workers' compensation laws and made recommendations to the president on its findings. This commission's work ended as of October 30, 1972.

Since it was instituted, OSHA has promulgated occupational health and safety standards. These are published in the *Code of Federal Regulations* (CFR) and updated on a regular basis. Having access to the most recent publication of these standards is a crucial responsibility of the occupational health nurse.

The occupational health nurse must be knowledgeable of Title 29 of the code, part 1910 (29 CFR 1910), and other sections of the code that apply to specific hazards in the workplace. For example, 29 CFR 1904 pertains to OSHA's record-keeping requirements and mandates the employer's responsibility to keep records of work-related injuries, illnesses, and deaths. These records must be posted in the workplace for 1 month per year and made available for review by OSHA at any time. In many cases, the occupational health nurse has full responsibility for compliance with this standard.

OSHA has ten regional offices throughout the United States. Inspectors are assigned to each region to enforce the standards and to provide consultation to industries. An OSHA inspection can be initiated in one of several ways. Each office plans a schedule of routine visits to the industries in their respective regions. In the past, funding has been an issue, and inspections have not taken place in the quantity or frequency originally intended. An inspection will occur if a major health or safety problem, such as a death, occurs at the worksite, or if three or more workers are sent to the hospital as a result of the same incident. Inspection also may occur by employer request. This is not usually done unless the employer has an exemplary occupational health and safety program and wishes to participate in OSHA's voluntary inspection program. Inspection also may be initiated by an employee request if there is concern about a suspected hazardous condition. In this case, OSHA is mandated to respond, and it must keep the employee's name confidential at the employee's request. In the past, penalties have been inconsequential, and sentences have rarely been served. However, recent events indicate that fines have increased, and OSHA has made public its intention to criminally prosecute company executives for serious and willful violations.

In many organizations, the occupational health nurse is the interface with the OSHA inspector. This requires the nurse to be knowledgeable about the potential hazards in the workplace and about the appropriate control measures designed to eliminate or minimize exposure. The nurse should know that employees or their union representatives have the right to accompany the OSHA investigators.

Workers' Compensation Acts

Workers' Compensation Acts are state mandated and state funded. These programs provide income replacement and pay for health care services for workers who sustain a work-related injury, temporary or permanent disability, or death. Workers' Compensation Acts also protect the employer if the compensation received by the employee precludes legal suits against the employer. Each state regulates its own workers' compensation program that is unique to that state. The employer can self-insure, contract with commercial insurance carriers, or purchase a policy with the state-operated insurance fund. Workers receive an average of 66% of their take-home pay before taxes, and some disabled workers and their families are eligible for other benefit programs, including old age, survivors, disability, and health insurance; supplemental security income (SSI); or any other disability program that they may have purchased through the company or on an individual basis.

In an era of high health care costs and a propensity for injured workers to engage the services of lawyers to represent them in negotiating financial settlements, many employers are claiming that workers' compensation costs are crippling their ability to compete in an international marketplace. The occupational health nurse has a unique opportunity to support both the employee and employer in this arena. For the employee, the nurse may be the initial person to whom the work-related injury or illness is reported. Accurate assessment of the injury or illness and appropriate treatment are essential. Community resources must be identified to ensure the injured worker is provided with high-quality health care and appropriate medical follow-up.

The occupational health nurse educates the employee regarding benefits under the Workers' Compensation Act and is often the one who files the claim. If the employee is disabled from work for a period of time, the nurse provides case management support and remains in contact with the employee until return to work. If the employer uses an insurance carrier, the nurse works closely with the claims adjuster to manage the case. The need for light duty or other workplace accommodations is determined before the employee's return. In most cases, the nurse facilitates this process with the employer.

For the employer, the occupational health nurse provides the expertise in early intervention and case management. The goal is to limit the worker's disability and provide an opportunity for early return to work through appropriate workplace accommodations. The desired outcome is a productive employee with optimum health and productivity, with reduced health care and workers' compensation costs.

Americans With Disabilities Act

The Americans With Disabilities Act (ADA), enacted by Congress in July 1990, is a comprehensive act that prohibits discrimination on the basis of disability. The core of this law requires employers to adjust facilities and practices for the purpose of making "reasonable accommodations" to enhance opportunities for individuals with disabilities (Kaminshine, 1991). Employment provisions of this act began on July 26, 1992, for employers with twenty-five or more employees and were revised in July 1994 to include employers with fifteen or more employees. Provisions regarding access to public transportation and accommodations became effective in January 1993.

The ADA defines disability as "physical or mental impairment that substantially limits one or more major life activities; having record of such an impairment; or being regarded as having such an impairment" (Kaminshine, 1991, p. 249). Physical or mental impairment guidelines are the same as those described in the Federal Rehabilitation Act and include "any physiologic disorder or condition, cosmetic disfigurement, anatomical loss affecting any of the major body systems, or any mental or psychological disorder" (Kaminshine, 1991, p. 249). Major life activities include caring for self, walking, seeing, hearing, and speaking. The ADA excludes conditions relating to sexual preference and gender identity, compulsive gambling, kleptomania, and pyromania. The ADA also denies protection for individuals who are currently involved in illegal drug use.

With regard to the ADA, the occupational health nurse has particular responsibility in two areas. The first involves the duty to provide or facilitate reasonable accommodations. This is facilitated by the nurse's familiarity with the physical requirements of jobs in the workplace. The second involves preplacement inquiries and health examinations. Preplacement health examinations will be permitted only if phrased in terms of the applicant's general ability to perform job-related functions rather than in terms of a disability and after a job offer has been made. The examination must be job related and consistently conducted for all applicants performing similar work.

As illustrated in this discussion of specific laws pertinent to occupational health, the legal context for occupational health nursing practice is broad and involves many arenas. The occupational health nurse must be knowledgeable about all laws and regulations that govern any industry where the nurse provides health care to employees (e.g., laboratories, transportation, and utilities).

LEGAL ISSUES IN OCCUPATIONAL HEALTH

In recognition of the dynamic nature of occupational health nursing practice, coupled with the influences and impact of larger policy issues, the occupational health nurse must know the legal parameters of practice and respond to legislative mandates that govern worker health and safety. The occupational health nurse is professionally primarily accountable to workers and worker populations and to the employer, the profession, and self (AAOHN, 2004). In particular, the occupational health nurse must be aware of liability and legal issues related to the following:

- The employee-nurse relationship
- The employment capacity of the occupational health nurse
- Any acts of negligence

The employee-nurse relationship can be confusing when the employer hires the nurse to provide services to the employee. The concern is whether a professional relationship exists under the law or the relationship is based on a co-worker status.

MULTIDISCIPLINARY TEAMWORK

As workplaces have become more complex, a diverse array of expertise has emerged in many functional and technical areas. To be successful, the occupational health nurse must recognize the need to work as part of an interdisciplinary team. The nurse may interact with occupational medicine professionals, industrial hygienists, safety professionals, employee assistance counselors, personnel professionals, and union representatives (Figure 30-2). Community health professionals, insurance carriers, and other support agencies in the community are also critical links.

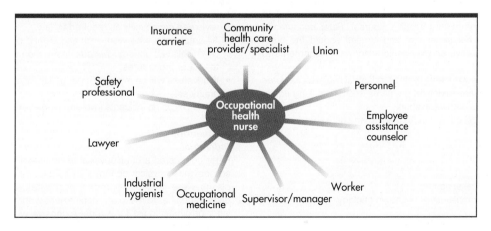

FIGURE 30-2 The occupational health nurse's professional links in the workplace and community.

SUMMARY

This chapter described the evolution of occupational health nursing during its first century of practice. Current and future demographics and business trends are highlighted as they relate to this nursing specialty area. Aging workers, escalating health care costs, increasing numbers of women and minorities in the workforce, and the competitive international marketplace are key factors shaping occupational health nursing practice.

The occupational health nursing role is challenging and can have a tremendous impact on the quality and delivery of health care to workers and their families. Nurses working in occupational settings should have an excellent understanding of all levels of prevention and possess the skills and competencies outlined here.

For the community health nurse who works in other settings such as home health, clinics, and schools, knowledge of occupational health nursing practice is also important. Many companies do not have on-site occupational health nurses and therefore must rely on community health nurses to support their occupational health and safety needs.

CASE STUDY   APPLICATION OF THE NURSING PROCESS

Leslie Johnston is a 23-year-old woman who was transferred by her employer into a job that required her to work with chemicals used in photolithography. Leslie became concerned when she noticed that the label on one of the pieces of equipment warned of possible adverse effects on reproduction. Because of her concern and related issues, she went to the on-site health clinic to talk with Peter Mitchell, the occupational health nurse.

Peter invited Leslie into his office to ask her questions and do a brief health history. Leslie reported that her health had been "excellent" until recently but that she had not felt well since transferring to her new position. She explained that she was newly married and thought she may be pregnant, but this was unconfirmed. She questioned whether her vague physical complaints (fatigue, headaches, occasional queasiness) might be related to working with chemicals, a pregnancy, or another reason.

Peter reassured Leslie that he had been employed at the company for 8 years, and he was aware that there were no restrictions in Leslie's work area for pregnant women. He pulled up her health file from his computerized database and gave her a set of health history forms to complete. He also had her read and sign several forms related to confidentiality and assured her that none of her health information would be shared with their employer without her consent.

Assessment

To obtain needed information, Peter:

- Completed general health and occupational health histories.
- Performed a modified physical assessment and discussed the symptoms Leslie was experiencing.
- Referred Leslie to her personal health care provider for further evaluation and to obtain a pregnancy test. (NOTE: In some cases, on-site clinics will be equipped for basic procedures such as this. If this is not a service provided by the occupational health nurse, referral must be made to the employee's health care provider. If the employee does not have one, referral must be made to an appropriate community health resource). Peter encouraged Leslie to inform her supervisor and himself should the pregnancy test be positive so they could adapt her assignments to her condition.
- Assessed Leslie's work area with an industrial hygienist to determine whether there might be problems such as leaking equipment or problems with ventilation.
- Reviewed the most current industrial hygiene data appropriate to the area.

Diagnosis
Individual

- At risk for chemical exposure
- Vague physical complaints of unknown etiology
- Possible pregnancy
- At risk for possible adverse pregnancy outcomes

- Stress related to concern regarding possible exposure to harmful chemicals

Community

- Potential for exposure of employees to unsafe chemicals and/or working conditions

Planning

Peter developed a plan of care based on Leslie's health history and concerns. Together they set the following goals:

Individual
Short-Term Goals

- Determine pregnancy status.
- Determine potential exposure levels and review side effects of chemicals.
- Determine reason for her vague physical complaints.
- Reduce stress experiences.

Long-Term Goals

- Ensure that the work environment is safe for future pregnancies (if Leslie is not pregnant at present).
- Collaborate with Leslie and her supervisor on possible work restrictions.

Community (Workplace)
Short-Term Goals

- Company personnel (e.g., the occupational health nurse, the industrial hygienist, and all others who are directly affected) will be knowledgeable in safe handling of all hazardous chemicals.
- All company policies will be followed regarding safety and exposure.

Long-Term Goals

- Policies on handling of chemicals and related information will be reviewed periodically as required by law.
- All employees who work with and around potentially hazardous chemicals will undergo periodic instruction and checkoff related to proper procedures.
- Work areas will be monitored per policy for compliance with safe practices.
- There will be no incidents involving worker exposure to chemicals.

Intervention
Individual

Peter conducted a brief physical examination and did not identify any obvious physical abnormalities. Because Leslie's chief complaints were fatigue, occasional headaches, and queasiness, he encouraged her to make an appointment with her primary care provider or gynecologist for a more extensive workup and to assess for pregnancy.

Continued

CASE STUDY APPLICATION OF THE NURSING PROCESS—cont'd

With her permission, he called the industrial hygienist to counsel with Leslie regarding the policies of the company and to explain what chemicals might potentially be hazardous and to review procedures and restrictions. The hygienist also stated that he would send a team to Leslie's work area to take air samples, check lighting, and perform other tests to ensure there were no problems.

Community (Workplace)

The assigned industrial hygiene team sampled the environment for chemical exposure per established procedure. They also set up a plan to add the area to more frequent observation pending the results of the tests. The hygienist assured Peter and Leslie that he would communicate any work restrictions or changes to the personnel department and Leslie's supervisor if needed.

Evaluation
Individual

Following the meeting with Peter and the industrial hygienist, Leslie stated that she felt reassured. She agreed to make an appointment as soon as possible with her doctor for an evaluation and pregnancy test. She also agreed to inform Peter and her direct supervisor if she learned that she was pregnant.

Community (Workplace)

The industrial hygienist and his assistants performed several tests in close proximity to Leslie's work station and found no abnormal readings and all equipment was in good working order. Per agency policy and following OHSA regulations, they charted all findings and submitted reports.

Levels of Prevention
Primary
- Teach about chemicals, exposures, etc.
- Instruct about chemical avoidance.
- Remove employee from environment through work restrictions.

Secondary
- Assess employee for signs and symptoms.
- Assess work environment for exposure.
- Refer for evaluation of possible health problems as needed.

Tertiary
- Provide reproductive counseling.

■ LEARNING ACTIVITIES

1. A large automobile manufacturer needs a program designed to control respiratory disease among foundry workers. Workers in different areas of ferrous foundries are exposed to different respiratory hazards. The main problems are exposure to silica and formaldehyde. The corporation would like to develop a pilot program for one of its foundries that will then be applied to its other foundries. Health and industrial hygiene data will be collected. Both the corporation and the workers support the project, and both see the project as having the following three purposes:
   - Detecting health effects in individuals who may benefit from intervention
   - Determining the relationship of health effects to environmental exposures
   - Identifying control strategies as appropriate
2. Outline a pilot program. Discuss the implications of discovering adverse health effects among current workers. Describe the roles of the occupational health nurse, physician, industrial hygienist, safety professional, manager, and employee.
3. A weight-loss program was conducted during August. Ten people participated in the 6-week program. The total weight loss for the group was 185 pounds. The following chart indicates the weight loss for the individuals:

Weight Before Program (lb)	Weight After Program (lb)
215	190
175	160
139	129
275	245
145	120
198	183
120	115
243	233
185	145
210	200

Is there a more effective way to show the results of the program? Assume a peer distributed this report for critique. Be creative, filling in any data, facts, figures, or other information that may be missing. Redesign a report to send to management.

4. Take an occupational history on five currently employed workers. Identify the occupation, associated job tasks, and potential health hazards. Describe control strategies that could minimize or eliminate the risk of adverse health effects.
5. Conduct a literature review to identify critical concepts in occupational health nursing, epidemiology, ergonomics, safety, industrial hygiene, and medicine, and describe how these disciplines work together to achieve optimal ends.

REFERENCES

American Association of Industrial Nurses: *The nurse in industry*, New York, 1976, The Author.

American Association of Occupational Health Nurses: *Standards of occupational and environmental health nursing*, Atlanta, GA, 2004, Author.

American Association of Occupational Health Nurses: Competencies in occupational and environmental health nursing, *AAOHN Journal* 55:442–447, 2007. http://www.aaohn.org.

American Association of Occupational Health Nurses: *AAOHN Code of ethics and interpretive statements*, 2009, www.aaohn.org.

American Cancer Society: *Cancer statistics*, 2009. http://www.cancer.org/downloads/stt/CFF2009_LeadingSites_Est_6.pdf. Accessed July 9, 2009.

Benner P: *From novice to expert: excellence and power in clinical nursing practice*, Menlo Park, Calif, 1984, Addison-Wesley.

Boden LI, Biddle EA, Spieler EA: Social and economic impacts of workplace illness and injury, *Am J Ind Med* 40:398–402, 2001.

Bureau of Labor Statistics: *Charting the labor market*, 2006, www.BLS.org. Accessed May 14, 2009, www.bls.gov/cps/labor2006/.

Byczek L, et al: Cardiovascular risk factors, *AAOHN J* 52:66–76, 2004.

Curtis J, Scott LR: Integrating disability management into strategic plans, *AAOHN J* 52:298–301, 2004.

Felton JS: The genesis of occupational health nursing: part I, *Occup Health Nurse* 30:45–49, 1985.

Felton JS: The genesis of occupational health nursing: part II, *AAOHN J* 34:210–215, 1986.

Fletcher M: Careful integration, management of disabilities helps hospitals trim millions from its corporate costs, *Bus Insur* 37:26–30, 2003.

Hecker DE: Occupational employment practices to 2010, *Mon Labor Rev* 124:21–38, 2001.

Intili H, Laws C: Delivering health care in a large urban hotel: cost-effective, quality care for an underserved and uninsured population, *AAOHN J* 51:306–309, 2003.

Kalina CM, Haag A, Tourigan R: Challenges and solutions in case management, *AAOHN J* 52:143–145, 2004.

Kaminshine S: New rights for the disabled: the Americans With Disabilities Act of 1990, *AAOHN J* 39:249–251, 1991.

Levy BS, et al: *Occupational and environmental health*, ed 5, Philadelphia, 2005, Lippincott Williams & Wilkins.

McGrath BJ: *Nursing in commerce and industry*, New York, 1946, The Commonwealth Fund.

National Institute for Occupational Safety and Health: *Worker health chartbook*, Washington, DC, 2004, DHHS (NIOSH) Pub No 2004-146.

O'Donnell M: Editor's notes: Definition of health promotion 2.0: Embracing passion, enhancing motivation, recognizing dynamic balance, and creating opportunities, *Am J Health Promot* 24:iv, 2009.

Parker-Conrad JE: A century of practice: occupational health nursing, *AAOHN J* 36:156–161, 1988.

Parker-Conrad JE: Celebrating our past, *AAOHN J* 50:537–541, 2002.

Randolph SA, Dalton PC: Limited duty work: an innovative approach to early return to work, *AAOHN J* 37:446–452, 1989.

Richlin D: *AAOHN guidelines for starting an occupational health and safety service*, Atlanta, 2003, The Author.

Rogers B: Establishing research priorities in occupational health nursing, *AAOHN J* 37:493–500, 1989.

Rogers B: Occupational health nursing expertise, *AAOHN J* 46:477–483, 1998.

Rogers B: Nursing: an ethic of caring, *AAOHN J* 51:155–157, 2003a.

Rogers B: *Occupational health nursing: concepts and practice*, ed 2, Philadelphia, 2003b, Saunders.

Rogers B, Randolph S, Mastrianno K: *Occupational health nursing guidelines for primary clinical conditions*, ed 4, Beverly, MA, 2009, OEM Press.

Rogers B, Franke J, Jeras J, et al: The Family Medical Leave Act: implications for occupational health nursing, *AAOHN J* 57(6):239–250, 2009.

Rogers B, Lawhorn E: Occupational health nursing strategies for health promotion. In Hickey J, Ovimetle R, Venegoni S, editors: *Advanced practice nursing*, Philadelphia, 2000, Lippincott Williams & Wilkins.

Rogers B, Livsey K: Occupational health surveillance, screening, and prevention activities in occupational health nursing practice, *AAOHN J* 48:92–99, 2000.

U.S. Department of Health and Human Services: *Healthy People 2010*, conference ed, Washington, DC, 2000, The Author.

Walz JA, Wehse KL: Wellness for welders: prevention strategies, *AAOHN J* 50:303–306, 2002.

Wyatt SN: Challenges of the working breast feeding mother: workplace solutions, *AAOHN J* 52:61–66, 2002.

Forensic and Correctional Nursing

Stacy Drake, Angela Snow

Additional Material for Study, Review, and Further Exploration

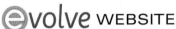 WEBSITE

http://evolve.elsevier.com/Nies
- Quiz
- Case Studies
- Glossary
- WebLinks

OBJECTIVES

Upon completion of this chapter, the reader will be able to do the following:
1. Define forensic nursing.
2. Describe the specialties of forensic nurses.
3. Explain issues important to each of the subspecialty areas of forensic nursing.
4. Describe interventions and services forensic nurses perform.
5. Discuss factors affecting health and wellness in a correctional setting.

KEY TERMS

child abuse
coroner
correctional nursing
elder abuse
forensic

forensic nurse death investigator
forensic nurse examiners
forensic nursing
forensic psychiatric nurse
legal nurse consultants

living forensics
medical examiners
nurse attorneys
nurse coroners
sexual assault forensic examiner (SAFE)

OUTLINE

Subspecialties of Forensic Nursing
Sexual Assault Forensic Examiner
Medicolegal Death Investigation
Legal Nurse Consultants and Nurse Attorneys
Clinical Forensic Nurse Examiner
Forensic Psychiatric Nurse
Correctional Nursing
Maintenance of a Safe Environment

Health Issues in Prison Populations
Chronic and Communicable Diseases
Women in Prison
Adolescents in Prison
Mental Health Issues in Correctional Settings
Education and Forensic Nursing

According to the Bureau of Justice Statistics National Crime Victimization Survey, in 2007 approximately 5,177,100 violent crimes were reported (U.S. Department of Justice/Bureau of Justice Statistics [USDOJ/BJS], 2007). These crimes ranged from vandalism and theft, to rape and sexual assault, to aggravated assault and murder. The estimated medical and productivity economic burden of interpersonal and self-directed violence (suicide, homicide, child maltreatment, youth violence, intimate partner violence, and other assaults) is estimated at $70 billion per year (Corso, Mercy, Simon et al., 2007). Because of the prevalence of violence and violent crimes in society, health care professionals are required to identify and assess victims of trauma, abuse, and/or neglect and provide proper care and referrals as needed. Indeed, screening for violence is now considered to be a minimum standard of care for all clients (American Association of Colleges of Nursing, 1999; Sekula, 2005).

The term forensic means "pertaining to the law; legal" (Venes, 2001). It refers to instances, activities, or information used in or suitable to courts of law. Health care providers, especially nurses, frequently care for both victims and perpetrators of crime (American Association of Colleges of Nursing, 1999).

Forensic nursing combines the disciplines of nursing science, forensic science, medical science, sociology, and psychology with law enforcement and the criminal justice system. Forensic nursing is one of the newest specialty areas recognized by the American Nurses Association (ANA) and is growing nationally and internationally. It was officially recognized by the ANA in 1995, and the *Scope and Standards of Forensic Nursing Practice* was published in 1997 (Burgess, Berger, and Boersma, 2004).

The International Association of Forensic Nurses (IAFN) defines forensic nursing as "the application of forensic science combined with the bio-psychological education of the registered nurse, in the scientific investigation, evidence collection and preservation, analysis, prevention and treatment of trauma and/or death medical-legal issues" (ANA, 1997, p. v). Thus the forensic nurse's role provides a vital link between the health care system, the investigative process, and courts of law (Lynch, 2006).

Forensic nurses practice in multiple areas and settings of the public health system. Their responsibilities may include screening, assessment and collection of evidence, and also include the documentation and expert testimony from victims and perpetrators in settings such as hospitals, community clinics, or death scenes. In addition to working with victims and perpetrators, forensic nurses may be involved in paternity disputes and cases involving workplace injuries, malpractice, vehicle accidents, food or drug tampering, and medical equipment defects (Burgess et al., 2004). The *Healthy People 2020* box lists some objectives related to this highly specialized practice area.

SUBSPECIALTIES OF FORENSIC NURSING

The IAFN recognizes core specialties within forensic nursing (Box 31-1). Each of the subspecialties will be briefly discussed.

Sexual Assault Forensic Examiner

Sexual assault forensic examiner (SAFE) is the most widely recognized subspecialty in forensic nursing. In the 1970s, emergency department (ED) registered nurses identified a special client population—sexual assault or rape victims—who were not receiving the appropriate, compassionate care after a terrifying traumatic event (Ledray and Arndt, 1994). They observed that the sexual assault victim would enter the ED, and in many cases the staff did not know how to compassionately approach the client, properly assess and collect evidence, or testify in court; therefore the SAFE role was developed.

A SAFE is a specially trained registered nurse who applies the nursing process during forensic examinations to victims or perpetrators of sexual assault. The SAFE collects forensic evidence related to a reported crime and frequently testifies as an expert witness at subsequent trials (Girardin, 2001; IAFN, 1996; Ledray, 2006). SAFEs are usually employed in EDs, labor and delivery departments, and community clinics dedicated to victims of interpersonal violence.

BOX 31-1   SPECIALTIES OF FORENSIC NURSES

- Sexual assault forensic examiner
- Nurse coroner and death investigator
- Legal nurse consultant and nurse attorney
- Forensic nursing educator and consultant
- Forensic psychiatric nurse
- Forensic nurse examiner
- Correctional nurse

 HEALTHY PEOPLE 2020

Proposed Objectives Related to Forensic Nursing

OBJECTIVE

IVP HP2020-12: Reduce physical assaults.

IVP HP2020-29: Reduce nonfatal child maltreatment.

IVP HP2020-32: Reduce sexual violence.

IVP HP2020-33: Increase the number of States and the District of Columbia with statewide emergency department data systems that routinely collect external-cause-of injury codes for 90 percent or more of injury-related visits.

IVP HP2020-35: Increase the number of States and the District of Columbia where 90 percent of sudden and unexpected deaths to infants are reviewed by a child fatality review team.

IVP 2020-40: Increase the number of States that link data on violent deaths from death certificates, law enforcement, and coroner and medical examiner reports to inform prevention efforts at the State and local levels.

MHMD-HP2020-7: Increase the proportion of juvenile residential facilities that screen admissions for mental health problems.

MHMD HP2020-8: Increase the proportion of counties served by community-based jail diversion programs and/or mental health courts for adults with mental health problems.

SA HP2020-17: Increase the number of Level I and Level II trauma centers that implement evidence-based alcohol screening and brief intervention.

USDHHS Healthy People 2020 Draft Objectives. 2009. http://www.healthypeople.gov/hp2020/Objectives/files/Draft2009Objectives.pdf.

BOX 31-2 TYPE OF EVIDENCE COLLECTED FROM A VICTIM OF SEXUAL ASSAULT

- Pubic combings
- Pubic hair controls (from the victim)
- Genital and thigh swabs
- Vaginal swabs and smears
- Rectal swabs and smears
- Oral swabs and smears
- Head hair
- Blood sample
- Fingernail scrapings
- Urine specimen
- All clothing worn at the time of the attack

From Saferstein R: Evidence collection and preservation. In Lynch VA, editor: *Forensic nursing*, St Louis, 2006, Mosby.

If the client is medically stable, the SAFE is responsible for conducting a thorough examination including obtaining a history, performing the physical assessment, and collecting forensic evidence (Box 31-2). If the client is medically unstable, he or she will be assessed and stabilized by a physician prior to the forensic examination (Antognoli-Toland, 1985). Other responsibilities of the SAFE are crisis intervention referral, evaluation for sexually transmitted infection, pregnancy risk assessment and interception as needed, and client referral for additional support (Ledray, 2006).

SAFE is the only forensic nursing subspecialty with a certification currently offered through the IAFN. Both adult and pediatric certifications are available. The requirements for a registered nurse to be eligible for the SAFE certification examination are that the nurse must (1) be in practice for a minimum of 2 years, (2) have successfully completed 40 hours of didactic instruction or 3 semester hours of academic credit from an accredited nursing program, and (3) demonstrate competency in sexual assault examinations (IAFN, 1998).

Medicolegal Death Investigation

According to Hanzlick (2007) there are four different types of death investigation: medicolegal, institution-based, private, and public health. Medicolegal death investigations are usually conducted to clarify the unnatural circumstances in which death occurred. Institution-based death investigations are usually those that occur in the hospital or nursing home setting. Private death investigations are family initiated and are focused on answering questions the family may have surrounding the death. Public health investigations are frequently conducted in cooperation with the medicolegal and/or are retrospective studies. An example of public health death investigation would be elderly mistreatment–related deaths. Typically the forensic nurse will be employed in the medicolegal death investigation or public health setting. The medicolegal death investigation system falls within the purview of the public health system as defined by the Centers for Disease Control and Prevention. One of the outputs of death investigation is death certificates. In the United States,

medicolegal death investigation systems are characterized as either medical examiner, coroner/justices of the peace, or mixed (Fulton, 2003; Hanzlick, 1996; Hanzlick and Combs, 1998; Lynch, 2006; Prahlow and Lantz, 1995).

Typically, medical examiners are licensed physicians who are board certified in anatomic and forensic pathology (Hanzlick, 2007). Usually medical examiners are appointed for an unspecified term and serve a county, district, region, or state as determined by law. The coroner/justices of the peace are usually elected laypersons; that is, persons who have little or no training in medicine or science who conduct medicolegal investigations and certify cause and manner of death. A mixed medicolegal system is a combination of medical examiner and coroner/justices of the peace systems, depending on state law (Hanzlick, 2007).

Most medicolegal death investigation agencies are responsible for issuing death certificates that state the cause and manner of death. These data are collected at city, county, state, and national levels and used to determine the health of the nation and how best to allocate financial resources. The cause of death is the event that initiated the progression of events that ended in death (Lynch, 2006). The manner of death is categorization that relates to the conditions in which the cause of death occurred (Hanzlick, 2007). The National Association of Medical Examiners (NAME) identifies five acceptable options for recording manner of death: natural, accident, suicide, homicide, and "undetermined" (Hanzlick, Hunsaker, and Davis, 2002).

Role of a Forensic Nurse Death Investigator

Forensic nurses enter the death investigation arena possessing essential knowledge of anatomy, physiology, pharmacology, growth and development, physical examination, and health history interviewing techniques that will be needed to conduct a comprehensive death investigation (Fulton, 2003). In most cases related to a death scene investigation, investigators are police officers or retired homicide detectives—professions without medical or science knowledge. The forensic nurse death investigator (FNDI) evaluates the death scene from a holistic nursing perspective and might interpret the scene differently. The requirements for being a forensic nurse death investigator vary; however, most employers ask for a minimum of 2 years of experience preferably in the setting of critical care or emergency.

Clinical Example

A police officer entering a house observes several pools of blood located throughout the residence and discovers a deceased male, nude and lying in bed; the police officer suspects murder. The FNDI entering the same death scene notices the same findings as the initial police officer, but also notes bloody emesis in the toilet, blood-soaked towels in the washing machine, and empty alcohol bottles in the trash. A preliminary examination of the decedent by the forensic nurse reveals ascites, jaundice, and multiple contusions on the body. Following communication with family members, the FNDI discovers the decedent was an alcoholic with many health problems; the FNDI suspects that he had ruptured esophageal varices. This was confirmed by an autopsy, and the manner of death was determined to be from natural causes rather than homicide as initially believed by the police officer.

Role of Nurse Coroner

In coroner systems where the chief medicolegal death investigator is elected and state laws do not have specific requirements of the office, nurses may decide to run for the position of coroner or nurse coroner. The nurse coroner would be responsible for ensuring that appropriate measures were taken to perform death investigations and certify death certificates. A nurse coroner's educational background and knowledge enables him or her to identify disease processes that the lay coroner may not recognize or may misinterpret as foul play, as in the preceding clinical example.

Forensic nurse death investigators and nurse coroners exhibit communication skills when dealing with grieving families. Nurses are provided the education in therapeutic communication and are able to practice those skills in any setting. They are acutely aware of the importance of using open-ended questions, attentively listening, and being fully present with family and friends. The use of these techniques allows family and friends to openly share the feelings and thoughts experienced with the death of a loved one (Potter and Perry, 2009).

Nurse coroners and FNDIs complement the medicolegal death investigation system by providing an understanding of nursing, forensic and medical science, sociology, psychology, and public health within the criminal justice system. The FNDI can contribute expertise and speak for the decedent through his or her existing knowledge in a holistic manner.

Legal Nurse Consultants and Nurse Attorneys

Legal nurse consultants (LNCs) and nurse attorneys are nurses who provide assistance within the legal system using specialized nursing knowledge and expertise when interaction of law and health issues arise (Geissler-Murr and Moorhouse, 2006; Saunders, 2000). Among many activities, LNCs evaluate, analyze, and render informed opinions on the delivery of health care and its outcomes (American Association of Legal Nurse Consultants, 1999). LNCs are hired by attorneys and insurers to review and interpret medical records and charts, provide objective opinions based on standards of care, and possibly to testify in court (Burgess et al., 2004; Raymond, 2002; Saunders, 2000).

Nurse attorneys are educated in both law and nursing. They may practice in health care, public health, or criminal or civil law, which would include malpractice cases. Malpractice cases may be from a plaintiff's or defendant's perspective, may involve licensure disciplinary action, or may involve agency oversight (Collins and Halpern, 2005). Some practitioners have differing opinions regarding LNCs and nurse attorneys. They may be perceived as either defending the profession or prosecuting peers by testifying against professional colleagues. Haas and Bradshaw (1999) observe that by providing services as experts and testifying, nurses serving as legal consultants help hold accountable poor practitioners who

are dangerous to clients. In contrast, meticulous practitioners who are wrongfully accused of negligence will be defended.

The number of LNCs is growing and totals around 4000 (Raymond, 2002). According to the American Association of Legal Nurse Consultants (1999), LNCs perform many different services and activities, including the following:

- Organizing and analyzing medical records and related materials
- Preparing chronologies of health care events
- Identifying standards of care
- Determining causation and damage issues
- Conducting literature research and summarizing medical literature
- Helping to determine the merits or defensibility of a case
- Providing education regarding facts and issues relevant to a case
- Identifying and determining damages and related costs of services
- Acting as a liaison among attorney, health care providers, clients, and experts

LNCs read reports and records and determine whether the standards of care were met or breached. In general, if working for a plaintiff in a malpractice case, the LNC will look for breaches in the standards of care; if working for the defense, the LNC will look for nursing care that is given within the standards of care related to the complaint. It is essential that the attorneys be kept informed of all findings—even those that might negatively affect their case (Meiner, 2005).

When providing services, the LNC may submit an affidavit, which is a written statement explaining the expert's credentials, background, and licensing or certification(s). It also provides a list of the materials read and considered in the case, and the findings of the review are summarized into a case analysis. Following the submission of an affidavit, the LNC may be asked to provide a deposition. The deposition is a pretrial discovery process that allows the attorneys on both sides to learn more about what the courtroom testimony will be. It is given to a court reporter, and the respondent is under oath.

During the deposition, the LNC will present the facts of the case and be questioned by attorneys from both sides. This process may be quite lengthy and stressful. It is essential that the LNC be prepared, having reviewed the case and all related materials very thoroughly. Following this process, the LNC will be given a written transcript of the deposition; this needs to be carefully reviewed for accuracy. If the case goes to trial, the LNC will then testify in court (Meiner, 2005; Ruiz-Contreras, 2005).

In some cases, the forensic nurse will be called on to testify in court, not as an expert witness as described above, but as a factual witness—one who has firsthand knowledge of the case in question. In these cases, the forensic nurse is present to provide factual statements about the evidence collected and what was observed (Ruiz-Contreras, 2005). Box 31-3 lists tips that will be helpful for nurses to review prior to testifying in court.

BOX 31-3 TIPS FOR TESTIFYING AT A DEPOSITION OR IN COURT

- Dress professionally and conservatively.
- Tell the truth at all times.
- Listen to the complete question before responding.
- Speak slowly, clearly, and concisely when answering.
- Avoid saying "I think" or "I believe."
- Never interrupt.
- Take a few seconds to formulate an answer before responding.
- Minimize "ums" or "uhs" by pausing at the end of sentences.
- If there is an objection, stop talking and wait for the judge to make a ruling.
- When answering questions, make eye contact with the jury members.
- Remain calm.
- Respond confidently.
- Do not answer a question that you do not understand; ask the attorney to repeat questions as needed.
- Practice difficult words.
- Do not become defensive or angry.
- Avoid nervous gestures; keep your hands in your lap.

Data from Ruiz-Contreras A: The nurse as an expert witness, *Top Emerg Med* 27(1):27-35, 2005.

Clinical Forensic Nurse Examiner
Emergency and Critical Care

Registered nurses may be employed in EDs and critical care units as forensic nurse examiners. In this role they deliver care to both living and deceased clients who are somehow involved with the legal system, and their services may include several subspecialties. The term living forensics refers to individuals who are subject to forensic investigations, including but not limited to survivors of rape, drug and alcohol addiction, domestic violence, nonfatal assaults, motor vehicle and pedestrian accidents, and police detainees (Lynch, 2006; Saunders, 2000).

The ED is frequently the initial location of the medicolegal investigation involving these individuals, both living and deceased (Fulton and Assid, 2006). It is imperative that ED registered nurses identify forensic cases and initiate the proper collection, preservation, and chain of command of evidence and provide accurate documentation for this unique population (Lynch, 1991). This collection of evidence plays an important role in the investigation of crimes and can have a major impact on legal decisions. Box 31-4 lists types of evidence.

BOX 31-4 TYPES OF EVIDENCE

- Direct evidence including eyewitness statements
- Documentation
- Trace evidence including hair fibers
- Photographs
- Weapons/tools
- Bullets, casing, wadding, gunshot residue
- Matches, lighters, or other ignition sources
- Toxicology (blood/biological samples)
- Clothing/personal effects
- Notes or messages made by patient

Data from Safertein R: *Criminalistics: an introduction to forensic science,* ed 6, Upper Saddle River, NJ, 1998, Prentice Hall.

Clinical Example

A 27-year-old female arrived at the emergency department (ED) with a circular defect on her head suggestive of a gunshot wound. Emergency medical technicians report to the ED nurse and doctor that the client was found by her boyfriend barely breathing. The boyfriend called 911, and the client was transported to the hospital. The client arrived at the hospital in asystole and was pronounced dead within 10 minutes of arrival. The ED nurse applied her forensic knowledge and placed brown paper bags on the client's hands, securing them with tape. This procedure is performed to preserve gunpowder or primer residue. Gunpowder or primer residue aids in the determination of the shooter and distance of the gun. When a gun is fired, residue is released and lands on the items close to the gun, specifically the hands and clothing of the person firing it.

The police agency investigated the death. The nurse's intervention, placing paper bags over the client's hands, preserved the presence or absence of gunshot or primer residue. The police agency performed a scanning electron microscope examination for gunpowder residue and did not find any on the client's hands. This finding led police to further investigate the incident and discover that the boyfriend shot the client instead of the first presumption of a self-inflicted gunshot wound.

Organ and Tissue Donation and Transplantation

Forensic nurses also have a role in providing a detailed physical examination of patients who may be organ and tissue donors. This area of care is incredibly complex and requires detailed understanding of related legal and ethical issues. When a patient is declared brain dead, federal law states that the legal next of kin shall be approached for organ and tissue donation. A forensic nurse is able to conduct and provide a detailed physical examination and collect any evidence that may be required. A thorough death investigation at the hospital may be required; reviewing medical records and documenting injuries are essential for the medicolegal investigation agency in identifying acceptable candidates and potential organs and tissues for harvest. The nurse involved in this process must be knowledgeable about legal specifications related to organ donation and have familiarity with agency policies and procedures for determining brain death. The nurse must also have excellent communication skills, as well as the ability to relate empathetically to grieving families. In this capacity, the forensic nurse working harmoniously with organ and tissue procurement agencies can obtain release authorization of lifesaving organs (Shafer, 2006).

Care of Vulnerable Populations

The youngest, oldest, and disabled populations are the most vulnerable to abuse and neglect. Nurses dedicating their practice to these vulnerable populations have an essential role of advocacy for individuals that cannot protect themselves.

Child abuse and neglect. Child abuse and neglect are major concerns for society; therefore the role of a forensic nurse examiner is especially imperative. The Federal Child Abuse Prevention and Treatment Act defines child abuse and neglect as:

Any recent act or failure to act on the part of a parent or caretaker which results in death, serious physical or emotional harm, sexual abuse or exploitation; or an act or failure to act which presents an imminent risk of serious harm. (U.S. Department of Health and Human Services Administration for Children and Families, 2008)

In 2006, approximately 905,000 children suffered some type of abuse or neglect, and nearly 80% of the perpetrators were the parents (U.S. Department of Health and Human Services Administration for Children and Families, 2008). Reported cases of child abuse or neglect resulting in death in 2006 were estimated to be 1530 children.

States have varying definitions of what constitutes or determines child abuse and neglect. The following definitions are provided by the U.S. Department of Health and Human Services Administration for Children and Families (2008):

- *Neglect:* Failure of a parent, guardian or caregiver to provide basic needs. Neglect may be physical (deprivation of adequate food, clothing, shelter, or supervision); medical (failure to provide necessary medical treatment); educational (failure to educate a child or attend to special education needs); or emotional (failure to attend to emotional needs or provide psychological care or allowing the usage of alcohol or other drugs).
- *Sexual abuse:* Range of activities from noncontact indecent exposure or production of pornographic materials, incest, rape, fondling, and genital contact to actual adult-child sexual intercourse.
- *Physical abuse:* Intentional physical injury including striking, kicking, burning, or biting.
- *Emotional abuse (or psychological abuse):* A pattern of behavior that impairs the child's emotional development or sense of self-worth including constant criticism, threats, or rejection.

For the well-being and safety of the child, a forensic nurse examiner ensures that abuse and neglect are swiftly identified and reported to proper authorities (LaSala and Lynch, 2006). The nurse obtains a thorough history and assessment, focusing on several facets of abuse and neglect. These include child-parent interaction, the child's appearance and behavior, child-child interaction, and the environment.

A forensic nurse may be employed in a variety of clinical settings that assess, diagnose, and treat children. These settings may include pediatric or general EDs, hospitals, physician offices, schools, home health, hospice, and child advocacy agencies.

Elder mistreatment. Forensic nurse examiners caring for the geriatric population play an important role similar to that of pediatric forensic nurses. Elder mistreatment is thought to be one of the most underdiagnosed and underreported crimes in the United States (Pearsall, 2005). Unfortunately, there is no exact accounting of elder mistreatment cases due to a lack of standardized reporting systems, no consistent definition of elder mistreatment, and lack of national data collection (Bonnie and Wallace, 2003; National Center on Elder Abuse, 2005c). The National Center on Elder Abuse

reported adult children are the most frequent abusers of the elderly (National Center on Elder Abuse, 2005b). Therefore the elderly client may be hesitant to report abuse, ask for assistance, or acknowledge the maltreatment because the abuser might be a son, daughter, or close relative (Moynihan, 2006), or the disclosure would possibly result in litigation and institutionalization (Pearsall, 2005). Forensic nurses may be employed in any setting, treating or seeing elder clients. Some settings include EDs, hospitals, physician offices, nursing homes, home health agencies, and geriatric day care centers.

There are several forms of elder mistreatment: physical, psychological or emotional, financial, neglect, and sexual abuse (McGann and Moynihan, 2006; Pearsall, 2005). Physical abuse is the intentional harm or injury of another person (McGann and Moynihan, 2006) resulting in bruises, abrasions, lacerations, fractures, or all of these (Pearsall, 2005). Psychological or emotional abuse occurs when there is mental or emotional anguish (e.g., humiliating, intimidating, or threatening comments directed toward the elder) (National Center on Elder Abuse, 2005a); this can be difficult to identify in an acute care setting. According to McGann and Moynihan (2006), more than 12% of verifiable elder abuse cases are financial abuse. Financial abuse occurs when the elder person's financial resources are utilized for another person's benefit without the elder's consent.

Neglect is the most common form of elder abuse, whether it is caregiver neglect or self-neglect. Caregiver neglect occurs when the caregiver does not provide appropriate clothing, food, or health services or in the case of abandonment of the elder client. Self-neglect occurs when the elder discounts personal well-being—this could be the result of medical or mental illnesses. Last, sexual abuse is the nonconsensual intimate contact between two people (Pearsall, 2005). The elder population is at risk for sexual abuse because of inability to resist pursuits or inability to recognize the abuse because of mental illness or other advanced disease process.

Disabled population. It is well documented that children and elderly with disabilities are more likely to be mistreated. Mandatory laws addressing the reporting of abuse or neglect of a disabled person aged 18 to 64 years varies within states. Across the life span, the risk for one or more forms of mistreatment increase at least four times with individuals having either mental illness or physical or intellectual disabilities (Heilporn, André, Didier et al., 2006).

Forensic Psychiatric Nurse

The forensic psychiatric nurse connects the gap between the criminal justice, legal, and mental health systems (Saunders, 2000). Forensic psychiatric nurses apply the nursing process to clients pending a criminal hearing or trial while maintaining a neutral, objective, and detached position (Coram, 2006). Forensic psychiatric nurses collect evidence by determining intent or diminished capacity in the client's thinking at the time of the incident. To do this, they often spend several hours interviewing and observing the client, carefully documenting conversations and observations.

Forensic psychiatric nurses may be called to court to testify as an expert witness in mental health issues; therefore it is imperative that the nurse have an exceptional understanding of mental illnesses and personality disorders. Roles filled by or activities provided by psychiatric forensic nurses include the following (Coram, 2006):

- Sanity or competency evaluation (for legal purposes)
- Assessment of violence potential
- Assessment of capacity to formulate intent
- Parole and probation considerations
- Assessment of racial or cultural factors in crime
- Assistance in jury selection
- Sexual predator screening
- Provision of expert witness testimony

CORRECTIONAL NURSING

Correctional nursing is a specialized subset of forensic nursing. It requires a significant amount of discrete knowledge, as well as an understanding and awareness of the unique needs and perspective of the clients served. Several issues specific to correctional nursing and related issues are described in this section.

Unlike any other care setting, clients are inmates, and care is negotiated and provided with recognition of safety and security issues for the nurse and the constitutional right of prisoners to receive adequate and timely health care. The primary goals in correctional facilities are to maintain a safe, secure, and humane environment for inmates. Health care, including nursing care, is a necessary and essential part of that environment.

Maintenance of a Safe Environment

Correctional facilities are, by nature, violent environments, and nurses practicing in correctional settings must continually negotiate personal safety and nursing care. Nurses in this setting must be aware that even medical supplies issued to inmates can be a safety threat to the environment. For example, a simple elastic bandage can be used to improve the grip on a homemade weapon. Virtually any prescribed medication can have value on the prison "black market." Further, nurses are subject to manipulation by inmates, who may seek nursing care for reasons other than health. Nurses may simply be someone to talk to in an inherently isolating environment.

As the following clinical example illustrates, in correctional settings, the nurse must maintain an escape route should a situation of personal violence be imminent. In addition, no nursing care in a correctional environment requires a nurse to be locked in an enclosed environment with an inmate. Although it might appear that providing humane, therapeutic nursing care in an environment of potential violence is contradictory, it is ultimately a prerequisite for nursing practice in correctional settings (Bell and Allen, 1998).

Clinical Example
Safety in Correctional Facilities
In a county jail in Georgia in 1996, two nurses were attacked and beaten by an inmate being held on aggravated assault charges. The deputy on duty responsible for protecting them was also subdued by the inmate. These nurses were locked inside the jail with the inmate with their freedom, mobility, and flight to safety limited. The nurses sued the sheriff and deputy for failing to protect them in their work environment. The lawsuit was dismissed because the court determined that the nurses did not have a constitutional right to protection from harm in the work environment (Cohen, 1999c, p. 34).

RESEARCH HIGHLIGHTS
Hearing-impaired Prisoners

Miller, Vernon, and Capella (2005) compared the incidence and types of violent offenses of a deaf prison population with a hearing prison population in the Texas correctional system. A total of ninety-nine individuals with severe-to-profound hearing loss were included in the study population. Of those 99 offenders, 64.6% were convicted of violent offenses including robbery, homicide, assault, and sexual assault.

The study found that compared with hearing violent offenders, a lower percentage of deaf violent offenders committed robberies. The authors speculated that this might be due to the circumstances involved in a robbery, such as communication issues. The findings also revealed that deaf offenders had a higher percentage of sexual assault convictions compared with hearing offenders. The researchers thought that one reason for this might be due to the offender being sexually assaulted as a child.

The authors proposed increasing education for the deaf population and developing regional centers for deaf defendants charged with a crime. It is hoped that the regional centers will allow the deaf defendant time to understand the linguistics of the criminal system and will allow for due process.

From Miller KR, Vernon M, Capella ME: Violent offenders in a deaf prison population, *J Deaf Stud Deaf Educ* 10(4):417-424, 2005.

HEALTH ISSUES IN PRISON POPULATIONS

Today's prison inmate often enters prison with significant health care issues. Nurses employed in the correctional setting are likely to see health care problems that are similar to those in an acute care setting or a community outpatient clinic. The daily operation of a correctional clinic includes management of acute and chronic illness. Most health care clinics in correctional environments screen each inmate upon entry into the facility. The health care triage process generally includes a physical health history and a mental health history. Many significant health care issues are recognized during the screening process, often for the first time.

Chronic and Communicable Diseases

The most critical heath care issues among the incarcerated population are chronic and communicable diseases. Of particular concern are human immunodeficiency virus (HIV), hepatitis, and tuberculosis (TB). According to the Bureau of Justice Statistics, the rate of HIV infection is 1.6% among male inmates and 2.4% among female inmates in the United States (Maruschak, 2008a). The high rate of HIV infection in this population is associated with high-risk behaviors common among inmates, including current and previous drug use, unprotected sexual intercourse, and tattooing (Hellard and Aitken, 2004; Macalino et al., 2004).

Hepatitis is a serious health care issue in correctional facilities. According to the Bureau of Justice Statistics in 2004, 5.3% of state inmates and 4.2% of federal inmates report hepatitis as a medical problem (Maruschak, 2008b). The National Commission on Correctional Health Care (NCCHC) recommends that all inmates be screened and, if indicated, treated for hepatitis upon incarceration.

Another serious health care issue in correctional facilities is TB. The 2004 Bureau of Justice Statistics indicated that 9.4% of state inmates and 7.1% of federal inmates reported having tuberculosis (Maruschak, 2008b). The rate of infection in correctional facilities is related to overcrowding, poor ventilation, and rapid movement of inmates into and out of jail, all conducive to the spread of the disease (Baillargeon et al., 2004). In 2006, the Centers for Disease Control and Prevention released general recommendations for the prevention and control of TB in correctional facilities, including the following:

- TB screening for all staff members and inmates, identifying persons with active TB disease and latent TB infection
- Containment by preventing transmission and providing adequate treatment to inmates with the disease
- Assessment, ongoing monitoring, and evaluation of screening and containment efforts
- Collaboration between correctional facilities and public health departments

As in the public domain, TB, especially in its antibiotic-resistant forms, will continue to be a major threat to the health of incarcerated people in the foreseeable future.

Women in Prison

In midyear 2007, there were 65,500 mothers in jail who reported having 147,400 children under the age of 18 years (Glaze and Maruschak, 2008). More than four in every ten women in prison admit to being abused before the current imprisonment: 34% physically abused and 34% sexually abused (Snell and Morton, 1994). Almost half of the women in prison report being under the influence of drugs or alcohol at the time of the offense and using drugs months prior to the offense.

Drug use and victimization, combined with the stress associated with being separated from their children, place incarcerated women at risk for many mental and physical health problems, including the risk of HIV infection and other sexually transmitted diseases. Unfortunately, health care providers in correctional facilities have limited experience and training to meet the health care needs of women in prison, and quality of care is adversely affected. For example, women who have been sexually assaulted are often reticent about obtaining regular gynecological examinations. The NCCHC confirms that routine gynecological examinations are not consistently a part of health screening for women upon entry into a correctional facility or a routine part of ongoing health care. The NCCHC (1999) offers the following to guide the provision of health care:

- Correctional institutions' health care intake procedures should include comprehensive gynecological examinations.

- Comprehensive health care services should be available to incarcerated women that give special consideration to the reproductive health needs of women, high rate of victimization among incarcerated women, counseling related to parenting issues, and accessibility to drug or alcohol treatment.

⚖ ETHICAL INSIGHTS
Inmates' Refusal of Medications

An inmate's right to refuse treatment is a legal and ethical issue that nurses working in a correctional environment will sometimes experience. The right to refuse treatment and the state's power to enforce treatment are both highly charged legal and political issues and have gained attention in state and local courts. The issue of forced medication and competence to stand trial is of particular concern. The legal and ethical principles that guide forced treatment against the will of an inmate have historically been potential for violence toward self or others and the capacity to understand the consequence of refusing medical treatment. A recent court decision determined that a judicial hearing is now required to forcibly treat a nondangerous incompetent offender to render competence to stand trial. The court decision was based on the following three-factor analysis (Cohen, 1999b, p. 17):
1. Individual's interests
2. State's interest
3. Value of the suggested treatment

Unlike nursing practice with the general population, prison inmates who refuse health care do not leave the facility and return home. Nurses practicing in correctional facilities continue to provide care and address the consequences of an inmate's refusal of treatment. For example, an inmate who refuses to adhere to treatment protocols for HIV infection may experience declining health status. Nurses are obliged to treat any resultant health issues. Individuals who are incarcerated by the state have a constitutional right to refuse and receive health care. Nurses practicing in correctional settings must respect the right to refuse care even if the result is an adverse outcome.

The correctional institute nurse must be mindful of the need to view incarcerated women holistically, realizing that many factors, such as early childhood trauma, violent victimization, gender discrimination, drug use, and a context of economic impoverishment, have often contributed to their current situations.

Adolescents in Prison

Increasing numbers of adolescents are committing violent crimes, and many states have lowered the age limit allowing adolescents to be tried and sentenced as adults. Consequently, adolescents who have been convicted of violent crimes are often incarcerated in adult facilities. Incarcerating adolescents in an adult population presents barriers to meeting the distinct developmental needs of adolescents. These developmental changes include rapid physical and emotional growth and unique nutritional needs, all influenced by environment, genetics, and family experiences. Adult correctional facilities are not generally equipped to deal with the challenges of adolescent development. Adolescents in an adult correctional facility are five times more likely to be sexually assaulted, three times more likely to be beaten by prison guards, and 50% more likely to be assaulted with a weapon, compared with adolescents held in a juvenile center (Coalition for Juvenile Justice, 2005). Juveniles in adult correctional facilities are five times more likely than the adult population and eight times more likely than juveniles in the juvenile center to commit suicide.

To ensure the safety of adolescents in an adult facility, the nurse must be aware of their individual vulnerability. A mechanism for adolescents to access medical and mental health care is essential. Services and interventions should be provided considering the developmental stage and experience of adolescence.

MENTAL HEALTH ISSUES IN CORRECTIONAL SETTINGS

Approximately 34% of state inmates, 24% of federal inmates, and 17% of jail inmates received treatment for mental health problems (James and Glaze, 2006). Being in prison with a mental illness such as schizophrenia, bipolar affective disorder, major depressive disorder, or personality disorder makes adjustment to incarceration extremely difficult. The great number of inmates with a mental illness in today's prisons makes it difficult to meet the needs of this population.

In the late 1950s and early 1960s, deinstitutionalization moved people with mental illness out of state hospitals into communities that were often ill-prepared to care for them. As a result, many people with a mental illness reside in nursing homes, residential homes, prisons, or jails. People with mental illness are often jailed for crimes committed in response to the symptoms of mental illness. With community services declining and increasing numbers of people with mental illness being incarcerated, the "criminalization of the mentally ill" has become a highly charged political topic (National Alliance for the Mentally Ill [NAMI], 1999).

According to NAMI, most jail inmates with symptoms of mental illness are charged with minor crimes. A far lesser number of inmates with severe mental illness commit more serious crimes, again frequently a consequence of either inadequate or no treatment. NAMI takes the position that many dangerous or violent acts by people with a severe mental illness are a result of inappropriate or inadequate treatment. The following strategies have been suggested to reduce the number of incarcerated people with severe mental illness:

- Diverting nonviolent offenders with severe mental illness away from incarceration to adequate treatment
- Convening mental health courts to address all cases involving offenders with severe mental illness
- Educating court judges and personnel about severe mental illness

Mental illness became increasingly understood as a neurobiological illness; therefore those prescribing psychiatric medications have changed their objective from attempting to control behavior to targeting the symptoms of mental illness. Antipsychotic medications, along with psychosocial support, have become the standard of treatment for people with a diagnosis of schizophrenia or other mental illnesses

that result in alterations in perception. Access to mental health treatment, including psychiatric medication, is a right for prison inmates. Correctional facilities must supply inmates with psychotropic medication after discharge for a time reasonable to seek community mental health treatment. Consequently, the state's responsibility for providing psychiatric medication extends beyond discharge from a correctional facility into the community (Cohen, 1999a, 1999c).

Nurses employed in correctional settings must always be aware of the vulnerabilities of people with mental illness who are incarcerated. Depression, schizophrenia, bipolar disorder, and other neurobiological disorders can be readily treated with new-generation psychiatric medications that radically reduce or ameliorate symptoms, but the unique vulnerabilities of incarceration often remain.

EDUCATION AND FORENSIC NURSING

According to Burgess and colleagues (2004), because of the amount and depth of knowledge and skills needed by forensic nurses, whatever their subspecialty area, simply completing a continuing education course is not adequate for practice. As a result, several colleges and universities offer a variety of programs to educate practitioners. This is the direct result of the identified need and growing knowledge base for practice of this specialty area. Table 31-1 gives an overview of basic curricula for forensic nursing programs. In addition, during the formal programs of study, the student usually completes a minimum specified number of supervised clinical hours; a clinical internship also may be required.

TABLE 31-1	BASIC CURRICULA FOR FORENSIC NURSING PROGRAMS
SUBJECT	**TOPIC**
Fundamentals for forensic nursing	Evidence collection
	Documentation
	Interviewing skills
	Basic criminal, procedural, and constitutional law
	Scope of practice
	Interdisciplinary collaboration
	Testifying in court as an expert witness
Forensic law	Legal concepts (culpability, burden of proof, rationale for punishment, mitigating circumstance)
	Defense issues (justification, insanity, entrapment, duress)
Forensic science	Collection and preservation of evidence
	Interpretation of DNA and laboratory reports
	Forensic chemistry and toxicology
	Cause of death
	Blood spatter interpretation
	Manner and mechanism of injury; wound identification and cause

Data from Burgess AW, Berger AD, Boersma RR: Forensic nursing: investigating the career potential in this emerging graduate specialty, *Am J Nurs* 104(3):58-64, 2004.

BOX 31-5	SCHOOLS OFFERING PROGRAMS IN FORENSIC NURSING (GRADUATE AND CERTIFICATE PROGRAMS)*

California
University of California at Riverside
  Riverside, California

Colorado
University of Colorado at Colorado Springs
Beth-El College of Nursing
  Colorado Springs, Colorado

Connecticut
Quinnipiac University
  Hamden, Connecticut

Florida
University of Florida
  Gainesville, Florida

Illinois
University of Illinois at Chicago, College of Nursing
  Chicago, Illinois

Maryland
Johns Hopkins University
  Baltimore, Maryland

Massachusetts
Boston College
  Chestnut Hill, Massachusetts
Fitchburg State College
  Fitchburg, Massachusetts

Nebraska
BryanLGH College of Health Sciences
  Lincoln, Nebraska

New Jersey
Monmouth University
  West Long Branch, New Jersey
Seton Hall University
  South Orange, New Jersey
Fairleigh Dickinson University
  Teaneck, New Jersey

New York
Kaplan College
  New York, New York—Online

North Carolina
Cabarrus College of Health Sciences
  Concord, North Carolina

Ohio
Cleveland State University
  Cleveland, Ohio
Xavier University
  Cincinnati, Ohio

Oklahoma
University of Central Oklahoma
  Edmond, Oklahoma

Pennsylvania
Duquesne University
  Pittsburgh, Pennsylvania
La Roche College
  Philadelphia, Pennsylvania
University of Pennsylvania
  Philadelphia, Pennsylvania
University of Pittsburgh
  Pittsburgh, Pennsylvania
University of Scranton
  Scranton, Pennsylvania

Tennessee
University of Tennessee Health Science Center
  Memphis, Tennessee
Vanderbilt University
  Nashville, Tennessee

Virginia
George Mason University
  Fairfax, Virginia

Washington
University of Washington
  Seattle, Washington

*As of 2009.

For those interested in seeking additional education in the growing and interesting specialty of forensic nursing, Box 31-5 lists nursing colleges and universities that have programs in forensic nursing. It should be noted that some of these programs offer a certificate in forensic nursing, whereas others provide a minor or concentration, and still others grant a graduate degree (typically a master of science in nursing degree).

▌ SUMMARY

Forensic nursing is an innovative, stimulating specialty that combines multiple aspects of nursing science into the care of patients and families with forensic or legal concerns. Most often, the forensic nurse will be employed in a hospital, clinic, correctional facility, or medicolegal death investigation office. Specialized skills (e.g., evidence collection, testifying in court) and knowledge (e.g., legal requirements for

determination of brain death) are essential to the practice and require advanced education and training.

As mentioned previously, assessing for evidence of violence and intervening as needed are fundamental requirements of care that all health professionals must perform. Therefore, every nurse has the potential to be a forensic nurse, regardless of the client population or setting of care. With the increase in violence in society, forensic nurses are faced with the challenge of advocating for victims of violence, living or deceased, and the need for practitioners in this specialty area is expected to grow.

▌ LEARNING ACTIVITIES

1. Spend a few hours of clinical time working with a forensic nurse in an ED. Observe the nurse's interventions and processes related to evidence collection and preservation and

CASE STUDY   APPLICATION OF THE NURSING PROCESS: CORRECTIONAL NURSING

Mr. Smith is a 65-year-old African-American male serving a sentence of 30 years for aggravated assault of a minor. He has served 15 years and is ineligible for parole. Mr. Smith has a medical history of diabetes mellitus, hypertension, coronary artery disease, and peripheral vascular disease. Three weeks ago, his right foot was amputated because of gangrene. Mr. Smith has been admitted to the infirmary six times since the surgery, stating, "I'm not feeling well; can you double-check my sugar?"

The incision site is healing well, and his diabetes mellitus is under control with medication. Mr. Smith takes his medications as prescribed, and his doctor believes he is doing well and continues with his current medication regimen.

Mr. Smith's daughter visits him only once every 6 months because she lives out of state. His son is also in prison but at another location. Mr. Smith's wife recently died from a motor vehicle accident, and he was unable to attend the funeral.

Assessment
Mr. Smith has a flat affect and does not make eye contact. He constantly looks at the ground and does not speak clearly when asked questions. Many times he is asked to repeat himself. According to medical records, he has lost approximately 18 pounds since surgery and he says, "I'm not hungry, that's why I don't eat." When asked about his sleeping habits, Mr. Smith states he sleeps all day except when the guards make him get up. He says he has not played cards with his buddies in more than a week. He also reports that he has been buying soma "from them" and has not taken a bath in 3 days.

Diagnosis
Individual
- Hopelessness related to deteriorating physiological condition
- Ineffective coping related to situational crises
- Powerlessness related to illness-related regimen

Family
- Ineffective coping related to situational crises

Community
- Lack of mental health services

Planning
Mr. Smith will set goals with the health care provider and will ask for assistance with communication with his daughter and son.

Individual
Long-Term Goal
- Client will reestablish positive relationships with fellow inmates within 2 weeks.

Short-Term Goal
- Client will verbalize and recognize his feelings.
- Client will participate in diversion activities of his choice (e.g., playing cards).

Family
Long-Term Goal
- Family will demonstrate coping skills appropriate to the situation.

Short-Term Goal
- Family will verbalize and recognize feelings.

Community
Long-Term Goal
- Program will be available for all individuals.

Short-Term Goal
- Begin mental health programs for individuals in need, utilizing forensic nurses.

Intervention
Individual
- Mr. Smith will be encouraged to express his feelings in an open and nonjudgmental environment, allowing for the development of a therapeutic relationship.
- The forensic nurse will schedule several visits to the clinic and encourage Mr. Smith to participate in activities, such as card playing, with his friends.
- Mr. Smith will be encouraged to discuss past achievements and conduct a life review with assistance from the nurse.

Family
- Mr. Smith's daughter will be included in the plan of care and encouraged to express her thoughts and feelings relating to her father's imprisonment.
- Mr. Smith's daughter also will be supported to convey her thoughts about her mother's death.

Community
- The forensic nurse will arrange several activities for inmates suffering from mental illnesses, including group activities and group talk.

Evaluation
Individual
Mr. Smith slowly engaged the forensic nurse individually and in group therapy. Mr. Smith gained 5 pounds over 2 weeks and was able to make eye contact. Mr. Smith expressed his grief for the death of his wife. He gradually stopped buying soma and spent more time with his friends.

Family
Mr. Smith's daughter continued to visit only once every 6 months but was able to fully explain her thoughts and feelings about her father's incarceration and her mother's death. The time the daughter spent with her father increased and was more meaningful.

Community
A forensic nurse was on constant duty to assist inmates with mental health illnesses.

Levels of Prevention
Primary
- Encourage interaction with colleagues and family.
- Promote participation in prison activities.

Secondary
- Screen for depression.
- Provide outreach services to inmates with mental illness.

Tertiary
- Encourage therapy to reduce symptoms of mental illness.

CASE STUDY   APPLICATION OF THE NURSING PROCESS: FORENSIC NURSING

Transcript of a 911 telephone call:

Emergency operator: "This is 911, what is your emergency?"

Caller: "My son isn't breathing, he's not moving, I need help!"

Emergency operator: "We will send an ambulance and police to assist you."

Caller: "Thank you, please hurry!"

Emergency medical personnel arrived at the house to discover James Oats, a 14-year-old white male, lying face up on his bed. The young man was unresponsive and not breathing. Emergency medical personnel immediately began lifesaving interventions, but, despite all efforts, they were unsuccessful. James Oats was pronounced dead at his house.

Police officers arrived at the residence during the rescue attempt and secured the scene. They then notified homicide detectives and the medical examiner's office. Teresa Fernandez, a forensic nurse death investigator (FNDI) employed by the medical examiner's office, was dispatched to the residence to work in collaboration with the homicide detective, Pete Smith, to investigate the house and crime scene.

The police determined that there was no indication of foul play: the house was in order, there was no ransacking of the residence and no evidence of a robbery, and all the doors and windows were locked. The decedent's room was typical for a 14-year-old boy. There were a PlayStation attached to the television, various clothes strewn about the room, and schoolbooks on the desk.

The decedent's mother, Jane Oats, informed the FNDI that James was in fine health. She explained that he had undergone a physical examination last week for athletics and that the findings were unremarkable. James had an older brother and younger sister, both in excellent health. James's father has hypertension and a history of heart disease, and diabetes and cancer were present in grandparents, but James was healthy.

Teresa (the FNDI) tried to comfort Mrs. Oats, who was extremely upset; she was crying and hyperventilating. Teresa turned to Mr. Oats, who was also present. In answer to Teresa's questioning, Mr. Oats reported that other parents and teachers had been concerned about rumors of increasing use of "bars" in area schools. Teresa was alarmed by this admission and questioned him further about what he meant; he confirmed that the school kids were reportedly using the antianxiety medication Xanax.

Assessment

Teresa performed an initial assessment of the decedent. James was wearing blue jeans, a yellow shirt, and socks. Her findings: "Livor mortis is consistent with body position and blanchable; rigor mortis is breakable in the jaw, arms, and legs. There are no visible signs of trauma."

The decedent was removed from the residence by technicians from the medical examiner's office, and an autopsy was performed the following day. The pathologist reported that the physical findings from the autopsy were unremarkable. During the autopsy, toxicology samples were collected from the heart, liver, and stomach.

Toxicology results were returned in 3 weeks and were positive for an extremely large amount of alprazolam (Xanax). The final, official cause of death for James Oats was alprazolam toxicity; the manner of death was accident.

Along with James's parents and Detective Smith, Teresa was informed of the cause and manner of death. Mr. and Mrs. Oats were devastated by the news and, upon questioning, stated that they did not understand how James had obtained the Xanax pills.

They assured the detective and the FNDI that the only prescription medications in the residence were locked in the master bedroom cabinet and that James had no access to them.

Mr. Oats reported that Mrs. Oats has not been eating and has lost 25 pounds in 3 weeks. She has not been able to return to work, cries continuously, and does not care for their other children. Mr. Oats reports the entire family is withdrawn; the younger child is misbehaving in school and has received detention several times. Mr. Oats expressed exasperation with the need to provide all child care, perform routine chores, and go to work; he admitted that he does not know how much more he can handle.

Mr. Oats told the investigators that community and church members have been extremely helpful and sensitive to the family. The school officials and area churches agreed to support and offer programs to encourage children to say no to drugs; these programs would focus more attention on prescription medications. Further, the school James attended is doing an investigation into drug and alcohol abuse. The school social worker told Mr. Oats that a support group is being formed to assist students with James's death.

Detective Smith interviewed several of James's classmates and discovered that Xanax is used by many of them. From the information that he was able to gather from other students, it appeared that this was the first time James had tried the drug. Detective Smith discovered that some of the students were obtaining Xanax from their parents and selling it in the schools to their peers. Further, he learned that students are trying the "bars" because "it's cool."

Diagnosis
Family
- Anxiety related to death of a child
- Complicated grieving, related to death of a child
- Compromised family coping related to situational crisis
- Caregiver role strain related to situational crisis

Community
- Readiness for enhanced coping related to social worker availability

Planning
Family
The Oats family will initiate counseling to assist with acceptance of and coping with James's death.

Long-Term Goal
- Family will identify need for outside support and seek such support.

Short-Term Goals
- Family will verbalize and recognize feelings surrounding the death.
- Family will express feelings honestly.

Community
Long-Term Goal
- Members of the community will establish a plan to deal with problems and stressors, including premature deaths.

Short-Term Goal
- Members of the community, including school personnel and students, will identify positive and negative factors affecting management of current and future problems and stressors.

Continued

CASE STUDY — APPLICATION OF THE NURSING PROCESS: FORENSIC NURSING—cont'd

Intervention

Family

Teresa Fernandez:

- Listened to the family's comments, remarks, and expression of concerns, noting nonverbal behaviors and responses
- Encouraged family members to verbalize feelings openly and clearly
- Referred family to appropriate resources for assistance as indicated (e.g., counseling, psychotherapy, spiritual guidance)

Community

With police, school personnel, and community leaders, Ms. Fernandez:

- Reviewed community plan for dealing with substance abuse problems among schoolchildren and assessed related stressors
- Determined community's strengths and weaknesses
- Identified available resources
- Established mechanism for self-monitoring of community needs and evaluation of efforts

Evaluation

Family

- The Oats family began family counseling and slowly accepted James's death.
- James's siblings began educating fellow classmates about the ill effects of abusing prescription medications.

Community

- The community implemented quarterly meetings for grieving families including licensed counselors.
- The community members employed "just say no" rallies focusing on school-aged children.

Levels of Prevention

Primary

- Initiate drug and prescription medication teaching in middle and high schools, focusing on long-term associated problems and side effects.
- Support programs that encourage students to role play and practice "just say no" to drugs.

Secondary

- Organize group sessions in school to discuss illegal prescription medication abuse.
- Provide information to school personnel and parents on how to identify or screen for evidence of use of drugs and alcohol among school-aged children.
- Provide information on area groups that provide support for students who want to avoid using drugs or want to stop using drugs.

Tertiary

- Reduce risk of additional students abusing prescription medication.

collaboration with, for example, police officers and court officials. Take note of the techniques used for interviewing and counseling.

2. Attend a session of local or state mental health court (court proceedings to determine the status of an individual's mental status and disposition—e.g., confinement to a mental institution or release in the care of a guardian or family member). Report on the experience to classmates.

3. Spend a clinical day in a jail or correctional facility working with a correctional forensic nurse. Pay particular attention to differences in care delivery related to legal and ethical issues unique to this subspecialty. Develop impressions into a paper.

REFERENCES

American Association of Colleges of Nursing: *Violence as a public health problem*, 1999. http://www.aacn.nche.edu/Publications/positions/violence.htm.

American Association of Legal Nurse Consultants: *Getting started in legal nurse consulting: an introduction to the specialty*, ed 2, Chicago, 1999, The Author.

American Nurses Association: *Scope and standards of forensic nursing practice*, Washington, DC, 1997, American Nurses Publishing.

Antognoli-Toland P: Comprehensive program for examination of sexual assault victims by nurses: a hospital-based project in Texas, *J Emerg Nurs* 11(3):132–135, 1985.

Baillargeon J, et al: The infectious disease profile of Texas prison inmates, *Prev Med* 38:607–612, 2004.

Bell K, Allen W: *Healthcare workers must be on constant guard*, St. Louis, Post-Dispatch September 27, 1998, A-12.

Bonnie RJ, Wallace RB: *Elder mistreatment: abuse, neglect and exploitation in an aging America*, 2003, www.nap.edu/catalog.php?record_id=10406#toc.

Burgess AW, Berger AD, Boersma RR: Forensic nursing: investigating the career potential in this emerging graduate specialty, *Am J Nurs* 104(3):58–64, 2004.

Centers for Disease Control and Prevention, MMWR Recommendations and Reports: *Prevention and control of tuberculosis in correctional and detention facilities: recommendations from CDC* 55(RR09):1–44; July 7, 2006, www.cdc.gov/mmwr/preview/mmwrhtml/rr5509a1.htm.

Coalition for Juvenile Justice: *Childhood on trial: the failure of trying and sentencing youth in adult criminal court*, 2005, www.juvjustice.org/media/resources/resource:115.pdf.

Cohen F: Deliberate indifference to detainee's serious medical needs shown, *Corrections Mental Health Rep* 1(4):65, 1999a.

Cohen F: Judicial hearing and strict scrutiny required to forcibly medicate incompetent detainees, *Corrections Mental Health Rep* 1(2):17, 1999b.

Cohen F: Prisons' duty to provide psychotropic medication includes post-release supply, *Corrections Mental Health Rep* 1(4):49, 1999c.

Collins SE, Halpern KJ: Forensic nursing: a collaborative practice paradigm, *J Nurs Law* 10(1):11–19, 2005.

Coram JW: Psychiatric forensic nursing. In Lynch V, editor: *Forensic nursing*, St. Louis, 2006, Mosby.

Corso PS, Mercy JA, Simon TR, Finkelstein EA, et al: Medical costs and productivity losses due to interpersonal and self-directed violence in the United States, *Am J Prev Med* 32(6):474–482, 2007.

Fulton DR, Assid P: Evidence collection in the emergency department. In Lynch V, editor: *Forensic nursing*, St. Louis, 2006, Mosby.

Fulton M: Forensic nurses as coroners and death investigators, *Forensic Nurse* Jan/Feb: 15–16, 2003.

Geissler-Murr A, Moorhouse MF: Legal nurse consulting. In Lynch V, editor: *Forensic nursing*, St. Louis, 2006, Mosby.

Girardin B: Is this forensic specialty for you? *RN* 64(12):37–41, 2001.

Glaze LE, Maruschak LM: *Parents in prison and their minor children*, Bureau of Justice Statistics Rep No NCJ 222984, August 2008, www.ojp.usdoj.gov/bjs/pub/pdf/pptmc.pdf.

Haas RE, Bradshaw MJ: The expert witness: defending the profession or prosecuting your peers, *CRNA* 10(2):71–79, 1999.

Hanzlick R: Coroner training needs, a numeric and geographic analysis, *JAMA* 276(21): 1775–1778, 1996.

Hanzlick R: *Death investigation systems and procedures*, Boca Raton, FL, 2007, CRC Press, Taylor Francis Group.

Hanzlick R, Combs D: Medical examiner and coroner systems, history and trends, *JAMA* 279(11):870–874, 1998.

Hanzlick R, Hunsaker JC, Davis GJ: *A guide for manner of death classification*, 2002, National Association of Medical Examiners, www.healthvermont.gov/hc/death_certificate/documents/mannerofdeath.pdf.

Heilporn A, André JM, Didier JP, et al: Violence to and maltreatment of people with disabilities: a short review, *J Rehabil Med* 38:10–12, 2006.

Hellard ME, Aitken CK: HIV in prison: what are the risks and what can be done? *Sex Health* 1(2):107–113, 2004.

International Association of Forensic Nurses: *Sexual assault nurse examiner standards of practice*, Pitman, NJ, 1996, The Author.

International Association of Forensic Nurses: *Sexual assault nurse examiner education guidelines*, Pitman, NJ, 1998, The Author.

James DJ, Glaze LE: *Mental health problems of prison and jail inmates*, Bureau of Justice Statistics Rep No NCJ 213600, September 2006, www.ojp.gov/bjs/pub/pdf/mhppji.pdf.

LaSala KB, Lynch VA: Child abuse and neglect. In Lynch V, editor: *Forensic nursing*, St. Louis, 2006, Mosby.

Ledray LE: Sexual assault. In Lynch V, editor: *Forensic nursing*, St. Louis, 2006, Mosby.

Ledray LE, Arndt S: Examining the sexual assault victim: a new model for nursing care, *J Psychosoc Nurs* 32(2):7–12, 1994.

Lynch V: Forensic nursing in the emergency department: a new role of the 1990s, *Crit Care Nurs Q* 14(3):69–86, 1991.

Lynch V: The forensic investigation of death. In Lynch V, editor: *Forensic nursing*, St. Louis, 2006, Mosby.

Macalino G, et al: Prevalence and incidence of HIV, hepatitis B virus, and hepatitis C virus infections among males in Rhode Island prisons, *Am J Public Health* 94(7):1218–1223, 2004.

Maruschak LA: *HIV in prisons, 2006*, Bureau of Justice Statistics Rep No NCJ 222179, April 2008a. http://www.ojp.gov/bjs/pub/pdf/hivp06.pdf.

Maruschak LA: *Medical problems of prisoners*, Bureau of Justice Statistics Rep No NCJ 221740, April 2008b. http://www.ojp.gov/bjs/pub/pdf/mpp.pdf.

McGann E, Moynihan BA: Elder abuse. In Lynch V, editor: *Forensic nursing*, St. Louis, 2006, Mosby.

Meiner SE: The legal nurse consultant, *Geriatr Nurs* 26(1):34–36, 2005.

Miller KR, Vernon M, Capella ME: Violent offenders in a deaf prison population, *J Deaf Stud Deaf Educ* 10(4):417–424, 2005.

Moynihan BA: Domestic violence. In Lynch V, editor: *Forensic nursing*, St. Louis, 2006, Mosby.

National Alliance for the Mentally Ill: *Position papers on criminalization of the mentally ill*, 1999, www.nami.org.

National Center on Elder Abuse: Elder abuse information series No. 1, 2005a, www.ncea.aoa.gov/ncearoot/Main_Site/pdf/basics/fact1.pdf.

National Center on Elder Abuse: Elder abuse information series No. 2, 2005b, www.ncea.aoa.gov/ncearoot/Main_Site/pdf/basics/fact2.pdf.

National Center on Elder Abuse: *Elder abuse prevalence and incidence*, 2005c, www.ncea.aoa.gov/ncearoot/Main_Site/pdf/publication/FinalStatistics050331.pdf.

National Commission on Correctional Health Care: *Standards for health services in corrections*, Chicago, 1999, The Author.

Pearsall C: Forensic biomarkers of elder abuse: what clinicians need to know, *J Forensic Nurs* 1(4):182–186, 2005.

Potter PA, Perry AG: *Fundamentals of nursing*, St. Louis, 2009, Mosby.

Prahlow JA, Lantz PE: Medical examiner/death investigator training requirements in state and medical examiner systems, *J Forensic Sci* 40(1):55–58, 1995.

Raymond L: Is a legal career for you? *RN* 65(3):63–64, 2002.

Ruiz-Contreras A: The nurse as an expert witness, *Top Emerg Med* 27(1):27–35, 2005.

Saunders L: Forensic nursing: formalizing a new role or recognizing existing practice? *Aust Nurs J* 8(3):49–50, 2000.

Sekula LK: The advance practice forensic nurse in the emergency department, *Top Emerg Med* 27(1):5–14, 2005.

Shafer TJ: Organ donation. In Lynch V, editor: *Forensic nursing*, St. Louis, 2006, Mosby.

Snell TL, Morton D: *Women in prison: survey of state inmates, 1991*, Bureau of Justice Statistics Special Rep No NCJ 145321, March 1994, www.ojp.gov/bjs/pub/pdf/wopris.pdf.

U.S. Department of Health and Human Services, Administration for Children and Families: *What is child abuse and neglect*, Washington, DC, 2008, The Author. www.childwelfare.gov/pubs/can_info_packet.pdf.

U.S. Department of Justice/Bureau of Justice Statistics: *Criminal victimization*, 2007, Bureau of Justice Statistics Rep No 224390 www.ojp.usdoj.gov/bjs/pub/pdf/cv07.pdf.

Venes D, editor: *Taber's cyclopedic medical dictionary*, ed 19, Philadelphia, 2001, FA Davis.

Faith Community Nursing

Beverly Cook Siegrist

Additional Material for Study, Review, and Further Exploration

evolve WEBSITE

http://evolve.elsevier.com/Nies

- Quiz
- Case Studies
- Glossary

- WebLinks
- Resource Tool
  - 32A: Guidelines for Simple Prayer Services

OBJECTIVES

Upon completion of this chapter, the reader will be able to do the following:

1. Understand the potential role of faith communities in improving the health of Americans.
2. Describe the philosophy and historical basis of faith community nursing.
3. Define the roles, functions, and education of the faith community nurse.
4. Discuss faith communities as clients of the community health nurse.

5. Describe the role of the faith community nurse in the spiritual health and wellness of faith communities.
6. Discuss contemporary issues in faith community nursing, such as working with vulnerable populations and facing ethical and legal issues.
7. Apply the nursing process to a case study related to a faith community practice.

KEY TERMS

CIRCLE Model of Spiritual Care
coordinator of volunteers
developer of support groups
facilitator
faith community

Granger Westberg
health advocate
health educator
integrator of health and healing
personal health counselor

referral agent
spiritual distress
spirituality

OUTLINE

Faith Communities: Role in Health and Wellness
Foundations of Faith Community Nursing
Roles of the Faith Community Nurse
Education of the Faith Community Nurse
The Faith Community Nurse and Spirituality

Issues in Faith Community Nurse Practice
  Providing Care to Vulnerable Populations
  End-of-Life Issues: Grief and Loss
  Family Violence Prevention
  Confidentiality
  Accountability

Nurses seem to have one foot in the sciences and one in the humanities; one foot in the spiritual world and one in the physical one....they [nurses] have insight into the human condition. (Maginnis and Associates, 1993, p. 1)

The purpose of this chapter is to present an overview of faith community nursing and to explore the challenges of providing nursing care to faith communities. On the basis of centuries-old philosophies from churches and religious groups, nurses are applying the science of nursing and caring to address the biopsychosocial health needs of individuals and groups in church congregations and faith communities across the country. The following scenarios illustrate models of faith community nursing found in the United States and suggest the unique ways that parish nurses provide nursing care.

Clinical Example
Faith Community Nursing Model 1

Sandra Mills began her faith community nurse (FCN) practice as a volunteer when her parish priest recruited her to help establish a cancer support group and coordinate classes for caregivers. Within 6 months, her church's social concerns committee established a paid position on their ministry team and employed her as a full-time, paid staff member. After completing a FCN program through a local university, she began to develop a health ministry in her church. She describes her days as full and rewarding. Each day, she visits ill or homebound parish members and provides support through prayer, education, and listening. She is challenged to locate and refer community resources, provide health education to church groups (e.g., mother's day out and the over-55 group), and coordinate the efforts of other volunteers in the church. She is practicing holistic nursing for the first time in her 15 years of practice. She found that the church, as a healing community, allows her to focus on the body-mind-spirit connection she believes is necessary to improve the health of congregation members.

Clinical Example
Faith Community Nursing Model 2

Marilyn Michaels is a former home care and hospice nurse who works as an FCN coordinator for St. Luke's Hospital, which is a 400-bed medical center serving a Midwestern rural population. Her position was created to assist community churches in developing and maintaining parish nurse programs. She coordinates educational programs, including a 30-hour preparation program for beginning FCNs, an advanced program for FCN coordinators in individual churches, and monthly educational programs offered through an FCN support group. Marilyn developed the support group and facilitates communication among the 200 nurses and 100 church communities that St. Luke's Hospital serves. She also assists the many faith community programs by connecting them with other services that the hospital and community agencies provide (e.g., screening, support groups, and speakers). The program at St. Luke's Hospital is self-supporting from grants and educational programs.

Clinical Example
Faith Community Nursing Model 3

Sue James is a member of an FCN group from five inner-city churches in south-central Indiana. This group of nurses came together from five different church denominations to meet their congregation members' health needs. The nurses are unpaid within their own congregations. They came together to share their resources because their churches are small in membership and they identified similar and unmet health needs in each of the churches. Primarily, the group serves an aging population that represents the few remaining individuals and families living in the inner-city area. Sue agreed to serve as the group coordinator, a position that has been shared among their group. In this position, she plans biweekly meetings for the nurses at alternating churches and serves as a community liaison for participating churches. The group's parish nurse effort began 2 years earlier, supported by a local hospital grant and matched with small donations from the participating churches. Each nurse volunteers at least 10 hours each week. On the basis of the health and wellness assessment completed in each church, they arranged a health fair that included health screening and referral information at one church and began educational classes on topics related to depression and healthy aging. They focus on health promotion, and their individual churches recognize them as the FCN, the congregational nurse, and the health minister.

The three clinical examples illustrate how faith nursing is evolving in the United States. From beginning as fewer than a dozen nurses in Chicago, the practice now includes thousands of nurses in more than twenty-three countries (International Parish Nurse Resource Center [IPNRC], 2009b). The growing number of registered nurses (RNs) in parish nursing documents this practice as a significant role for the community health nurse. Community health nursing has evolved from early church efforts to provide care for the sick and disenfranchised. Modern parish nursing focuses on the global health and wellness issues of all people and has its roots in more recent efforts to encourage the reemergence and blending of health care roles into the healing ministry of faith communities (Patterson, 2004; Solari-Twadell and McDermott, 1999).

FAITH COMMUNITIES: ROLE IN HEALTH AND WELLNESS

Former President Jimmy Carter, faculty and founding member of Strong Partners Interfaith Health Program at Emory University in Atlanta, Georgia, understands the importance of faith communities for Americans. President Carter is quoted on the Interfaith Health Program website (http://www.ihp-net.org):

What if churches, mosques, and temples worked together to improve the health of their communities? If faith groups adopted one small area and made sure that every single child were immunized...that every person had a basic medical exam...that every woman who became pregnant would get prenatal care? Are these possible? We believe the answer is yes. (Interfaith Health Program, 2005)

Throughout history, church communities have provided care for the indigent and disenfranchised, meeting basic human needs of food and clothing and basic health care. The majority of the world's populations belong to organized faith communities. Approximately one third of the people in

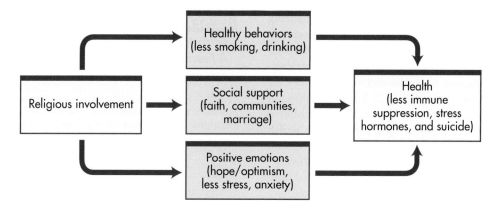

FIGURE 32-1 Possible explanations for the positive correlation between religious involvement and health and longevity. (From Myers DG: *Stress and health in psychology*, ed 7, New York, 2004, Worth Publishers.)

the world identify themselves as Christians (2 billion), followed by Muslims (1.5 billion), Hindus (900 million), and Buddhists (380 million) (IPNRC, 2009b). All of these religions have traditions and rituals related to health and healing, including specific prayers and practices. Some of the religions give specific guidelines for ministering to the ill, homebound, or dying members. All of the major religions describe the relationship between health, healing, and wholeness. The Old Testament discusses Shalom, or God's desire for health and wholeness for the earth and its people. The New Testament documents the healing activities of Jesus, restoring health to people. The Talmud describes the importance of maintaining physical health and vigor so that Jewish people will understand God's will in their lives. Followers of Buddhism believe that healing and recovery are promoted by awakening to the teachings of Buddha (IPNRC, 2009b).

Williams and Sternthal (2007) completed a meta-analysis of studies related to spirituality, religion, and health. In 17 studies, individuals who reported intrinsic religion (internalized or regularly practiced) and regular attendance at a religious service reported decreased stress. In 147 studies, it was found that there was an inverse relationship between religiosity and depression. The authors found evidence in another 49 studies that indicated people who practiced religious coping had lower levels of anxiety, depression, and stress and coped more positively with many chronic diseases such as human immunodeficiency virus (HIV), hypertension, and cancer. One reason for this variance may be that the people who reported the highest level of religious involvement also reported practicing healthier lifestyles, including exercising more and smoking less (Tsuang, Williams, and Lyons, 2002; Myers, 2004). Eckersley (2007) suggests that "religion provides things that are good for health and wellbeing, including social support, existential meaning, a sense of purpose, a coherent belief system and a clear moral code" (p. S54). Myers (2004) and Koenig and George (2004) suggest that faith communities contribute to the well-being of their members through support, prayer, and providing a sense of hope. The importance of stress management in health promotion and disease management is well documented. The interaction and possible

explanation for the positive correlation between religious involvement and health is visualized in Figure 32-1.

Organized religions are attempting to meet the needs of members in many nontraditional ways including exploring Internet church services, developing support groups, and including modern music and drama in traditional worship services to improve intergenerational communication. FCNs, because of their educational preparation and goals, are ideal health professionals to ensure that the health information provided in congregations is accurate and accessible. Parish nurses also understand the importance of spirituality in health and healing. The role of the FCN therefore complements the ministry of health found in faith communities.

FOUNDATIONS OF FAITH COMMUNITY NURSING

Reverend Granger Westberg, a Lutheran minister, is considered the founder of the modern FCN movement. Westberg, educated as a chaplain and minister, worked with nurses in hospitals, medical schools, and church communities. Impressed with the nurse's perspective of health and wholeness in viewing the physical, emotional, and spiritual challenges of human illness, he described parish nursing as the culmination of his lifelong work in relating theology and health care. In 1984, he first proposed a parish nurse program to Lutheran General Hospital (LGH) in Chicago, Illinois. Westberg envisioned a partnership between the hospital and all church congregations in the hospital's community. He proposed that participating churches would make contributions to fund a nurse's salary and identified seven roles the nurse could use to provide services to faith communities (Hickman, 2007; O'Brien, 2003; Patterson, 2004).

In 1985, six FCNs were hired in the Chicago area. Initially, LGH and the participating churches' contributions primarily funded the nurses' salaries. The churches assumed increasing responsibility for the nurses' salaries over a 4-year period. Westberg supported the development of an FCN training program and required the nurses to participate in a weekly educational session. Teaching chaplains, nurse educators, and physicians led the sessions, which were aimed at enhancing nurses' skills in counseling, education, spiritual assessment, and related nursing interventions. The meetings evolved into an ongoing support group for the nurses as they developed the faith community programs and identified self-care needs. LGH continued to provide FCN leadership through the IPNRC. Located in Park Ridge, Illinois, the center offered education, development guidance, and contact with parish nurses nationally and internationally. In 2001, ownership of the IPNRC moved from the Lutheran-rooted Advocate Health Care System to the Deaconess Foundation of St. Louis, Missouri. The Deaconess ministries in the United States have their roots in the Deaconess service movement founded in Germany in the mid-1800s. Deaconess has been involved in faith community nursing since the late 1980s and, as the Deaconess Parish Nurse Ministry, is a leader in the specialty in the United States. The Deaconess Parish Nurse Ministries is the current parent organization of the IPNRC (IPNRC, 2009a; Westberg, 2007).

In 1998, the American Nurses Association (ANA), in collaboration with the newly formed Health Ministries Association, Parish Nurse Division, published the first *Scope and Standards of Parish Nurse Practice*. This was a landmark publication for parish nurses, officially recognizing the practice as a nursing specialty. ANA revised the standards in 2005, providing a clearer definition of the practice including advanced nursing practice and changing the name of the specialty from parish nurse to FNC. While acknowledging the importance of the Judeo-Christian basis of the practice, the authors believed the change better reflected the diversity now found in the specialty. The IPNRC (2009b) reports that faith community nursing is now practiced in more than 23 countries including Australia, Bahamas, Canada, England, Ghana, Kenya, Korea, Madagascar, Malawi, Malaysia, New Zealand, Nigeria, Pakistan, Palestine, Scotland, Singapore, South Africa, Swaziland, Ukraine, United States, Wales, Zambia, and Zimbabwe serving Muslim, Jewish, and Christian faith communities. Many FCNs continue to identify themselves as parish nurses in deference to Dr. Westberg and the origins of the practice. For this reason, the terms are used interchangeably in the literature and at conferences. Other FCNs may be known as congregational nurses or church nurses, choosing to identify themselves in a manner most accepted by the individual faith communities.

Solari-Twadell and McDermott (1999) and Westberg (1990) described the philosophical basis of parish nursing as encompassing the following five key elements:
1. The spiritual dimension is central to the practice.
2. The role balances nursing science and technology with service and spiritual care.
3. The nurse's clients are members of the faith community defined by the church and its public service philosophy.
4. Parish nursing services are built upon principles of self-care and capacity building, with a focus on understanding the connection between health and the individual's relationship with God, faith traditions, nursing, and the broader society.

RESEARCH HIGHLIGHTS

Faith-Placed Cardiovascular Health Promotion: A Framework for Contextual and Organizational Factors Underlying Program Success

Best practices in planning and implementing programs related to cardiovascular health are a frequent topic among FCNs. Many comprehensive programs are being implemented to improve positive health behaviors among congregational members across all ethnic groups and ages. The purpose of this study was to review all current faith-placed cardiovascular health promotion programs and to construct a framework of factors to increase the effectiveness of existing programs. The sample included current, published reports of programs in the literature from 1984-2004. Variables were identified and characterized by identifying clusters from the literature that describe factors contributing to the success of any program. The significant variables for the model are defined as faith support, community support, community partnerships, faith organization capabilities, secular organization capabilities (other health care system support), and caring interventions. For example, the faith support variable required activation of family, peer, pastor, volunteer, and nurse support. Secular support includes increasing awareness through education, such as helping the community understand the connection among spiritual health, cardiovascular health, and success in a health promotion program. The construct of caring interventions is significant to FCNs implementing a cardiovascular health promotion program. The authors found that caring included "visible involvement" on many levels such as engaging staff and members in health conversations, providing group and individual support, and being highly visible to church members. The results of this study provide a useful model for successful implementation of health promotion programs for the nurse and health ministry team.

From Sternberg Z, Munchauer FE, Carrow SS et al: Faith-placed cardiovascular health promotion: a framework for contextual and organizational factors underlying program success, *Health Educ Res* 22(5):619-629, 2007.

5. The parish nurse understands that holistic health is a dynamic process that requires connections among the person's spiritual, psychological, physical, and social dimensions.

These beliefs direct the parish nurse in planning nursing care and defining health not only as wellness but also as wholeness of body and spirit. They also emphasize spiritual health as a motivating factor in seeking wellness care, participating in education, and enhancing self-care capabilities (Hickman, 2007; Patterson, 2004; Smith, 2003). The IPNRC (2009a) identifies a vision that "every faith community in the future will have access to a FNC."

A review of the historical foundations of community health nursing practice describes the significance of the church in early health care. In the Bible, the book of Romans (16:1-2) describes the early works of Phoebe, who is considered to be the first visiting nurse. In his 1786 sermon "On Visiting the Sick," John Wesley, the founder of the Methodist church, directed his believers to visit the sick to convey God's grace to others (Wesley, 1986). These selected examples illustrate the significance of the church as an influence on health and healing. The histories of all religions provide similar examples. The reemergence of these basic beliefs in health, healing, and spirituality are moving the church toward assisting members in wholeness; this is evidenced by the growing number of health ministries and FCN programs found in churches throughout the nation (Hickman, 2007; Patterson, 2004). The defining characteristics and roles of the FCN in any setting come from these philosophical foundations.

The current mission statement for parish nurses was developed and approved in 2000 by more than 600 attendees at the fourteenth annual Westberg Symposium.

> *Parish nursing is the intentional integration of the practice of faith with the practice of nursing so that people can achieve wholeness in, with, and through communities of faith in which the parish nurse serves. Parish nurses educate, advocate, and activate people to take positive action regarding wellness, prevention, appropriate treatment of illness, and social and spiritual connections with God, members of their congregations, and their wider community. (Patterson, 2004, p. 32)*

 HEALTHY PEOPLE 2020

Faith Community Nursing

Topic Area, Educational and community-based programs
Goal: Increase the quality, availability, and effectiveness of education and community-based programs designed to prevent disease and improve health and quality of life.
Parish nurse practice may vary depending upon the needs of the faith community served. Programs and services may contribute to many *Healthy People 2020* goals. The Topic Area, Educational and Community-Based Programs—directs public health agencies to form partnerships with many community-based organizations, including faith communities, to improve the quality and effectiveness of health education programs.

From US Department of Health and Human Services: *Healthy People 2010,* Washington, DC, 2000, Government Printing Office, www.healthy-people. gov/healthfinder.

ROLES OF THE FAITH COMMUNITY NURSE

The FCN practice focuses on health promotion and wellness. It is based on a holistic nursing practice that holds the spiritual dimension central to health and healing within the context of the faith community. In the nursing process, the FCN improves the health of a faith community by implementing interrelated roles including those of health educator, personal health counselor, referral agent, health advocate, coordinator of volunteers, developer of support groups, and integrator of health and healing (Hickman, 2007 IPNRC, 2009a).

As a health educator, the FCN provides or coordinates educational offerings for people of all ages and developmental stages. The educational efforts may target lifestyles, values, and wellness and incorporate the spiritual aspects of individual and community well-being. The educator role includes educating the church leaders and members about the roles and purposes of a parish nurse. Educational efforts are planned based on the church community's priorities and *Healthy People 2020* (USDHHS, 2009). Because the faith community membership includes people across the life span,

church-based educational programs can address all ten major health indicators (IPNRC, 2009a; King and Tessaro, 2009). Early in the development of a parish nurse program, and periodically thereafter, the parish nurse should assess the health status and needs of the congregation members to determine educational priorities. Figure 32-2 presents an example of an adult congregational health and wellness survey. The FCN should complete an assessment on each population group served by the congregation and include children grouped by developmental stages. Examples of educational efforts are teaching cardiopulmonary resuscitation to new mothers; teaching signs and symptoms of hypertension and stroke to adults in the congregation; educating lay church ministers in the signs and symptoms of acute illness when visiting homebound individuals; and teaching basic health and safety to school-aged children. With increasing frequency, FCNs are implementing comprehensive wellness programs. One such program is "Get My People Going" developed by the IPNRC. It provides an 8-week healthy lifestyle program based on the Exodus story that includes exercise, nutrition, and community support (IPNRC, 2008).

As a personal health counselor, the FCN discusses health problems with individuals and families within the church community. The nurse may focus on self-care issues such as explaining a prescribed medical regimen; assessing the need for further resources and referrals; or making visits to homes, nursing homes, or hospitals (McGinnis, 2008).

The FCN utilizes referral skills and knowledge of community resources to guide individuals as they access available resources. The nurse may function as a liaison and, with the client's approval, provide referrals to resources or health care providers. The FCN recognizes the difficulties encountered by vulnerable populations within the faith community and helps them maneuver the health care maze to access needed resources. These vulnerable populations may include non–English-speaking individuals, those who speak English as a second language (ESL), individuals living in poverty, individuals without health care insurance, and individuals living with complicated chronic or catastrophic illness.

In the role of health advocate, the FCN "facilitates clients' efforts in obtaining needed health services and appropriate care management plans, promotes community awareness of significant health problems, lobbies for beneficial public policy, and stimulates supportive action for health" (Clemon-Stone, McGuire, and Eigsti, 2002, p. 45). Advocacy can present challenges for the nurse in any setting. The nurse must always remember that the client (individual, family, or group) has the right to self-determination. The FCN's role may be that of educating clients to make the best choices or empowering them to speak for themselves. The nurse also must understand the policies and beliefs of the congregation related to specific health issues. Church doctrine may guide members to adopt values and beliefs that are in conflict with current health care recommendations. Individuals may request that the parish nurse provide education and support in making decisions related to issues of infertility, stem cell technology, birth control, and sex

Wellness Ministry Survey

Thank you for taking the time to complete this Wellness Survey. The results will be used to plan programs and activities that will meet the health care interests and needs of everyone in the congregation. Think of this as your survey to indicate the type of services you would like available to you, your family, and your brothers and sisters in Christ. Please do not sign your name. All information will be confidential.

Please complete the following:

My age is _____.
I am _____ female _____ male.
I am _____ White _____ Black _____ Hispanic _____ Asian.
I am _____ single _____ married _____ divorced _____ widowed.
I am _____ employed _____ unemployed _____ retired _____ homemaker _____ student.
I have health insurance. _____ yes _____ no
I have a family doctor. _____ yes _____ no
I think my health is _____ good _____ fair _____ poor.

Please place an "X" by those activities that you would benefit from now or might use in the future:

___ Visits to those individuals who are homebound
___ Visits to those who are experiencing loss
___ Visits to parishioners in hospitals or nursing homes
___ A nurse to assist parishioners in obtaining personal health counseling
___ Health education pamphlets or brochures
___ Classes held at church on health-related topics
___ Information on classes held elsewhere in our community

___ Health screening at our church
___ Flu shots or immunizations at our church
___ Volunteer training for parishioners to assist parishioners (e.g., respite and homebound visits)
___ Support groups at our church
___ Support groups elsewhere
___ Prayer and healing service
___ Other (please list):

Please place an "X" by those health topics listed below that you want to know more about

Heart Sense
___ Heart disease
___ Stroke
___ High blood pressure
___ Diet and cholesterol

Healthy Living
___ Nutrition and weight control
___ Exercise
___ Quitting smoking
___ Alcohol and drug issues

Emotional Health
___ Depression
___ Other mental illness
___ Reducing stress
___ Eating disorders
___ Self-esteem
___ Anger management

Women's Health
___ Breast cancer
___ Menopause
___ Estrogen replacement
___ Osteoporosis

An Ounce of Prevention
___ Cancer prevention
___ Protecting your back
___ Talking to your doctor
___ Understanding your medications
___ Safety at home and away
___ Understanding insurance

Healthy Families
___ Sexuality
___ Marriage
___ Pregnancy and childbirth
___ Parents through life stages
___ Teen issues
___ Single parenting

Chronic Concerns
___ Arthritis
___ Diabetes
___ Prostate trouble
___ HIV/AIDS
___ Pain management
___ Urinary incontinence
___ Life with a disability

As We Age
___ Our physical changes
___ Care of aging parents
___ Living well alone
___ Alzheimers
___ Loneliness
___ Getting "our affairs in order"

As Life Ends
___ Grief issues
___ Living wills and power of attorney
___ Hospice care
___ Organ donation

Other topics? _____

Put an "X" by days and times you would participate in an activity or class

Day of week	Mornings	Afternoon	Evenings
Monday	___	___	___
Tuesday	___	___	___
Wednesday	___	___	___
Thursday	___	___	___
Friday	___	___	___
Saturday	___	___	___
Sunday	___	___	___

FIGURE 32-2 Parish health assessment form. (Courtesy Holy Spirit Catholic Church, Bowling Green, KY.)

education for teens and youth. Although assuming the role of advocate implies a commitment to change, the parish nurse must understand that the politics of working within the faith system require acceptance of individual and system values and beliefs.

The role of coordinator of volunteers includes recruiting, training, and directing volunteers to work with the FCN program or health ministry. The nurse may work with other nurses and lay people within the congregation. The FCN program may encompass all programs related to the health of the church community. For example, the community needs assessment may identify the need for development of a transportation committee or respite program. These services affect the ability of church members to access health and related services; these programs may be delegated to the nurse. As a coordinator of volunteers, the nurse would plan, implement, and direct these programs. Many FCNs work through existing health ministry frameworks within their churches, such as health or social welfare committees. The membership of these committees may be interdisciplinary or representative of the entire church congregation. The FCN may be delegated the responsibility of developing specific health-related programs and activities. In the facilitator role, the nurse would also connect the church with existing resources and programs to meet identified health and educational needs. For example, the nurse might facilitate available health screenings, flu shots, or immunizations through the local public health department.

The role of developer of support groups requires skills in accessing, and the FCN uses community assessment and program evaluation skills. The nurse may practice within a community rich in resources and support groups or in a community with few health-related resources. Support groups are people who meet for support and sharing of issues related to common problems. Examples of support groups are bereavement groups or new mother groups. Support groups are different from self-help groups, which focus on personal growth (e.g., Alcoholics Anonymous). Some individuals prefer support groups to be physically located within their faith community where they have existing support systems and can network with individuals who share common values and beliefs. The FCN must evaluate the need for a support or self-help group within the faith community. Situations that might indicate the need for support groups include the increased incidence of a sudden and shared experience by members, for example, five or more members dying of cancer in a short timeframe; several incidences of suicide; or eating disorders within a teen group. A needs assessment of the faith community also might indicate the need for development of a support group. There are many models that the parish nurse may use as guidance in the development of groups. For example, "I Can Cope" is a program developed by the American Cancer Society that provides a series of educational programs related to cancer. This program can be adapted to meet the needs of individual groups (http://www.cancer.org). If acceptable to the client, an individual referral may be made to existing community groups. It is also important to remember that groups usually have an anticipated "life expectancy." After the needs of the groups are met through education or support, there may no longer be a need for a particular support group. The FCN should document the history of the group and move forward toward new goals.

As an integrator of health and healing, the nurse acknowledges and integrates spirituality as the basis of his or her nursing practice. For example, in teaching a class on healthy aging, the nurse will discuss lifestyle, compliance with prescribed medical treatment, attitudes, and values and their connections to well-being. In a home visit to a terminally ill person, the nurse will explore the meaning of healing versus cure and provide emotional support and encouragement. In certain faith communities, the nurse may lead, or contribute to, healing services as a member of the health ministry team. A basis for successful integration of health and healing in FCN practice is an understanding of spirituality as a foundation for parish nurse practice. The importance of spirituality to FCN practice and health is discussed later in this chapter.

These examples illustrate the diversity and autonomy found in faith community nursing. Depending on the needs of the church community and its members, the roles may be implemented in a variety of ways and through various organizational structures. Some organizational models use volunteer and paid nurses in the role of parish nurse. Hospitals provide parish nurses to community churches through grants, contracts, and public service. Many faith communities have incorporated positions for part-time and full-time nurses within their ministerial teams. Job descriptions and programs vary; examples can be found online at websites for individual parish nurse programs or at the IPNRC website (http://www.ipnrc.parishnurses.org).

EDUCATION OF THE FAITH COMMUNITY NURSE

A baccalaureate-prepared RN with several years of experience in clinical practice is best prepared to implement the roles of the FCN; however, many schools of nursing provide FCN education in baccalaureate prelicensure, RN to BSN (bachelor of science in nursing), and MSN (master of science in nursing) programs. The self-direction and independent decision making required by the autonomous roles of the FCN require a nurse experienced in clinical nursing and community-based nursing practice. The educational preparation of the baccalaureate nurse in community health nursing provides the theoretical basis needed to plan and implement programs for diverse populations in a congregational setting and to function as a beginning member of a pastoral team (IPNRC, 2009a). All FCNs should complete a formal program of study (IPNRC, 2009b; Smith, 2003; Solari-Twadell and McDermott, 1999; Westberg and McNamara, 1990). Universities, hospitals, or FCN programs now offer hundreds of programs that nurses may take for college credit, continuing education, or postgraduate certification. Courses are offered online, in seminars, and in regular classrooms. More than 136 international educational partners offer parish nurse courses. A list of these educational providers can be found on the IPNRC website.

Many universities are incorporating existing certificate programs into advanced nursing degree programs. Programs are generally offered at beginning and advanced levels and consist of approximately 30 contact hours of planned classroom instruction, self-study, or clinical experiences at each level. Box 32-1 provides an example of the curriculum content for a beginning FCN program as suggested by the IPNRC. The curriculum is currently being revised and is expected to be more flexible. The revised curriculum will include incorporation of other topics needed to provide comprehensive nursing care and health promotion for specific faith communities such as disaster management, care of families, and special needs of rural congregations. Andrea West, Nursing Director of the IPNRC, in a communication to FCN educators, described the anticipated changes expected in 2009: "as we look toward the future of parish nursing, the committee felt that limiting the focus only on the functions did not prepare the future parish nurse for this ministry. Therefore, the seven functions of parish nursing have to be broadened into the topics of Spirituality, Professionalism, Wholistic Health, and Community" (personal communication, May 11, 2009).

As faith community nursing programs grow in number and services provided to faith communities, continuing education programs will increase in availability and in diversity of content. The IPNRC conference held annually at the Westberg Symposium in St. Louis, Missouri, provides the greatest opportunity for education and networking among FCNs in the world.

Implementation of the FCN's roles requires the use of the nursing process to plan nursing interventions in wellness and physical, emotional, and spiritual health. Other chapters in this text provide useful information concerning health promotion and planning activities to promote physical and mental health. Spirituality, as a major focus of nursing care, presents different challenges for the nurse.

BOX 32-1   SUGGESTED CORE CURRICULUM CONTENT FOR BEGINNING PARISH NURSE PROGRAM

- Role of the church in health care
- History and philosophy of FCN nursing
- Models of faith community nursing
- Roles and functions of the faith community nurse
- Community assessment and resources
- Health promotion across the life span
- Philosophy of self-care
- Legal and ethical issues related to faith community nursing: confidentiality, accountability, documentation, end-of-life issues, and family violence
- Ministerial team and nursing role
- FCN's role in worship, prayer, and healing
- Starting a FCN program

From International Parish Nurse Resource Center: *Role of parish nurse, mission and resources*, Park Ridge, IL, 2009b, The Author.

THE FAITH COMMUNITY NURSE AND SPIRITUALITY

Westberg (1988) described the ideal FCN as one who is spiritually mature and able to apply spiritual aspects to the health care of congregation members. Many FCNs find the need for further education to develop spiritual assessment skills, acquire theological knowledge, and learn the nurse's role in healing.

Wright (2005) defines spirituality as "the human desire for a sense of meaning, purpose, connection, and fulfillment through intimate relationships and life experiences" (p. xviii). In nursing, spiritual distress is more often the focus of care. The North American Nursing Diagnosis Association (1992) defines spiritual distress as "a disruption in the life principle that pervades a person's entire being and that integrates and transcends one's biological and psychosocial nature" (p. 46). FCNs provide nursing interventions related to the nursing diagnosis as connected to spiritual distress (e.g., loneliness, isolation, and hopelessness). Spirituality is the basis of nursing care in the church setting. The Joint Commission, the International Council of Nursing, and the National Council of State Boards of Nursing and related NCLEX include as important "religious and spiritual influences on health" and include spiritual care as a characteristic in indicators of "quality care" (McEwen, 2005).

There are many models available to help nurses assess the spiritual dimensions of care including the HOPE Model and the JAREL Spiritual Well-Being Scale (McEwen, 2005). The FCN should learn to use a tested model that facilitates his or her practice because knowledge barriers are identified as a major barrier to spiritual nursing care (McEwen, 2005). Schnorr (1988, 2003) suggests the CIRCLE Model of Spiritual Care. This model illustrates the following concepts of care that guide nursing practice and interventions:

C aring
I ntuition
R espect for religious beliefs and practices
C aution
L istening
E motional support

Caring includes caring practices and attitudes. Nurse theorist Jean Watson described caring as "professional, ethical, scientific, esthetic, personalized giving-receiving behaviors that allow for contact between the nurse and client" (quoted in Dossey, 1999, p. 45). Intuition requires acting on instinct, hunches, or "gut feelings." Benner (1984) described intuitive abilities as responses that expert nurses have after several years of experience; these abilities enable the nurse to "read between the lines." Schnorr (1988) described respect as understanding the importance of religious beliefs and practices. The nurse allows time for prayer and sacrament and supports and encourages religious activities. Caution in spiritual care advises the parish nurse to avoid proselytizing or "preaching" religion to clients. The ANA's (2001) *Code of Ethics for Nurses* also provides the nurse with direction to avoid judgments and respect the client's right to self-determination. Listening is a skill that is highly developed in most experienced nurses. It allows an understanding of spoken and unspoken words and feelings, encourages open communication, and supports and empowers patients to communicate needs and desires. Emotional support is the link between the physical and spiritual. Among the emotional interventions, Schnorr (1988) includes working with feelings, showing love, and using appropriate touch and empathy.

Prayer is a commonly used spiritual intervention and can provide comfort and support. Many nurses are not comfortable with sharing individual or group prayer (see **Resource Tool 32A** on the book's website at http://evolve.elsevier.com/Nies/ for guidelines to assist nurses in the development of group prayer sessions). Clients may ask FCNs to offer prayer for healing or recovery. Many faith traditions, such as catholic or Jewish, have traditional prayers that the parish nurse can read or memorize. A guideline to follow is to keep the prayer simple and offer the request to the client's higher power. The nurse may have a poem for healing that is meaningful, which may be also be used. Silence may also be used after a simple prayer, or the nurse may request for the client to offer his or her own prayer. Hickman (2007) suggests that through prayer, spiritual assessment, and hope and faith, the FCN facilitates important client outcomes for spiritual health and well-being, including self-esteem, self-actualization, hope, trust, and peace.

Clinical Example

During a meeting of the health ministry committee, the FCN nurse learned that Mrs. James, a church member, had had end-stage breast cancer diagnosed. Mrs. James is a 45-year-old wife and mother of two school-aged children. She returned home following surgery and had to decide whether to seek further treatment within the following weeks. Her husband attended church with his family although he was a member of another faith community. A home health nurse was involved with Mrs. James' postoperative care, and it was possible that a referral to hospice would occur following her decisions regarding further treatment. The nurse called Mrs. James and offered to make a home visit to assess how the FCN and church community could support and care for the family's well-being. Mrs. James welcomed the visit. Showing respect for their faith beliefs, the nurse offered prayer and waited for a request from the couple. The nurse's instincts and experience working with patients with cancer and their families guided her in using listening as a nursing intervention during this initial visit and in using caution when Mrs. James asked for guidance in making treatment decisions. The nurse further explored the home situation, the needed educational support, and the physician's prognosis and treatment options with the patient. Emotional support was important for Mrs. James, and the FCN offered support through touch and words of concern. This model helped develop an initial nurse-client relationship of trust and open communication.

ISSUES IN FAITH COMMUNITY NURSE PRACTICE

The practice of faith community nursing is affected by many issues common to community health practice, as well as issues specific to parish nursing. Selected issues, which are discussed in this section, include working with vulnerable populations

and the legal and ethical issues of confidentiality and accountability. Other issues identified as important by the IPNRC are end-of-life and family violence issues; these are required content in faith community nursing courses.

Providing Care to Vulnerable Populations

The philosophical foundations of faith communities related to caring, outreach, and support of vulnerable populations place the parish nurse in a position to positively influence the health of diverse groups. Historically, churches have been among the first groups to sponsor and support refugees, develop programs for homeless individuals and families, provide assistance and resources to low-income families, and provide resources to entire communities during disasters (e.g., floods and tornadoes). FCNs are able to provide care for diverse populations using skills in assessment, planning, and interventions.

Boss (1994, 1996, 1999) suggests that parish nurses can be instrumental in helping diverse populations access services; however, nurses should not attempt to meet the populations' many needs alone. She reminds the nurse that in using available health resources, "more is not necessarily better." The nurse in the educator role can assess the needs of vulnerable populations and teach the faith community about the people and their spiritual, emotional, and physical needs. A community of caring that can collectively meet the many needs of vulnerable populations will emerge from the congregation. Boss (1999) called this the Nehemiah approach, which means that people collectively share their talents and desire to do the work. The parish nurse works as a member of a caring church community to meet the health and related needs of vulnerable populations.

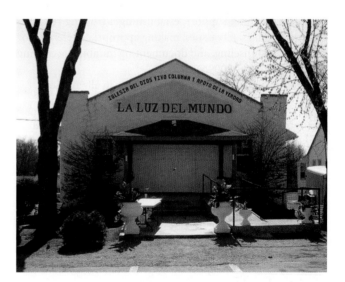

A Hispanic church located in a rural community. Established churches may provide resources for Hispanic populations to form their own churches. The parish nurse may serve an outreach church in addition to the parent church.

End-of-Life Issues: Grief and Loss

Faith communities have long been the first-line provider of support related to loss, grief, and dying. The aging population, increased prevalence in chronic diseases such as HIV and cancer, and public awareness have contributed to the need for improved end-of-life care. FCNs become partners with hospice and home care nurses in providing palliative care to congregation members. The IPNRC suggests that the FCN needs a theoretical base that includes an understanding of grief and loss from a developmental and social perspective, knowledge of manifestations of normal and complicated grief, and nursing interventions to facilitate healthy grieving.

FCN activities related to end-of-life care may include educational sessions on drawing up living wills, establishing health care surrogates, and understanding hospice and palliative care; providing home visits to dying congregational members and emotional support to family and survivors; and developing grief support groups.

Family Violence Prevention

Education and prevention of family violence directly relate to *Healthy People 2020* objectives, and all nurses must be informed in this area (IPNRC, 2009a; Smith, 2003). The FCN must have an understanding of risk factors for family, child, and elder abuse; knowledge of the cycle of abuse; and assessment skills to identify individuals and families at risk for violence. Family violence affects all racial, ethnic, religious, and socioeconomic classes in the United States.

In intimate partner violence (IPV) (also known as domestic abuse, spouse abuse, domestic violence, courtship violence, battering, marital rape, or date rape), it is important to understand that the main issue is an imbalance of power. There are no standard reporting laws (across the United States) related to IPV; however, it is essential that the FCN recognize signs and symptoms of IPV and have an intervention plan that includes providing support, establishing a trusting relationship, discussing safety issues, making appropriate referrals for shelter and counseling, and documenting the abuse according to policy (IPNRC, 2009b).

Child abuse and neglect are reportable in all 50 states.

All 50 States, the District of Columbia, and the U.S. territories have enacted statutes specifying procedures that a mandatory reporter must follow when making a report of child abuse and neglect. Mandatory reporters are individuals who are required by law to report cases of suspected child abuse or neglect. In most States, the statutes require mandatory reporters to make a report immediately upon gaining their knowledge or suspicion of abusive or neglectful situations. In all jurisdictions, the initial report may be made orally to either the child protection services agency or to a law enforcement agency. (U.S. Department of Health and Human Services, 2009)

Nursing interventions for suspected or actual child abuse include the following:
1. Report to the appropriate authority.
2. Provide resources and referrals.
3. Establish a trusting relationship with the child or adolescent.
4. Provide presence.
5. Listen.
6. Document according to policy, law, or both.

The National Research Council Panel on Risk and Prevalence of Elder Abuse and Neglect estimates that between 1 and 2 million people aged 65 years or older are victims of abuse or neglect each year and more than 5 million are victims of financial exploitation (National Center on Elder Abuse, 2009). Elder abuse includes not only physical abuse but also psychological neglect, with or without verbal threats; violation of personal choice or rights; financial theft or misuse of the elder's money; and failing to provide basic needs (food, shelter, clothing, and medical care). The parish nurse or another church volunteer may be the first individual to identify signs and symptoms of elder abuse. The nurse's role may also include educating church volunteers on identifying abuse and making reports and referrals. The nurse must have skill in recognizing symptoms of abuse and must possess assessment or screening questions to identify specific problems. Specific nursing interventions include the following:

1. Recognizing that all states have laws against elder abuse but that reporting varies from state to state so it is important to know state laws
2. Establishing a trusting relationship with the elder and a presence (being with the elder as needed)
3. Providing appropriate referral and resources
4. Documenting the abuse, according to policy, law, or both

⚖ ETHICAL INSIGHTS

Principles of Applied Ethics in a Faith Community

Applied ethics refers to the utilization of ethical principles in real-life situations. The values and beliefs of faith communities raise additional ethical considerations for the parish nurse. Actions of the parish nurse may result in a conflict between established nursing interventions and beliefs of the faith community. The IPNRC (2004) identifies these potential areas of ethical conflict:
- Infertility treatment
- Organ donations
- Blood transfusions
- Proper dress or behavior
- Withdrawal of and withholding nutrition
- DNR (do not resuscitate) orders
- Pro-life versus pro-choice
- Use of advance directives
- Distribution of scarce resources
- Competency for decision making
- Clergy sexual conduct (p. 319)

The FCN's roles include understanding the scope of practice for parish nurses related to ethical practice and the values and beliefs of the community served. The nurse must understand his or her own beliefs and values that are in conflict with the faith community's beliefs. It is necessary that the parish nurse know when to seek help, when to refer, and when to remove himself or herself from the ethical decision-making process (O'Brien, 2003).

Confidentiality

The *Code of Ethics for Nurses* (ANA, 2001 and the *Scope and Standards of Faith Community Nursing Practice* (Health Ministries Association and ANA, 2005) provide ethical guidance to parish nurses. Parish nurses are accountable to state boards of nursing, employing agencies (i.e., including churches), and the faith communities they serve. Many ethical and legal issues are generic to clinical practice settings; however, confidentiality issues have the potential to be problematic in a church community.

Concerned church members may identify individuals in need and refer them to the parish nurse. In the role of health minister, the parish nurse may receive private and sensitive information. The nurse does not act in the role of minister or priest. Congregation members should not relate information in the form of confession or repentance; however, the connection with the church ministry team may put the nurse in a position to hear this type of sensitive information.

The nurse should protect clients' rights to confidentiality in relation to information concerning their health or health-related condition. Although the nurse must share information with the church minister in certain instances, the nurse should share confidential information with other church ministry leaders (or prayer groups) only when given permission by the client. Exceptions are found in religious sects or congregations that require the public confession of members' behaviors or conditions so that members may benefit from divine intervention and forgiveness. As a care provider, the parish nurse should be aware of these rituals and practices before counseling members of the faith community (Fowler, 1999). General guidelines for medical record management should be followed by the FCN. Policies and procedures for managing and storing records and sharing and requesting medical information must be established. FCN programs within faith communities generally are not required to follow Health Insurance Portability and Accountability Act (HIPAA) guidelines related to medical records and confidentiality because churches are not in the category of identified health care providers. An exception is parish nurse services provided by a licensed health care provider such as a hospital; in this instance, HIPAA regulations do apply (IPNRC, 2009b).

Accountability

Sister Mary Angela Shaughnessy (1998) provides direction for the FCN by listing the following information related to church law:

1. Volunteers in a church are held to the same degree of accountability as are paid employees.
2. The doctrine of separation of church and state does not exempt churches from discrimination laws.
3. Ministers, both ordained and nonordained, may be required to disclose confidential information in court.

As volunteers or paid employees, nurses are accountable to the nursing standards and civil laws designed to protect individuals from abuse, neglect, and discrimination. FCNs, as nonordained ministers, do not have client-professional privileges and should be aware of appropriate standards in documenting provided services. In documenting parish nurse services, "less is better." Many churches may not have the facilities to store medical records in a secure locked area. In this instance the nurse should have a file storage system that locks and can be kept in a secure location. Simple records of blood pressure screenings or health education programs could include only numbers of attendees or blood pressure results categorized by American Heart Association standards as hypertensive, borderline, or normal. Also included in the documentation could be numbers of individuals referred for services. Faith community governing boards or committees need not have the names of individual clients but will be interested in the type of services and numbers of clients served. Individual client services will require a nurse's note or assessment and development of a nursing care plan. Prior to beginning an FCN program, the nurse should develop and follow general policies and guidelines for record keeping and storage. Shaughnessy (1998) provides further information related to contract law. The handbooks, brochures, or programs that church-related institutions offer are contracts. The FCN should ensure that health information is current and based on accepted practices and standards. These suggestions are not intended to limit the parish nurse's creativity or scope; rather, they emphasize that the professional nurse is accountable for his or her practice in any role.

CASE STUDY   APPLICATION OF THE NURSING PROCESS

Nancy Elliot, an FCN at Living Hope Baptist Church, recently completed a needs assessment of her faith community of 200 families. Nancy is new to the FCN role, having recently been hired. Living Hope, considered to be a moderate-sized church, is located in a rural community of 40,000. Nancy decided to complete the needs assessment of the congregation and community prior to planning programs and services for the faith community.

Assessment

The community has one hospital and a variety of voluntary and official community agencies. Many private practitioners are available, either in the town or within a 1-hour drive of a larger city. Recently the city was awarded a grant to develop community parks and recreational facilities. Nancy is surprised by the demographic picture she finds following completion of the assessment. Young families with toddlers to young school-aged children comprise more

than 70% of the congregation. She notes that these families are in the childbearing developmental stage of family growth and development. The remaining 30% of the members are elders with more than half being 80 years of age or older. The survey indicates that the members are most interested in health screening and educational opportunities presented at the church. Only 3% of the members reported having no health insurance.

A discussion with the minister provides additional information. Two new industries have recently relocated to the area. The parent home of both of these industries was formerly located in distant states. Many new members have relocated to the area. Nancy understands that these young families may have decreased family and social support and little knowledge of existing community resources. The minister also identifies that the current church ministries focus on the elderly members and that new services are needed. Nancy schedules a meeting with the

CASE STUDY APPLICATION OF THE NURSING PROCESS—cont'd

young parents following a church social gathering. Fifty mothers and fathers attend the session to discuss the health-related needs of the families. They identify that a "mother's-day-out" program is a priority and also request information on community resources, parenting classes, and health and wellness programs for the children and parents. On the basis of the needs assessment and sessions with the parents, the FCN identifies the following goals, nursing diagnoses, and population-focused nursing interventions.

Diagnosis
Individual
- Health-seeking behaviors, as evidenced by requests for health information related to parenting, health, and wellness
- Risk for altered parenting, as evidenced by developmental stage of families, requests for education, and presence of new community members with limited knowledge of community resources
- Risk for social isolation and role strain, as evidenced by individual concerns related to limited social support and lack of social networks

Family
- Delayed growth and development, related to stage of family development
- Risk for disabled family coping, related to recent relocation to new community and lack of social network

Community (Faith Community)
- Ineffective community coping, related to recent change in membership demographics, lack of developed resources, and new or developing FCN role

Planning
A plan of care is developed to address the needs of the individuals, families, and the Living Hope faith community. Goals suggested by the FCN are mutually agreed upon by the ministerial team and congregational members.

Individual
Long-Term Goals
- Monthly educational programs will be offered addressing current issues in parenting and health and wellness of young families.
- Congregation will establish a social network for young parents.
- Ministerial leaders will dedicate funds to increase resources for children and young adults.

Short-Term Goals
- Establish parent steering committee for educational program ideas, identification of parent talents (assist with education programs).
- Explore development of parents'-day-out program.

Family
Long-Term Goals
- Parent members will report increased social networks.
- Parent members will identify adequate resources to support growing family.

Short-Term Goal
- Identify community and congregation support for new and growing families.

Community (Faith Community)
Long-Term Goal
- Programs will be established to support growing families.

Short-Term Goal
- Implement one new program (educational, social) or resource for families each quarter of the church year.

Interventions
Nancy utilizes diverse interventions to meet the goals established for families of Living Hope.

Individual
Nancy asked the parents (men and women) to complete a talent survey to identify the resources available within the families of Living Hope. From this survey, Nancy identified two RNs willing to help provide educational programs and three previously certified early childhood teachers. The teachers were willing to develop a committee to explore the development of a mother's-day-out program, a playgroup, and a new parent support group. Additional members were willing to begin a ministry to provide meals to new parents. Community resources were identified at the local health department to help teach parenting classes and provide immunizations. A plan was established to begin the mother's-day-out program part-time within 2 months. The playgroup and educational programs were implemented immediately.

Family
The ministerial team and a parent advisory group were formed to identify family needs. Family social events were planned, including a church picnic. Planning was made for age-appropriate activities such as the development of a soccer team for the youth, a softball team for the young adults, and a literary club for those interested. The advisory committee developed a budget to submit to the ministerial team requesting financial support to develop a playground for the children attending the mother's-day-out program and the hiring of a part-time employee to supervise the related activities. The families reported increased feelings of support from the faith community, increased social support and networks, and a feeling of belonging to the greater community.

Community (Faith Community)
The faith community developed a budget to support individual and family requests. Monthly health education programs became the standard, with topics noted on the monthly calendar. Members reported increased feelings of "community" not only among the young families but also across generational lines, as new members increasingly participated in leadership roles within the congregation. The minister has documented an increase in weekly attendance, which had a positive impact on the long-range goals identified by the congregational members.

Evaluation
Individual and Family
Attendance at the health and wellness and parenting sessions increased with each educational session offered. Initial attendance was five to seven people for each session, and after 6 months the average attendance was fifteen to twenty people for each session. The request from attendees changed from offering additional educational sessions to planning intervention programs such as a yoga class and a weight reduction program. The playground was completed in less than the planned time because of the increased budget. The mother's-day-out program, which began as a part-time,

Continued

3-day per week program, grew to a Monday-through-Friday program within 12 months. The program became self-sufficient by the end of the year because of established fees, parent volunteers, and donations. Men and women verbalized an increased satisfaction with their spiritual growth and support from the faith community. Nancy developed a health ministry committee of volunteers from within the church and was able to increase the number and variety of related parish nurse activities.

Community (Faith Community)
The health and wellness activities attracted the attention of sister churches, and a grant was offered to increase the number of family support services and wellness programs offered within the church. Health and wellness programs were expanded to include additional methods for reaching congregational members, such as through a website. The increased attendance and participation of congregational members positively affected all members, who benefited from the leadership and positive environment. The educational offerings and intervention programs were developed based on *Healthy People 2020* goals, in particular increasing activity and exercise, healthy eating, and obesity prevention (USDHHS, 2009).

Levels of Prevention
The roles of the FCN direct the interventions and programs planned for faith communities. The following are examples of all three levels of prevention applied to this case study.

Primary
- Assessment and teaching about parenting, health, and wellness
- Development of programs and social support systems to prevent social isolation and increase resources for successful parenting and healthy behaviors

Secondary
- FCN assessment and screening to identify individuals and families at risk
- Congregational resources and educational programs developed to meet individual and family needs

Tertiary
- FCN provides, or refers to, resources for rehabilitation, for families coping with children with disabilities or chronic health problems (parents and children).

SUMMARY

This chapter provided an overview of the FCN's role in providing nursing care for faith communities, and it explored the historical and philosophical foundations of the modern FCN practice. Traditional roles of the nurse are used in unique ways to allow the FCN to provide nursing care to church communities. The FCN's role in the development of spiritual health and well-being becomes significant and requires the nurse to focus on the spiritual needs of congregation members. The CIRCLE model for planning spiritual nursing may be used to guide nursing interventions. Faith community nursing offers new opportunities for increasing the health and wellness of clients and requires the nurse to refocus skills and knowledge.

Many educational programs are available throughout the United States to provide FCN education after basic nursing education. These programs are offered as continuing education and through formal university courses as part of degree programs. Church law, nursing ethics, and standards are the basis for the legal and ethical FCN practice. As a relatively new area of community health nurse practice, FCN offers the RN many opportunities to improve the health of faith communities through a holistic nursing practice that connects the body, mind, and spirit in the celebration of health and healing.

LEARNING ACTIVITIES

1. Speak with an FCN in the community. Ask the nurse about congregational health needs and discuss how the roles of the parish nurse are implemented through the parish nurse programs and ministry. Observe the nurse in his or her daily activities and identify how spirituality is a basis for parish nursing care.
2. Speak with a minister, priest, rabbi, or church leader in the community from a faith belief system different from your own. Explore the philosophical basis for the church's role in health and healing.
3. Visit websites devoted to faith community nursing and identify the models of FCN programs or read the descriptions of their practice. Share these with the clinical group.

REFERENCES

American Nurses Association: *Code of ethics for nurses with interpretive statements*, Washington, DC, 2001, The Author.
Benner P: *From novice to expert*, Menlo Park, CA, 1984, Addison-Wesley.
Boss J: Being a professional caregiver can be dangerous to your health, *Health Dev* 4:10–14, 1994.
Boss J: Lesson learned over time: great teachers—St. Francis, St. Clare, and Eleanor, *Health Dev* 2:7–19, 1996.
Boss J: Parish nursing with underorganized, underserved, and marginalized clients. In Solari-Twadell PA, McDermott MA, editors: *Parish nursing: promoting whole persons health within faith communities*, Thousand Oaks, CA, 1999, Sage.
Clemon-Stone S, McGuire S, Eigsti D: *Comprehensive community health nursing*, ed 6, St. Louis, 2002, Mosby.
Dossey MD: *Dynamics of healing and the transpersonal self*. In Dossey MD et al, editors: *Holistic nursing: a handbook for practice*, Gaithersburg, MD, 1999, Aspen.
Eckersley RM: Culture, spirituality, religion and health: looking at the big picture, *Med J Aust* 186(Suppl 10):S54–S56, 2007.
Fowler M: Ethics as a context for the practice. In Solari-Twadell PA, McDermott MA, editors: *Parish nursing: promoting whole persons health within faith communities*, Thousand Oaks, Calif, 1999, Sage.
Health Ministries Association and American Nurses Association: *Faith community nursing: scope & standards*, Washington, DC, 2005, American Nurses Association.
Hickman JS: *Faith community nursing*, Philadelphia, 2007, Lippincott Williams & Wilkins.

Interfaith Health Program: *Strong partners: interfaith health program*, Atlanta, GA, 2005, Emory University: www.ihpnet.org.

International Parish Nurse Resource Center: *Basic parish nurse preparation curriculum*, St. Louis, 2004, Deaconess Parish Nurse Ministries.

International Parish Nurse Resource Center: Get my people going! Parish Nurse Perspectives 7:2, 2008.

International Parish Nurse Resource Center: *Role of parish nurse, mission and resources*, Park Ridge, IL, 2009a, The Author.

International Parish Nurse Resource Center: *International parish nursing*, St Louis, MO, 2009b, The Author.

King MA, Tessaro I: Parish nursing: promoting health lifestyles in the church. 26(1):22–24, 2009.

Koenig HG, George L: Religion, spirituality, and health in hospitalized older patients, *J Am Geriatr Soc* 52A:532–541, 2004.

Maginnis and Associates: *Combining health care and theology: the parish nurse, Maginnis Communique*, Louisville, KY, 1993, The Author.

McEwen M: Spiritual nursing care, *Holistic Nursing Practice* 19:161–168, 2005.

McGinnis DL: The emerging role of faith community nurses in prevention & management of chronic disease, *Policy Polit Nurs Pract* 9(3):173–180, 2008.

Myers DG: Stress and health: spirituality and faith communities. In Myers DG, editor: *Stress and health, psychology*, ed 7, New York, 2004, Worth Publishers.

National Center on Elder Abuse, US Administration on Aging: 2009, www.ncea.aoa.gov/ncearoot/Main_Site/pdf/publication/FinalStatistics050331.pdf.

North American Nursing Diagnosis Association: *NANDA nursing diagnosis: Definitions and defining characteristics*. Philadelphia, 1992, The Author.

O'Brien ME: *Parish nursing: healthcare ministry within the church*, Sudbury, MA, 2003, Jones and Bartlett.

Patterson D: Parish nursing: a beneficial partner for clergy, *The Clergy Journal* 32–33, 2004.

Schnorr MA: *Spiritual nursing care: theory and curriculum development*, Doctoral dissertation, 1988, Northern Illinois University, Dissert Abstr Int 50:601-A, DA8912525.

Schnorr MA: *Parish nurse pedagogy or andragogy Proceedings of the 17th Annual Westberg Parish Nurse Symposium*, St Louis, MO, 2003, International Parish Nurse Resource Center.

Shaughnessy MA: *Ministry and the law: what you need to know*, New York, 1998, Paulist Press.

Smith SD: *Parish nursing: a handbook for the new millennium*, New York, 2003, Haworth Pastoral Press.

Solari-Twadell PA, McDermott MA: *Parish nursing: promoting whole person health within faith communities*, Thousand Oaks, CA, 1999, Sage.

Tsuang MT, Williams WM, Lyons MJ: Pilot study of spiritual and mental health in twins, *Am J Psychiatry* 159:486–488, 2002.

U.S. Department of Health and Human Services: *Healthy people 2010*, Washington, DC, 2000, Government Printing Office, www.healthypeople.gov.

U.S. Department of Health and Human Services. Children's Bureau, Division of Children and Families: *Child welfare gateway*, Washington, DC, 2009, The Author, www.childwelfare.gov/.

Wesley J: On visiting the sick, 1786. In Outler AC, editor: *The works of John Wesley*, Nashville, TN, 1986, Abingdon.

Westberg G: *The parish nurse: Providing a minister of health for your congregation*, Minneapolis, 1990, Augsburg.

Westberg G: Parishes, nurses, and health care, *Lutheran Partners*: 34–36, 1988.

Westberg G: A personal historical perspective of whole person health and the congregation. In Williams DR, Sternthal MJ, editors: Spirituality, religion and health: evidence and research directions, *Med J Aust*, 186, (10 Suppl): S47–S50, 2007.

Westberg G, McNamara JW: *The parish nurse: providing a minister of health for your congregation*, Minneapolis, MN, 1990, Augsburg Fortress.

Williams DR, Sternthal MJ: Spirituality, religion and health: evidence and research directions, *Med J Aust* 186(Suppl 10): S47–S50, 2007.

Wright LM: *Spirituality, suffering and illness*, Philadelphia, 2005, FA Davis.

Home Health and Hospice

Carrie L. Abele, Mary A. Nies

Additional Material for Study, Review, and Further Exploration

evolve WEBSITE

http://evolve.elsevier.com/Nies
- Quiz
- Case Studies
- Glossary
- WebLinks

OBJECTIVES

Upon completion of this chapter, the reader will be able to do the following:

1. Discuss the purpose of home health services.
2. Define home health care.
3. Differentiate between the purpose of a public health nursing visit and that of a home health and hospice nursing visit.
4. Use the nursing process in outlining the steps involved in conducting a home visit.
5. Identify the types of home health agencies.
6. Apply the nursing process to a home health client situation.

KEY TERMS

advance directive
durable power of attorney

home health care
living will

OUTLINE

♥ **HEALTHY PEOPLE 2020**

2010 Objectives for Home Health and Hospice Care

- MICH HP2020 – 14 – Increase the proportion of children with special health care needs who receive their care in family-centered, comprehensive, coordinated systems.
- MICH HP2020 – 24 – Increase the percentage of women giving birth who attend a postpartum care visit with a health worker.
- OA – HP2020 – 2 – Reduce the proportion of unpaid caregivers of older adults who report an unmet need for caregiver support services.
- OA – HP2020 – 4 – Reduce the proportion of non-institutionalized older adults with disabilities who have an unmet need for long-term services and supports.

USDHHS Health People 2020 Draft Objectives. 2009. http://www.healthypeople.gov/hp2020/Objectives/files/Draft2009Objectives.pdf.

The purpose of home health services is to provide nursing care to individuals and their families in their homes. The specific objectives and services nurses offer vary depending on the type of agency providing services and the population served. Nurses who work for public health departments, visiting nurse associations, home health agencies, hospice agencies, or school districts usually provide home visits.

Nurses from clinics or health departments often conduct home visits as part of patient follow-up. These public health nurses make visits to follow patients with communicable diseases and provide health education and community referrals to patients with identified health problems. Home health nurses who work for home health agencies, which are affiliated with hospitals or nursing registries, often make home visits to assist patients in their transition from the hospital to home. In addition, health care providers in private practice may order these visits when patients experience exacerbation of chronic conditions.

The focus of all home visits is on the individual for whom the referral is received. In addition, the nurse assesses the individual-family interaction and provides education and interventions for the family and the client. The nurse evaluates how the individual and family interact as part of an aggregate group in the community. The nurse identifies the need for referrals to community services and performs the referrals as necessary.

Nurses who make home visits receive referrals from a variety of sources, including the patient's physician, nurse practitioner or nurse midwife, hospital discharge planner or case manager, schoolteacher, or clinic health care provider. The patient or the patient's family can also originate requests for nursing visits to assess and assist in the client's health care.

Home visits have been an integral part of nursing for more than a century, originating with Florence Nightingale's "health nurses" in England. In the United States in 1877, the Women's Branch of the New York City Mission sent the first trained nurses into the homes of the poor to provide nursing care. Under the direction of Lillian Wald, pioneering efforts were initiated to provide services to the poor in their homes in the late nineteenth century (Kelly and Joel, 1995).

HOME HEALTH CARE

The term *home health care* describes a system in which health care and social services are provided to homebound or disabled people in their homes rather than in medical facilities (U.S. Department of Commerce and International Trade Administration, 1990). The U.S. Department of Health and Human Services (USDHHS) set forth a definition of home health care that an interdepartmental work group developed, which follows:

Home health care is that component of a continuum of comprehensive health care whereby health services are provided to individuals and families in their places of residence for the purpose of promoting, maintaining or restoring health, or maximizing the level of independence, while minimizing the effects of disability and illness, including terminal illness. Services appropriate to the needs of the individual patient and family are planned, coordinated, and made available by providers organized for the delivery of home care through the use of employed staff, contractual arrangements, or combination of the two patterns. (Warhola, 1980)

Purpose of Home Health Services

The primary purpose of home health services is to allow individuals to remain at home and receive health care services that would otherwise be offered in a health care institution such as a hospital or nursing home setting. The home health industry grew tremendously in the 1980s but began to decline in the 1990s related to changes in Medicare home health reimbursement. However, with the development of the home health prospective payment system (PPS), the number of home care agencies has increased since 2001 (National Association for Home Care and Hospice [NAHC], 2008). Numerous factors generated the growth of home health services, including the increasing costs of hospital care and the subsequent introduction of the PPS by P.L. 98-21 of the Social Security Amendments in 1983. Under the PPS, hospitals receive a fixed amount of money based on the relative cost of resources used to treat Medicare patients within each type of diagnosis-related group (Guterman and Dobson, 1986). Moreover, many other third-party payers negotiate preferred provider programs or managed care systems. In a managed care arrangement, the health care provider is paid a set fee for providing care to clients enrolled in the program. Providing home care services contributes to cost containment in a managed care environment. This cost containment is accomplished through timely hospital discharges by providing nursing services in the home setting and supporting clients at home rather than in skilled facilities. Home care is also popular with consumers, who prefer to receive care in their own homes rather than in an institution.

Home health care services have changed to address the needs of the population. Home health nurses visit acutely ill clients, patients with acquired immunodeficiency syndrome, the elderly, terminally ill clients, high-risk pregnant women, and ill infants and children (Feldman, 1993). Home health care continues to focus on the care of sick patients and could expand to include health promotion and disease prevention interventions. Currently, most reimbursement for nursing services is based on the patient's need for skilled nursing. On each patient visit, the nurse must document that the care provided is of a skilled nature that requires the knowledge and assessment skills of a nurse and must verify that the patient or a family member could not provide the same level of care.

Services coordinated in the home include not only skilled nursing care provided by registered nurses (RNs), but also the services of physical, occupational, and speech therapists; social workers; and home health aides. The broader home care industry definition of home health care includes supportive social services, respite care, community nursing centers, group boarding homes, homeless shelters, adult day care, intermediate skilled extended care facilities, and assisted living facilities (American Nurses Association [ANA], 2008).

TYPES OF HOME HEALTH AGENCIES

Home health agencies differ in their financial structures, organizational structures, governing boards, and populations served. The most common types of home health agencies are official (i.e., public), nonprofit, proprietary, chains, and hospital-based agencies. The number of freestanding proprietary agencies has grown faster than any other type of Medicare-certified home health agency. Freestanding proprietary agencies now comprise 56% of all home health agencies, and hospital-based agencies comprise 18% of all certified home health agencies (NAHC, 2008).

There continues to be an increase in the number of managed care agencies, which may have any type of financial structure. Managed care agencies contract with payers, such as insurance companies, to provide specified services to the enrolled clients at a predetermined price. Managed care agencies receive payment before offering services and are responsible for taking the financial risk of providing care to patients within the budgeted allotment. This works well with large numbers of enrolled clients, where the financial risk is spread across a larger number of people, many of whom are healthy and will not require skilled services.

Official Agencies

Local or state governments organize, operate, and fund official (i.e., public) home health agencies. These agencies may be part of a county public health nursing service or a home health agency that operates separately from the public health nursing service but is located within the county public health system. Taxpayers fund official home health agencies, but they also receive reimbursement from third-party payers such as Medicare, Medicaid, and private insurance companies.

Nonprofit Agencies

Nonprofit home health agencies include all home health agencies that are not required to pay federal taxes because of their exempt tax status. Nonprofit groups reinvest any profits into the agency. Nonprofit home health agencies include independent home health agencies or hospital-based home health agencies. Not all hospital-based home health agencies are nonprofit, even if the hospital is nonprofit. The home health agency can be established as a profit-generating service and serve as a source of revenue for the hospital or medical center. In this situation, the home health agency is categorized organizationally as for-profit and it pays federal taxes on the profits.

Proprietary Agencies

Proprietary home health agencies are classified for-profit and pay federal taxes on the profits generated. Proprietary agencies can be individual-owned agencies, profit partnerships, or profit corporations. Providing the agencies make a profit, investors in corporate proprietary partnerships receive financial returns on their investments in the agencies. A percentage of the profits generated are also reinvested into the agency.

Chains

A growing number of home health agencies are owned and operated by corporate chains. These chains are usually classified as proprietary agencies and may be part of a proprietary hospital chain. Agencies within chains have a financial advantage over single agencies. The chains have lower administrative costs because a larger single corporate structure provides many services. For example, a multiagency corporation has greater purchasing power for supplies and equipment because it purchases a larger volume. A single corporate office can provide administrative services such as payroll and employee benefits for all chain employees, thereby reducing duplication of these services. Criticism of proprietary and chain agencies includes concerns over the quality of agency services that are profit driven.

Hospital-Based Agencies

Since the implementation of PPS in 1983, the number of hospital-based home health agencies has significantly increased (NAHC, 2008). This trend is not surprising in light of the fixed reimbursement under PPS and the hospitals' incentive to decrease length of stay. By establishing home health agencies, hospitals are able to discharge patients who have skilled health care needs, provide the necessary services to the patient, and receive reimbursement through third-party payers such as Medicare, Medicaid, and private insurance companies. The increasing number of home health agencies indicates that these agencies are profitable endeavors and provide hospitals with an additional revenue source.

CERTIFIED AND NONCERTIFIED AGENCIES

Certified home health agencies meet federal standards; therefore they are able to receive Medicare payments for services provided to eligible individuals. Not all home health agencies are certified. The number of Medicare-certified home health agencies increased to approximately 10,444 in 1997, decreased to 6861 in 2001, and increased to 9284 in 2007 (NAHC, 2008).

The noncertified home care agencies, home care aide organizations, and hospices remain outside the Medicare system. Some operate outside the system because they provide non–Medicare-covered services. For example, they do not provide skilled nursing care and are not eligible to receive Medicare reimbursement.

SPECIAL HOME HEALTH PROGRAMS

Many home health agencies offer special, high-technological home care services. Offering high-tech services at home is both beneficial to the patient's health and financially advantageous. Through the implementation of these special programs, patients who require continuous skilled care in an acute or skilled nursing institution are able to return to their homes and receive care at home. From the financial perspective, skilled services provided at home are less costly than hospitalization.

Examples of special services include home intravenous therapy programs for patients who require daily infusions of total parenteral nutrition or antibiotic therapy, pediatric services for children with chronic health problems, follow-up for premature infants who are at risk for complications, ventilator therapy, and home dialysis programs. The key to the success of all these programs is the patient's, family's, or caregiver's ability to learn the care necessary for a successful home program and the motivation of these individuals to provide the care. If family or caregiver support is not available in the home, the patient cannot be a candidate for any of these programs and other arrangements for care must be found.

REIMBURSEMENT FOR HOME CARE

Before the establishment of Medicare in 1965, individuals who required home health services paid cash for the services; donations to the service agency providers helped subsidize care services for patients who were unable to pay (Kent and Hanley, 1990). Since 1965, individuals who are eligible for Medicare benefits under Title XVIII of the Social Security Act or for Medicaid benefits under Title XIX and people with private health insurance are reimbursed by the federal government through the Medicare program to receive short-term, skilled health care services in their homes. Provided services include nursing care, social service, physical therapy, occupational therapy, and speech therapy, and the program is individualized to meet the patient's needs.

Any individual over 65 years old who is homebound, under the care of a physician, and requires medically necessary skilled nursing care or therapy services may be eligible for home care through a Medicare-certified home health agency. These services must be intermittent or part-time and require physician authorization and periodic review of the plan of care. The only exception is hospice care. Any individual over 65 years old who is terminally ill with a life expectancy of 6 months certified by a physician is eligible to receive the Medicare Hospice Benefit. There is no requirement for the individual to be homebound or in need of skilled care or

for the services to be intermittent or part-time. The physician must recertify the patient every 6 months to determine whether he or she is still eligible for hospice care (NAHC, 1996).

The rapid growth of the home health market is reflective of the following:
- Increasing proportion of people aged 65 years and older
- Lower average cost of home health care compared with institutional costs ($750 per month for routine skilled nursing care at home compared with $2000 for care in an institution)
- Active insurer support for home care
- Medicare promotion of home health care as an alternative to institutionalization

Patient or family payments comprised 46% of the private financing (12% of total spending) for home health services. Private health insurance and nonpatient revenue paid the remaining private financing.

Between 1967 and 1985, the number of home health agencies certified to provide care to Medicare recipients tripled from 1753 to 5983. In the mid-1980s, this number leveled off at 5900 resulting from an increase in the volume of paperwork required and unreliable payment policies. This led to a lawsuit against the HCFA charged by Representatives Harley Staggers (D-WV) and Claude Pepper (D-FL), and a coalition of members of the U.S. Congress, consumer groups, and the NAHC. The successful conclusion of the lawsuit gave NAHC the opportunity to participate in rewriting the Medicare home care payment policies. New payment policies brought an increase in the home health benefit and increased the number of Medicare-certified home health agencies to more than 10,000. The number is now declining as a direct result of the changes in Medicare home health reimbursement enacted as part of the Balanced Budget Act of 1997. However, because of this decline, the Centers for Medicare and Medicaid Services (CMS) enacted a new payment system where home care agencies are reimbursed on a prospective payment system based on the patient's diagnosis. The amount provided to home health agencies is determined on the basis of the average national cost of treating a home health client for 60 days. The goal of this system is to encourage efficient use of home health services without sacrificing quality (NAHC, 2008).

OASIS

The Outcome and Assessment Information Set (OASIS) is a data set that measures outcomes of adult home care patients to monitor outcome-based quality improvement. The data set includes sociodemographic, environmental, support system, health status, and functional status attributes of adult patients, as well as information about service utilization. These items are used to monitor outcomes, plan patient care, provide reports on patient characteristics for each agency, and evaluate and improve clinical performance. The use of OASIS is mandatory for all Medicare and Medicaid patients receiving skilled care (CMS, 2008).

NURSING STANDARDS AND EDUCATIONAL PREPARATION OF HOME HEALTH NURSES

The ANA (2008) has revised its standards for home health nursing practice. According to the ANA, the generalist home care nurse should be educated at the baccalaureate level because of the autonomy and critical thinking skills that are necessary in home care. The generalist home health nurse must have community health assessment skills to assess client and caregiver needs, provide client and caregiver education, perform nursing actions following the client's plan of care, manage resources to facilitate the best possible outcomes, provide and monitor care, collaborate with other disciplines and providers to coordinate client care, and supervise ancillary staff and caregivers. The responsibilities of the generalist home health nurse include, but are not limited to, performing holistic, periodic assessments of client and family/caregiver resources; participating in performance improvement activities; collecting and using research findings to evaluate the plan of care; educating clients and families on health promotion and self-care activities; being a client advocate; promoting continuity of care; using the *Scope and Standards of Home Health Nursing Practice* to guide clinical practice; and identifying ethical issues and exploring options with the necessary individuals and staff members to achieve resolution (ANA, 2008).

The advanced practice home health nurse has a master's or doctoral degree in nursing and can perform all of the duties of the generalist home health nurse. In addition, the advanced practice nurse contributes significant clinical expertise to home health patients and their families, demonstrates proficiency in care management and consultation, and is an expert in implementing and evaluating health programs, resources, services, and research for clients with complex conditions. The duties of the advanced practice home health nurse include, but are not limited to, prescribing pharmacological and nonpharmacological treatment to manage chronic illnesses, providing consultation and serving as a resource to the generalist home health nurse, participating at all levels of quality improvement and research, educating all members of the health care team about emerging trends in home health care, performing direct care of the client and family, managing and evaluating the care the client is receiving from caregivers, monitoring trends in reimbursement for home health services, consulting with staff about any ethical issues that may arise, managing an interdisciplinary team, and disseminating practice and research findings to colleagues (ANA, 2008).

Albrecht's conceptual model (1990) for home care clearly identifies educational content areas for students in undergraduate and graduate nursing programs that have specialties in home health care. An underlying premise of the model is that professional satisfaction and effective patient outcomes depend on the education and experience of the home health nurse. Implications that are apparent in the model include the following:

- Nursing programs at the undergraduate and graduate levels must prepare competent providers of home health care.

- Curricula must include concepts related to the suprasystem, health service delivery system, and home subsystem, which includes structural, process, and outcome elements.
- Students at the undergraduate level need at least one clinical observation or experience in a home care agency.
- Graduate-level students need specific courses that cover concepts present in the model, including knowledge of education; preventive, supportive, therapeutic, and high-tech nursing interventions for home health care; a multidisciplinary approach to home health care; health law and ethics; systems theory; economics covering supply, demand, and productivity; and case management and coordination (Albrecht, 1990, p. 125).

The home health nurse serves as a case manager for patients who receive care from the staff of the home health agency or receive care through contract services. The success of the case management plan is contingent upon the nurse's ability to use the nursing process to develop a plan of treatment that best fits the individual needs of the patient, the patient's family, or the caregiver. Patient and family assessment is the first step in developing the treatment plan and nursing care plan.

The Albrecht nursing model for home health care (Figure 33-1) provides a framework for nurses, patients, and their families to interact and identify mutual goals of interventions and promote the patient's self-care capability at home (Albrecht, 1990). Three major elements for measuring the quality of home health care patient outcomes include structural, process, and outcome elements.

Structural elements include the client, family, provider agency, health team, and professional nurse. The process elements include the type of care, coordination of care, and intervention. Outcome elements consist of patient and family satisfaction with care, quality of care, cost-effectiveness of care, health status, and self-care capability.

In the Albrecht model for home care, the relationship between the structural elements and the process elements directs the interventions. The nurse executes the nursing process, including assessment, nursing diagnosis, planning, intervention, and evaluation, and then the nurse coordinates patient care (Albrecht, 1990).

CONDUCTING A HOME VISIT

Visit Preparation

It is important that the nurse prepare for the home visit by reviewing the referral form including the purpose of the visit, the geographic residence of the family, and any other pertinent information. The first home visit gives the nurse the opportunity to establish a trust relationship with the client and family to establish credibility as a resource for health information and community referrals in a nonthreatening environment.

The Referral

The referral (Figure 33-2) is a formal request for a home visit. Referrals come from a variety of sources including hospitals,

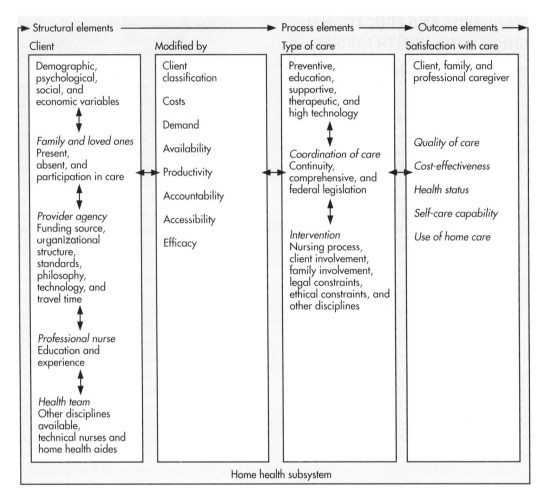

FIGURE 33-1 Albrecht nursing model for home health care. (Based on Albrecht MN: The Albrecht model for home health care: implications for research, practice, and education, *Public Health Nurs* 7:118-126, 1990. Reprinted by permission of Blackwell Scientific Publications, Inc.).

clinics, health care providers, individuals, and families. The type of agency that receives the referral will vary depending on the necessary client services. Public health referrals are made for clients who are in need of health education (e.g., infant care education and resource allocation) or for follow-up of clients with communicable diseases.

Home health referrals are requested to provide clients with short-term, intermittent, skilled services and rehabilitation. Visits can last from 30 to 90 minutes and are scheduled on an intermittent basis depending on the specific needs of the client. For example, a client who had a stroke requires skilled nursing assessments, physical therapy visits for gait training, speech therapy for speech deficit improvement, and occupational therapy for retraining in activities of daily living (ADL) such as bathing and cooking.

By reviewing the referral form before the first visit, the community health nurse (CHN), which includes the home health nurse and the public health nurse, obtains basic information about the client such as name, age, diagnosis or health status, address, telephone number, insurance coverage, and reason for the referral. The form also specifies the source of the referral such as a clinician, health care provider, communicable disease service, hospital, client, or client's family.

Public health referrals usually provide information on the client's condition that necessitates public health nurse (PHN) visits. For example, for a client who is positive for tuberculosis (TB), the PHN is notified of the client's place of residence, type and location of employment, and any known contacts, including family and friends. Another example of a public health referral is a 16-year-old girl who is referred for antepartum visits because she is 7 months' pregnant and has just initiated prenatal care.

Additional information provided in the home health referral includes current client medications, prescribed diet, physician's orders, care plan goals, and other disciplines involved in the client's care. This information is important because it helps the nurse become familiar with the client's condition.

Initial Telephone Contact

The nurse contacts the client and informs him or her about the service referral. The first telephone contact with the client or family consists of an exchange of essential information, including an introduction by the nurse, identification of the agency that received the referral, and the purpose of the visit. After the initial exchange of information, the nurse informs the client of his or her desire to make the home visit, the client

Patient number	☐ New ☐ Readmit	**Intake**	Date last seen by MD	Case manager

Name: Last   First   M.I. | Telephone no.: | Sex M F | Birthdate | Age | Date of first visit   MD auth. Yes____ No____

Street address: City: State: Zip: | Hosp/snf:

Adm. date:

Directions: | Dis. date:

Diagnoses: Primary #	Physician name: Specialty:	Hosp/snf:
1.	Address:	Adm. date:
2.	Tel. no:	Dis. date:
3.	Physician name: Specialty:	Medicare no.
4.	Address:	
DX known to pt?_____	Tel. no:	Medical no./ss#.

History:	Agency worker: Tel. no:	Ins. co.:
	Pay sources/service request:	Policy #: Grp:. #:
	PHN	PT	ST	OT	Cov. code:
	MSW	HHA	HCA	PD	Tel. no:

Religious/cultural patterns/ language/psychosocial	Emergency/family contacts (by priority) Name Rel. Home# Work#	Contact person:
	#1	
Medications	Address	
	#2	
	Address	

Pertinent hospital information

Date/time:_____
Skilled orders per:_____

Diet/fluids

Allergies

Equipment: DME Yes____ No____

| Intake source name   Agency   Tel. no: |
| How did you learn about our services? |
| Intake received by   Date |

FIGURE 33-2 Referral form. (Courtesy of Home Calls, Oakland, CA).

gives permission, and the group sets a mutually acceptable time for the visit. The nurse is a guest in the client's home; therefore, it is important that the client agrees to the visit. The nurse then verifies the client's address and asks for specific directions to the client's home.

During a home health visit, the nurse requests proof of insurance such as a Medicare, Medicaid, health maintenance organization membership identification, or insurance card. The nurse should forewarn the client so the client or family can locate the information before the visit. If the client is unable to provide this verification, the nurse assists with locating the information during the visit. Clients who receive a public health home visit do not require evidence of insurance coverage because these services are not billed directly.

A county public health budget or state or federally funded programs generally cover these visits.

Not all clients have a telephone. If that is the case, the nurse should check the referral for a telephone number where messages can be left. It is also worthwhile to contact the health care provider who made the referral to see whether the telephone number was omitted unintentionally. If the client does not have a telephone, the nurse may choose to make a drop-in visit. This type of visit consists of an unannounced visit to the client's home, during which the nurse explains the purpose of the referral, receives the client's permission for the visit, and appoints a time for a future visit with the client. The client may agree to the first visit while the nurse is there.

If the client is not at home for the drop-in visit, the nurse should leave an official agency card and a brief message asking the client to contact the agency to schedule a nursing visit. The nurse informs the referring agency that the visit was attempted, but that the client was not available for contact. A formal agency letter, identifying the agency and the reason for the referral, is often sent to clients who are difficult to contact. The nurse's primary responsibility when unsuccessful in locating the client is to keep the clinic, physician, or referring agency informed of efforts to establish contact with the client.

Environment

An environmental assessment begins as the nurse leaves the agency en route to the client's home. The nurse should make specific observations, which follow (Keating and Kelman, 1998):

- How does the client's neighborhood compare with other neighborhoods in the area?
- Are there adequate shopping facilities, such as grocery stores, close to the client's home?

The nurse should also note the client's dwelling; for example, whether the client lives in a single-family home, in a single room in a home or hotel, in an apartment, or in a shared apartment or house. Specific assessments include the following:

- Is the client's residence easily accessible by the client given the client's age and functional ability? For example, if the client has limited endurance, can he or she negotiate several flights of stairs when entering or leaving the dwelling?
- Are handicapped facilities available as necessary? Is the dwelling in an area with high rates of drug abuse or crime?
- Is the building or home secure? Does the client live alone? If so, how does the client get to the physician or clinic? How does the client purchase groceries?
- Does the client have food in the home? If so, who prepares the client's meals? Are the meals nutritious?
- Are there rodents, cockroaches, or other potential vectors of disease present in the client's home?
- Does the client's home have hot running water, heat, sanitation facilities, and adequate ventilation?
- Is the client's residence safe relative to the client's physical status, or is the home cluttered with debris and furniture?

Improving Communication

When the nurse meets with the client, whether in the home or at another mutually agreeable location, the initial conversation revolves around social topics. The nurse assumes a friendly manner and asks general questions about the client, the client's family, and health care services that will benefit the client. These questions help the nurse assess the client's needs and create a comfortable atmosphere for communication.

Building Trust

Many clients in need of nursing visits do not trust the health care system and are uncomfortable with the representative from an agency visiting their home. For example, a client who is pregnant and does not have legal status in the United States will be hesitant to allow a nurse to visit; the client will be afraid of being reported to immigration authorities. The nurse's role in visiting this client is to focus on the health and safety of the client and her fetus. The nurse must build a trust relationship early in the visit or the client will not allow additional visits. If a trust relationship is not established and the client believes that the nurse will report her to immigration authorities, it is highly probable that the client will move to another location to avoid future contact.

DOCUMENTATION OF HOME CARE

The nurse documents assessment data and interventions for all home visits. The patient record also contains a copy of the nursing care plan.

Many home health nurses would probably identify documentation issues as the most frustrating part of providing home health care. Medicare holds a prominent position as a home health care payer; therefore the HCFA's regulations determine the home health industry's documentation. Correct and accurate completion of required Medicare forms is the key to reimbursement. Payment or denial for visits is based on the information presented on the forms. If the nurse does not clearly document the provided skilled care in the nursing notes, the fiscal intermediaries will argue that the care was either unnecessary or not performed and will deny reimbursement. The home health nurse must have an excellent clinical foundation and the ability to identify and document actual and potential patient problems that require skilled nursing interventions (Morrissey-Ross, 1988).

Documenting the care provided to record the patient's quality of care is just as important as documenting for reimbursement purposes. The documentation of home visits records the nurse's observations, assessments of the patient's condition, provided interventions, and the patient's and family's ability to manage the care at home. In addition, documentation of patient visits serves as a formal communication system among other home health professionals who also interact with the patient and family.

APPLICATION OF THE NURSING PROCESS

Assessment

During the first home visit, the type of client assessment will vary depending on the purpose of the home visit. The home health nurse assesses the client's knowledge of his or her health status. The nurse identifies knowledge deficits and uses this information to develop a care plan.

Subjective information is obtained from the client and the client's family and includes the client's perception of the situation and what the client identifies as problems. The nurse assesses whether the client is isolated from others physically or socially and whether the client is a member of a close-knit, nurturing, supportive family or kinship network. The amount of support the client perceives as available may or may not be accurate; therefore the nurse asks several questions about the client's family, friends, and daily routine to assess the client's level of social support.

The home health nurse assesses the client's health knowledge; his or her physical, functional, and psychosocial status; physical environment; and social support during the first home visit. The nurse collects information through observations and questions the patient and family or caregivers in the home environment. It is not unusual to find inconsistencies between information the patient provides during hospitalization concerning the amount of physical and emotional support available to the patient in the home and the amount of help actually available to the patient in the home. The nurse validates or modifies the referral information to reflect the actual home situation. Home health nurses often use contracts that the nurse, patient, and family jointly develop to delineate the responsibilities of the patient in the home.

The client's physical assessment is generally performed in the home health visit and includes a review of all systems, with an emphasis on the systems affected by the client's present condition. The nurse obtains objective data through the use of essential physical assessment skills such as observation, palpation, auscultation, and percussion. The physical assessment also includes information regarding the client's functional status. Assessment of the functional status is important for Medicare reimbursement and for the development of an individualized plan of care. This assessment includes information regarding the client's ability to ambulate, to perform ADL independently, and to use assist devices such as a cane or wheelchair. Specific functional limitations, such as shortness of breath or muscle weakness, are assessed at this time.

Information obtained during the assessment phase is used to identify nursing diagnoses and develop a plan of care. Data collection continues while the patient receives home health services. Changes in the patient's condition, environment, or social structure necessitate modifications in the treatment plan and the nursing care plan.

There are differences between the treatment plan and the nursing care plan. The plan of treatment includes the type of home health services received, the projected frequency of visits by each discipline (Albrecht, 1991), and the necessary interventions. The nursing care plan addresses specific nursing interventions designed to treat the patient's actual or potential problems and includes identified goals with measurable outcomes.

Diagnosis and Planning
Develop a Plan for the Client and Family

After the assessment phase of the home visit, the nurse identifies the nursing diagnoses that address the patient's problems and identifies actual or potential problems. The identification of nursing diagnoses serves as the basis for the nursing care plan. This plan is developed in consultation with the client and the family. The plan identifies short-term and long-term goals and measurable outcomes for the patient. The plan identifies nursing interventions that are necessary and additional home health services that are appropriate to help the patient

achieve the identified goals. To maximize the plan's success, it is important that the patient and family are involved in the planning process and access community resources. Planning is a dynamic process that continues while the patient receives nursing services. The plan is modified as needed, depending on the patient's condition, until the identified goals are met.

Often the nurse will develop a contract with the client that delineates the role and responsibilities of the nurse regarding the client's health and the role of the client and family (Spradley, 1990). If the client expresses a disinterest in contracting to improve health during the planning phase, the nurse will be limited in possible interventions. Goals are identified that the client is willing to work toward with the nurse's assistance.

The goal of home visits for both public health and home health nursing is to involve the client and family in taking an active role in health promotion. The nurse is careful not to allow the client to become dependent on the nurse's interventions because the nurse's involvement is short term.

Outline the Client and Family Roles

Written contracts are helpful for both the nurse and the client because the client's role and the nurse's role in implementing the plan are clearly delineated (Spradley, 1990). If either the client or the nurse forgets his or her role in the plan, the written contract becomes a reference. The client and the nurse can modify the contract by mutual agreement.

Intervention

Implementation of the care plan begins during the first home visit. The nurse begins to provide the client and family with health information concerning the client's health status and informs them about the availability of and access to community resources. In the case of the home health visit, the nurse provides skilled nursing care. At the end of the initial home visit, the nurse discusses the need for another home visit. The nurse and client discuss the goal of the next visit; specifically, they discuss what the client should do before the visit. The nurse informs the client and family about any information or skills he or she will provide during the next visit, and the nurse and client agree on a day for the next visit.

Referral for Community Services

During the first visit, the nurse provides the client and family with information regarding community resources, including the purpose of the resources, their eligibility in the services provided, any involved expense, and agency telephone numbers. Referrals depend on the availability of community resources, the client's eligibility for the services, the client's and the family's willingness to use the services, and the resources' suitability for the client and family. Examples of such services include information about immunization clinics for children in the family; adult day care or senior centers for elderly clients who could benefit from socialization; adult education classes or continuation of high school for pregnant teen clients who have dropped out of high school; Meals on Wheels (MOW) services for clients who are not able to prepare meals;

homeless shelters for men, women, and families; soup kitchens; resources for clothing and housing; mental health clinics; resources for battered spouses; and primary care clinics for low-income clients with and without insurance.

If necessary, the client or client's family may request the nurse's assistance in contacting the community resources. The client and family are encouraged to make the contacts, but if the client and family are unable to make the calls or do not speak English, the nurse needs to intervene on behalf of the client. By providing referral information during the first home visit, the nurse can follow up on the client's or the family's success in contacting and using community services.

Terminating the Visit

The nurse terminates the first visit when the assessment is completed and a care plan is established with the client. The average visit should not exceed 1 hour. The client receives a great deal of information during that hour, and the nurse collects a great deal of information. Most clients are tired at the end of a 1-hour visit and often cannot retain additional information. It is preferable to set a date for another home visit to reinforce the information provided and work progressively toward achieving goals.

Evaluation
Evaluation of Progress toward Goals

The evaluation phase occurs when the nurse can determine whether the mutually established goals are realistic and achievable for the patient and the patient's family. The evaluation process is continuous and allows the nurse to determine the success or progress toward the patient's identified goals. The nurse can identify the need for revisions in the nursing care plan and treatment plan through the collection of additional data during the evaluation phase. The nurse can intervene to make necessary changes. An example is an elderly wife who, during the initial home visit, stated that she preferred to provide the physical care for her frail, nonambulatory husband. On a subsequent visit, the nurse assessed that the patient was not receiving the care required for the patient's personal care, specifically bathing. The nurse discussed the problem with the wife and presented her with available options. These included the services of a home health aide to provide personal care and bathing three times a week. A new plan was developed, and it included the home health aide. The plan was implemented and evaluated during future visits. Input from the client is critical to determine whether the goals established are realistic and achievable for the client.

Modification of the Plan as Needed

The evaluation process also allows the nurse and client or family to discuss what is working well and where modifications are necessary in the plan. Evaluation occurs through open communication between the nurse and client, and the nurse asks questions about specific parts of the care plan. If a trust relationship exists, the client feels comfortable telling the nurse about problems in the care plan.

When Goals Are Achieved

The overall purpose of home visits is to assist the client with necessary information and nursing care to enable the client to function successfully without nursing interventions. When the care plan goals are achieved, the client does not need the nurse any longer. The client knows what community resources are available and how to access health care services for primary, secondary, and tertiary interventions.

FORMAL AND INFORMAL CAREGIVERS

Formal caregivers include professionals and paraprofessionals who provide in-home health care and personal services. They are compensated for the services they provide. The largest number of employees consists of home care aides and RNs. Informal caregivers are family members who are caring for the client. The presence or absence of an involved family member can make the difference between the successful completion of the plan of treatment, with the patient remaining in the home, and the need to transfer the patient to an extended-care facility or board-and-care facility. When a capable family member or caregiver is available to assist the patient, the home health nurse spends much of the visit assessing the skills of the caregiver. The home health nurse instructs the caregiver in the correct procedures for providing care and in recognizing the signs and symptoms of problems that must be reported to the health care provider. The goal of the home health nurse's instruction is to provide the caregiver with the skills necessary to care for the patient successfully in the home without intervention of the nurse or other members of the home health team.

The home health nurse faces a special challenge in those patients who lack a family member or caregiver capable of learning and providing necessary care. When the patient lives alone and does not have caregivers, the nurse explores other resources available to supplement the patient's self-care activities in the home. For example, if the patient has extensive physical care needs and sufficient financial resources, the nurse may suggest hiring an attendant. Medicare and private insurance companies do not pay for attendant care. If the patient's income is low enough, in-home county support services may be an option. The nurse may consider other services for the patient such as MOW for nutritious meals delivered to the patient's home. Friendly Visitors, a volunteer service, sends a volunteer to the patient's home once a week or more to provide socialization for the patient. Other options that are available in some communities include adult day health centers or senior service centers. Both of these options require arranged patient transportation to and from the centers. A variety of transportation methods are available in different communities; volunteers may transport patients to the centers or public transportation systems may be available such as minivans that provide door-to-door service. Selected services and referrals are based on the patient's individual needs and on the patient's level of functional ability.

⚖ ETHICAL INSIGHTS

Ethics: Home Health and Hospice Care

- Most legal and ethical issues in home health care involve the care of terminally ill patients.
- Early education about these issues is essential in the prevention of problems.
- Early education also gives patients the opportunity to make decisions for themselves and communicate those decisions to family members and health care providers.
- All competent adults have the right to make decisions that will direct health care providers in the type of care they administer.
- This communication can occur through the completion of advance directives, durable power of attorney for health care, and living wills.

Advance Directive

- An advance directive is a written document in which a competent person gives instructions about future health care in the event that the individual is unable to make decisions. These directives are completed on a voluntary basis. Medicare-certified health care agencies must ask patients about advance directives and provide patients with the advance directive form if the patient is interested in completing the document.

Durable Power of Attorney for Health Care

- A durable power of attorney for health care is one type of advance directive. Also called a health care proxy, the durable power of attorney for health care gives another person the power to make medical decisions related to care. This person, as identified by the patient, acts as the patient's agent in all decisions regarding health care, personal care, and custody in the event that the patient becomes incompetent or disabled and unable to make decisions.

Living Will

- A living will is a written document in which a patient voluntarily informs doctors and family members about the type of medical care desired should the patient become terminally ill or permanently unconscious and unable to communicate. In the living will, the patient can describe the type of care desired, depending on the clinical situation. For example, if the patient is terminally ill and unconscious, the patient can direct the health care team to perform only those measures that will provide comfort and nothing further. The patient can specifically indicate his or her opposition to lifesaving measures; for example, the patient may request the denial of cardiopulmonary life support in the event of a cardiac arrest. Other examples include indicating the exclusion of chemotherapy, blood transfusions, and respirator use in an attempt to prolong life.

HOSPICE HOME CARE

Hospice and palliative nursing care is becoming increasingly important as there is a tremendous need to improve end-of-life care for the terminally ill. Nurses who work with the terminally ill seek to enhance the patient's quality of life by focusing on relieving suffering throughout the illness, supporting the patient and family through the dying process, and providing grief support to the family after the patient has died (ANA, 2007). Hospice and palliative care nurses have a holistic approach to their patients and are responsible for taking a comprehensive health history and physical examination including an evaluation of mental status; evaluating functional abilities; performing appropriate laboratory and diagnostic studies; determining effective pharmacological and nonpharmacological therapies to manage symptoms; identifying patient and/or family/caregiver goals; providing culturally competent care that is consistent with the patient's health beliefs, values, and practices; evaluating the patient's emotional state and the response to his or her illness and impending death; identifying coping strategies and support systems; evaluating financial resources; and conducting a spiritual assessment (ANA, 2007).

The advanced practice hospice and palliative nurse is an emerging role for nurses with a master's degree or higher in nursing. The advanced practice hospice and palliative nurse functions as an expert clinician who performs the duties of the generalist hospice nurse in addition to assuming the responsibilities of advanced-level care, which may include prescribing pharmacological treatment to manage symptoms. It is recommended that all advanced practice hospice and palliative nurses obtain certification in advanced practice hospice and palliative nursing (ANA, 2007).

Hospice and palliative nursing care is provided in a variety of settings including hospitals, nursing homes, residential homes, and palliative care clinics. For those patients receiving hospice services in the home, the goal is to keep the client as comfortable at home as long as possible and to provide support and instruction to caregivers. When the patient becomes terminally ill, the focus shifts from cure to comfort care. Some patients insist on staying home until they die, and others allow their caregivers to decide whether they should remain at home or be admitted to an extended-care facility or a hospital. Each family unit has different needs, and each must be supported in its decisions. Home death should not be the standard that determines excellence in any case, nor should home death be the ultimate measure of "successful" home care. It is vital to realize that caring for a terminally ill person also includes caring for the family or caregivers. Not all caregivers want their loved one to die at home, and not all caregivers are capable of allowing that to happen. The goal of having a home death must be the goal of the patient and family, regardless of the nurse's personal preference.

When caring for a terminally ill person at home, the hospice nurse must be skilled in physical and psychosocial care for both the patient and the caregiver. The patient is viewed as a whole person, not as an isolated disease. Caring for a terminally ill person at home demands that the nurse view the family system as a unit. In addition, the nurse is not the only member of the hospice team assigned to each patient. Each patient has a physician, a nurse, a social worker, a nurse assistant, and a spiritual counselor to provide a multidisciplinary, holistic approach to caring for that patient and his or her family. Furthermore, many hospice agencies have weekly interdisciplinary meetings where the various members of the hospice team meet to discuss the patients and work together to resolve issues and make sure the patients are receiving the best possible care.

Caring for the Caregiver

Although the dying patient is the focus of all skilled nursing care, the experienced home care nurse knows that a careful assessment of the caregiver's mental and physical health is important. The spouse, lover, children, friends, and neighbors who have made the commitment to stay until the end need the nurse's time and attention as much as, if not more than, the patient. Although the patient's wishes are important, all decisions regarding care are made considering the health of the caregivers. Gaynor (1990) found that women with more

caregiving experience had increased physical health problems compared with those with less caregiving experience; younger women found caregiving more psychologically burdensome than older women. Nursing interventions must be directed toward preventing a decline in the caregiver's health.

Caregivers need reassurance that their judgment is sound, and they need reminders that they cannot do anything "wrong" if it is done for the patient's comfort. The caregivers must understand that they will not mistakenly overdose the patient, and they must be reminded repeatedly that the patient will not die from something they did or did not do. Caring for the terminally ill requires that the home care nurse is willing to nurse the entire family. In addition, the nurse must involve all members of the hospice team to ensure that the caregivers receive the care they need.

CASE STUDY   **PUBLIC HEALTH VISIT: COMMUNICABLE DISEASE FOLLOW-UP**

The public health nurse received a referral from the county hospital to see Ray, a 57-year-old white man with newly diagnosed TB. The first purpose of the referral was for the public health nurse to meet with the client to ensure that he received the appropriate information about TB and received follow-up medical care on a regular basis. The second purpose of the referral was for the public health nurse to meet with Ray and identify the people with whom he had been in close contact. The nurse then established contact with these people, notified them that they had been exposed to TB, and encouraged them to have follow-up tests for TB.

The nurse contacted Ray and established a time for the home visit. The nurse noted that he resided in a residential hotel in a lower-middle-class neighborhood of a large urban area. During the initial visit, the nurse discovered that the client was an unemployed construction worker. He did not know where he might have contracted TB. Ray assured the nurse that he was taking his medication as directed. He gave the nurse the names of his friends he played poker with every week at a hotel and told the nurse that he advised his friends to be tested for TB. The nurse made a note of the names and later talked with them individually by telephone. During these subsequent conversations, the nurse was very careful to maintain the client's confidentiality. The nurse informed these individuals that they could have been exposed to TB and that they should seek testing through their health care providers or through their local health department.

Ray indicated that he did not have family and he had minimal contact with other people besides his friends at the hotel. The nurse recorded this information on the communicable disease form and returned the information to the public health department's communicable disease division.

Assessment

The public health nurse's assessment of the client with a communicable disease involved the individual, family, and community. The public health nurse assessed whether the client received appropriate information and regular medical care for TB and whether the client followed the prescribed treatment regimen.

Although Ray stated that he did not have family, his friends in the hotel constituted a working support network. The public health nurse was familiar with kinship networks and their importance as alternative family systems (Stack, 1974). Nursing assessment of Ray's kinship network involved determining whether the members were tested for TB. In addition, the public health nurse assessed the client's network for the following:

- Network composition
- Network's knowledge of TB
- Functional capacity
- Network stressors
- Network strengths and weaknesses
- Network's ability to provide support for Ray
- Health beliefs and practices
- Use of health services

The public health nurse was aware that the number of new cases of TB in the community had increased over the past 12 months. The public health nurse further noted that there was an increase in the number of area residents immigrating from various third-world countries, and this population might be at increased risk for development of TB (Dowling, 1991).

Diagnosis
Individual
- Deficient knowledge regarding the disease process and transmission of TB

Family
- Deficient knowledge related to the disease process and transmission of TB, location of communicable disease clinics, and the importance of screening those exposed to TB

Community
- Increased risk for development of TB among community residents as evidenced by increased incidence of new cases of TB over the past 12 months

Planning
A plan of care is established with mutually agreed-upon goals based on the nurse's assessment of the individual, family, and community.

Individual
Long-Term Goal
- Client will perform self-care activities related to treatment of TB and follow up as necessary with appropriate health care professionals.

Short-Term Goal
- Client will verbalize knowledge of transmission of TB; signs and symptoms of complications of TB; purpose, administration schedule, and side effects of medications.

Continued

CASE STUDY   PUBLIC HEALTH VISIT: COMMUNICABLE DISEASE FOLLOW-UP—cont'd

Family
Long-Term Goal
• Support network members with positive test results will receive appropriate treatment.

Short-Term Goal
• Support network members will demonstrate basic knowledge of cause and transmission of TB and will agree to be tested for TB.

Community
Long-Term Goal
• Incidence of TB in the community will decrease over the next 3 years.

Short-Term Goal
• Community members will demonstrate knowledge of increased incidence of TB in their community and of available community resources for treatment and prevention of TB.

Intervention
Implementation of the plan of care for the client with TB occurs at the individual, family, and community levels.

Individual
The public health nurse referred Ray to the communicable disease clinic at the local health department. TB is a reportable communicable disease; therefore the public health nurse obtained information from the client regarding people with whom he had been in close contact.

Family
The public health nurse contacted members of Ray's support network and referred them to the communicable disease clinic as appropriate. The nurse provided these people with information concerning TB transmission and the importance of early treatment and follow-up.

Community
The public health nurse met with professionals from the communicable disease clinic and the health department and with members of the community to establish a program to raise public awareness regarding the increased incidence of TB in the community. The public was informed about the importance of preventive measures, the availability of community screening services for TB, and the existing health care resources in the community.

Evaluation
Individual
The client's knowledge of the disease process, transmission, treatment, and signs and symptoms of TB are indicators in evaluating the care plan. Confirmation of the client's follow-up with the communicable disease clinic can also be used for evaluation.

Family
The support network's knowledge of the disease process, transmission, treatment, and signs and symptoms of TB are indicators in evaluating the care plan. Confirmation of the support network's follow-up with the communicable disease clinic can also be used for evaluation.

Community
The incidence rate of TB in the community and the rate at which TB clinics and related resources are used are measures that can be used to evaluate the effectiveness of interventions at the aggregate level.

Levels of Prevention
The public health nurse is actively involved in all three levels of prevention through education programs, early detection programs, and appropriate referrals for patients with TB. Examples of each of these levels of prevention are indicated as follows:

Primary
• Goal is the prevention of specific disease occurrence such as TB.
• Development of programs that increase public awareness of the disease process and of the transmission, diagnosis, and treatment of TB.

Secondary
• Goal is the early detection of existing conditions.
• Tuberculin skin testing and subsequent follow-up of positive test results.

Tertiary
• Goal is to reduce the effects and spread of TB.
• Referral for early, effective treatment and education of clients for self-care.

CASE STUDY   PUBLIC HEALTH HOME VISIT: ANTEPARTUM CLIENT

The public health nurse received a referral to see a 17-year-old African-American woman named Ali, who was referred by the county prenatal clinic. Ali was 5 months' pregnant with her third pregnancy within the past year. Ali miscarried the previous two pregnancies during the first trimester.

When the nurse made the home visit, she noted that Ali was 5 feet 9 inches tall and weighed 120 lb. She resided in a two-room apartment with her boyfriend, who was the father of the baby. The nurse began the first visit with social talk, asking Ali general questions about her employment, education, and the duration of her residence in the area. Ali appeared to be pleased that the nurse was interested in her. Once a trusting relationship was initiated, the nurse asked Ali how she felt about the pregnancy. Ali revealed that she was happy about the pregnancy but was worried that there would be problems because she had two previous miscarriages. She had not planned any of the pregnancies, but she did not use contraceptives to prevent the pregnancies either. Ali's boyfriend worked and was able to pay the rent and buy food for her. Ali dropped out of high school during her junior year, but she wanted to complete her high school education. She had Medicaid coverage for her health care.

During the initial home visit, the nurse assessed that Ali was underweight and had several knowledge deficits in the areas of prenatal nutrition, infant care, breastfeeding, and contraception. The nurse also identified the need for a referral to the public school for the continuation of Ali's high school education. The nurse briefly discussed her assessment with Ali in a nonthreatening, nonjudgmental manner. The nurse informed Ali that, if she was interested, she could schedule future home visits to provide Ali with more information and answer her questions. Ali agreed to receive future visits to discuss the topics the nurse identified during the assessment phase. They mutually agreed upon the plan for future visits.

As the visits progressed, the nurse and Ali modified the plan based on progress evaluation.

The nurse terminated home visits with Ali when the mutually established goals were achieved. The nurse scheduled a postpartum visit with Ali after the baby was born to assess infant care and answer any questions Ali had concerning infant care.

Assessment

Although it is important to perform an individual assessment of Ali, the public health nurse assessed Ali as a member of a family and as a member of the community. *Community* in this case referred to the aggregate of publicly insured adolescent pregnant women. Assessment of Ali revealed an underweight 17-year-old pregnant woman who was unable to demonstrate knowledge of nutrition in pregnancy, infant care, breastfeeding, contraception, and educational options for pregnant teenagers.

An individual assessment of Ali mandated the need for an assessment of the composition and function of Ali's family. The public health nurse assessed the following factors with regard to Ali's family (Logan, 1986):

- Family composition
- General support network
- Family and network patterns related to Ali's psychosocial and economic support
- Family and network attitude toward health
- Family and network beliefs regarding use of health-related services
- Beliefs and attitudes of family and network regarding infant care, breastfeeding, and nutrition
- Attitude of infant's father regarding involvement with Ali and their baby, health beliefs, ability to assume the role of parent, and knowledge of pregnancy and birth

The public health nurse was aware of the need to see the larger, aggregate picture. Identifying the aggregate as the pregnant adolescent community, the public health nurse used the following techniques in an ongoing assessment (Bayne, 1985):

- Observations
- Resource analysis
- Key informant interviews
- Environmental indexes

Using these techniques, the public health nurse gathered information regarding the following:

- Educational and employment options for pregnant teens and teens with infants
- Availability of health services targeting low-birth-weight infants
- Availability of support groups for this aggregate
- Availability of teen parenting classes

Diagnosis

The public health nurse formulated nursing diagnoses based on thorough individual, family, and community assessments.

Individual

- Deficient knowledge regarding nutrition in pregnancy, infant care and feeding, contraception, availability of community resources, and educational options for pregnant teenagers
- Imbalanced nutrition: less than body requirements related to low-income status and inadequate knowledge of nutritional requirement for pregnancy

Family

- Lack of family support related to Ali living away from home

- Altered family communication patterns related to role confusion among family members

Community

- Minimal availability of health care services, parenting classes, contraception counseling, and educational opportunities for pregnant teenagers
- Lack of coordination of existing services

Planning

Planning health services and interventions for pregnant teenagers involves formulation of mutually agreed-upon short-term and long-term goals for the individual, family, and community.

Individual
Long-Term Goal

- Ali will carry her infant to term without evidence of maternal or fetal complications.

Short-Term Goals

- Ali will gain at least 3 lb per month.
- Ali will demonstrate knowledge of community resources for pregnant adolescents by next nursing visit.

Family
Long-Term Goal

- Ali, her partner, and other family members will be able to perform mutually determined role responsibilities.

Short-Term Goal

- Ali and her partner will attend teen parenting classes.

Community
Long-Term Goals

- Establishment of effective, comprehensive prenatal health, contraception, and education services for pregnant teenagers
- Decline in rate of teen pregnancies and birth of compromised neonates over the next 24 months

Short-Term Goals

- Increased community awareness of resources for pregnant teenagers
- Increased awareness of contraception counseling services for adolescents

Intervention
Individual

Implementation of Ali's individual care plan involved visits by the public health nurse with a referral to existing prenatal services for pregnant teenagers.

Family

Family intervention was composed of Ali's and the father's referral to a support group for pregnant teenagers and partners.

Community

Implementation of the care plan for the aggregate of adolescent pregnant women included the following:

- Meeting with community leaders
- Meeting with local school administrators and faculty to disseminate information for pregnant teenagers
- Formation of community organizing groups (Bayne, 1985)

Continued

CASE STUDY   PUBLIC HEALTH HOME VISIT: ANTEPARTUM CLIENT—cont'd

Evaluation

Individual
Evaluation included measures of the client's nutritional status and her use of support groups and educational and nutritional services.

Family
Evaluation included measures of the family's use of support groups and educational and services.

Community
Evaluation of the effectiveness of interventions at the aggregate level focused on measurement of available options for pregnant teenagers, measures of teen awareness and use of services, and determination of changes in incidence rates of teen pregnancy and compromised neonates.

Levels of Prevention
The public health nurse not only works with the patient and the patient's support network but also provides care to the entire community through education and intervention programs. The public health nurse is actively involved in working with individual teenagers, their friends and families, and the community in reducing the incidence of teenage pregnancy and assisting pregnant teenagers with prenatal care and available resources. Examples of providing care at the three levels of prevention are listed below.

Primary
- Activities that prevent teen pregnancy from occurring such as individual and family counseling and school and community education programs

Secondary
- Interventions for early detection of teen pregnancy and early intervention such as counseling for prenatal care

Tertiary
- Goal is to reduce the effects of adolescent pregnancy.
- Provision of prenatal education in areas such as nutrition, parenting, and infant care.

CASE STUDY   HOME HEALTH VISIT

Susan Brown is a 40-year-old woman who was the driver in a single-car, rollover accident. She was airlifted to a trauma center and treated for multiple lacerations and abrasions, including a severe laceration to the left inner aspect of her arm. The hospital made a referral for home health services at the time of discharge. The referral requested the home health nurse to perform daily wound care to the infected left arm laceration. The specific wound care medical orders consisted of removing the arm brace, performing wet-to-dry dressing changes using one-fourth strength Dakin's solution, wrapping the arm with gauze, and reapplying the brace. Medications included one or two Vicodin tablets every 6 hours as needed for pain and 500 mg of Keflex four times a day.

Assessment
The home health nurse assessed the following related to Susan's wound:
- Amount, color, and odor of wound drainage (Susan had a moderate-to-large amount of yellow drainage from the laceration on her left arm.)
- Pain assessment including history, character, severity, location, effects on quality of life, precipitating factors, and relieving factors
- Patient's understanding of the wound care and the appropriate administration of the medication

The home health nurse assessed Susan's support network and found that Susan has a large, supportive family and a caregiver was available to assist her every day. However, there were problems between Susan's husband and Susan's sister that created tension and stress for Susan. Her family coordinated transportation to and from physician appointments without the nurse's intervention.

Diagnosis
In this case, the care plan revolves around Susan and her family. A community intervention was not necessary.

Individual
- High risk for infection related to left arm laceration as evidenced by large amounts of yellow drainage

- Severe arm pain related to the injury
- Deficient knowledge related to inadequate understanding of the self-administration of antibiotic

When the home health nurse asked Susan when she took the Keflex, Susan explained that she took the medication at 9:00 AM, 1:00 PM, 5:00 PM, and 9:00 PM because the drug was prescribed to be taken four times a day.

Family
- Anxiety related to family communication problems

Planning

Individual

Long-Term Goals
- Healed laceration without drainage or infection within 1 week
- Full range of motion of the affected arm within 2 weeks
- Pain free when arm injury is healed
- Infection resolved within 1 week

Short-Term Goals
- Keep the laceration clean, and débride the wound with daily wet-to-dry dressing changes.
- Encourage self-care in dressing changes within 24 to 48 hours.
- Pain control is initiated through medication and relaxation techniques within 24 hours.
- Patient will demonstrate correct self-administration of antibiotic within 24 hours.

Family

Long-Term Goals
- Anxiety is resolved or controlled within 1 week.
- Support network will remain intact and will provide care to patient as needed until injury is healed.

Short-Term Goal
- Decreased anxiety through verbalization of feelings within 24 to 48 hours

CASE STUDY   HOME HEALTH VISIT—cont'd

Intervention

Individual

Dressing changes were performed as ordered, and the nurse monitored the wound daily. When the large amount of drainage persisted more than 3 days after initiating the antibiotic therapy and the patient continued to have low-grade fevers (temperature 99.2° to 99.8° F), the home health nurse notified the physician and took a culture of the drainage. An alternative antibiotic was prescribed on the basis of the culture results. The nurse taught Susan and her mother how to change the dressings, and the nurse supervised them.

The assessment of Susan's arm pain included a history of when the pain was most severe and the frequency of pain medicine administration. The home health nurse assessed that the pain was most severe at night and recommended that Susan take two Vicodin tablets before going to bed and place her left arm in a position of comfort, supported by pillows to decrease edema. The nurse instructed Susan to lie down, rest, and listen to relaxing music during the day when the pain was intense to decrease the amount of arm pain through relaxation. In addition, the nurse explained the purpose of the antibiotic and the importance of taking it every 6 hours to maintain an optimum blood level. Susan and the nurse agreed on a schedule of 6:00 AM, 12:00 noon, 6:00 PM, and bedtime.

Family

Susan's sister arrived from out of state to assist with her care after the accident. Within 3 days of her arrival, Susan's husband and sister got into an argument, and the sister left abruptly and returned home. This altercation was very upsetting to Susan, who was distraught over the communication problems between her husband and sister. The home health nurse encouraged Susan to express her feelings concerning the dysfunctional relationship and discuss how she would address the situation with both her husband and her sister. The nurse stressed that the problem was between the husband and her sister and that Susan should not feel guilty or responsible for the disagreement.

Evaluation

Individual

The nurse remained involved with Susan until the infection cleared and the family learned how to provide the necessary wound care. Susan's pain was adequately controlled until the infection resolved and the arm healed. Susan took her antibiotics and pain medication as prescribed. Susan's internist and orthopedist referred her for follow-up. She was also referred for a gynecological appointment for evaluation of sudden onset of slight vaginal bleeding.

Family

Susan's sister returned to her home, and further confrontations did not occur. The nurse suggested counseling for Susan if the hostile relationship persisted between her husband and sister or if it continued to cause Susan anxiety.

Levels of Prevention

The following are examples of the three levels of prevention as applied to the individual and the family in this case:

Primary

- Intervening to ensure that the wound did not get infected, such as regular dressing changes, to keep the wound clean and monitoring for signs and symptoms of infection

Secondary

- Recognizing that the wound was infected and ensuring that the antibiotics were administered correctly

Tertiary

- The home health nurse taking steps to ensure that the infection does not spread and resolves in a timely manner

CASE STUDY   HOSPICE HOME VISIT

Anne McMillan is 80 years old and is terminally ill with metastatic breast cancer. She has been a widow for 5 years and has three daughters and two sons. All of her children are married with kids of their own except one son who is handicapped and lives with Anne. Anne is too weak to care for herself and is moving in with her youngest daughter. Her daughter's house is a colonial with all bedrooms upstairs. There is a first floor bathroom. During her first visit, the hospice nurse talks with Anne and her daughter and explains what hospice is all about. The nurse then admits Anne into the hospice program and begins her initial assessment. Anne's primary physical complaints are back pain and constipation. She is still eating and drinking regularly. The nurse immediately recognizes that Anne will need a hospital bed. Anne already has a walker, but the nurse informed Anne and her daughter that they could have a bedside commode if needed in the future as Anne becomes weaker. Anne's biggest concern is her handicapped son. "He can't be by himself for long and I don't know where he can go now that I can't take care of him." Except for the handicapped son, all of her children and many of her grandchildren are active in her care.

Assessment

On her initial visit, the hospice nurse collects the following data about Anne, her family, and her community. In this case, the community consists of Anne's social support outside of her family such as her neighborhood and church.

- Pain assessment including history, character, severity, location, effects on quality of life, precipitating factors, and relieving factors
- Other physical symptoms such as fatigue, nausea, vomiting, constipation, diarrhea, decreased appetite, and decreased mobility
- Client and family fears, anxiety about dying and the dying process
- Support network and family dynamics
- Client's anxiety about situation concerning handicapped son
- Additional support network outside of family
- Effect of diagnosis and prognosis on Anne's social support including her neighbors and her church community

Diagnosis

Individual

- Pain related to disease process
- Constipation related to decreased mobility
- Anxiety related to concerns about safety and well-being of handicapped son

Family

- Effective family coping as evidenced by active family participation in Anne's care

Community

- Anticipatory grieving related to social isolation secondary to leaving neighborhood and moving in with daughter

Continued

CASE STUDY HOSPICE HOME VISIT—cont'd

Planning

Individual

Long-Term Goals
- Pain will remain controlled until client expires.
- Client will have regular bowel movements for the next 2 months.
- Client will verbalize satisfaction about resolution of situation concerning handicapped son.

Short-Term Goals
- Pain will be well controlled within 24-48 hours.
- Client will have a bowel movement within 24-48 hours.
- Client will have decreased anxiety about handicapped son within 24-48 hours as the social worker will have found a place for the son to live.

Family

Long-Term Goals
- Family will remain active in Anne's care until she is buried.
- Family will provide a support network for each other and use hospice services for continued support through Anne's death and burial and for months afterward.

Short-Term Goal
- Family will actively participate in Anne's care.

Community

Long-Term Goal
- Client will continue to receive support from friends.

Short-Term Goal
- Client will verbalize feelings about moving in with daughter and leaving friends behind.

Intervention

Individual

After talking with the doctor, the hospice nurse starts Anne on methadone 10 mg every 8 hours and Roxanol 5 mg as needed for breakthrough pain. The nurse explains to Anne and her daughter that she is constipated because of her decrease in mobility. The nurse obtains an order for a stool softener and instructs Anne to take it twice daily. The nurse also explains to Anne and her daughter that, as Anne declines, her appetite will decrease and she will eat less and less and may not have bowel movements very frequently. Anne should let the nurse know if she ever feels uncomfortable because she has not had a bowel movement in a few days. The nurse talks to the social worker who finds a group home for Anne's handicapped son.

Family

The nurse and social worker talk with the family and help them develop a system so that Anne always has someone with her and to help ensure that all of the responsibility for Anne's care does not fall on one person. They also inform the family about resources to support the family.

Community

Anne has a nurse, social worker, spiritual counselor, and nurse assistant assigned to her care. Each of these hospice workers helps Anne discuss her feelings about her situation and works with her to continue to receive support from her friends and neighbors.

Evaluation

Individual

All of Anne's goals are met as she has good pain control until she dies, she no longer experiences discomfort and problems with constipation, and she expresses less anxiety and worries about her handicapped son. Although she still has some concerns, she feels much better about the situation.

Family

The family's goals are met as they remain active in Anne's care until she dies. In addition, they use hospice resources appropriately and as necessary, and they support each other through the entire process.

Community

The goals are met as Anne expresses her feelings about her situation, and her closest friends remain supportive to Anne through visits and phone calls.

Levels of Prevention

In this case, the three levels of prevention focus on assisting the client and family through all phases of hospice care from admission until death. Some examples are listed as follows.

Primary
- Anticipating needs and intervening early on to prevent problems such as skin breakdown and lack of pain control
- Educating the client and family about hospice and the dying process

Secondary
- Responding quickly to needs as they arise
- Continued education about the hospice and dying experience

Tertiary
- Assisting the client and family through the active phase of dying
- Providing follow-up bereavement support to the family

Pain Control and Symptom Management

Pain control is an important goal for hospice nurses and their patients. Hospice nurses perform regular pain assessments that involve asking patients the following questions about their pain: (1) history, (2) character (such as sharp, dull, aching), (3) severity or intensity (which is most commonly rated on a pain intensity scale from 0 to 10 with 0 being no pain and 10 being the worst pain imaginable), (4) location, (5) effects on quality of life, (6) precipitating factors, and (7) relieving factors (Norlander, 2008). It is vital that the hospice nurse not only performs regular pain assessments but also remembers that pain is highly subjective and every person experiences pain differently and uniquely; therefore, the patient's pain is whatever he or she says it is regardless of the nurse's objective evaluation of the situation.

Pain medication is administered in doses sufficient to keep the patient free of pain and is administered on a regular schedule to prevent pain from recurring before the next dose. Hospice methods of pain control are particularly well suited to home care. The vast majority of patients can be pain free until their deaths. The key to successful pain control for the terminally ill is to convince patients to take their medications on a regular basis, not just when they "cannot stand it any longer." Generally, these medications are long acting and are administered every 8 to 12 hours. In addition, patients will also have a fast-acting pain medication to take for "breakthrough pain," which happens when the patient experiences an increase in pain before it is time for the next dose of scheduled pain medication. The fast-acting medications are generally administered every 1 to 2 hours as needed.

Many patients, especially the elderly, are afraid of becoming "junkies" or "druggies" and want to delay using pain medication until they "get really bad." Many people believe that using these medications signals "the end of the line," and they are amazed to learn that patients do well while receiving this drug for months, even years, before death occurs. Almost every family must learn that addiction is not the same as tolerance and that their physicians will not "cut off their supply if they take too much."

In addition to pain control, hospice nurses help in managing other symptoms such as nausea and vomiting, constipation, diarrhea, fatigue, and decreased appetite. Nurses assist patients in managing these symptoms through medications and/or strategies to help cope with the symptoms. Strategies include such things as increasing fluids to prevent constipation, frequent rest periods to minimize fatigue, and eating small amounts as desired to cope with the decrease in appetite. In addition, the nurse educates the patient and family that some of these symptoms such as fatigue and decreased appetite are related to the dying process and are signs that the patient is declining.

Furthermore, the nurse, along with other members of the hospice team, provides emotional support to patients and families as they adjust to the patient's impending death. The nurse educates the patient and family about what physical symptoms the patient will most likely experience as he or she approaches death. In addition, the nurse, along with the social worker and spiritual counselor, provides emotional support and helps the patient and family work through any anxiety or fears they have about dying. Finally, the nurse is there to support the family immediately after the patient dies, and hospice provides bereavement support to families up to a year after the patient's death.

SUMMARY

This chapter presented information on performing public health, home health, and hospice nursing visits to clients in their homes. A general overview of the nursing process for clients in the home setting was presented and expanded to include the individual, family, and community. Case studies involving communicable disease, teen pregnancy, traumatic injury, and terminal cancer have been presented. The home visit is the foundation of community health nursing and provides a forum for important interventions with individuals, families, and communities. The CHN is responsible for bringing the concerns of individuals and families into the community.

LEARNING ACTIVITIES

1. Make arrangements to accompany a public health nurse, a home health nurse, and a hospice nurse on home visits.
2. Interview a public health nurse about the types of client referrals received, and ask what interventions are usually performed. Repeat this activity with a home health nurse and a hospice nurse. Ask the nurses what they like best about their jobs.
3. Contact a local home health agency and interview the agency director. Ask what type of agency it is, the profit status, and whether it is Medicare certified. Report findings to classmates.
4. Attend a team meeting in a home health agency or a hospice program to see how the roles of the various team members blend together to provide family-centered care.
5. Interview a public health nurse and home health nurse, and ask how the community impacts the care they provide.

REFERENCES

Albrecht MN: The Albrecht nursing model for home health care: implications for research, practice, and education, *Public Health Nurs* 7:118–126, 1990.

Albrecht MN: Home health care: reliability and validity testing of a patient-classification instrument, *Public Health Nurs* 8:124–131, 1991.

American Nurses Association: *Scope and standards of hospice and palliative nursing practice*, Washington, DC, 2007, The Author.

American Nurses Association: *Scope and standards of home health nursing practice*, Washington, DC, 2008, The Author.

Bayne T: The pregnant school-age community. In Higgs AR, Gustafson DD, editors: *Community as client: assessment and diagnosis*, Philadelphia, 1985, FA Davis.

Centers for Medicare and Medicaid Services: *Home health compare*, 2008, www.medicare.gov/HHCompare/Home.asp?dest=NAV|Home|Search#TabTop. Accessed April 28, 2009.

Dowling PT: Return of TB: screening and preventive therapy, *Am Fam Physician* 43:457–476, 1991.

Feldman R: Meeting the educational needs of home health care nurses, *J Home Health Care Pract* 5:12–19, 1993.

Gaynor SE: The long haul: the effects of home care on caregivers, *Image J Nurs Sch* 22:208–212, 1990.

Guterman S, Dobson A: Impact of the Medicare prospective payment system for hospitals, *Health Care Financing Rev* 7:97–114, 1986.

Keating SB, Kelman GB: *Home health care nursing: concepts and practice*, Philadelphia, 1998, JB Lippincott.

Kelly L, Joel L: *Dimensions of professional nursing*, ed 8, New York, 1995, McGraw-Hill.

Kent V, Hanley B: Home health care, *Nurs Health Care* 11:234–240, 1990.

Logan BB: Adolescent pregnancy. In Logan BB, Dawkins CE, editors: *Family-centered nursing in the community*, Menlo Park, CA, 1986, Addison-Wesley.

Morrissey-Ross M: Documentation. If you haven't written it, you haven't done it, *Nurs Clin North Am* 23(2):363–371, 1988.

National Association for Home Care and Hospice: *HomeCare online, Basic statistics about home care*, 2008, www.nahc.org/facts/08HC_Stats.pdf. Accessed April 28, 2009.

Norlander L: *To comfort always: a nurse's guide to end of life care*, Sigma Theta Tau International, 2008.

Spradley BW: *Community health nursing: concepts and practice*, ed 3, Glenview, IL, 1990, Scott, Foresman and Little, Brown.

Stack C: *All our kin.* New York, 1974, Harper & Row.

U.S. Department of Commerce and International Trade Administration: *U.S. industrial outlook*, Washington, DC, 1990, Government Printing Office.

Warhola C: *Planning for home health services: a resource handbook, USDHHS Pub No HRA 80-14017*, Washington, DC, 1980, Public Health Service, US Department of Health and Human Services.

Note: Page numbers followed by *b* indicates boxes, *f* indicates figures and *t* indicates tables.

Wald, Lillian *(Continued)*
 House on Henry Street and, 29, 30b
 legislation and politics, influence on, 199
 National Organization for Public Health Nursing and, 31
 nursing concepts of, 107
Walking, 64
War, effects of, 270
War on drugs, 526–527
Warts, 509t
Waste control
 environmental health and
  definition of, 248t
  example of, 249t
 problems relating to, 255
 recycling as, 255
 trash production/disposal and, 255
Waste incineration, 255–256
Waste management, medical, 263
Waste management program, 250f
Wastewater treatment plant, 250f
Water pollution, 270
Water quality
 environmental health and
  definition of, 248t
  example of, 249t
 problems in, 253
 water treatment technology and, 253
Water treatment technology, 253
Wealth, distribution of, 224
Weapons of mass destruction
 types of, 563
  biological organisms as, 564t
  chemical agents as, 564t
Wear-and-tear theory, 355
Weather, atmospheric quality and, 253
Web of causation model, 69–70, 71f
Weight, body, 62
Welfare Reform Act, 166
Well-being
 environmental determinants of, 246
 poverty influencing, 224, 235
 religion and, 637, 637f
Wellness Ministry Survey, 640f
Wesley, John, 638–639
Westberg, Reverend Granger, 637
Western population, 34
West Nile virus, 258
Wheel model
 characteristics of, 68
 of human-environment interaction, 70f
White Anglo-Saxon Protestant (WASP), 221
White House Fellowship, President's Commission on, 213
White population
 children as, 285–286
  in poverty, 395, 395f

White population *(Continued)*
 countries of origin for, 221
 culture-bound syndrome in, 234t
 death, leading cause of, 339t
  in older adult, 366t
 education and, 225
 as single parent family, 382t
 teen birth rate in, 383t
 See also Caucasian
Who Will Keep the Public Healthy?, 176
Wide range Achievement Test, 140–142
Widowhood, 358–359
Wife beating, 545
Wildfire, 577f
Windshield survey assessment
 example of, 95b
 purpose of, 94
 questions for, 97b
Wingspread Statement on Precautionary Principle, 246
Witchcraft, 232
Withdrawal syndrome, 522
 detoxification and, 528
Women
 acute illness in, 321
  pelvic inflammatory disease, 321
  toxic shock syndrome, 321
  UTI and dysuria in, 321
  vaginitis and vulvovaginitis, 321
 adoption and, 320
 breast cancer in, 323
 cancer in, 315–316
 cardiovascular disease in, 314–315
 chronic conditions/limitations in, 317
 chronic illness in, 321–325
  arthritis, 322
  coronary vascular disease/metabolic syndrome, 321–325
  diabetes, 322
  hypertension, 322
 death, cause of, 314t
 death and illness in, 313
 depression in, 318, 318b, 325
 diabetes in, 316
 disability and, 328
 domestic abuse in, 328, 546
 education of, 319
 employment of
  careers, 319
  hazardous occupations, 329t
  home life and, 319
  wages, 319, 319t
 examinations for, 363
 gynecological cancers in, 324–325
 as head of household, characteristics of, 320t
 health and safety issues, 611

Women *(Continued)*
 health promotion strategies for, 320–328, 330–331
 HIV and AIDS in, 327–328
 as homeless, 430–431
  with children, 432–433
  factors contributing to, 433
  health status of, 432–433
  prenatal care and, 437
 hospitalization of, 317
 illicit drug use by, 518
 life expectancy for, 313–314
 lung cancer in, 324
 mammography screening in, 454
 marriage and, 320
 maternal mortality in, 316–317
 mental disorder and stress in, 325
 mental health of, 318
 multiple family configurations and, 319–320
 networking and, 330
 as older adult, physiological changes, 359t
 osteoporosis in, 322–323
 population of, 313
 in prison, 628
 rape and, 547
 reproductive health of, 325–328
 STD in, types of, 327
 substance abuse in, 535–536
 suicide in, 546
 surgery and, 317–318
 as uninsured, 318–319
 violence against, 545
Women, Infants, and Children (WIC), 159, 303–304
Women for Sobriety, 531
Women's health, 312–336
 factors affecting, 318–320
 "health for all" and, 313
 Healthy People 2020, 312–336
 indicators of, 313–318
 legislation affecting, 328–330
  Civil Rights Act, 329
  Family and Medical Leave Act, 329–330
  Occupational Safety and Health Act, 329
  Public Health Service Act, 328
  Social Security Act, 329
 nursing process, application of, 331b
 Office of Research on, 333
 prevention in
  primary prevention and, 331
  secondary prevention and, 331
  tertiary prevention and, 331
 research in, 333
 unintentional injury/accidents in, 328
 working with, 326b
Women's health service, 330

Workers' Compensation Act, 616
Work Incentives Improvement Act, Ticket to Work and (TWWIIA), 410
Workplace
 health screening and education in, 171
 Occupational Safety and Health Act, 165
 shelter in place instructions at, 574t
Workplace health and safety, 213
Workplace rights, 213
Workplace violence, 552
Work-related disease/injury, 611t
Work risk
 environmental health and
  definition of, 248t
  example of, 249t
 environmental health problems relating to, 252
 job-related accidents/illnesses, 252
World Bank, 274
World Framework Convention on Tobacco Control, 272
World Health Organization (WHO)
 collaborating centers in nursing, 276
 Declaration of Alma-Ata, 272–273, 272b
 disability and, 405
 environmental health, goal of, 258
 goal of, 272
 health, definition of, 3, 51, 206
 HIV and, 206
 primary health care versus primary prevention, 172b
 "three by five Initiative", 271
 Tobacco Product Regulation, Study Group on, 272
 "two diseases, one patient" strategy, 271
World population
 distribution of, 270
 growth and urbanization, 270
World Trade Center attack, 257, 562
 picture of, 577f

Y

Yield, of screening test
 positive predictive value of, 79
 predictive value of, 79t
Yin-yang theory, 231
Youth-related violence, 552–553
 gangs and, 553
 risk factors for, 553t
Youth Risk Behavior Survey, 587
 purpose of, 588b
Youth Risk Surveillance System, 297–298
Youth. *See* Adolescent; Children

SPECIAL FEATURES